Manual of CRITICAL CARE NURSING

NURSING INTERVENTIONS AND COLLABORATIVE MANAGEMENT

Manual of CRITICAL CARE NURSING

NURSING INTERVENTIONS AND COLLABORATIVE MANAGEMENT

SEVENTH EDITION

MARIANNE SAUNORUS BAIRD, MN, RN, ACNS-BC
Corporate Director, Magnet Recognition Program
Magnet Program Director
Clinical Nurse Specialist
Emory Healthcare
Nursing Administration
Atlanta, Georgia

ELSEVIER

ELSEVIER

3251 Riverport Lane
St. Louis, Missouri 63043

MANUAL OF CRITICAL CARE NURSING: NURSING INTERVENTIONS
AND COLLABORATIVE MANAGEMENT, SEVENTH EDITION
ISBN: 978-0-323-18779-4

Notices

Knowledge and best practice in this field are constantly changing. As new research and experience broaden
our understanding, changes in research methods, professional practices, or medical treatment may become
necessary. Practitioners and researchers must always rely on their own experience and knowledge in evaluating and using any information, methods, compounds, or experiments described herein. In using such information or methods they should be mindful of their own safety and the safety of others, including parties
for whom they have a professional responsibility.

With respect to any drug or pharmaceutical products identified, readers are advised to check the most
current information provided (i) on procedures featured or (ii) by the manufacturer of each product to be
administered, to verify the recommended dose or formula, the method and duration of administration,
and contraindications. It is the responsibility of practitioners, relying on their own experience and knowledge of their patients, to make diagnoses, to determine dosages and the best treatment for each individual
patient, and to take all appropriate safety precautions.

To the fullest extent of the law, neither the Publisher nor the authors, contributors, or editors, assume
any liability for any injury and/or damage to persons or property as a matter of products liability, negligence
or otherwise, or from any use or operation of any methods, products, instructions, or ideas contained in the
material herein.

NANDA International, Inc. Nursing Diagnoses: Definitions & Classifications 2015-2017, Tenth Edition. Edited by
T. Heather Herdman and Shigemi Kamitsuru. 2014 NANDA International, Inc. Published 2014 by John Wiley
& Sons, Ltd. Companion website: www.wiley.com/go/nursingdiagnoses.

Previous editions copyrighted 2011, 2005, 2001, 1998, 1995, 1991.
International Standard Book Number: 978-0-323-18779-4

Executive Content Strategist: Lee Henderson
Content Development Manager: Jean Fornango
Content Development Specialist: Melissa Rawe

Publishing Services Manager: Julie Eddy
Senior Project Manager: Marquita Parker
Book Designer: Ashley Miner

Printed in the United States of America
Last digit is the print number: 9   8   7   6   5   4   3   2   1

Working together
to grow libraries in
developing countries

www.elsevier.com • www.bookaid.org

Contributors

Patrice C. Al-Saden, BS, RN, CCRC
Senior Clinical Research Associate
Comprehensive Transplant Center
Feinberg School of Medicine
Chicago, Illinois

Sonia Astle, RN, MS, CCNS, CCRN, CNRN
Clinical Nurse Specialist
Critical Care
Inova Fairfax Medical Campus
Falls Church, Virginia

Carol Ann Batchelder, MSN, RN, CCRN, ACCNS-AG BC
Clinical Nurse Specialist
Intensive Care Units, Tri-campus
Northside Hospital System
Atlanta, Georgia

Risa Benoit, DNP, CNS-BC
Advanced Practice Nurse
Perioperative Services
Sarasota Memorial Healthcare System
Sarasota, Florida

Cheryl L. Bittel, MSN, APRN, CCNS, NP-C, CCRN
Clinical Nurse Specialist
Emory Saint Joseph's Hospital
Atlanta, Georgia

Carolyn Blayney, BSN, RN
Clinical Operation Manager
Pediatrics
Harborview Medical Center
Seattle, Washington

Madalina Boitor, BScN, RN, PhD Student
Ingram School of Nursing
McGill University
Montreal, Canada

Jemma Brown, MSN-ED, RN, CCRN, CCM-BC
Stroke Program Coordinator
Emory University Hospital Midtown
Atlanta, Georgia

Susan B. Cali, MSN, RN, MHA
Infection Control Coordinator
Emory University Hospital Midtown
Atlanta, Georgia

Mimi Callanan, MSN, RN
Epilepsy Clinical Nurse Specialist
Stanford Comprehensive Epilepsy Center
Stanford Health Care
Stanford, California

Gretchen J. Carrougher, MN, RN
Research Nurse Supervisor
Department of Surgery, Harborview Medical Center
Seattle, Washington

Cynthia Rebik Christensen, MSN, CVN, ARNP-BC
Nurse Practitioner, Family Practice
Certified Vascular Nurse
Mobile Medical Professionals
Ankeny, Iowa

Janice C. Colwell, MS, RN, CWOCN, FAAN
Advanced Practice Nurse
University of Chicago Medicine
Chicago, Illinois

Alice E. Davis, PhD, GNP-BC, ACNP-BC, FNP-BC
Associate Professor
School of Nursing
University of Hawaii at Hilo
Hilo, Hawaii

Joni L. Dirks, MS RN-BC, CCRN-K
Manager Clinical Educators & ICU Educator
Providence Health Care
Spokane, Washington

Beverly George Gay, MSN, RN
Assistant Professor
Department of Nurse Anesthesia
School of Allied Health Professions
Virginia Commonwealth University
Richmond, Virginia

Céline Gélinas, PhD, RN
Associate Professor
Ingram School of Nursing
McGill University
Researcher
Center for Nursing Research and Lady Davis
Institute for Medical Research
Jewish General Hospital
Montreal, Quebec, Canada

Patricia R. Gilman, APRN, MSN, ACNS-BC
Adult Health Clinical Nurse Specialist
Cardiac ICU
Emory University Hospital (2012–2014)
Atlanta, Georgia
Robert Wood Johnson Nursing & Health
Policy Collaborative Fellow
University of New Mexico College of Nursing
Albuquerque, New Mexico

Vicki S. Good, RN, MSN, CENP, CPSS
System Director Quality/Safety
CoxHealth
Springfield, Missouri

Phyllis Gordon, MSN, APRN, ACNS-BC
Clinical Nurse Specialist, Vascular Surgery
Division
Clinical Assistant Professor, School of Nursing
University of Texas Health Science Center
San Antonio
San Antonio, Texas

Kimberly Graham, MSN, APRN, ACNS-BC
Clinical Nurse Specialist
General Medical
Emory University Hospital Midtown
Atlanta, Georgia

**Kiersten Henry, MSN, ACNP-BC, CCNS,
CCRN-CMC**
Acute Care Nurse Practitioner
Chief Advanced Practice Provider
MedStar Montgomery Medical Center
Olney, Maryland

Adina Hirsch, PharmD, BCNSP
Clinical Specialist–Nutrition Support,
Critical Care
Saint Joseph's Hospital of Atlanta;
Assistant Professor of Pharmacy Practice
School of Pharmacy
Philadelphia College of Osteopathic Medicine
Atlanta, Georgia

Beth Hundt, MS, APRN, NP-C, ACNS-BC
Clinical Nurse Specialist
Marcus Stroke & Neuroscience Center, Grady
Health System, Atlanta, GA (2012–2014);
Clinical Nurse Specialist
Neuroscience Center of Excellence, University
of Virginia Health System, Charlottesville,
Virginia (current)

Susie Hutchins, DNP, RN
Associate Clinical Professor
Coordinator
Simulation and Standardized Patient Lab for
MEPN
University of San Diego
Hahn School of Nursing
San Diego, California

Anne E. Hysong, MSN, APRN, CCNS
Clinical Nurse Specialist
Critical Care
Gwinnett Medical Center–Duluth
Duluth, Georgia

**Roberta Kaplow, PhD, APRN-CCNS,
AOCNS, CCRN**
Oncology Clinical Nurse Specialist
Emory University Hospital
Atlanta, Georgia

**Alice S. Kerber, MN, APRN, ACNS-BC,
AOCN, APNG**
Clinical Nurse Specialist
Oncology
Advanced Practice Nurse in Genetics
Georgia Center for Oncology Research and
Education (Georgia CORE)
Atlanta, Georgia

Kathleen Kerber, MSN, RN, ACNS-BC, CCRN
Clinical Nurse Specialist
Medical Intensive Care Unit/Critical Care
Step Down Unit
MetroHealth Medical Center
Cleveland, Ohio

**Barbara McLean, MN, RN, CCNS-BC, NP-BC,
CCRN, FCCM**
Critical Care Clinical Specialist
Critical Care Division
Grady Health Systems
Atlanta, Georgia

James P. McMurtry, MSN, APRN, CNS-BC, CCRN
Clinical Nurse Specialist
MICU; Pulmonary Critical Care
Emory University Hospital Midtown
Atlanta, Georgia

Maria Paulsen, BSN, RN
Critical Care Nurse
Coordinator, Trauma Outreach Education Program
Harborview Medical Center
Seattle, Washington

Lisa Reif, MSN, RN, APRN-CCNS, CCRN
Clinical Nurse Specialist, Neuroscience ICU
Emory University Hospital
Atlanta, Georgia

Alan Sanders, PhD
Director, Ethics
Trinity Health
Newtown Square Office, Pennsylvania

Paul E. Schmidt, RPh, BCPS
Clinical Pharmacist
Critical Care
Northside Forsyth Hospital
Cumming, Georgia

Elizabeth Scruth, PhD, RN, MPH, FCCM, CCNS, CCRN
Clinical Practice Consultant
Clinical Effectiveness Team
Kaiser Permanente Northern California
Regional Quality and Regulatory Services
Oakland, California
Critical Care Transport RN
Bayshore Ambulance
Foster City, California

Maureen A. Seckel, MSN, RN, APN, ACNS-BC, CCNS, CCRN, FCCM
Clinical Nurse Specialist
Medical Pulmonary Critical Care
Christiana Care Health System
Newark, Delaware

Kara A. Snyder, MS, RN, CCRN, CCNS
Director
Quality Improvement and Outcomes Management
Banner University Medical Center, Tucson and South Campuses
Tucson, Arizona

Monica Tennant, MSN, APRN, CCNS
Critical Care Clinical Nurse Specialist
Emory Saint Joseph's Hospital
Atlanta, Georgia

Daryl Todd, MS, APRN-CNS, CCCC, ACNS-BC
Certified Cardiovascular Care Coordinator
Clinical Nurse Specialist
Coordinator Bariatrics and Chest Pain
Centers of Excellence, Clinical Support for Hospice and Observation Units
Emory University Hospital Midtown
Atlanta, Georgia

Sharon Vanairsdale, MS, APRN, ACNS-BC, NP-C, CEN
Clinical Nurse Specialist
Emergency Department and Serious Communicable Disease Unit
Emory University Hospital
Atlanta, Georgia

Colleen Walsh-Irwin, DNP, RN, ANP, CCRN
Cardiology Nurse Practitioner
Northport VAMC
Northport, New York;
Cardiovascular Clinical Nurse Advisor
Department of Veterans Affairs
Washington, DC;
Clinical Assistant Professor
Stony Brook University
Stony Brook, New York

Joyce Warner, MN, RN, CCRN
Nurse Clinician
Surgical Intensive Care Unit
Emory Healthcare
Atlanta, Georgia

Karen E. Zorn, MSN, RN, ONC
Enterprise Solution Architect
Acute Care Integration
Emory Healthcare
Atlanta, Georgia

REVIEWERS

Bimbola Fola Akintade, PhD, ACNP-BC, MBA, MHA
Co-Specialty Director and Assistant Professor, Adult Gerontological Acute Care Nurse Practitioner/Clinical Nurse Specialist Program
University of Maryland Baltimore, School of Nursing
Baltimore, Maryland

David Allen, MSN, RN, CCRN, CCNS-BC
Deputy Chief, Center for Nursing Science and Clinical Inquiry
Brooke Army Medical Center
Fort Sam Houston, TX 78109

Penelope S. Benedik, PhD, CRNA, RRT
Associate Professor of Clinical Nursing
University of Texas Health Science Center at Houston
Houston, TX

Marcia Bixby, RN, MS, CCRN, APRN-BC
Critical Care Clinical Nurse Specialist
Consultant
Randolph, Massachusetts

Marylee Bressie, DNP, RN, CCRN, CCNS, CEN
Assistant Professor
University of Arkansas Fort Smith and Capella University
Ft Smith, Arkansas and Minneapolis, Minnesota

Diane Dressler, MSN, RN, CCRN
Clinical Assistant Professor
Marquette University College of Nursing
Milwaukee, WI

Jennifer L. Embree, DNP, RN, NE-BC, CCNS
Clinical Assistant Professor and Consultant
Indiana University School of Nursing - Indiana University Purdue University Indianapolis
Indianapolis, Indiana

Joyce Foresman-Capuzzi, MSN, RN, CCNS, CEN, CPN, CPEN, CCRN, CTRN, SANE-A, AFN-BC, EMT-P, FAEN
Clinical Nurse Educator
Lankenau Medical Center
Wynnewood, PA

David Goede, DNP, ACNP-BC
Assistant Professor of Nursing, Hospitalist Nurse Practitioner
University of Rochester School of Nursing
Rochester New York

Vinay Paul Singh Grewal, B.Sc.
Medical Student
Windsor University School of Medicine
Basseterre, Saint Kitts & Nevis

Elizabeth A. Henneman, PhD, RN, CCNS, FAAN
Associate Professor of Nursing
University of Massachusetts Amherst
Amherst, Massachusetts

Jennifer M. Joiner, MSN, RN, AGPCNP-BC, CCRN-CSC
Clinical Nurse Educator, CTICU and CCU
Robert Wood Johnson University Hospital
New Brunswick, NJ

Irena L. Kenneley, PhD, APHRN-BC, CIC
Assistant Professor/Faculty Development Co-ordinator
Case Western Reserve University
Cleveland, Ohio

Julene B. Kruithof, MSN, RN, CCRN
Nurse Educator
Spectrum Health
Grand Rapids, Michigan

Elaine Larson, PhD, RN, FAAN
Anna C. Maxwell Professor of Nursing Research, School of Nursing and Professor of Epidemiology, Mailman School of Public Health, Columbia University
Columbia University
NY, NY

Rosemary K. Lee, DNP, ARNP-BC, CCNS, CCRN
Clinical Nurse Specialist
Homestead Hospital
Homestead, FL

Justin Milici, MSN, RN, CEN, CPEN, CFRN, CCRN, TNS
RN III Emergency Department
Parkland Health and Hospital System
Dallas, Texas

Michaelynn Paul, MS, RN, CCRN
Assistant Professor
Walla Walla University
College Place, Washington

Julia Retelski, MSN, RN, CNRN, CCRN, CCNS
Clinical Nurse Specialist Neurosurgical Intensive Care Unit
Carolinas Health Care System
Charlotte, NC

Johnnie Robbins, MSN, RN, CCRN, CCNS
Critical Care Clinical Nurse Specialist
US Army Institute of Surgical Research
Fort Sam Houston, Texas

Tara L. Sacco, MS, RN, CCRN, ACNS-BC, ACCNS-AG
Visiting Assistant Professor
St. John Fisher College Wegmans School of Nursing
Rochester, New York

Diane Vail Skojec, MS, DNP, CRNP
Nurse Practitioner, Department of Surgery
The Johns Hopkins Hospital
Baltimore, Maryland

Scott C. Thigpen, DNP, RN, CCRN, CEN
Dean and Professor of Nursing
South Georgia State College
Douglas, Georgia

Judith A. Young, DNP, RN, CCRN
Clinical Assistant Professor
Indiana University School of Nursing
Indianapolis, Indiana

Preface

Manual of Critical Care Nursing is a clinical reference for both practicing nurses and students in critical care, progressive care, and complex medical-surgical units. It is the most comprehensive of the critical care handbooks available, yet is a concise and easy reference with an abbreviated outline format and a portable, trim size. This handbook provides quick information for more than 75 clinical phenomena seen in critical care and other high acuity care environments, which promotes evidence-based practice in planning goal-driven care.

WHO WILL BENEFIT FROM THIS BOOK?

Nurses from novice to expert will have access to key information used to perform appropriate assessments, plan and implement care, and evaluate the outcomes of interventions provided to critically ill and acutely ill patients. The textual information and numerous tables will serve as a focused review for the practicing nurse and advanced practice providers. Academicians may find the book helpful in teaching students to apply didactic classroom information to clinical practice. Students will have an excellent tool for assessing the patient systematically, and setting priorities for nursing interventions.

WHY IS THIS BOOK IMPORTANT?

The book provides information concisely, with emphasis on evidence-based practice and outcomes achievement. Goal-directed care is vital to patient safety, and promoting interdisciplinary collaboration. Both a collaborative plan of care, and specific nursing care plans are presented. Given the increasing acuity of hospitalized patients, problems previously managed in critical care such as using arterial blood gas interpretation to correct acid-base imbalances, medically managing dysrhythmias with medication infusions, or controlling blood pressure with vasoactive drugs can be part of daily care of patients in progressive care units, telemetry, stepdown units, and high-acuity medical-surgical units. Accordingly, the care plans presented are applicable across the spectrum of high-acuity care, from complex medical-surgical to critical care. The book addresses the highly technical life-support equipment as part of the care options for each condition, and in detail for those who are actively using the technology in separate, detailed sections.

BENEFITS OF USING THIS BOOK

The primary goal of this reference is to present the information necessary to provide patient- and family-centered care in a technologically advanced environment in a concise, easy-to-use format. The whole patient is addressed with care recommendations for physical, emotional, mental, and spiritual distress involved in illness. The prevention of potentially life-threatening complications is crucial to patient safety and addressed through collaborative, evidence-based care planning. The intent is to offer a thorough selection of prioritized actions that can be chosen as needed in planning individualized care.

HOW TO USE THIS BOOK

Manual of Critical Care Nursing is organized for easy access and logical presentation. Information regarding general concepts of patient care, including those unique to the critical care environment, is presented in the first two chapters, General Concepts in Caring for the Critically Ill and Managing the Critical Care Environment. Following is a chapter on Trauma and related disorders. Chapters 4 through 10 cover disorders classified by body systems, and Chapter 11 addresses Complex Special Situations, such as high-risk obstetrics and organ transplantation.

Each body system–specific chapter includes a general physical assessment, and several chapters include generic plans of care applicable to patients with all disease processes affecting that body system. Each disorder includes a brief review of pathophysiology, physical assessment, diagnostic testing, collaborative management, NANDA-approved nursing diagnoses and nursing interventions, patient/significant other teaching, desired outcomes, and disease-specific discharge planning considerations. Gerontologic icons highlight material relevant to the care of older adults, bariatric icons have been added for care specific to people of size, and safety alerts highlight key information needed to prevent complications. Desired nursing care outcomes and interventions are based on the University of Iowa's Nursing Intervention Classification (NIC) and Nursing Outcomes Classification (NOC) systems and are highlighted throughout the text. Nursing interventions are linked to nursing diagnoses, and suggested outcomes include specific measurement criteria for physical parameters and time frames for attainment of expected outcomes. The suggested time frames for outcomes achievement are guidelines. Each patient's response to the illness and interventions is unique.

For clarity and consistency throughout the book, normal values are given for hemodynamic monitoring and other measurements. All values should be individualized to each patient's baseline health status.

NEW TO THIS EDITION

The seventh edition has been revised to further emphasize evidence-based practices and patient safety and mirrors a practicing nurse's approach to patient care. Changes include:

- Enhanced patient safety information, including new patient safety alerts.
- Updated evidence-based guidelines, including evolving strategies for management of heart and respiratory failure, and advances in technology associated with mechanical ventilation, cardiac mechanical assist devices, and hemodynamic monitoring.
- Information to help assess and plan care for bariatric patients.
- Enhanced medical and nursing management information for correction of acid-base imbalances, management acute asthma, brain injury, burns, sepsis, organ transplantation, obstetric emergencies, cardiogenic shock, heart and respiratory failure, and the management of altered mental status including delirium.
- Appropriate resuscitation interventions within the section on Dysrhythmias and Conduction Disturbances.

I hope that critical care and high-acuity acute care providers, students, and academicians will find that the new edition of *Manual of Critical Care Nursing* provides a wealth of updated, concisely comprehensive, easy-to-access knowledge applicable to clinical practice as well as the classroom.

ACKNOWLEDGMENTS

I want to thank many individuals who supported the development of this manuscript. In particular, I am grateful for the time and efforts of the Elsevier Science staff, including Melissa Rawe, Content Development Specialist, and Marquita Parker, Senior Project Manager, Book Production. I appreciate the guidance of Lee Henderson, Executive Content Strategist. I thank all the contributors for their work, as well as all the reviewers whose comments helped guide our revisions. All are recognized as shining stars in their own right. Both perseverance and patience are the fundamental characteristics inherent in all participants.

Marianne Saunorus Baird

I acknowledge the support of my daughter Rachel, my best cheerleader, and my husband Thom for his patience. I also cannot thank the authors enough for your attention to detail; particularly all the new authors who "filled the gaps" from Emory Healthcare, Atlanta, Georgia. I would also like to acknowledge Savannah Davis, who helped the team begin our process with Elsevier Science.

MSB

Contents

1 General Concepts in Caring for the Critically Ill

ACID-BASE IMBALANCES

Cells must transport ions, metabolites, and gases to function appropriately in their respective roles in the body. For this to occur, the chemical environment of the bloodstream must be electrically stable. The stability of the environment is measured by the arterial pH and must be chemically neutral (pH 7.40) for all systems to function properly. The arterial blood gas (ABG) is the most commonly used analysis to measure acid-base balance and to assess the efficacy of oxygenation. Respiratory (CO_2) and metabolic acids (H^+) are generated as cells work and must be buffered or eliminated to maintain a neutral chemical environment. When the chemical environment is no longer neutral, the patient has an acid-base imbalance. Ineffective metabolism (tissue level), renal dysfunction, and/or problems with ventilation (breathing gasses effectively) are often the cause of acid-base imbalance.

There are two main types of acid-base imbalance: acidosis and alkalosis. The kidneys and lungs work in tandem to maintain chemical neutrality, but it is actually cellular function that produces acid. When either the kidneys or lungs are overfunctioning or underfunctioning, the other system is designed to have the opposite response to compensate and bring the pH back to a normal range. When the kidneys fail to regulate metabolic acids (H^+), the lungs must compensate. When the lungs fail to regulate respiratory acid (CO_2), the kidneys must compensate. Additional buffering mechanisms are also available to help regulate the accumulation of acids. Control of alkaline states, resulting from accumulation of bases or loss of acids, is maintained in a similar manner between the lungs and kidneys.

PATHOPHYSIOLOGY OF ACID-BASE REGULATION

Arterial pH is an indirect measurement of CO_2 and H^+ concentration, which reflects the overall level of acid and effectiveness of maintaining the balance. The normal acid-base ratio is 1:20—1 part acid (the H^+ and CO_2 component of H_2CO_3) to 20 parts base (HCO_3^-). If the ratio is altered through an increase or a decrease in either acid H^+, or CO_2, or the base, HCO_3^-, the pH changes. Chemically, the CO_2 does not contain H^+, but when dissolved in water (plasma), $CO_2 + H_2O$ yields H_2CO_3 (carbonic acid). CO_2, when combined with H_2O, becomes the largest contributor of H^+ (acids), which must be eliminated or buffered to maintain normal pH. Too many H^+ ions in the plasma create acidemia (pH less than 7.35), whereas too few H^+ ions create alkalemia (pH greater than 7.45).

Maintaining the 1:20 ratio ("the balance") depends on the ability of the lungs and kidneys to help normalize concentrations of carbonic acid (H_2CO_3), a product of hydrogen ion (H^+) plus bicarbonate buffer (HCO_3^-). Both the kidneys and lungs are designed to eliminate carbonic acid effectively, and therefore without the presence of lung or kidney disease, the pH should always be in the normal range. A pH change is a symptom that there is a significant problem with one or both of the systems.

- **Acidosis:** Extra acids are present or base is lost, with a pH less than 7.35.
  1. Cellular acidosis: When cells are hypoxic or processing proteins to yield glucose, there is an increase in lactic acid or ketoacid.
  2. Respiratory acidosis: If lung function is inadequate, such as in chronic obstructive pulmonary disease (COPD), the failure to effectively ventilate results in the inability to excrete CO_2, and that failure causes carbonic acid to increase (more acid) and pH to decrease.

   3. **Renal acidosis:** When the kidney function is inadequate, the ability to break down carbonic acid into H^+ and HCO_3^- is impaired. When this failure occurs, carbonic acid increases (more acid) and pH decreases.
- **Buffering of acid or compensation for acidosis** occurs in three primary ways:
   1. **Plasma and cellular buffering:** Using bicarbonate, proteins, intracellular electrolytes, and chloride to buffer H^+, the most common is the marriage of H^+ and HCO_3^-, which yields carbonic acid (H_2CO_3).
   2. **Hyperventilation (lungs):** The presence of increased carbonic acid stimulates a hyperventilation response. This allows for exhaling ("blow off") more of the CO_2 component of carbonic acid. This compensatory response for metabolic acidosis occurs within minutes and should bring the pH to a normal range.
   3. **Acid excretion (kidneys):** A functional kidney will use increased carbonic acid by breaking H_2CO_3 into bicarbonate and H^+, excreting H^+ and retaining bicarbonate. This should compensate for the increased respiratory acidosis but is very slow, taking 4 to 48 hours for compensation to occur.
- **Alkalosis:** Extra base is present or there is loss of acid, with a pH greater than 7.45.
   1. **Respiratory alkalosis:** When hyperventilation is the primary problem, there is a very rapid removal of CO_2, causing carbonic acid to decrease (less acid) and pH to increase.
   2. **Renal alkalosis:** If kidney function is overstimulated (e.g., with aggressive diuresis), there may be excessive loss of hydrogen ions (H^+), causing carbonic acid to decrease (less acid) and pH to increase.
   3. **Other contributors:** Gastric and intestinal removal of acids may occur when patients have diarrhea, vomiting, or when excessive gastric drainage influences the acid-base balance.
- **Compensation for alkalosis** occurs in two ways:
   1. **Hypoventilation:** The respiratory system responds by slowing ventilation and retaining CO_2 (acid) to help compensate for metabolic alkalosis from any cause. This response occurs within minutes.
   2. **Renal response:** The kidneys respond by retaining more acid (H^+) and excreting more bicarbonate to help correct respiratory alkalosis. This response occurs within 4 to 48 hours.

EXAMPLE OF COMPENSATION (pH REGULATION)

When metabolic acids accumulate, they are drawn to bicarbonate. The binding of H^+ and HCO_3^- buffers the acid. This yields an increase in carbonic acid (H_2CO_3) and causes the pH to decrease. Chemoreceptors are stimulated by the presence of this acid and the hypothalamus, if not damaged, triggers a hyperventilation response. Because H^+ is not measured directly, the indirect calculation of bicarbonate or the base is used to evaluate the presence or absence of metabolic acid. As H^+ increases, the bicarbonate or base decreases. When evaluating the acid-base balance, it is simplest to look at bicarbonate but to think of it in terms of how bicarbonate level also reflects the acid level. These values travel in completely opposite directions (when bicarbonate decreases, H^+ increases and vice versa).

The lungs increase buffering to compensate for a failure of the kidneys or a cellular excess acid production to keep the pH balanced. The lungs do this by effectively exhaling more CO_2 than usual, breaking down carbonic acid and therefore bringing the pH back toward normal.

When CO_2 is retained or increased because of respiratory failure, the kidneys should, in turn, respond by processing the increased H_2CO_3. The kidneys separate the carbonic acid into H^+ and HCO_3^- and excrete the H^+ while retaining HCO_3^- bicarbonate. If either the kidneys or lungs do not respond to a pH change (no compensation) or they provide an ineffective response (partial compensation), the patient will remain in acid-base imbalance. If the pH is outside the normal range, then there is a primary problem and compensation is inadequate or has failed. Patients may have a pure acidosis or alkalosis and the overall problem may be masked by compensation or two problems presenting at the same time.

Unless the patient has ingested acid (aspirin, ethanol, etc.), all acid in the bloodstream has been produced at the cellular level (Table 1-1). When evaluating patients, care providers must have a basic understanding of the acid-base balancing system. The main formula for maintenance of acid-base balance is:

$$CO_2 + H_2O \leftrightarrow H_2CO_3 \leftrightarrow HCO_3^- \text{ and } H^+$$

Table 1-1	PRODUCERS AND REGULATORS OF ACID	
Acid Pathways	**Cause**	**Measure**
Cells produce acid (acid production increases).	Hypermetabolic states, such as pain, hyperthermia, or inflammation. The respiratory and heart rates increase, and bicarbonate is initially consumed by buffering.	HCO_3^-
	Tissues are hypoxic; anaerobic metabolism ensues resulting in lactic acidosis.	Lactate level ↑
	Absolute insulin deficiency results in failure of glucose to be transported into cells.	Blood glucose level ↑ Ketoacids ↑
Cells regulate acids.	When acid production (H^+) increases, pH decreases, bicarbonate is initially consumed by buffering, and CO_2 is exhaled in larger amounts, and H^+ exchanges for K^+ as cells buffer acid.	pH ↓ HCO_3 ↓ K^+ ↑ Total serum CO_2 ↓
Lungs regulate acid.	When acid increases as a result of hypermetabolic states such as pain, hyperthermia, or inflammation, carbonic acid (H_2CO_3) increases and rapidly converts to CO_2 and H_2O. The respiratory rate increases to blow off CO_2.	$Paco_2$ ↓
Kidneys regulate acid.	When acid increases, tubules are affected by low blood pH, and work to neutralize increased carbonic acid (H_2CO_3) by separating it into H^+ and bicarbonate HCO_3. Kidneys excrete what is necessary to sustain normal pH if renal function is normal. If abnormal, kidneys may not perform this task.	HCO_3 ↑ Kidney function is assessed by serum blood urea nitrogen and creatinine; elevated blood urea nitrogen and creatinine indicate abnormal kidney function.

The most important component identified is H_2CO_3 or carbonic acid. As carbonic acid increases ("goes up"), the pH decreases ("goes down"), reflecting the presence of acid. If carbonic acid decreases ("goes down"), the pH increases ("goes up"), reflecting the absence of acid. The equation is constantly shifting from left to right and right to left to maintain a normal H_2CO_3 and therefore a normal pH. Whatever causes the change of carbonic acid concentration (may be related to a regulation failure by either the lungs or kidneys or a metabolic acid production state) is the "primary culprit." Identifying the origin or cause of the change in pH direction identifies the problem. Therefore, if the problem is too much acid (either increased CO_2 or H^+), carbonic acid increases and pH decreases. The primary problem is acidosis. Further evaluation is needed to determine whether failure to regulate the acid was ineffective regulation by the lungs, the kidneys, or an increase in cellular acid production (ketoacidosis or lactic acidosis).

Safety Alert   *Changes in pH are associated with changes in the potassium level. As the plasma level of nonvolatile or metabolic acid (H^+) increases, H^+ moves into the cells to reduce the acidemia. In this case, H^+ "exchanges places" with the intracellular potassium (K^+), resulting in a measured serum hyperkalemia but is actually an intracellular hypokalemia. The positively charged intracellular potassium ions are replaced by positively charged hydrogen ions. During an alkalotic state, K^+ may shift into cells as H^+ is released into the serum, creating a transient hypokalemia. As pH changes, it is imperative for the care providers to observe the corresponding changes in the K^+ level, and manage K^+ carefully. When the pH normalizes, the K^+ will shift back to its original location. If a transient K^+ change is managed too aggressively, the patient may experience dangerous hypokalemia or hyperkalemia when pH normalizes.*

UNDERSTANDING THE ARTERIAL BLOOD GAS (ABG)

The ABG is the most commonly used measurement to help assess the origin of problems with acid-base imbalance and to guide treatment designed to restore pH balance and effective oxygenation. "Perfect" values reflect chemical neutrality. There are normal variations or a range for each value.

ARTERIAL BLOOD GAS VALUES

Blood gas analysis is usually based on sampling of arterial blood. Mixed venous blood sampling from a pulmonary artery (PA) catheter (Svo_2) and central venous sampling from a central intravenous (IV) line ($Scvo_2$) may also be performed for patients who are very critically ill. Venous values are given for reference only.

Normal Arterial Values	Normal Venous Values
pH: 7.35–7.45	pH: 7.32–7.38
$Paco_2$: 35–45 mm Hg	$Pvco_2$: 42–50 mm Hg
Pao_2: 80–100 mm Hg	Pvo_2: 40 mm Hg
Sao_2: 95%–100%	Svo_2: 60%–80%
Base excess (BE): −2 to +2	BE: −2 to +2 (only calculated on ABG analyzer)
HCO_3^-: 22–26 mEq/L	Total serum CO_2^-: 23–27 mEq/L

pH (perfect 7.40, normal range 7.35 to 7.45): This reflects the level of respiratory and metabolic acids found in the blood during the continuous "balancing act" that regulates the acid environment. If this balance is altered, derangements in pH occur. Any alteration in pH should be evaluated. If the pH has changed from perfect, it can only be one of two reasons: normal variation or abnormality with compensation. When pH is less than 7.35 or greater than 7.45, it is considered an acute change that is uncompensated. When full compensation is attained for an acid-base imbalance, the pH normalizes. Failure to bring the pH into normal range means there is failure to compensate, despite the body attempting to mount a response. Traditionally, if the body made an attempt to compensate, this was known as partial compensation. This term is no longer advocated.

$Paco_2$ (perfect 40, normal range 35 to 45 mm Hg): This is a measure of pressure (partial pressure designated by the P) that the dissolved CO_2 exerts in the arterial blood. The dissolved gas exerts the pressure of CO_2, enabling it to diffuse across the capillary and alveolar cell wall. CO_2 is released during aerobic metabolism and is the main contributor to serum acid. CO_2 is controlled through ventilation. In the normal lung, CO_2 is regulated by changes in the rate and depth of alveolar ventilation. CO_2 is carried both bound to hemoglobin and dissolved in the blood. The measured CO_2 is termed $Paco_2$. $Paco_2$ is directly measured (not calculated) and is a reliable indicator of respiratory acid-base regulation. The correlation between $Paco_2$ and respiratory-based pH changes is direct, consistent, and linear. In other words, if $Paco_2$ is up and pH is down, the cause is respiratory deregulation. If the issue is metabolic, and respiratory compensation has occurred, the $Paco_2$ will decrease to bring pH back to normal levels. Respiratory compensation typically occurs rapidly in metabolic acid-base disturbances as long as respiratory function is not impaired. When a patient hyperventilates, $Paco_2$ decreases as it is "blown off" by rapid exhalations. During hypoventilation (slow and/or shallow breathing), $Paco_2$ increases. Although the only way to evaluate true lung function is by the gas exchange, the capacity of the lungs (CO_2 regulation response) is measured via the minute ventilation (V_E or MV). This measures the amount of volume exhaled per minute (V_E) calculated as respiratory rate (RR) multiplied by tidal volume (V_T). Normal MV is approximately 8 to 10 L/min.

Pao_2 (perfect 95 to 100 mm Hg, normal range 80 to 100 mm Hg): The partial pressure of oxygen (O_2), or Pao_2, is a measure of the dissolved (usable) gas in the arteries. The dissolved gas exerts the pressure of O_2, enabling it to diffuse across the capillary and cell wall to oxygenate cells. Pao_2 normally declines in the older adult.

- **Hypoxemia** (Pao_2 less than 80 mm Hg): Low partial pressure of O_2 affects the cellular levels of oxygen available and may result in cellular metabolic dysfunction reflected by lactic acid production and metabolic acidosis.
- **Fio_2:** Fraction of inspired O_2 or the percentage of the atmospheric pressure that is oxygenated. Room air is 21% or 0.21 O_2. O_2 delivery devices can increase the Fio_2 to 100% or 1.00.

P/F ratio (greater than 300): Pao_2 is evaluated in relationship to Fio_2, that is, the higher the percent O_2 pressure that is delivered to the lungs, the higher the O_2 in the blood should be.

$$Pao_2/Fio_2 \text{ (in the decimal)} = \text{the P/F ratio}$$
$$100/0.21 = 476$$
$$\text{Normal P/F} = 300$$
$$\text{Hypoxemia P/F} = 300 \text{ on} > 0.40 \, Fio_2$$

Sao$_2$ (perfect 100% or 1.0, normal range 95% to 100% or 0.95 to 1.0): O_2 saturation (Sao$_2$) reflects the loading of O_2 onto hemoglobin (Hgb) in the lungs. When Hgb is loaded with O_2, it is termed oxyhemoglobin. Hgb is the primary transporter of O_2 and supplies a reservoir (reserve) of O_2 for cellular use. Each Hgb molecule carries 1.34 to 1.36 mL of O_2. O_2 must be released from the Hgb, dissolve in blood (Pao_2), and exert pressure to diffuse across the cell wall. The uptake/use of O_2 by the tissues is measured by Svo_2 and/or $Scvo_2$ (mixed venous and/or central venous saturation of Hgb, respectively). Cellular metabolism and O_2 use are affected by changes in stress level, temperature, pH, blood flow, and $Paco_2$. When the Pao_2 falls to less than 60 mm Hg, there is a large drop in saturation, reflected in the oxyhemoglobin dissociation curve.

- **Pulse oximetry (Spo$_2$):** This can be used to noninvasively trend the arterial O_2 saturation and determine ventilation status using a probe fastened to the patient's finger, earlobe, or forehead. This monitoring technique is frequently used in critical care areas for patients at high risk of ventilation problems, in operating rooms, and in emergency departments. Spo$_2$ should be correlated with Sao$_2$ (or oxyhemoglobin) via blood gas analysis when pulse oximetry is initiated, to assess accuracy of Spo$_2$ readings. Pulse oximetry is a close correlate to Sao$_2$ under normal physiologic conditions, but if perfusion decreases, the pulse needed for accurate measurement by the Spo$_2$ probe is decreased, prompting inaccurate readings. Patients with anemia should have consistently high readings, thus what is usually considered a normal Spo$_2$ reading may be too low in a patient with anemia. The measure of true oxyhemoglobin (Hgb saturated with O_2) requires an ABG analysis. Many centers do not perform a correlation analysis when oximetry is initiated.

- **BE** (perfect 0, normal range –2 to +2): Base excess or base deficit uses a calculation to reflect the presence (excess) or absence (deficit) of buffers. The calculation reflects the tissue and renal tubular presence (or absence) of acid. As the proportion of acid rises, the relative amount of base decreases (and vice versa). Abnormally high values (greater than +2) reflect alkalosis, or an excess of base; low values (less than –2) reflect acidosis, or a deficit of base (base deficit).

  - **All buffers:** Absorb acids (H^+), but do so with a varying affinity. Buffers are present in all body fluids and cells and act within 1 second after acid accumulation begins. They combine with excess acid to form substances that may not greatly affect pH. Some buffers have a strong affinity to acid, others are weak. The three primary plasma buffers are bicarbonate (HCO_3^-), intracellular proteins, and chloride (Cl^-). All are negatively charged to facilitate attraction to positively charged hydrogen ions (H^+). Combining positively charged with negatively charged ions yields a neutral substance.

  - **Proteins:** Serum and intracellular proteins offer a significant contribution to buffering acids. Hgb not only transports O_2 but also provides a very strong buffer for hydrogen ions (H^+). Albumin is also a significant buffer, and hypoalbuminemia must be considered when performing anion gap calculations.

  - **HCO$_3^-$ (perfect 24, normal range 22 to 26 mEq/L):** Serum bicarbonate (HCO_3^-) is one of the major components of acid-base regulation by the kidney. Bicarbonate is generated and/or excreted by normally functioning kidneys in direct proportion to the amount of circulating acid to maintain acid-base balance. Because bicarbonate is affected by both the respiratory and metabolic components of the acid-base system, the relationship between metabolic acidosis and bicarbonate is not particularly linear or predictable. When the bicarbonate level changes, the acid level changes in the opposite direction. To determine the cause of bicarbonate changes (as the source of a pH problem versus compensation), the relationship to pH must be evaluated. The pH changes in the presence or absence of acid, and the directional relationship reflects what caused the pH alteration. The kidney is responsible for the regeneration of bicarbonate ions as well as excretion of the hydrogen ions. Although serum bicarbonate is a buffer, it is usually reported in the standard electrolyte panel from a venous blood sample as "CO_2 content" or "total CO_2" rather than as bicarbonate (HCO_3^-). The serum HCO_3^- concentration is usually calculated and reported separately with ABG analysis. Either value may be used as part of the assessment of acid-base balance (Table 1-2).

- **Chloride (Cl^-):** The number of positive and negative ions in the plasma must balance at all times. Aside from the plasma proteins, bicarbonate and chloride are the two most abundant negative ions (anions) in the plasma. To maintain electrical neutrality, any change in chloride must be accompanied by the opposite change in bicarbonate concentration. If chloride increases, bicarbonate decreases (hyperchloremic acidosis) and vice versa. However, the combination of H^+ and chloride actually creates hydrochloric acid (HCl). Chloride concentration may influence acid-base balance (see Anion gap). Chloride concentration should be observed closely when large amounts of normal saline are administered to patients.

Table 1-2	DIAGNOSTIC TESTS FOR ACID-BASE BALANCE	
Role of ABG	**Measures**	**Normals**
Evaluation of arterial oxygen (dissolved oxygen and oxygen bound to hemoglobin)	Arterial oxygen saturation (oxygen bound to hemoglobin)	SaO_2: 0.95 to 1.0 or 95% to 100%
	Partial pressure of arterial oxygen (dissolved oxygen)	PaO_2: 80 to 100 mm Hg (decreased over the age of 70 years)
Calculation of alveolar-arterial (A-a) oxygen gradient	Alveolar-arterial gradient	A-a DO_2: <20 mm Hg
	PaO_2/FiO_2 ratio	PF ratio: 300
Evaluation of cellular environment	pH (reflects H_2CO_3) i.e., ↑H_2CO_3 then pH↓	pH Perfect: 7.40 Normal range: 7.35 to 7.45
Evaluation of ventilation	$PaCO_2$	$PaCO_2$ Normal range: 35 to 45 mm Hg
Evaluation of tissue metabolism	H^+ inversely (indirectly) reflected by buffers: bicarbonate (HCO_3^-) Total CO_2 i.e., ↑H^+ then buffers ↑	pH Perfect: 7.40 Normal range: 7.35 to 7.45
		HCO_3^-: 22 to 26 mEq/L
		Total CO_2: 20 to 26
		Base Normal range: −2 to +2
		Anion gap: 12 ±2
Additional measures of tissue metabolism	Both contribute H^+ to blood Lactic acid Ketoacids	Lactic acid: 1 to 2 mmol/L
		Lactic acid: 1 to 2 mmol/L Ketoacids Blood: 0.27 to 0.5 mmol/L Urine levels Small: ≤20 mg/dL Moderate: 30 to 40 mg/dL Large: >50 mg/dL
Evaluation of renal clearance	Appropriate clearance of excessive components: H^+ or (HCO_3^-) Appropriate clearance of excessive components: BUN and creatinine	pH Perfect: 7.40 Range: 7.35 to 7.45 BUN: 0 to 20 mg/dL Creatinine: <2.0 mEq/L

ABG, Arterial blood gas; *BUN*, blood urea nitrogen.

- **Other buffers:** Other buffers, including phosphate and ammonium, are present in very limited quantities and have a lesser impact on acid regulation.
- **Cellular electrolytes:** The cells also offer protection in the metabolic acid environment. H^+ may exchange across the cell wall, attracted by negatively charged intracellular proteins in a cellular buffering process. When this happens, K^+ is released from the proteins and shifts out of the cell, causing an excess of K^+ in the blood.
- **Anion gap:** Anion gap is an estimate of the differences between measured and unmeasured cations (positively charged particles, such as Na and H^+, respectively) and measured and unmeasured anions (negatively charged particles, such as HCO_3^- and Cl^-). Normally, cations and anions are equally balanced in live humans (in vivo), but when measured in the laboratory (in vitro), the difference may be between 10 and 14 mmol/L. This difference is termed a normal gap (between number of + and – ions). Particles that possess charges tend to have high affinity to bind to other particles that possess charges that are opposite their own (hence the term "opposites attract"). Anion gap is used to determine if a metabolic acidosis is attributable to an accumulation of nonvolatile acids, such as lactic acid or ketoacids. Both contribute a positive charge as a result of excess H^+ or from net loss of bicarbonate (e.g., diarrhea). The gap is not affected when a patient has metabolic acidosis purely from kidney failure. The formula for the calculation of anion gap (AG) is:

$$AG = ([Na^+] + [K^+]) - ([Cl^-] + [HCO_3^-]) \text{ (normal value: } 12 \pm 2)$$

Unmeasured cations: Calcium, magnesium, gamma globulins, potassium, hydrogen ions (bind to negative-charged particles).
Unmeasured anions: Albumin, phosphate, sulfate, lactate (bind to positive-charged particles).

STEP-BY-STEP GUIDE TO ARTERIAL BLOOD GAS ANALYSIS

A systematic analysis is critical to the accurate interpretation of ABG values to determine the origin of acid-base imbalance and level of compensation (see Table 1-2).

Step 1: Check the pH: Determine if pH is perfect (7.40)

When there is a perfect balance of acid and buffer (base), the pH is termed neutral or perfect. If it is not perfect, determine if the direction of the difference is above or below 7.40. Next, determine if it is in the normal range (7.35 to 7.45). If it is abnormal, identify whether it is on the acidotic (less than 7.35) or alkalotic (greater than 7.45) side of normal. "Perfect pH" occurs when the system preserves neutrality (pH 6.8) inside the cells, where most chemistry occurs, and maintains the serum pH at 7.40. For the purposes of learning, the perfect pH is where all measurement begins. When the system contains too many acid ions (in the form of $\uparrow CO_2$ or $\uparrow H^+$), this causes acidemia. When the system contains too few acid ions (in the form of $\downarrow CO_2$ or $\downarrow H^+$), this causes alkalemia, and the pH will reflect the change. Any variation in the pH in relationship to perfect (7.40) must be noted by the provider. If the pH is in the range of 7.35 to 7.45, there are only two possibilities. First, the deviation is a normal variation, wherein no abnormalities exist on either the respiratory side ($Paco_2$) or the metabolic side (HCO_3^-) of the pH equation. Second, there is a problem with ventilation (respiratory), cellular acid production (metabolic), or the ability of the kidneys (metabolic) to balance the pH. Diagnosis of a problem with metabolic acid-base balance is more complex, because many conditions generate metabolic acids and renal failure creates an acid clearance deficit.

pH less than 7.35, Acidosis: Extra acids are present or base is lost. If pH is 7.35 to 7.39, the pH is normal but not perfect (7.40); the pH is considered "on the acidotic side."
- **Acidosis:** Extra acids are present or base is lost, with a pH less than 7.35.
  1. Cellular acidosis: When cells are hypoxic or processing proteins to yield glucose, there is an increase in lactic acid or ketoacid.
  2. Respiratory acidosis: If lung function is inadequate, such as in COPD, the failure to effectively ventilate results in the inability to exhale CO_2, and that failure causes carbonic acid to increase (more acid) and pH to decrease.
  3. Renal acidosis: If kidney function is inadequate, the ability to break carbonic acid from H_2CO_3 into hydrogen ions (H^+) and HCO_3^- is reduced or lost. When this failure occurs, carbonic acid increases (more acid) and pH decreases.

pH greater than 7.45, Alkalosis: Extra base is present or there is loss of acid. If pH is 7.41 to 7.45, the pH is normal but not perfect (7.40); the pH is considered "on the alkalotic side."

- **Alkalosis:** Extra base is present or there is loss of acid, with a pH greater than 7.45.
    1. Respiratory alkalosis: When hyperventilation is the primary problem, there is a very rapid removal of CO_2, causing carbonic acid to decrease (less acid) and pH to increase.
    2. Renal alkalosis: If kidney function is overstimulated (e.g., with aggressive diuresis), there may be excessive loss of hydrogen ions (H^+), causing carbonic acid to decrease (less acid) and pH to increase.
    3. Other contributors: Gastric and intestinal removal of acids may occur when patients have diarrhea, vomiting, or when excessive gastric drainage removes acidic secretions and influences the acid-base balance.

Step 2: Check the $Paco_2$

Check $Paco_2$ for perfect levels (40 mm Hg). If not perfect, determine if the direction of change is above or below 40 mm Hg. Next, determine if CO_2 is in the normal range (35 to 45 mm Hg). If abnormal, identify whether it is on the acidotic (> 45 mm Hg) or alkalotic (< 35 mm Hg) side of normal. If $Paco_2$ has been retained as a result of hypoventilation or overly removed through hyperventilation, the change in pH will be in the opposite direction of the $Paco_2$. Elevated CO_2 lowers pH, whereas decreased CO_2 increases pH. If the change in pH is in the normal range but not perfect, or is out of range, with a $Paco_2$ value that has traveled in the opposite direction, respiratory acid retentions caused the imbalance. Using this technique helps determine whether the primary problem is respiratory (involving $Paco_2$) or metabolic (reflected by HCO_3^-). The $Paco_2$ has to be outside the normal range for there to be a problem.

Step 3: Check for base (deficit or excess)

Check bicarbonate (HCO_3^-) (24 mEq/L) and base (0) for perfect levels. If not perfect, determine if the direction of change is above or below perfect. Next, determine if HCO_3^- (22 to 26 mEq/L) and/or base (–2 to +2) is in the normal range. If the values are abnormal, relate the two values to metabolic acid (H^+). If bicarbonate and base are decreased (a deficit), metabolic acid is increased. If bicarbonate and base are increased (in excess), metabolic acid is decreased. If the change in pH is in the normal range but not perfect, or out of range and the assumed H^+ is in the opposite direction (meaning that the HCO_3^- and/or base are in the same direction as the pH), metabolic issues caused the imbalance. Using this technique helps determine whether the primary problem is respiratory (involving $Paco_2$) or metabolic (reflected by HCO_3^-), or both.

Step 4: Evaluate both $Paco_2$ and HCO_3^-

Correlating the direction of the pH change with the direction of change in $Paco_2$ and H^+ (HCO_3^-) is essential. The value that deviates in the opposite direction from the pH suggests that the primary disturbance is responsible for the altered pH. Assess pH for acidosis or alkalosis, and then evaluate whether the change in CO_2 or H^+ (HCO_3^-) is most reflective of the "direction" of the pH change.

A mixed metabolic-respiratory acid-base imbalance or compensation may be responsible for the values reflected by the ABG.

Step 5: Check Pao_2 and Sao_2

Check Pao_2 and O_2 saturation to determine whether they are decreased, normal, or increased. Decreased Pao_2 and O_2 saturation may signal the need for increased concentrations of O_2 or alveolar recruitment strategies. Conversely, high Pao_2 may indicate the need to decrease delivered concentrations of O_2. Oxygen evaluation is the same for all ABG values, although in the presence of metabolic acidosis, a more in-depth investigation will require evaluation of tissue metabolic functions.

RESPIRATORY ACIDOSIS
PATHOPHYSIOLOGY
Evaluation of an abnormal arterial blood gas resulting in a decreased pH attributable to hypoventilation
Example: pH 7.28, $Paco_2$ 55, HCO_3^- 24, Pao_2 92 mm Hg, Sao_2 91%.

Step 1: pH is 7.28, not perfect or neutral (7.40) and outside the normal range of 7.35 to 7.45

Ideally the pH should always be perfect (7.40), but a small variation is acceptable (range of 7.35 to 7.45). One must remember that pH changes are a symptom of a problem. Thus, the first issue is to identify the problem.

pH: The primary problem with pH regulation is identified by the direction of the pH change with regard to perfect: Is it on the acid side (less than 7.40) or the alkaline side (greater than 7.40)?

1. pH 7.28: Acid side, outside the normal range.
2. Question: Is there a problem? YES, acidosis (identified by the pH).
3. Where is the acid being generated? Are the acids respiratory or metabolic?
4. $Paco_2$: 55 (elevated outside the normal range) ↑ respiratory acid is accumulating.
5. (HCO_3^-)—: 24 (perfect) ↑ metabolic acid is not present, perfect HCO_3.

Step 2: $Paco_2$ is 55 mm Hg, not perfect (40 mm Hg) and above the normal range of 35 to 45 mm Hg, indicating an excess of respiratory acid

Investigation Begins

1. Hypercapnia/elevated $Paco_2$ ($Paco_2$ greater than 45 mm Hg): Signals alveolar hypoventilation. This problem occurs when alveoli are not recruited, there is poor blood flow, the RR rate or tidal volume is inadequate, or there is fluid or an increase in the space between the alveoli and blood vessel. These conditions may be chronic or acute.
2. If this is the causative problem, the pH has to be below 7.40, reflecting excess acid (CO_2) or an increase in carbonic acid (H_2CO_3), which is a primary acidosis. Therefore, one must now investigate what caused the increase in carbonic acid (H_2CO_3). For every 10 mm Hg increase in CO_2, the pH will acutely decrease 0.08 (on the acid side).
3. **Problem: Respiratory acidosis**

   Respiratory acidosis (hypercapnia, hypoventilation) is always related to a ventilation problem caused by inadequate therapeutic interventions or lung pathophysiology, resulting in retention of $Paco_2$. $Paco_2$ derangements are direct reflections of the degree of ventilatory function or dysfunction. The degree to which the increased $Paco_2$ alters the pH depends on the rapidity of onset and the ability of the blood and kidney to compensate via the blood buffer and renal regulation systems. The pH may be profoundly affected initially because of the time required (hours to days) for kidney compensation to occur. The most common cause of inadequate CO_2 excretion (CO_2 retention) is inadequate alveolar ventilation or alveolar hypoventilation. Alveolar hypoventilation can occur when there is airway obstruction, loss of alveolar recoil, or inadequate time for exhalation affecting the ability to express carbon gas into the environment. For CO_2 to be removed from the blood, the partial pressure of CO_2 in the alveoli must be less than that in the blood. In air-trapping syndrome (loss of alveolar recoil or elasticity or airway obstructive disease) or profound hypoventilation states, the alveolar concentration of CO_2 increases, which then limits the removal of CO_2 from the blood. If the problem is not properly managed, the patient may deteriorate into acute respiratory failure.

Step 3: The HCO_3^- in the example is perfect at 24 mEq/L

The normal range of bicarbonate is 22 to 26 mEq/L.

Investigation Begins

1. Normal HCO_3^- indicates that there is not a metabolic problem, although compensation should begin within 4 to 48 hours, as opposed to respiratory compensation for metabolic pH imbalances, which happens in minutes.
2. Problem: No apparent kidney or metabolic problems.

Is there compensation for the respiratory acidosis? For compensation to occur, the carbonic acid must be presented to the kidney and separated into H^+ and HCO_3^-. In other words, the excess CO_2 will be processed into carbonic acid and ultimately into H^+ (which will be excreted in a functional kidney state) and HCO_3^-. Kidney or renal compensation for accumulation of respiratory acids is a slow process. After 48 hours if there continues to be an acidotic pH, one must assume that the kidneys have lost the ability to eliminate H^+ or retain HCO_3^-.

Step 4: Diagnosis begins

1. Only the CO_2 is elevated, without a change in the HCO_3^-.

2. pH is down and outside the range reflecting the presence of acid in the blood.
3. Problem: The patient has acute respiratory failure, causing an accumulation of respiratory acid (CO_2). There is no compensation, but no evidence is available at this time.

Diagnosis: Acute Respiratory Acidosis

Step 5: Pao_2 92 mm Hg (not perfect 98 to 100 mm Hg but within normal range 80 to 100 mm Hg), Sao_2 91% (not perfect 100% and below normal range of 95% to 100%)

Investigation begins: Slight decrease is apparent in Pao_2 and Sao_2

1. Use of O_2: If O_2 is not in use on a patient with reduced Pao_2 and Sao_2, applying O_2 often corrects the readings. If O_2 is in use, changing to a device that delivers a higher concentration of O_2, such as changing from a nasal cannula to a face mask, may be sufficient to correct the alveolar levels of O_2. If the Pao_2 and Sao_2 do not respond to the first device change or values further deteriorate, a 100% nonrebreather mask may be applied to provide close to 100% O_2. Note: All ABG readings must be recorded with consideration of the mode of O_2 delivery recorded, as well as the Fio_2 or concentration of O_2. Otherwise, evaluation of the Pao_2 and Sao_2 values is meaningless. If the values are NOT recorded, the assumption is made that the readings are done on room air, without O_2 in place.
2. Evaluating risk for poor tissue oxygenation: Thus far, ventilation has been evaluated using the ABG, but both ventilation and perfusion must be evaluated as part of O_2 delivery to the cell level. To objectively and proactively identify the patient at risk for tissue hypoxia, early signs of the perfusion changes that precede increases in serum lactate and the widening anion gap associated with lactic acidosis may be noted. Changes in heart rate (HR), blood pressure (BP), respiratory rate (RR), urine output, saturation of continuous central or mixed venous Hgb, and serum creatinine are common. In the shock setting, normal or near normal Pao_2 and Sao_2 readings are possible on an ABG while capillary bed dysfunction ensues. Normal readings indicate that O_2 is being provided in adequate amounts to saturate Hgb effectively, but the ABG is unable to assess whether all tissue beds are receiving O_2 or whether the cells are able to use the O_2. Until metabolic acidosis ensues resulting from accumulation of lactic acid byproducts of anaerobic metabolism caused by hypoperfusion, the ABG and Spo_2 readings may be misleading.

COLLABORATIVE MANAGEMENT: ACUTE RESPIRATORY ACIDOSIS

CARE PRIORITIES
1. Restore effective alveolar ventilation

- Symmetrical lung expansion: Always check for symmetrical lung expansion, particularly if the patient was recently admitted for trauma, has recently had central line placement, or has recently been intubated or extubated. A pneumothorax may be present, which may cause ineffective ventilation.
- Support ventilation: If $Paco_2$ is greater than 50 to 60 mm Hg, there may be a need to intubate and place the patient on mechanical ventilation, or if already ventilated, there may be a need to reevaluate the ventilation settings. The primary mechanism to treat respiratory acidosis is to increase the tidal volume (V_T) and/or the respiratory rate (F), to increase minute ventilation ($V_T \times F$). Care must be taken to ensure the adequate minute ventilation; therefore, if low tidal volumes are applied, the respiratory rate may need to be increased. If lung compliance allows, the flow rate (how rapidly the volume is delivered) may also be increased. This will prolong exhalation time and allow adequate time for CO_2 excretion.
- Bronchodilation: Consider the use of inhaled beta-agonists to maintain open airways.

2. Normalize the pH

- Although a life-threatening pH must be corrected to an acceptable level promptly, a normal pH is not the immediate goal. Generally, the use of bicarbonate is avoided because of the risk of alkalosis when the respiratory disturbance has been corrected and the secondary effect of blocking the signal to the hemoglobin to release the oxygen (shift to the left). Note: If lactic acidosis is present, the patient has metabolic acidosis, which has resulted from ineffective tissue oxygenation. Supporting ventilation will not resolve lactic acidosis. Further, bicarbonate may temporarily neutralize the pH, but may actually worsen tissue hypoxia.

3. Evaluate compensation (occurs in the presence of normal renal function)

- Although the response of the kidneys to an abnormal pH level is slow (4 to 48 hours), they are able to facilitate a nearly normal pH level by excreting or retaining large quantities of HCO_3^- or H^+ from the body. Note that the level of available HCO_3^- is always opposite the level of H^+ present in the plasma. HCO_3 is partnered as it buffers H^+ which yields carbonic acid.

Compensatory response for acute respiratory acidosis

When the respiratory acid level (CO_2) increases, carbonic acid increases and the pH decreases. The increased H_2CO_3 (carbonic acid) is presented to the kidney, where the H^+ is separated from the bond, yielding HCO_3^-. The "free" bicarbonate (HCO_3^-) provides additional buffer. In addition, the kidneys excrete the "free" H^+ (hydrogen ions) in the urine to reduce the acid level. When the kidneys are functional, the pH decrease seen from increased respiratory acid is less dramatic. The decrease in pH is modified to a small degree by intracellular buffering. To compensate for the acidosis created by increased CO_2, K^+ ions are released from cellular proteins and H^+ ions take their place, bound to the proteins. The result is frequently serum hyperkalemia (reflective of intracellular hypokalemia). This is much more common and dangerous in the presence of metabolic acidosis (particularly diabetic ketoacidosis [DKA]).

Renal or kidney compensation via synthesis and retention of HCO_3 regulates much of the acid; however, the pH will not be returned to perfect. When carbonic acid is converted into HCO_3^- (bicarbonate buffer), the pH will be decreased only by approximately 0.03 for every 10 mm Hg increase in CO_2.

1. **Uncompensated respiratory acidosis:** pH 7.28, $Paco_2$ 55, HCO_3^- 24 [Pao_2 92 mm Hg, Sao_2 91%]

$$\uparrow CO_2 + H_2O \rightarrow \uparrow H_2CO_3 \rightarrow HCO_3^- + H^+$$

Compensation for respiratory acidosis

Over time, if ventilation is not effectively managed, the HCO_3^- will increase to 32, which will correct the pH to 7.35 if kidneys are functioning normally. The CO_2 remains 55. O_2 provided at 4 L/min by nasal cannula increases the Pao_2 to 100% and the Sao_2 to 100%.

With the same $Paco_2$, the pH is corrected, primarily by the kidneys, to 7.35: on the acid side of the normal range. Whenever the pH is less than 7.40, it reflects either a normal variation OR abnormality with compensation.

2. **Respiratory acidosis with kidney compensation:** pH 7.35, $Paco_2$ 55, HCO_3^- 32 (Pao_2 100 mm Hg, Sao_2 100%)

$$\uparrow CO_2 + H_2O \rightarrow \uparrow H_2CO_3 \rightarrow \uparrow HCO_3^- + \downarrow H^+$$

pH 7.35: Acid side but in normal range.
$Paco_2$ 55 mm Hg: Acid and outside normal range.
Problem: Respiratory acidosis, but pH is in normal range.
HCO_3^- 32 mEq/L: The kidneys took the H_2CO_3, separated it into HCO_3^- and H^+, and then excreted the H^+ and retained the end product, the bicarbonate (made from the CO_2).

Ultimately, the increase in $Paco_2$, which created an increase in carbonic acid, made the pH decrease. When the increased carbonic acid was presented to the kidney, it was separated into $\uparrow$bicarbonate ($H^+\downarrow$) and yielded the end diagnosis: compensated respiratory acidosis. The kidneys must be functional for compensation to occur in the presence of respiratory acidosis.

CHRONIC RESPIRATORY ACIDOSIS

The compensated scenario just described is what is often seen with chronic hypercapnia, which occurs with chronic obstructive pulmonary disorders (e.g., chronic emphysema and bronchitis, cystic fibrosis), restrictive disorders (e.g., pneumothorax, hemothorax, Pickwickian syndrome), neuromuscular abnormalities (e.g., myasthenia gravis, Guillain-Barré syndrome, amyotrophic lateral sclerosis), respiratory center depression (e.g., brain tumor, stroke, bleed, head injury), and poor ventilation management. In patients with a chronic lung disease, a near-normal pH is the result of kidney compensatory mechanisms, as discussed earlier.

Patients with chronic lung disease can experience acute increases in $Paco_2$ or lose their metabolic compensation (increased production of metabolic acid or loss of renal function) secondary to superimposed disease states, such as pneumonia, hypermetabolic cellular hypoxia, or renal dysfunction. If the chronic compensatory mechanisms in place (e.g., elevated) are inadequate to meet the sudden increase in $Paco_2$ or if the circulation of metabolic acids increases, pH may change rapidly. In fact, these patients frequently have normal HCO_3^- measures upward of 30. As an acute (on top of chronic) process begins, the pH decreases, but the bicarbonate may be slower to reflect the real problem. Care must be taken when evaluating patients with chronic respiratory acidosis who have secondary issues.

CLINICAL PRESENTATION
Patients may have possible increased work of breathing, anxiety, pallor, sweating, reflective of respiratory distress. In advanced respiratory acidosis, somnolence and inability to awaken the patient are common. CO_2-based acidosis has a sedative-like effect on patients. Sleep may ensue following distress, giving the false impression that the problem has resolved, when in reality, the problem has resulted in sufficient CO_2 accumulation for the patient to lose consciousness from the sedative effect of severe hypercapnia. Patients with obstructive sleep apnea are at risk for developing respiratory acidosis.

PHYSICAL ASSESSMENT
Patients have decreased depth of respirations with an initially increased rate or decreased rate and depth of respirations in severe respiratory acidosis. With obstructive lung disease or acute asthma exacerbation, audible wheezing may be present. With severe asthma, the chest can become silent, indicative gas exchange is extremely impaired, and the patient is close to respiratory arrest.

MONITORING PARAMETERS
Use pulse oximetry to assess if hypoxemia ensues because of ineffective ventilation. The patient needs close observation for deterioration, so appropriate steps can be taken to provide noninvasive positive-pressure ventilation (NPPV), such as bilevel positive airway pressure (BiPAP) or endotracheal (ET) intubation with mechanical ventilation.

CARE PLAN: RESPIRATORY ACIDOSIS
Impaired gas exchange related to alveolar-capillary membrane changes secondary to pulmonary tissue destruction

Goals/Outcomes: Within 24 hours of initiation of treatment, the patient improves and is reevaluated. The ultimate goal of adequate gas exchange is evidenced by $Paco_2$, pH, and Sao_2 that are normal or within 10% of the patient's baseline.
NOC Respiratory Status Ventilation, Vital Signs Status, Respiratory Status: Gas Exchange, Symptom Control Behavior, Comfort Level, Endurance, Acid-Base Management: Respiratory Acidosis.

Respiratory Monitoring
1. Monitor serial ABG results to assess the patient's response to therapy. Consult the provider for significant findings: Increasing $Paco_2$ with decreasing pH, Pao_2, and Sao_2 values.
2. Monitor O_2 saturation via pulse oximetry (Spo_2). Compare Spo_2 with Sao_2 values to assess reliability. Watch Spo_2 closely, especially when changing Fio_2, and evaluate the patient's response to activities (e.g., repositioning, chest physiotherapy).
3. Assess and report on the respiratory response to exertion and treatments: Respiratory rate and rhythm, work of breathing, and breath sounds. Compare findings before and after (e.g., O_2 therapy, physiotherapy, medications) for improvement.
4. Assess and report on changes in the patient's level of consciousness (LOC). If $Paco_2$ increases, be alert to subtle, progressive changes in mental status. A common progression is agitation $\rightarrow$ insomnia $\rightarrow$ somnolence $\rightarrow$ coma. To avoid creating a comatose state caused by increasing CO_2 levels, regularly awaken patients with elevated $Paco_2$. Consult the advanced practice provider if the patient is difficult to awaken.

Oxygen Therapy
1. Carefully monitor the patient's response to prescribed O_2 therapy. Assess respiratory status after every change in Fio_2. Patients with chronic CO_2 retention may be very sensitive to increases in Fio_2, resulting in respiratory depression. If the patient is no longer able to breathe effectively enough to exhale an adequate amount of CO_2,

mechanical ventilation may be needed. Be aware of the importance of maintaining the compensated acid-base status. If the $Paco_2$ is rapidly decreased by excessive mechanical ventilation (dropping $Paco_2$, but a remaining excess of bicarbonate), a severe metabolic alkalosis (posthypercapnic metabolic alkalosis) could develop. The sudden onset of metabolic alkalosis may cause hypocalcemia, which can result in tetany (see Hypocalcemia), or hypokalemia, which coupled with severe alkalosis may precipitate cardiac dysrhythmias.

Ventilation Assistance
1. Assess for presence of bowel sounds and monitor for gastrointestinal (GI) distention, which can impede movement of the diaphragm and further restrict ventilatory effort.
2. Assess for presence of symmetrical lung expansion and normal resonance of lung fields. Hyperresonance and asymmetry indicate pneumothorax; dullness and asymmetry indicate solid tissue or fluid occupation of lung or pleural space (e.g., hemothorax, pleural effusion, and hyperplasia).
3. In patients who have obstructive lung disease and are not intubated, encourage use of pursed-lip breathing (inhalation through nose, with slow exhalation through pursed lips), which helps airways to remain open and allows for better air excursion. Optimally, this technique will diminish air entrapment in the lungs and make respiratory effort more efficient.

NIC Cough Enhancement, Acid-Base Management, Respiratory Acidosis, Mechanical Ventilation, Artificial Airway Management, Oral Health Maintenance.

ADDITIONAL NURSING DIAGNOSES AND INTERVENTIONS
Nursing diagnoses and interventions are specific to the pathophysiologic process. See Acute Pneumonia (Chapter 4), Acute Lung Injury and Acute Respiratory Distress Syndrome (Chapter 4), and Acute Respiratory Failure (Chapter 4), along with Mechanical Ventilation later in this chapter.

RESPIRATORY ALKALOSIS
PATHOPHYSIOLOGY
The problem is alveolar hyperventilation, which results in an increased pH.
Example: pH 7.48, $Paco_2$ 30, HCO_3 23.

Step 1: The pH is not perfect
The problem is named by the direction of the pH with regard to perfect: Is the pH on the alkaline side greater than 7.40 or the acid side less than 7.40? The pH of 7.48 is on the alkaline side.

Step 2: The $Paco_2$ has decreased to 30 mm Hg, reflecting hypocapnia ($Paco_2$ less than 35 mm Hg)
This signals alveolar hyperventilation (decreased respiratory acid causing an alkaline pH). When minute ventilation is increased, CO_2 decreases, which causes H_2CO_3 to also decrease (production of carbonic acid decreases) and the pH becomes alkalotic. Question: Is there a problem? The CO_2 has decreased and the pH has increased. The problem is respiratory alkalosis.

Step 3: The HCO_3^- is 23, which is less than perfect but still in the normal range
It must be determined if there is a metabolic contribution to the alkalosis or if there is compensation provided by the kidney retaining acid and excreting bicarbonate. The BE is –1, within the normal range.

Step 4: The Pco_2 is low, the pH is high, and the HCO_3 is normal
The patient is exhibiting a rapid respiratory rate, with deep breaths.

Step 5: The Spo_2 may be normal because the patient is breathing very rapidly but effectively
However, when the respiratory rate is very rapid, there is less time for oxygen diffusion, thus it is possible that the patient's oxygen levels may decrease.
Problem: $\downarrow CO_2 + H_2O \rightarrow \downarrow H_2CO_3 \rightarrow HCO_3^- + H+$

ACUTE RESPIRATORY ALKALOSIS

Respiratory alkalosis occurs as a result of an increase in the minute ventilation (alveolar hyperventilation). Defined as $Paco_2$ less than 35 mm Hg, acute alveolar hyperventilation results most frequently from anxiety and is commonly referred to as hyperventilation syndrome. Caution must be applied to evaluate whether hyperventilation is actually a compensatory mechanism for primary metabolic acidosis. Although it may become necessary to control the patient's minute ventilation, in the presence of metabolic acidosis, loss of the hyperventilation compensation may create a life-threatening acidotic pH and profound refractory hypotension and asystole.

In the alkalotic environment, cells release H^+ and K^+. The result is frequently serum hypokalemia (low serum K^+ with intracellular hyperkalemia). Kidney compensation for the respiratory alkalosis is not clinically apparent for 4 to 48 hours. Acute respiratory alkalosis progresses to chronic respiratory alkalosis if it persists for longer than 6 hours and/or renal compensation occurs.

COMPENSATORY RESPONSE TO RESPIRATORY ALKALOSIS

The kidneys, within 4 to 48 hours, should excrete bicarbonate and retain additional H^+ in an attempt to compensate for the lack of respiratory acid.

- Acute respiratory alkalosis: First 4 to 48 hours HCO_3^- (and therefore the increase in H^+) will decrease 2 mEq/L for every 10 mm Hg decrease in Pco_2.
- Chronic respiratory alkalosis: After approximately 48 hours, the amount of bicarbonate should decrease 4 mEq/L of HCO_3 for every 10 mm Hg decrease in Pco_2.

1. Uncompensated respiratory alkalosis: pH 7.48, $Paco_2$ 30, HCO_3^- 23

$$\downarrow CO_2 + H_2O \rightarrow \downarrow H_2CO_3 \rightarrow HCO_3^- + \downarrow H^+$$

2. Compensated respiratory alkalosis: pH 7.44, $Paco_2$ 30, HCO_3^- 19

$$\downarrow CO_2 + H_2O \rightarrow \downarrow H_2CO_3 \rightarrow \downarrow HCO_3^- + \uparrow H^+$$

If there is only one problem contributing to the pH abnormalities, the pH should function as expected. In other words, a removal of acid by the problem system should be compensated by acid retention by the opposing system.

CHRONIC RESPIRATORY ALKALOSIS

Chronic respiratory alkalosis is a state of chronic hypocapnia caused by stimulation of the respiratory center. The decreased $Paco_2$ stimulates the renal compensatory response and results in a proportionate decrease in plasma bicarbonate (and retention of H^+) until a new, steady state is reached. Maximal renal compensatory response requires several days to occur and can result in a normal or near-normal pH. Chronic respiratory alkalosis is not commonly observed in patients who are acutely ill but, when present, it can signal a poor prognosis.

Safety Alert *In alkalotic environments*

- Sodium and potassium: May be decreased slightly to profoundly (potassium will shift from the extracellular space to the intracellular space in exchange for H^+).
- Serum calcium: May be decreased because of increased calcium and bicarbonate binding. Signs of hypocalcemia include muscle cramps, hyperactive reflexes, carpal spasm, tetany, and convulsions.
- Serum phosphorus: May decrease (less than 2.5 mg/dL), especially with salicylate intoxication and sepsis, because the alkalosis causes increased uptake of phosphorus by the cells. No symptoms occur, and treatment usually is not required unless a preexisting phosphorus deficit is present.

CLINICAL PRESENTATION

Presentation includes lightheadedness, anxiety, paresthesias (especially of the fingers), and circumoral numbness. In extreme alkalosis, confusion, tetany, syncope, and seizures may occur.

PHYSICAL ASSESSMENT

Increased rate and depth of respirations (hyperventilation) are present.

MONITORING PARAMETERS
Cardiac dysrhythmias are present.

CARE PLAN: RESPIRATORY ALKALOSIS
Ineffective breathing pattern *related to anxiety, tissue hypoxia, or work of breathing.*

Goals/Outcomes: If the respiratory alkalosis is primary, within 4 hours of initiating treatment the patient has improved. Final outcome is that the patient's breathing pattern is effective, as evidenced by $Paco_2 \geq 35$ mm Hg and pH 7.45.
NOC Respiratory Status: Ventilation, Vital Signs Status, Respiratory Status: Gas Exchange, Symptom Control Behavior, Comfort Level, Endurance; Electrolyte and Acid-Base Balance.

Ventilation Assistance
1. Manage anxiety: Reassure the patient that a staff member will remain in the room.
    Encourage slower, deeper breathing. Have the patient mimic your own breathing pattern. Administer sedatives or tranquilizers if prescribed. Report the patient's response to the advanced practice provider.
2. Monitor for and manage dysrhythmias: Consult the advanced practice provider for new or increased dysrhythmias. Slight alkalosis can sometimes cause dysrhythmias in those with preexisting heart disease requiring inotropic drugs (see Appendix 6). Hypokalemia associated with alkalosis increases the probability of dysrhythmias.
3. Manage fatigue: Provide uninterrupted rest after the breathing pattern has stabilized. Hyperventilation can result in fatigue.

Safety Alert *Hyperventilation may lead to hypocalcemic tetany despite a normal or near-normal calcium level because of increased binding of calcium. For chronic respiratory alkalosis, nursing diagnoses and interventions are specific to the pathophysiologic process.*

ADDITIONAL NURSING DIAGNOSES AND INTERVENTIONS
Nursing diagnoses and interventions are specific to the pathophysiologic process.

METABOLIC ACIDOSIS

PATHOPHYSIOLOGY
Accumulation of metabolic acids, reflected by decreased HCO_3^- (less than 22 mEq/L) with a pH decreased below 7.40. Metabolic acids are circulating acids that cannot be exhaled. These acids should be neutralized by buffers, excreted by the kidneys, or metabolized.
　　Example: pH 7.28, $Paco_2$ 39, HCO_3^- 16, Pao_2 98 mm Hg, Sao_2 99%.

Step 1: The pH is not perfect
The problem is named by the direction of the pH with regard to perfect: Is the pH on the alkaline side greater than 7.40 or the acid side less than 7.40? The pH of 7.28 is on the acid side.
*   Increased acid production: Excessive lactate and ketones cause acidosis and contribute more unmeasured positives (H^+) into circulation. When an increase in H^+ occurs, HCO_3^- decreases because the role of bicarbonate is to buffer H^+. The conjugation of H^+ and HCO_3^- yields an increase in carbonic acid. As carbonic acid (H_2CO_3) increases, the pH decreases.
*   Decreased renal tubular function (acute tubular necrosis [ATN] or chronic failure): If the kidney is unable to excrete H^+, or if the load is beyond tubular transport capabilities, an increase in H^+ occurs. HCO_3^- decreases because the role of bicarbonate is to buffer H^+ and the kidney has lost the capability to regulate and create appropriate bicarbonate. The conjugation of H^+ and available HCO_3^- yields an increase in carbonic acid. As carbonic acid (H_2CO_3) increases, the pH decreases.

- Ingestion of exogenous acids: Certain medications can cause an increase in circulating acids. Alcohols and other ingested acids can facilitate a wide anion gap.

Step 2: The Paco$_2$ is slightly decreased to 39 but within the normal range

The patient does not have respiratory alkalosis or acidosis. The lungs are not retaining CO_2 and are not exhaling excessive amounts of CO_2.

Step 3: The HCO$_3^-$ is 16, which is less than perfect and below the normal range

This means that the metabolic acid (H^+) is increased. The BE is -6, below the normal range. It must be determined if the acidosis is the problem or a compensatory mechanism for respiratory alkalosis. We have determined respiratory alkalosis is not present.

Problem: Metabolic acidosis is caused by any/or any combination thereof:
- Failure of the kidneys to regulate and excrete acid appropriately (acute or chronic kidney failure).
- Cellular production of acid increases beyond normal regulatory capacity resulting from metabolic alterations (lactic acidosis or ketosis).
- Ingestion of acids (aspirin, methanol).

 Safety Alert   *Metabolic acidosis is much more difficult to diagnose than the simple presence or absence of acid. One must first diagnose the cause of the acid-base imbalance.*

Step 4: The Pco$_2$ is normal, whereas the HCO$_3^-$ is decreased

The patient is exhibiting a normal respiratory rate, with normal depth. With a decreased HCO_3^- and normal Paco$_2$, the patient is not compensating for a respiratory alkalosis. The Paco$_2$ would be decreased with respiratory alkalosis if the decreased HCO_3^- was a compensatory response. The decreased HCO_3^- is the primary problem; an acute metabolic acidosis. Question: What is the problem? The HCO_3^- has decreased and no compensation is apparent by the lungs. The respiratory rate and depth have not increased.

Step 5: The Pao$_2$ and Sao$_2$ are normal because the patient is breathing normally

The patient has normal oxygenation.

Step 6: Performed only in metabolic acidosis: Evaluate glucose, ketones, lactate, chloride level, anion gap and tissue oxygenation (if necessary)

Example: pH 7.28, Paco$_2$ 39, HCO$_3^-$ 16, Pao$_2$ 98 mm Hg, Sao$_2$ 99%.

One must investigate why H^+ is increased and bicarbonate is decreased.
- Is it a compensatory response? If so, the $H_2CO_3\uparrow$ ($H^+\uparrow$) and the patient would have a pH on the alkaline side, indicating compensatory response for respiratory alkalosis.
- Is it a kidney problem? In this case, blood urea nitrogen (BUN) and/or creatinine would be elevated.
- Is it a high chloride (inadequate buffer) problem? If so, the chloride would have to be high.
- Did the patient ingest acids?
- Is it a tissue metabolism issue? In this case, the patient will have high ketones and/or lactic acidosis.

If the answer to the first four questions is no, or those problems do not seem significant enough to cause the pH change, a further investigation must be performed.

Evaluation of glucose and ketones may be reviewed (see Diabetic Ketoacidosis, Chapter 8). If glucose is elevated, a serum ketone level should also be drawn to evaluate for ketoacidosis. If the patient is not found to be in hyperglycemic crisis, lactic acidosis may be present. Evaluation of tissue perfusion and oxygenation requires more testing. Consideration must be allowed for glucose and ketones.

If lactic acid is elevated, it may become necessary to find the cause by using measures to evaluate tissue oxygenation.

Glucose 120, Ketones negative, Lactate 6.8.

This then points to acute metabolic (lactic) acidosis.

METABOLIC LACTIC ACIDOSIS (LACTATE LEVEL >4 MMOL/L)

ASSESSING PERFUSION AND OXYGEN CONSUMPTION AT THE CELLULAR LEVEL

Since the early work of Dr. William Shoemaker, it has been well identified that global tissue hypoxia accompanies all categories of shock, including both O_2 delivery and O_2 use shock. The work of the Surviving Sepsis Campaign to establish early goal-directed therapy validated the role of lactate measurement as a guide to therapy. When cells are in a shock state, O_2 delivery shock is present. Shock effects the mechanics of delivery, whereas systemic inflammatory response or severe sepsis, with the secondary effects of endothelial dysfunction, vasodilation, inflammatory mediation, and unopposed procoagulation, interfere with the use of O_2 at a microcirculatory and cellular level. Large areas of the capillary beds may be hypoperfused, resulting in cells resorting to anaerobic metabolism to survive.

Anaerobic metabolism results in the production of lactic acid, a metabolic acid that can create acidosis if compensation fails. The ABG reflects a decreased pH but does NOT always reflect a markedly decreased PaO_2 and SaO_2. Persistent tissue-level hypoxia further exacerbates the systemic inflammatory response and may lead to multi-organ dysfunction syndrome (MODS) and eventually death.

Arterial lactate concentration is dependent on the balance between its production and consumption. In the critically ill septic population, increased glucose metabolism, increased energy expenditures, and profound catabolism are the norm. The corresponding lactic acidosis signals physiologic stress but may not necessarily be evidence of tissue hypoxia. The concomitant energy expenditures, along with metabolic dysfunction, will increase lactate production, but high levels of clearance may mask this disturbing trend.

These conditions, coupled with an out-of-control inflammatory response and increasing oxygenation dysfunction at the tissue level, combine to produce a profound tissue acidosis. The lactate production is further increased via other abnormal pathways that are specifically related to metabolic dysfunction, even in the absence of tissue hypoxia (type B lactic acidosis).

The main cause of the significantly increased lactate is still a puzzle. One factor is the failure of adenosine triphosphate (ATP) production, which clearly occurs in the presence of a profound O_2 supply/demand imbalance (type A lactic acidosis). This in turn affects the mitochondrial ability to use pyruvate, and the increased pyruvate is indicative of a profound metabolic hyperlactatemia, an elevated lactate/pyruvate ratio, increased glucose, and low energy production. Ultimately, as severe sepsis progresses, it evolves into a mediator-induced cardiac failure state, with profound intraarterial hypovolemia.

SPECIAL CONSIDERATIONS FOR PATIENTS WITH LACTIC ACIDOSIS

In 2004, Nguyen et al., in their work related to early goal-directed therapy when treating sepsis, validated that the higher the clearance of lactate in the first 6 hours after resuscitation, the lower the mortality. In those first hours of evaluation and resuscitation, achieving a normal $ScvO_2$ along with an increasing lactate clearance is the desired therapeutic end point, reducing the potential for MODS.

MEASURING LACTIC ACIDS

In any patient whose condition arouses suspicion (e.g., with tachycardia, tachypnea, hyperventilation, and/or hypotension), it is essential to directly measure acid.

1. Lactate level: All patients who run the risk of cellular hypoxia must have a sample drawn for a lactate level to evaluate for lactic acidosis. An arterial lactate sample should be placed on ice and taken as soon as possible to the laboratory. Any lactate greater than 4 mmol/L needs to be investigated for severe tissue hypoxia and hypoperfusion. Lactates greater than 2 mmol/L should be observed along with the clinical conditions of the patient. Serial lactates should be performed to evaluate therapy effectiveness and follow the clearance level. A lactate clearance greater than 10% in 24 hours is considered a successful measure of therapeutic intervention for severe sepsis.
   a. Limitations to lactate level: The value of lactate is obviously limited as a result of lactate concentrations that are affected by both production and elimination. Liver dysfunction, ketosis, and many medications administered in the critical care unit may affect the measured lactate levels. Therefore, lactate levels by themselves will not give

as much beneficial information as those in the presence of wide anion gap and low or normal Scvo$_2$.

COLLABORATIVE MANAGEMENT: METABOLIC LACTIC ACIDOSIS
CARE PRIORITIES

Key concepts to keep in mind when managing the patient with lactic acidosis, including specific additional monitoring used in refining the plan of care.

1. Manage perfusion first

Lactic acidosis IS NOT respiratory acidosis! Respiratory acidosis is primarily a ventilation problem, whereas lactic acidosis is primarily a perfusion-, metabolic stress-, or cellular O$_2$ consumption or extraction–related problem.

2. Do not rely on Sao$_2$ to assess oxygenation

Reflects reservoir bound O$_2$ and very indirectly reflects oxygen delivery. Normal Sao$_2$ is 0.95 to 1.00.

3. Implement additional monitoring for tissue hypoxia

Supplemental measures may be used in patients who are critically ill for evaluation of tissue hypoxia. Mixed venous and/or central venous saturation of Hgb evaluates the amount of O$_2$ being used by the cells. The comparison of arterial (precellular) saturation to central or mixed venous (postcellular) is most commonly used to evaluate the tissue O$_2$ consumption compared with O$_2$ delivery.

- **Mixed venous (Svo$_2$) or central venous oxygen saturation (Scvo$_2$):** This value is measured by an indwelling O$_2$ probe/sensor on the tip of a catheter placed in the central vein (CV catheter) or PA (PA catheter). Measurement may provide an early indication of perfusion failure or increased tissue demands for O$_2$, reflected by a decreased mixed venous saturation of Hgb. If this saturation is normal or high, but the patient has an increased lactate level, the cells may be unable to extract or use O$_2$, which frequently occurs in the later stages of severe sepsis.
- **Mixed venous saturation values (Svo$_2$):** This value should always be correlated with other tissue indicators of hypoxia, base deficit, widening anion gap, serum bicarbonate, and lactate levels. The difference between arterial and venous blood gases is reflective of global O$_2$ consumption. The following standard parameters are based on mixed venous blood gas and have not yet been standardized for central venous gases; however, the basic principles are the same.
- **Svo$_2$ or Scvo$_2$:** Reflect unused O$_2$ or remaining reservoir after release of needed O$_2$ has occurred. Normal Svo$_2$ is 0.60 to 0.80 OR Scvo$_2$ of 0.65 to 0.85.
- **Oxygen consumption:** Sao$_2$ minus Scvo$_2$ reflects O$_2$ consumption.
  Example: Sao$_2$ 1.00 – Svo$_2$ 0.70 = 0.30, approximately 30% consumption.
- **O$_2$ extraction ratio:** Sao$_2$ minus Svo$_2$ divided by Sao$_2$ reflects O$_2$ extraction ratio:
  Example: (Sao$_2$ 1.00 – Svo$_2$ 0.70) ÷ 1.00 = 30% oxygen extraction ratio.

Normal oxygen extraction ratio is 20% to 30%: In other words, the patient should normally use between 20% and 30% of their total available O$_2$. O$_2$ extraction is a mathematical formula that assists in evaluating the compensatory mechanisms. The first line of compensation is to increase the delivery of O$_2$ (increase the cardiac output [CO], amount of Hgb, and O$_2$ saturation), and the second line is to release O$_2$ from Hgb to provide more dissolved O$_2$ at the cell level, resulting in a shift to the right in the dissociation curve (Figure 1-1).

4. Recognize unusual findings, such as persistent lactic acidosis with normal Svo$_2$

Patients presenting with a normal Svo$_2$ and persistent lactic acidosis are NOT normal. Patients who are using more than 20% to 30% are signaling inadequate O$_2$ delivery, dipping into second-line compensation by removing abnormally high levels of oxygen from the hemoglobin. Second line compensation may be short lived, resulting in acute celluar hypoxia when desaturation of oxyhemoglobin fails.

ACUTE METABOLIC ACIDOSIS

Example: pH 7.28, Paco$_2$ 39, HCO$_3^-$ 16, Pao$_2$ 98 mm Hg, Sao$_2$ 99%.

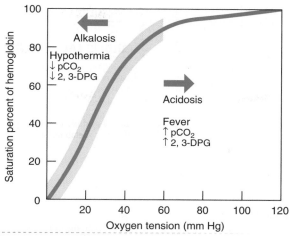

Figure 1-1 **The oxyhemoglobin dissociation curve.** (From Stillwell SB: *Mosby's critical care nursing reference*, ed 4, St Louis, 2006, Mosby).

Bicarbonate is decreased, which always means that H^+ is elevated. If H^+ is elevated, resulting in increased carbonic acid, and the pH is decreased even slightly, the problem is acid accumulation. In this case, it is acute metabolic acidosis, without compensation.

> **Safety Alert** As the nonvolatile acid H^+ increases, it will displace the intracellular potassium, resulting in a serum hyperkalemia but an intracellular hypokalemia. The lungs should increase the rate and depth of respirations to exhale CO_2, to compensate for the excess metabolic acid, so that the pH can return to normal range.

COMPENSATORY RESPONSE TO ACUTE METABOLIC ACIDOSIS

When H^+ (acid) increases, pH decreases in the plasma. The central respiratory center in the brain responds by increasing the rate and depth of ventilation to four to five times the normal level to exhale significant amounts of CO_2 and returning the carbonic acid; therefore, the pH is back to normal (but never perfect if there is a problem). The decrease in pH (high presence of H^+) stimulates respirations. Attempts to compensate occur rapidly, as manifested by lowering of the $Paco_2$, which may be reduced to as little as 10 to 15 mm Hg. The most important mechanism for ridding the body of excess H^+ is the increase in acid excretion through ventilation. In addition, if the kidney is functional, acid will be excreted and bicarbonate reabsorbed. Nonvolatile acids, however, may accumulate more rapidly than the body's buffers can neutralize them, compensated for by the respiratory system, or excreted by the kidneys.

1. Uncompensated acute metabolic acidosis: pH 7.28, $Paco_2$ 39, HCO_3^- 16.

$$CO_2 + H_2O \leftarrow \uparrow H_2CO_3 \leftarrow \downarrow HCO_3^- + H^+\uparrow$$

2. Compensated metabolic acidosis: pH 7.36, $Paco_2$ 30, HCO_3^- 16, Sao_2 99%, Pao_2 100%.

$$\downarrow CO_2 + H_2O \leftarrow \uparrow H_2CO_3 \leftarrow \downarrow HCO_3^- + H^+\uparrow$$

Step 1: pH 7.36: Acid side but in normal range

- *Question:* Is there a problem? Normal variation in pH from perfect, OR a compensated acid-base imbalance?
- *Answer:* Yes, there is a problem. The pH decrease is not a normal variation because the $Paco_2$ and HCO_3 are out of range.

Step 2: Paco₂ 30 mm Hg

Level is decreased, which should reflect toward the alkaline side, which does not coincide with the direction of the pH change.

Step 3: HCO₃⁻ 16 mEq/L

Level is decreased and beyond the low normal range, which means the metabolic acid (H^+) is increased. Here is the cause of the problem that decreased the HCO_3^-.

Step 4: The Paco₂ is decreased in the presence of a decreased HCO₃⁻

Acid reduced the pH, and the lungs compensated by separating the H_2CO_3 into CO_2 and H_2O and, with the help of the respiratory center, exhaled the CO_2. The problem is compensated metabolic acidosis.

Step 5: The Pao₂ and Sao₂ are normal because the patient is breathing normally

The patient has normal oxygenation.

COLLABORATIVE MANAGEMENT: ACUTE METABOLIC ACIDOSIS

CARE PRIORITIES

1. It is most important to treat the underlying disorder, if possible

- **Diabetic ketoacidosis:** Insulin and fluids. If acidosis is severe (with a pH of less than 7.15 or HCO_3^- 6 to 8 mEq/L), judicious administration of $NaHCO_3$ may be necessary.
- **Alcoholism-related ketoacidosis:** Glucose and saline.
- **Diarrhea:** Usually occurs in association with other fluid and electrolyte disturbances; correction addresses concurrent imbalances.
- **Acute renal failure:** Hemodialysis or peritoneal dialysis to maintain an adequate level of plasma HCO_3^-.
- **Renal tubular acidosis:** May require modest amounts (less than 100 mEq/day) of bicarbonate.
- **Poisoning and drug toxicity:** Treatment depends on drug ingested or infused. Hemodialysis or peritoneal dialysis may be necessary.
- **Lactic acidosis:** Correction of underlying disorder related to hypoxia and/or hypoperfusion. Mortality associated with lactic acidosis is high. Unless pH is life threatening, treatment with $NaHCO_3$ is generally not indicated and may actually be harmful.

2. Measure anion gap

Anion gap is an estimate of the differences between measured and unmeasured cations (positively [+] charged particles, such as Na and H^+, respectively) and measured and unmeasured anions (negatively [-] charged particles, such as HCO_3^- and Cl^-). A thorough discussion was provided earlier in this chapter. The gap is not affected when a patient has metabolic acidosis purely from kidney failure. The formula for calculation of anion gap (AG) is:

$$AG = ([Na^+] + [K^+]) - ([Cl^-] + [HCO_3^-]) \text{ (normal value: } 12 \pm 2)$$

3. Treat the pH

Treat the pH only if the patient's life is threatened. Sodium bicarbonate ($NaHCO_3$) may be indicated when arterial pH is ≤7.15. The usual mode of delivery is IV drip: 2 or 3 ampules (44.5 mEq/ampule) in 1000 mL D₅W, although $NaHCO_3$ may be given by IV push in emergencies. Deficit should be calculated and replaced accordingly. Concentration depends on severity of the acidosis and presence of any serum sodium disorders. $NaHCO_3$ must be given very cautiously to avoid metabolic alkalosis and pulmonary edema as a result of the sodium load. Dose (mmol) = BE × weight/10 to replace half of the loss. Usual dose for full replacement is 1 mmol/kg IV (repeated as required).

4. Manage hyperkalemia

Usually serum hyperkalemia is present, but an intracellular potassium deficit may be present. If a potassium deficit exists (K^+ less than 3.5), it must be corrected before $NaHCO_3$ is administered, because when the acidosis is corrected, the potassium shifts back to intracellular spaces. This shift in K^+ could result in a profound serum hypokalemia with serious consequences, such as cardiac irritability with fatal dysrhythmias and generalized muscle weakness. See Hypokalemia for more information.

5. Support ventilation

If mechanical ventilation is required on the basis of ABG results and clinical signs, it is important that the patient's compensatory hyperventilation be allowed to continue to prevent acidosis from becoming more severe. Therefore, the respiratory rate on the ventilator should not be set lower than the rate at which the patient has been breathing spontaneously, and the tidal volume should be large enough to maintain compensatory hyperventilation until the underlying disorder can be resolved.

NURSING DIAGNOSES AND INTERVENTIONS

Nursing diagnoses and interventions are specific to the pathophysiologic process. See nursing diagnoses and interventions in the section on Mechanical Ventilation, Acute Respiratory Failure (Chapter 4), Emotional and Spiritual Support of the Patient and Significant Others (Chapter 2), Acute Renal Failure/Acute Kidney Injury (Chapter 6), and Diabetic Ketoacidosis (Chapter 8).

CHRONIC METABOLIC ACIDOSIS

ASSESSMENT
History and risk factors

Affected patients generally include those with chronic renal failure, renal tubular acidosis, loss of alkaline fluid (e.g., with diarrhea or pancreatic or biliary drainage) for greater than 3 to 5 days.

Clinical presentation

Usually the process leading to chronic metabolic acidosis is gradual and the patient is symptom-free until serum HCO_3^- is ≤ 15 mEq/L. Fatigue, malaise, and anorexia may be present in relation to the underlying disease. Findings vary, depending on underlying disease states and the severity of the acid-base disturbance and the speed with which it developed. There may be changes in LOC that range from fatigue and confusion to stupor and coma.

Physical assessment

Tachycardia (until pH is less than 7.0, then bradycardia), decreased BP, tachypnea leading to alveolar hyperventilation (may be Kussmaul respirations), dysrhythmias, and shock state. Depending on the type of shock and the vascular response, skin temperature and color will be affected. Mild metabolic acidosis (HCO_3^- 15 to 18 mEq/L) may result in no symptoms, whereas symptoms will develop with a pH less than 7.2.

Monitoring parameters

A waveform suggestive of hyperkalemia (prolonged PR interval, widened QRS, and peaked T waves) may occur. Persistent tachycardia may indicate tissue hypoperfusion.

Electrocardiography (ECG): Detects dysrhythmias, which may be caused by metabolic acidosis or hyperkalemia. Changes seen with hyperkalemia include peaked T waves, depressed ST segment, decreased size of R waves, decreased or absent P waves, and widened QRS complex. Ventricular fibrillation may occur.

COLLABORATIVE MANAGEMENT:
CHRONIC METABOLIC ACIDOSIS

CARE PRIORITIES
1. Normalize the pH with alkalizing agents

- For serum HCO_3^- levels less than 15 mEq/L, oral alkalis may be administered ($NaHCO_3$ tablets or sodium citrate and citric acid oral solution [Shohl solution]). They are used cautiously to prevent fluid overload and tetany caused by hypocalcemia.

- Caution: Be alert to the possibility of pulmonary edema if bicarbonate is administered parenterally to patients with renal insufficiency or cardiovascular disorders.

2. Manage hypophosphatemia with oral phosphates
- These are given if hypophosphatemia is present; it is not common with chronic renal failure but may result from overuse of phosphate binders given to treat hyperphosphatemia (very common with chronic renal failure).

3. Provide renal replacement therapies
- Hemodialysis, citrated blood and renal replacement therapy (CRRT), or peritoneal dialysis may be indicated for chronic renal failure or other disease processes (see Acute Renal Failure, Chapter 6).

NURSING DIAGNOSES AND INTERVENTIONS FOR CHRONIC METABOLIC ACIDOSIS
Nursing diagnoses and interventions are specific to the underlying pathophysiologic process.

METABOLIC ALKALOSIS
PATHOPHYSIOLOGY
Elevated HCO_3^- levels (greater than 26 mEq/L) reflect decreasing circulating metabolic acids (H^+). Caution must be applied to differentiate compensatory alterations in response to respiratory acidosis versus primary disorder. The diagnosis is made by the presence of elevated serum HCO_3^- (up to 45 to 50 mEq/L). Acute metabolic alkalosis most commonly reflects:
- Excessive loss of hydrogen ions: Loss of gastric acid from vomiting or gastric suction, diuretic therapy.
- Excessive resorption of bicarbonate: Posthypercapnic alkalosis (which occurs when chronic CO_2 retention is corrected rapidly).
- Ingestion or administration of alkaline: Excessive $NaHCO_3$ administration (i.e., overcorrection of a metabolic acidosis) or ingestion of over-the-counter antacids.

Even when the causative factors have been removed, the alkalosis will be sustained until volume and electrolyte disturbances that are contributing to the alkalosis have been corrected. Severe alkalosis (pH greater than 7.6) is associated with high morbidity and mortality. Acidosis is better tolerated than alkalosis. SpO_2 will be used for Step 5, because a discussion of PaO_2 and SaO_2 does not add to knowledge of metabolic alkalosis.

Example: pH 7.58, $PaCO_2$ 40 mm Hg, HCO_3^- 35, SaO_2 99%, PaO_2 99 mm Hg.

Problem: $CO_2 + H_2O \leftarrow H_2CO_3 \downarrow \leftarrow \uparrow HCO_3^- + H^+ \downarrow$

Step 1: The pH is not perfect
The problem is named by the direction of the pH with regard to perfect: on the acid side less than 7.40 or the alkaline side greater than 7.40.

Example: pH 7.58 on alkaline side, outside normal range.

Question: Is there a problem? YES.

Step 2: The $PaCO_2$ is 40 mm Hg, which is perfect
This indicates $PaCO_2$ is not driving the increase in pH.

Step 3: HCO_3^- has increased to 35 mEq/L, indicating that the kidneys are retaining bicarbonate (H^+ is decreased)
Here is the cause of the problem: acute metabolic alkalosis.

HCO_3^- is 35 (up and out of range), which means that the metabolic acid and H^+ is decreased.

Step 4: The $PaCO_2$ has not increased in an attempt to help correct or compensate for the increased HCO_3^-
The patient is exhibiting a normal respiratory rate, with normal depth. With an increased HCO_3^-, and normal $PaCO_2$, the patient is not compensating for a metabolic alkalosis.

Step 5: The Pao_2 and Sao_2 are normal because the patient is breathing normally

The patient has a normal oxygenation, but has an abnormal response to alkalosis. The respiratory rate and depth should decrease to promote CO2 retention to compensate.

COMPENSATORY RESPONSE TO METABOLIC ALKALOSIS

When H^+ (acid) decreases, pH increases. The central respiratory center in the brain responds by decreasing the rate and depth of ventilation (in the normal lung) to 50% to 75% of the normal level. This method of compensation is very poorly tolerated, because patients will almost stop breathing.

Uncompensated metabolic alkalosis: pH 7.58, $Paco_2$ 40 mm Hg, HCO_3^- 35.

$$CO_2 + H_2O \leftarrow H_2CO_3 \leftarrow \uparrow HCO_3^- + \downarrow H^+$$

Compensated metabolic alkalosis: pH 7.45, $Paco_2$ 59 mm Hg, HCO_3^- 35.

$$\uparrow CO_2 + H_2O \leftarrow H_2CO_3 \downarrow \leftarrow \uparrow HCO_3^- + \downarrow H^+$$

In this example: pH 7.45, $Paco_2$ 59 mm Hg, HCO_3^- 35, Sao_2 99%, Pao_2 99 mm Hg.

Step 1: pH 7.45

Alkaline side, inside the normal range.

* Question: Is there a problem, despite the normal pH? Yes! Other values are abnormal.

Step 2: $Paco_2$ 59 mm Hg

Increased level, which reflects toward the acid side; change is opposite the pH, which is toward the alkaline side. The $Paco_2$ is not the problem but rather a compensation. The increased $Paco_2$ would not increase the pH to alkaline. This measure is in the wrong direction to be the cause.

Step 3: HCO_3^- 35 mEq/L

Increased and out of range. Here is the cause of the problem. Metabolic alkalosis is present because the metabolic acid (H^+) is decreased.

Step 4: The $Paco_2$ is elevated at 59 mm Hg

The $Paco_2$ has increased response to an increased HCO_3^- level. When HCO_3^- increases, the pH increases, indicating that less H^+ is present in the body. The pH has normalized on the alkaline side, thus the patient has fully compensated metabolic alkalosis.

Step 5: The Sao_2 is normal

The patient has a normal rate and depth of respirations.

COLLABORATIVE MANAGEMENT: ACUTE METABOLIC ALKALOSIS

Management will depend on the underlying disorder. Mild or moderate metabolic alkalosis usually does not require specific therapeutic interventions. Correction of chloride deficits is a priority for treatment with many underlying disorders.

CARE PRIORITIES
1. Manage chloride deficit

Normal saline infusion may correct volume (chloride) deficit in patients with gastric alkalosis because of gastric losses. Metabolic alkalosis is difficult to correct if hypovolemia and chloride deficit are not corrected.

2. Correct hypokalemia

Potassium chloride (KCl) is indicated for patients with low potassium levels. KCl is preferred over other potassium salts because chloride losses can be replaced simultaneously.

3. Sodium and potassium chloride

Effective for posthypercapnic alkalosis, which occurs when chronic CO_2 retention is corrected rapidly (e.g., via mechanical ventilation). If adequate amounts of chloride and potassium are not available, renal excretion of excess HCO_3^- is impaired and metabolic alkalosis continues.

4. Cautious IV administration of isotonic hydrochloride solution, ammonium chloride, or arginine hydrochloride

May be warranted if severe metabolic alkalosis (pH greater than 7.6 and HCO_3^- greater than 40 to 45 mEq/L) exists, especially if chloride or potassium salts are contraindicated. The medication is delivered via continuous IV infusion at a slow rate, with frequent monitoring of IV insertion site for signs of infiltration. Ammonium chloride and arginine hydrochloride may be dangerous to patients with renal or hepatic failure.

NURSING DIAGNOSES AND INTERVENTIONS FOR ACUTE METABOLIC ALKALOSIS

Nursing diagnoses and interventions are specific to the underlying pathophysiologic process.

CHRONIC METABOLIC ALKALOSIS

PATHOPHYSIOLOGY

Chronic metabolic alkalosis results in a pH greater than 7.45 and HCO_3^- greater than 26 mEq/L. $Paco_2$ will be elevated (greater than 45 mm Hg) to compensate for the loss of H^+ or excess serum HCO_3^-. The three clinical situations in which this can occur are:

1. Abnormalities in the excretion of HCO_3^- of the kidneys related to a mineralocorticoid effect.
2. Loss of H^+ through the GI tract.
3. Long-term diuretic therapy, especially with the thiazides and furosemide. A compensatory increase in $Paco_2$ (up to 50 to 60 mm Hg) may be seen. Respiratory compensation is very limited because of hypoxemia, which develops as a result of decreased alveolar ventilation.

Compensatory response to chronic alkalosis

When extracellular fluid is alkalotic, the kidneys conserve H^+ and eliminate HCO_3^-, resulting in excretion of alkalotic urine. Renal excretion of acid load and increase in circulating buffer represent the major compensation for respiratory deficits and require a normally functioning kidney. Although the response of the kidneys to an abnormal pH level is slow (4 to 48 hours), they are able to facilitate a nearly normal pH level by excreting or retaining large quantities of HCO_3^- or H^+ from the body. Acid-base balance is regulated by increasing or decreasing H^+ and bicarbonate (HCO_3^-) concentration in body fluids. A series of complex reactions with H^+ secretion, sodium ion (Na^{2+}) resorption, HCO_3^- retention, and ammonia synthesis (excretes H^+ in the urine) occurs.

CLINICAL PRESENTATION

Muscular weakness, neuromuscular instability, and hyporeflexia because of accompanying hypokalemia are present. Decrease in GI tract motility may result in an ileus. Severe alkalosis can result in apathy, confusion, and stupor. Seizures may occur.

PHYSICAL ASSESSMENT

Decreased respiratory rate and depth, periods of apnea, and tachycardia (atrial or ventricular) are present.

MONITORING PARAMETERS

Atrial and ventricular dysrhythmias as a result of cardiac irritability secondary to hypokalemia; prolonged QT intervals are present (see Hypokalemia).

- Urinalysis: Urine chloride levels can help identify the cause of the metabolic alkalosis. Urine chloride level will be less than 15 mEq/L if hypovolemia and hypochloremia are present, and greater than 20 mEq/L with excess retained HCO_3^-. This test is not reliable if diuretics have been used within the previous 12 hours.
- ECG findings: To assess for dysrhythmias, especially if profound hypokalemia or alkalosis is present.

COLLABORATIVE MANAGEMENT: CHRONIC METABOLIC ALKALOSIS

The goal is to correct the underlying acid-base disorder via the following interventions.

CARE PRIORITIES
1. Fluid management
If volume depletion exists, normal saline infusions are given.

2. Potassium replacement
If a chloride deficit is also present, KCl is the drug of choice. If a chloride deficit does not exist, other potassium salts are acceptable.
- IV potassium: If the patient is undergoing cardiac monitoring, up to 20 mEq/h of KCl is given for serious hypokalemia. Concentrated doses of KCl (greater than 40 mEq/L) require administration through a central venous line because of blood vessel irritation.
- Oral potassium: Unpleasant flavor if mixed as a liquid; 15 mEq/glass is the most patients can tolerate, with a maximum daily dose of 60 to 80 mEq. Slow-release potassium tablets are an acceptable form of KCl. All forms of KCl may be irritating to gastric mucosa.

3. Dietary
The normal diet contains 3 g or 75 mEq potassium but not in the form of KCl. Dietary supplementation of potassium is not effective if a concurrent chloride deficit is also present.

4. Potassium-sparing diuretics
These may be added to treatment if thiazide diuretics are the cause of hypokalemia and metabolic alkalosis.

CLINICAL PRESENTATION
The patient may be symptom-free. With severe potassium depletion and profound alkalosis, the patient may experience weakness, neuromuscular instability, and a decrease in GI tract motility, which can result in ileus.

PHYSICAL ASSESSMENT
Decreased respiratory rate and depth, and tachycardia (atrial or ventricular) are present.

MONITORING PARAMETERS
Frequent *premature ventricular contractions* (PVCs) or U waves with hypokalemia and alkalosis are present.

NURSING DIAGNOSES AND INTERVENTIONS FOR CHRONIC METABOLIC ALKALOSIS
Nursing diagnoses and interventions are specific to the underlying pathophysiologic process.

ALTERED MENTAL STATUS
PATHOPHYSIOLOGY
Consciousness is a state of awareness of the self and environment composed of three aspects: arousal (ability to awaken), ability to perceive internal and external stimuli, and ability to perform goal-directed behavior. Alterations are noted when a person has difficulty focusing, sustaining, or shifting attention. Mental status is the salient feature of consciousness and a direct measure of brain function. Mental status encompasses orientation, thought processing, memory and learning, attention, and judgment. Changes in mental status occur as a result of direct injury to brain tissue resulting from perfusion defects (ischemia), brain injury, and tumors. Mental status change also occurs as a result of systemic problems, including infection, metabolic, or endocrine problems. A change in mental status is also associated with dementia, delirium, coma, encephalopathy, and psychiatric disorders. Mental status change may be as subtle as a variation in behavior or as profound as loss of consciousness. Whatever the cause, confusion, memory loss, change in alertness, disorientation, lack of judgment or insight, emotional dysregulation, anxiety, agitation, restlessness, and change in psychomotor skills or behavior are critical clues to a changing condition.

Factors precipitating various alterations in consciousness or mental status are listed in Table 1-3. These precipitating factors arise from intrinsic causes (medical condition and

Table 1-3	FACTORS PRECIPITATING ALTERATIONS IN CONSCIOUSNESS OR CHANGE IN MENTAL STATUS			
Acute Behavior Change	**Delirium**	**Coma**	**Cognitive Dysfunction**	**Others**
CNS infection (meningitis, encephalitis) CNS trauma Drug interactions Drug overdose Drug toxicity Drug withdrawal Dehydration Exacerbation of metabolic or endocrine disease (DKA, myxedema) Exacerbation of psychiatric illness Hypoxia Hypoglycemia Sepsis/infection	Age Aggressive/ dominant personality Anesthesia time Arrhythmias Body temperature change Cardiac dysrhythmia or failure Cerebral disorders Dehydration Disease severity ICU admission Drug interactions Toxic ingestions Electrolyte imbalances End-stage disease (renal, liver) Impaired communication Infection Metabolic disturbances Neuropsychiatric disorders Pulmonary disorders Sleep deprivation Surgery (hip, cardiac, neurologic) Toxins Use of physical restraints Withdrawal syndromes Sensory impairment (hearing and vision)	Cerebral structural changes (brain injury) Cerebrovascular impairment (hemorrhage, ischemia, or edema) CNS dysfunction Metabolic conditions (liver/renal failure, diabetic coma, ketoacidosis)	Chronic alcohol (ethanol) abuse Intravenous or oral substance abuse Dementia Huntington disease Hydrocephalus Hypoxic/anoxic injury Parkinson disease Stroke Thiamine, vitamin B deficiencies Traumatic brain injury	Coma related to cerebral or metabolic disorders Diffuse organic cerebral dysfunction (confused with the catatonic behavior of schizophrenia or severe depressive reaction) Drug overdose Alcohol (ethanol) intoxication Locked-in syndrome Stupor Supranuclear motor deafferentation related to brainstem injury Vegetative state (coma vigil)

CNS, Central nervous system; *DKA*, diabetic ketoacidosis; *ICU*, intensive care unit.

associated problems) and extrinsic causes (environmentally produced). Impaired consciousness or change in mental status, regardless of etiology, results in higher complication rates, puts the patient's safety at risk, causes longer hospital stays, and is linked to higher morbidity and mortality. Three states of mental status change or impaired consciousness, coma, delirium, and cognitive dysfunction, can be recognized in emergency department and hospitalized patients. Although each of these conditions may arise from distinct medical problems, the clinical features are often similar and may be superimposed on each other, making diagnosis and treatment more complex. Change in mental status or change in behavior are often the early warning signs of a medical emergency. The differential diagnosis is crucial to the proper treatment of these mental status changes. The following are descriptions of common mental status variants that require further evaluation.

ABNORMAL BEHAVIOR

Often a precursor to alterations in consciousness, acute change in behavior is a frequent predictor of an underlying medical or psychiatric problem. Abnormal behavior described as an objective change in a person's normal activity pattern is often associated with confusion. Although there are no specific medical definitions of abnormal behavior or confusion, subtle changes in normal routine are identified by family members and caregivers. Reported behavioral changes may be simply a variation in daily pattern, inability to articulate a common word or do a familiar task, failure to recognize danger, fear, euphoria, somnolence, or change in interaction with a known person (friend, family member, caregiver, or authority figure). Individuals do not have insight into their change in behavior, thus the reports of others must be recognized as valid. Although the causes of abnormal behavior and associated confusion are varied, the first step in the evaluation of abnormal behavior is to identify life-threatening causes. Screening for vital sign changes (BP, HR, RR, and temperature), hypoxia, and hypoglycemia provide initial data to differentiate acute medical conditions such as sepsis, DKA, and respiratory compromise that require immediate attention or hypovolemia caused by dehydration. For elderly persons and persons with existing chronic conditions, behavior change may be the single indicator of declining medical status. The second step in evaluation of a patient with change in behavior is determining if the problem is disorientation and memory (linked to medical or neurologic problems) or changes in thought content (linked to psychiatric problems). In addition to the history of the present illness, taking a thorough medical and substance abuse history is imperative. Quick bedside tests such as the Six-Item Screen, Quick Confusion Scale, or Vigilance A Test provide reliable information for cognitive function, attention, and confusion.

DELIRIUM

This is a state of disordered attention that reflects an underlying acute or subacute process. It is usually a transient condition (may be prolonged) that develops along a continuum including a clouding of consciousness, confusion, attention deficit, global cognitive impairment, and psychosis. Symptoms include disorientation to time, place, and person; disorganized thinking; fear; irritability; misinterpretation of sensory stimuli (e.g., pulling at tubes and dressings); appearance of being distracted; altered psychomotor activity; altered sleep-wake cycles; memory impairment; hallucinations; inappropriate communication (e.g., yelling, swearing, nonsensical speech); and dreamlike delusions. Lucid intervals alternate with episodes of delirium. Patients may have difficulty following commands. Daytime drowsiness is contrasted with nighttime agitation. Clinical variants of delirium include the hyperactive-hyperalert form, the quiet form, and a combination form that combines the hyperactive-hyperalert and quiet forms to produce both lethargy and agitation (Figure 1-2).

COMA

Coma is an alteration in arousal and diminished awareness of self and environment. No understandable response to external stimuli or inner need is elicited. No language is spoken. There are no covert or overt attempts at communication or eye opening. Spontaneous purposeful movement and/or localizing movements are absent. Motor responses to noxious stimuli are reflexive and do not result in recognizable defensive movements. Sleep-wake cycles are absent on the electroencephalogram (EEG). The extent of coma is difficult to quantify because limits of consciousness are difficult to define. Self-awareness can only be inferred from appearance and actions. Coma occurs when normal central nervous system (CNS) function is disrupted by alteration in the cerebral structure (brain injury), cerebrovascular impairment (hemorrhage, ischemia, or edema), or metabolic conditions (hepatic encephalopathy). If coma persists for longer than 4 weeks, it is defined as transitioning to a vegetative state.

Differential diagnosis of coma

The characteristics of syndromes or mental states described as follows are useful in determining the differential diagnosis because many have similar presentations.

- **Stupor:** Deep sleep with responsiveness only to vigorous and repeated stimuli with return to unresponsiveness when the stimulus is removed. Stupor usually is related to diffuse organic cerebral dysfunction but may be confused with the catatonic behavior of schizophrenia or the behavior associated with a severe depressive reaction.

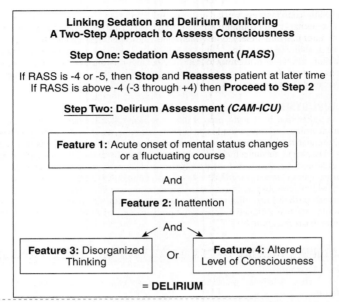

Figure 1-2 Linking sedation and delirium monitoring; a two-step approach to assess consciousness.
(Copyright © E. Wesley Ely, MD, MPH, and Vanderbilt University, 2002.)

- **Minimally conscious state (MCS):** Describes patients who demonstrate inconsistent but reproducible behavior indicating awareness of self and environment. Generally, they cannot reliably follow commands or communicate but show visual fixation and tracking and have emotional and/or behavioral responses to external stimuli. Once the patient consistently follows commands, can reliably communicate, and uses objects in a functional way, the minimal conscious state ends. Although the etiology is uncertain, MCS seems to be related to diffuse, bilateral, subcortical, and hemispheric damage.
- **Akinetic mutism (AM):** Subcategory of MCS in which a decrease in spontaneity and initiation of actions, thoughts, speech, or emotion is present. Sensory motor function is normal. Visual tracking and eye movements are intact, and there is occasional speech and movement to commands. However, internally guided behavior is absent because cortical activation is inadequate. AM is associated with orbitomedial frontal cortex, limbic system, and reticular formation lesions.
- **Vegetative state (VS):** VS is a subacute or chronic condition that may follow coma from brain injury or occur independently of coma (e.g., dementia). Transition from coma to VS occurs if coma without detectable awareness of environment persists for longer than 4 weeks. Onset of VS is signaled by a return of wakefulness (eyes are open and sleep patterns may be observed) with return of spontaneous control of autonomic function but without observable signs of cognitive function. The patient cannot follow commands, offers no comprehensible sounds, and displays no localization to stimuli. There is complete loss of meaningful interaction with the environment. When the VS continues for weeks or months, it is considered persistent vegetative state (PVS). PVS may exist for many years because the autonomic and vegetative functions necessary for life have been preserved. PVS generally resolves more quickly in patients with a traumatic brain injury than in patients with no trauma.
- **Locked-in syndrome (LIS):** Characterized by paralysis of all four extremities and the lower cranial nerves but with preservation of cognition. Associated with deafferentation (disruption of the pathways of the brainstem motor neurons), this condition prevents the patient from communicating with a full range of language and body movement.

Generally, consciousness, vertical eye movement, and eyelid blinking are intact and provide a mechanism for communication. LIS is classified by the degree of voluntary speech and motor function preservation. In complete LIS, there is total immobility and anarthria (inability to speak). In incomplete LIS, there is vertical eye movement and blinking function. LIS can be distinguished from a VS because patients give appropriate signs of being aware of themselves and their environment. Often, sleep patterns are disrupted (see Spinal Cord Injury).

COGNITIVE DYSFUNCTION

This is an alteration in thought process involving many of the following brain functions: memory, learning, language, attention, judgment, reasoning, reading, and writing. Aphasia, or difficulty understanding language or with responding with the proper words, may also be present. Dysphagia, or difficulty swallowing, occurs because of attention deficits or muscle weakness. These cognitive impairments, whether permanent or transitory, if overlooked, underdiagnosed or incorrectly diagnosed may result in failure to correct a new acute illness or an exacerbation of a chronic illness. See Table 1-3 for factors contributing to cognitive dysfunction in acute, critical, or chronic illnesses. Acute changes in behavior or mental status superimposed on chronic cognitive dysfunction (dementia) is a harbinger of an underlying condition that needs immediate attention.

ASSESSMENT: MENTAL STATUS OR ALTERATION IN CONSCIOUSNESS

GOAL OF ASSESSMENT

- Identify changes in behavior, including ability to both understand and comply with directions.
- Determine if different or altered behaviors have occurred in the past or occur regularly; new-onset changes in mental status should be evaluated very closely. Considerations of cause may include withdrawal from abused substances, a reaction to a new medication, hypoxia, and hypoglycemia.
- Determine the severity of the change in behavior from baseline; acute changes require prompt action.
- An acute or unexpected change in mental status that occurs should be investigated immediately and requires an extensive medical evaluation with laboratory analysis, physical examination, and neuroimaging. These patients may need immediate transfer to a higher level of care. Change in mental status is often the earliest warning sign of a medical emergency!
- Resist the temptation to sedate an agitated patient before completing a full assessment, to ensure the patient is not hypoxic or hypoglycemic. Assessment for hypoxia should include both a ventilation and perfusion assessment. The ABG includes an estimated Hgb level, which can prove to be invaluable to determine if the patient may have internal bleeding or an unrecognized anemia.

HISTORY AND RISK FACTORS

- Age: Older adults (age 60 years and older) are more prone to alterations in consciousness, especially with changes in the environment, subclinical response to infection or other medical conditions including myocardial infarction (MI), and prescription drug toxicity.
- Brain injury: Lesions of the cortex, subcortex, and brainstem caused by global or focal ischemia, stroke, or traumatic brain injury (see Traumatic Brain Injury, Chapter 3).
- Cerebral disorders: Deteriorating brain conditions, such as expanding lesions, hydrocephalus, Parkinson disease, dementia, or mental health disorders (bipolar, depression, schizophrenia).
- Cardiovascular status: Disorders that lower CO (heart failure, MI, shock states), procedures that cause postcardiotomy delirium, intraaortic balloon pump sequelae, and hypoperfusion states (altered cerebral perfusion pressure and dysrhythmias).
- Pulmonary disorders: Those causing hypoxia and hypoxemia such as pneumonia, acute respiratory distress syndrome (ARDS), and pulmonary emboli.
- Drug therapy: Sedation, analgesia, drug toxicity, drug interactions, drug withdrawal, or drug sensitivity.

- Medication review
  - Full review of all prescription medications currently being taken.
  - When prescribed (new or old) dose, last time taken, reason for taking.
  - Be alert to the following medication classifications that may cause behavioral change or alterations in consciousness: Sympathomimetics, anticholinergics, hallucinogens, opioid, sedative-hypnotic, cholinergic, and serotonin uptake inhibitors.
- Surgical factors: Nature (hip, cardiac, neurosurgery patients at increased risk) and extent of surgery and anesthesia time.
- Infection: Bacteremia, urinary tract infections, pneumonia, or sepsis.
- Perceptual/sensory factors: Sleep deprivation, sensory overload, sensory deprivation, impaired sensation (hypesthesia, decreased hearing or vision), impaired perception (inability to identify environmental stimuli), and impaired integration (inability to integrate environmental stimuli).
- Metabolic factors: Changes in glucose level, hypermetabolism, hypometabolism, renal insufficiency, and endocrine crises (diabetic coma, ketoacidosis, pituitary dysfunction or injury, myxedema).
- Fluid and electrolyte disturbances: Sodium and potassium imbalances, hypovolemia, or dehydration.

VITAL SIGNS
All of the following vital sign changes may be associated with an alteration in consciousness:
- Fever may indicate possible sepsis and/or bacteremia. Subnormal or absence of fever may also indicate sepsis.
- Tachycardia may indicate hypovolemia, resulting from dehydration or bleeding. If the patient has undergone a recent invasive procedure, evaluation for internal bleeding is warranted. Tachycardia is also present with fever and hypoglycemia.
- Cardiac Output (CO) = Heart Rate (HR) × Stroke Volume (SV). Any change in SV will increase HR to maintain CO and decrease CO will cause a change in HR initially.
- Tachypnea, if coinciding with tachycardia, may reflect the same findings but is also a compensatory mechanism to help control acidosis. Tachypnea is also present during a panic attack, as well as hypoxia.
- Bradypnea may be associated with high doses of narcotics used for pain control.
- Patients with a head injury may exhibit signs of increased intracranial pressure (ICP), which vary depending on the degree of pressure elevation (see Traumatic Brain Injury, Chapter 3). Often changes in behavior including restlessness and agitation or a decrease in agitation (increasing somnolence) herald worsening injury and require immediate attention.
- Hypotension may indicate a later sign of shock or may be associated with higher doses of antihypertensive medications, narcotics, or other medications that can slow the HR or reduce the BP.

OBSERVATION AND NEUROLOGIC EVALUATION
- The patient's normal baseline neurologic status must be documented and used for comparison. This evaluation may begin with simple scales, such as the Six-Item Screen or Quick Confusion Scale, often used in the emergency department.
- Baseline neurologic findings elicited from each component of the examination must be documented.
- Requires a thorough evaluation of mental/emotional status, cranial nerve function, motor function, sensory function, and reflex activity. When changes in mental status are noted, the mental/emotional component of the examination is of particular importance. Is there a behavioral change without other focal signs or symptoms?
- In patients who are unconscious or demonstrate low-level function, assessment techniques are used that do not require patient participation, such as coma and cognitive functioning scales. The purpose of assessment is to determine the extent of wakefulness and cognition through observed responses, such as eye opening, movement of the head and body, verbalization, and ability to follow commands. These observations alone will not fully discriminate the subtle differences in altered states of arousal.
- Assessment should be accompanied by an in-depth history focusing on the possible etiology of the change in mental status. Extensive cognitive testing including attention,

concentration, memory, and learning assessments is performed when the patient is arousable and aware.

SCREENING LABWORK

- ABGs evaluate ventilation, perfusion, estimated Hgb, and acid-base status.
- Point-of-care blood glucose readings evaluate for hypoglycemia or extreme hyperglycemia.
- Biochemical panel analysis evaluates for electrolyte imbalances, such as hyponatremia, which are associated with alterations in behavior.
- Urine analysis and urine drug screen for detection of renal function and drug use.
- Serum lactate levels if systemic inflammatory response syndrome (SIRS) or sepsis is suspected.

NEUROLOGIC EVALUATION

- **Mental status testing:** Subjective assessment requiring patient cooperation for best results (Box 1-1).
- **Quick Confusion Scale:** Consists of six items and is used for screening impaired mental status in the emergency department. Total points are 15 with a total score of 11 suggesting the need for further evaluation and a score of ≤7 confirming impairment (Box 1-2).
- **Mini-Mental Status Examination (MMSE):** Objective neuropsychological tool used to measure orientation, recall, attention, calculation, and language. Scores less than 23 (total 25) indicate cognitive dysfunction. Patient participation is necessary for this examination (Box 1-3).
- **Six-Item Screen:** Used for assessing cognitive function, attention, and confusion, and was developed from the MMSE. Six items related to cognition, attention, and short-term memory are scored using a nine-point scale. Scores less than 5 indicate cognitive impairment (Box 1-4).
- **Vigilance A Test:** This is a quick bedside test for attention and concentration. Given a series of 60 random letters, patients are asked to identify all the A's in the sequence. Omission of more than two A's is suggestive of attention deficit (Box 1-5).
- **Glasgow Coma Scale:** Quantitative, three-part scale that assesses the patient's ability to open his or her eyes, to move, and to speak/communicate. Scores range from 3 to 15, with 3 being unresponsive to all stimuli and 15 being awake, alert, and oriented. Patients who are unable to cooperate can be evaluated using this scale (see Appendix 1).
- **Coma Recovery Scale:** Quantitative 35-item scale used to assess brain function at four levels (generalized, localized, emergent, cognitively mediated). Seven responses are evaluated: arousal and attention, auditory perception, visual perception, motor function, oromotor ability, communication, and initiative. Patients who are unable to cooperate can be evaluated using this scale.
- **Confusion Assessment Method (CAM, CAM-Intensive Care Unit):** Four-part scale used to evaluate confusion. Onset and course, inattention, disorganized thinking, and LOC are assessed (Box 1-6).
- **Intensive Care Delirium Screening Checklist (ICDSC):** Eight-item scale that rates behavioral responses exhibited by patients in intensive care; delirium is indicated with scores *greater than* 4 to 8 (Table 1-4).
- **Richmond Agitation-Sedation Scale (RASS):** Scores sedation and agitation with a 10-point scale using verbal and physical stimulation to determine the patient's response, and used to titrate medications (Table 1-5).
- **Rancho Los Amigos (RLA) Cognitive Functioning Scale:** Seven-level scale that describes levels of cognitive functioning. Levels range from unresponsive to sensory stimuli to purposeful/appropriate actions. Patients who cannot cooperate can be evaluated using this scale (Table 1-6).

DIAGNOSTIC TESTS
NEURODIAGNOSTIC TESTING
See the section on Traumatic Brain Injury in Chapter 3.

| **Box 1-1** | **MENTAL STATUS COMPONENT OF THE NEUROLOGIC EXAMINATION** |

1. General appearance
2. Behavior (with and without stimulation)
3. Language and speech characteristics (organization, coherence, and relevance)
4. Mood and affect
5. Judgment
6. Abstract thinking
7. Orientation (time, place, person)
8. Attention and concentration
9. Memory (recent, remote)
10. Cognition (following commands, fund of knowledge, interpretation of information, problem solving)

| **Box 1-2** | **QUICK CONFUSION SCALE** |

Quick Confusion Scale

Item number	Question	Scoring	Points
1	What is the year?	1 point if correct 0 if incorrect	
2	What is the month?	1 point if correct 0 if incorrect	
3	What time is it?	1 point if correct 0 if incorrect	
Introduce Memory Phrase: John Brown, 42 Market Street, New York			
4	Count backwards from 20 to 1	2 point if no errors 1 point if 1 error 0 if more than 1 error	
5	Say the months backwards (in reverse)	2 point if no errors 1 point if 1 error 0 if more than 1 error	
6	Repeat memory phrase	1 point for each underlined portion remembered	

Total Score 15: Score of 11 points needs further evaluation
Score of ≤7 points certain cognitive impairment

Adapted from Huff J, Farace E, Brady W, et al: The Quick Confusion Scale in the emergency department: comparison with the Mini-Mental State Examination. *Am J Emerg Med* 19:461-464, 2001.

| **Box 1-3** | **MINI-MENTAL STATUS EXAMINATION** |

1. What is the year, season, date, day, month? (5 points)
2. Where are we: state, county, town, hospital, room? (5 points)
3. Name three objects. (3 points)
4. Count backward by sevens (e.g., 100, 93, 86, 79, 72). (5 points)
5. Repeat same three objects from item number 3 above. (3 points)
6. Name a pencil and watch. (2 points)
7. Follow a three-step command. (3 points)
8. Write a sentence. (1 point)
9. Follow the command "close your eyes." (1 point)
10. Copy a design (e.g., two hexagons). (1 point)

Box 1-4	SIX-ITEM SCREEN

Six-Item Screen (Used to detect problems with cognition, attention, short-term memory, and orientation; subset of the MMSE, the Blessed Dementia Rating Scale (BDRS), and the Word List Recall)
1. Examiner names three items and asks patient to repeat each item. (3)
2. Examiner asks what year, what month, what day of the week? (3)
3. Examiner asks patient to recall the three items (3) in number 1 above.
   Total score is 9. If score <5, then patient has cognitive impairment

Adapted from Callahan C, Unverzagt F, Hui S, et al: Six-item screener to identify cognitive impairment among potential subjects for clinical research. *Med Care* 40(9):771-781, 2002.

Box 1-5	VIGILANCE A TEST
Vigilance A Test	**Scoring**
Random list of 60 letters with the letter A appearing greater than random frequency. The patient is asked to tap or indicate when the target letter (A) is spoken by the examiner.	Count number of omissions or commission of the target letter (A). Greater than two missed is abnormal

NEUROPSYCHOLOGICAL TESTING
Although not a routine part of critical care, neuropsychological testing should be planned and implemented for patients with brain injury or altered consciousness when they enter the recovery phase. This testing provides a comprehensive baseline for rehabilitation by evaluating higher cortical functions, such as memory, learning, and language.

LABORATORY STUDIES
If there is an acute or unexpected mental status change, laboratory studies include complete blood count (CBC), electrolytes, cardiac profile, blood and sputum cultures, urinalysis and culture, ABG, chest radiograph, ECG, and other tests as determined by signs and symptoms.

COLLABORATIVE MANAGEMENT
CARE PRIORITIES
When evaluating alteration in consciousness or a change in mental status, there are two primary targets: (1) recognize that the disorder is present and (2) uncover the underlying cause. Acute and/or life-threatening problems must be ruled out before proceeding. Therefore, signs and symptoms such as lethargy, somnolence, fatigue, anxiety, or sleeplessness should not be normalized as part of illness behavior but as signs and symptoms prompting further investigation. Although severe agitation is difficult to manage, it is imperative that physiologic causes of agitation are ruled out before sedating the patient. Once acute causes of the problem are ruled out, the following measures may be implemented for other causes of behavioral changes:

1. Delirium
- Determine and correct physiologic imbalances and drug interactions.
- Correct sensory/perceptual deficits (e.g., provide hearing aid, eyeglasses).
- Reorient the patient to self and environment.
- Implement appropriate medications to help control behavior.
- Consider consultation with a geriatrician.
- Manage pain and assess effectiveness.
- Minimize sedative medications; benzodiazepines are not recommended.
- Check bowel and bladder function.
- Establish sleep-wake cycle.

Box 1-6	CONFUSION ASSESSMENT METHOD-INTENSIVE CARE UNIT (CAM-ICU) WORKSHEET

Feature 1: Acute onset or fluctuating course

Positive if you answer "yes" to either 1A or 1B.

Positive or Negative

1A: Is the patient different than his/her baseline mental status?

Or

1B: Has the patient had any fluctuation in mental status in the past 24 hours as evidenced by fluctuation on a sedation scale (e.g., RASS), GCS, or previous delirium assessment?

Yes or No

Feature 2: Inattention

Positive if either score for 2A or 2B is less than 8.

Attempt the ASE Letters first. If the patient is able to perform this test and the score is clear, record this score and move to Feature 3. If the patient is unable to perform this test or the score is unclear, then perform the ASE Pictures. If you perform both tests, use the results of the ASE Pictures to score the feature.

Positive or Negative

2A: ASE Letters: Record score (enter NT for not tested)

Directions: Say to the patient, "*I am going to read you a series of 10 letters. Whenever you hear the letter 'A,' indicate by squeezing my hand.*" Read letters from the following letter list in a normal tone.

S A V E A H A A R T

Scoring: Errors are counted when patient fails to squeeze on the letter "A" and when the patient squeezes on any letter other than "A."

Score (out of 10): _____

2B: ASE Pictures: record score (enter NT for not tested)

Directions are included on the picture packets.

Score (out of 10): _____

Feature 3: Disorganized thinking

Positive if the combined score is less than 4

Positive or Negative

3A: Yes/No Questions

(Use either Set A or Set B, alternate on consecutive days if necessary):

Set A	Set B
1. Will a stone float on water?	1. Will a leaf float on water?
2. Are there fish in the sea?	2. Are there elephants in the sea?
3. Does one pound weigh more than two pounds?	3. Do two pounds weigh more than one pound?
4. Can you use a hammer to pound a nail?	4. Can you use a hammer to cut wood?

Score ____ (Patient earns 1 point for each correct answer out of 4)

3B: Command

Say to patient: "Hold up this many fingers" (Examiner holds two fingers in front of patient). "Now do the same thing with the other hand" (Not repeating the number of fingers). (If patient is unable to move both arms, for the second part of the command ask patient "Add one more finger"). Score____ (Patient earns 1 point if able to successfully complete the entire command)

Combined Score (3A + 3B):_____ (out of 5)

Feature 4: Altered level of consciousness

Positive if the Actual RASS score is anything other than "0" (zero)

Positive Negative

Overall CAM-ICU (Features 1 and 2 and either Feature 3 or 4): Positive Negative

Table 1-4	INTENSIVE CARE DELIRIUM SCREENING CHECKLIST
Symptom Checklist (total 0 to 8)	**Level of Consciousness Scoring**
Level of Consciousness	*Level of Consciousness*
Inattentiveness	
Disorientation	A: No response: none
Hallucination, delusion, psychosis	B: Response to intense, repeated stimuli (loud voice or pain): none
Agitation	C: Response to mild or moderate stimulation: 1
Inappropriate speech or mood	D : normal wakefulness: 0
Sleep/wake cycle disturbance	E : exaggerated response to normal stimulation: 1
Symptom fluctuation	(if A or B above do not complete evaluation for the day)

Adapted from Bergeron N, Dubois M-J, Dumont M, et al: Intensive care delirium screening checklist: evaluation of a new screening tool. *Intensive Care Med* 27(5):859-864, 2001.

Table 1-5	RICHMOND AGITATION-SEDATION SCALE (RASS)
+4 Combative	Overtly combative or violent, immediate danger to staff
+3 Very agitated	Pulls on or removes tubes or catheters, aggressive behavior toward staff
+2 Agitated	Frequent nonpurposeful movement or patient-ventilator dyssynchrony
+1 Restless	Anxious or apprehensive but movements not aggressive or vigorous
0 Alert and calm	
−1 Drowsy	Not fully alert, sustained ($\geq$10 seconds) awakening, eye contact to voice
−2 Light sedation	Briefly ($<$10 seconds) awakens with eye contact to voice
−3 Moderate sedation	Any movement (but no eye contact) to voice
−4 Deep sedation	No response to voice, any movement to physical stimulation
−5 Unarousable	No response to voice or physical stimulation
Procedure	

1. Observe the patient. Is patient alert and calm (score 0)?
   Does the patient have behavior that is consistent with restlessness or agitation?
   Assign score +1 to +4 using the criteria listed above.

2. If the patient is not alert, in a loud-speaking voice state the patient's name and direct the patient to open his or her eyes and look at the speaker. Repeat once if necessary. Can prompt the patient to continue looking at the speaker.
   The patient has eye opening and eye contact, which is sustained for more than 10 seconds (score −1).
   The patient has eye opening and eye contact, but this is not sustained for 10 seconds (score −2).
   The patient has any movement in response to voice, excluding eye contact (score −3).

3. If the patient does not respond to voice, physically stimulate the patient by shaking shoulder and then rubbing sternum if there is no response.
   The patient has any movement to physical stimulation (score −4).
   The patient has no response to voice or physical stimulation (score −5).

Continued

Table 1-5	RICHMOND AGITATION-SEDATION SCALE (RASS) — cont'd
Score Term Description	
+4 Combative	Overtly combative, violent, immediate danger to staff
+3 Very agitated	Pulls or removes tube(s) or catheter(s); aggressive
+2 Agitated	Frequent nonpurposeful movement, fights ventilator
+1 Restless	Anxious but movements not aggressive or vigorous
0 Alert and calm	
−1 Drowsy	Not fully alert, but has sustained awakening (eye opening/eye contact) to voice (≥10 seconds)
−2 Light sedation	Briefly awakens with eye contact to voice (<10 seconds)
−3 Moderate sedation	Movement or eye opening to voice (but no eye contact)
−4 Deep sedation	No response to voice, but movement or eye opening to physical stimulation
−5 Unarousable	No response to voice or physical stimulation
Procedure for RASS Assessment	

1. Observe the patient
   - The patient is alert, restless, or agitated (score 0 to +4).

2. If not alert, state the patient's name and say to open eyes and look at the speaker.
   - The patient awakens with sustained eye opening and eye contact (score −1).
   - The patient awakens with eye opening and eye contact, but not sustained (score −2).
   - The patient has any movement in response to voice but no eye contact (score −3).

3. When no response to verbal stimulation, physically stimulate the patient by shaking shoulder and/or rubbing sternum.
   - The patient has any movement to physical stimulation (score −4).
   - The patient has no response to any stimulation (score −5).

Reproduced, with permission, from Sessler CN, Gosnell M, Grap MJ, et al: The Richmond Agitation-Sedation scale: validity and reliability in adult intensive care unit patients. *Am J Respir Crit Care Med* 166(10):1338-1344, 2002. Copyright © 2002 American Thoracic Society. From Ely EW, Truman B, Shintani A, et al: Monitoring sedation status over time in ICU patients: the reliability and validity of the Richmond Agitation-Sedation Scale (RASS). *JAMA* 289(22):2983-2991, 2003.

- Treat agitation.
- Perform neuropsychological testing.
- See Sedation and Neuromuscular Blockade, Chapter 2.

 Safety Alert *For mild confusion, good outcomes have been reported with the use of reorientation techniques and observation (use of "sitters"), especially by family members. Prophylactic low-dose haloperidol did not prevent delirium but was noted to reduce the severity of delirium in one study. Newer atypical antipsychotic medications, those with fewer extrapyramidal side effects such as quetiapine, olanzapine, and risperidone, have been shown to have an efficacy similar to haloperidol.*

2. Coma
- Assess cognitive function using the RLA score or Coma Recovery Scale.
- Initiate a sensory stimulation program for patients with low-level cognition.
- Minimize stimulation for patients who are confused or agitated.
- Plan care to prevent or minimize problems related to the injury (e.g., spasticity, swallowing disorders) and complications of immobility (e.g., disuse syndrome, contractures, and pressure ulcers).
- Consult with rehabilitation services including physical, occupational, and speech therapy.

Table 1-6		COGNITIVE REHABILITATION GOALS
Level	**Response**	**Goal/Intervention**
I	None	Goal: Provide sensory input to elicit responses of increased quality, frequency, duration, and variety.
II	Generalized	
III	Localized	Intervention: Give brief but frequent stimulation sessions, and present stimuli in an organized manner, focusing on one sensory channel at a time; for example: Visual: Intermittent television, family pictures, bright objects. Auditory: Tape recordings of family or favorite song, talking to the patient, intermittent television or radio. Olfactory: Favorite perfume, shaving lotion, coffee, lemon, orange Cutaneous: Touch or rub skin with different textures, such as velvet, ice bag, warm cloth. Movement: Turn, range-of-motion exercises, up in chair. Oral: Oral care, lemon swabs, ice, sugar on tongue, peppermint, chocolate.
IV	Confused, agitated	Goal: Decrease agitation and increase awareness of environment. This stage usually lasts 2 to 4 weeks. Intervention: Remove offending devices (e.g., nasogastric tube, restraints), if possible. Do not demand the patient to follow through with task. Provide human contact unless this increases agitation. Provide a quiet, controlled environment. Use a calm, soft voice and manner around the patient.
V	Confused, inappropriate	Goal: Decrease confusion and incorporate improved cognitive abilities into functional activity.
VI	Confused, appropriate	Intervention: Begin each interaction with introduction, orientation, and interaction purpose. List and number daily activity in the sequence in which it will be done throughout the day. Maintain a consistent environment. Provide memory aids (e.g., calendar, clock). Use gentle repetition, which aids learning. Provide supervision and structure. Reorient as needed.
VII	Automatic, appropriate	Goal: Integrate increased cognitive function into functional community activities with minimal structuring. Intervention: Enable practicing of activities. Reduce supervision and environmental structure. Help the patient plan adaptation of activities of daily living and home living skills to home environment.

Modified from the Rancho Los Amigos Levels of Cognitive Functioning Scale (scale based on behavioral descriptions or responses to stimuli). From Swift CM: Neurologic disorders. In Swearingen PL, editor: *Manual of medical-surgical nursing care*, ed 4, St Louis, 1999, Mosby.

3. Locked-in syndrome

- Provide a normal day/night routine to help minimize sleep-wake cycle disturbances.
- Establish a communication system/pattern.
- Consult a mental health professional to assess the psychological impact of this syndrome.
- Consult with rehabilitation (see preceding section on Coma).

4. Vegetative state

- Perform neurodiagnostic and neuropsychological testing to confirm the diagnosis.
- Provide essential supportive care to minimize complications such as pressure ulcers and aspiration.
- Initiate a sensory stimulation program for low-level cognitive function, including visual, auditory, tactile, gustatory, and vestibular stimuli (Figure 1-3).

Safety Alert *Research has demonstrated positive outcomes from two interventions designed to reduce delirium in the intensive care unit—one was to reduce delirium in postoperative patients by controlling disturbances in the sleep-wake cycle. The second involved the daily visit of a geriatric consult service, which provided targeted recommendations using a 10-item protocol. The protocol included (1) maintenance of central nervous system O_2 delivery, (2) fluid and electrolyte corrections, (3) pain management, (4) removal of unnecessary medications, (5) bowel/bladder regulation, (6) establishing adequate nutrition, (7) mobilization and rehabilitation, (8) detection/prevention and treatment of surgical complications, (9) sensory stimulation, and (10) treatment of agitational variant of delirium.*

SENSORY STIMULATION (SS) PROGRAMS AS AN INTERVENTION TECHNIQUE IN THE CRITICALLY ILL

STRONG EVIDENCE	INSUFFICIENT EVIDENCE	RECOMMENDATIONS
SS programs appear to be safe to administer.	There is still no clear evidence that increased arousal is brain injury recovery or SS program enhanced recovery.	SS programs can be initiated as an adjustment therapy.
SS programs do not increase ICP or CPP and do not affect HR or BP. A positive trajectory of recovery has been documented in all studies.	It is unclear how the time when SS was started (early or late) influences outcome. It is unclear how the type of program (multimodal or unimodal) influences outcome.	SS program can be incorporated into daily nursing routine. Use rest periods between sessions to diminish fatigue.
	It is unclear what type of stimulation is most useful for increasing arousal (e.g., novel, familiar music, voices). It is unclear how long daily stimulation should last (concentrated or multiple short sessions).	Stop intervention if an unstable medical status develops, and resume when patient is stable. Include family in intervention program.

BP, blood pressure; CPP, cerebral perfusion pressure; HR, heart rate; ICP, intracranial pressure

Figure 1-3 Sensory stimulation (SS) programs as an intervention technique in the critically ill. (From Kater K: Response of head-injured patients to sensory stimulation. *West J Nurs Res* 11[1]:20-33, 1989; Lewinn E, Dimancescu M: Environmental deprivation and enrichment in coma. *Lancet* 2[8081]:156-157, 1978; Mackay L, Bernstein BA, Chapman PE, et al: Early intervention in severe head injury: long-term benefits of a formalized program. *Arch Phys Med Rehabil* 73[7]:635-641, 1992; Mitchell S, Bradley VA, Welch JL, et al: Coma arousal procedure: a therapeutic intervention in the treatment of head injury. *Brain Inj* 4[3]: 273-279, 1990; Schinner K, Chisholm AH, Grap MJ, et al: Effects of auditory stimuli on intracranial pressure and cerebral perfusion pressure in traumatic brain injury. *J Neurosci Nurs* 27[6]:336-341, 1994; and Wilson S, Powell GE, Brock D, et al: Vegetative state and response to sensory stimulation: an analysis of 24 cases. *Brain Inj* 10[11]:807-818, 1996.)

CARE PLANS: ALTERATION IN CONSCIOUSNESS

Acute confusion   *related to physiologic changes; psychological changes; environmental changes; sensory deprivation; sensory overload; drug interactions.*

Goals/Outcomes: If the cause of alteration in consciousness is an extracerebral event, within 72 hours of this diagnosis, the patient's level of arousal and cognition improves and the patient responds consistently and appropriately to stimuli. If the cause is cerebral, increased arousal and improvement in cognition may take days to weeks.

NOC Cognitive Orientation, Distorted Thought Self-Control, Information Processing.

Neurologic Status: Consciousness

Cognitive ability: Ability to execute complex mental processes; ability to identify person, place, and time.
Information Processing: Ability to acquire, organize, and use information.

1. Priority care is to identify the cause of the change in mental status. Perform laboratory and diagnostics tests to identify the cause of the problem and correct it. This may include limiting sedation or pain medication, monitoring for withdrawal syndromes, drug interactions, or impending sepsis (SIRS, see Chapter 11).
2. Eliminate environmental causes of sensory/perceptual deficit.
   * Assess patient for potential causes of sensory/perceptual deficits. For the hearing-impaired or vision-impaired patient, wearing eyeglasses or hearing aids will decrease misinterpretation of visual and auditory stimuli.
   * Assess environment for potential causes of disorientation and confusion. Maintain day/night environment as much as possible. Keep clocks and calendars within the patient's field of vision.
3. Develop a plan of care consistent with sensory/perceptual deficit.
4. Assess the patient for sensory deprivation and sensory overload. Decrease or increase stimulation based on RLA assessment (see Figure 1-3) and the patient's needs. For example, individuals who are agitated and confused require structure and reorientation interventions, whereas those who are comatose or stuporous require stimulation techniques.
   * Orient the patient to time, place, and person during all interactions. Explain procedures in terms the patient can understand.
   * Teach significant others reorientation and sensory stimulation strategies, and provide liberal visitation to facilitate their assistance.
   * Assess underlying cause of confusion or delirium before using sedation, anxiolytic, analgesic, or antipsychotic drug therapy (see Sedation and Neuromuscular Blockade).

NIC Cognitive Restructuring; Cognitive Stimulation; Environmental Management; Reality Orientation; Dementia Management; Electrolyte Management; Delirium Management.

Impaired verbal communication   *related to neurologic deficits*

Goals/Outcomes: If the cause of alteration in consciousness is an extracerebral event, within 72 hours of this diagnosis, the patient communicates needs and feelings and exhibits decreased frustration and fear related to communication barriers. If the cause is cerebral, improvement in communication may take days to weeks.
NOC Communication: Expressive; Communication; Communication: Receptive.

Communication Enhancement

1. Determine the underlying cause of impaired communication, including physiologic (cortical, brainstem, or cranial nerve injury) or psychological (depression, fear, or anger).
2. When communicating with patients, use their name, face them, use eye contact if they are awake, speak clearly, and use a normal tone of voice.
3. Be alert to nonverbal messages, especially eye movement, blinking, facial expressions, and head and hand movements. Attempt to validate these signals with the patient.
4. Assure the patient that you are attempting to find methods that promote communication if the patient's needs cannot always be understood.
5. For the patient who does not respond to or acknowledge verbal stimulation, continue communication attempts.
6. Teach significant others methods of communication and encourage them to continue attempts at communication.

7. Brainstem-evoked potentials and audiometry (hearing test) can provide useful information related to the patient's ability to receive and process auditory stimuli. Detection and treatment of otitis media in patients who have ET tubes will improve hearing.
8. Obtain a speech therapy consultation to assess nature and severity of communication impairment and assist in developing a communication plan. Special attention is required for individuals with locked-in syndrome.
9. Obtain a mental health consultation to assist with a patient who is angry, frustrated, and fearful because of the communication impairment.

NIC Communication Enhancement: Speech Deficit; Support System Enhancement.

Impaired physical mobility *related to perceptual or cognitive impairment; imposed restrictions of movement*

Goals/Outcomes: By the time of discharge from the critical care unit, the patient demonstrates range of motion (ROM) and muscle strength within 10% of maximal normal function.
NOC Mobility, Ambulation.

Exercise Therapy: Joint Mobility
1. Assess muscle strength and tone to determine type of interventions required. Consult physical therapy and occupational therapy for evaluation and treatment plan.
2. Manage decreased muscle tone (flaccidity):
   • Maintain body alignment and positioning.
   • Perform passive ROM and stretching exercises.
   • Avoid prolonged periods of limb flexion.
   • Apply splints and other adaptive devices to maintain functional position of the extremities.
   • Turn patient every 2 hours.
   • Consider chair sitting as the patient stabilizes.
3. Manage increased muscle tone (spasticity):
   • Avoid supine position; use side-lying, semiprone, prone, and high Fowler positions.
   • Position limbs opposite flexion posture.
   • Use skeletal muscle relaxant, such as baclofen (Lioresal), as prescribed for decreasing tone.
4. Monitor calcium and alkaline phosphatase levels. Increased levels can lead to the development of heterogeneous ossification, which is often seen with states of impaired mobility, such as spinal cord injury. See Fluid and Electrolyte Disturbances.
5. Maintain the patient's skin integrity. See Wound and Skin Care.
6. Prevent pulmonary complications in the following ways:
   • Encourage deep breathing if the patient is able, or suction as needed. Coughing is warranted only if sputum is present.
   • Assess swallowing ability before initiating oral feedings. Obtain dysphagia consultation (usually from a speech therapist) if swallowing reflexes are impaired.
   • Initiate enteral feeding protocol for patients with feeding tubes to prevent aspiration. See Nutritional Support.

NIC Bed Rest Care; Positioning; Exercise Promotion; Self-Care Assistance.

ADDITIONAL NURSING DIAGNOSES

Also see nursing diagnoses and interventions under Nutritional Support, Sedation and Neuromuscular Blockade, Prolonged Immobility, and Risk for Disuse Syndrome, in Traumatic Brain Injury, Acute Spinal Cord Injury, and SIRS, Sepsis, and MODS.

FLUID AND ELECTROLYTE DISTURBANCES

The volume and composition of body fluids and electrolytes are affected by hormonal, renal, vascular, and exogenous factors. An understanding of the complexity of chemical currents, cellular function, and distribution of water between the cells and vessels provides the information used to facilitate the best patient outcome.

Water is the major constituent of the human body, comprising 55% to 72% of body mass. Body water decreases with both age and increasing body fat. The average male adult is approximately 60% water by weight, whereas the average female adult is 55% water by weight. Two thirds of body fluid is within the intracellular fluid compartment (ICF) accounting for approximately 40% of body weight. ICF contains a high concentration of potassium (K^+), magnesium (Mg^+), phosphates (PO_4^-), proteins, and sulfates. The extracellular fluid compartment (ECF) is composed of interstitial fluid, which surrounds the cells (14% of body weight), intravascular fluid, contained within blood vessels (5% of body weight), and transcellular fluid, which includes cerebral spinal fluid and fluid contained in other body spaces such as joint spaces, pleural, peritoneal, and pericardial spaces (1% to 2% of total body weight.) ECF contains the remaining one third of body fluid and has a high concentration of the plasma ions sodium (Na^+), chloride (Cl^-), and bicarbonate (HCO_3^-).

The composition and concentration of ECF are primarily regulated by the concentration of Na^+, which defines the relative relationship of sodium and water. Although ECF is altered and then modified as the body reacts with its surrounding environment, ICF remains relatively stable. Intracellular stability is important for maintaining normal cellular function.

In addition to water, body fluids contain two types of dissolved substances: electrolytes and nonelectrolytes. Electrolytes are substances that carry an electrical current and can dissociate into ions, which have either a positive or a negative charge. They are measured by their capacity to combine (milliequivalents/liter [mEq/L]) or by the molecular weight in milligrams (millimoles/liter [mmol/L]). Nonelectrolytes are substances such as glucose and urea that do not dissociate in solution and are measured by weight (milligrams per 100 milliliters, or mg/dL) and mmol/L. The intravascular and extravascular components of the ECF are separated by a semipermeable or porous capillary membrane, which allows movement of dissolved substance/particles between compartments, and slow passage of albumin (5% per hour), which is returned to the circulation via the lymphatic system at the same rate. The unique composition of each compartment is maintained (Table 1-7) in a state of equilibrium. Whereas the hydrostatic pressure within the circulation tends to drive fluid out, the oncotic pressure of the plasma proteins (e.g., albumin) draws fluid in and maintains the relative constancy of the plasma volume.

OSMOLALITY

Osmolality is the number of particles in solution. This concentration of particles determines the relationship of fluid between the ICF and ECF. Normal osmolality is regulated by a wide variety of mechanisms, which include arterial BP, sympathetic stimulation, renal regulation, and hormonal outflow.

Osmolality = $2(Na^+)$ + Glucose/18 + BUN/2.8 (normal value: 265 to 285 mOsm/L)

Table 1-7	PRIMARY CONSTITUENTS OF BODY WATER COMPARTMENTS*		
Element	**Intravascular**	**Interstitial**	**Intracellular (Skeletal Muscle Cell)**
Na^+	142 mEq/L	145 mEq/L	12 mEq/L
Cl^-	104 mEq/L	117 mEq/L	4 mEq/L
HCO_3^-	24 mEq/L	27 mEq/L	12 mEq/L
K^+	4.5 mEq/L	4.5 mEq/L	150 mEq/L
HPO_4^-	2 mEq/L	2 mEq/L	40 mEq/L

*This is a partial list. Other constituents include calcium (Ca^{2+}), magnesium (Mg^{2+}), and proteins.
Cl^-, Chloride; HCO_3^-, bicarbonate; HPO_4^-, phosphate; K^+, potassium; Na^+, sodium.

HORMONAL INFLUENCE

Three hormones are responsible for fluid volume regulation:

- Antidiuretic hormone (ADH) or vasopressin: Released by the posterior pituitary in response to a reduction in intravascular volume (hypovolemia) or an increase in extracellular osmolality, which acts on the kidney at both the glomerulus and the tubules to conserve water by increasing urine concentration. The hormone regulates the electrolyte and fluid balance to keep serum in "perfect" concentration (osmolality). Thirst is stimulated by hypovolemia and increased osmolality.
- Aldosterone: Released by the adrenal cortex in response to an increased plasma renin level, acts on the kidney to conserve sodium (along with water), and increases potassium and hydrogen excretion.
- Atrial natriuretic peptide (ANP): Released by the cardiac atria in response to increased atrial pressure (e.g., acute volume expansion). ANP reduces BP and vascular volume by increasing excretion of sodium and water by the kidneys, decreasing release of aldosterone and ADH, and by direct vasodilation.

FLUID DISTURBANCES

Fluid changes affect the volume status, regulation, and the composition of body fluids. Fluid loss or gain changes the concentration of particles in fluid compartments.

HYPOVOLEMIA

PATHOPHYSIOLOGY

ECF volume depletion or hypovolemia may be caused by abnormal skin losses, GI losses, polyuria/diuresis, bleeding, decreased intake, and movement of fluid into a third space (e.g., pleura, peritoneum, interstitium). Depending on the type of fluid lost or "third-spaced," hypovolemia may be accompanied by acid-base, osmolar, or electrolyte imbalances. Severe ECF volume depletion can lead to hypovolemic shock and cellular dehydration, which causes alterations in electric potentials (the ability to conduct impulse) throughout the body.

Compensatory mechanisms in hypovolemia include increased sympathetic nervous system stimulation: increased HR, increased force of cardiac contraction (positive inotropic effect), vasoconstriction to maintain perfusion to O_2-dependent organs (i.e., heart, lungs, brain), increased thirst, and increased release of aldosterone and ADH (vasopressin). Reduced perfusion to high-flow, low O_2–consuming organs (i.e., kidney, mesenteric bed, skeletal muscles) may lead to acute renal failure, ischemic bowel, and skeletal muscle cell rupture.

Hypovolemic shock develops when the intravascular volume decreases to the point where compensatory mechanisms can no longer maintain the perfusion needed for normal, aerobic cellular function. Without normal levels of O_2, cellular metabolism becomes anaerobic, resulting in acidosis, cardiac depression, intravascular coagulation, increased capillary permeability, and release of toxins. If shock is not adequately treated, it may become irreversible, leading to death.

HYPOVOLEMIA ASSESSMENT

GOAL OF ASSESSMENT

Identify the signs and symptoms of hypovolemia.

HISTORY AND RISK FACTORS

The following list of factors may be associated with loss of intravascular fluids or overall blood volume:

- Abnormal GI losses: Vomiting, nasogastric suctioning, diarrhea, intestinal drainage.
- Abnormal skin losses: Excessive diaphoresis secondary to fever or exercise, burns.
- Abnormal renal losses: Diuretic therapy, polyuria/osmotic diuresis seen with DKA, hyperglycemic hyperosmolar nonketotic syndrome (HHNS), nephrotoxicity, rhabdomyolysis, diabetes insipidus, diuretic phase of acute renal failure/acute kidney injury, adrenal insufficiency.

Table 1-8	WEIGHT LOSS AS AN INDICATOR OF EXTRACELLULAR FLUID DEFICIT IN THE ADULT	
Acute Weight Loss	**Severity of Deficit**	
2% to 5%	Mild	
5% to 10%	Moderate	
10% to 15%	Severe	
15% to 20%	Fatal	

- Third-spacing or plasma-to-interstitial fluid shift: Peritonitis, intestinal obstruction, burns, ascites, severe sepsis.
- Hemorrhage: Major trauma, GI bleeding, obstetric complications, postoperative bleeding, high dosage of anticoagulants or antiplatelet medications.
- Altered intake: Coma, fluid deprivation.

VITAL SIGNS
Evaluate BP, HR, temperature, weight, central venous pressure (CVP), pulmonary artery wedge pressure (PAWP), and urine output to determine the extent of volume depletion.
- Check BP lying, sitting, and standing to determine presence of orthostasis.
- HR will be increased (tachycardia).
- Narrowed pulse pressure.
- Low CVP (less than 2 mm Hg).
- Low PAWP (less than 3 mm Hg).
- Urine output decreased and may be less than 0.5 mL/kg/h.
- Increased temperature.
- Acute weight loss unless third spacing is occurring (Table 1-8).

OBSERVATION
Evaluate the skin, mucous membranes, and clinical presentation for signs of dehydration including furrowed tongue, dry mucous membranes, sunken eyeballs, flat neck veins, clinical pallor, dizziness, weakness, fatigue, syncope, anorexia, nausea, vomiting, thirst, confusion, and constipation.

PALPATION
Chest and abdominal palpation are performed to elicit pain in the abdomen or chest.

SCREENING LABWORK
Blood studies can reveal the extent of hypovolemia, because the blood becomes more concentrated as fluid is lost. If bleeding is present, studies will reveal blood loss.
- Hematocrit levels are elevated with dehydration and decreased with bleeding.
- BUN values may be elevated, with a BUN/creatinine ratio of greater than 20:1 suggesting hypovolemia.
- Electrolyte levels will vary depending on the type of fluid lost.
- ABG values depend on the type of fluid lost.
- Serum and urine osmolality depend on the type of fluid lost and a comparison assists in the diagnosis of renal insufficiency.

 Safety Alert *Early hypovolemic shock is often missed. Blood pressure (BP) may be compensated and remain normal or slightly elevated. Narrowing of pulse pressure (systolic BP − diastolic BP = pulse pressure) is a more accurate tool in early shock.*

A narrow pulse pressure in a patient with hypovolemic shock indicates a decreasing cardiac output and an increasing peripheral vascular resistance. Reduced venous blood volume from blood or fluid loss stimulates the sympathetic nervous system to increase or maintain the falling BP through systemic vasoconstriction. Stimulation of beta receptors increases heart rate and myocardial contractility, which temporarily correct the rate of decline in systolic BP. Vasoconstriction increases diastolic BP and thus pulse pressure can be reduced. A BP of 104/88 mm Hg appears "normal," but perfusion requires further assessment.

Safety Alert

As shock progresses, pulse pressure may widen as the compensatory response fails. Heart rate decreases, ventricular compliance is reduced, and with impaired ventricular relaxation during diastole, ventricular filling time is reduced, resulting in decreased central venous pressure and pulmonary artery pressure. Volume status may be underestimated. If the difference in systolic and diastolic blood pressure is less than 25% of the systolic blood pressure, the pulse pressure is considered to be narrow. A wide pulse pressure is considered to be greater than 50% of the systolic blood pressure.

COLLABORATIVE MANAGEMENT

CARE PRIORITIES

Identification of patients at risk for volume loss and prevention of continued losses and fluid replacement guide the care plan for these patients.

1. Restore tissue perfusion with fluid volume replacement and correct electrolyte disturbances: Administer and monitor fluid replacement with crystalloids, colloids, or blood.
2. Document response to fluid administration.
3. Maintain a safe environment for patients with neurologic symptoms.
4. Monitor for signs and symptoms of dehydration.
   - Monitor urine output.
   - Moisten mucous membranes.
5. Protect skin with lotions and egg crate or alternating pressure mattress.

Management of Hypovolemia

1. Restore Normal Fluid Volume and Correct Acid-Base and Electrolyte Disturbances

The type of fluid replacement depends on the type of fluid lost and the severity of the deficit and on serum electrolytes, serum osmolality, and acid-base status. Intravenous (IV) fluids are provided to expand intravascular volume or to correct an underlying imbalance in fluids or electrolytes. Fluids should be infused at a rate resulting in a positive fluid balance (e.g., 50 to 100 mL in excess of all hourly losses).

Replacement fluids

- Isotonic solutions (normal saline 0.9%): Expand the extracellular fluid compartment (ECF) only; do not enter the intracellular fluid compartment (ICF). Appropriate for rapid volume replacement.
- Hypotonic saline solutions (0.45% saline): Expand the ECF and provide some free water to the cells. Used in the management of the patient who is both volume-depleted and hyperosmolar (e.g., in cases of hypernatremia or hyperglycemia).
- Dextrose and water (5% dextrose in water): Provide free water only that will be distributed evenly through both the ICF and ECF; used to treat water deficit.
- Mixed isotonic saline/electrolyte solutions: Provide additional electrolytes (e.g., potassium and calcium) and a buffer (e.g., lactate or acetate). *Example:* Lactated Ringer solution (Ringer lactate): Isotonic solution containing a small amount of K^+ and lactate, which metabolizes to bicarbonate in the liver to assist blood buffering.
- Blood and albumin: Expand only the intravascular portion of the ECF. Both packed red blood cells and fresh-frozen plasma expand the intravascular volume.
- Dextran or hetastarch, hypertonic saline, hextend: Synthetic colloidal solutions used to expand the intravascular volume.

2. Restore Tissue Perfusion (Hypovolemic Shock)

- *Rapid volume replacement with crystalloids:* Fluids may be given rapidly as long as cardiac filling pressures and blood pressure remain low. Overaggressive fluid resuscitation in uncontrolled hemorrhage can increase the risk of secondary hemorrhage as the intravascular hydrostatic pressure increases.
- *Volume replacement with colloids:* Use of volume replacement with colloids to prevent the development of pulmonary edema secondary to rapid volume replacement remains controversial. Solutions include albumin and synthetics such as hetastarch.
- *Blood:* Administered only if necessary to maintain oxygen-carrying capacity. Hematocrit should not be raised greater than 35%.
- *Vasopressors:* Used to reduce the size of blood vessels while volume infusions continue to increase blood pressure. Effective for false hypovolemia induced by vasogenic (septic, anaphylactic, neurogenic) shock to control severe vasodilation.

CARE PLANS FOR HYPOVOLEMIA

Deficient fluid volume *related to loss of body fluid or blood*

Goals/Outcomes: Within 24 hours of starting fluid therapy, the patient becomes normovolemic, as evidenced by urine output $\geq$0.5 mL/kg/h, specific gravity 1.010 to 1.030, stable weight, no clinical evidence of hypovolemia (e.g., furrowed tongue), BP within the patient's normal range, HR and pulse pressure normalized, CVP 2 to 6 mm Hg, pulmonary artery pressure (PAP) 20 to 30/8 to 15 mm Hg, CO 4 to 7 L/min, mean airway pressure (MAP) 70 to 105 mm Hg, HR 60 to 100 beats per minute (bpm), and systemic vascular resistance (SVR) 900 to 1200 dynes/s/cm^5.
NOC Fluid Balance, Hydration, Kidney Function.

Fluid Monitoring
1. Monitor input and output (I&O) hourly: During initial therapy, intake should exceed output. Consult the advanced practice provider for urine output less than 0.5 mL/kg/h for 2 consecutive hours. Measure urine specific gravity every 4 hours as available. Normal range is 1.010 to 1.030. Expect it to decrease with therapy.
2. Monitor vital signs and hemodynamic pressures for continued hypovolemia: Be alert to decreased BP, CVP, PAP, CO, and MAP and to increased HR and SVR.
3. Weigh the patient daily: Daily weight measurements are the single most important indicator of fluid status, because acute weight changes usually indicate fluid changes. A decrease in daily weight of 1 kg is equal to the loss of 1 L of fluid. The adult who is not eating or receiving enteral nutrition or parenteral nutrition (PN) may lose 0.25 kg of nonfluid weight daily because body tissues are used for glucose production. Weigh patient at the same time of day (preferably before breakfast) on a balanced scale, with the patient wearing approximately the same clothing. Document type of scale used (i.e., standing, bed, chair).
4. Monitor for signs of fluid overload or too-rapid fluid administration: Crackles (rales), decreased O_2 saturation (pulse oximetry/SpO_2), shortness of breath (SOB), tachypnea, tachycardia, increased CVP, increased PA pressures, neck vein distention, and edema.
5. Monitor the patient for hidden fluid losses: Measure/record abdominal girth or limb size if indicated.
6. Monitor for signs of abdominal compartment syndrome: Acute increase in ventilator pressures and a decrease in SpO_2.
7. Monitor for signs of bleeding: Decreased hematocrit (Hct), Hgb, tachycardia. Note that Hct, serum Na^+, and BUN may decrease in dehydrated patients as rehydration progresses.
8. Monitor for hypocalcemia: May develop in patients who are rapidly transfused as a result of the citrate used in banked blood (citrate binds calcium, making it unavailable for cellular uptake). Sudden symptoms may include refractory hypotension (see Hypocalcemia. Calcium chloride or gluconate may be prescribed.

Fluid Management
1. Place hypotensive patients in supine position with legs elevated to 45 degrees to increase venous return. Avoid the Trendelenburg position, which causes abdominal organs to lean on the diaphragm, thereby impairing ventilation.
2. Administer oral (per os, PO) and IV fluids as prescribed. Ensure adequate intake, especially in older adults, a population at higher risk for volume depletion. Give water with enteral feedings and supplements.
3. Ensure a patent IV access and availability of blood products if needed.

NIC Fluid Monitoring; Hypovolemia Management; Fluid Resuscitation; Intravenous (IV) Therapy; Invasive Hemodynamic Monitoring; Shock Management; Volume.

Ineffective peripheral tissue perfusion *related to lack of blood volume*

Goals/Outcomes: Within 12 hours after initiation of volume resuscitation, the patient has adequate perfusion, as evidenced by alertness, warm and dry skin, BP within the patient's normal range, HR ≤100 bpm, urinary output ≥0.5 mL/kg/h, and capillary refill less than 2 seconds.

NOC Circulation Status, Tissue Integrity: Skin and Mucous Membranes.

Circulatory Care: Arterial Insufficiency
1. Monitor for signs of decreased cerebral perfusion: vertigo, syncope, confusion, restlessness, anxiety, agitation, excitability, weakness, nausea, and cool and clammy skin. Consult the physician or midlevel practitioner for worsening symptoms.
2. To avoid unnecessary vasodilation, treat fevers promptly.
3. Cover the patient with a light blanket to maintain body temperature.
4. Palpate peripheral pulses bilaterally in arms and legs (radial, brachial, dorsalis pedis, posterior tibial). Use a Doppler ultrasonic device if unable to palpate pulses. Rate pulses (0 to 4+ scale). Consult the physician for weak/absent pulses.

Safety Alert   *Abnormal pulses may also be caused by a local vascular disorder.*

5. Consult the advanced practice provider for urinary output less than 0.5 mL/kg/h for 2 consecutive hours.

Positioning
1. Protect patients who are at high risk for falling: those who are confused, dizzy, or weak. Keep side rails up and bed in lowest position with wheels locked. Assist with ambulation. Raise the patient to sitting or standing positions slowly.
2. Monitor for orthostatic hypotension: decreased BP, increased HR, dizziness, and diaphoresis. If symptoms occur, return the patient to supine position.

NIC Neurologic Monitoring

ADDITIONAL NURSING DIAGNOSES

For additional nursing diagnoses, see specific medical disorder, electrolyte imbalance, or acid-base disturbance.

HYPERVOLEMIA
PATHOPHYSIOLOGY

Hypervolemia is a state of higher-than-normal intravascular volume that occurs in four situations: (1) excessive retention of sodium and water caused by a chronic renal stimulus to conserve sodium and water; (2) abnormal renal functioning causing reduced excretion of sodium and water; (3) excessive administration of IV fluids; and (4) interstitial-to-plasma fluid shifting. Hypervolemia may lead to heart failure and pulmonary edema, especially in the patient with cardiovascular dysfunction.

HYPERVOLEMIA ASSESSMENT
GOAL OF ASSESSMENT

*   Evaluate the potential causes and sequelae of hypervolemia.

HISTORY AND RISK FACTORS

*   Retention of sodium and/or water: Heart failure, hepatic failure, nephrotic syndrome, excessive administration of glucocorticosteroids, and syndrome of inappropriate antidiuretic hormone (SIADH).
*   Abnormal renal function: Acute or chronic renal failure, oliguria, anuria, and excessive administration of IV fluids.
*   Interstitial-to-plasma fluid shifting: Remobilization of fluid after burn treatment, excessive administration of hypertonic solutions (i.e., mannitol, hypertonic saline), and excessive administration of colloid oncotic solutions (i.e., albumin).

OBSERVATION

* Evaluate for the clinical signs of volume overload: SOB, orthopnea, peripheral edema, distended neck veins, and moist skin.

VITAL SIGNS

* HR, BP, and hemodynamic measurements to evaluate volume status.
* Increased BP.
* BP: will decrease as the heart fails.
* HR: tachycardia.
* Respirations: tachypnea.
* O_2 saturation decreased.
* Increased CVP, PAP, PAWP.
* MAP: increased unless heart failure is present.
* Pulse pressure: may be narrow early in development of cardiogenic shock.

PALPATION

* Pulse assessment to evaluate tissue perfusion: Bounding pulses, ascites, and peripheral and sacral edema.

AUSCULTATION

* Heart and lung assessment to evaluate signs of volume overload: Tachycardia, gallop rhythm, crackles, rhonchi, and wheezes.

SCREENING LABWORK

* Blood studies are variable and nonspecific: Hematocrit, BUN and creatinine, ABGs, serum sodium and osmolality, urinary sodium, and urine specific gravity.

RADIOLOGY

* Chest radiograph may reveal signs of pulmonary vascular congestion.

Diagnostic Tests for Hypervolemia		
Test	**Purpose**	**Abnormal Findings**
Hematocrit	Assess for anemia	Decreased: As a result of hemodilution by excess fluids in the vasculature
Blood urea nitrogen	Evaluate for presence of renal dysfunction	Decreased: In pure hypervolemia. Increased: With renal failure
Arterial blood gases	Assess for hypoxemia and acid-base imbalance (acidosis or alkalosis)	Hypoxemia with alkalosis: May be present as a result of tachypnea associated with early pulmonary edema. Respiratory acidosis: May be present in severe pulmonary edema. Diffusion of oxygen is difficult across the edematous alveolar-capillary membrane
Serum sodium and serum osmolality	Assess for water retention	Decreased: If hypervolemia is from water retention (i.e., chronic renal failure)
Urinary sodium	Evaluate efficacy of renal handling of sodium	Elevated: Results from kidneys excreting excess sodium. Sodium excretion prompts fluid excretion. Note: Urinary sodium is not elevated with secondary hyperaldosteronism (e.g., heart failure, cirrhosis, nephrotic syndrome) because hypervolemia occurs secondary to a chronic renal stimulus; the aldosterone increases resorption of Na^+
Urine specific gravity	Evaluate the solute concentrating ability of the kidney	Decreased: If the kidney is excreting excess volume. May be fixed at 1.010 in acute renal failure
Chest radiograph	Assess for pulmonary edema	May reveal signs of pulmonary vascular congestion ("whiter" appearance)

Box 1-7	FOODS HIGH IN SODIUM
Bouillon	Pickles
Celery	Preserved meat
Cheeses	Salad dressings and prepared sauces
Dried fruits	Sauerkraut
Frozen, canned, or packaged foods	Snack foods (e.g., crackers, chips,
Monosodium glutamate (MSG)	pretzels)
Mustard	Soy sauce
Olives	

COLLABORATIVE MANAGEMENT
CARE PRIORITIES
The priorities include prevention of further volume overload and returning the patient to a euvolemic state.

1. **Restrict intake of sodium and water:** Monitor intake of oral, enteral, and parenteral fluids. Prevent the intake of high sodium foods. Box 1-7 lists foods high in sodium.
2. **Administer diuretics:** May be given IV or PO. Loop diuretics (i.e., furosemide) are indicated for severe hypervolemia or heart failure. Diuresis may prompt profound electrolyte loss.
3. **Monitor weight and output:** Assess the response to diuretics. Monitor for electrolyte loss.
4. **Renal replacement therapy:** Used in renal failure or life-threatening fluid overload (see Acute Renal Failure/Acute Kidney Injury, Chapter 6).
5. **Patient education:** Signs and symptoms of volume overload. Information provided regarding high sodium-containing foods.
6. **Vital signs:** Monitor for changes in BP and CO with diuresis.

> **Safety Alert**   *Also see specific discussions under Burns (Chapter 3), Acute Lung Injury and Acute Respiratory Distress Syndrome (Chapter 4), and Acute Renal Failure/Acute Kidney Injury (Chapter 6).*

CARE PLANS FOR HYPERVOLEMIA
Excess fluid volume   *related to the patient's disease state(s), medications, and/or other therapies*

Goals/Outcomes: Within 24 hours of starting treatment, the patient is improved, as evidenced by reduced edema, BP approaching the patient's normal range, HR 60 to 100 bpm, CVP 2 to 6 mm Hg, PAP 20 to 30 mm HG systolic, 8 to 15 mm Hg diastolic, MAP 70 to 105 mm Hg, and CO 4 to 7 L/min.
 NOC Electrolyte and Acid-Base Balance, Fluid Balance, Fluid Overload Severity.

Fluid/Electrolyte Management
1. Monitor intake and output hourly. Urine output should be ≥0.5 mL/kg/h unless the patient is in oliguric renal failure.
2. Measure urine specific gravity or urine osmolality if available, every 4 hours. If the patient is receiving diuretic therapy, specific gravity should be 1.010 to 1.020 with osmolality less than 500 mOsm/L.
3. Monitor and manage edema (pretibial, sacral, periorbital), using a 0 to 4+ rating scale.
4. Weigh patient daily. Daily weight measurements are the single most important indicator of fluid status.
5. Limit oral, enteral, and parenteral sodium intake as prescribed. Be aware that medications may contain sodium (e.g., penicillin, bicarbonate). See Box 1-7 for some foods high in sodium.
6. Limit fluids as prescribed. Offer a portion of allotted fluids as ice chips to minimize the patient's thirst. Teach the patient and significant others the importance of fluid restriction and how to measure fluid volume.
7. Provide oral hygiene at frequent intervals to keep oral mucous membranes moist and intact.
8. Document response to diuretic therapy (e.g., increased urine output, decreased CVP/PAP, decreased adventitious breath sounds, decreased edema). Many diuretics (e.g., furosemide, thiazides) cause hypokalemia.

Observe for indicators of hypokalemia: muscle weakness, dysrhythmias (especially PVCs and ECG changes such as flattened T wave, presence of U waves). (See Hypokalemia) Potassium-sparing diuretics (e.g., spironolactone, triamterene) may cause hyperkalemia: signs include weakness, ECG changes (e.g., peaked T wave, prolonged PR interval, widened QRS complex). (See Hyperkalemia) Consult the advanced practice provider for significant findings.

9. Observe for indicators of overcorrection and dangerous volume depletion. Vertigo, weakness, syncope, thirst, confusion, poor skin turgor, flat neck veins, and acute weight loss.

10. Monitor vital signs and hemodynamic parameters for volume depletion occurring with therapy. Decreased BP, CVP, PAP, MAP, and CO; increased HR. Consult the advanced practice provider for significant changes or findings.

11. Monitor appropriate laboratory tests (e.g., BUN and creatinine in renal failure). Consult with the advanced practice provider for abnormal trends.

NIC Fluid Monitoring; Hypervolemia Management; Fluid/Electrolyte Management; Invasive Hemodynamic Monitoring; Hemodialysis Therapy.

Impaired gas exchange *related to fluid volume overload*

Goals/Outcomes: Within 12 hours of initiating treatment, the patient has improved gas exchange, as evidenced by RR <20 breaths/min with normal depth and pattern (eupnea), HR <100 bpm, PaO_2 >80 mm Hg; pH 7.35 to 7.45, $PaCO_2$ 35 to 45 mm Hg, and SpO_2 >92%. The patient exhibits reduction in or absence of crackles, gallops, or other clinical indicators of pulmonary edema. PAP is ≤30/15 mm Hg and PAWP is 6 to 12 mm Hg.
NOC Respiratory Status: Gas Exchange; Respiratory Status: Ventilation.

Respiratory Monitoring
1. Monitor the patient for signs of acute pulmonary edema, a potentially life-threatening complication of hypervolemia: air hunger, decreased pulse oximetry, anxiety, cough with production of frothy sputum, crackles, rhonchi, tachypnea, increasing ventilator pressures, tachycardia, gallop rhythm, and elevation of PAP and PAWP. Administer diuretics and other medications to reduce venous return to the heart, as prescribed.
2. Monitor ABG values for hypoxemia and respiratory alkalosis. Monitor O_2 saturation. Administer O_2 to maintain SpO_2 >92%. Increased O_2 requirements may signal increased pulmonary vascular congestion.
3. Keep the patient in semi-Fowler position or position of comfort to minimize dyspnea.

NIC Ventilation Assistance, Positioning.

Impaired skin integrity *related to edematous, possibly friable tissue*

Goals/Outcomes: The patient's skin and tissue remain intact.
NOC Tissue Integrity: Skin and Mucous Membranes.

Pressure Management
1. Assess and document circulation to extremities at least each shift. Note color, temperature, capillary refill, and peripheral pulses. Consult the physician or midlevel practitioner if capillary refill is delayed or if pulses are diminished or absent.
2. Turn and reposition the patient at least every 2 hours to minimize tissue pressure.
3. Check tissue areas at risk with each position change (e.g., heels, sacrum, areas over bony prominences).
4. Use pressure-relief mattress as indicated.
5. Support arms and hands on pillows and elevate legs to decrease dependent edema. Do not elevate legs in the presence of pulmonary congestion.
6. Treat pressure ulcers per unit protocol. Consult the advanced practice provider if sores, ulcers, or areas of tissue breakdown are present, especially with patients who are at high risk for infection (i.e., those with diabetes mellitus or renal failure or who are immunosuppressed).
7. Consult a skin/wound care nurse specialist for advanced tissue breakdown or any alteration in tissue integrity in high-risk patients.

NIC Circulatory Care; Skin Surveillance.

HYPONATREMIA (serum sodium less than 135 mEq/L)

PATHOPHYSIOLOGY

Hyponatremia occurs from a net gain of water or a loss of sodium-rich fluids that have been replaced by water (net gain fluid > net gain Na^{2+}). The most common cause of hyponatremia is water gain from renal dysfunction. The kidneys should increase output if intake increases. As serum osmolality decreases, fluid shifts into cells, causing swelling and sometimes compartment syndromes.

There are three types of hyponatremia: hypovolemic, hypervolemic, and euvolemic. Dilutional states are the most frequent cause of hyponatremia in the critically ill. Clinical indicators and treatments depend on the cause of hyponatremia and whether it is associated with normal, decreased, or increased ECF volume. For more information, see Burns (Chapter 3), Heart Failure (Chapter 5), Acute Renal Failure/Acute Kidney Injury (Chapter 6), and Syndrome of Inappropriate Antidiuretic Hormone (Chapter 8).

 Safety Alert *Hyperlipidemia, hyperproteinemia, and hyperglycemia may cause a pseudohyponatremia. Pseudohyponatremia reduces the Na^{2+} content but also causes a reduction in volume. Actual osmolality may be normal or high. If blood glucose, lipids, or proteins are elevated, an osmolality calculation or laboratory determination should be performed. Hyperlipidemia and hyperproteinemia reduce the percentage of plasma water. With hyperglycemia, the osmotic action of elevated glucose causes water to shift out of the cells into the extracellular fluid compartment, thus diluting the serum sodium. For every 100 mg/dL that glucose is elevated, sodium is diluted by 1.6 mEq/L. The sodium-to-water ratio of plasma is unchanged, but the amount of sodium in the plasma is reduced.*

HYPONATREMIA ASSESSMENT

GOAL OF ASSESSMENT
- Evaluate for the signs and symptoms of hyponatremia.

HISTORY AND RISK FACTORS
- Decreased ECF volume. GI losses: diarrhea, vomiting, fistulas, and nasogastric suction; renal losses: diuretics, salt-wasting kidney disease, and adrenal insufficiency; skin losses: burns, wound drainage, and excessive diaphoresis.
- Normal/increased ECF volume. Hypothyroidism, SIADH, edematous states: heart failure, cirrhosis, and nephrotic syndrome; vigorous administration of hypotonic IV fluids; very dilute enteral feedings; oliguric renal failure; primary polydipsia; any patient with impaired ability to excrete free water (e.g., those being treated with thiazide diuretics) is at risk if given hypotonic fluids.

VITAL SIGN ASSESSMENT
- BP and HR will vary based on the state of ECF volume.
  - Postural hypotension with decreased ECF volume.
  - Elevated BP with normal or increased ECF volume.
  - Weight gain with normal or increased ECF volume.
- Hemodynamic measurements.
  - Decreased ECF volume: decreased CVP, PAP, CO, MAP; increased SVR.
  - Increased ECF volume: increased CVP, PAP, MAP.

OBSERVATION
- Hyponatremia with decreased ECF volume: Irritability, apprehension, dizziness, personality changes, poor skin turgor, dry mucous membranes, tremors, seizures, and coma.
- Hyponatremia with normal or increased ECF volume: Headache, lassitude, apathy, confusion, weakness, edema, convulsions, and coma.

PALPATION
- Cold clammy skin with decreased ECF volume.
- Hyperreflexia and muscle spasms with normal on increased ECF volume.

SCREENING LABWORK

- Serum sodium.
- Serum osmolality.
- Urine specific osmolality.
- Urine sodium.

Diagnostic Tests for Hyponatremia		
Test	Purpose	Abnormal Findings
Serum sodium	Evaluate sodium level	Decreased: Less than 135 mEq/L.
Serum osmolality	Assess hydration status	Decreased: Except in cases of pseudohyponatremia.
Urine specific osmolality	Assess renal concentrating ability	Elevated: Usually greater than 100 mOsm/kg, but less than the plasma level. SIADH: The urine will be inappropriately concentrated.
Urine sodium	Assess renal ability to conserve sodium	Decreased: Usually less than 20 mEq/L EXCEPT with SIADH, salt-wasting kidney disease, adrenal insufficiency, or excessive diuretic therapy.

SIADH, Syndrome of inappropriate antidiuretic hormone.

COLLABORATIVE MANAGEMENT

CARE PRIORITIES

1. Replace sodium and fluid losses with reduced ECF volume

Adequate replacement of fluid volume is essential to stop the physiologic stimulus to ADH release and enable the kidneys to restore sodium and water balance. Administer IV fluids while monitoring for further signs and symptoms of hyponatremia and I&O.

2. Replace other electrolyte losses

Other electrolytes include potassium and bicarbonate.

3. Administer IV hypertonic saline (3% NaCl)

Use if serum sodium is dangerously low or the patient has extreme symptoms. The therapeutic goal is to slowly shrink the cerebral cells. The dose is based on the patient's response. Therapy is sufficient when symptoms resolve and may be discontinued. Therapy MUST BE administered carefully, because too rapid correction can result in a life-threatening demyelination syndrome.

4. Monitor rate of sodium replacement to prevent too rapid correction of hyponatremia

Mild symptoms/no symptoms of hyponatremia: Strive to increase serum sodium 0.5 to 1 mEq/L/h. Severe symptoms, including seizures: Increase serum sodium no more than 1 to 2 mEq/L/h for 3 to 4 hours. Sodium should not increase more than 10 mEq/L in any 24-hour period, and no more than 6 mEq/L during the first 3 to 4 hours.

5. For Hyponatremia with expanded ECF volume

- Remove or treat the underlying cause.
- Administer diuretics.
- Restrict fluid intake to 1000 mL/day to establish a negative water balance and increase sodium levels.

6. Assess for resolution of the signs and symptoms of neurologic changes.

7. For dilutional hyponatremia

Administer diuretics and restrict water intake.

See Syndrome of Inappropriate Antidiuretic Hormone, Chapter 8, for specific treatment of hyponatremia.

HIGH ALERT! Osmotic Demyelination Syndrome

Overly aggressive or inappropriate treatment of hyponatremia can also cause permanent neurologic damage secondary to osmotic demyelination syndrome. Osmotic demyelination is poorly understood but should always be suspected after hypertonic resuscitation when patients display bilateral neurologic deficits, flaccidity, and quadriparesis. Initially, sodium levels should not increase at a level greater than 0.5 to 1.0 mEq/L/h in patients being treated for symptomatic hyponatremia with hypertonic NaCl. For those symptomatic with severe hyponatremia (less than 120 mEq/L), the rate of correction should be 1 to 2 mEq/h for 3 to 4 hours. After an initial 6 to 8 mEq/L increase in the serum sodium level, the rate of increase should not be greater than 0.5 mEq/L/h. Levels should not increase at an average rate of greater than 0.5 mEq/L/h in patients without symptoms. The total increase in the first 24 hours of treatment should not exceed 12 mEq/L.

CARE PLANS FOR HYPONATREMIA

Readiness for enhanced fluid balance *related to the dynamic fluid and electrolyte changes that prompt sodium imbalance*

Goals/Outcomes: Within 24 hours of initiating treatment, the patient's volume status is improving, as evidenced by normalization of the heart and respiratory rates (HR 60 to 100 bpm, RR 12 to 20 breaths/min), BP within the patient's normal range, CVP 2 to 6 mm Hg, and PAP 20 to 30 mm HG systolic, 8 to 15 mm Hg diastolic or within the patient's normal range.

NOC Fluid Balance, Kidney Function, Hydration.

Fluid Monitoring

If the patient is receiving hypertonic saline, assess carefully for signs of intravascular fluid overload: tachypnea, tachycardia, acute SOB, crackles (rales), rhonchi, increased CVP and PAP, gallop rhythm, and increased BP. For other interventions, see Hypovolemia or Hypervolemia.

NIC Electrolyte Management: Hyponatremia; Fluid/Electrolyte Management; Intravenous (IV) Therapy; Invasive Hemodynamic Monitoring.

Acute confusion *related to hyponatremia*

Goals/Outcomes: Within 48 hours of treatment, the patient more consistently verbalizes orientation to time, place, and person and has not sustained physical injury related to altered sensorium. Serum sodium level should ideally increase to greater than 125 mEq/L in the first 48 hours after treatment.

NOC Cognitive Orientation; Distorted Thought Self-Control; Information Processing; Neurologic Status: Consciousness.

Neurologic Monitoring

1. Assess and document LOC, orientation, and neurologic status with each vital sign check. Reorient the patient as necessary. Consult the advanced practice provider for significant changes.
2. If seizures are expected, pad side rails and keep an appropriate-size airway at the bedside.
3. Inform the patient and significant others that altered sensorium is temporary and will improve with treatment.
4. Keep side rails up and bed in lowest position with wheels locked.
5. Use reality therapy such as clocks, calendars, and familiar objects; keep these items at the bedside within the patient's visual field.
6. Monitor serum sodium levels closely. Permanent neurologic damage may occur with untreated, severely symptomatic hyponatremia secondary to cerebral edema.

HIGH ALERT! Overly rapid correction of chronic hyponatremia may result in permanent neurologic damage.

NIC Electrolyte Management: Hyponatremia; Seizure Precautions, Reality Orientation, Fall Prevention.

HYPERNATREMIA (serum sodium greater than 145 mEq/L)

PATHOPHYSIOLOGY

Hypernatremia may occur with either free water loss or sodium gain. Hypernatremia always causes hypertonicity because sodium is the major determinant of ECF osmolality. Hypertonicity causes a shift of water out of the cells, which leads to intracellular dehydration. Hypernatremia usually results from volume depletion (hypovolemia) and is rarely caused by increased sodium intake.

HYPERNATREMIA ASSESSMENT

GOAL OF ASSESSMENT

Evaluate the risk factors and clinical symptoms of hypernatremia.

HISTORY AND RISK FACTORS

- Water (volume) loss: Increased diaphoresis, respiratory infection, mechanical ventilation, diabetes insipidus, osmotic diuresis (e.g., hyperglycemia), and osmotic diarrhea.
- Sodium gains: IV administration of hypertonic saline or sodium bicarbonate, increased oral intake, primary aldosteronism, and drugs such as sodium polystyrene sulfonate (Kayexalate).

OBSERVATION

- Symptoms related to hypertonicity, intracellular dehydration, and electrolyte imbalance: Intense thirst, fatigue, restlessness, agitation, coma, flushed skin, and peripheral edema.

VITAL SIGNS

- Low-grade fever.
- Postural hypotension.
- Increased CVP and PAP: with sodium excess.
- Decreased CVP and PAP with water loss: may be minimized by the extracellular shift of fluid that occurs with hypernatremia.
- Tachycardia may be present.

 Symptoms of hypernatremia occur only in individuals who do not have access to water or who have an altered thirst mechanism (e.g., infants, older adults, those who are comatose).

 Symptoms are most likely to develop with a sudden increase in plasma sodium. After 24 hours, brain cells adjust to extracellular fluid hypertonicity by increasing intracellular osmolality. The mechanism of action is unclear, but the increased osmolality helps to rehydrate the cells. Individuals with chronic hypernatremia exhibit few symptoms. This adaptive mechanism plays a key role in the treatment of hypernatremia.

HIGH ALERT! *Overly aggressive water administration may cause rapid movement of water into the cells, which can result in dangerous cerebral edema caused by a too-rapid reduction of sodium.*

Diagnostic Tests for Hypernatremia

Test	Purpose	Abnormal Findings
Serum sodium	Assess level of sodium	Increased: Greater than 145 mEq/L.
Serum osmolality	Determine concentration of solutes	Increased: As a result of elevated serum sodium; greater than 300 mOsm/kg.
Urine specific gravity	Assess the ability of the kidneys to retain water	Increased: Greater than 1.030. Lower than expected in diabetes insipidus and too dilute in early osmotic diuresis (e.g., hyperglycemia).

COLLABORATIVE MANAGEMENT

CARE PRIORITIES

1. Assess the patient for fluid losses or gains.
2. Administer IV or PO water replacement: Used for water loss. If sodium is greater than 160 mEq/L, IV 5% dextrose or hypotonic (0.45%) saline is given to replace pure water deficit (see Diabetes Insipidus, Chapter 8).
3. Monitor intake to prevent too rapid correction of water loss.
4. Administer diuretics with water replacement: Use for sodium gain.
5. Provide information to the patient to help decrease sodium intake.

 Safety Alert *Hypernatremia is corrected slowly, over approximately 2 days, to avoid too great a shift of water into brain cells.*

CARE PLANS FOR HYPERNATREMIA

Acute confusion *related to hypernatremia*

Goals/Outcomes: Within 48 hours after treatment, the patient more consistently verbalizes orientation to time, place, and person and has not sustained an injury caused by altered sensorium or seizures. Serum sodium level has decreased and is approaching high normal (145 mEq/L).

NOC Cognitive Orientation; Distorted Thought Self-Control; Information Processing; Neurologic Status: Consciousness.

Fluid/Electrolyte Management

1. Monitor serial serum sodium levels (sodium should not decrease at a rate greater than 0.5 to 1.0 mEq/L/h); consult the physician for rapid decreases. Cerebral edema may occur if hypernatremia is corrected too rapidly.
2. Assess the patient for signs of cerebral edema: lethargy, headache, nausea, vomiting, increased BP, widening pulse pressure, decreased HR, altered sensorium, and seizures.
3. Assess and document LOC, orientation, and neurologic status with each vital sign check. Reorient the patient as necessary. Consult the advanced practice provider for deterioration.
4. Inform the patient and significant others that altered sensorium is temporary and will improve with treatment.
5. Keep side rails up and bed in lowest position with wheels locked.
6. Use reality therapy such as clocks, calendars, and familiar objects; keep these items at the bedside within the patient's visual field.
7. If seizures are anticipated, pad side rails and keep an appropriate-size airway at the bedside.
8. Provide comfort measures to decrease thirst.

NIC Neurologic Monitoring; Electrolyte Management: Hypernatremia; Seizure Precautions; Surveillance: Safety.

ADDITIONAL NURSING DIAGNOSES

See Hypovolemia for Fluid Volume Deficit and Hypervolemia for Fluid Volume Excess.

POTASSIUM IMBALANCE (normal serum K⁺ level 3.5 to 5 mEq/L)

Potassium is the primary intracellular cation ($^+$ or positive ion), with normal levels inside cells of 150 mEq/dL. Of total potassium, 98% is inside the cell and markedly affects cell metabolism. Abnormal serum K⁺ levels may adversely affect neuromuscular and cardiac function, because they affect resting membrane potential and conduction velocity of nerve and cardiac cells. A relatively small amount of potassium is present in the ECF, and concentrations are maintained within a narrow range. Potassium is constantly moving into and out of the cell. Distribution of potassium between the ECF and ICF is maintained by the sodium-potassium pump located in the membrane of all body cells and is affected by ECF pH, glucose and protein metabolism, insulin levels, and stimulation of beta₂-adrenergic receptors. Acute changes in serum pH are accompanied by reciprocal changes in serum potassium concentration as the exchange of K⁺ and H⁺ takes place.

The body gains potassium through foods (primarily meats, fruits, and vegetables) and medications. The ECF also gains potassium from breakdown or death of cells, when a large amount of intracellular K⁺ is released from the cell contents. Potassium is eliminated from the body through the kidneys, the GI tract, and the skin. The potassium level may decrease in the serum (ECF) when K⁺ shifts inside the cells. The serum potassium level increases when renal function decreases, when circulation is reduced to a large amount of cells causing cell death, with cellular lysis, and with rhabdomyolysis. Changes in insulin production, insulin and other receptor activity, and catecholamine level affect the movement of K⁺ across the cell wall. The kidneys are the primary regulators of potassium balance.

 Safety Alert   *Disorders of potassium balance are potentially life threatening because of the effects of altered potassium levels on neuromuscular and cardiac function. Suspected alterations in potassium balance require prompt consultation with the advanced practice provider.*

HYPOKALEMIA (serum potassium level less than 3.5 mEq/L)

PATHOPHYSIOLOGY

Hypokalemia occurs because of a loss of potassium from the body or a movement of potassium into the cells. Acid-base imbalances are associated with changes in serum potassium level. Management of shifts in the K⁺ level must be done judiciously if an acid-base imbalance is present. Hypokalemia is sometimes associated with alkalosis (see *Acid-Base Imbalances*). Serum K⁺ levels are an inadequate measure of intracellular K⁺, but intracellular measurement is not clinically available.

 Safety Alert   *Changes in serum potassium levels reflect changes in extracellular fluid potassium—not necessarily changes in total body levels.*

HYPOKALEMIA ASSESSMENT

GOAL OF ASSESSMENT

Evaluate for the risk factors and signs and symptoms of hypokalemia and use the information to manage the symptoms. The patient is at risk for torsades de pointes and ventricular tachycardia.

HISTORY AND RISK FACTORS

- Reduction in total body potassium: Hyperaldosteronism, diuretic therapy or abnormal urinary losses, increased GI losses, increased loss through diaphoresis, decreased intake, and dialysis.
- Intracellular shift: Increased insulin (e.g., from total parenteral nutrition [TPN] or aggressive IV insulin), acute alkalosis: K⁺ moves into the cells in exchange for H⁺ to

electrically and pH balance the serum; stress causing a loss of potassium in the urine secondary to increased release of aldosterone; intracellular shift of potassium secondary to increased stimulation of beta$_2$-adrenergic receptors.

VITAL SIGNS
- Postural hypotension.
- Irregular respiratory pattern resulting from respiratory muscle weakness.

AUSCULTATION
- Decreased bowel sounds.

PALPATION
- Weak and irregular pulse.
- Decreased reflexes.
- Decreased muscle tone.
- Paresthesias.

SCREENING
12-Lead ECG: Evaluate changes typically seen with hypokalemia, including ST segment depression, flattened T waves, presence of U waves; with severe hypokalemia, P wave amplitude is increased, PR interval is prolonged, QRS and QT complexes widen, and patient is at risk for torsades de pointes.

Safety Alert	*An inadequate diet may contribute to but will rarely cause hypokalemia. Large amounts of potassium are contained in many common foods. Hypokalemia sometimes develops when patients are maintained on parenteral fluid therapy with inadequate replacement of potassium or when increased losses occur when oral intake is poor.*

Diagnostic Tests for Hypokalemia

Test	Purpose	Abnormal Findings
Serum potassium	Determine if hypokalemia is present	Decreased: Less than 3.5 mEq/L.
Arterial blood gases	Evaluate for the presence of alkalosis	Increased pH and bicarbonate. Hypokalemia is associated with metabolic alkalosis.

Safety Alert	*Hypokalemia potentiates the effect of digitalis. Electrocardiography may reveal signs of digitalis toxicity despite a normal serum digitalis level.*

COLLABORATIVE MANAGEMENT
CARE PRIORITIES
1. Replace potassium (K$^+$)
Administer IV potassium as an infusion if less than 3.0 mEq/L. IV infusion is 40 to 80 mEq/L given in divided doses. Generally, 10 mEq of K$^+$ is diluted in 50 mL IV solution and given over 30 minutes. The process is repeated until the K$^+$ is normalized. If K$^+$ level is 3.0 to 3.5 mEq/L, increase dietary intake and use oral supplements (see Box 1-8 for high-potassium foods).

Safety Alert	*Never give potassium IV push to avoid lethal dysrhythmias.*

2. Document dietary intake of potassium

3. Administer potassium-sparing diuretics
This is done in place of thiazide or loop diuretics, which promote potassium loss. Diuretics are often associated with hypokalemia.

Box 1-8   FOODS HIGH IN POTASSIUM

Apricots	Nuts
Artichokes	Oranges, orange juice
Avocados	Peanuts
Bananas	Potatoes
Cantaloupes	Prune juice
Carrots	Pumpkins
Cauliflower	Spinach
Chocolate	Swiss chard
Dried beans, peas	Sweet potatoes
Dried fruit	Tomatoes, tomato juice, tomato sauce
Mushrooms	

4. Monitor for signs of hyperkalemia
When replacing K^+ monitor for signs of hyperkalemia.

HIGH ALERT! Patients receiving 10 to 20 mEq/h should be on a continuous cardiac monitor.
If potassium is administered via a peripheral line, the rate of administration may need to be decreased to prevent irritation of vessels. The development of tall, peaked T waves suggests the presence of hyperkalemia and should be reported to the advanced practice provider. Intravenous potassium may be administered as potassium chloride or potassium phosphate.

CARE PLANS FOR HYPOKALEMIA
Decreased cardiac output *related to dysrhythmias caused by hypokalemia*

Goals/Outcomes: Within 2 hours of treatment, the patient is normalizing cardiac conduction, as evidenced by normal T wave configuration and normal sinus rhythm without ectopy on ECG.
NOC Cardiac Pump Effectiveness, Circulation Status.

Electrolyte Management
1. Administer potassium supplement as prescribed. Avoid giving IV potassium chloride at a rate faster than recommended, because this can lead to life-threatening hyperkalemia. K^+ supplements for symptomatic hypokalemia may be given in isotonic saline, as sometimes D_5W increases the insulin-induced intracellular shift of potassium. Concentrated solutions of potassium may be administered in limited volumes (i.e., 20 mEq in 100 mL of isotonic NaCl), administered at less than 20 mEq/h. Concentrated solutions are used only with severe hypokalemia.

 Safety Alert *Potassium chloride should not be added to intravenous (IV) bags while they are hanging on a pole, to avoid accumulation of K^+ at the bottom of the IV bag. The solution container should be inverted before adding the medication and mixed well.*

2. Be aware that IV potassium chloride (KCl) can cause local irritation of veins and chemical phlebitis. Assess IV insertion site for erythema, heat, or pain. Irritation may be relieved by applying an ice bag, giving mild sedation, or numbing insertion site with a small amount of local anesthetic. Phlebitis may necessitate changing of IV site.
3. Oral supplements may cause GI irritation. Administer with a full glass of water or fruit juice; encourage the patient to sip slowly. Consult the advanced practice provider for symptoms of abdominal pain, distention, nausea, or vomiting. Do not switch potassium supplements without consulting with the advanced practice provider.
4. Monitor I&O hourly. Report urine output less than 0.5 mL/kg/h. Unless severe symptoms of hypokalemia are present, potassium supplements should not be given to patients with low urine output; hyperkalemia may develop in patients with oliguria (output less than 15 to 20 mL/h). High urine output (diuresis or polyuria) increases the risk of hypokalemia.

5. Monitor ECG for signs of continuing hypokalemia (i.e., ST segment depression, flattened T wave, presence of U wave, ventricular dysrhythmias) or hyperkalemia during potassium replacement (i.e., tall, thin T waves; prolonged PR interval; ST depression; widened QRS complex; loss of P wave).
6. Monitor serum potassium levels in patients at risk for hypokalemia, such as patients taking diuretics or undergoing gastric suction.
7. Administer potassium cautiously in patients at risk for hyperkalemia, such as patients receiving potassium-sparing diuretics (e.g., spironolactone or triamterene) or angiotensin-converting enzyme (ACE) inhibitors (e.g., captopril).
8. Monitor patients on digitalis, because hypokalemia potentiates the effects. Signs of increased digitalis effect include multifocal or bigeminal PVCs, paroxysmal atrial tachycardia with atrioventricular block, and other heart blocks.

NIC Electrolyte Management: Hypokalemia; Medication Administration; Dysrhythmia Management.

Ineffective breathing pattern *related to respiratory muscle weakness associated with severe hypokalemia*

Goals/Outcomes: Within 2 hours of treatment, the patient has an effective breathing pattern, as evidenced by normal respiratory depth and pattern and rate of 12 to 20 breaths/min.
NOC Respiratory Status: Ventilation; Vital Signs.

Respiratory Monitoring
1. If the patient has worsening hypokalemia, if respirations become rapid and shallow, notify the advanced practice provider. Severe hypokalemia causes respiratory muscle weakness. Shallow respirations, apnea, and respiratory arrest may occur.
2. Keep manual resuscitator (Ambu bag) at the patient's bedside when severe hypokalemia is present. Reposition the patient every 2 hours to prevent stasis of secretions; suction airway as needed.
3. Encourage deep breathing (and coughing if indicated) every 2 hours.

NIC Ventilation Assistance.

HYPERKALEMIA (serum potassium level greater than 5 mEq/L)
PATHOPHYSIOLOGY
Hyperkalemia results from increased intake of potassium, decreased urinary excretion of K^+, or sudden movement of K^+ out of cells. The rate of change in serum K^+ is as important as the level. Rapid increases do not allow time to compensate. Hyperkalemia is often associated with acidosis.

 Safety Alert *Changes in serum potassium levels reflect changes in extracellular fluid potassium—not necessarily changes in total body levels of potassium.*

HYPERKALEMIA ASSESSMENT
GOAL OF ASSESSMENT
Evaluate for the risk factors and signs and symptoms of hyperkalemia. Information should be used immediately to manage potentially life-threatening dysrhythmias. Hyperkalemia is often associated with acidosis.

HISTORY AND RISK FACTORS
- Inappropriately high intake of potassium: IV potassium delivery, aggressive red blood cell administration, and symptomatic hyperkalemia may develop when doses of IV potassium are administered too rapidly.
- Decreased excretion of potassium: Renal disease both acute and chronic, potassium-sparing diuretics and ACE inhibitors, and Addison disease (hypoaldosteronism).

- Movement of potassium out of the cells: Acidosis, insulin deficiency particularly in patients on dialysis, and tissue catabolism (e.g., fever, sepsis, trauma, surgery).

OBSERVATION
- Irritability.
- Abdominal distention.
- Diarrhea.
- Ascending weakness.
- Parethesias.

VITAL SIGNS
- Irregular pulse.
- Cardiac arrest at levels greater than 8.5 mEq/L.
- Hypotension.

SCREENING
- 12-Lead ECG: Tall, thin T waves, prolonged PR interval, ST depression, widened QRS complex with progression to cardiac arrest, loss of P wave; eventually, QRS widens further and cardiac arrest occurs.

Diagnostic Tests for Hyperkalemia		
Test	**Purpose**	**Abnormal Findings**
Serum potassium	Evaluate potassium level	Elevated: Greater than 5 mEq/L.
Arterial blood gases	Evaluate acid-base status	Decreased pH and bicarbonate. Hyperkalemia associated with acidosis.

Safety Alert *Pseudohyperkalemia may occur with mechanical trauma during venipuncture or incorrect handling of the laboratory specimen. If red blood cells hemolyze (are injured), potassium is released from damaged cells while or after specimen has been drawn.*

COLLABORATIVE MANAGEMENT
CARE PRIORITIES
1. Administer calcium gluconate to decrease myocardial irritability for severe hyperkalemia
IV calcium gluconate is given to counteract the neuromuscular and cardiac effects of hyperkalemia. Serum K^+ may remain elevated.

2. Administer insulin and IV glucose and bicarbonate to move potassium into the cell for severe hyperkalemia
This strategy provides a temporary reduction in serum potassium. Sodium bicarbonate shifts K^+ into the cells.

3. Administer beta$_2$-adrenergic agonists (albuterol) to shift K^+ back into the cells
This provides a temporary reduction in K^+ level.

4. Take precautions when drawing blood to prevent hemolysis.
Damaged cells release intracellular contents into the blood sample, which elevates the K^+ level of the sample. Most laboratories can provide information about whether the sample was hemolyzed.

5. Administer cation exchange resin orally or rectally
Cation exchange resin (e.g., Kayexalate) is given orally, or as a retention enema to exchange sodium for potassium in the gut. The oral form is combined with sorbitol to promote rapid transit through the gut and to induce diarrhea. Recommended rectal dose is 30 to 60 g every 6 hours.

6. Provide hemodialysis to lower K⁺ level if rapid removal for K⁺ is needed

7. Monitor for signs of hypokalemia

Hypokalemia may result from aggressive management of hyperkalemia.

 The effects of calcium, glucose and insulin, sodium bicarbonate, and beta₂-adrenergic agonists are temporary, lasting only a few hours. These medications should be followed by therapy to remove potassium from the body (i.e., hemodialysis or administration of cation exchange resins).

CARE PLANS FOR HYPERKALEMIA

Decreased cardiac output *related to dysrhythmias induced by hyperkalemia*

Goals/Outcomes: Within 6 hours after initiation of treatment, the patient's CO is adequate, as evidenced by PAP 20 to 30/8 to 15 mm Hg, CVP ≤6 mm Hg, CO 4 to 7 L/min, HR ≤100 bpm, BP within the patient's normal range, and absence of the clinical signs of heart failure or pulmonary edema (e.g., crackles, SOB). ECG shows normal sinus rhythm without ectopy or other electrical disturbances. Serum K⁺ levels normalize.

NOC Cardiac Pump Effectiveness, Circulation Status.

Fluid/Electrolyte Management

1. Monitor I&O: Consult the advanced practice provider for urine output less than 0.5 mL/kg/h. Oliguria increases the risk for development of hyperkalemia.
2. Monitor for signs of hyperkalemia: Irritability, anxiety, abdominal cramping, diarrhea, ascending weakness, paresthesias, and irregular pulse. Assess for hidden sources of potassium: medications (e.g., potassium penicillin G), banked blood, salt substitute, GI bleeding, or catabolic conditions (i.e., infection or trauma).
3. Monitor for signs of hypokalemia after treatment: Muscle weakness, cramps, nausea, vomiting, decreased bowel sounds, paresthesias, and weak and irregular pulse.
4. Monitor serum potassium levels, especially in high-risk patients (i.e., those with renal failure): Monitor other laboratory values associated with conditions that alter potassium levels (e.g., BUN, creatinine, ABGs, glucose). Consult the advanced practice provider for abnormal values.
5. Monitor ECG for signs of hypokalemia (i.e., ST segment depression, flattened T waves, presence of U wave, ventricular dysrhythmias) or continuing hyperkalemia (i.e., tall, thin T waves, prolonged PR interval, ST depression, widened QRS complex, loss of P wave): Report changes to the advanced practice provider as soon as possible.
6. Administer insulin and glucose in the order prescribed.
7. Administer calcium gluconate as prescribed: Use caution in patients receiving digitalis. Monitor for digitalis toxicity. Do not add calcium gluconate to solutions containing sodium bicarbonate, because precipitates may form. For more information about calcium administration, see Hypocalcemia.
8. If administering cation exchange resins by enema, encourage the patient to retain the solution for at least 30 to 60 minutes to ensure therapeutic effects: Administer Kayexalate (without sorbitol) via a Foley catheter inserted into the rectum. The balloon is filled with sterile water to keep the catheter in place, and the catheter is clamped. Cleansing enemas may be done before administering Kayexalate to enhance absorption, and after to reduce the risk of bowel complications.

NIC Electrolyte Management: Hyperkalemia; Dysrhythmia Management; Hemodialysis Therapy.

CALCIUM IMBALANCE (normal serum Ca²⁺ level: 8.5 to 10.5 mg/dL, ionized 4.5 to 5.5 mg/dL)

Calcium, one of the body's most abundant ions, combines with phosphorus to form the mineral salts of the bones and teeth. Calcium exerts a sedative effect on nerve cells and has important intracellular functions, including development of the cardiac action potential and contraction of muscles. Only 1% of the body's calcium is contained within the ECF, yet this concentration is regulated carefully by the hormones parathyroid hormone (PTH) and calcitonin.

Slightly less than half of the calcium in the plasma is free or ionized calcium. The percentage of ionized calcium is affected by plasma pH and the albumin level. Approximately 40% of calcium is bound to protein, primarily albumin. Calcium bound to albumin is not ionized and cannot be used. Albumin releases calcium to the ionized state when needed. Only the ionized calcium exerts physiologic effects and combines with nonprotein anions such as phosphate, citrate, and carbonate. Patients with alkalosis may show signs of hypocalcemia because of increased calcium binding. Changes in the plasma albumin level will affect the total serum calcium level without changing the level of ionized calcium.

 Safety Alert *To determine the "true calcium level" or calcium correction factor: For every gram of albumin less than 4, add 0.8 to the serum calcium value.*

PTH is released by the parathyroid gland in response to low serum Ca^{2+} levels to increase movement of Ca^{2+} and phosphorus out of the bone (resorption of bone); to activate vitamin D (increases the absorption of calcium from the GI tract); and to stimulate the kidneys to conserve calcium and excrete phosphorus. Calcitonin is produced by the thyroid gland when serum Ca^{2+} increases to inhibit bone resorption.

Calcium regulates skeletal and cardiac muscle contractions, is part of the clotting cascade, and has other essential functions. It is imperative to maintain the Ca^{2+} balance.

HYPOCALCEMIA (serum calcium less than 8.5 mg/dL, ionized less than 4.5 mg/dL)
PATHOPHYSIOLOGY
Symptoms of hypocalcemia result from decreased total body calcium or a decreased percentage of ionized calcium. Low total calcium levels may be caused by increased calcium loss, reduced intake secondary to altered intestinal absorption, altered regulation (i.e., hypoparathyroidism), and aggressive infusion of citrated blood or CRRT if citrate is used for anticoagulation. Elevated phosphorus levels and decreased magnesium levels may precipitate hypocalcemia.

HYPOCALCEMIA ASSESSMENT
GOAL OF ASSESSMENT
Evaluate the signs and symptoms of hypocalcemia.

HISTORY AND RISK FACTORS
- Decreased ionized calcium.
  - Alkalosis.
  - Rapid administration of citrated blood. Citrate added to the blood to prevent clotting may bind with calcium, causing hypocalcemia.
  - Hemodilution (e.g., occurring with volume replacement with normal saline after massive hemorrhage).
- Increased calcium loss in body fluids.
  - Large volume diuresis from loop diuretics.
- Decreased intestinal absorption: Decreased intake, impaired vitamin D metabolism, chronic diarrhea, and postoperatively following a gastrectomy.
- Other causes: Acute and chronic renal failure, hypoparathyroidism, hyperphosphatemia, hypomagnesemia, acute pancreatitis, chemotherapy, and treatment with bisphosphonates.

OBSERVATION
- Numbness with tingling of fingers and circumoral region.
- Tetany.
- Convulsions.
- Alteration in mental status (anxiety, depression, frank psychosis).

VITAL SIGNS
- Hypotension secondary to vasodilation.
- Heart failure secondary to decreased myocardial contractility.

PERCUSSION
- Positive Trousseau sign: Ischemia-induced carpopedal spasms. Elicited by applying a BP cuff to the upper arm and inflating it past systolic BP for 2 minutes.
- Positive Chvostek sign: Unilateral contraction of facial and eyelid muscles. Elicited by stimulating the facial nerve during percussion of the face just in front of the ear.

SCREENING
- 12-Lead ECG: Prolonged QT interval caused by elongation and elevation of ST segment.

Diagnostic Tests for Hypocalcemia

Test	Purpose	Abnormal Findings
Total serum calcium level	Evaluate total calcium level	Decreased: Less than 8.5 mg/dL. Evaluate with serum albumin. For every 1 g/dL drop in the serum albumin level there is a 0.8 to 1 mg/dL drop in the total calcium level.
Ionized calcium level	Evaluate the free calcium level	Decreased: Less than 4.5 mg/dL.
Parathyroid hormone level	Evaluate for hyperpara-thyroidism or hypopara-thyroidism	Hypoparathyroidism: Less than 150 pg/mL. Hyperparathyroidism: Greater than 70 pg/mL. Varies among laboratories.
Magnesium level	Evaluate for hypomagnesemia	Decreased: Less than 1.5 mEq/L.
Phosphorus level	Evaluate for hyperphosphatemia	Increased: More than 4.5 mg/dL.

COLLABORATIVE MANAGEMENT

CARE PRIORITIES

1. Administer IV calcium by continuous infusion over 4 to 6 hours
May give PO or IV calcium. Tetany is treated with 10 to 20 mL of 10% calcium gluconate administered IV or by continuous infusion of 100 mL of 10% calcium gluconate diluted in 1000 mL D_5W over at least 4 to 6 hours.

2. Administer vitamin D therapy
Provide additional vitamin D (e.g., dihydrotachysterol, calcitriol) to increase vitamin D absorption from the GI tract. Use of oral vitamin D_3 (activated vitamin D, available over the counter) is helpful to maintain calcium levels over time.

3. Administer magnesium replacement
Used for magnesium depletion; hypomagnesemia-induced hypocalcemia is often refractory to calcium therapy alone.

4. Administer phosphate binders if needed
Used to reduce elevated phosphorous before treating hypocalcemia. Used primarily in renal failure.

5. Monitor for signs of hypercalcemia during calcium replacement therapy
Lethargy, weakness, anorexia, nausea, vomiting, constipation, itching, polyuria, confusion, personality changes, stupor, and coma.

CARE PLANS FOR HYPOCALCEMIA
Ineffective protection *related to the potential complications of hypocalcemia*

Goals/Outcomes: The patient is not permanently harmed by severe hypocalcemia.

NOC Electrolyte and Acid-Base Balance; Nutritional Status: Food and Fluid Intake; Kidney Function; Fluid Balance.

Electrolyte Management: Hypocalcemia
1. Monitor the patient for worsening hypocalcemia and consult the advanced practice provider promptly for symptoms that occur before overt tetany: Numbness and tingling of fingers and circumoral region, hyperactive reflexes, and muscle cramps. Positive Trousseau or Chvostek sign also signals latent tetany. Monitor total and ionized calcium levels as available.

HIGH ALERT! *Administer intravenous (IV) calcium slowly.* Undiluted IV 10% calcium should not be given faster than 0.5 to 1 mL/min. Diluted calcium given in an infusion is preferred. *Rapid administration can cause hypotension.* Observe IV insertion site for infiltration; calcium will slough tissue. *Concentrated calcium solutions (calcium chloride) should be administered through a central line.* Do not add calcium to solutions containing sodium bicarbonate or sodium phosphate to avoid dangerous precipitates. Digitalis toxicity may develop, because calcium potentiates digitalis. Monitor for hypercalcemia: lethargy, confusion, irritability, nausea, and vomiting.

 Safety Alert *Always clarify the type of intravenous (IV) calcium to be given. Both calcium chloride and calcium gluconate come in 10-mL ampules. One ampule of calcium chloride contains 13.6 mEq of calcium, whereas one ampule of calcium gluconate contains 4.5 mEq of calcium.*

---

2. For patients with chronic hypocalcemia, administer oral calcium supplements and vitamin D preparations as prescribed. Administer oral calcium 30 minutes before meals or at bedtime for maximal absorption. Administer phosphorus-binding antacids with meals. If calcium carbonate is being administered primarily to bind phosphorus, administer with food.
3. Consult the advanced practice provider if response to calcium therapy is ineffective. Tetany that does not respond to IV calcium may be caused by hypomagnesemia.
4. Maintain seizure precautions for affected patients.
5. Avoid hyperventilation if hypocalcemia is suspected. Respiratory alkalosis may cause tetany if pH increases when ionized calcium is low.
6. Monitor for calcium loss (e.g., with loop diuretics, renal tubular dysfunction) or conditions that place the patient at risk for it (e.g., acute pancreatitis).
7. Inform the patient and significant others that the neuropsychiatric symptoms of hypocalcemia will improve with treatment.

NIC Neurologic Monitoring; Seizure Precautions; Medication Administration.

Decreased cardiac output *related to abnormal action of calcium in myocardial contractile tissues*

Goals/Outcomes: Within 12 hours of initiation of treatment, the patient's CO is improving, as evidenced by readings approaching normal baseline or PAP 20 to 30/8 to 15 mm Hg, CVP less than 6 mm Hg, CO 4 to 7 L/min, HR 100 bpm, BP within the patient's normal range, and diminishing clinical signs of heart failure or pulmonary edema (e.g., crackles, SOB). ECG shows a sinus rhythm without ectopy or other electrical disturbances.
NOC Cardiac Pump Effectiveness.

Cardiac Care: Acute Hemodynamic Regulation
1. Monitor ECG for signs of worsening hypocalcemia (e.g., prolonged QT interval) or of digitalis toxicity with calcium replacement: multifocal or bigeminal PVCs, paroxysmal atrial tachycardia with AV block, and other heart blocks.
2. Hypocalcemia may decrease cardiac contractility. Monitor patient for signs of heart failure or pulmonary edema: crackles, rhonchi, SOB, decreased BP, increased HR, increased PAP, or increased CVP.

NIC Dysrhythmia Management; Cardiac Care.

Ineffective breathing pattern *related to abnormal rigidity of upper airway and respiratory muscles*

- -

Goals/Outcomes: Within 1 hour of initiation of treatment, the patient is regaining an effective breathing pattern, as evidenced by more comfortable work of breathing with RR 12 to 20 breaths/min and absence of the indicators of laryngeal spasm: laryngeal stridor, dyspnea, or crowing.

NOC Respiratory Status: Ventilation; Respiratory Status: Airway Patency.

Respiratory Monitoring
1. Assess the patient's respiratory rate, character, and rhythm. Be alert to laryngeal stridor, dyspnea, and crowing, which occur with laryngeal spasm, a life-threatening complication of hypocalcemia.
2. Keep an emergency tracheostomy tray at the bedside of all patients with symptoms of hypocalcemia.

NIC Airway Management; Ventilation Assistance.

HYPERCALCEMIA (serum calcium level greater than 10.5 mEq/L, ionized greater than 5.5 mg/dL)

PATHOPHYSIOLOGY

Hypercalcemia is caused by increased total serum calcium or increased percentage of free, ionized calcium. If hypercalcemia is accompanied by a normal or elevated serum phosphorus level, calcium phosphate crystals may precipitate in the serum and deposit throughout the body. Soft tissue calcifications usually occur when the product of the serum calcium and serum phosphorus (i.e., calcium level $\times$ phosphorus level) exceeds 70 mg/dL.

HYPERCALCEMIA ASSESSMENT

GOAL OF ASSESSMENT

Evaluate the signs, symptoms, and risk factors for hypercalcemia.

HISTORY AND RISK FACTORS

- Hyperparathyroidism: May be stress-related in critical illness.
- Lymphoproliferative disorders: Which prompt parathyroid protein production.
- Increased intake of calcium: Excessive administration during cardiopulmonary arrest; milk-alkali syndrome.
- Increased intestinal absorption: Vitamin D overdose or hyperparathyroidism. Increased release of calcium from bone: hyperparathyroidism, malignancies, prolonged immobilization; Paget disease.
- Decreased urinary excretion: Renal failure, thiazide diuretics, and hyperparathyroidism.
- Increased ionized calcium: Acidosis.

OBSERVATION

- Symptoms absent unless serum calcium is greater than 11 mg/dL.
- Behavioral changes: Personality changes and depression.
- Neurologic changes: Lethargy, weakness, confusion, paresthesias, stupor, and coma.
- GI/digestive changes: Anorexia, nausea, vomiting, and constipation.
- Other: Polyuria, itching, and bone pain.

VITAL SIGNS

- Hypertension.
- Heart block.
- Cardiac arrest.

12-LEAD ECG

- Shortening ST segment and QT interval.
- PR interval is sometimes prolonged.
- Ventricular dysrhythmias.

Diagnostic Tests for Hypercalcemia

Test	Purpose	Abnormal Findings
Total serum calcium	Evaluate total calcium level; calcium is bound to albumin; if albumin is low, calcium is low.	Elevated: More than 10.5 mg/dL. Evaluate with serum albumin level to avoid false lows.
Ionized calcium	Evaluate free calcium level.	Elevated: More than 5.5 mg/dL.
Parathyroid hormone	Assess for hyperparathyroidism or hypoparathyroidism.	Elevated: More than 70 pg/mL.
Radiographs (bone scan, DEXA scan, KUB)	Evaluate for bone changes or urinary calculi.	Osteoporosis, bone cavitations, or urinary calculi.

DEXA, Dual energy x-ray absorptiometry; *KUB*, kidney, ureter, and bladder.

COLLABORATIVE MANAGEMENT

CARE PRIORITIES

1. Administer loop diuretics and isotonic saline

Administered rapidly to increase urinary calcium excretion. Concomitant administration of furosemide prevents the development of fluid volume excess and further increases urinary calcium excretion.

2. Discontinue vitamin supplements and thiazide diuretics

If the patient has been taking vitamin supplements and thiazide diuretics, then discontinue them.

3. Treat the underlying cause

May include antitumor chemotherapy for malignancy, partial parathyroidectomy for hyperparathyroidism, discontinuation of calcium supplements, vitamins A and D, and thiazide diuretics.

4. Facilitate rebuilding of bone

- Increase activity level: Weight-bearing stimulates bone deposition; increased activity decreases bone resorption.
- Administer bisphosphonates (etidronate and pamidronate): Act directly on bone to reduce decalcification; used primarily to treat hypercalcemia associated with neoplastic disease. May take several days to work but the effects last for days to weeks.
- Mithramycin: Is a cytotoxic antibiotic that decreases bone resorption.
- Calcitonin: Reduces bone resorption and increases bone deposition of calcium and phosphorus; increases urinary calcium and phosphate excretion.
- Gallium nitrate: Inhibits osteoclasts and increased bone calcium. Used in the treatment of malignancy-induced hypercalcemia.

5. Reduce calcium intake and intestinal absorption

Administer steroids to compete with vitamin D, thereby reducing intestinal absorption of calcium.

6. Monitor for signs of hypocalcemia

May result from hypercalcemia therapies.

CARE PLANS FOR HYPERCALCEMIA

Ineffective protection *related to the inability to guard self from internal and external threats attributable to acute confusion.*

Goals/Outcomes: Within 24 to 48 hours of initiating treatment, the patient more consistently verbalizes orientation to time, place, and person. The patient does not exhibit evidence of injury caused by neurosensory changes.
NOC Cognitive Orientation; Distorted Thought Self-Control; Neurologic Status.

Neurologic Monitoring

1. Monitor the patient for worsening hypercalcemia: disorientation to time, place, and person; and deterioration in neurologic status.
2. Note personality changes, hallucinations, paranoia, and memory loss. Inform the patient and significant others that altered sensorium is temporary and will improve with treatment. Use reality therapy: clocks, calendars, and familiar objects; keep them at the bedside within the patient's visual field.

Electrolyte Monitoring: Hypercalcemia

1. Administer fluids and diuretics as prescribed. Evaluate response to therapy. Monitor serum calcium levels and albumin levels. Observe for signs of fluid volume excess that develop with treatment.
2. Hypercalcemia causes neuromuscular depression with poor coordination, weakness, and altered gait. Provide a safe environment. Keep side rails up and bed in lowest position with wheels locked. Assist with ambulation.
3. Monitor for signs of digitalis toxicity (hypercalcemia potentiates digitalis): multifocal or bigeminal PVCs, paroxysmal atrial tachycardia with AV block, and other heart blocks.
4. Monitor serum electrolytes: calcium, potassium, and phosphorus (normal range is 2.5 to 4.5 mg/dL). Note changes that result from therapy. Consult the advanced practice provider for abnormal values.
5. Encourage increased mobility to reduce bone resorption. Ideally, the patient should be out of bed and up in a chair for at least 6 hours a day.

NIC Fluid Monitoring; Dysrhythmia Management; Fluid Management.

Impaired urinary elimination *related to hypercalcemia decreasing the ability of the kidneys to concentrate urine, which can lead to polyuria and possible fluid volume deficit. Hypercalcemia can impair renal function.*

Goals/Outcomes: Within 24 hours of initiation of treatment, the patient exhibits a voiding pattern and urine characteristics that are moving toward normal for the patient.
NOC Urinary Elimination.

Fluid Management

1. Monitor I&O hourly. Consult the advanced practice provider for unusual changes in urine volume (e.g., oliguria alternating with polyuria, which may signal urinary tract obstruction, or continuous polyuria). This is a type of nephrogenic diabetes insipidus (see Diabetes Insipidus, Chapter 8). Monitor for signs of volume depletion when giving diuretics: decreased BP, CVP, PAP, and increased HR.
2. Monitor the patient's renal function carefully: urine output, BUN, and creatinine values (see Acute Renal Failure/Acute Kidney Injury, Chapter 6).
3. Provide the patient with a low-calcium diet and avoid use of calcium-containing medications (e.g., antacids such as Tums). Encourage intake of fruits (e.g., cranberries, prunes, plums) that leave an acid ash in the urine. Acidic urine reduces the risk of calcium stone formation. Also increase fluid intake (at least 3 L in nonrestricted patients) to reduce the risk of renal stone formation.
4. Assess the patient for indicators of kidney stone formation: intermittent pain, nausea, vomiting, and hematuria.

NIC Fluid Monitoring; Urinary Elimination Management; Electrolyte Management: Hypercalcemia.

PHOSPHORUS IMBALANCE (normal serum level 2.5 to 4.5 mg/dL or 1.7 to 2.6 mEq/L)

Phosphorus, the primary anion ($^-$ or negative ion) of the ICF, has a wide variety of vital functions: formation of energy-storing substances (e.g., ATP); formation of red blood cell 2,3-diphosphoglycerate (2,3-DPG) (facilitates the release of O_2 from the Hgb to be used by the cells); metabolism of carbohydrates, protein, and fat; and maintenance of acid-base balance. In addition, phosphorus is critical to normal nerve and muscle function and provides structural support to bones and teeth.

Plasma phosphorus levels vary with diet and acid-base balance. Glucose, insulin, or sugar-containing foods cause a temporary drop in phosphorus because of a shift of serum phosphorus into the cells. Phosphorous and calcium have an interdependent effect on each other and share many of the common causes of abnormalities. Alkalosis, particularly respiratory alkalosis, may cause hypophosphatemia as a result of an intracellular shift of phosphorus. Although the exact mechanism for this shift is not fully understood, it may be related to an alkalosis-induced cellular glycolysis, with increased formation of phosphorus-containing metabolic intermediates. Respiratory acidosis may cause a shift of phosphorus out of the cells and contribute to hyperphosphatemia.

Although the level of ECF phosphate is affected by a combination of factors, including dietary intake, intestinal absorption, and hormonally regulated bone resorption and deposition, phosphorus balance depends largely on renal excretion.

HYPOPHOSPHATEMIA (serum phosphate level less than 2.5 mg/dL or less than 1.7 mEq/L)

PATHOPHYSIOLOGY

Hypophosphatemia (serum phosphorus less than 2.5 mg/dL) may occur because of transient intracellular shifts, increased urinary losses (most common), decreased intestinal absorption, or increased use (see History and Risk Factors that follow). Severe phosphorus deficiency may also develop because of a combination of factors in conditions such as chronic alcohol abuse and DKA.

HYPOPHOSPHATEMIA ASSESSMENT

GOAL OF ASSESSMENT

Evaluate the signs, symptoms, and risk factors for hypophosphatemia. Acute, severe hypophosphatemia can be a life-threatening condition. Symptoms can be so profound that care providers focus on extensive workups while sometimes overlooking the hypophosphatemia.

HISTORY AND RISK FACTORS

- Intracellular shifts: Carbohydrate load, respiratory alkalosis, and treatment of DKA.
- Increased use because of increased tissue repair: TPN with inadequate phosphorus content; recovery from protein-calorie malnutrition. Hypophosphatemia is common in the critical care patient largely because of nutritional deficiency.
- Increased urinary losses: Hypomagnesemia, ECF volume expansion, hyperparathyroidism, use of thiazide diuretics, diuretic phase of ATN, and glucosuria.
- Reduced intestinal absorption or increased intestinal loss: Use of phosphorus-binding medications; vomiting and diarrhea; malabsorption disorders such as vitamin D deficiency; and prolonged gastric suction.
- Other conditions: Chronic alcohol abuse, DKA, severe burns, and sepsis.
- Resulting from interventions: Postoperative patients, patients on mechanical ventilation, and postoperative renal transplant patients.

OBSERVATION

Symptoms may be caused by sudden decreases in serum phosphorus, or they may develop gradually because of chronic deficiency. The majority of symptoms are secondary to decreases in ATP and 2,3-DPG; therefore, the patient will become acutely hypoxic at the cellular level, producing a high lactate and metabolic acid load, resulting in poor coordination, confusion, seizures, and coma. Other acute symptoms include:

- Chest pain as a result of poor oxygenation of the myocardium.
- Muscle pain and weakness.
- Increased susceptibility to infection.
- Numbness and tingling of the fingers.
- Numbness of the circumoral region.
- Respiratory alkalosis from hyperventilation.
- Difficulty speaking as a result of decreased strength.
- Bruising and bleeding because of platelet dysfunction.
- Rhabdomyolysis, hemolysis.

Chronic symptoms include memory loss, lethargy, weakness, bone pain, joint stiffness, arthralgia, cyanosis, osteomalacia, and possible pseudofractures.

VITAL SIGNS
- Decreased respiratory rate.
- Increased PAWP.
- Decreased CO.
- Decreased BP with decreased response to pressor agents.

 Safety Alert *Respiratory alkalosis causes phosphorus to move intracellularly, aggravating the existing hypophosphatemia.*

Diagnostic Tests for Hypophosphatemia		
Test	**Purpose**	**Abnormal Findings**
Serum phosphate level	Determine the severity of hypo-phosphatemia	Decreased: Less than 2.5 mg/dL (1.7 mEq/L). Mild: 1 to 2.5 mg/dL. Severe: Less than 1 mg/dL.
Parathyroid hormone	Evaluate for hyperparathyroidism	Elevated: In hyperparathyroidism, to greater than 70 pg/mL.
Serum magnesium	Evaluate loss of magnesium	Decreased because of increased urinary excretion of magnesium in hypophosphatemia.
Skeletal radiographs	Evaluate bone changes	Skeletal changes of osteomalacia.

COLLABORATIVE MANAGEMENT

CARE PRIORITIES

1. Discontinue use of phosphate binders
Phosphate binders include aluminum, magnesium, or calcium gels of antacids.

2. Correct respiratory alkalosis if present
See Acid-Base Balance.

3. Increase phosphorus intake
Mild hypophosphatemia may respond to increased intake of foods high in phosphorus, such as milk (Box 1-9).

4. Administer oral phosphate supplements
Moderate hypophosphatemia is treated with phosphate supplements including Neutra-Phos (sodium and potassium phosphate) or Phospho-Soda (sodium phosphate).

5. Administer IV sodium phosphate or potassium phosphate
Severe hypophosphatemia is treated with sodium phosphate or potassium phosphate. IV infusions are also used for patients with a nonfunctional GI tract.

6. Monitor for resolution or progression of neurologic and hematologic signs and symptoms

Box 1-9 FOODS HIGH IN PHOSPHORUS	
Dried beans and peas	Nuts (e.g., Brazil nuts, peanuts)
Eggs and egg products (e.g., eggnog, soufflés)	Poultry
Fish	Seeds (e.g., pumpkin, sesame, sunflower)
Meats, especially organ meats (e.g., brain, liver, kidney)	Whole grains (e.g., oatmeal, bran, barley)
Milk and milk products (e.g., cheese, ice cream, cottage cheese)	

CARE PLANS FOR HYPOPHOSPHATEMIA

Ineffective protection *related to inability to guard self from internal and external threats attributable to impaired decision-making resulting from acute confusion*

Goals/Outcomes: Within 24 hours of initiation of treatment the patient exhibits improvement of acute confusion and normalization of associated electrolyte imbalances.

NOC Cognitive Orientation; Distorted Thought Self-Control; Neurologic Status.

Neurologic Monitoring
1. Monitor the patient for worsening hypophosphatemia: disorientation to time, place, and person; and deterioration in neurologic status.
2. Note personality changes, hallucinations, paranoia, and memory loss. Inform the patient and significant others that altered sensorium is temporary and will improve with treatment.
3. Apprehension, confusion, and paresthesias are signals of developing hypophosphatemia. Assess and document LOC, orientation, and neurologic status with each vital sign check. Reorient the patient as necessary. Alert the advanced practice provider to significant changes.
4. Inform the patient and significant others that altered sensorium is temporary and will improve with treatment.
5. Keep the side rails up and the bed in its lowest position with wheels locked.
6. Use reality therapy: clocks, calendars, and familiar objects. Keep these articles at the bedside within the patient's visual field.
7. If the patient is at risk for seizures, pad the side rails and keep an appropriate-size airway at the bedside.

Electrolyte Management: Hypophosphatemia
1. Monitor serum phosphorus levels in patients at increased risk. Consult the advanced practice provider for decreased levels. Monitor for signs of associated electrolyte and acid-base imbalances: hypokalemia, hypomagnesemia, respiratory alkalosis, and metabolic acidosis.
2. When IV phosphorus is administered as potassium phosphate, the infusion rate should not exceed 10 mEq/h. Monitor IV site for signs of infiltration, because potassium phosphate can cause necrosis and sloughing of tissue.

HIGH ALERT! *Do not administer intravenous (IV) phosphate at a rate greater than that recommended by the manufacturer. Potential complications of IV phosphorus administration include tetany as a result of hypocalcemia (serum calcium levels may drop suddenly if serum phosphorus levels increase suddenly; see Hypocalcemia, for additional information); soft tissue calcification (if hyperphosphatemia develops, the calcium and phosphorus in the extracellular fluid compartment may combine and form deposits in tissue); and hypotension, caused by a too-rapid delivery.*

---

3. Encourage intake of foods high in phosphorus (see Box 1-9). Teach the patient and significant others the importance of using phosphorus-binding antacids only as prescribed.

NIC Medication Administration.

Impaired gas exchange *related to respiratory muscle weakness, coupled with the inability of red blood cells to off-load O_2 at the cellular level resulting from decreased 2,3-dpg levels*

Goals/Outcomes: Within 12 hours of initiation of treatment, the patient has increasingly normal gas exchange, as evidenced by RR 12 to 20 breaths/min with normal depth and pattern; orientation to time, place, and person; SpO_2 at least 92%; and absence of the indicators of hypoxia (e.g., restlessness, somnolence).

NOC Respiratory Status: Gas Exchange.

Safety Alert *With decreased 2,3-diphosphoglycerate levels, the oxyhemoglobin dissociation curve will shift to the left. At a given PaO_2 level, more O_2 will be bound to hemoglobin and less will be available to the tissues.*

Respiratory Monitoring
1. Assess the patient for signs of hypoxia: restlessness, confusion, increased respirations, complaints of chest pain, and cyanosis (a late sign).
2. Monitor Spo$_2$ as available. Administer O$_2$ as prescribed to maintain Spo$_2$ at $\geq$92%.
3. Monitor rate and depth of respirations in patients with severe hypophosphatemia. Assess for decreased tidal volume or decreased minute ventilation. Consult the advanced practice provider for changes.
4. Monitor ABG values for evidence of hypoxemia or hypercapnia. Consult the advanced practice provider for significant changes.
5. Monitor serum phosphate levels in patients who are mechanically ventilated; they exhibit a high incidence of hypophosphatemia. Hypophosphatemia may contribute to difficulty in weaning patients from ventilators.

NIC Oxygen Therapy.   Impaired physical mobility related to muscle weakness resulting from hypophosphatemia

Goals/Outcomes: Within 24 hours of initiation of therapy, the patient is able to move purposefully and has full or baseline ROM and muscle strength.
NOC Mobility; Transfer Performance.

Exercise Promotion: Strength Training
1. Monitor all patients with suspected hypophosphatemia for decreasing muscle strength. Perform serial assessments of hand grasp strength and clarity of speech. Consult the advanced practice provider for changes.
2. Monitor serum phosphorus levels if mobility or strength decreases. Consult the advanced practice provider for changes.
3. Assist the patient with ambulation and activities of daily living (ADLs).
4. Medicate for pain as prescribed.

NIC Energy Management; Pain Management.

Decreased cardiac output *related to cardiac muscle weakness related to hypophosphatemia*

Goals/Outcomes: Within 12 hours of initiation of treatment, the patient's CO is increasingly adequate, as evidenced by CO at least 4 L/min, cardiac index (CI) at least 2.5 L/min/m^2, CVP 4 to 6 mm Hg, PAP 20 to 30 mm Hg systolic, 8 to 15 mm Hg diastolic, HR <100 bpm, BP within the patient's normal range, and absence of the clinical signs of heart failure or pulmonary edema.
NOC Cardiac Pump Effectiveness.

Cardiac Care
1. Monitor the patient for signs of heart failure or pulmonary edema: crackles, rhonchi, SOB, decreased BP, increased HR, increased PAP, or increased CVP.
2. Prevent the patient from hyperventilating. Metabolic alkalosis causes increased movement of phosphorus into cells, which will reduce CO.
3. For additional interventions if decreased CO develops, see Heart Failure.

NIC Cardiac Care: Acute Hemodynamic Regulation; Vital Signs Monitoring.

Ineffective protection *related to compromised immunity resulting from hypophosphatemia*

Goals/Outcomes: The patient is free of infection, as evidenced by normothermia and absence of erythema, swelling, warmth, and purulent drainage at invasive sites.
NOC Immune Status.

Infection Protection
1. Monitor temperature every 4 hours for evidence of infection. Obtain cultures of wounds and drainage as prescribed if infection is suspected.
2. Use meticulous aseptic technique when changing dressings or manipulating indwelling lines (e.g., TPN catheters, IV needles).

3. Provide oral hygiene and skin care at regular intervals. Intact skin and membranes are the body's first line of defense against infection.

NIC Risk Identification.

HYPERPHOSPHATEMIA (serum phosphate level greater than 4.5 mg/dL or greater than 2.6 mEq/L)

PATHOPHYSIOLOGY

Hyperphosphatemia is common in patients with renal insufficiency/failure whose kidneys are unable to effectively excrete excess phosphorus. Other causes of hyperphosphatemia include increased intake of phosphates, extracellular shifts (i.e., movement of phosphorus out of the cell and into the ECF), cellular destruction with concomitant release of intracellular phosphorus, and decreased urinary losses that are unrelated to decreased renal function. As serum phosphorus levels increase, serum calcium levels often decrease, leading to hypocalcemia. Hypocalcemia is most likely to occur in sudden, severe hyperphosphatemia (e.g., after IV administration of phosphates) or in patients prone to hypocalcemia (e.g., those with chronic renal failure).

The primary complication of hyperphosphatemia is metastatic calcification (i.e., the precipitation of calcium phosphate in the soft tissue, joints, and arteries). Chronic hyperphosphatemia in the patient with chronic renal failure may contribute to the development of renal osteodystrophy.

Precipitation of calcium phosphate occurs when the product of the serum calcium and serum phosphorus (i.e., calcium $\times$ phosphorus) exceeds 70 mg/dL.

HYPERPHOSPHATEMIA ASSESSMENT

GOAL OF ASSESSMENT

Evaluate the signs, symptoms, history, and risk factors for hyperphosphatemia.

HISTORY AND RISK FACTORS

- Renal failure: Acute and chronic; may signal declining glomerular filtration rate.
- Increased intake
  - Excessive administration of phosphorus supplements.
  - Vitamin D excess with increased GI absorption.
  - Excessive use of phosphorus-containing laxatives or enemas.
  - Massive transfusion.
- Extracellular shift: Respiratory acidosis, DKA (before treatment).
- Cellular destruction
  - Neoplastic disease (e.g., leukemia, lymphoma) treated with cytotoxic agents.
  - Increased tissue catabolism.
  - Rhabdomyolysis.
- Decreased urinary losses: Hypoparathyroidism, volume depletion.

OBSERVATION

- GI symptoms: Anorexia, nausea, and vomiting.
- Neuromuscular symptoms: Muscle weakness, hyperreflexia, and tetany.

VITAL SIGNS

- Hypotension secondary to vasodilation.
- Heart failure secondary to decreased myocardial contractility.
- Tachycardia.

PERCUSSION

- Positive Trousseau sign: Ischemia-induced carpopedal spasms. Elicited by applying a BP cuff to the upper arm and inflating it past systolic BP for 2 minutes.
- Positive Chvostek sign: Unilateral contraction of facial and eyelid muscles. Elicited by stimulating the facial nerve during percussion of the face just in front of the ear.

Usually patients experience few symptoms with hyperphosphatemia. The majority of symptoms relate to development of hypocalcemia or soft tissue (metastatic) calcifications. Indicators of metastatic calcification include oliguria, corneal haziness, conjunctivitis, irregular heart rate, and popular eruptions.

SCREENING

- 12-Lead ECG: Deposition of calcium phosphate in the heart may lead to dysrhythmias and conduction disturbance; prolonged QT interval caused by elongation and elevation of ST segment.

Diagnostic Tests for Hyperphosphatemia		
Test	**Purpose**	**Abnormal Findings**
Serum phosphate level	Determine severity of hyperphosphatemia	Elevated: Greater than 4.5 mg/dL (2.6 mEq/L)
Parathyroid hormone	Evaluate for hypoparathyroidism	Decreased: In hypoparathyroidism
Skeletal radiographs	Assess for bony changes	May show skeletal changes of osteodystrophy

COLLABORATIVE MANAGEMENT
CARE PRIORITIES

1. Reduce severely elevated phosphate level
Hemodialysis may be used for acute, severe hyperphosphatemia accompanied by symptoms of hypocalcemia.

2. Administer phosphate binders
Aluminum, magnesium, or calcium antacids.

3. Monitor for symptoms of hypocalcemia
Positive Chvostek and/or positive Trousseau sign.

 Calcium carbonate and calcium acetate are the preferred preparations for the patient with chronic renal failure. Magnesium antacids are avoided in renal failure because of the risk of hypermagnesemia. Aluminum-containing antacids are contraindicated because they may lead to aluminum accumulation and contribute to the development of bone disease.

CARE PLANS FOR HYPERPHOSPHATEMIA
Deficient knowledge *related to medications that may induce hyperphosphatemia*

Goals/Outcomes: Within the 24-hour period before discharge from the intensive care unit (ICU), the patient describes the potential complications of uncontrolled hyperphosphatemia and preventive measures.
NOC Health Promoting Behavior; Health Promoting Behavior Medication.

 Prevention of long-term complications relies primarily on adequate patient education, because symptoms of hyperphosphatemia may be minimal.

Teaching: Prescribed Medication
1. Teach patients the purpose of phosphate binders. Stress the need to take binders as prescribed with or after meals to maximize effectiveness.
2. Educate patients about possible constipation from phosphate binders. Encourage use of bulk-building supplements or stool softener if constipation occurs. Phosphate-containing laxatives and enemas must be avoided (i.e., Fleet's Phospho-Soda products).

3. Phosphate binders are available in liquid, tablet, or capsule form. Confer with the physician or midlevel practitioner regarding an alternate form or brand for individuals who find binders unpalatable or difficult to take. Phosphate binders vary in aluminum, magnesium, or calcium content. One may not be exchanged for another without first ensuring that the patient is receiving the same amount of elemental aluminum, magnesium, or calcium.
4. Discuss avoiding or limiting foods high in phosphorus (see Box 1-9).
5. Review the importance of avoiding phosphorus-containing over-the-counter medications: certain laxatives, enemas, and mixed vitamin-mineral supplements. Instruct the patient and significant others to read the label for the words "phosphorus" and "phosphate."

NIC Teaching: Prescribed Medication; Electrolyte Management: Hyperphosphatemia.

Ineffective protection *related to the inability to avoid internal complications associated with* *hyperphosphatemia*

Goals/Outcomes: The patient does not develop symptoms of physical injury caused by precipitation of calcium phosphate in the soft tissue or joints, or by hypocalcemic tetany.
NOC Activity Tolerance; Mobility; Energy Conservation.

Electrolyte Management: Hyperphosphatemia
1. Monitor serum phosphorus and calcium levels. Calculate the calcium-phosphorus product (calcium $\times$ phosphorus). Values greater than 70 mg/dL are associated with precipitation of calcium phosphate in the soft tissue. Consult the advanced practice provider for abnormal values. Phosphorus values may be kept slightly higher (4 to 6 mg/dL) to ensure adequate levels of 2,3-DPG in patients with chronic renal failure, to minimize effects of chronic anemia on O_2 delivery to the tissues.
2. Vitamin D products and calcium supplements (taken between meals) may be limited until serum phosphorus approaches a normal level.
3. Consult the advanced practice provider if the patient develops indicators of metastatic calcification: oliguria, corneal haziness, conjunctivitis, irregular HR, and papular eruptions.
4. Monitor the patient for symptoms of increasing hypocalcemia that may precede overt tetany: numbness and tingling of the fingers and circumoral region, hyperactive reflexes, and muscle cramps. Positive Trousseau or Chvostek sign may signal latent tetany. Consult the advanced practice provider promptly if these symptoms develop (See Hypocalcemia.)
5. Because hyperphosphatemia can impair renal function, monitor renal function carefully: urine output, BUN, and creatinine values.

NIC Neurologic Monitoring; Energy Management.

MAGNESIUM IMBALANCE (normal serum magnesium level 1.5 to 2.5 mEq/L)
Approximately 60% of the body's magnesium is located in the bone, and approximately 1% is located in the ECF. The remaining magnesium is contained within cells. Mg^{2+} is the second most abundant intracellular cation (+ or positive ion) after potassium. Magnesium is regulated by a combination of factors, including vitamin D–regulated GI absorption and renal excretion.

Because magnesium is a major intracellular ion, it plays a vital role in normal cellular function. Specifically, it activates enzymes involved in the metabolism of carbohydrates and protein, and it triggers the sodium-potassium pump, thus affecting intracellular potassium levels. Magnesium is also important in the transmission of neuromuscular activity, neural transmission within the CNS, and myocardial functioning.

HYPOMAGNESEMIA (serum magnesium level less than 1.5 mEq/L)
PATHOPHYSIOLOGY
Hypomagnesemia usually results from decreased GI absorption, increased urinary loss, or excessive GI loss (e.g., vomiting, diarrhea), and with prolonged administration of magnesium-free parenteral fluids. Chronic alcohol abusers (see History and Risk Factors that

follow) and patients who are critically ill most commonly experience low magnesium. Hypomagnesemia is associated with increased mortality in the critical care setting. Dysrhythmias and sudden death increase when decreased magnesium levels occur in combination with MI, heart failure, or digitalis toxicity. Hypomagnesemia is usually associated with hypocalcemia and hypokalemia (see Hypokalemia and Hypocalcemia for additional information). Symptoms of hypomagnesemia tend to develop once the serum magnesium level drops below 1 mEq/L. Decreased magnesium intake has been identified as a risk factor for hypertension, cardiac dysrhythmias, ischemic heart disease, and sudden cardiac death.

HYPOMAGNESEMIA ASSESSMENT
GOAL OF ASSESSMENT
Evaluate for the signs, symptoms, and risk factors for hypomagnesemia and investigate further whether the patient may also have hypokalemia and/or hypocalcemia.

HISTORY AND RISK FACTORS
- Chronic alcoholism: Poor dietary intake, decreased GI absorption, and increased urinary excretion.
- Decreased GI absorption: Cancer, colitis, pancreatic insufficiency, surgical resection in the GI tract, use of laxatives, and diarrhea.
- Increased GI losses: From prolonged vomiting or gastric suction.
- Administration of low-magnesium or magnesium-free parenteral solutions: Especially with refeeding after starvation.
- Poorly controlled diabetes including DKA: A result of movement of magnesium out of the cell and loss in the urine because of osmotic diuresis.
- Increased urinary excretion: Use of diuretics, diuretic phase of ATN.
- Medications: Amphotericin, tobramycin, gentamicin, cisplatin, cyclosporine, or digoxin.
- Protein-calorie malnutrition.
- Cardiopulmonary bypass.

OBSERVATION
- Behavioral changes: Mood changes, lethargy, hallucinations, and confusion.
- Neuromuscular symptoms: Weakness, fatigue, paresthesias, tremors, convulsions, and tetany.
- GI symptoms: Anorexia, nausea, and vomiting.

VITAL SIGNS
- Hypotension.
- Tachycardia.
- Shallow respirations with respiratory muscle weakness.
- Laryngeal stridor.

PERCUSSION
- Increased reflexes.
- Positive Chvostek sign.
- Positive Trousseau sign.
- Skeletal muscle weakness.

SCREENING
- 12-Lead ECG: PVCs, possible torsades de pointes, prolonged PR interval, widened QRS complex, prolonged QT interval, depressed ST segment, flattened T wave, prominent U wave, atrial fibrillation, paroxysmal atrial tachycardia with variable block, or other heart blocks related to digitalis effect (in those taking digitalis derivatives).

Diagnostic Tests for Hypomagnesemia		
Test	**Purpose**	**Abnormal Findings**
Serum magnesium level	Evaluate for low magnesium	Decreased: Less than 1.5 mEq/L
Magnesium tolerance test	Identify those with or at risk	Results based on the amount of magnesium retained after an infusion of magnesium
Serum potassium level	Evaluate the sodium potassium pump	Possibly decreased: Possible failure of the cellular sodium potassium pump to move potassium into the cell and the accompanying loss of potassium in the urine. This hypokalemia may be resistant to replacement until the magnesium deficit has been corrected
Serum calcium level	Assess for hypocalcemia	Possibly decreased: Magnesium deficit may lead to hypocalcemia because of a reduction in the release and action of parathyroid hormone

COLLABORATIVE MANAGEMENT
CARE PRIORITIES
1. Increase magnesium level
- Administer IV or intramuscular (IM) magnesium: To manage severe hypomagnesemia and related symptoms.
- Administer magnesium supplements: Chronic loss is treated with magnesium oxide or chloride. Magnesium-containing antacids (e.g., Mylanta, Maalox, Milk of Magnesia, Gelusil) may be used.
- Encourage food high in magnesium: See Box 1-10.

2. Monitor for ECG changes and manage changes with IV magnesium
Check for hypokalemia and manage hypomagnesemia before treating hypokalemia.

3. Monitor for hypotension, shallow respirations, and laryngeal stridor

CARE PLANS FOR HYPOMAGNESEMIA
Ineffective protection *related to the inability to control the internal effects of hypomagnesemia*

Goals/Outcomes: Within 8 hours of initiation of treatment, the patient verbalizes orientation to time, place, and person. The patient does not exhibit evidence of cardiac or brain injury caused by complications of severe hypomagnesemia. **NOC** Neurologic Status: Consciousness; Neurologic Status.

Electrolyte Management: Hypomagnesemia
1. Monitor serum magnesium levels in patients at risk for hypomagnesemia and its deleterious effects (e.g., those who are alcohol abusers or experiencing heart failure, cases of recent MI or digitalis toxicity). Normal range for serum magnesium is 1.5 to 2.5 mEq/L. Consult the physician or midlevel practitioner for abnormal values.

Box 1-10	FOODS HIGH IN MAGNESIUM
Bananas	Molasses
Chocolate	Nuts and seeds
Coconuts	Oranges
Grapefruits	Refined sugar
Green, leafy vegetables (e.g., beet greens, collard greens)	Seafood
Kelp	Soy flour
Legumes	Wheat bran

Symptoms of hypomagnesemia may be mistakenly attributed to delirium tremens of chronic alcoholism. Be alert to indicators of magnesium deficit in these patients.

2. Administer IV MgSO₄ slowly. Refer to the manufacturer's guidelines. Too-rapid administration may lead to dangerous hypermagnesemia, with cardiac or respiratory arrest. Patients receiving IV magnesium should be monitored for decreasing BP, labored respirations, and diminished patellar reflex (knee jerk). An absent patellar reflex signals hyporeflexia (seen with dangerous hypermagnesemia). Should any of these changes occur, stop the infusion and consult the physician or midlevel practitioner immediately (see Hypermagnesemia). Keep calcium gluconate at the bedside in the event of hypocalcemic tetany or sudden hypermagnesemia.
3. For patients with chronic hypomagnesemia, administer oral magnesium supplements as prescribed. All magnesium supplements should be given with caution in patients with reduced renal function because of an increased risk of the development of hypermagnesemia. Caution the patient that oral magnesium supplements may cause diarrhea. Administer antidiarrheal medications as needed.
4. When it is appropriate, encourage intake of foods high in magnesium (see Box 1-10). For most patients, a normal diet is usually adequate.
5. Maintain seizure precautions for patients with symptoms (i.e., those who have hyperreflexia). Decrease environmental stimuli (e.g., keep the room quiet; use subdued lighting).
6. For patients in whom hypocalcemia is suspected, caution against hyperventilation. Metabolic alkalosis may precipitate tetany as a result of increased calcium binding.
7. Dysphagia may occur in hypomagnesemia. Test the patient's ability to swallow water before giving food or medications.
8. Assess and document LOC, orientation, and neurologic status with each vital sign check. Reorient the patient as necessary. Notify the physician or midlevel practitioner for significant changes. Inform the patient and significant others that altered mood and sensorium are temporary and will improve with treatment.
9. See Hypokalemia, Hypocalcemia, and Hypophosphatemia for nursing care of patients with these disorders.

 Because magnesium is necessary for the movement of potassium into the cell, intracellular potassium deficits cannot be corrected until hypomagnesemia has been treated.

NIC Neurologic Monitoring; Electrolyte Management: Hypomagnesemia; Electrolyte Management: Hypokalemia; Electrolyte Management: Hypocalcemia; Seizure Precautions; Medication Administration.

Decreased cardiac output *related to abnormal contraction of myocardial tissues resulting in heart failure*

Goals/Outcomes: Within 24 hours of initiating treatment, the patient's CO is adequate, as evidenced by CO at least 4 L/min, CI at least 2.5 L/min/m², normal configurations on ECG, and HR within the patient's normal range. The patient has urinary output of at least 0.5 mL/kg/h.
NOC Cardiac Pump Effectiveness; Circulation Status.

Cardiac Care
1. Monitor HR and regularity with each vital sign check. Consult the advanced practice provider for changes. Be alert to decreased CO and CI.
2. Assess ECG for evidence of hypomagnesemia. Consider hypomagnesemia as a possible cause if the patient develops sudden ventricular dysrhythmias.
3. Because hypomagnesemia (and hypokalemia) potentiate the cardiac effects of digitalis, monitor for digitalis-induced dysrhythmias. ECG changes may include multifocal or bigeminal PVCs, paroxysmal atrial tachycardia with varying AV block, and other heart blocks.
4. Monitor for and report decreased urinary output and delayed capillary refill.

NIC Dysrhythmia Management.

Imbalanced nutrition: less than body requirements *related to a diet lacking in magnesium or poor overall food intake*

Goals/Outcomes: Within 24 hours of resumption of oral feeding, the patient receives a diet adequate in magnesium.

NOC Knowledge: Diet; Nutritional Status: Nutrient Intake.

Teaching: Prescribed Diet
1. Encourage intake of small, frequent meals.
2. Teach the patient about foods high in magnesium content (see Box 1-10) and encourage intake of these foods during meals.
3. Include the patient, significant others, and the dietitian in meal planning as appropriate.
4. Provide oral hygiene before meals to enhance appetite.
5. As with the other major intracellular electrolyte levels, magnesium depletion may develop with refeeding after starvation. Anticipate hypomagnesemia with refeeding and ensure increased dietary intake or supplementation.
6. Consult the physician or midlevel practitioner for patients receiving magnesium-free solutions (e.g., TPN) for prolonged periods.

NIC Nutritional Monitoring; Nutrition Management; Nutrition Therapy; Nutritional Counseling.

HYPERMAGNESEMIA (serum magnesium level greater than 2.5 mEq/L)

PATHOPHYSIOLOGY

Hypermagnesemia occurs almost exclusively in individuals with renal failure who have an increased intake of magnesium (e.g., those who use magnesium-containing medications). It may also occur in acute cases of adrenocortical insufficiency (Addison disease) or in obstetric patients treated with parenteral magnesium for pregnancy-induced hypertension. In rare cases hypermagnesemia occurs because of excessive use of magnesium-containing medications (e.g., antacids, laxatives, enemas). The primary symptoms of hypermagnesemia are the result of depressed peripheral and central neuromuscular transmission. Symptoms usually do not occur until the magnesium level exceeds 4 mEq/L.

HYPERMAGNESEMIA ASSESSMENT

GOAL OF ASSESSMENT

Evaluate the signs, symptoms, and risk factors for the development of hypermagnesemia.

HISTORY AND RISK FACTORS

- Decreased magnesium excretion: Renal failure or adrenocortical insufficiency.
- Increased intake of magnesium: Excessive use of magnesium-containing antacids, enemas, or laxatives.
- Excessive administration of magnesium sulfate: In the treatment of hypomagnesemia or pregnancy-induced hypertension.

OBSERVATION

- Neurologic/neuromuscular symptoms: Altered mental status, drowsiness, coma, muscular weakness or paralysis, sensation of warmth, diaphoresis, flushing, and thirst.
- Paralysis of respiratory muscles: When magnesium level exceeds 10 mEq/L.
- Nausea and vomiting.

VITAL SIGNS

- Hypotension.
- Bradycardia.
- Decreased arterial pressure caused by peripheral vasodilation.

PALPATION

- Soft tissue calcification (metastatic).
- Decreased deep tendon reflexes.
- Loss of patellar reflex when level exceeds 8 mEq/L.

SCREENING

- 12-Lead ECG: Prolonged PR interval, prolonged QRS and QT intervals with levels greater than 5 mEq/L, complete heart block, cardiac arrest in severe hypermagnesemia.

Diagnostic Tests for Hypermagnesemia		
Test	Purpose	Abnormal Findings
Serum magnesium level	Evaluate severity	Elevated: Greater than 2.5 mEq/L
Electrocardiogram	Assess for presence of abnormalities	Magnesium levels greater than 5 mEq/L: Prolonged PR, QRS, and QT intervals Magnesium levels greater than 15 mEq/L: Complete heart block and cardiac arrest

COLLABORATIVE MANAGEMENT

CARE PRIORITIES

1. Discontinue magnesium-containing medications
Especially in patients with renal failure (see Box 1-10).

2. Administer diuretics and IV fluids
Use loop diuretics and 0.45% NaCl solution to promote magnesium excretion in patients with adequate renal function.

3. Administer IV calcium gluconate
Use 10 mL of 10% solution to antagonize the neuromuscular effects of magnesium for patients with potentially lethal hypermagnesemia.

4. Consider use of hemodialysis
A magnesium-free dialysate may be used for patients with severely decreased renal function, who may not respond as readily to other magnesium-lowering strategies. Patients must be very closely monitored for other electrolyte changes during treatment.

5. Monitor ECG for changes and manage dysrhythmias
Manage according to Advanced Cardiac Life Support (ACLS) guidelines, bearing in mind the special considerations related to correcting the hypermagnesemia while using additional recommended strategies.

6. Monitor hypotension and bradycardia
Manage according to ACLS guidelines, bearing in mind the special considerations related to correcting the hypermagnesemia while using additional recommended strategies.

7. Monitor for neurologic and neuromuscular status changes
To help gauge efficacy of treatment.

CARE PLANS FOR HYPERMAGNESEMIA

Ineffective protection *related to inability to control internal changes caused by hypermagnesemia*

Goals/Outcomes: Within 12 hours of initiation of treatment, the patient verbalizes orientation to time, place, and person. The patient does not exhibit evidence of injury as a result of complications of hypermagnesemia, including no symptoms of soft tissue (metastatic) calcifications: oliguria, corneal haziness, conjunctivitis, irregular HR, and papular eruptions.
NOC Neurologic Status.

Neurologic Monitoring
1. Monitor serum magnesium levels in the patient at risk for hypermagnesemia (e.g., those with chronic renal failure). Normal range for serum magnesium levels is 1.5 to 2.5 mEq/L.

Table 1-9	MAGNESIUM-CONTAINING MEDICATIONS
Brand Name Antacids	**Laxatives**
Aludrox Camalox Di-Gel Gaviscon Gelusil and Gelusil II Maalox and Maalox Plus Mylanta and Mylanta-II Riopan Simeco Tempo	Magnesium citrate Magnesium hydroxide (Milk of Magnesia, Haley M-O) Magnesium sulfate (Epsom salts) Magnesium-containing mineral supplements

2. Assess and document LOC, orientation, and neurologic status (e.g., hand grasp) with each vital sign check. Assess patellar (knee jerk) reflex in patients with a moderately elevated magnesium level (greater than 5 mEq/L). With the patient lying flat, support the knee in a moderately fixed position and tap the patellar tendon firmly just below the patella. Normally the knee will extend. An absent reflex suggests a magnesium level of greater than 7 mEq/L. Consult the advanced practice provider for significant changes.
3. Reassure the patient and significant others that altered mental functioning and muscle strength will improve with treatment.
4. Keep side rails up and the bed in its lowest position with the wheels locked.
5. Assess the patient for the development of soft tissue calcification. Consult the advanced practice provider for significant findings.
6. Monitor for cardiopulmonary effects of hypermagnesemia: hypotension, flushing, bradycardia, and respiratory depression.

NIC Electrolyte Management: Hypermagnesemia.

Deficient knowledge *related to magnesium-containing medications*

Goals/Outcomes: Within the 24-hour period before discharge from ICU, the patient verbalizes the importance of avoiding unusual magnesium intake and identifies potential sources of unwanted magnesium.
NOC Knowledge: Medication.

Teaching: Individual
1. Caution patients with chronic renal failure to review all over-the-counter medications with the physician or mid-level practitioner before use.
2. Provide a list of common magnesium-containing medications (Table 1-9).
3. Caution patients to avoid combination vitamin-mineral supplements because they usually contain magnesium.

NIC Teaching: Prescribed Diet; Teaching: Prescribed Medication.

HEMODYNAMIC MONITORING

Hemodynamic monitoring is continuous monitoring of the pressures being exerted on or within the veins, arteries, and heart. Hemodynamic monitoring is a diagnostic tool, not a treatment or therapy. The information gained from hemodynamic monitoring is used to evaluate cardiovascular performance, which includes information about the cardiac output (CO), tissue perfusion, blood volume, tissue oxygenation, and vascular tone. Hemodynamic monitoring readings encompass a broad array of measurements, depending on the technology used. Understanding hemodynamic values and the trends of the information provided is important in determining actions used to improve cardiac function, oxygenation, oxygen use, overall circulation, and tissue perfusion. Accurately determined hemodynamic values are used to guide fluid and occasionally blood administration and cardiovascular drug–based and device-based therapies provided to patients who are critically ill.

The three overarching assessment parameters provided by hemodynamic monitoring are calculation of preload (end-diastolic volume and pressure in both ventricles before contraction), afterload (pressure created by blood volume and arterial tone, which the heart must overcome to open the aortic and pulmonic heart valves), and contractility (ability of the heart muscle to pump/contract effectively). Preload, afterload, contractility, and HR ultimately determine stroke volume (SV), CO, and BP. Changes in any of the four determinants of CO (preload, afterload, contractility, or HR) may produce significant adverse effects on BP with resulting adverse changes in cellular function and energy production as a result of altered tissue perfusion. Hemodynamic monitoring helps to assess these parameters in the patient who is critically ill so that appropriate treatment with medications or devices can be provided. Usage guidelines were developed to outline when use of hemodynamic monitoring provides the most benefit (Box 1-11).

PATHOPHYSIOLOGY
DETERMINANTS OF CARDIAC OUTPUT AND BLOOD PRESSURE

The most powerful determinant of CO is tissue oxygen (O_2) demand. The primary function of circulation is to provide a medium for exchange of oxygen, nutrients, and waste products between the blood and tissues. The flow of blood throughout the microcirculation, where the exchange occurs, is dependent on arterioles (regulate blood flow through changing level of resistance), capillaries (primary exchange vessels), and venules (collect and exchange vessels). As metabolism and O_2 consumption increase or decrease, the heart responds, and CO increases or decreases in direct response to increased or decreased need. The heart works as a two-sided pump, with the right side pumping deoxygenated blood into the lower pressure pulmonary circulation (reflected by PA pressure) and the left side pumping oxygenated blood into the higher pressure systemic circulation (reflected by BP). Evaluation of CO requires an assessment of the components that determine SV (preload, afterload, and contractility) for both sides of the heart and factors affecting the HR.

In the absence of underlying pathology, such as intracardiac right-to-left or left-to-right shunting, the output of the ventricles should be the same. If the output of one of the ventricles changes, the other ventricle should adjust its output to compensate for the difference. The right and left sides of the heart are connected by the pulmonary arteries and veins. Many specialized types of central vessel and arterial catheters are available to measure the pressures within the cardiopulmonary circulation and provide a means to calculate CO. The original PA catheter was known as the Swan-Ganz catheter named after the physicians who developed it. All PA catheters provide information about the right side and left side of the heart, as well as systemic circulation. Options for measurements vary with each uniquely configured catheter. Once the hemodynamic data are evaluated, strategies may be implemented to manipulate preload, afterload, contractility, and HR.

Preload

Understanding Frank Starling's law is fundamental to understanding preload. Starling's law of the heart states, "The greater the ability of the myocardial muscle to stretch at the end of diastole, the greater is the force of myocardial contraction." However, if the stretch becomes consistently excessive, the force of contraction will diminish. Preload is determined by the compliance (ability to stretch) of the ventricles during diastole as the blood volume fills the ventricles. As the blood volume increases, the heart must "stretch" with each heartbeat to accommodate it. As the blood volume decreases, the heart stretches much less but must still generate the force needed to propel the blood volume forward during systole. This mechanism enables the heart to adjust ventricular size to varying blood volumes. Preload coupled with the electrical conduction system of the heart coordinates the output of the right and left ventricles.

Factors that affect ventricular blood volume include venous return, circulating blood volume, condition of the heart valves, and atrial contractility. Ventricular compliance is affected by stiffness and thickness of the cardiac muscle. Any stressor that influences one of these factors will result in a change in preload, with a concomitant change in CO. Heart disease affects preload. Patients with biventricular heart failure and/or "stiff ventricles" are not able to handle increased intravascular volume. Their preload is always high because the heart cannot

| Box 1-11 | OPTIMAL USE OF PULMONARY ARTERY CATHETERS |

Rajaram et al., in 2013, published a review of studies of pulmonary artery catheter (PA catheter) use in adult patients in intensive care units (ICUs). The total number of patients included in the review was 5686. The authors concluded that there was no difference in ICU or hospital length of stay, mortality, or cost between patients who had a PA catheter and those that did not. The evidence does not support the argument that the PA catheter is costly and unnecessary. However, the authors remind their readers that hemodynamic monitoring is a diagnostic tool not a treatment.

A 2013 guideline for the management of heart failure from the American College of Cardiology Foundation and the American Heart Association (ACCF/AHA) gave a Class I recommendation for use of a PA catheter. The report indicated that the PA catheter should be used to guide therapy in patients who have respiratory distress or clinical evidence of impaired perfusion such that cardiac filling pressures could not be determined via clinical assessment.

The ACCF/AHA 2011 guideline for coronary bypass surgery included placement of a PA catheter as a Class I recommendation for patients in cardiogenic shock undergoing coronary bypass surgery.

In 2007, the ACCF/AHA produced guidelines on perioperative cardiovascular evaluation and care for patients undergoing noncardiac surgery. The following excerpts concern their recommendations on the use of hemodynamic monitoring.

The use of a PA catheter may be helpful in the surgical patient at risk for hemodynamic disturbances detectable using a PA catheter. The guideline suggests that three parameters should be assessed before use: patient disease (incidence of fluid shifts), surgical procedure (anticipate fluid shifts), and practice setting (presence of skilled personnel to maintain the PA catheter and interpret data). Routine use of a PA catheter perioperatively, especially in patients at low risk of developing *hemodynamic* disturbances, is not recommended.

In 2003, *Practice Guidelines for Pulmonary Artery Catheterization: An Updated Report by the American Society of Anesthesiologists Task Force on Pulmonary Artery Catheterization* was published.

The task force recommended looking at the patient, surgery, and setting before making a clinical decision to use hemodynamic monitoring. "Patients at increased risk for hemodynamic disturbances are those with clinical evidence of significant cardiovascular disease, pulmonary dysfunction, hypoxia, renal insufficiency, or other conditions associated with hemodynamic instability (e.g., advanced age, endocrine disorders, sepsis, trauma, burns).

Low-risk patients: Include those with an American Society of Anesthesiologists (ASA) physical status score of 1 or 2, with hemodynamic disturbances unlikely to cause organ dysfunction. *Moderate-risk patients*: Category ASA 3 who have hemodynamic disturbances that occasionally cause organ dysfunction. *High-risk patients*: Category ASA 4 or 5 who have hemodynamic disturbances with a great chance of causing organ dysfunction or death. "The assessment of risk should be based on a thorough analysis of the medical history and physical examination findings, rather than on exclusive consideration of specific laboratory results or other quantitative criteria. Surgical procedures associated with an increased risk of complications from hemodynamic changes, including damage to the heart, vascular tree, kidneys, liver, lungs, or brain, may increase the chance of benefiting from PA catheterization."

stretch normally to accommodate more volume. The diseased heart has little ability to compensate for volume changes. Patients with a right ventricular (RV) infarction are in a difficult position, as they require a higher preload to maintain a normal CO because the infarct zone cannot stretch. Extra ventricular blood volume, or higher preload, creates more stretch in the normal RV tissues to promote better RV output but can result in excessive work for the left ventricle. All patients with heart disease may develop heart failure, thus expert monitoring by the clinician is required to optimize CO (see Heart Failure, Chapter 5).

Clinically, preload is measured as ventricular end-diastolic pressure (VEDP), because pressure in the ventricles correlates closely with volume. For the right side of the heart, RV end-diastolic (filling) pressure (RVEDP) is reflected by right atrial (RA) pressure (RAP) or CVP. Left ventricular (LV) end-diastolic (filling) pressure (LVEDP) is reflected by left atrial (LA), PA diastolic (PAD), or PA occlusive (PAOP) or wedge (PAWP) pressure measurements. If preload begins to increase in a patient with heart disease, appropriate medications, including diuretics, may be given to help decrease CVP and PAOP. Vasodilating drugs with strong venodilating properties may also be used to decrease venous return so that a heart with limited ability to stretch can accommodate and pump the lesser blood volume. An increase in preload signals that the ventricles may be unable to eject enough of the end-diastolic volume, causing more blood to be retained in the ventricles. As a result, venous congestion and fluid overload occurs, leading to the clinical signs of congestive heart failure. Conversely, decreased preload is seen with hypovolemia and certain types of shock where vasomotor tone is affected causing vasodilation. Decreased preload can lead to a decrease in CO related to the decrease in SV. Hypovolemia may be difficult to assess, because the patient may have pitting edema but is deficient of fluid volume within the blood vessels. The CVP may not always provide a complete picture of volume status. Stroke volume variability (SVV) can assist the clinician in assessment of the need for fluid replacement and the adequacy of the volume delivered. SVV is determined using the arterial waveform to calculate the change in SV from beat to beat of the heart (see Septic Shock).

Afterload

Afterload refers to the pressure or force that must be generated within the right and left ventricles/ventricular myocardium during systole to overcome the vascular resistance to ejection. The pressures created by the blood volume and vascular tone within the pulmonary, aortic, and systemic circulation create resistance against the aortic and pulmonic valves, which can impede ventricular ejection. Other resistant forces include increased blood viscosity, reduced distensibility of the vascular system (created by atherosclerosis or "hardening of the arteries"), and diseased heart valves. The clinician should be aware that diseased ventricles are extremely sensitive to abrupt changes in afterload because the diseased tissue cannot readily generate additional force to overcome additional resistance to ejection. Paying close attention to PA pressures, as well as systemic arterial pressure, is of paramount importance. If blood volume starts to be retained in the ventricles, rather than being normally ejected, VEDP increases, followed by increases in PA pressure. When these changes are observed, measures such as administration of diuretics or vasodilating drugs with strong arterial dilating properties may be initiated to decrease afterload and help improve ventricular ejection. Medications used for management of hypertension are administered to reduce afterload.

Because vascular resistance plays a major role in determining pressures throughout the heart and lungs, RV afterload is evaluated by calculating pulmonary vascular resistance (PVR), whereas LV afterload is reflected by SVR. The higher the afterload, the greater the myocardial wall tension/pressure must be to open the aortic and/or pulmonic valves, and the greater is the work of the heart to overcome resistance to flow. This explains why hypertension is called "the silent killer," because the constantly increased afterload strains the heart. Increased cardiac work requires increased myocardial blood flow to deliver additional O_2. When blood flowing through the coronary arteries is diminished by atherosclerosis, the demand for the increased blood flow required to manage energy needs created by increased afterload may not be met, resulting in myocardial ischemia, injury, and possibly infarction.

Contractility

This is the inherent capacity of the myocardium to contract during systole. This mechanism functions independently of variations in preload and afterload. Changes in ventricular contractility have a significant effect on tissue perfusion and the shape/slope of the ventricular function curves generated during CO measurement. Although contractility is not measured directly, a change in contractility can be inferred when CO is decreased and other variables that affect CO (i.e., preload, SV, afterload, HR) remain the same. Changes in ventricular function curves infer changes in contractility. Several factors positively influence contractility: sympathetic stimulation, calcium, and positive inotropic agents, such as digitalis, dobutamine, milrinone, and beta-adrenergic drugs. Factors such as acidemia, hypoxia, myocardial ischemia, myocardial infarct, cardiomyopathies, beta-blocker drugs, and antidysrhythmic drugs can decrease contractility.

Heart Rate

Changes in HR affect myocardial functioning significantly. Slight increases in HR with a constant SV result in increased CO. Very rapid HRs are associated with a reduction in CO as the duration of diastole is shortened, resulting in decreased coronary perfusion and reduced ventricular filling time. Patients who are critically ill often manifest sinus tachycardia to maintain a CO that meets the demand for O_2 and nutrients at the cellular level. The heart requires more O_2 when the HR increases, and as long as coronary artery perfusion is adequate, HR increases provide compensation needed for increased metabolic demands. Tachycardia can, however, reach a critical point where the heart is receiving less O_2 if filling time becomes too brief to provide appropriate coronary artery perfusion. Bradycardia often results in decreased CO unless there are increases in SV during the longer ventricular filling times. Athletes are able to maintain excellent CO with slower HRs, but the patient who is critically ill may not be as fortunate when HR decreases. Algorithms have been created for advanced cardiac life support, which include both pharmacologic and electrical therapies to manage HR.

HEMODYNAMIC ASSESSMENT

The goal of hemodynamic monitoring is to obtain accurate measurements and to observe trends in values that are used in combination with physical assessment findings to provide appropriate, effective therapies to maintain adequate BP, CO, and tissue perfusion. The hemodynamic measurements listed in Table 1-10 are considered the values needed in a complete hemodynamic profile.

SYSTEMIC ARTERIAL PRESSURE OR BLOOD PRESSURE MAY BE MEASURED INDIRECTLY AND/OR DIRECTLY

- Indirect measurement: A "spot check" or "snapshot" of the BP in a moment of time, performed with a manually inflated BP cuff and manometer. Arterial pressure is auscultated over a pulse point using a stethoscope or Doppler ultrasound device. A noninvasive automatic BP cuff (NIBP or NBP) may be used, in lieu of manually inflating the cuff and auscultating the pressure using a stethoscope and manometer. Manual or auscultatory BP readings are wrought with pitfalls that cause false-high and false-low readings. Proper cuff size, proper cuff position, arm position being level with the heart, and skill in determining the onset of the first Korotkoff sound are imperative components for accurate readings.
    - Bariatric consideration: Proper cuff size may require a special large and/or long cuff for proper fit. Alternate BP measurement sites may be required such as the forearm or lower leg, and the site used must be documented with the BP reading. Alternate sites also require correct cuff size for accurate readings (refer to the manufacturer's instruction for proper fit and placement). Regardless of the site used, the cuff should be at the level of the patient's heart. If using a lower extremity, the patient should be in a supine position.
    - Geriatric consideration: Comparison of BP readings from each arm on initial encounter is best practice, because it may provide information about the vascular status of the individual. Both BP measurements are recorded with the site noted, and it is recommended that the site with the higher pressure be used and documented. This practice is not limited to the elderly. Measurement of BP with the individual lying or sitting rather than taken when standing is used to determine if the individual has orthostatic hypotension (sometimes called postural hypotension). Orthostatic hypotension is indicated when the systolic BP drops 20 mm Hg and/or the diastolic BP falls by 10 mm Hg, or greater change when in the standing position. Clinically the patient may be dizzy or light-headed. Prepare to safely assist the patient back to a sitting or lying position to prevent a fall.
- Direct measurement: Continuous monitoring of BP that requires insertion of a hollow, semirigid catheter into an artery to create an arterial line (A-line). When an arterial line is used to measure BP, it is labeled ABP to distinguish this from a noninvasive measurement. BP is a dynamic or ever-changing event and the continuous monitoring of ABP reflects the beat-to-beat changes that occur. Cardiovascular dynamics are assessed through

Table 1-10	HEMODYNAMIC NORMAL VALUES AND DERIVED VALUES	
Parameter	**Formula**	**Normal Values**
Arterial blood pressure (BP) systolic (SBP)/diastolic		90 to 130/50 to 80 mm Hg
Mean arterial pressure (MAP)	$SBP + (D \times 2)/3$	70 to 100 mm Hg
Central venous pressure (CVP)*		2 to 6 mm Hg
Right atrial pressure (RAP)*		2 to 6 mm Hg
Left atrial pressure (LAP)		8 to 12 mm Hg
Right ventricular pressure (RVP)		15 to 25/0 to 8 mm Hg
Pulmonary artery systolic (PAS) pressure		15 to 25 mm Hg
Pulmonary artery diastolic (PAD) pressure		8 to 15 mm Hg
Pulmonary artery occlusive pressure (PAOP) Same as wedge (pulmonary capillary wedge pressure [PCWP] or pulmonary wedge pressure [PWP])		6 to 12 mm Hg
Mean pulmonary artery pressure (MPAP, PAM)	$PAS + (PAD \times 2)/3$	10 to 20 mm Hg
Cardiac output (CO)	$HR \times SV$	4 to 8 L/min
Cardiac index (CI)		2.5 to 4 L/min/m²
Systemic vascular resistance (SVR)	$MAP - RAP/CO \times 80$	800 to 1200 dynes/s/cm⁵
Pulmonary vascular resistance (PVR)	$MPAP - PAOP/CO \times 80$	150 to 250 dynes/s/cm⁵
Coronary perfusion pressure (CPP)	Diastolic BP $-$ PAOP	50 to 70 mm Hg
Stroke volume (SV)	$CO/HR \times 1000$	55 to 100 mL/beat
Stroke volume index (SVI)	SV/BSA	30 to 60 mL/beat/m²
Right ventricular stroke work index (RVSWI)	$SVI (PAM - RAP) \times 0.0136$	4 to 8 g/m²/beat
Left ventricular stroke work index (LVSWI)	$SVI (MAP - PAOP) \times 0.0136$	40 to 75 g/m²/beat
Arterial oxygen content (Cao_2)	$(Hgb \times 1.34) \times Sao_2$	18 to 20 mL/vol%
Venous oxygen content (Cvo_2)	$(Hgb \times 1.34 \times Svo_2)$	15.5 mL/vol%
Oxygen delivery (Do_2)	$Cao_2 \times CO \times 10$	800 to 1000 mL/min
Oxygen delivery index (Do_2I)	$Cao_2 \times CI \times 10$	500 to 600 mL/min/m²
Arteriovenous oxygen content difference ($C[a - v]o_2$)	$Cao_2 \times Cvo_2$	4 to 6 mL/vol%
Oxygen consumption (Vo_2)	$CO \times 10 \times C(a - v)o_2$	200 to 250 mL/min
Oxygen consumption index (Vo_2I)	$CI \times 10 \times C(a - v)o_2$	115 to 165 mL/min/m²
Arterial oxygen saturation (Sao_2)	95% to 98%	
Mixed venous oxygen saturation (Svo_2) (Global venous return)	$(CO \times Cao_2 \times 10) - Vo_2$	60% to 80% Values should be trended for optimal clinical assessment
Mixed venous oxygen saturation-regional ($Scvo_2$) (Head and neck venous return)		65% to 85% Values should be trended for optimal clinical assessment
Stroke volume variation (SVV)		10% to 15%

*CVP and RAP are used interchangeably at times.
BSA, Body surface area; *Hgb*, hemoglobin; *HR*, heart rate.

a review of pressure waveforms and analysis of trends in arterial pressure readings. Arterial lines are used to obtain arterial blood samples for labwork, including blood gas determinations, without repeated arterial punctures.

ARTERIAL OXYGEN SATURATION

* The percentage of oxyhemoglobin (Hgb bound with O_2) compared with the total amount of Hgb can be measured directly using blood samples from the arterial line or approximated indirectly by photoelectric technology using an external pulse oximetry probe placed on the patient's finger, ear, or forehead.

CENTRAL VENOUS PRESSURE OR RIGHT ATRIAL PRESSURE

* CVP can be monitored continuously or "spot checked" using a central line.
* CVP and RAP may be used interchangeably to assess intravascular fluid volume, efficacy of venous return to the right side of the heart, and RVEDP or preload.
* RAP is obtained using the RA port of a PA catheter.
* Specialized CV catheters allow continuous venous oximetry ($Scvo_2$) monitoring that provides information on oxygen use.

PULMONARY ARTERY PRESSURES

* PAPs are measured continuously using a flow-directed, multilumen catheter placed in the PA. PA catheters vary in technology. More sophisticated catheters provide information about O_2 delivery and O_2 consumption (Svo_2) and may provide continuous cardiac output (CCO) measurements. Basic PA catheters provide measurement of RAP, PAP, PAOP or "wedge pressures," and CO.
* The RAP, PAP, PAOP, and CO provide information that helps in calculating preload, afterload, and contractility. Waveform analysis helps to identify any pathology or abnormality of the heart valves and other cardiac disorders.
* The hemodynamic measurements paired with the data gathered about oxygen delivery and oxygen use give the clinician information about tissue perfusion.

CARDIAC OUTPUT

CO can be calculated using several methods.

* **Fick oxygen consumption method:** The original, or "gold standard," mathematical method used to calculate CO. The formula for CO uses arteriovenous O_2 content difference to calculate the value. A number of technical problems can interfere with obtaining accurate results, and because of the cumbersome nature of the procedure, the formula is generally used in research laboratories, rather than routinely in clinical practice.

$$\text{Cardiac Output (CO)} = \frac{\text{Oxygen Consumption (VO}_2)}{\text{Arteriovenous Oxygen Difference (Ca} - \text{Cv)}}$$

* **Thermodilution (TD) method:** Measurement method using a PA catheter to determine the flow rate of a room temperature IV solution (injectate) passing through the heart. The temperature of the injectate is lower than the temperature of the blood in the central circulation. IV solution is injected into a more proximally located port in the PA catheter and travels through the heart to a more distally located port. A temperature sensor is used to track the flow rate of the injectate. The speed of the flow from the proximal to the distal port is used to calculate CO. It is considered accurate and reliable. The TD method of CO determination is now used as the standard for comparing other methods of CO determination.
* **Continuous cardiac output measurement:** Performed using a specialized PA catheter using thermal technology that allows the user to obtain readings that are averaged over 3-minute periods and updated every 30 to 60 seconds.
* **Arterial pressure–based cardiac output measurement (APCO):** This method of CO calculation assesses the aortic pulse pressure using the arterial waveform to calculate the SV and is a beat-to-beat measurement.
* **Impedance cardiography (ICG) method of CO measurement:** ICG is a noninvasive measurement that uses transthoracic bioimpedance to determine CO. Currently, BioZ and Task Force monitoring have proven to accurately determine CO compared with the

TD method in medical cardiac patients. ICG measurements are less reliable in patients with valvular disease, aortic vessel disease, cardiac shunts, or states with fluid accumulation in the thorax. Therefore, this method is not recommended for use in cardiac surgery patients.

- **Transthoracic echocardiograms (TTE) and transesophageal echocardiograms (TEE):** Can determine CO as a calculation of SV. TTE is noninvasive and is used for short-term diagnostics. TEE is minimally invasive and is often used in the surgical setting.

TISSUE OXYGENATION

Adequate tissue oxygenation is the goal of therapy for patients in critical care. The regulation of oxygenation is dependent on regulation of blood flow. The cardiovascular system controls blood flow by maintaining the appropriate perfusion pressure throughout the arterial system supplying blood to each organ, and by allowing each organ to regulate vascular resistance based on the needs of the organ. CO can be redistributed at the organ or tissue level based on need. Vasoregulation occurs at the local level by the arterioles or resistance vessels. Vasoactive medications used to support perfusion pressure require careful titration based on an analysis of meaningful data. To assist the clinician in meeting this goal, oxygen use is measured via specialized catheters.

- The Svo_2 PA catheter not only gives a CCO but also measures the venous O_2 saturation (Svo_2) via a fiber optic tip in the PA, and is used for determination of the balance between O_2 delivery and O_2 use. O_2 delivery is the result of CO multiplied by the arterial O_2 content (CaO_2). The arterial O_2 content is determined by Hgb and arterial O_2 saturation (Sao_2). The balance between oxygen delivery (DO_2) and oxygen use (VO_2) is reflected by the Svo_2.
- The $Scvo_2$ is measured via a specialized CV catheter, usually placed in the subclavian vein. The $Scvo_2$ reflects the mixed venous oxygen use as does the Svo_2. However, the $Scvo_2$ measurement is taken from the superior vena cava and does not include the inferior vena cava contribution. The $Scvo_2$ trends with the Svo_2 and the same factors influence the findings. The factors that affect tissue oxygenation include CO, Sao_2, Hgb, oxygen delivery (DO_2), and oxygen use (VO_2). Oxygen use is dynamic and Svo_2 and $Scvo_2$ can normally change 5%. Therefore, the clinician should act on changes of greater than 5% to 10% that are sustained greater than 5 minutes. Both Svo_2 and $Scvo_2$ should be used with CO, Hgb, and Sao_2 monitoring to give the clinician a complete picture of oxygen use (see Table 1-10).

PROMOTING ACCURACY OF HEMODYNAMIC VALUES: SETTING UP EQUIPMENT

Ensuring proper setup and maintenance of the pressure monitoring system will prevent most inaccuracies. Normal waveform configurations must be understood for all readings so that abnormal waveforms can be readily identified. Abnormal waveforms can sometimes reflect a problem with the system setup or maintenance.

General considerations related to the hemodynamic monitoring setup

1. Use rigid pressure tubing from the transducer to the patient. Most monitoring kits have the proper setup prepackaged with disposable transducers to assure proper use. Flexible tubing may be used from the flush bag to the transducer.
2. During the initial setup, flush or prime the monitoring system (all tubing and the transducer[s]) without pressure applied to the flush bag to help prevent formation of air bubbles from turbulent flow within the empty tubing. Slower priming allows for more even fluid dispersion throughout the system.
3. Remove excess air from the flush bag before flushing to help prevent an air embolus from entering the patient's vasculature. The excess air can be accidentally introduced into the patient.
4. Flush all stopcocks and apply sterile dead-end caps to seal the system. Vented caps are not recommended, because the venting offers an entry point for organisms and could create a leak in the system.
5. Maintain a minimum of 100 mL in the flush bag and change the bag according to institutional guidelines. Many institutions focus on maintaining a closed system to minimize the chance of contamination. The Centers for Disease Control and Prevention (CDC) recommends that the tubing be changed every 96 hours.

6. Apply and maintain 300 mm Hg of pressure to the pressure bag enclosing the flush bag.
7. Maintain electrical safety guidelines to avoid microshocks entering the heart via the fluid column created by the monitoring system.
8. Normal saline is the recognized flush solution of choice for hemodynamic monitoring systems. Heparinized saline is no longer recommended for routine use, to avoid the risk of inducing heparin-induced thrombocytopenia (HIT positive).

Leveling and zeroing the system

1. All monitoring systems must be leveled before use. To level the system, the transducers are positioned at the phlebostatic axis to provide the most accurate pressure readings. Transducers must remain leveled to provide accurate pressure readings. The phlebostatic axis is located at the intersection of the fourth intercostal space and the line that denotes half the anteroposterior diameter of the chest. Readings are accurate with the head of the bed (HOB) elevated from 0 to 60 degrees. Higher HOB elevation will result in false-low readings.
2. Transducers must be "zeroed" before using the monitoring system. Newer computerized bedside monitors remind the nurse to zero the system. Zeroing the transducer requires opening the transducer to air while possibly pressing a button on the bedside monitor to establish a referenced atmospheric pressure of zero.
3. Leveling and zeroing should be done at least once a shift, for any change in patient position, when the system has been opened to air, and/or if there is a question of accuracy in values or waveforms obtained.

Square wave testing (also called fast flush or dynamic response test)

1. This is done to test the compliance of the monitoring system to provide a common measure of accuracy. Hemodynamic systems are constructed differently in each monitoring setting, but, minimally, each should have a flush system pressurized at 300 mm Hg and a continuous fluid column contained within rigid tubing between the transducer and the patient. The number of transducers, and type and length of tubing may vary. Flaws within the system directly affect the accuracy of pressure readings. The test indicates if the system is normal, overdamped, or underdamped.
2. Overdamping causes the systolic pressure to be falsely low and the diastolic pressure to be falsely high. Large air bubbles, loose connections, no or low amount of flush solution in the system, low pressure on the flush bag, or a kinked catheter causes overdamping.
3. Underdamping causes the systolic pressure to be falsely high and the diastolic pressure to be falsely low. Small air bubbles, a defective transducer, or pressure tubing that is too long causes underdamping.
4. Testing should be done when the system is set up, once every shift, when the system is opened to air for any reason (including blood sampling), and when waves appear distorted from the usual appearance.
5. To perform the square wave test:
   - Fast flush the monitoring system by pulling the pigtail or pressing the appropriate button for each transducer. The flush should be pressurized to 300 mm Hg.
   - When the system is being flushed, a large, square wave appears on the monitor. Stop flushing abruptly (snap the flush mechanism) and observe the shape of the square wave, and wait for the pressure waveform to normalize.
   - An acceptable response is the waveform normalizing and returning to baseline following 1.5 to 2 oscillations (Figure 1-4, A). If the resulting waveform is abnormally shaped, lacks shape, lacks amplitude, or does not return to baseline, the response is abnormal.
   - In optimally damped systems, one small undershoot (negative deflection) and one small overshoot (exaggerated positive deflection or bounce) are seen, followed by a return of the normal waveform.
   - Overdamped systems (Figure 1-4, B) demonstrate less than 1.5 oscillations or bounces, and a slurring of the square wave upstroke. Waves are blunted, sluggish, and falsely wide.
   - Underdamped systems (Figure 1-4, C) have greater than 2 oscillations, sharp bounces with waves that are exaggerated, narrow, and falsely peaked.

Square wave test configuration

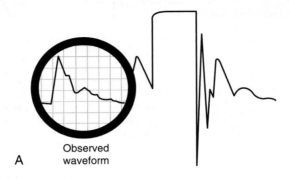

Observed
A   waveform

Square wave test configuration

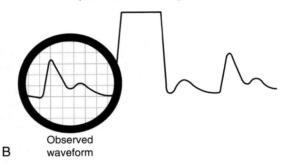

Observed
B   waveform

Square wave test configuration

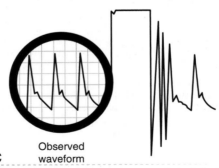

Observed
C   waveform

Figure 1-4 Dynamic response testing (square wave, frequency response testing) using the fast-flush system. A, Optimally damped system. B, Overdamped system. C, Underdamped system.

- If overdamping or underdamping is present, troubleshoot the monitoring system. If troubleshooting is ineffective, the monitoring system should be checked by the biomedical engineer or technician. If these problems cannot be resolved, another monitor may be needed to obtain accurate readings. Also see Troubleshooting (Table 1-11).

Table 1-11 | **MECHANICAL PROBLEMS AFFECTING HEMODYNAMIC MEASUREMENTS**

Problem	Waveform Appearance	Cause	Corrective Action
Overdamping*	Smaller than usual with a slow rise; diminished or absent dicrotic notch (arterial and pulmonary artery catheters). Square wave test will have less than 1.5 deflections.	Tubing too long	Remove extra length of tubing
		Nonpressure tubing used	Replace with pressurized tubing
		Air bubbles in system	Flush air out of system
		Thrombus formation	Consider changing catheter
		Lodging of catheter against vessel wall	Flush line for at least 10 seconds. Ensure pressure bag inflated to 300 mm Hg.
		Loose connection in tubing or transducer	Tighten all connections on initial setup, and if any leakage is noted, then flush air from system. (Initially flushing lines without pressure will result in fewer air bubbles.)
		Incorrect calibration	Recalibrate (zero) transducer
		Spontaneous catheter migration into a near-wedged position (PA catheter only)	Flush PA line; if PA catheter wedges with 0.5 mL of air or less, notify the advanced practice provider for repositioning
		Kinking or knotting of catheter or tubing	Externally ensure lines are straight; if internal jugular sites tend to kink at insertion site, neck may need to be supported for prevention. If internally PA catheter kink or knot is seen on chest radiograph, notify the advanced practice provider.
Catheter whip or fling. Underdampening.	Erratic, "noisy" waveform with highly variable and inaccurate pressures. Square wave test may be hyperdynamic or more than 2 deflections.	Spurious movement of the catheter tip within the vessel lumen (may require repositioning). Catheter too long for vessel (arterial). Pressure tubing too long.	Assess proper position of PA catheter with chest radiograph and determine if PA catheter will wedge with 0.5 to 1.5 mL of air. Minimize length of pressure tubing. Rezero monitor. Notify the advanced practice provider if improper placement is found or if catheter whip (fling) is uncorrected despite above measures.
No waveform.	Complete absence of waveform.	PEA, absence of pulse, with electrical activity.	Check patient condition. Check pulse (PEA); begin CPR.
		Stopcock turned to wrong position	Most common; if patient stable, check system; start at patient and work back to transducer
		Large leak in the system, usually with blood backing up into the tubing. Loose or cracked transducer or air in transducer.	Turn system off to patient at nearest stopcock until leak can be found and corrected.† If system has been contaminated, change setup.
		Catheter tip or lumen totally occluded by clot	Notify the advanced practice provider

Continued

Table 1-11	MECHANICAL PROBLEMS AFFECTING HEMODYNAMIC MEASUREMENTS—cont'd		
Problem	**Waveform Appearance**	**Cause**	**Corrective Action**
		Inadequate pressure (< 300 mm Hg) on pressure bag	Ensure bag is inflated and maintaining pressure. If flush bag has less than 100 mL, change the bag.
		Defective transducer or amplifier	Assess monitor cable first, then amplifier, and then change transducer.
Inability to obtain a PAOP reading (PA catheter only).	Absence of wedge waveform after balloon inflation of up to 1.5 mL of air. If when instilling air (1.5 mL or less) into the balloon, the waveform goes up and off the screen; this is overwedging.	Retrograde catheter slippage Balloon rupture Migration of PA catheter into smaller vessel	Assess waveform; ensure it is a PA waveform and not already in wedge position or an RV waveform. If it is a PA waveform, the catheter needs to be repositioned for proper placement. If it is an RV waveform, the catheter should immediately be pulled back to the RA to prevent ventricular dysrhythmias. If when less than 0.5 mL of air is instilled the waveform goes up and is lost at high range, the catheter is overwedging and needs to be repositioned. The catheter level should be assessed to see if it has changed positions since insertion. If in wedge position, notify the advanced practice provider. If unable to wedge, the physician should be notified. If balloon rupture is suspected, notify the advanced practice provider immediately and do not attempt any further PAOP readings; close balloon port.

*Whenever the amplitude of an arterial or PA waveform decreases, the patient should first be assessed for hypovolemia or shock.
†If line has become disconnected or a portion open to air, the patient must be assessed for any potential air embolus; then, the line should be changed to prevent sepsis. PA catheters must always be transduced, as it is necessary to assess catheter migration through waveform analysis. Catheter migration may result in pulmonary infarction if not identified and managed.
CPR, Cardiopulmonary resuscitation; *PA*, pulmonary artery; *PAOP*, pulmonary artery occlusive pressure; *PEA*, pulseless electrical activity; *RV*, right ventricular.

HEMODYNAMIC MONITORING: CONSIDERATIONS DURING SETUP, LINE INSERTION, AND PLACEMENT
Arterial pressure monitoring
- The most common sites used for intraarterial catheter insertion are the radial, brachial, or femoral arteries. Arterial catheters are inserted via the radial artery, because this artery is readily accessible and collateral blood flow is usually adequate. The arterial catheter may also be inserted in the femoral or brachial artery. The arterial pressure waveform is displayed on a bedside monitor to provide continuous observation of systolic, diastolic, and mean arterial pressures (Figure 1-5). The appearance of the arterial waveform is influenced by variations in BP, dysrhythmias, hypovolemia, vasoconstriction, and mechanical factors. Mechanical factors that influence the waveform include overdamping, catheter whip, and inaccurate calibration/zeroing (Table 1-12).

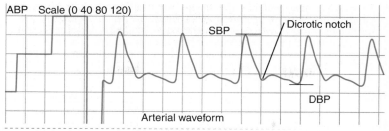

Figure 1-5 Arterial pressure waveform. (Redrawn from Daily E, Schroeder J: *Techniques in bedside hemodynamic monitoring,* ed 4, St Louis, 1989, Mosby.)

Table 1-12	ABNORMAL PULMONARY ARTERY PRESSURES	
Hemodynamic Pressure	**Normal Range**	**Clinical Conditions**
Pulmonary artery systolic (PAS) pressure	20 to 30 mm Hg	*Increased:* Right ventricular failure, chronic left ventricular failure, constrictive pericarditis, cardiac tamponade, pulmonary hypertension (primary or related to lung disease). *Decreased:* Hypovolemia, preload reduction.
Pulmonary artery diastolic (PAD) pressure*	8 to 15 mm Hg	*Increased:* Left ventricular failure, mitral stenosis, left-to-right shunts, pulmonary hypertension (primary or related to lung disease). *Decreased:* Hypovolemia, preload reduction.
Pulmonary artery occlusive pressure (PAOP)†	6 to 12 mm Hg	*Increased:* Left ventricular failure, cardiac tamponade, mitral valve regurgitation, mitral valve stenosis, acute ventricular septal defect, fluid volume overload. *Decreased:* Hypovolemia, afterload reduction.

*PAD may exceed PAOP by ≥5 mm Hg in patients with pulmonary hypertension, hypoxemia, acidosis, pulmonary emboli, and other lung disease.
†PAOP > PAD signals a mechanical problem (i.e., overwedging or improper identification of PAD).

- Potential complications include decreased perfusion distal to the insertion site, which can cause limb ischemia. Slower blood flow can lead to thrombus formation. If air inadvertently enters the system during line insertion, through a crack or other flaw in the closed system, an air embolus may result, which, if lodged in the hand, can render distal tissues anoxic. Rarely, patients have needed to have fingers amputated because of prolonged lack of perfusion. If the closed system is cracked or becomes disconnected, exsanguination may occur. With any invasive procedure the risk of infection is present. Follow strict adherence to invasive line insertion procedures to decrease the risk of infection.

Pulmonary artery pressure monitoring

- The most common sites used for PA catheter insertion are the internal jugular or subclavian veins. Femoral and brachial veins may also be used. The most common PA catheter placement technique is percutaneous insertion of the catheter introducer/introducing needle using the Seldinger technique for insertion, in combination with waveform analysis provided by the hemodynamic monitoring system as the catheter passes through the heart. Waveform analysis and pressure readings provide the practitioner with the information needed to know the position of the catheter. Insertion may also be done using a cutdown to expose the vessel but is rarely needed. Catheter placement is occasionally done under fluoroscopy for patients with abnormal cardiac or vasculature structures.

- Potential complications include decreased perfusion distal to end of the PA catheter if the catheter is inserted too far or migrates out of position. This can cause pulmonary tissue ischemia or infarction, if it is severe. Slower blood flow can lead to thrombus formation. If air inadvertently enters the system during line insertion, through a crack or other flaw in the closed system, an air embolus may result. If the closed system is cracked or becomes disconnected, exsanguination may occur. The cardiac chambers can be perforated during insertion, resulting in hemorrhage into the mediastinum and cardiac tamponade. The vasculature can be perforated during insertion, resulting in the extravascular catheter tip causing fluid or blood accumulation in the pleural space or the mediastinum and/or a pneumothorax. Dysrhythmias may occur, particularly when the catheter passes through the right ventricle.

Diagnostic Tests Associated with Pulmonary Artery Catheter Placement for Hemodynamic Monitoring

Test	Purpose	Abnormal Findings
Noninvasive Cardiology		
Continuous cardiac monitoring (electrocardiography [ECG]): The ECG should be monitored continuously during insertion of pulmonary artery (PA) catheters and throughout use of hemodynamic monitoring using a 5-lead or 3-lead system.	Assess for dysrhythmias during PA catheter insertion. ECG tracings are used to correlate pressure waveforms with the cardiac cycle as part of acquiring accurate measurements.	During insertion: Premature ventricular contractions (PVCs) may occur as the catheter passes quickly through the ventricle on the way to the PA. If ventricular ectopy persists, the catheter should be withdrawn into the right atrium (RA) and refloated. The balloon on the catheter should remain inflated throughout the procedure so that the blood flow moves the catheter through the heart.
Radiology		
Chest x-ray (CXR) A CXR should be done upon insertion to assess central catheter position. Central venous pressure (CVP) placement: Tip at the superior vena cava/atrial junction. PA catheter placement: Tip should be in the middle third of lung fields within the PA and within or barely outside of the sternal border. Most PA catheters are inserted into the right PA. Routine daily CXR is not recommended. CXR should be driven by clinical indications.	Assess for abnormal findings following PA catheter or central venous catheter insertion or manipulation. If catheters are positioned improperly in the blood vessels, ischemia may occur distally from the catheter, or the catheter may cause erosion of vessel walls. Medication administration should not be done until it is confirmed that the catheter is in the proper position.	Pneumothorax or hemothorax: May occur with central line placement in the internal jugular, external jugular, or subclavian insertion sites. Widening mediastinum: Indicative of acute cardiac tamponade, which may indicate rupture of a chamber of the heart during PA catheter insertion. Subclavian insertion: If a CVP catheter is not readily seen, inspect upper portion of film to make sure the catheter is not in the internal jugular vein. RA catheter positioning: A CVP line positioned in the RA is more likely to cause atrial perforation and cardiac tamponade, although rare. Happens more often with peripherally inserted central catheters (PICC lines) resulting from arm movement. Left PA positioning: PA catheters can be placed in the left PA. On the anteroposterior film, the catheter appears to be pointing distally. When seen, assess for knotting or coiling of the PA catheter within the right ventricle, which may have caused the catheter to be directed toward the left PA.

Test	Purpose	Abnormal Findings
Fluoroscopy radiographic method wherein catheter can be visualized as it passes through the heart and blood vessels.	Used during PA catheter insertion to ensure accurate placement. Used at varying frequencies, depending on provider practice patterns. If not used often, may cause a delay insertion.	Some centers use fluoroscopy only for anticipated "difficult" PA catheter insertions, whereas others use it frequently. Abnormal vasculature or structural abnormality of the heart may be visualized as the catheter passes into position.

Diagnostic Tests Associated with Pulmonary Artery Catheter Placement for Hemodynamic Monitoring—cont'd

DIAGNOSTIC TESTS

FACTORS AFFECTING HEMODYNAMIC MEASUREMENTS

Systolic blood pressure

This is determined by (1) the amount of blood ejected by the ventricle per beat (SV), (2) wall compliance of the arterial system, and (3) peripheral resistance. Elevations in systolic pressure produce large, steep waveforms, often reflective of changes in vascular compliance, such as the hypertension seen in patients with atherosclerosis. A decrease in systolic pressure producing smaller, slightly wider waveforms is seen in connection with heart disorders that result in decreased SV. The use of arterial vasodilators such as nitroprusside, hydralazine, and nifedipine will cause a rapid upstroke and steep decline with a drop in diastolic pressure related to the potent arterial dilation.

Diastolic blood pressure

This is determined by (1) volume of blood within the arterial system, (2) compliance of the arterial wall, and (3) peripheral resistance. Coronary artery blood flow occurs during diastole, and a drop in diastolic pressure may result in myocardial ischemia as flow is reduced with lower diastolic pressure. Monitoring of diastolic BP is critical, especially when vasodilating drugs are administered, because diastolic BP generally decreases from the effect of these medications.

 Safety Alert

Caution must be used in managing hypertension or decreasing afterload with sodium nitroprusside (e.g., Nipride), because this medication causes both venous and arterial vasodilation and can rapidly decrease the blood pressure (BP), causing hypotension with rapid decrease in delivery of O_2 and nutrients to the cells. Nitroprusside may also induce deterioration in arterial O_2 saturation if ventilation cannot increase enough to "match" the increased blood in the lungs caused by pulmonary vasodilation. If the BP is extremely labile, the patient may be intravascularly volume-depleted or hypovolemic. Replacing fluid volume or blood (if hemorrhage is the cause) will help stabilize the BP.

Mean arterial pressure (MAP)

The normal MAP value is 70 to 100 mm Hg. MAP is the average pressure within the arterial tree throughout the cardiac cycle, reflecting the average force that pushes blood through the systemic circulation to the tissues. MAP is the product of CO × SVR. An increase in CO or SVR will increase MAP. A decrease in either value will decrease MAP. MAP is the most accurate noninvasive measurement of central aortic pressure. The intraaortic balloon provides the most accurate invasive measurement as it is taken from the catheter tip located just after the aortic arch in the descending aorta. MAP can be calculated by the following formula: MAP = SBP + (DBP × 2)/3.

Central venous pressure (CVP)

The normal CVP value is 2 to 6 mm Hg. CVP is the measurement of systemic venous pressure at the level of the superior vena cava just before it enters the right atrium. CVP can be measured

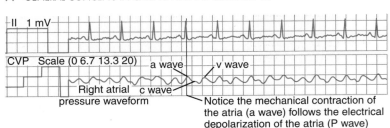

Figure 1-6   **Right atrial pressure waveform with electrocardiography (ECG).** (Redrawn from Daily E, Schroeder J: *Techniques in bedside hemodynamic monitoring,* ed 4, St Louis, 1989, Mosby.)

by a catheter threaded into the jugular, subclavian, or other large vein, by the use of a CV catheter; often, these are multilumen catheters. RAP correlates with CVP because the normal values and waveforms (Figure 1-6) are the same and the terms are used interchangeably in practice. Using a PA catheter, RAP is measured through the proximal port, which lies in the right atrium. Because 60% of total blood volume resides in the venous system, CVP is valuable in assessing for fluid volume excess or deficit and venous tone. CVP also provides indirect information regarding RV function. RV failure, cardiac tamponade, fluid volume overload, pulmonary hypertension, tricuspid valve disease, and chronic LV failure may increase CVP. Decreased CVP is most often caused by hypovolemia. Venous dilation caused by sepsis, drugs, or neurogenic dysfunction may also decrease CVP. Complications of CV catheters include venous air embolism, dysrhythmias, hemorrhage, infection, vascular erosion, perforation of cardiac chambers, pneumothorax, and thromboembolic problems.

Safety Alert   *Be alert for air embolism during central catheter insertion and maintenance of the central venous pressure monitoring system. This is an uncommon but potentially fatal event. As little as 20 mL of air may cause a problem for patients who are critically ill. Entry of 200 to 300 mL of air into the vessel over a short period of time (seconds) has a 50% mortality rate. Prevention is the key. During insertion, ensure the practitioner inserting the catheter does not allow ports to be uncapped or uncovered (open to air) once inside the vessel. Air can be entrained down the port by the blood flow during inspiration (when intrathoracic pressure is negative), resulting in embolization. If air embolism is suspected, place the patient with head of the bed down (Trendelenburg position) in the left lateral decubitus position immediately (see Suspected Air Embolism in the Collaborative Management section).*

Right atrial pressure (RAP)

The normal mean RAP is 2 to 6 mm Hg. RAP is measured via the proximal catheter port and is essentially the same as CVP. With the PA catheter, RAP can be monitored continuously and displayed on a bedside screen (see Figure 1-6). In addition, the catheter lumen can be used for fluid or drug administration.

Right ventricular pressure (RVP)

The normal RVP is 15 to 25 mm Hg systolic, 0 to 8 mm Hg diastolic. RVP is measured only during catheter insertion and provides information about the function of the right ventricle and the tricuspid and pulmonic valves. Elevation of RV systolic pressure may be seen in pulmonic stenosis, pulmonary hypertension, or ventricular septal defect (VSD) with left-to-right shunt. Elevation of RV diastolic pressure may occur with RV failure, cardiac tamponade, or constrictive pericarditis.

Safety Alert   *It is important for the nurse to identify the normal right ventricular waveform (Figure 1-7), because a complication of the pulmonary artery (PA) catheter is potential displacement of the catheter tip into the right ventricle, causing ventricular ectopy. Immediate action to reposition the PA catheter should be performed. Some institutions*

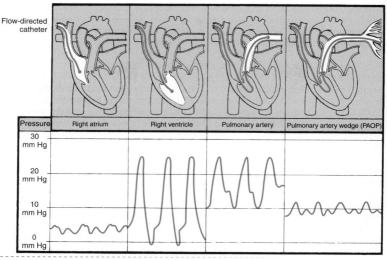

Figure 1-7 Location of catheter tip and waveforms obtained during insertion of pulmonary artery catheter. *PAOP*, Pulmonary artery occlusion pressure. (From Urden LD, Stacy KM, Lough ME: *Priorities in critical care nursing,* ed 5, St Louis, 2008, Mosby.)

may allow nurses to reposition the patient and inflate the PA catheter balloon so blood flow into the PA carries the catheter back into position, whereas others may be required to immediately pull the PA catheter back into the right atrium.

Pulmonary artery (PA) pressures

Multiple values are measured via the use of a PA catheter (see Table 1-10). PAP monitoring is used to evaluate heart function and pulmonary vascular status. PA catheters (e.g., Swan-Ganz, Opticath, and others) provide valuable information used to assess and treat life-threatening illness or injury. Blood volume, heart function, and tissue oxygenation can be assessed using various available pressures. PA catheters are inserted via the jugular, subclavian, brachial, or femoral vein and passed through the right side of the heart into the PA, where the tip of the catheter is positioned in the distal PA. The PA catheter should be positioned in zone 3 of the lung field, below the level of the left atrium to promote maximal accuracy of readings, given the effects of gravity on blood flow through the lungs.

PA pressures are normally one fifth of systemic BP. PA systolic (PAS), PA mean (PAM), and PA diastolic (PAD) pressures are monitored continuously by the distal port of the PA catheter, after the catheter is passed out of the right side of the heart, through the pulmonic valve, and into the PA. PAOP can be assessed after inflating the balloon on the distal end of the catheter, which allows it to float and "wedge" into a smaller branch of the PA. Once the artery is occluded by the balloon, the filling pressures of the left side of the heart can be indirectly measured. PAOP is often referred to as the PA wedge (PAW) pressure or occasionally the pulmonary capillary wedge pressure (PCWP) or, in general conversation, as the "wedge."

If a more sophisticated Svo_2 PA catheter is used, mixed venous O_2 saturation levels are also continuously monitored. CO can be measured intermittently using TD or, with some PA/Svo_2 catheters, is measured continuously. A full hemodynamic profile can also be calculated for the patient, including SV, stroke work, PVR, and SVR (see Table 1-10). All values are helpful in determining how to manage the patient's fluid balance, heart function, and vascular tone and can be individualized to the patient's body size (index values). There is ongoing research on the usefulness of indexing hemodynamic values to body weight in the morbidly obese population; no consensus has been formed. Abnormal PA pressures are discussed in

Table 1-12. Complications of PA catheters include ventricular or atrial dysrhythmias, pulmonary ischemia or infarction, valvular damage (tricuspid, pulmonic), PA rupture, infection, emboli (thrombotic, air, balloon), and pneumothorax. The incidence of PA catheter complications ranges from less than 1% to 3% and most are related to insertion.

PA systolic (PAS), diastolic (PAD), and mean pressures (PAM)

Normal PA pressures are 15 to 25/8 to 15 mm Hg (PAS/PAD) with PAM 10 to 20 mm Hg (Figure 1-8). The PA pressures are used to evaluate heart function and pulmonary vascular disease. In patients with healthy pulmonary vasculature, the PAD pressure corresponds closely to the PAOP and reflects the LVEDP. A significant difference (i.e., greater than 5 mm Hg) between the PAD and PAOP is seen with pulmonary disease or a pulmonary embolus. When this occurs, PA systolic and diastolic pressures are elevated, whereas the PAOP remains normal. Specific disease states that result in elevated PA pressures include pulmonary hypertension, pulmonary embolism, hypoxia, and LV failure resulting from valve disease, MI, cardiomyopathy, and left-to-right intracardiac shunt. Decreased PA pressures are seen with hypovolemia and pharmacologic preload reduction.

Pulmonary artery occlusive pressure (PAOP)

Normal mean PAOP is 6 to 12 mm Hg (Figure 1-9). The PAOP ("wedge pressure") reflects the LVEDP and is used to evaluate cardiac performance. PAOP does not accurately reflect LVEDP in patients with severe pulmonary hypertension. An elevated PAOP may be seen with LV failure, acute mitral regurgitation, acute VSD, and acute cardiac tamponade. A decreased PAOP is seen with hypovolemia and afterload reduction. On patients who are mechanically ventilated, positive end-expiratory pressure (PEEP) or continuous positive airway pressure (CPAP) settings of greater than 10 cm H_2O may result in falsely elevated PA pressures and PAOP. Regardless of the inaccuracy, patients should not be disconnected from the ventilator to measure PA pressures, because significant hypoxemia and inaccurate measurements can result. Correlation of measured pressures with the respiratory cycle improves the accuracy of these measurements.

Cardiac output (CO) and cardiac index (CI)

The normal CO value is 4 to 8 L/min. CO is the volume of blood in liters ejected by the heart each minute and is calculated as the product of the SV and the HR (CO = SV × HR). SV is the volume of blood ejected by the heart per beat. Normal SV is 55 to 100 mL/beat. The CO is commonly individualized in relation to body size by dividing the CO by the body surface area (BSA) to obtain the value known as the CI. The normal CI is 2.5 to 4 L/min/m². If continuous CO monitoring is done, the machine obtains an average CO that is recorded over 3-minute intervals and updated every 30 to 60 seconds. CCO monitoring closely and accurately monitors the patient's hemodynamic profile. Benefits of CCO monitoring may improve response to changes in output, resulting in improved outcomes for patients who are severely ill (e.g., cardiomyopathy, ejection fractions less than 20%). CO reflects the overall management of preload, afterload, contractility, and HR. The presence of intracardiac shunts renders CO measurements invalid, because pulmonary and systemic blood flows are erratic and unequal.

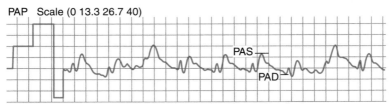

PAP   Scale (0 13.3 26.7 40)

PAS

PAD

Note: measurement at end expiration with patient receiving positive pressure ventilation

Figure 1-8 **Pulmonary artery pressure waveform.** (Redrawn from Daily E, Schroeder J: *Techniques in bedside hemodynamic monitoring*, ed 4, St Louis, 1989, Mosby.)

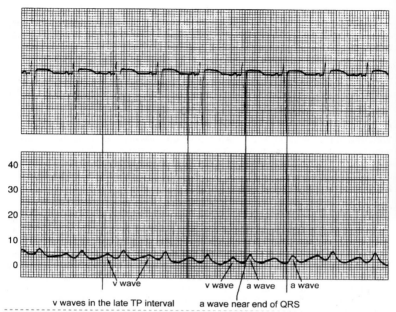

Figure 1-9 Pulmonary artery occlusive pressure waveform. (From American Association of Critical-Care Nurses (AACN): *AACN procedure manual for critical care,* ed 5, Philadelphia, 2005, Saunders.)

Left atrial pressure (LAP)

The normal value for LAP is 8 to 12 mm Hg. LAP is the most direct measure of the volume within the left ventricle at the end of diastole (LVEDP). LAP monitoring is not commonly used. A small, semirigid catheter is inserted into the left atrium during cardiac surgery and brought through the chest wall or epigastric area. Continuous monitoring of LVEDP may be indicated for the cardiac surgery patient with significant pulmonary hypertension. PAOP is no longer reflective of left-side heart function when severe pulmonary hypertension is present. Because the catheter enters directly into the left atrium, the patient is at high risk for air or tissue emboli. An in-line air filter should be added to the flush system to reduce the risk of air emboli. If the waveform pattern dampens, the catheter should be aspirated until blood is seen. If there is no blood return, consult the physician. It is not advisable to flush the LA catheter because of the risk of inducing arterial air embolism.

CALCULATED OR DERIVED MEASUREMENTS

All hemodynamic readings can be adjusted to body size by dividing the direct reading by the BSA. It is sometimes beneficial to use indexed values to gain a clearer idea of the normalcy of the hemodynamic profile. On first glance, a profile may appear relatively normal, but when indexed, numerous values are found out of normal range (see Table 1-10).

In addition to indexed values, various other calculations are done to help guide therapies (as follows).

Systemic vascular resistance (SVR)

The normal value for SVR is 800 to 1200 dynes/s/cm⁵. SVR is the major factor that determines LV afterload or resistance that must be overcome before LV ejection. The formula for SVR is: SVR = (MAP − CVP)/CO × 80.

Any factor that increases SVR will increase the workload of the heart and may reduce CO. Vasodilator therapy is used to reduce SVR to normal limits. A low SVR can indicate systemic vasodilation, commonly seen with septic, anaphylactic, and neurogenic shocks, and seen immediately postoperatively when recovering vascular tone. Vasopressors and IV fluids are administered to manage vasodilatation along with medications directed at the cause. Patients with low SVR often have high CO as a result of low resistance to ventricular ejection. Medications may affect SVR: norepinephrine, vasopressin, and phenylephrine (Neo-Synephrine) increase it, whereas isoproterenol, nifedipine, prostaglandins, sodium nitroprusside, and acetylcholine decrease it.

Pulmonary vascular resistance (PVR)

The normal value is 150 to 250 dynes/s/cm^5. PVR measures RV afterload or the resistance the right ventricle must overcome to eject into the pulmonary circulation. The formula for PVR is: PVR = (PAM − PAOP)/CO × 80.

PVR may be elevated as a result of primary pulmonary hypertension or secondary pulmonary hypertension resulting from mitral or aortic valve disease, congenital heart disease, long-standing LV heart failure, hypoxia, COPD, or pulmonary embolus. Medications may affect PVR: norepinephrine, vasopressin, and phenylephrine increase it, whereas isoproterenol, nifedipine, prostaglandins, sodium nitroprusside, and acetylcholine decrease it.

Mixed venous oxygen saturation

The normal range for Svo_2 is 60% to 80%. Svo_2 is defined as the average percentage of Hgb bound with O_2 in the venous blood, which infers the balance of O_2 supply and demand at the tissue level. Svo_2 reflects the global mixed venous oxygen saturation. Other specialized catheters can measure the venous oxygen saturation regionally. Svo_2 measures the mixed venous oxygen saturation from blood returned from the head and neck. This regional measurement correlates with Svo_2 and all of the considerations discussed with Svo_2 also apply to $Scvo_2$. Traditional belief was that hemodynamic stability and normal ABG levels meant O_2 delivery (DO_2) to tissues was adequate to meet and address cellular O_2 needs. As technology developed, it became clear that conventional methods were unable to measure cellular O_2 needs (O_2 demand) or use (O_2 consumption) by assessing O_2 delivery alone. With the development of monitors displaying Svo_2 continuously, the onset of O_2 supply/demand/consumption imbalance can be more readily identified. Svo_2 can be measured intermittently using mixed venous blood samples from the distal port of the PA catheter or continuously using a specialized fiber optic Svo_2 PA catheter. CO, Hgb level, and arterial O_2 saturation impact O_2 delivery. Svo_2 is reflective of O_2 delivery and consumption. If O_2 delivery is inadequate, or O_2 demand is high, more O_2 will be extracted from Hgb. If the patient is anemic, there are fewer red blood cells carrying oxyhemoglobin, thus more O_2 is extracted. If the patient has pulmonary disease, such as ARDS, O_2 saturation is less, thus less O_2 is delivered. Normal O_2 delivery is 600 mL O_2/min/m^2 if CO, Hgb level, and O_2 saturation (Sao_2 or Spo_2) are normal. Normal O_2 consumption ($\dot{V}o_2$), which should mirror demand, is 150 mL/min/m^2, which means 450 mL/min/m^2 of O_2 should be left in the red blood cells returning to the heart. In other words, approximately 25% of O_2 is used, leaving behind approximately 75%. The textbook normal value for Svo_2 is 0.75, or 75%. Very low levels (less than 30%) indicate poor perfusion and are often associated with lactic acidosis (see Acid-Base Balance). If the Svo_2 value changes by more than 10% for longer than 10 minutes, the nurse should evaluate Sao_2, CO, Hgb, and $\dot{V}o_2$. Svo_2 monitoring can be used to evaluate the effects of medical and nursing interventions on tissue O_2 use. By examining the variables involved in tissue oxygenation, the nurse can help determine which parameters may need to be better managed to meet the current metabolic demands (Table 1-13).

Stroke volume variability (SVV)

SVV is determined using the arterial waveform to calculate the change in SV from beat to beat of the heart. SVV can assist the clinician in assessment of the need for fluid replacement and the adequacy of the volume delivered. The normal range for SVV is 10% to 15% with the goal of therapy 13% or less.

Safety Alert   *The accuracy of stroke volume variability (SVV) has only been studied on patients with mechanically controlled ventilation. The SVV is not an accurate measurement when the patient is having dysrhythmias.*

Table 1-13	FACTORS AFFECTING MIXED VENOUS OXYGEN SATURATION

Svo_2 is a sensitive indicator of oxygen supply/demand balance. $Scvo_2$ will respond in the same manner as Svo_2. If Svo_2 decreases to less than 50%, the patient should be rapidly assessed for the cause of an increased oxygen demand, or decrease in supply. Anemia, hypoxemia, and decreased CO may result in markedly reduced oxygen delivery. In the presence of the high metabolic demands imposed by critical illness, a reduction in O_2 delivery or further increase in O_2 demand can produce profound instability in the patient. Changes in Svo_2 often precede overt changes reflective of physiologic instability.

Factor	Effect on Svo_2	Clinical Examples
Arterial Oxygen Saturation		
↑Sao_2	↑Svo_2	Supplemental oxygen
↓Sao_2		
	↓Svo_2	Reduced oxygen supply (e.g., ARDS, ET suctioning, removal of supplemental oxygen, pulmonary disease, asthma, respiratory failure, obstructive sleep apnea)
Cardiac Output		
↑CO	↑Svo_2	Administration of inotropes to increase contractility
↓CO	↓Svo_2	Dysrhythmias, increased SVR, MI, hypovolemia, ↑HR, or ↓HR
Hemoglobin		
↓Hgb	↓Svo_2	Hemorrhage, hemolysis, severe anemia in patients with cardiovascular disease
Oxygen Consumption		
↑Vo_2	↓Svo_2	States in which metabolic demand exceeds oxygen supply (e.g., shivering, seizures, hyperthermia, hyperdynamic states)
↓Vo_2	↑Svo_2	States in which there is failure of peripheral tissue to extract or use oxygen. Significant peripheral arteriovenous shunting: cirrhosis, renal failure. Redistribution of blood away from beds where oxygen extraction occurs: sepsis, acute pancreatitis, major burns. Blockage of oxygen uptake or use: cyanide poisoning (including nitroprusside toxicity), carbon monoxide poisoning.
Mechanical problems	↑Svo_2	Wedged PA catheter creates falsely elevated Svo_2

ARDS, Acute respiratory distress syndrome; *CO,* cardiac output; *ET,* endotracheal; *Hgb,* hemoglobin; *HR,* heart rate; *MI,* myocardial infarction; *PA,* pulmonary artery; *SVR,* systemic vascular resistance.

COLLABORATIVE MANAGEMENT

The need for accuracy of hemodynamic values cannot be stressed enough. Making clinical decisions based on these values and the calculations derived from them is the reason for using hemodynamic monitoring in patients who are critically ill. Continuous monitoring of hemodynamic and oxygen use values allow the clinical team to see trends so that they can intervene earlier and accurately monitor response to treatment.

CARE PRIORITIES

1. Promote patient safety by meticulously managing the monitoring system, assessing the pressure readings/waveforms, and assessing the patient (see Table 1-11).

- Ensure proper setup and maintenance of the pressure monitoring system. Assessment of PAOP provides information about the blood being pumped from the left side of the heart, as does the CO. In combination with BP readings, the values frame the treatment plan. Configuration of normal waveforms must be understood so that abnormalities can be recognized, analyzed, and managed.
- Assess for proper system compliance. Before initiating monitoring, and any time over-damping or underdamping is suspected, square wave testing is done to assess proper compliance within the system, which is essential for accurate readings.
- Prevent pulmonary infarction. A continuous PAOP waveform with the balloon deflated indicates that the catheter has migrated distally and is lodged in a small pulmonary vessel. The chest radiograph may reveal that the catheter is visible beyond the mediastinal structures, which indicates that the catheter has passed too far into the distal pulmonary circulation. The catheter should be repositioned immediately according to institutional protocol to avoid damage to the surrounding lung tissues.
- Prevent limb ischemia. Before radial artery catheter insertion, the practitioner should perform the Allen test to ensure that the ulnar artery is pulsatile. Maintaining all arterial lines should include a neurovascular assessment distal to the catheter.
- Prevent RV irritation by the catheter. RV waveform instead of the PA wave indicates improper positioning. The catheter should be repositioned according to institutional protocol to avoid ventricular dysrhythmias.

2. Recognize and manage the complications associated with hemodynamic monitoring equipment.

- Complications of arterial catheters: Arterial thrombosis with ischemia, infection, infiltration, and blood loss caused by disconnection. Continuous observation of the arterial line insertion site for infection and leakage is an essential nursing responsibility. Monitor and document pulses distal to the catheter site every 1 to 2 hours. It is important to note the patient's baseline BP and to compare left and right cuff BPs with arterial BPs. Meticulous care should be taken with setup and maintenance of the arterial pressure monitoring system. If air enters a peripheral arterial catheter, the distal structures (e.g., hand, leg) are at highest risk for ischemic complications caused by air bubbles lodging in smaller arterial vessels.
- Suspected air embolus: Complications are seen more frequently from venous air emboli, which may happen during any central catheter insertion, including PA catheters. Symptoms include acute respiratory distress, apnea, possible wheezing, sudden hypotension, syncope, hypoxia, cyanosis, possible murmur, elevated CVP, neurologic deficits, cardiac arrest with asystole, pulseless electrical activity (PEA), or ventricular fibrillation. Arterial monitoring systems connected to intraaortic balloon catheters can cause life-threatening air embolism in the central circulation, including the aorta, but this is rarely seen in clinical practice.

HIGH ALERT! Suspected Air Embolus

The patient should immediately be placed in left lateral Trendelenburg (head down) position and 100% O_2 administered. Have the patient try to perform a Valsalva maneuver. Aspirate air from the system: intravenous tubing, arterial line tubing, or the catheter itself. If severe complications ensue, hyperbaric O_2 treatment using the Diving Accident Protocol may be used if available. Perform cardiopulmonary resuscitation if necessary. Air can cause stroke or death in the patient.

---

3. Recognize the characteristics of normal waveforms and pressure readings.

- **Arterial pressure waveform:** The upstroke on arterial pressure waveform represents the rapid ejection phase of ventricular systole. The anacrotic shoulder (rounded peak) is where the systolic pressure is measured. The descent represents slowed ventricular ejection followed by aortic valve closure represented by the dicrotic notch, followed by runoff of flow systemically during diastole. Diastolic pressure is measured as the end-diastolic pressure just before the next systole (see Figure 1-5).

- **PA waveform:** Has the same waveform components as arterial pressure, except that the dicrotic notch represents pulmonic valve closure, followed by runoff flow in the pulmonary vasculature during diastole. The PA pressure measurements are taken at the peak systolic and end-diastolic pressures (see Figure 1-8).
- **End-expiratory pressures:** Care must be taken to measure and record all end-expiratory pressures. With positive-pressure ventilation, these will be at the low point of the wave. With spontaneous ventilation, end-expiratory pressures are higher than pressure during inspiration. One must be careful not to import or just assume that the digital average is an accurate reading. Readings must be done at end expiration; as with respiratory fluctuations, values can be off 10 to 20 mm Hg. To assure accuracy, measurements should be obtained from a graphic tracing with simultaneous ECG tracing for proper waveform identification.
- **RAP, CVP, and PAOP waveforms:** Are composed of an *a-wave*, followed by an *x* descent; a *c-wave* may look like a notch on the *a-wave* or may be a separate wave, followed by a *v-wave*, and this is followed by the *y* descent (see Figure 1-6). The a-wave represents atrial systole, the *c-wave* if present represents valvular closure, the *x* descent is atrial relaxation, and the *v-wave* is produced by atrial filling during ventricular systole as the atrioventricular valve bulges toward the atrium when the ventricle contracts. The *c-wave* is not commonly seen in the PAOP waveform as a result of the time of retrograde transmission (see Figure 1-9).
- **Timing waveforms with the ECG:** The a-wave and v-wave are distinguished by their timing with the ECG. The electrical conduction of the heart occurs before mechanical contraction. This is why the RAP/CVP a-wave is found just before the QRS and the v-wave is found at the T wave. The PAOP wave has farther to travel to be transmitted; therefore, the a-wave follows the QRS and the v-wave is found after the T wave and before the next P wave (see Figure 1-6).
- **Cannon waves and large v-waves:** ECG correlations are important diagnostic adjuncts, because a-waves are absent in an atrioventricular junctional or idioventricular rhythm. Large, abnormal a-waves called cannon waves are caused by the atria trying to contract against a closed AV valve, which may occur during atrial fibrillation and complete heart block. PAOP with a large v-wave is an indication of mitral insufficiency.
- **Inflating the PAOP balloon:** When obtaining the PAOP, the PA catheter balloon should be inflated slowly with no more than 1.5 mL of air. The PA waveform should be observed changing to a smaller PAOP/wedge waveform. No additional air should be used once the change has begun. Once the PAOP has been obtained, the balloon should be deflated passively; the syringe is removed and emptied of air, and then reattached to prevent accidental balloon inflation (see Figures 1-7 and 1-9).

HIGH ALERT!   Pulmonary Artery Rupture and Occlusion

Overwedging or rapid balloon inflation can cause pulmonary artery (PA) rupture. Prolonged balloon inflation or PA catheter migration can lead to balloon rupture, as well as clot formation and pulmonary infarction. Pulmonary artery occlusive pressure (PAOP) may be assessed less frequently if a strong correlation is established between the PAOP and the PA diastolic to avoid repeated trauma to the pulmonary vessels and to prolong the life of the balloon. The PA waveform must be continually monitored to observe for distal migration of the catheter, or proximal displacement resulting from pulling on the catheter or movement of the external monitoring system during patient care procedures (see Table 1-11).

CARE PLANS FOR HEMODYNAMIC MONITORING

Deficient knowledge *related to the rationale for hemodynamic monitoring and procedure for catheter insertion*

- -

Goals/Outcomes: Before and during catheter placement, the patient or significant other states that they are comfortable with the rationale for hemodynamic monitoring, procedure for insertion of lines, and sensations that are experienced during and after the procedure.

NOC Knowledge: Treatment Regimen.

Teaching: Procedure/Treatment
1. Assess the patient's knowledge about hemodynamic monitoring. As indicated, explain to the patient/family that hemodynamic monitoring measures BP within the body and BP within the heart and lungs, and gives information about the pumping action of the heart, which is useful in guiding therapy.
2. Teach the patient about the insertion procedure, emphasizing that a local anesthetic agent will be used, he or she will not be able to move during the procedure, and, following the procedure, a dressing will be applied to the insertion site. For radial arterial lines, explain that an arm board or other device may be used to immobilize the wrist. For PA and central lines, explain that a large drape is placed over the body and face during insertion and a chest radiograph will be obtained following the procedure.
3. Explain that unusual sensations may be felt during the procedure and that a nurse will be present to hold his or her hand, offer support should they have questions, and be able to administer supplemental medications to promote their comfort. Depending on the situation, a clue to the next sensation anticipated is best rendered during the procedure, such as, "You may feel coolness from the cleansing solution" or, "You may feel a 'bee sting' from injection of the local anesthetic" or, "You may feel pressure as the catheter advances."

Risk for ineffective cardiac tissue perfusion *related to complications from PA catheter presence in the pulmonary circulation*

This includes circulatory impairment from migration of PA catheter into a wedged position, "overwedging" of the catheter balloon, PA rupture, pulmonary vascular thrombosis, or other patient safety hazards associated with the monitoring system.
Goals/Outcomes: Within 15 minutes of recognizing a complication with the hemodynamic monitoring system, the problem is addressed and resolved.
NOC Tissue Perfusion: Cardiac; Tissue Perfusion: Peripheral; Tissue Perfusion: Pulmonary.

Hemodynamic Regulation
1. Monitor the PA waveform continuously. Report any change in configuration, particularly if the waveform becomes decreased in amplitude and flattened in appearance (see Table 1-11).
2. Assess the patient for decreased pulmonary arterial blood flow, as evidenced by acute onset of pleuritic chest pain, SOB, tachypnea, and hemoptysis.
3. Evaluate the position of the catheter via chest radiograph according to institutional protocol. Never push the PA catheter forward in the PA to avoid possibility of PA rupture or lodging the catheter in a small vessel.
4. Record the position of the PA catheter when inserted. Assess and record this level every shift. If there is a change in the waveform, catheter position should be reassessed. The advanced practice provider should be notified for catheters that are out of position or fail to wedge.
5. Exercise care in taking PAOP measurements. Prolonged and repeated readings can cause trauma to the vessel wall. The catheter can also be "overwedged." Proper wedging entails slow injection of enough air to obtain a wedge configuration, but no more than the amount recommended by the catheter manufacturer. Never pull back on the plunger of a balloon syringe to remove air; rather, disconnect the syringe and allow passive deflation of the balloon.
6. Verify and document PAD and PAOP* every 4 to 8 hours. PAD may exceed PAOP by ≥ 5 mm Hg in patients with acidosis, hypoxemia, pulmonary emboli, lung disease, and pulmonary hypertension. If the PAD approximates the PAOP, the frequency of PAOP readings may be able to be reduced in some practice settings, to preserve the catheter balloon and reduce the possibility of vessel erosion. *Note: In some institutions routine PAOP readings are not performed and in certain settings the nurse may not perform this function. Please refer to the institutional policy concerning hemodynamic monitoring.
7. Consult the advanced practice provider if the PA waveform remains in wedged position after balloon deflation. This may indicate that the catheter has lodged in the vessel, which can lead to pulmonary infarction resulting from lack of perfusion distal to the lodged catheter.
8. Pay special attention to the PA waveform when the patient is moved (e.g., when being taken to the radiology department; getting into a chair, when position is changed or bed is made). The monitoring system may no longer be appropriately leveled with the patient's phlebostatic axis (RA level) after the patient has changed position. Assess the catheter position to ensure that the catheter has not moved. Also ensure the catheter is not pulled on when moving the patient.

Ineffective protection *related to inability to control internal responses and external threats posed by the presence of invasive hemodynamic catheters*

Goals/Outcomes: The patient is free of infection, as evidenced by normothermia, white blood cell (WBC) count <11,000/mm³, negative culture results, and absence of erythema, heat, swelling, or purulent drainage at the insertion site.

NOC Immune Status Uncompromised.

Infection Protection

1. Before insertion, full barrier precautions should be in place according to institution protocol. Central line catheter insertion and dressing changes are to be done with strict adherence to sterile technique. Following a central line bundle checklist is recommended.
2. On a daily basis, monitor for temperature elevations >37.7° C (100° F) and WBC count elevation.
3. Monitor the catheter insertion site for erythema, tenderness to the touch, local warmth, and purulent drainage.
4. Use normal saline rather than D₅W for hemodynamic flush solution, because dextrose solutions better support bacterial growth.
5. Change hemodynamic tubing, transducer, and flush solution according to hospital protocol.
6. Maintain a closed system from the transducer to the flush solution and the patient. Keep all external openings and stopcocks securely capped at all times.
7. Use a closed system for CO injection fluid.
8. Maintain an occlusive, dry sterile dressing over the insertion site. As prescribed, obtain a culture of any suspicious drainage and report positive findings.
9. Change the central/PA line dressing according to hospital protocol, using aseptic technique.
10. Record the date of catheter insertion: Ensure that the catheter is changed according to agency protocol.
11. If the line becomes infected, notify the advanced practice provider. The catheter should be removed and the catheter tip cut off and then sent in a sterile container for a culture and sensitivity test.

Safety Alert *Central venous pressure monitoring is the recommended monitoring strategy during early goal-directed therapy recommended by the Society of Critical Care Medicine, for patients with sepsis. Line sepsis may be masked as a potential cause of current infection. The lines should be changed only as needed unless reddened, white blood cells are increasing, or the patient is febrile. Most central lines are able to remain in place for 7 days; but should be removed as soon as possible when central access or monitoring is no longer needed.*

Ineffective peripheral tissue perfusion (involved extremity) *related to interrupted blood flow secondary to presence of arterial catheter or thrombosis caused by the catheter.*

Goals/Outcomes: Within 15 minutes of this diagnosis, the patient has adequate perfusion to affected extremity, as evidenced by brisk capillary refill (less than 2 seconds), natural color, warm skin, normal sensation, and the ability to move the fingers.

NOC Circulation Status.

Circulatory Precautions

1. Continuously monitor capillary refill, color, temperature, sensation, pulses, and movement. Be alert to indicators of ischemia and teach them to the patient, stressing the importance of notifying staff members promptly if they occur.
2. Maintain arterial line on continuous flush at 3 mL/h with normal saline with the pressure bag inflated to 300 mm Hg. Heparinized saline is infrequently used, as it has not been shown to be significantly more effective at maintaining patency, when all other measures of pressure monitoring are done.
3. Ensure tight connections of tubing throughout the system.
4. Support the patient's wrist or appropriate extremity with an arm board or other supportive device to prevent flexion and movement of the catheter.

Ineffective protection *related to potential for insertion complications secondary to ventricular irritability, patient movement during insertion procedure, or difficult anatomy.*

Goals/Outcomes: The patient has no complications from PA or CVP catheter insertion, as evidenced by normal sinus rhythm on ECG, BP within the patient's normal range, HR <100 bpm, RR <20 breaths/min with normal pattern and depth, normal breath sounds, and absence of adventitious breath sounds or muffled heart sounds.

NOC Circulation Status.

Risk Identification

1. Use patient safety precautions used for any invasive procedures to conduct a preprocedure verification process; mark the correct site and use of "Time Out" to assure patient safety.
2. During preprocedure teaching, caution the patient about the importance of remaining still during insertion of the catheter. Provide sedation and analgesics as prescribed.
3. Perform a baseline assessment, monitoring BP, HR, RR, breath sounds, heart sounds, and ECG.
4. Be alert to decreased BP, pulsus paradoxus, increased HR or RR, diminished or absent breath sounds, and muffled heart sounds, as well as dysrhythmias on ECG. Report any significant findings to the physician or midlevel practitioner.
5. Perform a postprocedure assessment, comparing it with baseline findings. After the procedure, obtain a chest radiograph as prescribed.
6. Monitor for catheter-related complications (see Table 1-11).
7. Keep amiodarone or lidocaine at bedside for immediate IV injection if the patient has sustained ventricular dysrhythmias. This precaution should be rarely required.

MECHANICAL VENTILATION

Mechanical ventilation provides assistance with movement of gases in and out of the lungs to facilitate blood-alveolar clearance of CO_2 and uptake of O_2 into the blood. For ventilation to be effective, the nervous system must be intact, the diaphragm and respiratory muscle groups must contract, the rib cage must be intact, the external fibrous level of the pleural sac must be attached to the rib cage, and intrapleural or intraalveolar pressures should be normal. This combination of conditions decreases the alveolar resting pressures, promoting a pressure gradient that facilitates gas movement into the conducting tubes that ultimately distends (recruits) the alveoli.

Spontaneous ventilation (whether or not supported) depends on the ability to generate alveolar distention, or negative pressure, and therefore increases compliance. This is referred to as increasing alveolar compliance (static compliance), a decreasing alveolar pressure (p_{Plat}), or negative pressure breathing. There are other conditions required for patients to generate negative pressure and breathe spontaneously (Box 1-12). When patients are too weak to generate adequate force (negative pressure), too weak to maintain their airway, too sick or sedated to stimulate and contract the diaphragm, or when the conducting airways or the alveolar units are constricted, collapsed, or congested (Box 1-13), ventilator support may be unavoidable. To ensure optimal care of the patient who requires mechanical ventilation, the practitioner must have adequate knowledge of the equipment and processes involved in mechanical ventilation. An exhaustive review of mechanical ventilation is not possible in this chapter; however, basic concepts must be addressed.

REVIEW OF BASIC VENTILATION TERMS

RESPIRATORY RATE (RR OR f [FREQUENCY OF BREATHING])

- Charted as breaths per minute.
- The frequency of breaths enabled by the patient and/or delivered by the ventilator may range from 10 to 50 bpm depending on ventilation strategies, except during weaning, when the frequency of breaths may be less than 10 to augment, rather than fully support, breathing.

Box 1-12	FACTORS AFFECTING NORMAL SPONTANEOUS VENTILATION

1. Having intact phrenic nerve innervation of the diaphragm
2. Ability of the diaphragm and external intercostals to maintain the appropriate contractile force
3. Ability to maintain a patent airway
4. Diameter of the airway
5. Ability of the alveoli to open during inspiration

Box 1-13	CONDITIONS THAT MAY REQUIRE VENTILATOR SUPPORT

Acute obstructive disease: acute severe asthma; airway mucosal edema

Altered ventilatory drive: hypothyroidism; intracranial hemorrhage; dyspnea-related anxiety

Atelectasis: acute respiratory distress syndrome; pneumonia

Burns and smoke inhalation: inhalation injury, surface burns

Cancer: malnutrition; infections

Cardiopulmonary problems: congestive heart failure; pulmonary hemorrhage

Chest trauma: blunt injury; flail chest; penetrating injuries

Chronic obstructive pulmonary disease: emphysema, chronic bronchitis, asthma; cystic fibrosis; bronchiectasis

Fatigue/atrophy: muscle overuse; disuse

Head/spinal cord injury: medullary brainstem injury; Cheyne-Stokes breathing; neurogenic pulmonary edema

Neuromuscular disease: amyotrophic lateral sclerosis; Guillain-Barré syndrome; myasthenia gravis

Postoperative conditions: cardiac and thoracic surgeries

Pharmacologic agents/drug overdose: muscle relaxants; barbiturates; Ca^{2+} channel blockers; long-term adrenocorticosteroids; aminoglycoside antibiotics

TIDAL VOLUME (V_T)

* Volume (amount) of gas delivered with each preset breath. Controversy exists regarding use of lung protective tidal volumes on all patients, versus those solely with noncompliant lung conditions. Predicted body weight (PBW) is often used to calculate Vt, rather than ideal body weight (IBW). The formula is as follows: Males: PBW (kg) = 50 + 2.3 (height [in] – 60); Females: PBW (kg) = 45.5 + 2.3 (height [in] – 60). PBW and IBW are similar values.
* In patients who are mechanically ventilated, V_T is usually set at 8 mL/kg PBW according to the National Heart, Lung, and Blood Institute ARDS Network (www.ardsnet.org).
* V_T decreases to 6 mL/kg IDBW or PBW if the patient has a noncompliant lung condition.
  * Many clinicians have successfully used strategies to treat ARDS by reducing the delivered tidal volume (from 8 to 10 mL/kg IBW to 4 to 6 mL/kg IBW) balanced with an RR (12 to 35) necessary to maintain adequate minute ventilation. Lung-protective ventilator strategies are considered standard practice in the care of patients with ARDS. Level of positive end expiratory pressure (PEEP) and fraction of inspired oxygen (FIO_2) are adjusted in tandem with Vt to provide the most effective gas exchange, while helping to reduce the incidence of ventilator induced lung injury.
* Charted as: V_T or tidal volume (i.e., 375 mL/breath).

MINUTE VENTILATION (V_E V_{TE} or $\dot{MV}$)

* The amount of volume exhaled per minute (V_E or V_{TE}).
* Measured as: Respirations $\times$ V_{TE} (MV).
* Normal is 8 to 10 L/min.

FRACTION OF INSPIRED OXYGEN (FIO_2)

* Percent of atmospheric pressure (760 mm Hg) that is O_2.
* For example, 0.21 or 21% is calculated as: 0.21 $\times$ 760 mm Hg = 159 mm Hg P_{atmos} O_2.
* For simplicity, documented as FIO_2 use the decimal (0.21) in P/F calculations or the calculated pressure in $A\text{-}aDo_2$ calculations.

PEAK INSPIRATORY PRESSURE (PIP)

* Peak pressure measured when the tidal volume is pushed into the airways. The value is also called peak airway pressure (PAP).
* Value used to set high-pressure and low-pressure alarm limits.

- In normal lungs (resistance and compliance normal) less than 35 cm H_2O.
- In any condition that increases resistance or decreases compliance, may be greater than 35 cm H_2O.

MEAN AIRWAY PRESSURE
- Average proximal airway pressure during the entire respiratory cycle; a major determinate for oxygenation and a focus for the settings of alternative ventilation.

PRESSURE MEASURED DURING INSPIRATORY HOLD ($p_{Plateau}$ or P_{Plat})
- Airway pressure measured during an inspiratory hold after a volume-controlled breath.
- Used to determine the patient's static lung compliance.
- Normally less than 25 cm H_2O.

FLOW RATE (V̇)
- The delivery method and rate of speed for the tidal volume breath (also affects time spent in inspiration versus exhalation, as well as pressure reached).
- Normally 40 to 60 L/min.

 Safety Alert *All airway pressures, including peak inspiratory pressure, pulmonary artery wedge pressure, and $p_{Plateau}$, are measured by changing the tidal volume, airway resistance, and peak inspiratory flow rate. Pressures are also significantly affected by alterations in lung compliance.*

TRIGGER: WHAT STARTS A BREATH? INSPIRATORY FLOW BEGINS
- Elapsed time: How many breaths per minute?
- Patient effort: Negative inspiratory force: The patient's effort can be "sensed" as a change in pressure or a change in flow (in the circuit).

SENSITIVITY
- A setting on the ventilator that adjusts how much negative inspiratory pressure the patient must generate (see Patient effort) before the ventilator delivers a breath. Is activated only in assist-control ventilation (ACMV) or synchronized intermittent mandatory ventilation (SIMV).

CYCLE: WHAT STOPS A BREATH? INSPIRATORY FLOW ENDS
1. Pressure cycle: A predetermined and preset pressure terminates inspiration. Pressure is constant/volume is variable. Used for pressure control ventilation.
2. Volume cycle: A predetermined and preset volume when delivered terminates the inspiration. Volume is constant/pressure is variable. Used for volume control ventilation.
3. Time cycle: Delivers air/gas over a set time after which the inspiration ends (affects the I:E)—inspiratory time/exhalation time (I:E).
   - Directly related to how rapidly or slowly the flow of tidal volume occurs.
   - Directly related to the pressure achieved when volume is delivered at a certain rate of speed.
4. I:E time examples.
   - If an assumed tidal volume of 400 mL/breath is delivered at a flow rate (rate of speed) of 80 L/min, either volume or pressure control limits will be reached rapidly and "inspiratory (I) time" will be shorter and "exhalation (E) time" will be longer. This strategy is used in compliant lungs when CO_2 retention or ventilator dyssynchrony is evaluated.
   - If an assumed tidal volume of 400 mL/breath is delivered at a flow rate (rate of speed) of 40 L/min, either volume or pressure control limits will be reached over a longer period of time and "I time" will be longer and "E time" will be shorter. This strategy may be used to recruit alveoli when lungs are noncompliant and hypoxemia is the problem, that is, low oxygen and high pressures are an issue. The expectation is that the pressure generated when the tidal volume flows will be lower.

- If an assumed tidal volume of 400 mL/breath is delivered at a flow rate (rate of speed) of 100 L/min, either volume or pressure control limits will be reached over a shorter period of time and "I time" will be shorter and "E time" will be longer. This strategy may be used to allow for more time to exhale and is generally used if the expectation is that the pressure generated when the tidal volume flows will be lower, but that the patient's major problem is alveolar recoil (i.e., COPD disease).

NEGATIVE PRESSURE VENTILATION

Normal intrapleural pressure ranges from -2 (rest) to -10 cm H_2O (inspiration). Negative pressure ventilators generate subatmospheric pressure to the thorax and trunk (similar to applying an external vacuum) to initiate respiration and do not require intubation for use. The iron lung, chest cuirass shell, and poncho chest shell are examples. Because these devices are noninvasive and do not require intensive monitoring, there has been a resurgence of interest in their use for long-term home therapy. They are not discussed here.

POSITIVE-PRESSURE VENTILATION

All methods of mechanical ventilation require a means of administering positive pressure for delivery of a predetermined volume of gas. Positive-pressure ventilation creates a super atmospheric pressure (greater than 760 mm Hg), which is generated at the upper airway. The resultant pressure gradient between the upper airway and the alveoli then allows for the "pushing" gas volume. This delivery system may be administered via a mask system (noninvasive) or invasively via an ET tube or tracheostomy. The concept, put very simply, is to decrease the need for the development of a significant negative pressure or force, supplanting that requirement with the super atmospheric pressure.

NONINVASIVE POSITIVE-PRESSURE VENTILATION (NiPPV or NPPV)

Positive-pressure support may be administered via a face mask, nasal mask, helmet, or mouth seal. This may also be presented as CPAP or BiPAP. The early application of NPPV or noninvasive mechanical ventilation (NIMV) may enhance respiratory rescue and may be applied by trained providers outside of ICU. Indications include airway obstruction disorders, chest wall disease, neuromuscular weakness, and sleep-related breathing disorders. Currently, NPPV is contraindicated in patients who cannot protect their airway or clear secretions and those with severe agitation or shock. NPPV may allow patients to maintain normal functions, such as speaking and eating, and assists in the avoidance of the risks and complications of intubation and sedation. Patients who are severely distressed may be dependent on the system, and may be unable to remove the system to eat or drink without deterioration. Consideration for additional support is needed when patients cannot remove the system for short periods of time.

1. CPAP: A mode of assistance with positive pressure via application of a constant pressure to the airways. This method does not supply any volume breath, but rather maintains airway and alveolar opening to facilitate inspiration and decrease collapse during exhalation. Very similar in concept and design to methods applied for sleep apnea.
2. BiPAP: A mode of ventilatory assistance that uses alternating inspiratory positive pressures (IPAP) and expiratory positive pressures (EPAP) to enhance variable spontaneous tidal volumes. The resistance and compliance of the airways will determine the IPAP "driving pressure" necessary to produce a desired tidal volume. The level of EPAP needed is based on the oxygenation status of the patient. The physician determines a tidal volume goal (usually 8 to 12 mL/kg) and an oxygenation goal the clinician will use to determine the titration range for IPAP, EPAP, and FIO_2. BiPAP (may be referred to as BiLevel) mode can be found on many conventional ventilators and on freestanding units used for NPPV.

INVASIVE MECHANICAL VENTILATION

When endotracheal intubation is required (Box 1-14), the oral route is generally preferred to nasal, to reduce incidence of sinusitis. After intubation, the nurse or respiratory therapist should do the following:

1. Confirm the placement of the ET tube using a CO_2 detector and then auscultate for bilateral breath sounds.
2. Mark and chart the centimeter mark on the tube using the teeth as a reference point.

Box 1-14	REASONS TO CONSIDER INTUBATION
Severe acidosis or hypoxemia	Aspiration risk
Severe dyspnea	Copious/viscous secretions
Respiratory arrest	Recent facial trauma
Cardiovascular instability	Extreme obesity

3. Secure the tube to the face and head.
4. Cut/shorten the tube to reduce dead space, taking care not to cut the pilot balloon, so only 4 cm protrudes from the teeth.
5. Over the next 4 hours, monitor for the development of a life-threatening tension pneumothorax, by assessing for hypoxia, bradycardia, tachycardia, and moderate to life-threatening hypotension.

BASIC VENTILATION MODES

ASSIST-CONTROL VENTILATION (A/C or ACV)

This mode can be used with either volume of gas or pressure within the patient/ventilation system as the limit used to end inspiration, or breath limit. In assist-control (often labeled "volume control," or "pressure control"), patients may receive either ventilator-controlled or ventilator-assisted breaths. The set rate will deliver breaths in a time line (i.e., rate of 12 ventilator delivers breaths 12 times per minute). In addition, when the patient generates a natural breath, the machine senses the negative-pressure event (sensitivity set on the ventilator), which triggers the ventilator to deliver a breath of identical duration and magnitude as the mandatory breath. The patient receives a breath each time a spontaneous breath is initiated, regardless of actual minute ventilation requirement. The "interactive" feature of this mode is that the patient receives a breath when he or she generates enough negative pressure to turn the ventilator on. The advantage of this mode is that patients breathe spontaneously with small amounts of work. Conventional assist-control (A/C) delivers a preset breath based on time intervals (defined by frequency). The inspiratory flow rate is measured in liters per minute, and it determines how quickly the breath is delivered. The time required to complete inspiration is determined by the tidal volume delivered and the flow rate: $T_i = V_T/Flow$ rate. The breath is limited by reaching either the preset volume (volume control [VC]) or pressure (when volume is delivered reaching a predetermined pressure [pressure control, PC]). Every breath is controlled (either pressure or volume), but the patient may take more breaths than the mandatory rate determines (Table 1-14).

ALL breaths in ACMV are ventilator-assisted: Set rate plus patient-generated request (effort).

Ventilator rate + Patient request rate = Total respiratory rate

Every breath, whether ventilator-determined or patient-requested, is a ventilator breath and predetermined for either pressure or volume control.

Table 1-14	VOLUME-CONTROLLED VERSUS PRESSURE-CONTROLLED MECHANICAL VENTILATION	
Volume Control	**Pressure Control**
Volume delivery constant	Volume delivery varies
Inspiratory pressure varies	Inspiratory pressure constant
Inspiratory flow constant	Inspiratory flow varies
Inspiratory time determined by set flow and V_T	Inspiratory time set by clinician

> **Safety Alert** *Control mode should never be deliberately set because ventilators should never be insensitive to a patient's inspiratory effort. New ventilators do not incorporate a pure "control" method, although the rate predetermined by the provider in conjunction with sedation and analgesic management will essentially "control" the patient. Controlling ventilation is related to the context and must be attributable to the loss of sympathetic and parasympathetic drive (i.e., spinal cord injury) or pharmacologic control.*

SYNCHRONIZED INTERMITTENT MANDATORY VENTILATION (SIMV)

Delivers a preset mandatory volume-controlled or pressure-controlled breath at a preset rate. The patient can also breathe spontaneously (at his or her own rate with a variable tidal volume and pressure) between mandatory ventilator breaths from a flow-by circuit. The difference between ACMV and SIMV is that in SIMV the patient may take spontaneous nonventilated breaths between the required ventilator breaths. In addition, the ventilator is synchronized to deliver the mandatory breath (controlled volume or pressure) when the patient initiates inspiration; however, if time is reached when mandatory breath must be administered, it will be done even if the patient has not initiated his or her own negative inspiratory effort. SIMV is generally administered in conjunction with pressure support, which is applied on spontaneous flow-by breaths.

Only set rate breaths in SIMV are ventilator-assisted: Set rate plus patient-generated request (effort).

Ventilator rate + Patient request rate = Total respiratory rate

Only set breath is a ventilator breath and predetermined for either pressure or volume control. All patient breaths are volume/pressure variable.

> **Safety Alert** *All providers should analyze the methods and modes of ventilation support and consider the use of synchronized intermittent mandatory ventilation and the flow rate before administration of sedatives to control the patient and/or reduce their efforts. Frequently, agitation will be present if the flow rate of the gas is too low or if the patient feels like he or she cannot control his or her own breathing. After consideration of flow and mode, sedation may be used to decrease respiratory drive, and machine sensitivity should be adjusted to prevent hyperventilation in patients whose respiratory rate increases because of mild anxiety or neurologic factors. Assist-control ventilation has effectively replaced controlled ventilation, because the control of respiratory efforts must be performed pharmacologically and not mechanically.*

PRESSURE SUPPORT VENTILATION (PSV)

PSV augments or supports the patient's spontaneous inspiration with a preselected pressure level. Pressure is applied (via flow of gas) at the initiation of inspiration and ends when a minimum inspiratory flow rate is reached. The patient retains control over inspiratory and expiratory time, frequency, tidal volume, and spontaneous minute ventilation. PSV creates less patient discomfort and diaphragmatic stress than assist-control or SIMV alone. Compensating for resistance created by the demand valve or ET tube size decreases inspiratory work. PSV MUST be combined with SIMV to improve patient tolerance of mechanical ventilation, to overcome the resistance offered by the ET tube (tube compensation), and to decrease the work of breathing through the ET tube. PSV is often used to facilitate weaning from mechanical ventilation.

These two methods are flow-triggered/limited and (pressure) and volume-controlled. In ACMV when the patient takes a breath, the controlled method (volume) turns on. In SIMV when the patient takes a breath, the breath may either be a synchronized ventilator breath or a spontaneous volume breath.

Mode and method of ventilation should be determined by patient need and provider expertise rather than by individual bias.

BREATH LIMIT

- Time limited or cycled: Relates to time that inspiratory flow is administered and is determined by a preset time or percent of cycle that relates to inspiration. Inspiratory time is increased to deliver a volume-controlled or pressure-controlled breath over a longer time of the breath cycle. Depending on the manufacturer, inspiratory (I) and expiratory (E) times or flow rate may be the direct setting to adjust. In either case, the provider may maintain the tidal volume, minute ventilation, and frequency when adjusting the E time. I time is increased to deliver a volume-controlled or pressure-controlled breath over a longer time of the breath cycle. This will affect the frequency and therefore the tidal volume delivered. This may be used for noncompliant lungs and alveolar recruitment to promote better oxygenation and is referred to as inverse I to E.
- Pressure controlled (PC): The peak inspiratory pressure (PIP) is preset based on the estimated tidal volume requirements. A smaller tidal volume may be given if the preset pressure is reached too soon, such as in a state of low compliance or high airway resistance.
- Volume control (VC): Volume is preset and the pressure is variable to deliver the preset volume. The PIP seen at the end of inspiration is higher under conditions of low compliance and/or high airway resistance.

A comparison of ventilator strategies and variables is available in Table 1-15.

Safety Alert *Airway pressure and lung volumes have a DIRECT impact on the intrathoracic pressure, which then may decrease blood flow and blood pressure and INDIRECTLY affect different organ systems.*

BASIC VENTILATION ADJUNCTS

POSITIVE END-EXPIRATORY PRESSURE (PEEP) AND ALVEOLAR MECHANICS

The application of trapping of fresh gas (flow) is known as PEEP. PEEP increases functional residual capacity (FRC) and compliance while decreasing dead space ventilation, shunt fraction, and is very effective for recruitment of atelectatic alveoli, as well as for equalizing opening pressures in alveoli that are filled with fluid. PEEP does not improve lung function as a result of poor perfusion and may affect the perfusion of lung capillaries. As the alveolar pressure rises, the vessels are compressed and pulmonary blood flow is reduced. There may be a decrease in RA filling, which also affects overall perfusion. In hemodynamically unstable patients, application of or increase in PEEP may prompt a decrease in BP.

Generally, PEEP pressures range from 2.5 to 20 cm H_2O. Higher pressures (greater than 24 cm H_2O) may be used if the patient can tolerate the increase and if the condition is warranted. Tolerance is primarily determined by monitoring BP and regularly assessing for a pneumothorax.

Table 1-15	MODES OF MECHANICAL VENTILATION			
Type	**Volume**	**Pressure**	**Flow**	**Inspiratory Time**
Spontaneous (patient-dependent)	Variable	Variable	Variable	Variable
VCV	Fixed	Variable or limited	Fixed	Fixed
PCV	Variable or targeted	Fixed	Variable	Fixed
PSV (patient-dependent)	Variable	Fixed	Variable	Variable
SIMV				
Combination of spontaneous, PS, and the mandatory breath type	Any	Any	Any	Any

PCV, Pressure-controlled ventilation; *PSV*, pressure support ventilation; *SIMV*, synchronized intermittent mandatory ventilation; *VCV*, volume-controlled ventilation.

The role of PEEP in lung ventilation is to stabilize alveoli, decreasing alveolar collapse, and promoting better gas exchange. PEEP is applied when the exhalation valve in the circuit closes, promoting lung trapping of gas (refreshed), which is then measured as pressure sustained at the end of expiration. When PEEP is increased, the valve closes earlier. In lung-protective ventilation, PEEP allows for better distribution of gas over a larger open lung surface, while preventing alveolar over distention. Gattinoni et al. showed that injured lungs have less lung surface, which participates in ventilation, and the application of PEEP in this diagnosis can open collapsed alveoli and prevent the shear stresses caused by alveolar recruitment/derecruitment. In the open lung approach, alveoli and small airways are stented open with a constant airway pressure. This allows the breath to reach more functional surface area early in inspiration, as alveolar opening is maintained by the application. PEEP promotes better gas exchange, increases the P/F ratio, and allows for reduction of F_{IO_2}, and is frequently used in conjunction with mechanical ventilation to improve oxygenation. Clinical improvements are reflected by increased partial pressure of O_2 in arterial blood (Pao_2) and the ability to decrease F_{IO_2}.

Application of PEEP increases intrathoracic pressure and can compromise the patient's hemodynamic status by compressing the heart and great vessels. Increased intrathoracic pressure decreases venous return, RV-filling pressures, and CO, which may cause or potentiate hypotension and shock. Patients with intravascular volume depletion are at higher risk for associated hemodynamic instability. High levels of PEEP can cause pneumothorax, particularly if lung compliance is diminished. The understanding gained through the study of alveolar mechanics would suggest that an open lung approach might minimize shear stress and improve oxygenation. Multiple modes of ventilation will allow for open lung ventilation: high-frequency oscillatory ventilation (HFOV), airway pressure-release ventilation (APRV), and alveolar recruitment maneuvers (high levels of PEEP applied for short times to open collapsed alveoli), followed by the application of PEEP. The decision-making strategies for patient management are discussed in Table 1-16.

> **Safety Alert**   *Clinicians should be prepared for a narrowing pulse pressure, decreasing stroke volume, blood pressure, and cardiac output when positive end-expiratory pressure levels are increased. Hemodynamic changes may include volume resuscitation and/or inotropic support to correct the decrease in blood pressure and cardiac output.*

LOW TIDAL VOLUME/PROTECTIVE LUNG VENTILATION/ PERMISSIVE HYPERCAPNIA

The strongest evidence-based methods for mechanically supported ventilation are reflected in the work of the ARDS Network. Low tidal volumes used with PEEP levels high enough to

Table 1-16	FACTORS CONSIDERED WHEN CHOOSING MODES OF VENTILATION	
Gas Exchange	**Ventilation Effect**	**Airway Compliance**
$F_{IO_2} > 0.35$	Vital capacity >10 to 15 mL/kg body weight	Tidal volume >325 mL
$Pao_2 > 60$ mm Hg	Maximal negative inspiratory pressure	Tidal volume/body weight >4 mL/kg
A-a Pao_2 gradient <350 mm Hg	< -30 cm H_2O	Dynamic compliance >22 mL/ cm H_2O
Pao_2/F_{IO_2} ratio >200	Minute ventilation <10 L/min	Static compliance >33 mL/cm H_2O
	Maximal voluntary ventilation more than twice resting minute ventilation	

open a possibly recruitable lung may allow the most injured portions of the lung to "rest" until the resolution of the underlying lung injury.

A methodolog approach to low tidal volume, FIO_2, and PEEP can be accessed at http://www.ardsnet.org/system/files/Ventilator+Protocol+Card.pdf.

Calculation of predicted or ideal body weight (PBW or IBW) can be performed with the automatic calculator at ARDSnet: http://www.ardsnet.org/node/77460.

Formulas:

$$\text{Males: PBW (kg)} = 50 + 2.3 \text{ (height [in]} - 60)$$
$$\text{Females: PBW (kg)} = 45.5 + 2.3 \text{(height [in]} - 60)$$

RESEARCH BRIEF BOX 1-1

Higher positive end-expiratory pressure (PEEP) should be used for moderate and severe acute respiratory distress syndrome (ARDS), whereas lower PEEP may be more appropriate in patients with mild ARDS. PEEP should be set to maximize alveolar recruitment while avoiding overdistention. Volume and pressure limitation during mechanical ventilation can be described in terms of stress and strain. Fraction of inspired oxygen and PEEP are typically titrated to maintain arterial oxygen saturation (SpO_2) of 88% to 95% (PaO_2 55 to 80 mm Hg).

From Biehl M, Kashiouris MG, Gajic O: Ventilator-induced lung injury: minimizing its impact in patients with or at risk for ARDS. *Respir Care* 58(6):927-937, 2013.

ADDITIONAL MODES OF MECHANICAL VENTILATION TO PROMOTE ALVEOLAR RECRUITMENT

This discussion is designed to introduce alternative ventilatory methods. It is beyond the scope of this book to perform a substantive manual of alternative techniques.

When FIO_2 is at a toxic level (levels of oxygen that promote radical byproducts, which may actually cause alveolar lining destruction), it may be of vital importance to consider alternative strategies designed to increase the functional lung surface available for gas exchange. The following list is a small sample of current and experimental ventilator modes designed to optimize MAP and alveolar recruitment.

INVERSE RATIO VENTILATION (IRV)

During IRV, the inspiratory phase is prolonged (as the flow rate is low for a given volume or pressure) and the expiratory phase is shortened. Normal inspiration/expiration (I/E) ratio is 1:2 to 1:4. During IRV, the inspiratory phase of the I:E ratio is increased to greater than 1:1 (e.g., 2:1), thereby promoting alveolar recruitment through achieving a more constant MAP (at the level required for alveolar opening), which improves oxygenation by keeping alveoli open for longer periods of time. The patient will require administration of sedation, analgesia, and possibly a paralyzing agent to minimize the discomfort and anxiety associated with this unusual breathing pattern.

AIRWAY PRESSURE-RELEASE VENTILATION (APRV or BiVent)

APRV is basically a set level of CPAP that intermittently releases (valve open) to a lower level using a time-controlled release valve. High CPAP and lung volumes are reestablished when the release valve closes. The principle of reducing lung volume distinguishes this technique from other modes of ventilation. APRV always implies a reverse I:E ratio because it uses a very short low-pressure time (for removal of CO_2) for pressure release. APRV is a mode with two basic methods applied: PC/IRV (via a BiPAP method) and SIMV. First, it appears similar to PC/IRV as it used a high-pressure time that may be relatively long and a low-pressure time that is profoundly short. The inverse times promote a constant airway pressure and an intrinsic PEEP (auto-PEEP) to optimize oxygenation. An inspiratory time (T HIGH) and an expiratory time (T LOW) are set, as well as inspiratory pressure (P HIGH) and expiratory pressure

(P LOW). During the high time, the patient may breathe spontaneously as well as receive ventilator breaths, which will be synchronized whenever possible (SIMV). Spontaneous breathing is not required, but facilitated. No breathing occurs during low time until weaning begins.

BILEVEL VENTILATION
BiLevel is a method of switching between low-pressure and high-pressure limits based on the patient's inspiration and exhalation. In BiPAP, the circuit switches between a high-airway and low-airway pressure in an adjustable time sequence. If the patient is not breathing spontaneously, the I:E ratio and the ventilatory frequency can be adjusted to optimize ventilation and oxygenation. If the I:E ratio is reversed, then APRV has to be set up, and mandatory breaths can be applied. Breathing is allowed during both high-pressure and low-pressure times. Airway pressure is not as well controlled. BiLevel can be used initially as pressure-controlled ventilation, can be weaned to BiPAP, and then weaned to CPAP before extubation.

HIGH-FREQUENCY OSCILLATORY VENTILATION (HFOV)
Recently, this mode of ventilation has received much more attention for use in the adult population. HFOV uses very small tidal volumes (not really tidal volume, but rather amplitude, termed Delta P:P) usually equal to, or less than, the dead space (150 mL) to maintain a continuously high alveolar opening pressure. "Breaths" are administered at a very fast rate (Hertz [Hz] set at 4 to 5 breaths per second). Given that large tidal volumes in ARDS cause alveolar stress (via continuously opening and closing alveoli), in theory, very small, rapid tidal volumes used in HFOV should be protective because alveoli are no longer fully closing, and are continuously recruited by the higher constant airway pressure.

ADJUNCTS TO MECHANICAL VENTILATION
Autoflow is an advance in volume-controlled modes of mechanical ventilation. The ventilator automatically regulates inspiratory flow. This autoregulation works in conjunction with the set tidal volume and the patient's lung compliance.

Mandatory minute ventilation or minimum minute ventilation (MMV) provides a predetermined minute ventilation to augment the patient's spontaneous minute ventilation (breathing efforts). It is used to prevent hypoventilation and respiratory acidosis during ventilator weaning when SIMV is supporting the patient.

In proportional-assist ventilation (PAV), the ventilator automatically adjusts airway pressure in response to the patient's ventilatory patterns. The ventilator frequently adjusts needed support based on the patient's inspiratory flow rate, exhaled tidal volume, compliance, and resistance.

Other methods such as tracheal gas insufflation, extracorporeal membrane oxygenation, and methods that may be used for patients with refractory hypoxemia are currently used in less than 5% of institutions and therefore will not be discussed further here.

Diagnostic Evaluation of Appropriate Ventilation		
Test	**Purpose**	**Abnormal Findings**
Noninvasive Pulmonary Volumes and Pressures		
Pulmonary pressures measured during volume control breath	Measure the relationship of volume delivered and the compliance of the surface, which contains it. Normal PAWP or PIP when receiving a 10-mL/kg/IBW breath is 35 cm H_2O. Normal $p_{Plateau}$ when holding a 10-mL/kg/IBW breath at the end of inspiration is 25 cm H_2O.	Patients presenting with lung injury and distress will have significant increases in $p_{Plateau}$ pressures to >25 cm H_2O. This increase may or may not manifest as a proportional increase in PIP. For example, with a 350-mL breath, the patient with ARDS may have a PIP of 48 and a $p_{Plateau}$ of 43.

Continued

Diagnostic Evaluation of Appropriate Ventilation—cont'd		
Test	**Purpose**	**Abnormal Findings**
Static compliance	Measure the distensibility of the lungs and chest wall when gas has been delivered into the lung, but no exhalation has occurred (inspiratory hold). $V_{TE}/p_{Plateau}$ Normal compliance$_{stat}$ 50 to 80 mL/cm H_2O.	Patients presenting with loss of lung compliance will have significant decrease in measures of static compliance as well as increasing $p_{Plateau}$ pressures. Subtract PEEP from $p_{Plateau}$ before performing calculation.
Blood Studies		
Arterial blood gas (ABG) analysis	Evaluate the oxygenation of the arterial blood as well as the presence or absence of acid and the effect on the pH (environment of the cells). See ABGs.	Although not always predictable when in the disease process changes will occur, generally patients will develop hypoxemia that may initially be resolved with increasing the F_{IO_2}, but eventually will require great increases in F_{IO_2}, and ultimately will no longer respond to oxygen therapy.
Pao_2/F_{IO_2} ratio	The Pao_2 divided by the F_{IO_2} (Pao_2/F_{IO_2} ratio, or more simply P/F) can be used to more simply assess the severity of the gas exchange defect. The normal value for the ratio of the partial pressure of oxygen in arterial blood to F_{IO_2} (Pao_2/F_{IO_2}) (F_{IO_2} is expressed as a decimal ranging from 0.21 to 1.00) is 300 to 500.	A value of less than 300 indicates gas exchange derangement, and a value less than 250 is indicative of severe impairment, and compliance calculations should be performed to encourage alveolar recruitment strategies.
Radiology		
Chest x-ray (CXR)	Assess size of lungs, presence of fluids, abnormal gas or fluids in the pleural sac, diaphragmatic margins, the pulmonary hilum, as well as integrity of the rib cage.	Presence of fluids in the lung parenchyma initially presents as pulmonary edema. The continuous accumulation differentiates this edema formation to one that is not cardiac.
Computed tomography (CT) lung scan	Assess the three-dimensional lung capacities, fluid load, and the primary displacement of the fluid.	Normally a large gas-filled surface, the ALI/ARDS lung when seen on CT is frequently seen as fluffy and white as a result of fluid that has extravagated through the endothelial deficits (capillary leak).

ALI, Acute lung injury; *ARDS*, acute respiratory distress syndrome; *IBW*, ideal body weight; *PEEP*, positive end-expiratory pressure; *PAWP*, pulmonary artery wedge pressure; *PIP*, peak inspiratory pressure.

COMPLICATIONS RELATED TO MECHANICAL VENTILATION

BAROTRAUMA, VOLUTRAUMA, AND PNEUMOTHORAX

Barotrauma can occur when ventilatory pressures increase intrathoracic and intrapleural pressures, causing damage to the lungs, the major vessels, and possibly all organs in the thorax, with referred damage to the abdomen. If severe, barotrauma can lead to pneumothorax: a partially or totally collapsed lung. Symptoms vary depending on the amount of lung collapsed.

TENSION PNEUMOTHORAX

This develops when pressurized air escapes from the lungs and enters and collects in the thoracic cavity, causing one or both lungs to collapse. High pressure from mechanical positive-pressure ventilation may tear diseased or fragile lung tissue, leading to this life-threatening complication. Symptoms include respiratory distress, fluctuations in BP, shifting of the trachea toward the unaffected side, and sudden and sustained increases in PIP.

HIGH ALERT! If tension pneumothorax is suspected, the patient should be disconnected from the ventilator immediately and ventilated using a bag/valve/tube device (Ambu bag). While the primary nurse/therapist is using tube/mask ventilation, others will facilitate an emergency physician call and set up the patient for immediate chest tube insertion/placement.

GASTROINTESTINAL COMPLICATIONS

Peptic ulcers with profound hemorrhage may develop as a result of physiologic pressures and stress. Histamine H_2-receptor antagonists (e.g., ranitidine) or proton-pump inhibitors (e.g., omeprazole [Prilosec], lansoprazole [Prevacid], rabeprazole [Aciphex], pantoprazole [Protonix], esomeprazole [Nexium], and Zegerid), or sucralfate (Carafate) may be administered to prevent these ulcers from developing. A great deal of controversy surrounds the best strategy for peptic ulcer prevention and the evidence is evolving. In addition, gastric dilation can occur as a result of the large amounts of air swallowed in the presence of an artificial airway. If gastric dilation is left untreated, paralytic ileus, vomiting, and aspiration may develop. Extreme dilation can compromise respiratory effort because of the restriction of diaphragmatic movement. Treatment includes insertion of a gastric tube orally or nasally (oral placement may be preferred) connected to low intermittent suction to remove air from the GI tract.

HYPOTENSION WITH DECREASED CARDIAC OUTPUT

This develops as a result of decreased venous return secondary to increased intrathoracic pressure caused by positive-pressure ventilation. Unless associated with tension pneumothorax, this phenomenon is transient and is seen immediately after the patient has been placed on mechanical ventilation. This may require aggressive volume resuscitation.

SUSTAINED HYPOTENSION WITH DECREASED CARDIAC OUTPUT

PEEP, especially at levels greater than 20 cm H_2O, and MAP strategies to open the alveoli (lung) may increase the incidence and severity of the phenomena resulting from compression of the heart and large blood vessels from increased intrathoracic pressure. This produces an arterial hypovolemic state. Aggressive IV fluid therapy and occasionally inotropic support may be used with PEEP to maintain adequate intravascular volume for sufficient CO to perfuse vital organs. HR and BP should be monitored frequently if the patient is unstable.

INCREASED INTRACRANIAL PRESSURE (ICP)

Increased ICP occurs as a result of decreased cerebral venous return to the heart resulting from compression of intrathoracic blood vessels when using PEEP greater than 5 cm H_2O or mean airway pressure management strategies. This may limit cerebral venous outflow, therefore increasing the ICP. See the section on Traumatic Brain Injury in Chapter 3 for additional information.

FLUID IMBALANCE

Increased production of ADH occurs as a result of increased pressure on baroreceptors in the thoracic aorta, which causes the system to react as if the body were volume-depleted. ADH stimulates the renal system to retain water. Patients may need diuretics if signs of hypervolemia are present. Be alert to new symptoms of dependent edema or adventitious breath sounds.

VENTILATOR-ASSOCIATED EVENT (VAE)

Patients with mechanical ventilation are at high risk for developing healthcare-associated pneumonia or ventilator associated pneumonia (VAP). In 2012, the National Healthcare Safety Network facilities reported greater than 3957 VAP cases. The incidence for various hospital units ranged from 0.0 to 4.4 per 1000 ventilator days. Providers continually disagreed on criteria for VAP, prompting the reportable benchmark to be changed to VAE. Studies indicate that 70% to 90% of patients who are mechanically ventilated colonize hospital-acquired bacteria in the oropharynx, trachea, or digestive tract. Aspiration of bacteria from the oropharynx is a leading cause of VAP. The onset of infection may have several mechanisms:

- Presence of an ET/tracheostomy tube creates a bypass of upper respiratory tract defense mechanisms of cough and mucociliary clearance action.
- Contaminated secretions pool above the ET/tracheostomy tube cuff promoting colonization of bacteria and ultimately leak into the lower respiratory tract.
- Use of endotracheal tubes with subglottic secretion drainage is effective for the prevention of VAP and may be associated with reduced duration of mechanical ventilation.
- Supine positioning, the presence of a nasogastric tube, or reflux of bacteria from the stomach contribute to oropharyngeal colonization. The medications that patients who are mechanically ventilated may receive to prevent GI bleeding also alter the gastric pH. Use of sucralfate, which does not increase gastric pH, decreases the incidence of pneumonia compared with antacids alone or in combination with hydrogen ion antagonists.
- Use of contaminated equipment/supplies, inadequate hand washing, or poor infection control practices may directly inoculate the tracheobronchial tree with pathogens.

ANXIETY

Many individuals experience anxiety related to the discomfort associated with loss of control over their ventilatory process and the perception that their health status is threatened. Hypoxemia and air hunger, if present, contribute to anxiety and prompt rapid, shallow, and often irregular respiratory efforts. The first approach is always to evaluate mode and method of ventilation to insure appropriate ventilatory support. The flow rate of the volume must be considered, and can best be evaluated with a volume-pressure loop. Coordinated and effective ventilation may not be possible with severe anxiety and agitation. Diligent administration of anxiolytic drugs and analgesics, along with close monitoring of the patient's response to potent medications, may be necessary to reduce the work of breathing and facilitate effective mechanical ventilation. The use of an approved sedation scale is also recommended (see Sedation and Neuromuscular Blockade). In extreme cases, if the patient is unable to tolerate the ventilator mode most appropriate for his or her condition and cannot be managed using high-dose anxiolytic agents, sedatives, and analgesics, the advanced practice provider may consider use of neuromuscular blockade (induced paralysis) to facilitate more effective ventilation. Neuromuscular blockade should be reserved for only the most extreme situations, wherein the patient's life is threatened by the overall energy expenditure related to fear, anxiety, or inability to attain control over his or her breathing pattern despite other efforts (see Sedation and Neuromuscular Blockade).

WEANING THE PATIENT FROM MECHANICAL VENTILATION

Weaning patients from mechanical support requires skill, knowledge, and patience. This goal may take many forms ranging from abrupt cessation to gradual withdrawal from ventilatory support. Successful weaning depends primarily on the patient's overall condition as well as the techniques used. Patients for whom attempts at weaning fail constitute a unique problem in critical care. Physiologic factors (cardiovascular status, fluids and electrolyte balance, acid-base balance, nutritional status, comfort, and sleep pattern) and emotional factors (fear, anxiety, coping skills, general emotional state, ability to cooperate) are important and must be evaluated both before and during the weaning process. Adequate pulmonary function parameters must be attained before the weaning process is begun (Table 1-17). To begin the weaning process, patients must be hemodynamically stable and able to initiate a spontaneous breath. A weaning assessment tool that is chosen for use in patients who are critically ill should be well designed and supported by evidence, and thus strategies have a better opportunity for success. The most well evaluated and internationally used is the Burns Wean Assessment Program (BWAP). A series of predictors for weaning success is listed in Table 1-17, and a listing of ventilator adjustments during weaning is included in Table 1-18.

TRADITIONAL WEANING METHODS

Two weaning protocols are generally used: incremental reduction of ventilator support or progressively longer periods of spontaneous breathing trials. Physical rehabilitation is an important component of weaning protocols. Success depends on comorbidities, hospital culture, level of knowledge of the care providers, availability of physical therapy, use of weaning

Table 1-17	PARAMETERS FOR WEANING FROM MECHANICAL VENTILATION	
Pulmonary Function	**Optimal Parameters**	**Definition**
Minute ventilation	>10 L/min	Tidal volume $\times$ respiratory rate; if adequate, it indicates that the patient is breathing at a stable rate with adequate tidal volume
Negative inspiratory force	>-20 cm H_2O	Measures respiratory muscle strength; maximum negative pressure indicates that the patient is able to generate and initiate spontaneous respirations; indicative of the patient's ability to initiate inspiration independently
Maximum voluntary ventilation	$2 \times$ resting minute ventilation	Measures respiratory muscle endurance; indicates the patient's ability to sustain maximal respiratory effort
Tidal volume	5 to 10 mL/kg	Indicates the patient's ability to ventilate lungs adequately
Arterial blood gases Fractional concentration of inspired oxygen (Fio_2) 0.40	$Pao_2 > 60$ mm Hg $Pao_2 < 45$ mm Hg pH 7.35 to 7.45 or patient's baseline	

Table 1-18	COMMON ADJUSTMENTS DURING WEANING TO IMPROVE GAS EXCHANGE	
Ventilation Strategies		**Oxygenation Strategies**
When CO_2 retention is the problem		When refractory oxygenation is the problem
Increase minute ventilation	Increase f (RR)	Increase Fio_2
	Increase V_T	When Fio_2 is >0.40 (40%), consider PEEP
Increase flow rate		When PEEP is >12 to 15, consider MAWP strategies

MAWP, Mean airway pressure; *PEEP*, positive end-expiratory pressure; *RR*, respiratory rate; V_T, tidal volume.

protocols, and patient autonomy. Methods for incremental reduction of ventilator support include:
1. SIMV mode: The patient is switched to SIMV from assist-control mode, or respiratory rate and pressure support are decreased if the patient is already on SIMV.
   Patients with nonchronic pulmonary disease decrease rate every 30-minute interval. After 2 hours at a mandatory rate of zero with CPAP, if the patient is clinically stable, he or she may be extubated.
   Patients with chronic pulmonary disease begin with an RR of 8 breaths per minute and decrease SIMV rate by 2 breaths per hour unless the patient experiences clinical deterioration. If stable after at least 1 hour of a mandatory rate zero with CPAP, the patient may be extubated.
2. Pressure support ventilation (PSV): Start with 25 cm of pressure support and no mandatory breaths.
   Patients with Nonchronic Pulmonary Disease decrease pressure support every 30 minutes; if the patient is able to tolerate PSV of zero for 2 hours, he or she can be extubated.
   Patients with Chronic Pulmonary Disease decrease pressure support by 2 to 4 cm H_2O every hour as long as the patient is stable.

When PSV is zero for at least 1 hour, fit the patient with a T-piece or initiate CPAP and observe.

3. T-piece method: A T-shaped adapter is placed on the end of the ET tube. The patient is taken off the ventilator and allowed to initiate spontaneous breaths for increasingly longer periods of time. The T-piece method may be used by starting with 1 to 2 minutes off the ventilator, followed by 58 to 59 minutes on, with a gradual reversal of this ratio until the patient breathes independently. In this manner, the patient builds strength and endurance for independent respiratory effort.

SPONTANEOUS BREATHING TRIALS

The patient is closely monitored for a period of time while disconnected from the ventilator. Respiratory pattern, gas exchange, hemodynamic stability, and patient comfort should be monitored closely. If the patient tolerates the spontaneous breathing trial for 30 to 120 minutes, extubation should be considered.

HIGH ALERT! Apnea
Frequent patient assessments with vigilant monitoring must be done, because there may not be ventilator backup or an apnea program to support the patient if the patient fails to breathe.

FAILURE TO WEAN

Patients who need prolonged mechanical ventilation are increasing in numbers. These complex patients require high resource use and achieve suboptimal outcomes, especially if elderly. Patients who fail the transition from ventilator support to sustained spontaneous breathing do so primarily because of weakness of the respiratory muscles, including the diaphragm. Considerations regarding the following parameters should be evaluated before attempting weaning. The following parameters should be evaluated when patients are unable to be weaned from the ventilator.

- Nutrition and metabolic deficiencies: K, Mg, Ca, phosphate, and thyroid hormone.
- Complications related to use of corticosteroids or need for corticosteroids.
  - Left ventricular dysfunction, cardiomyopathy, and myocardial ischemia.
- Chronic renal failure, which alters capacity for compensation.
- Systemic diseases that affect protein synthesis, degradation, and glycogen stores.
- Hypoxemia and hypercapnia.
  - Critical illness–related neuromuscular abnormalities.

TROUBLESHOOTING MECHANICAL VENTILATOR PROBLEMS

The most important assessment factor in troubleshooting a mechanical ventilator is the effect on the patient. Regardless of which alarm sounds, always assess the patient first to evaluate his or her physiologic response to the problem. (See Table 1-19 and Box 1-15 for processes that contribute to high-pressure and low-pressure alarm situations.) If at any time the patient is not receiving the proper volumes or the nurse is unable to properly assess and manage the alarm situation, take the patient off the ventilator, ventilate with a bag-valve tube system, and ask someone to contact the respiratory therapist immediately.

CARE PLANS FOR MECHANICAL VENTILATION

Impaired gas exchange *related to altered oxygen supply resulting from an abnormal tidal volume distribution associated with mechanical ventilation.*

- -

Goals/Outcomes: The patient has adequate gas exchange, as evidenced by PaO_2 greater than 60 mm Hg, $PaCO_2$ 35 to 45 mm Hg, SpO_2 greater than 92%, SvO_2 greater than 60%, and RR 12 to 20 breaths/min.
NOC Respiratory Status: Gas Exchange.

Mechanical Ventilation
1. Observe for, document, and report any changes in the patient's condition consistent with increasing respiratory distress (see Acute Respiratory Failure, Chapter 4).

Table 1-19	CAUSES OF HIGH-PRESSURE ALARMS DURING MECHANICAL VENTILATION	
Increased airway resistance	Decreased lung compliance
Patient requires suctioning	Pneumothorax
Kinks in ventilator circuitry	Pulmonary edema
Water or expectorated secretions in circuitry	Atelectasis
Patient coughs or exhales against ventilatory breaths	Worsening of underlying disease process
Patient biting ET tube	ARDS
Bronchospasm	
Herniation of airway cuff over end of artificial airway	
Change in patient position that restricts chest wall movement	
Breath stacking	

ARDS, Acute respiratory distress syndrome; *ET,* endotracheal.

Box 1-15	CAUSES OF LOW-PRESSURE ALARMS

Patient disconnected from machine
Leak in airway cuff
   Insufficient air in cuff
   Hole or tear in cuff
   Leak in one-way valve of inflation port
Leak in circuitry
   Poor fittings on water reservoirs

Dislodged temperature-sensing device
Hole or tear in tubing
Poor seal in circuitry connections
Displacement of airway above vocal cords
Loss of compressed air source

2. Position the patient to allow for maximal alveolar ventilation and comfort. Remember that the dependent lung usually receives more ventilation and more blood flow than the nondependent lung; however, during mechanical ventilation the dependent portion of the lung receives less distribution of tidal volume than the nondependent areas.
   - Analyze SpO_2, SvO_2, and ABG results with the patient in different positions to determine adequacy of ventilation.
   - Use postural drainage principles where appropriate.
   - In unilateral lung disease, position the patient with the healthy lung down.
   - In bilateral lung disease, position the patient in the right lateral decubitus position, inasmuch as the right lung has more surface area. If ABG results show that the patient tolerates left lateral decubitus position, alternate between the two positions. Rotational therapy (rotating the patient and/or use of a chest percussion bed) may be effective.

3. Turn the patient at least every 2 hours if signs of deteriorating pulmonary status occur.

4. Auscultate the upper chest over the artificial airway to assess for leaks.

5. Assess the ventilator for proper functioning and parameter settings, including FIO_2, tidal volume, rate, mode, PIP, and temperature of inspired gases. In addition, ensure that connections are tight and alarms are set. A thorough ventilator check is generally done every 2 hours in best practice settings. Ventilator checks should be systematically documented in the medical record by the respiratory care practitioner. Assessing the ventilator for proper function and the patient's response to therapy is most often a collaborative effort between the nurse and the respiratory therapist.

6. Keep the ventilator circuitry free of condensed water and expectorated secretions. Not all ventilators have a problem with condensation. Fluids present in the circuit may obstruct the flow of gases to and from the patient. Water is a warm, moist environment that is ideal for the growth of microorganisms. Gloves should be worn any time the ventilator circuit is manipulated.

7. Monitor serial ABG results. Be alert for hypoxemia (decreases in PaO_2) or hypercapnia (increases in $PaCO_2$) with concomitant decrease in pH (less than 7.35), which can signal hypoventilation and/or inadequate oxygenation. Also observe for decreased $PaCO_2$ (less than 35 mm Hg) with increased pH (greater than 7.45), which may signal mechanical hyperventilation.
8. Notify the advanced practice provider of dysrhythmias, which can occur even with modest alkalosis if the patient has heart disease or is receiving inotropic medications (see Appendix 6).
9. If changes in patient status are noted, note the SpO_2 reading and end-tidal CO_2, if used, or follow institutional protocol for addressing deterioration in the status of a patient receiving mechanical ventilation. An ABG analysis may be warranted.
10. Keep manual resuscitator or bag-valve device at the bedside for ventilation in case of malfunctioning equipment.

Ineffective airway clearance (or risk for same) *related to altered anatomic structure secondary to the presence of ET or tracheostomy tube.*

Goals/Outcomes: The patient maintains a patent airway, as evidenced by the absence of adventitious breath sounds or signs of respiratory distress, such as restlessness and anxiety.
NOC Respiratory Status: Airway Patency.

Airway Management
1. Assess and document breath sounds in all lung fields at least every 2 hours. Note quality and presence or absence of adventitious sounds.
2. Monitor the patient for restlessness and anxiety, which can signal early airway obstruction and hypoxia.
3. Avoid routine or scheduled suctioning. Use aseptic technique (including use of sterile gloves) for suctioning based on the needs of the patient. The decision to suction is based on assessment findings, and is done to maintain a patent airway when the patient is unable to cough out secretions. Document the amount, color, and consistency of tracheobronchial secretions and the patient's tolerance of the procedure. Collaborate with the respiratory care practitioner and report significant changes (e.g., increase in production of secretions, tenacious secretions, bloody sputum) to the physician or midlevel practitioner. Maintain the artificial airway in a secure and proper alignment.
4. Maintain the correct temperature (32° C to 36° C [89.6° F to 96.8° F]) of inspired gas. Cold air irritates the airways, and hot air may burn fragile lung tissue.
5. Maintain humidification of inspired gas either using the ventilator or an alternative device, to prevent drying of tracheal mucosa. Without humidification, tracheobronchial secretions may become thick and tenacious, creating mucous plugs that place the patient at risk for development of atelectasis and infection.

Ineffective breathing pattern *related to anxiety resulting from the need for mechanical ventilation.*

Goals/Outcomes: The patient exhibits a stable respiratory rate of 12 to 20 breaths/min (synchronized with ventilator) without restlessness, anxiety, lethargy, or sounding of the high-pressure ventilator alarm.
NOC Mechanical Ventilation Response: Adult.

Ventilation Assistance
1. Monitor for evidence of ventilator dyssynchrony: Frequent sounding of high-pressure alarm when the patient breathes against mechanical inspiration or mismatch of the patient's respiratory rate and ventilatory cycle.
2. Monitor the respiratory rate and quality, and for early signs of respiratory distress (e.g., tachypnea, hyperventilation, anxiety, restlessness, lethargy). Cyanosis is a late sign of respiratory insufficiency.
3. Teach the patient the technique for progressive muscle relaxation (see Appendix 7). When the patient becomes anxious, remain at the bedside until the respirations are under control. Reassure the patient that they have the best opportunity to synchronize respirations with the ventilator if he/she relaxes.

HIGH ALERT! Restlessness Management
Administer prescribed medication for restlessness only after any physiologic causes, including hypoxia and hypoglycemia, have been ruled out. Restlessness, if attributable to a nonphysiologic cause such as anxiety or unrelieved pain, should be managed with either sedation or analgesia, because it increases O_2 demand and consumption and can interfere with adequate ventilation.

Ineffective protection *related to increased environmental exposure (contaminated respiratory equipment); tissue destruction (during intubation or suctioning); invasive procedures (intubation, suctioning, presence of ET tube); immunocompromised state; and/or the physiologic stress resulting from a critical illness.*

Goals/Outcomes: The patient is free of infection, as evidenced by normothermia, WBC count ≤11,000/mm³, clear sputum, and negative sputum culture results.

NOC Immune Status.

Infection Protection

1. Assess the patient for signs and symptoms of infection, including temperature greater than 38° C (100.4° F), tachycardia (HR greater than 100 bpm), erythema of tracheostomy, and foul-smelling sputum. Document all significant findings.
2. To minimize the risk of cross-contamination, wash hands before and after contact with the respiratory secretions of any patient (even though gloves were worn) and before and after contact with the patient who is undergoing intubation.
3. Maintain appropriate seal on artificial airway cuff to prevent aspiration of oral secretions.
4. Implement the Institute for Healthcare Improvement Ventilator bundle:
   - Keep the HOB elevated 30 to 45 degrees.
   - Perform daily sedation vacations (interruption of sedation) and assessment for readiness to extubate.
   - Implement peptic ulcer disease prophylaxis.
   - Provide daily oral care with chlorhexidine.
   - Implement venous thromboembolism (VTE) prophylaxis.
5. Monitor the patient for reflux of feedings, as well as for signs of intolerance to feedings (absence of bowel sounds, abdominal distention, residual feedings of greater than 100 mL), which can precipitate vomiting and result in pulmonary aspiration of gastric contents.
6. Consider the use of a postpyloric feeding tube if the patient is at high risk for aspiration or is intolerant of conventional feeding strategies.
7. Recognize that bacteria and spores can be introduced easily during suctioning. Follow standard techniques:
   - Use aseptic technique during suctioning process, including use of sterile catheter and gloves. Use of lavage solutions is not recommended.
   - Suction the tracheobronchial tree before suctioning the oropharynx if using the same suction catheter, to avoid introducing oral pathogens into the tracheobronchial tree. Ideally, a separate tonsil suction device is dedicated to use exclusively in the oropharynx.
   - Never store or reuse a single-use suction catheter. Consider use of closed system for suctioning.
   - Change suction canisters and tubing within the time frame established by the agency and/or always when filled. Change canisters and tubing between patients.
8. Wash hands and use sterile gloves when performing tracheostomy care to prevent colonization of stoma with bacteria from the practitioner's hands.
9. Provide oral hygiene at least every 4 hours to prevent overgrowth of normal flora and aerobic gram-negative bacilli. Suction the oropharynx and posterior pharynx to prevent pooling of secretions. Endotracheal tubes with subglottic secretion drainage are available to provide continuous suctioning of the posterior pharynx. Oral rinse products with chlorhexidine have been used to help control bacteria. Specialized suctioning toothbrushes may be used to brush the teeth and tongue every 12 hours.
   - Change the entire ventilator circuit (ventilator tubing) within the time frame established by policy, or sooner if soiled with secretions or blood.
   - When disconnecting the patient from ventilatory circuits, keep ends of connectors clean. Avoid unnecessary disconnection.
   - Keep connectors on manual resuscitator bags clean and free of secretions between uses. Although no data suggest that disposable bags be changed with any frequency, reusable bags should not be used between patients without sterilization.
10. Be aware of special risk factors for patients with tracheostomy tubes, and intervene accordingly:
    - Maintain the tracheostomy tube in a secure and proper alignment to avoid irritation of stoma from too much movement.
    - Change the tracheostomy ties daily, or more frequently if heavily soiled with secretions or wound exudate.
    - Perform stoma care at least every 8 hours, using aseptic technique until the stoma is completely healed. Keep the area around the stoma dry at all times to prevent maceration and infection. Change the stoma dressing as needed to keep it dry.

- Avoid use of cotton-filled gauze or other material that may shed small fibers. The patient may aspirate fibers, which in turn can lead to infection.
- Use aseptic technique (including use of sterile gloves and drapes) when changing the tracheostomy tube.
- Culture secretions or wound drainage; administer antibiotics as prescribed.

Anxiety *related to actual or perceived threat to health status as a result of the need for or the presence of mechanical ventilation.*

Goals/Outcomes: During the interval of mechanical ventilation, the patient relates the presence of emotional comfort and exhibits a decrease in irritability, with an HR within the patient's normal range.
NOC Anxiety Level.

Anxiety Reduction
1. Reassure the patient and significant others that ventilatory support may be a temporary measure until the underlying pathophysiologic process has resolved. The patient may be weaned from the ventilator at that time. Some in the general public equate ventilator placement with a hopelessly chronic, vegetative state. Set time lines for reevaluation of the patient's progress.
2. Reassure the patient that he or she will not be left alone.
3. Explain all procedures before they are initiated to the patient and significant others. Inform the patient of his or her progress.
4. Describe and point out the alarm system, explaining that it will alert staff in the event of any problem with the ventilator, including an accidental disconnection.
5. Provide the patient with a mechanism for communication (e.g., picture board, erasable marker board, pen and paper).
6. If aggressive sedation is used, perform a "sedation vacation" at least every 24 hours to assess if the patient can tolerate mechanical ventilation without sedation. Weaning the patient from sedation is an important step in the weaning from mechanical ventilation process. Sedatives can also mask symptoms of pain.
7. Evaluate the patient's need for pain control, particularly during the daily sedation vacation. Analgesics should be administered to control pain.

Impaired gas exchange *related to decreasing support or ventilation during weaning from mechanical ventilation.*

Goals/Outcomes: The patient has adequate gas exchange, as evidenced by Pao_2 less than 60 mm Hg, $Paco_2$ less than 45 mm Hg, Spo_2 greater than 92%, Svo_2 greater than 60%, and pH 7.35 to 7.45 (or values within 10% of the patient's baseline).
NOC Mechanical Ventilation Weaning Response: Adult.

Mechanical Ventilatory Weaning
1. Maintain the patient in a comfortable position to enhance ventilation. Many patients find that a semi-Fowler position, with the HOB elevated 30 to 45 degrees, promotes more effective ventilation. Studies support these findings and recommend that the HOB remains elevated throughout mechanical ventilation, to reduce the risk of aspiration.
2. Observe for indicators of hypoxia, including tachycardia, tachypnea, cardiac dysrhythmias, pain, anxiety, and restlessness.
3. Assess and record vital signs every 15 minutes for the first hour of weaning, then hourly if the patient is stable. Report significant findings to the advanced practice provider such as increased respiratory effort, hyperventilation, anxiety, lethargy, and cyanosis.
4. Check the patient's tidal volume after the first 15 minutes of weaning and as needed. Optimally, it will be within 5 to 10 mL/kg.
5. Obtain a specimen for ABG analysis during weaning as indicated and per hospital protocol. Monitor Spo_2 continuously and, as available, Svo_2 for values outside the normal range.

Anxiety *related to perceived threat to health status secondary to the weaning process*

Goals/Outcomes: During the weaning process, the patient expresses the attainment of emotional comfort and is free of the signs of harmful anxiety, as evidenced by HR less than 100 bpm, RR less than 20 breaths/min, and BP within the patient's normal range.

NOC Anxiety Self-Control.

Anxiety Reduction
1. Before the weaning process is initiated, discuss plans for weaning with the patient and significant others. Explain that the patient's condition will be assessed at frequent intervals during the weaning procedure. Provide time for questions and answers about the procedure.
2. Stay with the patient during the initial phase of weaning, keeping the patient informed of progress being made. Provide positive feedback for positive efforts.
3. Teach the patient progressive muscle relaxation technique, which may reduce anxiety and fear, and thus relax chest muscles (see Appendix 7).
4. Instruct the patient to take deep breaths if he or she is capable of doing so. This may provide the confidence of knowing that he or she can initiate and sustain respirations independently.
5. Encourage the patient to sit in the chair or to move about in the bed as much as possible.
6. Leave call light within the patient's reach before leaving bedside. Reassure the patient that help is nearby.

NIC Acid-Base Management; Acid-Base Monitoring; Airway Management; Airway Suctioning; Anxiety Reduction; Aspiration Precautions; Bedside Laboratory Testing; Infection Control; Laboratory Data Interpretation; Mechanical Ventilation; Mechanical Ventilatory Weaning; Oxygen Therapy; Positioning; Respiratory Monitoring; Vital Signs Monitoring.

ADDITIONAL NURSING DIAGNOSES

Also see nursing diagnoses and interventions under Prolonged Immobility *and* Emotional and Spiritual Support of the Patient and Significant Others, Chapter 2.

NUTRITION SUPPORT

Malnutrition in patients who are hospitalized is common, with an incidence ranging from 24% to over 50% in different studies. The impact of malnutrition on patient outcomes is significant, including decreased wound healing, immune dysfunction, increased infection, and increased mortality. Length of stay and costs can be as much as three times higher in patients with a diagnosis of malnutrition than in patients who are well nourished. The patient who is critically ill is at high risk for malnutrition and its negative sequelae. The metabolic response to critical illness includes increased energy expenditure, protein catabolism, oxidation of stored lipids, and altered carbohydrate metabolism. Because the body has no protein stores, protein is transported from the periphery (muscle mass) to the liver during critical illness for production of acute phase proteins and gluconeogenesis and to the gut for preservation of the GI lining and gut-associated lymphoid tissue. The resting energy expenditure in patients who are critically ill can be elevated by up to 120% to 160% and remains elevated for up to 21 days in patients with sepsis or trauma, even when these conditions are being adequately managed. In patients with sepsis and trauma, 13% of total body protein stores are lost in the first 21 days of illness despite the provision of adequate nutrition support. In the patient who is unfed, stressed, and critically ill, up to 250 g (~0.5 lb) of lean body mass can be broken down daily. Patients who are critically ill are often admitted to ICU with some degree of malnutrition. Those who were not previously suffering from malnutrition have poor volitional intake in ICU. The role of nutrition support in the management of patients who are critically ill cannot be overestimated.

Nutrition support is defined as the administration of parenteral or enteral nutrition. The goals of nutrition support therapy in the patient who is critically ill are to preserve lean body mass, maintain immune function, prevent metabolic complications, and in certain instances to attenuate the disease process. Since the publication of the last edition of this handbook, the American Society of Parenteral and Enteral Nutrition (ASPEN) and the Society of Critical Care Medicine (SCCM) have published joint guidelines for the provision of nutrition support in the adult patient who is critically ill. The Canadian Critical Care Nutrition (CCCN) guidelines were updated in 2013 to include additional recommendations for the administration of nutrition support in patients who are critically ill. The revised guidelines underscore the importance of nutrition support in improving patient outcomes. The recommendations will be discussed throughout this chapter.

NUTRITION ASSESSMENT

Multiple sources of information are used for the assessment of nutritional status in the hospitalized patient who is critically ill including medical and nutrition history, anthropometric data (body measurements), biochemical analysis of blood and urine, and type and duration of the disease process. With an individual who is critically ill, the medical and nutrition history may be obtained from significant others. Although clinical dietitians in ICU are responsible for a complete nutrition assessment during the patient's stay, according to The Joint Commission, screening for nutrition risk should be done within 48 hours of admission and is usually performed by the nurse.

MEDICAL/DIET HISTORY

A diet history identifies individuals who are or may be at risk for malnutrition resulting from inadequate intake or an imbalance in food intake. It should describe the adequacy of both usual and recent food intake, as well as focus on factors that may have impaired adequate selection, preparation, ingestion, digestion, absorption, and excretion of nutrients. The medical history is included to assess diseases or conditions affecting nutritional status. The following should be included in the medical and diet history assessment:

- Comprehensive review of usual dietary intake, including food allergies, food aversions, use of nutritional supplements including vitamins, supplements, and alternative/complementary therapies.
- Recent weight loss or gain; intentional or unintentional.
- Chewing or swallowing difficulties.
- Nausea, vomiting, or pain with eating.
- Altered pattern of elimination (e.g., constipation, diarrhea).
- Diseases/conditions increasing energy needs (e.g., burns, extensive wounds, decubitus ulcers, sepsis, surgery, trauma).
- Chronic disease affecting use of nutrients (e.g., malabsorption, pancreatitis, diabetes mellitus).
- Use of medications (e.g., laxatives, antacids, antibiotics, antineoplastic drugs).
- How food is obtained and meals are prepared (and by whom).
- Cultural preferences restricting specific nutrient intake or causing excessive intake.
- Alcohol or drug use.
- Recent fad or vegetarian diets.
- Other influences on nutritional status, such as living environment, functional status, dependency on caregivers, and financial resources.

RISK FACTORS FOR MALNUTRITION

The following factors may place a patient at risk of or indicate the presence of nutritional deficiencies:

- Age younger than 18 years or older than 65 years (increased risk at older than 75 years).
- Recent unintentional weight loss of more than 5% in 1 month or more than 10% in 6 months. Weight loss is calculated as follows:
  Percent weight loss = (UBW − CBW)/UBW, where UBW is usual body weight and CBW is current body weight.
- Excessive alcohol intake or other substance abuse.
- Living conditions: Homelessness or living with limited access to food.
- Limited capacity for oral intake resulting from physical problems, such as dysphagia, odynophagia, stomatitis, or mucositis.
- NPO (nil per os [nothing by mouth]) status for more than 3 days.
- Increased metabolic demands induced by extensive burns, major surgery, trauma, fever, infection, draining abscesses or wounds, fistulas, pregnancy.
- Protracted nutrient losses associated with malabsorption syndromes, short gut syndrome, draining abscesses, wounds, or fistulas; effusions, renal dialysis.
- Requires intake of catabolic drugs including corticosteroids, immunosuppressants, and antineoplastic agents.
- Protracted emesis from conditions such as anorexia nervosa, bulimia, hyperemesis gravidarum, radiation, or oncologic chemotherapy.

- Presence of chronic disease such as acquired immune deficiency syndrome (AIDS), diabetes, cystic fibrosis, or cancer.
- Patients with obesity who are critically ill experience more complications than patients with normal body mass index (BMI), including length of stay, infectious morbidity, mortality, and attainment of nutritional goals.

PHYSICAL ASSESSMENT

Most physical findings are not conclusive for particular nutritional deficiencies. It is important to compare current assessment findings with past assessments, especially related to the following:
- Loss of muscle and adipose tissue.
- Work and muscle endurance, neuromuscular function.
- Changes in hair and nails and the presence of skin lesions.

ANTHROPOMETRIC DATA

Anthropometrics is the measurement of the body or its parts. Pounds and inches are converted to metric measurements using the following formulas:
Divide pounds by 2.2 to convert to kilograms (kg).
Multiply inches by 2.54 to convert to centimeters (cm).
- Height: Used to determine ideal weight and BMI; if unavailable, obtain estimate from family or significant others.
- Weight: A readily available and practical indicator of nutritional status that can be compared with previous weight and ideal weight or used to calculate BMI. Large changes may reflect fluid retention (edema, third spacing), diuresis, dehydration, surgical resections, traumatic amputations, or weight of dressings or equipment. Note: 1 liter (L) of fluid equals approximately 2 pounds (lb). Frequent monitoring of patient weight is essential to detect significant weight loss and weight gain in patients who are critically ill.
- Body mass index (BMI): Used to evaluate adult weight. One calculation and one set of standards apply to both men and women:
  - BMI $\leq$ 15: Severely underweight
  - BMI $<$ 18.5: Underweight
  - BMI 18.5 to 24.9: Normal
  - BMI 25 to 29.9: Overweight
  - BMI 30 to 34.9: Obesity Class I
  - BMI 35 to 39.9: Obesity Class II
  - BMI $>$ 40: Obesity Class III (morbid obesity)

Although obesity is usually associated with poor health outcomes, several metaanalyses of the effects of obesity on patient outcomes in the critical care setting have actually shown no difference in mortality between patients who are obese and their counterparts who are not obese. This phenomenon has been given the term "the ICU conundrum." However, BMI values less than 18.5 and greater than 40 are associated with an increase in morbidity and are associated with longer ICU stay, increased postoperative complications, and higher readmission rates.
- Midarm muscle circumference (MAMC): Measures muscle mass of the mid-upper arm using a formula.
- Triceps skinfold thickness (TSF): Measured at the midpoint of the upper arm by taking half the distance between the olecranon and the acromion process and grasping the skin and subcutaneous tissue at the back of the arm approximately 1 cm from the midpoint. Surgical calipers are used to measure the skinfold. A TSF measurement of less than 3 mm signals severely depleted fat stores.

Specially trained clinicians and dietitians should perform this assessment for more accurate and consistent results. The skill level and technique used vary among clinicians.

See Table 1-20 for height and weight determinations in men and women.

DIAGNOSTIC TESTS

No laboratory test specifically measures nutritional status. Status can be estimated, however, using the following parameters.

VISCERAL PROTEIN STATUS

Normal values may vary with different laboratory procedures and standards. If the hydration status is normal and anemia is absent, albumin and transferrin levels may be the initial

Table 1-20	HEIGHT AND WEIGHT GUIDELINES FOR MEN AND WOMEN					
	Men (Weight in lb)			Women (Weight in lb)		
Height	Small Frame	Medium Frame	Large Frame	Small Frame	Medium Frame	Large Frame
4 ft 10 in	—	—	—	102–111	109–121	118–131
4 ft 11 in	—	—	—	103–113	111–123	120–134
5 ft	—	—	—	104–115	113–126	122–137
5 ft 1 in	—	—	—	106–118	115–129	125–140
5 ft 2 in	128–134	131–141	138–150	108–121	118–132	128–143
5 ft 3 in	130–136	133–143	140–153	111–124	121–135	131–147
5 ft 4 in	132–138	135–145	142–156	114–127	124–138	134–151
5 ft 5 in	134–140	137–148	144–160	117–130	127–141	137–155
5 ft 6 in	136–142	139–151	146–164	120–133	130–144	140–159
5 ft 7 in	138–145	142–154	149–168	123–136	133–147	143–163
5 ft 8 in	140–148	145–157	152–172	126–139	136–150	146–167
5 ft 9 in	142–151	148–160	155–176	129–142	139–153	149–170
5 ft 10 in	144–154	151–163	158–180	132–145	142–156	152–173
5 ft 11 in	146–157	154–166	161–184	135–148	145–159	155–176
6 ft	149–160	157–170	164–188	138–151	148–162	158–179
6 ft 1 in	152–164	160–174	168–192	—	—	—
6 ft 2 in	155–168	164–178	172–197	—	—	—
6 ft 3 in	158–172	167–182	176–202	—	—	—
6 ft 4 in	162–176	171–187	181–207	—	—	—

parameters used for a general assessment of nutritional status. The following are all visceral proteins:

- Serum albumin (3.5 to 5.5 g/dL): An indicator associated with increased morbidity in critical illness if the level is less than 3.5 g/dL. It has a long half-life (14 to 21 days) and changes slowly in response to nutrition support when protein-calorie malnutrition is present.
- Prealbumin (20 to 30 mg/dL): A reliable indicator of response to nutritional therapy. It has a short half-life (2 to 3 days) and may not be reliable if the patient is severely stressed or ill, has an elevated C-reactive protein (CRP) level, is on steroid therapy, or has renal failure.
- Retinol-binding protein (4 to 5 mg/dL): The indicator with the shortest half-life (12 hours) used to assess the response to nutritional therapy. It is not as reliable in patients who are severely stressed or those with inflammation, vitamin A deficiency, and renal failure.
- Transferrin (180 to 260 mg/dL): The indicator with a longer half-life (8 to 10 days), used as a baseline indicator of protein intake and synthesis. Similar to prealbumin, it may not be reliable when the patient is severely stressed and is also affected by changes in iron status.

It is important to note that none of these markers of nutritional status are validated in the patient who is critically ill because they are all affected by the acute phase response.

The Academy of Nutrition and Dietetics (AND) in conjunction with the American Society of Parenteral and Enteral Nutrition recently published recommended clinical characteristics for identifying patients with moderate to severe malnutrition. These characteristics include energy intake, weight loss, body fat and muscle loss, edema, and reduced grip strength, as well as the presence or absence of acute illness or injury, chronic illness, or social or environmental circumstances that would predispose patients to malnutrition. Regarding interpretation of weight loss, percent of weight change over time is used to differentiate between moderate and severe malnutrition. Of note, both the AND-ASPEN guidelines and the ASPEN-SCCM guidelines do not recommend using visceral protein markers to identify malnutrition.

NITROGEN BALANCE

Nitrogen balance is used in the clinical setting to measure protein metabolism and protein status. Nitrogen balance is calculated as follows: Nitrogen balance = Nitrogen in (calculated from total protein intake) − Nitrogen out (the sum of nitrogen lost in urine, stool, and body fluids). Most nitrogen loss occurs through the urine, with a small, constant amount lost via the skin and feces. Nitrogen balance studies should be performed by nutrition support specialists, because accurate calculation is important to determine the patient's protein status and protein requirements. Nitrogen balance studies require a 24-hour urine collection and accurate measurement of protein intake. Heavy losses of protein in the presence of ascites, large wounds, malabsorption, and excessive chest tube drainage are difficult to measure but are considered by the nutrition support specialist when calculating the nitrogen balance. A positive or neutral nitrogen balance is optimal, but is sometimes difficult to attain during critical illness because of the catabolic nature of the disease.

ESTIMATING NUTRITION REQUIREMENTS

ENERGY NEEDS

The primary goals of nutrition support are to preserve lean body mass, preserve immune functioning, and to prevent metabolic complications while also preventing worsening of malnutrition in the patient who is critically ill. The nutrition support plan should avoid overfeeding and underfeeding and the complications associated with both. Energy needs can be estimated using the following options.

CALCULATION BASED ON PATIENT WEIGHT

Estimated energy requirements are 25 to 35 kcal/kg daily for the patient who is not stressed. Patients who are highly stressed or malnourished may require up to 40 kcal/kg daily. Patients who are obese may require 11 to 14 kcal/kg daily or 22 to 25 kcal/kg of IBW. Although this is not a preferred method for determining energy needs in patients who are critically ill, calculation based on weight is often used because of its simplicity.

INDIRECT CALORIMETRY

Indirect calorimetry is the "gold standard" for calculating energy needs in the patient who is critically ill and mechanically ventilated. This test measures O_2 consumption and CO_2 production as a byproduct of metabolism and gives the resting metabolic rate (RMR) and the respiratory quotient (RQ). The RMR is slightly higher than the basal metabolic rate (BMR). The RQ is the ratio of carbon dioxide produced relative to oxygen consumption, and can determine if the patient is being adequately fed (RQ 0.85), underfed (RQ < 0.82), or overfed (RQ > 1). Indirect calorimetry accuracy can be affected by many factors including $F_{IO_2} \geq 60$, leaking chest tubes, bronchopleural fistulas, and renal replacement therapy. Specialized personnel and access to a metabolic cart are required to provide accurate results.

PREDICTIVE EQUATIONS

Many predictive equations have been validated over the years. The Harris Benedict Equation was formerly the most common and accepted formula used to determine RMR. Published originally in 1919, it was widely accepted until 2003 when the American Dietetic Association recommended other more reliable equations.

Currently, there are many available equations for estimating energy needs. We will focus on the two equations that are commonly endorsed and are validated for use for patients who are critically ill, including the patient with obesity who is critically ill.

Mifflin St Jeor (MSJ)

The MSJ formula is based on patient age, height, weight, and gender. The MSJ formula has been shown to be one of the most accurate formulas for predicting RMR in both obese and nonobese patients. It has been endorsed by the American Dietetic Association and by the American Society of Parenteral and Enteral Nutrition. The MSJ formula is appropriate for most healthy patients. For critically ill hospital patients who are not mechanically ventilated, adding a stress factor of 1.2 to 1.3 × MSJ is recommended.

$$\text{Males: BMR} = 10 \times \text{weight (kg)} + 6.25 \times \text{height (cm)} -5 \times \text{age (year)} + 5$$
$$\text{Females: BMR} = 10 \times \text{weight (kg)} + 6.25 \times \text{height (cm)} -5 \times \text{age (year)} - 161$$

Modified Penn State Formula

The Modified Penn State Formula is intended for patients who are mechanically ventilated. It is based on the MSJ formula (it was formerly based on the Harris Benedict Equation) and includes additional measures including temperature and minute ventilation (a function of tidal volume and respiratory rate). If it is not possible to perform indirect calorimetry or to calculate the Modified Penn State Formula, then the MSJ formula can be used.

$$\text{RMR (kcal/day)} = (\text{Mifflin St Jeor}) \, (0.71) + V_E \, (64) + T_m \, (85) - 3085$$

where V_E = minute ventilation (Tidal volume [L] × Rate) and $T_m = T_{max}$ (centigrade)

PROVISION OF MACRONUTRIENTS (CARBOHYDRATE, FAT, AND PROTEIN)

- Carbohydrate: Carbohydrates should comprise 45% to 65% of the total caloric intake. Dextrose is the carbohydrate source in PN. Increased dextrose loads can lead to hyperglycemia, excessive CO_2 production, hypophosphatemia, fat deposits in the liver, and transient elevated liver enzymes. A minimum of 50 g of carbohydrate daily is required to prevent ketosis.
- Protein: Protein requirements are generally calculated based on g/kg of IBW unless the patient's actual weight is less than his/her IBW, when actual body weight is used. ASPEN-SCCM guidelines recommend using actual body weight for patients whose BMI is less than 30. For BMI > 30, IBW should be used to calculate protein needs. Protein requirements for maintenance therapy are 0.8 to 1.2 g/kg/day. Patients who are critically ill, as well as patients with fever, infection, and wounds, may need an estimated 1.5 to 2 g/kg/day. Patients on hemodialysis or continuous renal replacement therapy have even higher protein requirements, up to 2 g/kg/day. Whereas in the past, protein has been restricted for patients with advanced liver disease, currently higher protein is recommended for such patients (1 to 1.5 g/kg) unless the patient has refractory hepatic encephalopathy in which case protein restriction is recommended until resolution of hepatic encephalopathy. Severe stress or burns may increase protein requirements up to 4 g/kg/day.
- Fat requirements: Fat requirements range from 25% to 55% of total calories. Fat should not exceed 60% of total caloric intake. Fat can be administered in minimal quantities to satisfy needs for essential fatty acids, or it can be provided in larger quantities, as tolerated, to meet energy needs. In patients receiving PN, the maximum recommended amount of IV fat emulsion in patients who are critically ill is 1 g/kg/day. A minimum of 100 g IV fat emulsion per week is necessary to prevent essential fatty acid deficiency (EFAD). Signs and symptoms of EFAD include dry, scaly skin and rash, impaired wound healing, and rarely neurologic symptoms.

VITAMIN AND ESSENTIAL TRACE MINERAL REQUIREMENTS

In general, the recommended dietary allowances (RDAs) for vitamins, minerals, and trace elements should be followed to provide minimum quantities of vitamins and minerals. For specific patients, supplements of specific vitamins or minerals are needed in increased amounts for existing disease states (e.g., zinc and vitamins A and C for burns; thiamine, folate, and vitamin B_{12} for chronic alcohol ingestion). Patients who are malnourished and who are at increased risk of refeeding syndrome should receive additional thiamine (B_1). Enteral formulas contain the RDA for most vitamins and minerals. However, it is not uncommon for patients who are tube fed to receive additional multivitamin preparations. Parenteral multivitamin infusion (MVI) is added to TPN. Trace elements include zinc, copper, manganese, chromium, and selenium. Trace elements are usually included in enteral or oral multivitamin preparations. They are available as a separate multitrace element preparation for IV administration in TPN. For a list of common signs and symptoms of vitamin and mineral deficiency and toxicity, see Table 1-21. For a list of common signs and symptoms of trace element deficiencies, see Table 1-22.

Table 1-21	**SIGNS AND SYMPTOMS OF VITAMIN DEFICIENCY AND TOXICITY**		
	Other Names	**Common Signs of Deficiency**	**Common Signs of Toxicity**
Fat-Soluble Vitamins			
A	beta-Carotene, retinol	Impaired wound healing, night blindness, xerophthalmia	Hip fracture, hepatotoxicity, alopecia, ataxia, lipids, cheilitis
D	Ergocalciferol (D_2) Cholecalciferol (D_3)	Hypocalcemia, osteomalacia, osteoporosis, rickets	Hypercalcemia, hypercalciuria, soft tissue calcification
E	alpha-Tocopherol	Asymptomatic early, ↑ platelet aggregation, hemolytic anemia, ataxia, weakness, vision changes	Skeletal muscle lesions, inclusion bodies in bone marrow, impaired coagulation
K		Bleeding, bruising, ↑ fractures, low bone density	Toxicity rare
Water-Soluble Vitamins			
B_1	Thiamine	Wernicke disease: ocular abnormalities, gait ataxia, mental status changes Beriberi, Korsakoff syndrome	Uncommon
B_2	Riboflavin	Sore throat, angular cheilitis, magenta tongue, anemia (normochromic/normocytic), visual disturbances, seborrheic dermatitis	Rare
B_3	Niacin, niacinamide	Pellagra (dermatitis, diarrhea, dementia), neurologic changes	Flushing of skin, hepatotoxicity, hyperglycemia, myopathy, hyperuricemia, gout
B_5	Pantothenic acid	Very rare	Rare
B_6	Pyridoxine	Anemia, convulsions, confusion, angular stomatitis, glossitis, cheilosis	Sensory neuropathy and ataxia, areflexia, impaired cutaneous and deep sensation, skin lesions
B_7	Biotin	Rare: dermatitis, glossitis, electrocardiography changes, anorexia, muscle pain	None
B_9	Folate	Megaloblastic anemia, diarrhea, smooth, sore tongue, nervous instability	Rare
B_{12}	Cyanocobalamin, cobalamin	Cognitive impairment, depression, psychosis, glossitis, paresthesias, megaloblastic anemia	None

Continued

Table 1-21	SIGNS AND SYMPTOMS OF VITAMIN DEFICIENCY AND TOXICITY—cont'd		
	Other Names	**Common Signs of Deficiency**	**Common Signs of Toxicity**
C	Ascorbic acid	Anorexia, fatigue, muscle pain, ↑ infection Scurvy: anemia, bleeding gums ↓ wound healing, weakening of bone/teeth	Oxalate stones at doses >100 to 500 per day (especially with renal failure) N/V, ↓ B_{12} bioavailability

From Clark SF. Vitamins and Trace Elements. The A.S.P.E.N. Adult Nutrition Support Core Curriculum, 2nd Edition. Charles M. Mueller, Editor. 2012.

Table 1-22	SIGNS AND SYMPTOMS OF TRACE ELEMENT DEFICIENCY AND TOXICITY	
Trace Element	**Signs of Deficiency**	**Toxicity**
Chromium	Glucose intolerance, hyperlipidemia, peripheral neuropathy, encephalopathy	Renal failure, anemia, thrombocytopenia, liver failure
Copper	Common: hypochromic, microcytic anemia and neutropenia (similar to signs and symptoms of vitamin B_{12} deficiency) Central nervous system dysfunction, hypotonia	Gastrointestinal symptoms, hepatic failure Biliary excretion — caution in liver failure
Manganese	Weight loss, transient dermatitis Rare: nausea and vomiting	Parkinson-like motor dysfunction, neuro-logic and psychiatric symptoms (irritability, hallucinations)
Selenium	Cardiomyopathy, myalgia, myositis, hemolysis, and impaired cellular immunity	Chronic: nail and hair changes, N/V, weight loss, paresthesias, fatigue, garlic odor on breath, ↑ incidence of diabetes Acute (rare): cardiac abnormalities, hypotension
Zinc	Dermatitis, alopecia, anorexia, growth failure, reduced taste sensitivity, poor night vision, immune compromise, impaired wound healing	Gastrointestinal symptoms, copper deficiency, renal failure, neuropathy, metallic taste

From Vanek VW, Borum P, Buchman A, et al. A.S.P.E.N. position paper recommendations for changes in commercially available parenteral multivitamin and multi-trace element products. *Nutr Clin Pract.* 2012;27:440-491. Jensen GL and Binkley J. Clinical manifestations of nutrient deficiency. *JPEN J Parenter Enteral Nutr.* 2002;26:S29-S33

FLUID REQUIREMENTS

Many factors affect fluid balance. All sources of intake (oral, enteral, intravenous, and medications), as well as output (urine, stool, drainage, emesis, fluid shifts, and respiratory and evaporative losses), must be considered. Fluid intake is closely associated with energy provided. Approximately 1 mL fluid per calorie is one method to calculate fluid requirements; however, this often underestimates fluid needs. Another method to determine fluid requirements is according to patient weight. Most patients require between 30 and 40 mL/kg of fluid daily. For patients with fluid restriction, use less than 25 mL/kg or 1.4 to 1.9 L daily. It is important to remember to calculate fluid received from enteral nutrition and PN to avoid fluid overload. Fever increases fluid needs, and fluid intake should be closely monitored in renal and cardiac dysfunction.

NUTRITION SUPPORT MODALITIES
ENTERAL NUTRITION

Enteral feedings (tube feedings) are the preferred strategy for nutrition support in the critically ill. Studies indicate that enteral feedings prevent the passage of bacteria from the GI tract into the lymphatic system (bacterial translocation) and other organs, reducing a major source of sepsis and possible organ failure. Cost, safety, and convenience considerations have been the rationale for using enteral over parenteral support, because the potential physiologic benefits justify that every effort be made to use enteral feeds. Enteral feedings promote wound healing and immune competence and preserve gut function. Current ASPEN-SCCM guidelines for nutrition support in the patient who is critically ill recommend enteral nutrition as the preferred route of therapy. According to these guidelines, enteral nutrition should be initiated as soon as possible in the patient who is critically ill: within 24 to 48 hours after admission once the patient is fully resuscitated and the patient is hemodynamically stable. The guidelines further recommend that enteral feedings be advanced to the goal rate over the next 48 to 72 hours. Despite these recommendations and the benefits of enteral nutrition, patients in the ICU setting frequently receive only up to 50% of their goal calories. This is as a result of unnecessary holding of enteral feeds around procedures, ordering inadequate calories, or tube feeding intolerance. It is also attributable to a common misconception that enteral feeding cannot be started until bowel sounds are present. According to the ASPEN-SCCM 2009 guidelines, as well as the CCCN guidelines, neither the presence of bowel sounds nor the presence of flatus or stool is necessary to initiate tube feeding in the patient who is critically ill. The rationale for this is that bowel sounds are indicators of gut contractility and do not necessarily correlate with gut function or absorptive capacity. The reasons for patient intolerance of enteral feeds in the critical care setting are multifactorial and can be attributed to inappropriate enteral formula selection, enteral access, mode of enteral feeding (e.g., bolus versus continuous tube feeding), medications, or the patient's underlying disease process. A dedicated interdisciplinary nutrition support team can address these issues and prevent tube feeding intolerance in many if not most circumstances.

RESEARCH BRIEF BOX 1-2

Early enteral nutrition in patients who are critically ill

Another recent trial, by Elke et al., was a secondary analysis of pooled data that were collected prospectively from nutrition studies. This trial looked at clinical outcomes of critically ill mechanically ventilated patients with sepsis and/or pneumonia ($N = 2207$) who were enterally fed at either close to goal calories or hypocaloric or trophic feeding. The study results showed that an increase of 1000 kcal daily was associated with a statistically significant reduction in 60-day mortality (odds ratio 0.61, 95% confidence interval 0.53 to 5.08, $P = 0.02$) and a statistically significant increase in ventilator-free days (2.81 days, 95% confidence interval 0.48 to 0.77, $P < 0.001$). Similar results were found regarding an increase of 30 g daily of protein

From Elke G, Wang M, Weiler N, et al: Close to recommended caloric and protein intake by enteral nutrition is associated with better clinical outcome of critically ill septic patients: secondary analysis of a large international nutrition database. *Crit Care* 18(1):R29, 2014.

Whether one chooses to base clinical practice on the EDEN trial or the trial by Elke et al., it is important to note that both trials implemented early enteral nutrition in patients who were critically ill.

Enteral formulas

Enteral formulas are composed of a wide variety of standard and modular formulas. See Table 1-23 for a more detailed discussion of currently available enteral formulas.

Table 1-23	TYPES OF ENTERAL FORMULATIONS
Enteral Formula	**Description**
Blenderized Diet	
Compleat, Compleat Modified	Nutritionally complete, requiring complete digestive capabilities; composed of natural foods, including meat, vegetables, milk, and fruit
Standard Lactose-Free Formulas	
Nutren, Isosource, Osmolite	Nutritionally adequate, liquid preparation; used for non–disease-specific nutrition support; standard isotonic; low residue formulas
Specialty Formulas	
Hepatic failure	
Nutrihep	Nutritionally complete; has a greater ratio of branched chain to aromatic amino acids while restricting total amino acid concentrations and adding nonprotein calories. Calorie-dense to prevent fluid overload.
Renal failure	
Suplena Renalcal	Low-protein, calorie-dense, low-electrolyte (no electrolytes in Renalcal) formulas designed for patients with reduced kidney function but not yet on dialysis; restricted total protein content may reduce or postpone need for dialysis. High in vitamin B_6 and folic acid.
Nepro Novasource Renal	Calorie-dense, high-protein, low-electrolyte formulas designed for patients on dialysis. High in vitamin B_6 and folic acid.
Respiratory Insufficiency	
Pulmocare Novasource Pulmonary	Nutritionally complete; contains a higher proportion of fat to carbohydrates; may help prevent an increase in CO_2 production. Helpful in patients with COPD, cystic fibrosis, or respiratory failure.
Oxepa	Specialized formula with unique blend of patented oils (EPA and GLA) to help modulate the inflammatory response in patients who are critically ill and ventilated, especially those with ALI, ARDS, and sepsis.
Hypermetabolic and Trauma States	
Impact Peptide 1.5, Pivot 1.5	Very-high protein, calorie-dense, immune-enhancing formulas with added arginine for the patient who is metabolically stressed and immunosuppressed.
Impact, Impact with fiber, Impact glutamine, Pivot 1.5	Specialized nutrition for surgical and trauma patients.
Peptamen bariatric	Very-high protein, low-calorie to meet the needs of patients who are critically ill and obese.
Oxepa	Specialized formula with unique blend of patented oils (EPA and GLA) to help modulate the inflammatory response in patients who are critically ill and ventilated, especially those with ALI, ARDS, and sepsis.
Diabetes or Hyperglycemia	
Diabetisource AC, Glucerna products, Glytrol	Reduced carbohydrate, fiber-containing formulas to help minimize glycemic response. Lactose-free.
Fiber-Enhanced	
Compleat, FiberSource Replete fiber, Promote with Fiber Jevity, Nutren Fiber, Impact with Fiber, Peptamen 1.5 with Prebio, Glucerna products, Diabetisource AC, Glytrol	Fiber blends help to support digestive health and normal bowel function. Products contain soluble or insoluble fiber or a blend of both. Insoluble fiber is NOT recommended in critically ill patients in the ICU setting.

Table 1-23	TYPES OF ENTERAL FORMULATIONS—cont'd
Enteral Formula	**Description**
Calorie-Dense Products	
TwoCal HN, Nutren 2.0	Calorie content is 2 calories/mL to provide adequate nutrients in lower volume for volume-restricted patients; some standard products also come in 1.5 calories/mL concentration.
High-Protein Formulas	
Promote, Replete	Increased protein to help support wound healing. Meets or exceeds 100% of recommended daily intake for vitamins and minerals.
Soy-Based Products	
FiberSource HN, Isosource HN	Soy protein isolate and soy fiber for patients who cannot tolerate milk protein. Not suitable for patients with galactosemia.
Elemental or Semielemental	
Vivonex, Optimental, Peptamen products, Perative, Impact Peptide 1.5, Vital products	Designed for easy absorption for the patient who has malabsorption or intestinal atrophy; protein source is free amino acids or protein hydrolysates (peptides) or both; fat sources are oils easily absorbed: MCT, soybean, canola, safflower; some formulas contain fiber; some have flavor packets for oral use.

ALI, Acute lung injury; *ARDS,* acute respiratory distress syndrome; *COPD,* chronic obstructive pulmonary disease; *EPA,* eicosapentaenoic acid; *GLA,* gamma linolenic acid; *MCT,* medium chain triglycerides.

- Standard: Consist of intact proteins and a caloric source; most are lactose-free; all are sterile, and suitable for small-bore feeding tubes and have a fixed nutrient composition. Vitamins and trace elements and minerals are included.
- Modular: Consist of a single nutrient that may be combined with other modules (nutrients) for a formula tailor-made for an individual's specific deficits (e.g., carbohydrate, fat, protein, specific amino acids). The most common modular product is protein powder.
- Specialty: Enteral formulas that are disease-specific, as described in the following section on special diets for organ-specific pathology and in Table 1-23.

Nutritional composition of enteral formulas

- Carbohydrates are the most abundant macronutrient and energy source, comprising between 40% and 90%, in enteral formulas. Carbohydrates are broken down and absorbed as monosaccharides (glucose, galactose, and fructose) in the small intestine. Nearly all enteral formulas are lactose-free to avoid problems in individuals with lactase deficiencies. However, these formulas are not appropriate for patients with galactosemia.
- Fiber is a polysaccharide that is found in plant foods and is not digested in the human GI tract. There are two types of fiber: soluble and insoluble. Soluble fiber is fermented by gut bacteria to produce short-chain fatty acids, which help maintain gut integrity and promote water and sodium absorption. Insoluble fiber is not fermented in the gut. Both soluble and insoluble fiber are included in many enteral formulas to decrease incidence of diarrhea by increasing water and sodium absorption, decreasing transit time, and increasing fecal weight. Fiber may also help with glucose control in patients with diabetes mellitus.

Some enteral formulas contain prebiotics (such as FOS [fructooligosaccharides]). Prebiotics promote the growth of beneficial bacteria in the gut (such as bifidobacteria and lactobacillus).

Care should be used when administering high-fiber (especially insoluble fiber) formulas to patients who are critically ill, because this can lead to bowel ischemia. Current ASPEN-SCCM guidelines recommend avoiding insoluble fiber in patients who are critically ill and at high risk for gut dysmotility and ischemia. Adverse side effects of fiber and prebiotics include bloating, abdominal pain, and flatulence.

- Protein: Enteral formulas contain either intact protein, hydrolyzed protein, or free amino acids.
  - Intact protein: Most standard enteral formulas contain intact protein, which is the protein found in complete and original form (e.g., commercial and blenderized whole food diets). The most common types of intact protein in enteral formulas are casein and whey (derived from milk) and soy.
  - Hydrolyzed protein: Formulas that contain hydrolyzed proteins are called semielemental or elemental formulas. Hydrolyzed protein has been broken down to smaller peptides to aid absorption. It is better absorbed in patients with GI dysfunction or pancreatic insufficiency.
  - Free amino acids (FAAs) have been broken down completely to single amino acids and, therefore, require no additional digestion before absorption. Similar to elemental and semielemental formulas, FAAs are intended for use in patients with GI dysfunction or pancreatic insufficiency.
- Fat generally comprises between 30% and 50% of enteral formulas. Fat provides energy, essential fatty acids, and is a source of fat-soluble vitamins (A, D, E, and K). Most enteral formulas contain both long-chain triglycerides (LCTs) and medium-chain triglycerides (MCTs). LCTs are a source of essential fatty acids and calories. MCTs are more easily absorbed and digested because they do not require pancreatic enzymes for digestion and are absorbed immediately into the GI tract without having to be absorbed via the lymph system. However, MCTs do not contain essential fatty acids and are therefore not a sole fat source in enteral formulas. Some enteral formulas contain "structured" lipids. Structured lipids have been chemically modified to contain both LCTs and MCTs on the same lipid backbone.

Specialized enteral formulas for organ-specific pathology
These formulas are costly, and the metabolic advantages of some of these products remain unproved.
- Hepatic failure: Branched-chain amino acids (BCAAs) in combination with reduced aromatic amino acid concentrations may help alleviate encephalopathy associated with hepatic failure. However, data with regard to the efficacy of BCAAs are very limited, and these formulas are not currently routinely recommended for patients with liver failure. These formulas should be reserved for patients with hepatic encephalopathy that is refractory to lactulose and antibiotics.
- Renal disease: Predialysis formulas contain lower protein content and are low in phosphorus and potassium. These formulas are calorie dense (fluid restricted). Some formulas have no electrolytes. Dialysis formulas are higher in protein, are calorically dense, are lower in phosphorus and potassium, and have vitamin and mineral profiles that are designed for patients on hemodialysis.
- Respiratory disease: It was previously thought that high-carbohydrate load exacerbated pulmonary dysfunction in patients with chronic pulmonary diseases. It is now accepted that avoidance of overfeeding any substrate (fat, carbohydrate, or protein) in this patient population prevents an increase in CO_2 production and, consequently, prevents an increase in the work of breathing. Pulmonary formulas are lower in carbohydrate and are higher in fat. The high-fat content can lead to intolerance in some patients. Although these formulas are still available, they are not widely used, and nutrition support clinicians prefer to use standard formulas and to avoid overfeeding. There are specific formulas for ARDS and acute lung injury (ALI) that have an antiinflammatory lipid profile (borage oil and omega-3 fatty acids) and high amounts of antioxidants. The ASPEN-SCCM guidelines for nutrition support in the patient who is critically ill recommend these formulas for ICU patients with ALI/ARDS, with a high level of recommendation. However, recent randomized, controlled trials failed to show any benefit of these products in patients with ALI, thus these recommendations may be downgraded in updated guidelines. The recently updated CCCN guidelines did downgrade the recommendation for use of these formulas in patients with ALI/ARDS from "recommended" to "should be considered."
- Diabetes: Diabetic formulas, designed to maintain good glycemic control, contain reduced carbohydrates, higher fat content, and higher fiber content. Some of these products contain high amounts of insoluble fiber and should be avoided in patients who are critically ill and at high risk for GI dysmotility and bowel ischemia (ASPEN-SCCM

guidelines). According to the AND, there is insufficient evidence to determine whether diabetes-specific formulas have an impact on mortality in the patient with diabetes who is critically ill. Current guidelines for nutrition support in the adult ICU patient with hyperglycemia do not make specific recommendations regarding use of diabetes-specific formulas for patients who are critically ill. Current practice is to use a standard formula with insulin coverage for hyperglycemia, reserving the diabetic formulas for patients who have problems maintaining good glucose control despite insulin.

Enteral access

There are many different options for enteral access based on length of therapy desired (short term versus long term), site of entry (nasal versus enterostomy), and terminal site (stomach, duodenum, jejunum).

Site of delivery

Stomach: The stomach is the easiest site for enteral tube placement; gastric feeding simulates normal GI function, and may be used for bolus, intermittent, cyclic, or continuous feedings. Entry site into the stomach is nasal (NG), oral (OG), percutaneous (PEG), laparoscopic, or surgical (open gastrostomy).

Postpyloric: Postpyloric placement includes anywhere distal to the pylorus but before the ligament of Treitz. The most common site of entry for postpyloric feeding tubes is the nose, and these tubes can be placed at the bedside, endoscopically, or under fluoroscopy.

Jejunal: Jejunal tubes are placed distal to the ligament of Treitz. These tubes are more difficult to place at the bedside, although specially trained personnel can place nasojejunal (NJ) tubes at the bedside. Generally, NJ placement is done endoscopically or under fluoroscopy. Direct jejunal feeding tubes can be placed either percutaneously, under fluoroscopy, laparoscopically, or surgically.

Site of Entry

Nasoenteric feeding tubes: Nasoenteric tubes are indicated for short-term enteral nutrition. Nasoenteric tubes are measured by their external diameter, but flow through these tubes is determined by their internal diameter. Therefore, a tube with a small internal diameter will be more prone to clogging even if its external diameter is larger. Nasoenteric tubes are available in different lengths, depending on the desired site of delivery of enteral nutrition. Nasogastric tubes are the shortest, whereas nasoenteric tubes are longer for placement into the duodenum or jejunum. Nasoenteric feeding tubes are most commonly used in the ICU setting. It is vital that feeding tube placement be verified either by x-ray, fluoroscopy, or electromagnetic imaging before initiation of enteral feeding.

Complications of nasoenteric feeding tube placement

Procedure-related: The most common procedure-related complications are epistaxis, aspiration, and circulatory or respiratory arrest. The most serious complication is misplacement into the bronchi. For this reason, verification of feeding tube placement is imperative when placing a nasoenteric feeding tube.

Postprocedure-related: The most common postprocedural complication of nasal feeding tubes is feeding tube clogging. One of the most effective methods to prevent feeding tubes from clogging is to flush the feeding tube regularly with water (at least 30 mL every 6 hours). Other complications include dislodgment of the feeding tube or feeding tube malfunction (kinking or breaking of the tube).

Enterostomy tubes: Enterostomy tubes are indicated for long-term enteral nutrition support (usually defined as greater than 4 weeks) and include gastrostomy tubes, gastrojejunostomy tubes, and jejunostomy tubes. Gastrojejunostomy tubes are intended for patients with GI dysmotility who require simultaneous gastric decompression and jejunal feeding. As stated earlier, gastrostomy and jejunostomy tubes can be placed percutaneously, under fluoroscopy, laparoscopically, or surgically (open G or J tube).

Enterostomy tube placement complications

Procedure-related: Procedure-related complications of enterostomy tubes are less common than those associated with nasoenteric tubes. Complications include perforation of the GI lumen, hemorrhage, aspiration, and ileus.

Postprocedure-related: Minor postprocedural complications include infection and leakage around the site of the feeding tube. Major complications include necrotizing fasciitis and buried bumper syndrome. This syndrome occurs when gastric mucosa grows over the internal bumper of the enterostomy tube. Risk factors for buried bumper syndrome include poor wound healing and significant weight gain. Another complication is feeding tube dislodgement. Dislodged feeding tubes must be replaced immediately to prevent closure of the entry site.

Methods of administration of enteral nutrition

Enteral nutrition can be delivered either as continuous infusion, cyclic infusion, intermittent feeding, or bolus or gravity drip feeding. For patients with feeding tubes terminating in the jejunum, only continuous or cyclic infusion is appropriate because the jejunum cannot tolerate large boluses of fluid.

Continuous, pump-assisted, tube feeding is the most common and preferred method of enteral nutrition delivery in ICU patients. Other indications for continuous infusion are patients at risk for refeeding syndrome, patients receiving feeding via a jejunostomy tube, patients with poor glycemic control, or those who have not tolerated bolus or intermittent feeding. Continuous tube feeding is usually started at a low rate (10 to 25 mL/h) and is advanced slowly every 4 to 6 hours to the goal rate. The goal rate can be calculated by determining the total daily volume to be infused and dividing by 24 hours.

Cyclic tube feeding is almost the same as continuous tube feeding, but the total volume is infused over a shorter amount of time, usually 12 to 16 hours, but sometimes as little as 8 hours. This method is also used to infuse tube feeds at night (nocturnal tube feeding) as a method to help the patient transition to an oral diet.

Intermittent tube feeding can be delivered via a pump or by the gravity drip method. Larger volumes of formula (240 to 720 mL or 1 to 3 cans) are infused over a shorter period of time (usually from 20 to 60 minutes) several times a day, depending on the volume needed to meet the patient's caloric needs.

Bolus or gravity drip feedings are similar to intermittent tube feeding, but the volume of enteral formula is given over a shorter period of time (5 to 10 minutes) several times a day instead of being allowed to infuse over a longer period of time. Bolus feeding is most similar to normal feeding, and is the least expensive and cumbersome method of tube feeding. It is generally not used in patients who are critically ill and who cannot tolerate such rapid infusion of large amounts of volume (Table 1-24).

Monitoring tolerance of enteral feeding

Tolerance of enteral feedings should be monitored based on physical assessment, measurement of gastric residuals, and by radiographic confirmation (abdominal x-ray) if ileus or obstruction is suspected.

Gastric residual volumes should be checked approximately every 4 hours in continuously enterally fed patients. According to the current ASPEN-SCCM guidelines (2009), holding tube feeding for gastric residuals less than 500 mL in the absence of other signs of intolerance should be minimized. Recently published Canadian Nutrition Support guidelines (2013) for patients who are critically ill recommend holding enteral feeding for gastric residuals of greater than 250 mL (approximately 8 oz or one cup). It is important to monitor physical symptoms, such as abdominal pain or distension, and by passage of stool or flatus.

For patients receiving bolus or intermittent bolus enteral feeding, gastric residuals should be checked before initiation of the bolus feeding.

To minimize aspiration, the following factors should be considered:

1. Keep the HOB elevated at 30 to 45 degrees.
2. For patients at high risk of aspiration, use continuous infusion.
3. Use prokinetic agents (metoclopramide, erythromycin, alvimopan for opiate-induced dysmotility).
4. Consider postpyloric placement of the feeding tube.
5. Maintain good oral hygiene.

Management of feeding tube complications

For management of feeding tube complications, see Table 1-25.

Medication administration via feeding tubes

Medication administration via feeding tubes is a very complex issue. Administration of medications via feeding tubes can change the effectiveness of the drug (either decreasing efficacy or increasing toxicity), can be incompatible with enteral feeding, can cause diarrhea, or can cause

	Table 1-24	METHODS OF ADMINISTRATION FOR ENTERAL PRODUCTS
Type	**Typical Rate of Administration**	**Comments**
Bolus	250 to 400 mL four to six times daily. Administer using an open-ended, 60-mL catheter-tipped syringe allowing infusion by gravity. Do not push until feeding tolerance is well established.	Recommended for stable, ambulating patients. May cause cramping, bloating, nausea, diarrhea, aspiration; not recommended for unstable critically ill patients. Higher risk for aspiration.
Intermittent	Bolus feeding infused by pump: Begin with 120 mL formula (half a can) over 1 hour, with 30 to 50 mL water flush before and after feeding. *Advancement:* Increase formula by 60 mL every 8 to 12 hours if residual is less than half the volume of the previous feeding to a maximum of 450 mL of feeding.	*Starting regimen* Should not exceed 30 mL/hr; may cause cramping, nausea, bloating, diarrhea, aspiration; may need to reduce infusion rate to decrease discomfort and increase tolerance.
Cyclic	Continuous tube feeding generally infused over 12 to 20 hours daily. Rate to be determined by formula and caloric needs. Full-strength formula should be used to afford the patient the best opportunity to receive maximal support from the feeding.	Recommended for patients who cannot tolerate bolus or intermittent feeding and patients with J-tubes. Allows more time for absorption of nutrients while also allowing time for gut rest and allowing time for patient to ambulate freely.
Continuous	Rate to be determined by formula and caloric needs. Full-strength formula should be used. If not well tolerated, reducing the infusion rate may be warranted. Be mindful of the number of interruptions in feedings, as each interruption reduces the amount of nutrition support the patient receives.	Allows more time for absorption of nutrients. Less risk of aspiration. Recommended for patients who are critically ill and patients with J-tubes.

drug interactions by administering multiple medications at the same time. In addition, there is always the concern that medications administered via syringe can be accidentally administered via an IV line causing catastrophic consequences.

In 2003, a case report was published of a 38-year-old woman who received both extended-release nifedipine and labetalol via a feeding tube. The nifedipine caused a profound decrease in her BP and the labetalol prevented a compensatory increase in her HR. The patient went into cardiac arrest (asystole) and was resuscitated. However, the underlying reason for her arrest was not clarified. The next day, she received the same medications via her feeding tube, again went into cardiac arrest, and died.

To ensure safe administration of medications via feeding tubes, the following steps are recommended.

1. Use oral route when possible (if the patient is taking some PO, PO administration is preferred).
2. Liquid preparations (solutions, suspensions, elixirs) are the preferred dosage form via feeding tubes. Dilute thick liquid preparations with water (1:1) before administration to prevent clogging of feeding tube.
3. Check osmolality and sorbitol content if the patient experiences diarrhea. If medication has high osmolality, dilute before administration.
4. If solid dosage form is used, make sure tablets can be crushed or capsules can be opened. Not all immediate-release tablets and capsules can be administered via feeding tubes.
5. In general, sustained-release tablets and capsules cannot be administered via feeding tubes. Sustained-release preparations will usually have the following acronyms: CD, CR, ER, LA, SA, SR, TD, TR, XL, XR.
6. Flush feeding tube BEFORE AND AFTER drug delivery with at least 15 mL (preferably 30 mL) of water.
7. Administer medications ONE AT A TIME via feeding tube to prevent drug-drug interactions.

Table 1-25	MANAGEMENT OF COMPLICATIONS IN THE TUBE-FED PATIENT
Complication/Possible Causes	**Suggested Management Strategy**
Nausea and Vomiting	
Fast rate Fat intolerance Fiber content Delayed gastric emptying Gastrointestinal intolerance (high residuals, abdominal pain and distension)	Decrease rate Change to a low-fat formula Change to a low-fiber formula Change from bolus to continuous or cyclic tube feeding Decrease rate or hold tube feeding, consult the physician to rule out ileus, gut ischemia
Clogged Tube	
Inadequate flushing	Flush tube with at least 30 mL water after each feeding and before and after medication administration. Flush every 4 hours with a minimum of 30 mL water as ordered. For clogged feeding tubes, flush with warm water (60 to 100 mL), repeat as necessary. If feeding tube is still clogged, consider an enzyme solution to unclog feeding tube, such as Viokace or Clog-Zapper. Do not use Coca-Cola or pineapple juice to unclog feeding tube because this can further denature the protein and exacerbate the clog.
Instillation of crushed medications	Do not instill crushed medications in small-bore tubes. Substitute liquid preparations after consulting the pharmacist and prescriber. Some medications may be crushed into a fine powder and dissolved. Check with the pharmacist, because crushing can alter medication characteristics. **Never crush time-released medications.** Incompatibilities between drugs and feeding formulas are possible. Some medications that require that tube feeding be held around administration include phenytoin, warfarin, fluoroquinolone, and tetracyclines.
Viscous medications	Dilute viscous medications with water before administering.
Dislodged feeding tube (enterostomy tube)	If a standard tube for replacement is not immediately available, insert a Foley catheter of suitable size to keep the entry site open until a feeding tube is available.

8. Do NOT mix medications directly into feeding formulas.
9. Certain medications require that tube feeding be held around administration to prevent decreased efficacy. A list of common specific drug-nutrient interactions is provided in the following section.
10. Consult pharmacy to review medications for all patients who are tube fed, to determine if they can be safely administered via feeding tubes.
11. DO NOT use Luer-Lock syringes to administer medications or flush feeding tubes to prevent inadvertent IV administration.

Specific drug-nutrient interactions
1. Phenytoin: Hold tube feeding for 2 hours before and after drug administration.
2. Fluoroquinolones (levofloxacin, ciprofloxacin, moxifloxacin) and tetracyclines (doxycycline, minocycline, tetracycline): Hold tube feeding 1 hour before and 2 hours after drug administration.
3. Warfarin: QUICKLY administer warfarin dose OR hold tube feedings 1 hour before and after warfarin administration.

For a noncomprehensive list of medications that cannot be crushed, see Table 1-26.
For a list of common medications that can cause or exacerbate diarrhea, see Table 1-27.

PARENTERAL NUTRITION
Parenteral (IV) nutrition provides some or all of the patient's required nutrients using either a peripheral venous catheter (PIV) or central venous catheter (CVC). TPN or hyperalimentation

Table 1-26	SELECTED "DO NOT CRUSH" MEDICATIONS AND MEDICATIONS THAT REQUIRE CAUTION WITH CRUSHING
"Do Not Crush"	**Comments**
Aggrenox	Sustained release
Alendronate	Mucous membrane irritant, use solution
Benzonatate	Local anesthesia of mucosa
Bisacodyl	Sustained release
Diltiazem (sustained action and immediate release)	Immediate-release formulation has coating that releases the drug over 3 hours
Pancreatic enzymes (Creon, Zenpep, Pancrelipase)	Sustained release — Viokace is an immediate-release alternative
Dabigatran	Increased toxicity
KCl tablet	Use liquid formulation
Lopinavir/ritonavir tablet	Use liquid formulation
Mycophenolate mofetil capsule	Use suspension
Nifedipine (immediate release and sustained release)	DO NOT administer via feeding tube! Request alternative calcium-channel blocker
Ritonavir tablet/capsule	Use liquid formulation
Sevelamer carbonate	Tablets expand and can clog feeding tubes; use liquid formulation
Sirolimus	Pharmacokinetic, nanocrystal technology may be affected
Tamsulosin	Request alternative selective or nonselective alpha-blocker
Caution when crushing	**Comments**
Dutasteride, finasteride	Women who are or may become pregnant should NOT handle this drug
Hydroxyurea	Skin toxicities can occur with exposure; wear gloves when handling

Table 1-27	SELECTED MEDICATIONS THAT CAN CAUSE OR EXACERBATE DIARRHEA
Common Medications with High Osmolality		**Common Medications with High Sorbitol Content**
Acetaminophen liquid	Hydroxyzine HCl syrup	Acetaminophen liquid
Acetaminophen with codeine elixir	Lithium citrate syrup	Guaifenesin/dextromethorphan syrup
Dexamethasone solution	Metoclopramide HCl syrup	Lithium citrate syrup
Diphenoxylate HCl-atropine sulfate suspension	Multivitamin infusion liquid	Metoclopramide HCl syrup
Docusate sodium syrup	KCl liquid,	Pseudoephedrine syrup
Ferrous sulfate liquid	Promethazine HCl syrup	Pseudoephedrine/triprolidine syrup
		Theophylline oral solution

(HAL) are interchangeable terms referring to the administration of IV nutrition. TPN that is administered via a peripheral vein is called peripheral parenteral nutrition (PPN). TPN administered via a central line is called central parenteral nutrition (CPN). CPN can meet total nutritional needs in patients who cannot be given enteral support safely or whose GI tract cannot be accessed. Parenteral nutrition is also used when the GI tract is unable to function, such as in the case of motility disorders, for example, postoperative ileus or small bowel obstruction. PPN, by contrast, usually does not meet the nutritional needs of the patient and is generally reserved for short-term IV nutrition.

Parenteral nutrition solutions are compounded from a combination of dextrose, amino acids, electrolytes, vitamins, trace elements, sterile water for injection (SWFI), and IV fat emulsion (IV lipids). Total nutrient admixtures (TNAs) are formulated by combining dextrose, fat, and amino acids together in one container. 2-in-1 TPN admixtures combine dextrose and amino acids, and are combined with electrolytes, vitamins, and minerals, and IV fat emulsion is given separately. A 0.22-micron in-line filter must be used with 2-in-1 TPN formulas (amino acids and dextrose solutions). The 0.22-micron filter cannot be used for TNA solutions because it can disrupt the lipid emulsion. Instead, a 1.2-micron filter should be used with TNA. In-line filters are not required for IV fat emulsion hung separately. TPN can be infused as a continuous infusion or as a cyclic TPN. Cyclic TPN is usually infused over 8 to 16 hours and is beneficial in long-term TPN patients to increase patient mobility and to allow for organ rest.

Components of TPN

- **Carbohydrates:** Dextrose solutions are used to meet the majority of the patient's energy needs. Dextrose provides 3.4 kcal/g in contrast to dietary carbohydrate that provides 4 kcal/g. PPN contains less than 10% dextrose, but CPN can contain up to 25% dextrose. Administration of excess dextrose can lead to hyperglycemia, hyperlipidemia, increased liver function tests, steatosis, and refeeding syndrome. Refeeding syndrome occurs in previously malnourished patients who receive a significant amount of dextrose. This is manifested by significant electrolyte shifts (hypophosphatemia, hypokalemia, and hypomagnesemia) and fluid shifts that can be life threatening if not treated. If high dextrose containing TPN is stopped abruptly, this can lead to rebound hypoglycemia; therefore, CPN should always be tapered by 50% for 1 to 2 hours before discontinuing the infusion.
- **Protein:** Protein in TPN is provided by crystalline amino acid solutions. They provide 4 kcal/g similar to dietary protein. Amino acid stock solutions are available in different concentrations (from 3% to 20%) and are available as standard amino acid solutions or disease-specific (hepatic failure, metabolic stress, renal failure, pediatric). Excessive protein administration without adequate nonprotein calories and/or fluid can lead to prerenal azotemia.
- **Fat:** IV fat emulsion (lipids) are available as 10%, 20%, and 30% emulsions. The 10% and 20% emulsions can be administered as part of TPN or separately; 30% fat emulsion can only be used to compound TNA and cannot be administered separately. IV fat emulsions (IVFEs) are isotonic solutions that provide essential fatty acids and a source of concentrated calories. IVFEs in the United States have traditionally consisted of polyunsaturated LCTs only. Recently, a new IVFE has been approved by the U.S. Food and Drug Administration (FDA) that also contains olive oil (a monounsaturated LCT). Outside of the United States, IVFEs containing MCTs and fish oil are also available. As stated earlier, an IVFE that is administered separately can be infused without an in-line filter. However, for TNA, a 1.2-micron filter (not a 0.22-micron filter) should be used.
  - When IVFEs are administered separately, infusion should not exceed 12 hours and should not be infused too quickly to avoid adverse reactions. Symptoms of adverse reactions include febrile response, hypertriglyceridemia, chills and shivering, and pain in the chest and back. A delayed type of adverse reaction occurs with prolonged use of IVFEs and may result in a transient increase in liver enzyme levels, eosinophilia, and hypertriglyceridemia. IVFE should be held in patients with triglyceride levels greater than 400 mg/dL. In addition, IV lipids are contraindicated in patients with egg, soy, and peanut allergies, because the emulsion contains egg phospholipids, soy, and peanuts (in some formulations). CDC guidelines for the prevention of fungemia recommend that when IV lipids are given as a separate infusion, the IV lipids should be infused over 12 hours (as opposed to a 24-hour infusion). In addition, any unused portion of the IVFE infusion should be discarded immediately. When in

a TNA, the admixture may infuse over 24 hours. Patients receiving propofol (Diprivan), which is lipid-based, should receive fat emulsion with caution, not to exceed 60% of total calories from fat. Current recommendations for patients who are critically ill recommend no more than 1 g/kg of IVFE daily.

- **Multivitamins:** Multivitamins for TPN are available as MVI-12 and MVI-13. The IV MVI contain fat-soluble vitamins (A, E, D, and K) and water-soluble vitamins (B complex and C). The only difference between the two formulations is that MVI-12 does not contain vitamin K. Usually 10 mL of MVI is added to the TPN daily.
- **Trace elements:** Trace elements include zinc, copper, manganese, chromium, and selenium. Parenteral trace elements are available as MTE-4 or MTE-5 in the United States. MTE-4 does not contain selenium. There is currently a severe shortage of parenteral trace elements in the United States, and many hospitals are unable to obtain parenteral trace elements. The FDA has temporarily allowed for the importation of trace elements from Europe. These trace elements differ from commercially available trace elements in the United States in that they contain the following additional trace elements: iodine, fluoride, iron, and molybdenum. Some recommendations for managing the current shortage include:
  1. Use oral formulations of trace elements whenever possible if patients can tolerate PO.
  2. Give individual trace elements separately if available.
  3. Administer parenteral trace elements three times weekly instead of daily.
  4. Use imported products if use is approved by the specific institution.
  5. Increase awareness of signs and symptoms of specific trace element deficiencies (see Table 1-22).

Parenteral feeding: selection of catheter insertion site

Types of catheters: See Table 1-28.

Table 1-28	CATHETERS USED IN PARENTERAL NUTRITION
Catheter	**Description**
Temporary/Short-Term Use	
Peripherally inserted central catheter (PICC)	May be inserted into a peripheral vein and threaded into a central vein at bedside by a physician or specially trained infusion therapy nurse. May be a single or double lumen. May be used for total parenteral nutrition (TPN) administration at home. Catheter may remain in place for several months. Multiple uses of a single lumen for blood sampling, nutrition support, and medication administration increase the risk of infection, especially in patients who are immunocompromised. *Note:* A midline PICC is NOT a central catheter and only peripheral parenteral nutrition should be infused via this type of line.
Multilumen central venous catheter (CVC)	Inserted at bedside. May have up to four lumens. Subclavian or jugular vein accessed. Dedicate one lumen, preferably the most distal, for administration of TPN. Other lumen(s) are used for medication administration and drawing of blood samples.
Permanent/Long-Term Use	
Right atrial catheter (e.g., Hickman, Broviac)	Generally placed surgically by a physician into the subclavian or jugular vein with the catheter tunneled and exiting from the skin. The catheter usually includes a Dacron cuff from which the catheter exits the vessel. This type of catheter is associated with the lowest infection rates of all central lines.
Implantable venous access device (IVAD, such as Infuse-a-Port, or Port-a-Cath)	May be placed by a radiologist or surgeon. Designed for repeated access, making the need for repeated venipuncture unnecessary.

Modified from Eisenberg P. In Swearingen PL, editor: *Manual of medical-surgical nursing care*, ed 6, St Louis, 2007, Mosby Elsevier.

Central venous IV catheter (CVC): Used for infusion of large amounts of nutrients or electrolytes with smaller fluid volumes (hypertonic solutions) than those in PPN. The solution is usually delivered through a large-diameter vein (e.g., superior vena cava via the subclavian vein). The volume of blood flow rapidly dilutes the hypertonic solutions and decreases irritation of vein walls. Nontunneled catheters are usually placed in the ICU for short-term infusion of medications and TPN. Tunneled catheters are more difficult to insert, but are better suited for long-term TPN. For a list of complications associated with central lines, refer to Table 1-29.

Peripheral venous access: Peripheral IV (PIV) lines are generally not as effective for TPN infusion as central venous administration. The need for low osmolality of solutions (less than 900 mOsm/L) means that PPN will not meet the caloric and protein requirements of most patients. PPN is usually prepared in a higher volume of fluid because of the necessity of low osmolality, which can be problematic with patients who require fluid restriction. PPN can be infused either as a TNA or a 2-in-1 TPN with IV lipids infused separately. PPN is usually reserved for individuals who need partial or total nutrition support for short periods (5 to 7 days, no more than 2 weeks) when CVC access is unavailable or not warranted. Adverse reactions to PPN include phlebitis and burning at the infusion site. Because PPN solutions are hyperosmolar and can irritate peripheral veins, PIV sites should be changed every 48 to 72 hours.

Table 1-29	LINE COMPLICATIONS IN PATIENTS RECEIVING PARENTERAL NUTRITION
Potential Complications	**Management Strategy**
Upon Central Line Insertion	
Pneumothorax	Position a rolled towel under the patient's back, parallel to the spine before the temporary catheter is inserted. Ensure that x-ray is done immediately after insertion to determine placement of catheter before initiating total parenteral nutrition (TPN). Monitor for diminished or unequal breath sounds, tachypnea, dyspnea, and labored breathing. The greater the number of catheter attempts, the greater the chance for pneumothorax.
Accidental subclavian artery penetration leading to hemothorax	If pulsatile, bright red blood returns into the syringe during central catheter insertion into the subclavian vein, assist with immediate removal of the needle and apply pressure for 10 minutes anteriorly and posteriorly at the point of penetration. If internal bleeding is unable to be controlled, the patient will develop a hemothorax and hemorrhagic shock.
During Catheter Maintenance	
Catheter occlusion	If solution is infusing sluggishly, flush line using positive pressure with saline. Check to see if line or tubing is kinked. If line is occluded, try to aspirate clot and contact the physician or midlevel practitioner who may prescribe a thrombolytic agent, such as Cathflo TPA, TPA (tissue plasminogen activator), or urokinase, according to agency protocol.
Leakage or catheter puncture	Do not insert needles into central line port lumen caps to avoid damaging the catheter. If the lumen is accidentally punctured and begins leaking, notify the physician or midlevel practitioner immediately for further action.
Air embolism (a medical emergency)	If signs of air embolism occur, examine the catheter to determine whether an open port enabled air to enter the infusion system. Clamp the catheter distal to any opening discovered. Turn the patient onto their left side and place in the Trendelenburg position (head down, feet up) and notify the physician or midlevel practitioner immediately while administering oxygen.
Central line–related thrombosis leading to upper extremity deep vein thrombosis	Assess for swelling of the upper extremities and perform a neurovascular assessment. If limb is swollen, is cool, and has reduced or absent pulses, the physician or midlevel practitioner should be notified and consideration given to removing the central venous catheter. The extremity should be elevated and the thrombosis managed as ordered to address anticoagulation.

TPN Administration: Continuous TPN is infused at a constant rate using an infusion pump. When initiating cyclic TPN, the infusion rate is gradually increased to avoid hyperglycemia. Then when stopping TPN, the rate is similarly gradually decreased (usually by 50%) to prevent rebound hypoglycemia. Discontinuation of CPN should never be done abruptly, but is accomplished by tapering the CPN by reducing the rate by half for 2 hours, then stopping the CPN. PPN usually has a low concentration of dextrose and can, therefore, be stopped without tapering the infusion.

Indications for TPN

Parenteral nutrition is indicated for patients who are unable to meet their nutrition requirements with enteral or oral nutrition and who are at risk for malnutrition. PPN can be used when patients require nutrition support for up to 2 weeks. CPN should be used when patients require more than 2 weeks of nutrition support. Specific indications for TPN include paralytic ileus, small bowel obstruction, mesenteric ischemia, and high-output fistula when enteral feeding cannot be administered distal to the fistula. Other indications include failure of enteral nutrition despite trials of postpyloric placement and elemental feedings, and other GI dysfunction that precludes oral or enteral intake.

Although the initiation of enteral nutrition support in the patient who is critically ill is highly recommended within the first 24 hours of admission to ICU, early initiation of TPN in the patient who is critically ill and cannot maintain volitional oral intake or who is not a candidate for enteral nutrition is no longer routinely recommended. In general, it is recommended to wait at least 5 days before initiating TPN in patients who are critically ill. These recommendations were based on studies that found a decreased risk of infectious morbidity and complications in patients who were NPO compared with those who received TPN.

Early initiation of TPN in patients who are critically ill is recommended for patients who are already malnourished on admission (10% to 15% recent weight loss or a patient weighing less than 90% of his or her IBW), especially those who are going to undergo major GI surgery. Some clinicians will recommend holding IVFE for the first week of PN therapy in patients who are critically ill because fat metabolism is impaired in critical illness and soy-based IVFE may have immunosuppressive properties. It is important to note that TPN therapy that is provided for a very short time period (less than 5 to 7 days) is not recommended because it will not improve the patient's nutritional status and only puts the patient at risk for complications. It is also important that patients who are receiving TPN be reassessed frequently for the possibility of transitioning to either enteral or oral nutrition.

TPN complications

Complications with TPN can be divided into two categories: early complications and late complications. Early complications from TPN include hyperglycemia, hyperlipidemia, line infections, phlebitis, azotemia, refeeding syndrome, and electrolyte abnormalities. Late complications include trace element deficiencies, hepatobiliary disorders (hepatic steatosis, PNALD (PN-associated liver disease), metabolic bone disease, and central line infections.

For information regarding managing macronutrient-related and micronutrient-related complications, see Table 1-30.

For information regarding signs and symptoms of vitamin, mineral, and trace element deficiencies, see Tables 1-21 and 1-22.

Electrolyte imbalances

Electrolyte imbalances can occur during the administration of both enteral nutrition and PN (Table 1-31).

TRANSITIONAL FEEDING

A period of adjustment is needed before discontinuing nutrition support. It is good practice to taper enteral nutrition and PN as oral intake increases instead of discontinuing nutrition support as soon as the patient is able to take a PO diet. Often, parenteral or enteral nutrition can be cycled over a period of hours as a means of tapering. For example, the nutrition support clinician may cycle the enteral or parenteral feeding at night to allow the patient to increase PO intake during the day. If nutrition support is not tapered when the patient begins an oral diet, this can interfere with the patient's appetite and minimize his or her PO intake, keeping him or her on nutrition support for longer than necessary.

Table 1-30	MACRONUTRIENT AND MICRONUTRIENT COMPLICATIONS IN PATIENTS ON TOTAL PARENTERAL NUTRITION
Complication	**Management Strategy**
Macronutrient-Related	
Hyperglycemia	Consider insulin therapy (exogenous insulin or insulin added to total parenteral nutrition [TPN]). Monitor blood glucose every 4 to 6 hours initially. Patients with diabetes or at risk for hyperglycemia should start with lower dextrose concentrations in TPN.
Hypoglycemia	Avoid stopping TPN abruptly (rebound hypoglycemia). May be related to excessive insulin in TPN. Ensure that all physicians and midlevel practitioners are aware about insulin being added to TPN so that excess insulin is not prescribed.
Hypertriglyceridemia	Can result from either excessive intravenous (IV) fat emulsion or by infusing IV fat emulsion too quickly. Hypertriglyceridemia can also result from excessive dextrose administration. Monitor triglycerides weekly. Hold IV fats for triglycerides >400 mg/dL.
Essential fatty acid deficiency (EFAD)	Usually seen in patients who are not receiving IV fat emulsion with TPN. Can occur within 1 to 3 weeks of IV fat emulsion-free TPN. Minimum IV fat emulsion necessary to prevent EFAD is 100 g weekly (500 mL of 20% IV fat emulsion)
Azotemia	Usually occurs because the patient is either receiving excessive protein, inadequate fluid, or both. Monitor input and output for signs of dehydration. Ensure adequate fluid intake.
Micronutrient and Fluid and Electrolyte Disturbances: See Tables 1-21, 1-22	
Refeeding syndrome	Usually attributable to carbohydrate administration in patients who are malnourished or prolonged NPO (nil per os) status. Initiate TPN slowly (lower % dextrose). Monitor electrolytes (especially phosphorus, potassium, and magnesium). Consider the addition of thiamine in TPN to prevent thiamine deficiency and subsequent lactic acidosis, beriberi, and Wernicke encephalopathy.

From Kumpf VJ, Gervasio J. Complications of Parenteral Nutrition. The A.S.P.E.N. Adult Nutrition Support Core Curriculum, 2nd Edition. Charles M. Mueller, Editor. 2012.

CARE PLANS: PATIENTS RECEIVING ENTERAL AND PARENTERAL NUTRITION

Imbalanced nutrition: less than body requirements *related to the inability to ingest, digest, or absorb nutrients.*

Goals/Outcomes: Within 7 days of initiating parenteral/enteral nutrition, the patient's nutritional status is improving, as evidenced by stable weight or steady weight gain (weight gain is not often seen in the acute care setting); malnutrition is improved, as indicated by increasing or normal measures of protein stores (serum albumin, transferrin, prealbumin, and retinol-binding protein) — usually not seen in the critical care setting; positive nitrogen balance; presence of wound granulation; and absence of infection (see Risk for Infection).

NOC Nutritional Status: Nutrient Intake.

Nutrition Monitoring
1. Ensure nutrition screening and assessment of the patient within 24 to 48 hours of admission by nursing staff and within 72 hours by a dietitian; document nutrition assessment. See Nutrition Assessment. Reassess weekly.
2. Monitor electrolytes and blood glucose levels daily until stabilized. Ensure that serum albumin, transferrin, or prealbumin are monitored weekly. Ensure that trace elements are monitored periodically (quarterly).
3. Monitor hemoglobin and hematocrit, as the patient may have an iron-deficiency anemia or a macrocytic anemia (B_{12} or folate deficiency).
4. Weigh the patient daily.
5. Monitor for dry, flaky skin with depigmentation (sign of vitamin/trace element deficiency or EFAD).
6. Monitor for pale, reddened, and dry conjunctival tissue (sign of vitamin/trace element deficiency).

Table 1-31	POSSIBLE ELECTROLYTE IMBALANCES OCCURRING IN ENTERAL AND PARENTERAL NUTRITION

Sodium: Daily requirement is 1 to 2 mEq/kg. Sodium is the primary extracellular cation in maintaining concentration and volume of extracellular fluid.

Complication	Pathophysiology and Management
Hypernatremia	May result from free water deficit, overdiuresis, excessive water loss, hypertonic total parenteral nutrition (TPN) solutions, inadequate volume of TPN solutions, or inadequate water flushes via feeding tube. May be attributable to nephrogenic or central diabetes insipidus, uncontrolled diabetes mellitus, or use of sodium penicillin, heparin sodium, or corticosteroids. Management *Parenteral:* Increase free water, decrease sodium in TPN, increase volume of TPN. *Enteral:* All enteral formulas are low sodium. Change tube feeding formula to less concentrated formula and increase water flushes.
Hyponatremia	Most common cause in patients receiving TPN is administration of hypotonic fluids or volume overload. In patients who are tube-fed, hyponatremia may be caused by excessive fluid administration or excessive water flushes. Other causes of hyponatremia include adrenal insufficiency, renal insufficiency, SIADH (syndrome of inappropriate antidiuretic hormone), cirrhosis, and chronic heart failure. Management Parenteral: Decrease fluid and/or increase sodium in TPN. Enteral: Switch to calorie-dense, fluid-restricted tube-feeding formula, decrease water flushes via feeding tube or flush with normal saline as directed.

Potassium: Daily requirement is 1 to 2 mEq/kg. Potassium is the major intracellular cation required for neurotransmission, protein synthesis, cardiac and renal function, and carbohydrate metabolism.

Complication	Pathophysiology and Management
Hyperkalemia	May be caused by excessive parenteral or enteral potassium supplementation, metabolic acidosis, increased tissue catabolism, and renal insufficiency. Medications that can cause elevated potassium levels include angiotensin-converting enzyme inhibitors, angiotensin receptor blockers, heparin, cyclosporine, and potassium-sparing diuretics. Management Parenteral and Enteral: Decrease potassium in TPN or switch to low electrolyte tube-feeding formula. Decrease other sources of exogenous potassium (in intravenous [IV] fluids, potassium supplementation). Consider stopping or reducing dose of potassium-sparing medications. Correct metabolic acidosis with sodium bicarbonate if present. May require administration of glucose with insulin, IV calcium gluconate (if electrocardiography changes are present), beta$_2$-adrenergic agents (e.g., albuterol), or hemodialysis in severe cases.
Hypokalemia	May occur during anabolism (tissue synthesis) in patients or in refeeding syndrome causing potassium to shift into the intracellular space. Other causes include excessive gastrointestinal (GI) losses, diuretic use, or inadequate potassium intake. In metabolic alkalosis, potassium is also decreased (potassium is decreased by 0.4 to 1.5 mEq/L for every 0.1 increase in pH). Management Parenteral: Increase potassium in TPN, provide potassium supplementation in patients receiving tube feeding. Potassium given via a peripheral line can be irritating to the peripheral vein. Administration via a peripheral line should not exceed 10 mEq/h. Enteral: PO (per os) potassium supplementation can be irritating to GI mucosa and may cause diarrhea. If hypomagnesemia is present, it should be corrected before potassium supplementation. Both: Initiate tube feeding or TPN slowly to avoid refeeding syndrome. Correct metabolic alkalosis if present.

Phosphorus: Daily requirement is approximately 20 to 40 mmol/day. Phosphorus is required for release of oxygen from hemoglobin in the form of 2,3-diphosphoglycerate and for bone deposition, calcium regulation, and synthesis of carbohydrates, fats, and protein.

Continued

Table 1-31	POSSIBLE ELECTROLYTE IMBALANCES OCCURRING IN ENTERAL AND PARENTERAL NUTRITION—cont'd
Complication	**Pathophysiology and Management**
Hyperphosphatemia	Occurs in catabolic stress, renal failure, and hypocalcemia or excessive exogenous administration of phosphorus. Medications that can cause hyperphosphatemia include phosphorus-rich solutions, antacids, diuretic agents, and steroids. Associated with metabolic acidosis. Management Parenteral: Decrease phosphate in TPN or other exogenous phosphate administration. Enteral: May require treatment with phosphate binders such as sevelamer (Renvela) and calcium acetate (PhosLo). Change to a renal tube-feeding formula.
Hypophosphatemia	A complication with a high mortality, often found in malnourished patients with refeeding syndrome. As the patient receives fluids containing dextrose, phosphorus shifts rapidly into the intracellular space, causing hypophosphatemia. Refeeding syndrome also affects other intracellular electrolytes, particularly potassium and magnesium. Associated with metabolic alkalosis. Management Parenteral and Enteral: Initiate tube feeding or TPN slowly to avoid refeeding syndrome. Parenteral: Increase phosphorus in TPN or provide other sources of phosphorus (sodium phosphate, potassium phosphate) in patients with low phosphorus levels.

Magnesium: Daily requirement is 18 to 30 mEq/day. Magnesium is required for carbohydrate and protein metabolism and enzymatic reactions.

Complication	**Pathophysiology and Management**
Hypermagnesemia	Generally seen with excessive magnesium supplementation including magnesium-containing antacids or renal failure. Medications include Milk of Magnesia and magnesium citrate. Management Parenteral: Decrease magnesium in TPN or IV fluids. Parenteral and Enteral: Discontinue any medications that contain magnesium. May require diuresis or hemodialysis in severe cases.
Hypomagnesemia	Low levels commonly occur in patients with severe malnutrition, patients with refeeding syndrome, or in patients with lower GI losses, prolonged nasogastric suctioning, and diabetic ketoacidosis. Often occurs in alcoholics, malabsorption syndromes, and the critical care population. Medications that can cause hypomagnesemia include diuretics, insulin, and cyclosporine. Management Parenteral: Increase magnesium in TPN, give supplemental magnesium. Parenteral magnesium should be used to treat moderate to severe hypomagnesemia in patients receiving parenteral and enteral nutrition. Enteral: Give oral magnesium supplements. Monitor for diarrhea.

Calcium: Daily requirement is 1000 to 1500 mg (10 to 15 mEq/day) of elemental calcium. Calcium is a necessary ingredient of the cells that plays a major role in neurotransmission and bone formation.

Complication	**Pathophysiology and Management**
Hypercalcemia	Occurs in prolonged immobilization, malignancy, hyperparathyroidism, tumor lysis syndrome, adrenal insufficiency, and renal failure. Medications that can cause hypercalcemia include thiazide diuretics, lithium, calcium supplements, and aluminum-containing and magnesium-containing antacids. Management Parenteral and Enteral: Volume expansion with normal saline, which disrupts the stimulus for calcium reabsorption in the kidney. Loop diuretics are calcium wasting and may be used in cases of severe hypercalcemia. Bisphosphonates can be used to treat chronic hypercalcemia. Parenteral: Decrease calcium in TPN.
Hypocalcemia	Occurs with reduced vitamin D intake, hypoparathyroidism, and hypomagnesemia. Medications that can cause hypocalcemia include loop diuretics, bisphosphonates, calcitonin, phenobarbital, and phenytoin. Management Parenteral and Enteral: Calcium supplementation (parenteral or oral). Ionized calcium level should be used as a guide to replacement, because serum calcium is bound to albumin. If albumin level is low, calcium level will appear falsely low.

7. Evaluate energy level for malaise, weakness, and fatigue indicative that the patient is not receiving adequate nutrition to promote strength and mobility.
8. Monitor for spoon-shaped, brittle, ridged nails (sign of vitamin deficiency).
9. Record I&O carefully, tracking fluid balance trends. Check volume enteral nutrition or PN infused and rate of infusion hourly.
10. Ensure that the patient receives the prescribed amount of nutrients.
11. Be aware that residual volumes of gastric feedings include not only feeding but also gastric secretions. The amount of residual feeding is NOT purely feeding. More recent studies indicate that caregivers may not need to be concerned about residual volumes of less than 250 to 500 mL. Patient positioning also effects the amount of residual volume that may be found by the caregiver.

Ineffective protection resulting in risk for aspiration *related to GI bleeding, delayed gastric emptying, or location/type of feeding tube.*

Goals/Outcomes: The patient is not aspirating, as evidenced by auscultation of clear breath sounds; vital signs within the patient's baseline; and absence of signs of respiratory distress.
NOC Immune Status, Respiratory Status.

Enteral Tube Feeding
1. Check the radiograph to assess the position of the feeding tube before the first feeding (Note: Radiographic confirmation is not required for PEG tubes or surgically placed feeding tubes). Mark and secure the tube for future reference. Insufflation with air and aspiration of stomach contents are commonly used to confirm position thereafter but do not guarantee correct position and are no longer recommended by the American Association of Critical Care (AACN) guidelines.
2. Assess the respiratory status at least every 4 hours, observing respiratory rate and effort, and presence of adventitious breath sounds.
3. Monitor temperature at least every 4 hours.
4. Auscultate for bowel sounds, and assess abdominal contour and girth every 8 hours. Consult the advanced practice provider if the abdomen becomes distended, or nausea and vomiting occur.
5. Elevate the HOB at least 30 degrees during and for 1 hour after feeding. If the patient is receiving continuous enteral nutrition, the HOB should always be elevated at least 30 degrees.
6. Notify the advanced practice provider if gastric residual is greater than 250 to 500 mL (per institution protocol) or if the patient is having any signs of abdominal pain or distention. The patient should be positioned on their right side for 20 minutes before aspirating the enteral tube for residual volume to ensure that feeding is being directed toward the small bowel. False high volumes may be reported if feeding has pooled in the body of the stomach in a supine patient. If the caregiver is certain that the residual volume was properly obtained, hold feeding for 1 hour, and then recheck residuals.
7. Stop the enteral feeding 0.5 to 1 hour before chest physical therapy or lowering the HOB when the patient is supine.
8. Discuss with the advanced practice provider the possibility of placing the feeding tube beyond the pylorus to help minimize the risk for aspiration in patients at higher risk for aspiration.
9. As prescribed for delayed gastric emptying, administer prokinetic agents such as metoclopramide HCl, erythromycin, or other agents that promote gastric motility.

Diarrhea *related to adjustment to formula, method of administration, and volume of enteral feeding.*

Goals/Outcomes: The patient has begun to form normal stools within 24 to 48 hours of intervention.
NOC Bowel Elimination, Electrolyte and Acid-Base Balance; Nutritional Status: Food and Fluid Intake

Diarrhea Management
1. Assess abdomen and GI status, including bowel sounds, distention, consistency and frequency of bowel movements, characteristics of stools, cramping, skin turgor, and indicators of hydration such as skin turgor, thirst, and presence or absence of sunken eyes.
2. Obtain daily weights and monitor I&O status carefully to prevent dehydration.
3. Cramping or diarrhea associated with bolus feeding: Evaluate whether proper technique is used for bolus feeding, including a slow infusion of a room temperature feeding. If proper technique is used and cramping results, switch to an intermittent, cyclic, or continuous feeding method.
4. Evaluate the patient for presence of *Clostridium difficile* if diarrhea is present with any patient who is critically ill. Diarrhea is often blamed on tube feeding intolerance, when the actual cause is inappropriate use of antibiotics resulting in antibiotic-associated diarrhea or *C. difficile*-associated diarrhea.
5. Avoid lactose-containing products. Most enteral products are lactose-free.

6. Bacterial contamination:
   - Use clean technique in handling feeding tube, enteral products, and feeding sets.
   - Wear disposable gloves when administering enteral nutrition.
   - Change administration sets every 24 hours.
   - Hang time for reconstituted formula, enteral nutrition with additives, or mother's milk is 4 hours.
   - Use sterile water for reconstitution of powdered formula.
   - Hang time for sterile decanted formula is 8 hours.
   - Hang time for closed-system enteral formulas is 24 to 48 hours per manufacturer's guidelines.
   - Refrigerate all opened products but discard them after 24 hours.
   - A feeding pump with a drip chamber is recommended because it can prevent retrograde contamination of the enteral formula from the feeding tube.
7. Osmolality intolerance:
   - Determine osmolality of feeding formula. Most are isotonic (plasma osmolality 300 mOsm). If hypertonic, change to an isotonic formula.
   - Determine the osmolality of medications administered via feeding tube. If hyperosmolar, dilute the medications before administration.
8. Medications:
   - Monitor use of antibiotics, antacids, potassium chloride, and sorbitol in liquid medications. Dilute liquid medications with water. Use sterile water for dilution of medication.
   - The use of probiotics to restore GI flora is controversial and should only be given as prescribed by the physician or midlevel practitioner. ASPEN-SCCM guidelines do not have a recommendation for administration of probiotics in patients in ICU. The 2013 CCCN guidelines currently recommend that probiotics be considered in patients who are critically ill. There have been reports of gut ischemia with probiotic use in patients with acute pancreatitis (PROPATRIA trial) and there have been several cases of fungemia associated with the use of *Saccharomyces boulardii* (Florastor). Therefore, it would be prudent to avoid use of probiotics in patients with acute pancreatitis and to avoid the use of Florastor in patients in ICU or those with CV catheters.

Impaired tissue integrity *related to mechanical irritant presence of enteral tube, intolerance of tube feeding, diarrhea, or hyperglycemia.*

Goals/Outcomes: At time of discharge from critical care, the patient's tissue is intact with absence of erosion around orifices, excoriation, skin rash, or mucous membrane breakdown.

NOC Bowel Elimination, Nutritional Status: Food and Fluid Intake, Tissue Integrity: Skin and Mucous Membranes.

Skin Surveillance
1. Initiate appropriate strategies to manage diarrhea, control blood glucose, and assess tolerance of tube feeding. Changing the site of feeding/feeding tube insertion and type of feeding may assist with tolerance of feedings and diarrhea, which will facilitate improvement of skin integrity.
2. Maintain blood glucose goal ranges of 140 to 180 mg/dL in patients who are critically ill to enhance wound healing.

Nasoenteric Tube/Postpyloric Feeding Tube
3. Assess nares for irritation or tenderness every 8 hours and alter position to avoid pressure. Use hypoallergenic tape to anchor tube.
4. Use a small-bore tube if possible.
5. Provide frequent oral care to maintain integrity of teeth and oral mucosa.
6. If long-term support is needed (> 4 weeks), discuss using gastrostomy or jejunostomy tube with the physician or midlevel practitioner.
7. Give ice chips, chewing gum, or hard candies PRN (pro re nata [when necessary]) if permitted.
8. Apply petroleum jelly to lips every 2 hours.
9. Brush teeth and tongue every 8 hours.

Gastrostomy Tube/PEG
10. Assess site for erythema, drainage, tenderness, and odor every 4 hours.
11. Monitor placement of tube every 8 hours.
12. Secure tube so that there is no tension on the patient's tissue and skin.
13. After insertion, clean skin with mild soap and water. Rinse and dry the area thoroughly. Routine use of antibiotic ointment and hydrogen peroxide is no longer recommended.

Jejunostomy Tube/PEJ
14. Assess site for erythema, drainage, tenderness, and odor every 4 hours.
15. Secure tube to avoid tension. Coil tube on top of dressing if necessary.
16. Provide frequent oral care to maintain integrity of teeth and oral mucosa.
17. Skin care for a PEG tube is the same as for gastrostomy tube.
18. Avoid large-volume water flushes (greater than 120 mL) as this may cause small bowel necrosis.
19. Avoid bolus feeding via a jejunal feeding tube as this can cause abdominal pain and can lead to small bowel necrosis.

Risk for infection *related to the presence of central line for TPN*

Goals/Outcomes: The patient does not acquire a bloodstream infection, as evidenced by temperature and vital signs within normal limits, total lymphocytes 25% to 40% (1500 to 4500 mL), WBC count less than 11,000/mm^3, and absence of clinical signs of sepsis, including erythema and swelling at insertion site, chills, fever, and hyperglycemia.
NOC Immune Status, Respiratory Status.

Infection Protection
1. When the central line is inserted, ensure that the CDC central line insertion guidelines are followed, including use of full barrier precautions.
2. Twice weekly and PRN, monitor CBC and differential for values outside the normal range.
3. Check blood glucose at least every 6 hours initially or using the facility's guidelines for values outside the normal range.
4. Examine catheter insertion site(s) every 8 hours for erythema, swelling, or purulent drainage.
5. Use sterile technique when changing central line dressing, containers, or lines.
6. Avoid using the nutrition support port on the central IV or PIV catheter for blood drawing, pressure monitoring, or administration of medications or other fluids.
7. Change all IV administration sets and rotate insertion site within the time frame per institutional protocol.
8. Do not allow parenteral solutions to hang longer than 24 hours.
9. If infection or sepsis is suspected, take blood specimens for culture and administer antibiotics as prescribed. Remove catheter and culture catheter tip if prescribed.
10. Routine use of antibiotic ointments at catheter insertion site is not recommended.

Risk for injury *related to central line insertion.*

Goals/Outcomes: The patient has adequate gas exchange, as evidenced by stable vital signs, stable ABG values, normal bilateral chest excursion, and arterial oximetry within normal limits, and absence of dyspnea, tachypnea, cyanosis, chest pain, tachycardia, and hypotension.
NOC Neurological Status: Consciousness, Respiratory Status.

IV Insertion
1. When central line is inserted, place the patient in the Trendelenburg position.
2. Observe central line insertion procedure and remind the practitioner inserting the line to avoid leaving the catheter open to air once blood vessel has been entered.
3. If the patient experiences SOB, tachypnea, chest pain, hypotension, or cyanosis during line insertion, place on his or her left side in the head down position to facilitate trapping any air introduced in the right ventricle, and administer high-flow O_2 by face mask.
4. Check chest radiograph film to determine catheter position following insertion.

IV Therapy
1. Use the Trendelenburg position when changing tubing or when CV catheters are inserted or removed.
2. Teach the patient the Valsalva maneuver (if possible) for implementation during tubing changes.
3. Use Luer-Lock connectors on all connections.
4. Use occlusive dressing over insertion site for 24 hours after the catheter is removed to prevent air entry via catheter-sinus tract.
5. Monitor the patient for chest pain, tachycardia, tachypnea, cyanosis, and hypotension.
6. If air embolus is suspected, clamp the catheter and turn the patient to left side-lying Trendelenburg position to trap air in the right ventricle. Administer high-flow O_2 and contact the physician immediately.

Risk for imbalanced fluid volume   *related to overhydration or underhydration.*

Goals/Outcomes: The patient's hydration status is adequate, as evidenced by baseline vital signs, glucose less than 300 mg/dL, balanced I&O, urine specific gravity 1.010 to 1.025, and electrolytes within normal limits.

NOC Fluid Balance, Electrolyte and Acid-Base Balance; Nutritional Status: Food and Fluid Intake, Hydration

Fluid Monitoring
1.   Weigh the patient daily; monitor I&O hourly.
2.   Consult advanced practice provider for urine output less than 0.5 mL/kg/h.
3.   Check urine specific gravity; consult the physician or midlevel practitioner for elevated specific gravity according to institutional guidelines.
4.   Monitor serum osmolality and electrolytes daily and PRN; consult the physician or midlevel practitioner for abnormalities.
5.   Monitor for circulatory overload during fluid replacement. Ensure that IV fluids are adjusted when TPN or enteral nutrition is initiated to prevent volume overload.
6.   Monitor for indicators of hyperglycemia and manage appropriately to avoid osmotic diuresis. Perform point-of-care blood glucose reading at least every 6 hours or using institutional guidelines until blood glucose is stable. Administer insulin according to institutional guidelines to control blood glucose. Targets for blood glucose during critical illness may range from 140 to 180 mg/dL.
7.   Assess rate and volume of nutrition support hourly. For HHNS, discontinue infusion until blood glucose and fluid balance is normalized. Reset to prescribed rate as indicated (see Hyperglycemia, Ch 8).
8.   Provide 1 to 2 mL water for each calorie of enteral formula provided (or 30 to 40 mL/kg body weight). For patients with fluid restriction, provide either less than 25 mL/kg water or 1.4 to 1.9 L daily. Make sure to include the free water provided by the enteral formula to prevent fluid overload.

ADDITIONAL NUTRITION-RELATED NURSING DIAGNOSES
For other nursing diagnoses and interventions, see Fluid and Electrolyte Disturbances, which includes a discussion of electrolyte abnormalities listed in Table 1-31.

PAIN

Advances in pharmacologic and complementary therapies, ongoing research in pain management and numerous guidelines, position statements, and practice recommendations have flourished over the past decades. Despite these innovations and national and international efforts, pain remains a common phenomenon in ICU. Patients who are critically ill experience moderate to severe pain at rest and during procedures such as turning, drain removal, coughing, and endotracheal suctioning. Removal of endotracheal tubes, a common procedure in ICU, is a substantial trigger of severe pain in patients in ICU, and the majority of patients who are mechanically ventilated experience moderate to severe pain despite an unrestricted use of fentanyl and morphine. In addition to procedure-induced pain, pathologic conditions, tissue damage, and immobility are common sources of pain. The acuity and care requirements of patients admitted in ICU expose them to multiple sources of pain. These are presently addressed with pharmacologic and nonpharmacologic treatments, yet pain remains undertreated in most of these patients.

Advances in medical technology and an aging population have resulted in an increased demand for intensive care services including the use of invasive procedures such as endotracheal intubation. Ultimately, the need for better pain relief of patients in ICU will only continue to grow.

Unrelieved pain is not benign but affects every aspect of the patient's experience with critical care. It is a significant stressor for patients who are critically ill and contributes to and potentiates other problems such as confusion, inadequate ventilation, immobility, sleep deprivation, depression, and immunosuppression, which can lead to extended healing times. The cardiovascular effects of unrelieved pain are increased HR, BP, SVR; increased myocardial O_2 consumption; altered regional blood flow; and deep vein thrombosis (DVT). The pulmonary effects noted of uncontrolled pain are decreased lung volumes, atelectasis, decreased cough effort, increased sputum retention, and hypoxemia. GI and genitourinary effects are decreased gastric and bowel motility and urinary retention. The neuroendocrine response to uncontrolled pain is to release more of the stress hormones such as catecholamines, cortisol, and glucagon. Psychological effects are anxiety, fear, and sleeplessness.

Unrelieved pain can also lead to multisystem complications, anatomic changes, and physiologic changes in the nervous system contributing to the development of chronic disabling pain and posttraumatic stress disorder, which in turn may seriously impact the patient's functioning, quality of life, and well-being. The negative impacts of pain are not only experienced by the patient admitted in ICU but they also extend to family members and significant others. Admission of a relative who is critically ill to ICU causes both stress and anxiety to family members. They are exposed to a number of potential stressors including deterioration in the patient's condition, uncertain prognosis, an unfamiliar environment loaded with mechanical equipment, and pain and suffering experienced by the patient. Posttraumatic stress disorder, anxiety, guilt, frustration, and depression are some of the emotional reactions of families to such stressors.

PATHOPHYSIOLOGY

Pain is a warning signal to which the body responds to prevent further injury. Nociception represents the neural processes of encoding and processing noxious stimuli that can be perceived as painful. Four processes are involved in nociception: (1) transduction, (2), transmission, (3) perception, and (4) modulation.

In summary, *transduction* refers to the mechanical (e.g., surgical incision), thermal (e.g., burn), or chemical (e.g., toxic substance) noxious stimuli that damage tissues. These noxious stimuli lead to the release of excitatory neurotransmitters that stimulate nociceptors and thus serve to initiate *transmission*. Afferent nerve fibers such as A delta (Aδ) and C fibers respond to pain stimuli peripherally and relay this information to the spinal cord entering through the dorsal horn. Aδ fibers are small, myelinated, fast-conducting fibers that transmit pain sensation that is well localized. C fibers are small, unmyelinated, slow-conducting fibers that transmit poorly localized, dull, aching pain sensations. In the dorsal horn, neurotransmitters such as substance P are released in response to the nociceptive input that activates the second-order dorsal horn neurons. The activation of the second-order neurons results in (1) spinal reflex responses such as muscle spasm, and increased sensitization; and (2) activation of the ascending tracts, which transmits the nociceptive input to several regions within the brain. This is where several responses to pain occur, including the *perception* of pain and the emotional and behavioral responses. *Modulation* refers to the release of endogenous opioids, which inhibit, through the descending pathways, the transmission of the nociceptive signal in the spinal cord and produce analgesia.

ASSESSMENT
DEFINITION AND TYPES OF PAIN

Pain is described as an unpleasant sensory and emotional experience associated with actual or potential tissue damage. Such a definition highlights the subjectivity of a complex multidimensional pain experience. Indeed, the "gold standard" measure for pain is the patient's self-report. However, in the critical care setting, many patients are unable to self-report their pain. In such a situation, behavioral changes caused by pain are valuable forms of self-report and should be considered as alternative measures of pain. The inability to self-report does not negate the possibility that an individual is experiencing pain and is in need of appropriate pain-relieving treatment, and pain assessment methods must be adapted to the patient's cognitive capacity and condition.

Pain can be classified as acute or chronic, and nociceptive or neuropathic. Acute pain implies tissue damage that is usually from an identifiable cause that lasts for the healing process, which is approximately 30 days. Chronic pain persists for more than 3 to 6 months following the healing process. Pain can be nociceptive or neuropathic. Nociceptive pain arises from the activation of nociceptors and can be of somatic or visceral origin. Somatic pain involves peripheral tissues such as the skin, muscles, joints, and bones. Visceral pain involves organs such as the heart, stomach, and liver. Neuropathic pain arises as a direct consequence of an injury or disease affecting the somatosensory system. It can originate from the peripheral (e.g., neuropathy) or central (e.g., phantom pain, stroke) somatosensory system.

GOAL OF ASSESSMENT

Pain assessment is an integral part of nursing care and is a prerequisite for adequate pain management. Pain is a subjective and multidimensional concept that requires complex assessment.

Many factors may alter verbal communication in patients who are critically ill, making pain assessment more difficult. The American Society for Pain Management Nursing has described a stepwise approach for pain assessment in vulnerable patients including the critically ill:

1. Attempt to obtain the patient's self-report of pain: A comprehensive initial assessment of pain, whenever possible, is important in accurately evaluating and managing pain. Regular follow-up pain assessments are necessary postoperatively and during ICU stay until the pain is well controlled. A simple yes or no for presence or absence of pain communicated verbally or using signs (e.g., head nodding, hand grasping) should be considered as a valid self-report.

2. Identify potential causes of pain: Pathologic conditions requiring admission to ICU and care procedures (e.g., turning, endotracheal suctioning, drain/tube removal, wound care) known to be painful in patients who are critically ill should trigger an intervention. If there is reason to suspect pain, the critical care nurse may assume that pain is present and attempt an analgesic trial (according to the 2008 American Pain Society guidelines). Other problems that may be causing pain or discomfort should be identified and adequately treated (e.g., infection, constipation).

3. Observe changes in the patient's behaviors: When it is not possible to obtain the patient's self-report of pain, behavior observation is an alternative and valid approach to pain assessment. Although behaviors are useful in detecting if pain is present or not, it is not an accurate reflection of pain intensity. Indeed, a behavioral pain score of 5/10 is not equal to a patient's self-report of pain intensity of 5/10 as these two measures assess different aspect of the pain experience. Awareness of the patient's baseline and changes that occur during care procedures are useful in differentiating pain from other causes.

4. Use of proxy reporting: Relevant information can be obtained from a family member or relative who knows the patient well. Their familiarity with the patient and knowledge of their behaviors can assist the critical care nurse in identifying changes in behaviors that may be indicative of pain. Discrepancies exist between the patient's self-report and the external observer's evaluations of pain intensity.

RESEARCH BRIEF BOX 1-3

Puntillo et al. compared patient, family member, nurse reports, and physician reports of the perceived intensity and distressing aspects of pain in patients in the intensive care unit. Family members' reports of both the intensity and distress of the patient's pain was positively moderately correlated with the patient's self-report. Interestingly, these family members were more accurate at determining the intensity and distress of their loved one's pain than that of the physicians and nurses currently in charge of the patient's care. Proxy pain assessments should be combined with other evidence such as direct observation using validated behavioral pain scales, and the patient's diagnosis, health history and physical examination, and evaluation of treatment response.

Derived from Puntillo KA, White C, Morris AB, et al: Patients' perceptions and responses to procedural pain: results from Thunder Project II. *Am J Crit Care* 10(4):238-251, 2001.

HISTORY AND RISK FACTORS
Origins for undertreated pain in the intensive care unit

Interferences with optimal pain management persist and are often attributed to the patient, the healthcare team, and the healthcare system. In the critical care context, clinician-related barriers such as knowledge deficits regarding pain assessment and management principles, personal and cultural bias, and communication difficulties between the patient and the healthcare team have been the main contributors to suboptimal pain management. Specific professional and patient-related barriers include (1) societal expectations concerning pain (e.g., unrelieved pain is expected and accepted in certain situations such as during surgical or invasive procedures, treatment for malignant conditions, or as a normal part of aging); (2) professionals' knowledge deficits regarding the pharmacokinetics and equianalgesic dosing; (3) patients' lack of knowledge concerning the side effects of unrelieved pain and the lack of knowledge of pain management in general; (4) inadequate pain assessment techniques by healthcare professionals (failure to assess and acknowledge the existence of pain); (5) inappropriate professional attitudes and beliefs (e.g., certain patients do not have pain [e.g., neonates], pain management is low priority); (6) inappropriate patients' attitudes and beliefs (e.g., pain builds character, pain is a part of procedures); (7) cultural norms that frame the expected response to pain (e.g., succumbing to pain is a sign of weakness); (8) views of the spiritual significance of enduring suffering (e.g., suffering on earth will entitle the person to more rewards in the afterlife); and (9) fear of tolerance, addiction, and analgesic side effects by both professionals and patients.

ASSESSMENT
Vital signs to use with caution in pain assessment
Vital signs such as BP, HR, and RR are easily accessible through continuous monitoring and are widely used by critical care nurses for pain assessment. However, their validity for this purpose is not supported because vital signs have been found to increase, decrease, or remain stable in patients in ICU. Fluctuations in vital signs may also occur with physiologic or emotional distress, or may be a medication effect (e.g., vasodilation and decreased BP following the administration of morphine). No vital signs have been found to predict the presence of pain. Considering that vital sign use for pain assessment remains poor, they are not considered valid pain indicators and should only be used as cues to begin further assessment of pain.

Self-report pain assessment tools
Whenever possible, the patient's self-report of pain should be obtained. Mechanical ventilation should not be a barrier for critical care nurses to document patients' self-reports of pain. Indeed, many patients who are intubated can use pain scales by pointing to them. Attempts should be made before concluding that a patient is unable to self-report. Sufficient time must be allowed for the patient to respond with each attempt. Various self-report pain scales exist such as 0 to 10 Numeric Rating Scale (NRS; where 0 refers to "no pain" and 10 to "worst possible pain"), 100 mm Visual Analog Scale, Verbal Descriptor Scale (VDS; no pain, mild, moderate, severe), and Faces Scales (Figure 1-10). The use of a tool must take into account the patient's preference. A vertical pain intensity scale seems to be easier to use for patients who are elderly because it reminds them of a thermometer. Also, in a recent study, an enlarged, readable horizontal 0 to 10 NRS-Visual was the most feasible scale in patients in ICU. Once the nurse determines which scale the patient can use, the same scale should be used for the duration of clinical care so that accurate comparisons can be made regarding the patient's pain intensity, effectiveness of pain management strategies, and to guide further alterations in pain relief efforts.

Behavioral pain scales
Several behavioral pain assessment tools have been developed in recent years. The Behavioral Pain Scale (BPS) and the Critical-Care Pain Observation Tool (CPOT) are the two suggested scales for clinical use in patients in ICU in the recent practice guidelines of the SCCM. A cut-off score is useful to identify the presence of significant pain and can help to evaluate the effectiveness of pain management interventions. The cut-off of the 3 to 12 BPS is greater than 5, and greater than 2 for the 0 to 8 CPOT. Following appropriate training, the use of these scales has led to increased frequency of pain assessments, a better use of analgesic and sedative agents, and better patient outcomes.

COLLABORATIVE MANAGEMENT
1. Ethical obligation: Nurses' role in pain management
Nurses have an ethical obligation to relieve pain and reduce associated physiologic and psychological risks of untreated pain, which may be poorly understood by the patient. In line with the ethical principles of beneficence and nonmaleficence, healthcare professionals are held responsible to provide pain management and comfort to all patients, including those vulnerable individuals who are unable to speak for themselves. Ensuring that adequate pain management is also provided to patients unable to self-report, their pain is directed by the principle of justice that demands the provision of quality and comparable care to all individuals. The American Society for Pain Management Nursing insists that all persons with pain

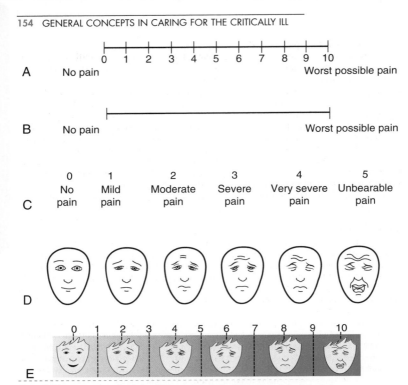

Figure 1-10 Pain intensity scales. A, 0 to 10 Numeric Scale. **B,** Visual Analog Scale. **C,** Descriptive Scale. **D,** Faces Pain Scale—Revised (From Hicks et al., 2001; www.painsourcebook.ca). **E,** Faces Pain Thermometer (From Hicks et al., The Faces Pain Scale-Revised: toward a common metric in pediatric pain measurement. Pain. 2001 Aug;93(2):173-83) (From Gelinas C: Management of pain in cardiac surgery intensive care unit patients: have we improved over time? *Intensive Crit Care Nurs* 23(5):298-303, 2007).

deserve prompt recognition and treatment such that pain is routinely assessed, reassessed, and documented to facilitate treatment and communication among healthcare clinicians. A standard for pain assessment using valid and reliable pain assessment tools is identified to be essential for the recognition and prompt treatment of pain. Moreover, the use of pain assessment tools is needed to reassess pain relief and guide analgesia readjustments that may include upward titration of treatment as well as tapering of the analgesics and implementation of adjuvant therapies. In the recent clinical guidelines of the SCCM, the use of nonpharmacologic interventions is recommended for the management of pain in adults who are critically ill, and nurses should attempt to employ these interventions in their efforts to promote optimal pain relief.

- There are many sources of pain in ICU and unrelieved pain can have multiple negative impacts on the patient's recovery.
- Nurses have an ethical responsibility to provide comfort to all their patients by systematically assessing for the presence of pain, administering the appropriate pharmacologic and nonpharmacologic treatments, and reassessing if optimal pain relief was achieved.
- In assessing pain, patient self-report should be attempted first. However, when self-report is not available, the use of behavioral indicators is considered a valid approach to pain assessment.
- Pain assessment findings are to be communicated with the multidisciplinary team to ensure an optimal care plan for pain management.

2. Pharmacologic therapies

The pharmacologic management of pain is widely used in the critical care setting. Pain pharmacology can be divided into three main categories of action: opioids, nonopioids, and adjuvants. The mechanism of action of these different agents in association with nociception, their administration routes, therapeutic uses, and side effects are described in Table 1-32. Pain can be managed using a combination of the available agents, and must consider the type of pain and the patient response to treatment.

Opioids: The opioids most commonly used are agonists, and their IV administration is recommended as first-line analgesics to treat acute nonneuropathic pain in patients who are critically ill. The agonist opioids bind to mu (μ) receptors (transmission process), which appear to be responsible for pain relief. They are used to manage moderate to severe acute pain. For the most effective therapy, titrate in small increments to produce the desired analgesia with minimal side effects. "As needed" dosing provides poor pain management because of delays in administration and fluctuations in the patient's analgesic blood levels. Patient-controlled analgesia (PCA) pumps, continuous peripheral or epidural infusions, and small, frequent IV bolus dosing are effective methods used for patients in critical care settings. Opioid tolerance, physiologic or psychological dependence, and addiction are unusual when opioids are used to manage acute pain in patients without a history of chemical dependency. Parenteral opioids may cause hypotension in patients with hypovolemia. Restore fluid volume before or concurrently with administration. Some patients are at a greater risk for respiratory depression such as the opioid naïve, those with compromised pulmonary status or neuromuscular disease, the extremely young (neonates), and older adults. Opioid-induced respiratory depression can be prevented with careful titration and monitoring.

- Morphine: Most frequently used opioid for the treatment of moderate to severe acute pain. With its vasodilatory effects and little effect on CO and HR, morphine is beneficial for patients with LV failure, pulmonary hypertension, or pulmonary edema. Rapid IV injection may trigger histamine release with related vasodilation, decreased preload, and decreased BP. Continuous opioid infusion minimizes hemodynamic changes that can occur with bolus dosing. Epidural administration may result in reduced responsiveness of the respiratory center in the brainstem to CO_2. This results in gradual decrease in the depth and rate of respiration, increase in $Paco_2$, increase in sedation level, and respiratory acidosis.

- Hydromorphone (Dilaudid): Highly effective opioid; substitute analgesic for patients with morphine allergy or intolerance. Care must be taken to modify the dose of hydromorphone in comparison to morphine, because hydromorphone is approximately 5 to 7 times stronger than morphine (see Table 1-32).

- Meperidine (Demerol): Not suggested for routine analgesia use in the critical care unit, it may be indicated for brief courses (i.e., < 48 hours, < 600 mg/24 h) in patients with allergy or intolerance to morphine, hydromorphone, or other opioids, and for the treatment of postoperative shivering. Morphine is approximately 7 to 10 times stronger than meperidine, thus meperidine doses are much higher (see Table 1-32). The drug is not well tolerated by older adults. Its toxic metabolite, normeperidine, is a cerebral irritant and may cause seizures, which has decreased its usage in both older adults and the critically ill. Some patients report little pain relief from meperidine, despite stating a strong feeling of intoxication.

| **Safety Alert** | *Use of naloxone on patients receiving chronic or high-dose therapy may result in seizures caused by predominance of convulsant activity from normeperidine overriding the central nervous system depressant effects of meperidine.* |

- Fentanyl: Potent synthetic opioid. IV preparation is especially useful in critical care because of minimal cardiovascular effects, short duration of action, and rapid onset of action. Duration of action increases with repeated doses. Caution must be taken if large doses of fentanyl are given rapidly. This may cause chest wall muscle rigidity requiring ventilatory support and rapid-acting muscle relaxants. Other forms for chronic pain are available such as a transdermal patch.

Table 1-32	EQUIANALGESIC DOSES OF NARCOTIC ANALGESICS		
Class/Name	**Route**	**Equianalgesic Dose (mg)***	**Average Duration (h)**
Morphine-Like Agonists			
Codeine	IM, SC	130†	3
	PO	180†	3
Hydromorphone (Dilaudid)	IM, SC	1.5	4
	PO	6-7.5	4
Levorphanol (Levo-Dromoran)	IM, SC	2	6
	PO	4	6
Morphine	IM, SC	10	4
Oxycodone (Percodan)	PO	30†	4
Oxymorphone	IM, SC	1	4
(Numorphan)	Rectal	15-20	4
Meperidine-Like Agonists			
Fentanyl (Sublimaze)	IV, IM, SC	0.1	3-4‡
Meperidine (Demerol)	IM, SC	100	3
Methadone-like agonists			
Methadone (Dolophine)	IM, SC	10	6
	PO	10-20	6
Propoxyphene (Darvon)	PO	130-250†	4
Mixed Agonist-Antagonist			
Buprenorphine (Buprenex)	IM	0.3-0.4	4
Butorphanol (Stadol)	IM, SC	2	3
Nalbuphine (Nubain)	IM, SC	10	3-4
Pentazocine (Talwin)	IM	150	33
	PO	60	

Modified from Hazard V, Hopfer DJ: *Davis' drug guide for nurses*, ed 5, Philadelphia, 1997, Davis; Macintyre PE, Ready LBN: *Acute pain management: a practical guide*, London, 1996, Saunders; and Salerno E: Pharmacologic approaches. In Salerno E, Willens JS, editors: *Pain management handbook: an interdisciplinary approach*, St Louis, 1996, Mosby.

*Recommended starting dose; actual dose must be titrated to patient response.
†Starting doses lower (codeine 30 mg, oxycodone 5 mg, meperidine 50 mg, propoxyphene 65 to 130 mg, pentazocine 50 mg).
‡Respiratory depressant effects persist longer than analgesic effects.
IM, Intramuscular; *IV*, intravenous; *PO*, oral; *SC*, subcutaneous.

HIGH ALERT! A fentanyl patch may be used for continuous analgesia, usually with supplemental doses of morphine or another opiate titrated to produce analgesia for breakthrough pain but should be used only for patients with opiate tolerance. A fentanyl patch is not recommended for mild pain, acute postoperative pain, or intermittent pain because of its slow onset (12 to 16 hours) and long duration, and because it is difficult to reverse its side effects and adverse effects. Respiratory depression with hypoventilation occurs, as with morphine. Transdermal fentanyl absorption can be increased in patients with elevated temperatures.

Nonopioids: Nonopioids can be used to treat mild pain, and as coanalgesics for the treatment of moderate to severe pain. Their use can help decrease the amount of opioids administered and to decrease opioid-related side effects.
• Acetaminophen: Acetaminophen is a safe nonopioid agent, and side effects are rare at therapeutic doses. The critical care nurse must consider the other products containing

acetaminophen that the patient may receive when calculating the total daily dose of acetaminophen. Total daily dose of acetaminophen should be reduced to not exceed 2 g in patients with liver dysfunction, malnutrition, or a history of excess alcohol consumption.

- Nonsteroidal antiinflammatory drugs (NSAIDs): The use of NSAIDs is indicated in the patient with acute musculoskeletal and soft tissue inflammation. NSAIDs can be grouped as first-generation (COX-1 and COX-2 inhibitors, such as aspirin, ibuprofen, naproxen, and ketorolac) or second-generation (COX-2 inhibitors, such as celecoxib) agents. The inhibition of COX-1 is thought to be responsible for many of the side effects, such as gastric ulceration, bleeding as a result of platelet inhibition, and acute renal failure. In contrast, the inhibition of COX-2 is responsible for the suppression of pain and inflammation. Second-generation NSAIDs are associated with minimal risks of serious adverse effects, but their role in patients who are critically ill remains unknown. Most NSAIDs are given orally (e.g., ibuprofen, aspirin), but injectable NSAIDs such as ketorolac are available.
- Ketorolac (Toradol): Effective for short-term use in relieving mild to moderate pain. The effect on ventilation is minimal, and the drug has been effective when given on an alternate schedule with morphine or another opioid analgesic during ventilator weaning of postoperative patients. Renal toxicity is possible, which limits use to patients with normal renal function. Bleeding complications are more likely with high-dose therapy and in older adults.

Adjuvants: According to Barr et al. (2013), anticonvulsants, either enterally administered gabapentin or carbamazepine, should be considered for the treatment of neuropathic pain. Antidepressants administered at lower doses are also considered as adjuvant analgesics in a variety of chronic pain syndromes, such as headache, fibromyalgia, low back pain, neuropathy, central pain, and cancer pain. They are usually divided into two main groups: tricyclic antidepressants (e.g., amitriptyline, imipramine, desipramine), and biogenic amine reuptake inhibitors (e.g., venlafaxine, paroxetine, sertraline).

Other agents: Ketamine: Ketamine is a dissociative anesthetic agent that has analgesic properties, and is commonly used for specific procedural pain. In comparison to opioids, ketamine has the benefit of sparing the respiratory drive. However, it has many side effects related to the release of catecholamines and delirium. Before administering the drug, the dissociative state should be explained to the patient. Dissociative state refers to the feelings of separateness from the environment, loss of control, hallucinations, and vivid dreams. The use of benzodiazepines (e.g., midazolam) can help reduce the incidence of this unpleasant effect.

Dexmedetomidine (Precedex): Dexmedetomidine is a short-acting alpha$_2$-agonist used for sedation in patients who are critically ill and mechanically ventilated or not. This drug has sedative, analgesic, and anxiolytic effects. It is ideal for mild to moderate sedation, often referred to as conscious sedation. The analgesic effect of dexmedetomidine is attributable to spinal antinociception via binding to nonnoradrenergic receptors located on the dorsal horn neurons of the spinal cord. It can help reduce opioid requirements and spares the respiratory drive. Its main side effects are hypotension and bradycardia.

Older adults

Older adults are more sensitive to the therapeutic and toxic effects of analgesics. The distribution of medications is altered by age. With aging, lean body mass decreases and body fat increases. Also, muscle and soft tissue mass decrease, and body water declines. This results in water-soluble opioid analgesics such as morphine having a lower volume of distribution. This causes an increased rate of the onset of action and raises the peak concentration, which is associated with increased toxicity. Lipid-soluble opioid analgesics (e.g., fentanyl) may be more widely distributed, resulting in a delayed onset of action and accumulation with repeated doses. Because of age-related changes in metabolism and elimination, older adults are also at risk for drug-accumulation toxicity.

In treating older adults, it is best to start at lower doses (50% to 75% of recommended younger adult doses). The interval between doses can be increased, using opioids with shorter half-lives (morphine, hydromorphone, oxycodone). All older adults should be monitored for signs of opioid toxicity, including increased sedative effects, inability to awaken the patient easily, and respiratory depression. With careful assessment, proper dosing and titration, knowledge of analgesic onset and peak times, and careful monitoring, the risk for respiratory depression is low. However, naloxone (Narcan), an opioid antagonist, should be immediately available to reverse respiratory depression.

Safety Alert *Naloxone reduces respiratory depression but also reverses analgesia—dilute 0.4 mg ampule in 10 mL 0.9% normal saline and administer 0.5 mL (0.02 mg) by direct intravenous push every 2 minutes; titrate to effect patient response to avoid withdrawal, seizures, and severe pain; onset occurs within 1 to 2 minutes with a duration of approximately 45 minutes. Patients can sometimes exhibit aggressive and sometimes violent behavior when the naloxone takes effect. See Table 1-32 for equianalgesic doses of narcotic analgesics.*

NONPHARMACOLOGIC INTERVENTIONS

In light of the recognition of the high prevalence of pain in the critically ill despite the administration of standard pharmacologic treatments, a multimodal approach to pain management in patients in ICU is recommended. A multimodal approach supports the combination of nonopioid with opioid analgesics for optimal pain relief versus an increase in the dosage of opioids administered to prevent the adverse effects of high opioid doses on patients. Moreover, the recent clinical practice guidelines of the SCCM for the management of pain in ICUs suggest the use of complementary, nonpharmacologic interventions for pain management (massage, music therapy, relaxation techniques) in addition to a multimodal approach.

The general belief of ICU nurses is that pain is primarily managed with pharmacologic treatments such as indicated in most ICU pain management protocols, but when this type of treatment is not sufficient, they try different nonpharmacologic approaches. Several nonpharmacologic interventions such as deep breathing exercises, massage, and positioning were reported to be already used by nurses for the management of pain in ICU.

These nonpharmacologic interventions are intended to supplement pharmacologic treatments to maximize pain relief. Even though they are commonly used in clinical practice, there is still limited evidence to support their effectiveness in critical care settings. These interventions include sensory, emotional, and cognitive interventions, such as massage, relaxation, distraction, guided imagery, repositioning, and transcutaneous electrical nerve stimulation, and are used for mild pain and anxiety and as adjuncts to pharmacologic management of moderate to severe pain.

Physical techniques

- Massage: Massage has been identified to be advantageous in its opioid-sparing and analgesia-enhancing properties, but also because it is recognized to be low cost, easy to provide, and safe to administer. Several therapeutic benefits have already been documented for the administration of massage in various clinical settings. It has been shown to reduce fatigue and improve sleep quality, to promote relaxation and decrease muscle tension, and to impact vital signs by decreasing systolic and diastolic BP, cardiac, and respiratory rates.

  Patients and family members with a previous experience of ICU hospitalization and ICU nurses identified massage as a nonpharmacologic intervention to be useful, relevant, and feasible for pain management in ICU. Feasibility results of a randomized controlled trial and a pilot study revealed that hand-massage and hand-holding by an interventionist were feasible in ICU, especially if clinicians (i.e., nurses and physicians) supported its administration. Also, participants receiving massage reported enjoying the experience and further recommended its delivery to other patients. Thus, massage is viewed favorably by both patients and clinicians, and has gained more consideration in its regular delivery in ICU.

- Cold Application: This therapy is used to alter the pain threshold, reduce muscle spasm, and decrease vascular congestion, particularly in the area of injury. Ice is believed to relieve pain by inducing local anesthesia around the treatment area. Ice therapy was found to reduce pain in the critically ill after chest tube removal when ice packets were placed around the site for 10 minutes before removal. Cold is also known to decrease initial tissue injury response.

Cognitive-behavioral techniques

- Relaxation: This nonpharmacologic technique is defined as the absence of physical, mental, and emotional tension, and can impact pain levels both physiologically and psychologically. At the physiologic level, it can reduce the sympathetic response to pain with subsequent decreases in oxygen consumption, BP, HR, and respiration. Psychologically, through distraction, this technique decreases the cognitive awareness of pain by encouraging the patient to focus on something unrelated to the pain. Examples include conversing, reading, watching television or videos, and listening to music.
- Guided imagery: Using this nonpharmacologic treatment, the patient employs a mental process that uses images to alter a physical or emotional state. This technique promotes relaxation and decreases pain sensations. Several barriers might interfere with the patient's ability to direct attention away from pain in the critical care environment, yet the successful use of guided imagery may be beneficial to maximize pain relief.

RESEARCH BRIEF BOX 1-4

Owens and Flom indicate that family members of patients in the intensive care unit are able to predict when their loved one is in pain approximately 75% of the time, but the severity is usually underestimated

From Owens D, Flom J: Integrating palliative and neurological critical care. *AACN Clin Issues* 16(4):542-550, 2005.

CARE PLANS FOR PAIN MANAGEMENT

Pain *related to biophysical injury secondary to pathology: surgical, diagnostic, treatment or intervention; or related to trauma.*

Goals/Outcomes: Within 1 hour of initiating therapy, the patient's pain levels improve. Those able to self-report will express a decrease in pain, and the use of valid and reliable scales for pain assessment in patients who are noncommunicative will indicate lower pain scores.

NOC Pain Control.

Pain Management
1. Develop a systematic approach to pain management for each patient. The primary nurse should collaborate with the physician and patient for optimal management of pain.
2. Monitor the patient at frequent intervals for the presence of discomfort. Use a formal, patient-specific method of assessing pain. One method is to have the patient rate discomfort on a scale of 0 (no discomfort) to 10 (worst pain imaginable). Other methods may be used, but the method selected should be used consistently and the patient's report should be respected and documented as reported.
3. Evaluate patients with acute and chronic pain for nonverbal indicators of discomfort.
4. Evaluate health history for evidence of alcohol and drug (prescribed and nonprescribed) use. Individuals with a history of chemical dependence may require a higher dose for effective analgesia. Persons with evidence of chronic or acute hepatic insufficiency may require a reduced dose and careful selection of appropriate analgesics. Consult pain control team if available. All care providers must be consistent in setting limits while providing effective pain control through pharmacologic and nonpharmacologic methods. Psychiatric consultation may be warranted. Be aware that some opioid agonist–antagonist analgesics (e.g., butorphanol, buprenorphine, pentazocine) have strong narcotic antagonist activity and may trigger withdrawal symptoms in individuals with opiate dependency.

Analgesic Administration
1. Administer opioid and related mixed agonist–antagonist analgesics as prescribed. Monitor for side effects, such as excessive sedation, respiratory depression, nausea, vomiting, and constipation.

Opioid-induced sedation precedes respiratory depression, thus frequent assessment is warranted to determine patient arousability, especially in patients who are opioid-naive or receiving opioids by intravenous or epidural routes. Opioids should be stopped if the patient is difficult to arouse. Be aware that meperidine (Demerol) may produce excitation, muscle twitching, and seizures, especially in conjunction with phenothiazines. Do not administer mixed agonist-antagonist analgesics concurrently with morphine or other pure agonists, because reversal of analgesic effects may occur. Meperidine is poorly tolerated by older adults.

2. Assess patients receiving opioid analgesics at frequent intervals for evidence of excessive sedation when awake or respiratory depression (i.e., RR less than 10 breaths/min or SaO_2 less than 92%). In the presence of respiratory depression, reduce the amount or frequency of the dose as prescribed. Have naloxone (Narcan) readily available to reverse severe respiratory depression.
3. If the patient is receiving an epidural or intrathecal opioid, monitor closely for side effects and complications.
4. Check the patient's analgesia record for the last dose and amount of medication given during surgery and in the postanesthesia care unit. Be careful to coordinate timing and dose of postoperative analgesics with previously administered medication.

Medication Management
1. Administer nonnarcotics and NSAIDs as prescribed for relief of mild-to-moderate pain or on alternating schedule with opiate analgesics for moderate-to-severe pain.

Long-term use of acetaminophen is associated with hepatotoxicity and nephrotoxicity. Daily dose restrictions are recommended: 4000 mg/day for short-term use in normal, healthy adults, up to 3600 mg/day for chronic, long-term use, and no more than 2000 mg for older adults. Total daily doses should be calculated on a running 24-hour clock and include all combination products such as hydrocodone (e.g., Lortab, Vicodin) and propoxyphene (e.g., Darvocet). Patient teaching should include attention to products containing acetaminophen and cumulative daily doses (e.g., maximum total number of pills taken per day). Nonsteroidal antiinflammatory drugs are especially effective when pain is associated with inflammation and soft tissue injury. Ketorolac (Toradol) may be given intramuscularly or intravenously when oral agents are contraindicated. Monitor for excessive bleeding, gastric irritation, and renal compromise in patients receiving all nonsteroidal antiinflammatory drugs, including all products containing ibuprofen and naproxen.

2. Administer PRN analgesics before pain becomes severe. Assess pain and offer the patient PRN pain medication around-the-clock based on the PRN schedule to achieve better and more even pain relief. Prolonged stimulation of pain receptors results in increased sensitivity to painful stimuli and will increase the amount of drug required to relieve pain.
3. Administer intermittently scheduled or supplemental analgesics before painful procedures (e.g., suctioning, chest tube removal) and ambulation and at bedtime, scheduling them so that their peak effect is achieved at the inception of the activity or procedure.
4. Augment analgesic therapy with sedatives and tranquilizers to prolong and enhance analgesia. Avoid substituting sedatives and tranquilizers for analgesics.
5. Wean the patient from opioid analgesics by decreasing dosage or frequency of the drug. When changing route of administration or medication, be certain to use equianalgesic doses of the new drug (see Table 1-32). Remember doses listed on the table are ratios of one drug to another and one route to another; these ratios should be used as estimates for a new starting dose along with pain intensity, patient pain assessment, and patient response to the drug. The current total 24-hour dosage will need to be calculated first; include scheduled and rescue doses.

Self-Responsibility Facilitation
1. Augment action of medication by using nonpharmacologic methods of pain control. Many of these techniques may be taught to and implemented by the patient and significant others.
2. Sudden or unexpected changes in pain intensity can signal complications such as internal bleeding or leakage of visceral contents. Carefully evaluate the patient's report of pain, compare to previous pain reports, and consult the surgeon immediately.

3. Educate patients about their medications, including asking for medications when in pain and declining them if offered when not in pain.

Environmental Management: Comfort
1. Maintain a quiet environment to promote rest. Plan nursing activities to enable long periods of uninterrupted rest at night.
2. Evaluate for and correct nonoperative sources of discomfort (e.g., position, full bladder, infiltrated IV site).
3. Position the patient comfortably, and reposition at frequent intervals to relieve discomfort caused by pressure and to improve circulation.
4. Document efficacy of analgesics and other pain control interventions, using the pain scale or other formalized method.

NIC Analgesic Administration; Analgesic Administration: Intraspinal; Patient-Controlled Analgesia (PCA) Assistance.

Ineffective breathing pattern *related to neuromuscular impairment secondary to central respiratory depression; pain-induced splinting.*

Goals/Outcomes: The patient exhibits effective ventilation within 30 minutes of this diagnosis, as evidenced by relaxed breathing, RR 12 to 20 breaths/min with normal depth and pattern (eupnea), clear breath sounds, normal color, $PaO_2 \geq 80$ mm Hg, pH 7.35 to 7.45, $PaCO_2$ 35 to 45 mm Hg, HCO_3^- 22 to 26 mEq/L, and $SpO_2 \geq 92\%$.
NOC Respiratory Status: Ventilation.

Respiratory Monitoring
1. Assess and document respiratory rate and depth hourly. Note signs of respiratory compromise, including RR less than 10 or greater than 26; shallow or grunting respirations; use of accessory muscles of respiration; prolonged I:E ratio; pallor or cyanosis; decreased vital capacity; and increased residual volume. Consult the physician for evidence of respiratory compromise.
2. Monitor SpO_2 and ABG values. Consult the physician for decreased SpO_2 (less than 92%) or increased $PaCO_2$ (greater than 45 mm Hg).
3. Assess and document LOC every 1 to 2 hours.
4. Use apnea monitor as indicated.
5. Keep naloxone (Narcan) at the patient's bedside during and for 24 hours after epidural or intrathecal administration.
6. Maintain IV access for immediate administration of naloxone to reverse respiratory depression.
7. Respiratory depression may persist for as long as 24 hours after the last dose of epidural morphine. Monitor for respiratory depression during and for 24 hours after the patient has received epidural or intrathecal opioids.

NIC Airway Management; Oxygen Therapy; Aspiration Precautions.

Urinary retention *related to inhibition of reflex arc secondary to opioid action*

Goals/Outcomes: Within 4 hours of this diagnosis, complete bladder emptying is achieved. Overflow incontinence is absent.
NOC Urinary Elimination.

Urinary Retention Care
1. Monitor for symptoms of urinary retention: bladder distention, frequent voiding of small amounts of urine, sensation of bladder fullness, residual urine, dysuria, and overflow incontinence.
2. Monitor I&O precisely.
3. Catheterize bladder intermittently or insert indwelling catheter as prescribed.
4. Administer IV naloxone as prescribed.

NIC Urinary Catheterization.

Risk for impaired skin integrity *related to itching secondary to alteration in sensory modulation from opioid effects.*

Goals/Outcomes: The patient's skin remains intact.

NOC Tissue Integrity: Skin and Mucous Membranes.

Medication Management
1. Decrease the opioid dose via epidural or PCA infusion.
2. Administer diphenhydramine or hydroxyzine as prescribed. Monitor sedation when antihistamine is added.
3. Maintain comfortably cool environment.
4. Apply cool, moist compresses.
5. If relief from the above measures is inadequate, administer small amounts of IV naloxone as prescribed and until RR is at least 8/min, continue to assess patient closely and frequently because naloxone may need to be repeated as effect of opioid is of longer duration than the effect of naloxone.

See also Prolonged Immobility in the following section.

NIC Skin Surveillance; Positioning; Pressure Ulcer Prevention.

PROLONGED IMMOBILITY

Prolonged immobility is a common consequence of prolonged hospitalization for severe and critical illness. Morbidity related to prolonged immobility is often profoundly impacted by nursing care. Nurses attend to patients continuously, providing ongoing, expert assessments and interventions. Significant adverse outcomes of prolonged immobility have been demonstrated to be preventable (Box 1-16).

Illnesses or diseases that may necessitate prolonged bed rest include:
- Neurologic disorders such as stroke/cerebrovascular accident and Guillain-Barré syndrome.
- Cardiovascular disorders such as severe heart failure and cardiomyopathy.
- Pulmonary disorders such as chronic obstructive lung disease and pneumonia.
- Musculoskeletal disorders such as postmotor vehicle accident and joint contractures.
- Others:
  - Complications from surgery.
  - Severe sepsis.
  - Failure to thrive.

Box 1-16	**PHYSIOLOGIC EFFECTS AND COMPLICATIONS OF BED REST (DECONDITIONING)**

Cardiovascular
- Increased heart rate and blood pressure for submaximal workload
- Decrease in functional capacity
- Decrease in circulating volume
- Orthostatic hypotension
- Reflex tachycardia
- Deep vein thrombosis

Pulmonary
- Modest decrease in pulmonary function
- Atelectasis
- Pneumonia
- Pulmonary embolus

Gastrointestinal
- Ileus
- Deficient protein state
- Negative nitrogen state

Musculoskeletal
- Loss of muscle mass
- Loss of muscle contractile strength
- Bone demineralization
- Joint contractures

Skin
- Decubitus ulcers

SAFE PATIENT HANDLING

Healthcare workers are needlessly injured on the job. During 2011, workers in the healthcare sector suffered a higher rate of musculoskeletal injuries and disorders than construction, mining, or manufacturing workers. Also, "in 2011, registered nurses ranked fifth among all occupations for the number of cases of musculoskeletal disorders resulting in days away from work, with 11,880 total cases. Nursing assistants reported 25,010 cases, the highest for any occupation."

The following are the Interprofessional Standards of Safe Patient Handling and Mobility (SPHM) as established by the American Nurses Association (ANA).

STANDARD 1. ESTABLISH A CULTURE OF SAFETY

The employer and healthcare workers partner to establish a culture of safety that encompasses the core values and behaviors resulting from a collective and sustained commitment by organizational leadership, managers, healthcare workers, and ancillary/support staff to emphasize safety over competing goals.

1.1 Employer

1.1.1 Establish a statement of commitment to a culture of safety Organizational policy will include a written commitment to a culture of safety that will be used to guide the organization's priorities, resource allocation, policies, and procedures. The written statement regarding SPHM will describe layers of accountability across sectors and settings.

1.1.2 Establish a nonpunitive environment Organizational policy will support a system to encourage healthcare workers to report hazards, errors, incidents, and accidents, so that the precursors to SPHM errors can be better understood and organizational issues can be changed to prevent future incidents and injuries. Healthcare workers know that they are accountable for their actions, but will not be held accountable for problems within the system or environment that are beyond their control.

1.1.3 Provide a system for right of refusal Organizational policy will provide the healthcare worker the right to accept, reject, or object to any healthcare recipient transfer, repositioning, or mobility assignment that puts the healthcare recipient or the healthcare worker at risk for injury. The refusal shall be made in writing, without fear of retribution. The policy will describe steps for resolving the hazard.

1.1.4 Provide safe levels of staffing An evidence-based system will be used to determine safe and appropriate caseloads. Adequate staffing levels will support safe patient handling and mobility, including allocated time for training and education.

1.1.5 Establish a system for communication and collaboration Collaboration among all sectors and settings is critical. The organization will use a variety of communication systems to inform and engage the healthcare workers and healthcare recipients about SPHM.

1.2 Healthcare worker

1.2.1 Participate in creating and maintaining a culture of safety The healthcare worker will actively participate in creating and maintaining a culture of safety.

1.2.2 Notify the employer of hazards, incidents, near misses, and accidents The healthcare worker will notify the employer of hazards, near misses, incidents, and accidents related to SPHM as soon as possible, using the reporting procedures defined by the employer.

1.2.3 Use the system to communicate and collaborate The healthcare worker will engage, verbally and in writing, with others about SPHM.

The Patient's Ability to Assist with Transfer (U.S. Department of Veterans Affairs):
1. Assess the patient's height and weight. Weight alone may be the determining factor in deciding how much assistance is needed or if an assistive device is needed.
2. Assess the patient's level of independence with turning and transferring.
   - Independent: Can the patient independently perform turning or transferring (e.g., bed to stretcher, bed to chair) safely, with or without assistive devices (e.g., cane or walker), without staff assistance?
   - Some Assistance Required: Can the patient partially assist with transfer, needing one caregiver to observe or assist? Remember to assess upper and lower extremity strength, mobility, and ability to cooperate and comprehend instructions.
   - Total Dependence: Is the patient unable to assist with turning or transfer?

Assistive Devices Assistive devices are very helpful in preventing injury and decreasing the number of staff needed to assist. There are many assistive devises on the market, usually in the form of slings. Some types of slings may be independent, roll on wheels, and be able to be moved from one patient to another. Another type of sling, which is not portable, may be attached to the ceiling and slide.

It is important to know how to use the sling properly and to have enough staff to assist with the use safely. Read the instructions before using any new device that is not familiar.

The following set of nursing care plans frames the care of those who require prolonged periods of bed rest and/or those who are immobile.

CARE PLANS FOR PROLONGED IMMOBILITY

Activity intolerance   *related to prolonged bed rest; generalized weakness; and imbalance between O_2 supply and demand.*

Goals/Outcomes: Within 48 hours of discontinuing bed rest, the patient exhibits cardiac tolerance to low-intensity exercise (defined later), as evidenced by:
- HR $\leq$ 20 bpm over resting HR.
- Systolic BP $\leq$ 20 mm Hg over or under resting systolic BP.
- SaO_2 greater than 90%.
- SvO_2 $\geq$ 60%.
- RR $\leq$ 20 breaths/min.
- Normal sinus rhythm.
- Skin warm and dry.
- Absence of crackles, murmurs, and chest pain.

NOC Activity Tolerance; Endurance.

Exercise Promotion: Strength Training
1. Perform low-intensity exercise 2, 3, or 4 times daily: ROM exercises on each extremity. Individualize the exercise plan on the basis of the following guidelines. Depending on the degree of debility of the patient, it may be necessary to begin with passive exercises, moving the joints through the motions of abduction, adduction, flexion, and extension.
2. Progress to active-assisted exercises, in which the nurse supports the joints while the patient initiates muscle contraction. When the patient is able, supervise him or her in active exercises and then isotonic exercises, during which the patient contracts a selected muscle group, moves the extremity at a slow pace, and then relaxes the muscle group. Have the patient repeat each exercise 3 to 10 times.

HIGH ALERT!   Avoid isometric exercises in patients with cardiac disease. Stop any exercise that causes muscular or skeletal pain. Consult with a physical therapist for necessary modifications to allow for exercise without causing muscular or skeletal pain.

---

3. Assess exercise tolerance:
   - Be alert to signs and symptoms that the cardiovascular and respiratory systems cannot meet the demands of the low-level ROM exercises. Excessive SOB may occur if:
     - Transient pulmonary congestion occurs secondary to ischemia or LV dysfunction.
     - Lung volumes are decreased.
     - O_2-carrying capacity of the blood is reduced.
     - There is shunting of blood from the right to the left side of the heart without adequate oxygenation.
   - If CO does not increase to meet the body's needs during modest levels of exercise, look for:
     - A fall in the systolic BP.
     - Dysrhythmias.
     - Crackles that can be auscultated.
     - A new S_3 or a systolic murmur indicating mitral regurgitation that may occur.
   - If the patient tolerates the exercise, increase the intensity or number of repetitions each day.
     - Ask the patient to rate perceived exertion (RPE) using the scale shown in Table 1-33. The patient should not experience an RPE greater than 3 while performing ROM exercises. Reduce the intensity of the exercise and increase the frequency until an RPE of $\leq$ 3 is attained.

Table 1-33	RATING PERCEIVED EXERTION
Rating	**Perceived Exertion**
0	Nothing at all
1	Very weak effort
2	Weak (light) effort
3	Moderate
4	Somewhat stronger effort
5	Strong effort
6	
7	Very strong effort
8	
9	Very, very strong effort
10	Maximal effort

From Borg G: Psychophysical bases of perceived exertion. *Med Sci Sports Exerc* 14(5):377-381, 1982.

4 Monitor the intensity of the activity:
- Begin with 3 to 5 repetitions, as tolerated by the patient.
- Assess exercise tolerance by measuring HR and BP at rest, peak exercise, and 5 minutes after exercise.
    - If HR or systolic BP increases more than 20 bpm or more than 20 mm Hg over the resting level, decrease the number of repetitions.
    - If HR or systolic BP decreases more than 10 bpm or more than 10 mm Hg at peak exercise, this could be a sign of LV failure, denoting that the heart cannot meet this workload.
- Plan to increase duration:
    - Begin with 5 minutes or less of exercise.
    - Gradually increase the exercise to 15 minutes as tolerated.
- Plan to increase frequency:
    - Begin exercises 2 to 4 times daily.
    - As the duration increases, the frequency can be reduced.
5. Increase activity as the patient's condition improves:
- Progress to sitting in a chair as soon as possible.
    - Assess for orthostatic hypotension, which can occur as a result of decreased plasma volume and difficulty in adjusting immediately to postural change.
- Prepare the patient by increasing the amount of time spent in a high-Fowler position and moving the patient slowly and in stages as follows:
    - Level I/bed rest: Allow flexion and extension of extremities 4 times daily with 15 repetitions per extremity. Deep breathing should occur 4 times daily, 15 breaths each time. Reposition the patient every 2 hours.
    - Level II/out of bed to chair: The patient sits in the chair 2 or 3 times daily for 20 to 30 minutes as tolerated. ROM exercises may be performed 2 times daily while sitting in the chair.
    - Level III/ambulate in room: The patient ambulates for 3 to 5 minutes, 3 times daily as tolerated.
    - Level IV/ambulate in the hall: The patient initially walks 50 to 200 feet 2 times daily, and progresses to 600 feet 4 times daily. Slow stair climbing may be incorporated in preparation for hospital discharge.
    - If the patient is able, have him or her independently perform self-care activities, such as eating, mouth care, and bathing, as tolerated.
6. Teach and involve significant others in interventions for preventing deconditioning.
7. Provide emotional support to help allay fears of failure, pain, or medical setbacks.

NIC Exercise Therapy: Ambulation; Energy Management; Cardiac Care: Rehabilitative.

Risk for disuse syndrome *related to mechanical or prescribed immobilization; severe pain; altered LOC.*

Goals/Outcomes: The patient displays full ROM without verbal or nonverbal indicators of pain.
NOC Mobility.

Exercise Promotion
1. Prevent joint contractures by performing ROM exercises. The following areas are at high risk for joint contractures:
   - Shoulders can become "frozen," which would limit abduction and extension.
   - Wrists can "drop," prohibiting extension.
   - Fingers can develop flexion contractures that limit extension.
   - Hips can develop flexion contractures that affect the gait by shortening the limb or can develop external rotation or adduction deformities that affect the gait.
   - Knees can develop flexion contractures that limit extension and alter the gait.
   - Feet can "drop" as a result of plantar flexion, which limits dorsiflexion and alters the gait.
2. Change the patient's position at least every 2 hours. Post a turning schedule at the patient's bedside. Position changes will:
   - Maintain all joints in a neutral position.
   - Reduce strain on the joints.
   - Prevent contractures.
   - Minimize pressure on bony prominences.
   - Promote maximal chest expansion.
3. Position to achieve proper standing alignment and maintain with pillows, towels, or other positioning aids.
   - Head neutral or slightly flexed on neck.
   - Hips extended.
   - Knees extended or minimally flexed.
   - Feet at right angles to the legs.
   - HOB elevated 30 degrees.
   - The patient's shoulders and arms extended using pillows for support.
   - Fingertips to extend over the edge of the pillows to maintain normal arching of hands.
   - Hip flexion contracture prevention. Ensure that when the patient is in the side-lying position, the hips are extended for the same amount of time the patient is in the supine position.

HIGH ALERT! Because elevating the head of the bed promotes hip flexion, ensure that the patient spends equal time with the hips in extension. When the patient is in the side-lying position, extend the lower leg from the hip to help prevent hip flexion contracture.

---

4. Maintain the joints in neutral position by using:
   - Pillows, rolled towels, blankets, sandbags, antirotation boots, splints, and orthotics.
   - When using adjunctive devices, monitor the involved skin at frequent intervals for alterations in integrity. Implement measures to prevent skin breakdown.
5. Prevent foot drop.
   - Foot posture is naturally in plantar flexion, thus be alert to the patient's inability to pull the toes up. Document this assessment daily.
   - Foam boots or "high top" tennis shoes may be used to support the feet.
   - Teach the patient the rationale and procedure for ROM exercises, and have the patient return the demonstrations, if able.
6. Ensure that the patient does not exceed his or her tolerance by performing constant assessment of activity tolerance. Provide passive exercises for patients unable to perform active or active-assistive exercises. Incorporate exercising all joints with ADLs, such as changing position, giving bed baths, using bedpan, and changing the patient's gown.
7. Assess the patient's existing muscle mass, strength, and joint motion.
   - Perform and document limb girth measurements.
   - Use dynamography, hand-grip device to measure muscle strength.
   - Establish exercise baseline limits.
   - Perform ROM.

8. Educate the patient. Maintaining or increasing muscle strength and tissue elasticity surrounding joints is impera-tive. Consult with the physician about the form and extent of the exercise. Muscle atrophy occurs from disuse leading to decrease in muscle mass, decrease in blood supply, loss of tissue elasticity surrounding joints, pain, and further difficulty moving.

9. Reinforce progress.
   - Post the exercise regimen at the patient's bedside to ensure consistency by all healthcare personnel.
   - Provide a chart to show the patient's progress.
   - Provide large amounts of positive reinforcement.

10. Balance rest and activity. Provide periods of uninterrupted rest between exercises/activities to enable the patient to replenish energy stores.

11. Consult rehabilitation services. Seek a referral to a physical therapist or occupational therapist as appropriate.

NIC Positioning; Pressure Management; Exercise Therapy: Joint Mobility; Exercise Therapy: Muscle Control.

Impaired skin integrity of the oral mucous membrane *related to ineffective oral hygiene*

Goals/Outcomes: The patient's oral mucosa, lips, and tongue are intact within 24 hours before discharge from ICU.
NOC Tissue Integrity: Skin and Mucous Membranes.

Oral Health Maintenance
1. Assess the patient's oral mucous membrane, lips, and tongue at least every 4 hours, noting the presence of dry-ness, exudate, swelling, blisters, and ulcers.
2. Perform oral care every 2 to 4 hours.
   - Use a soft-bristle toothbrush (premade mouth care kits are available) to cleanse the teeth. This is particu-larly important for patients who are intubated because evidence shows that pneumonia can be reduced or prevented. Suction mouth continuously during oral hygiene to remove fluid and debris.
   - Use a moistened cloth or sponge-tip applicator to moisten and help remove crusty areas or exudate on tongue and oral mucosa.
3. Offer sips of water or ice chips to prevent dryness if the patient is alert and able to take oral fluids.
4. Apply lip balm every 2 hours and as needed to prevent cracking of lips.
5. Consider using an artificial saliva preparation to assist in keeping mucous membrane moist.
6. Have the patient wear dentures as possible, to improve communication and enhance comfort.
7. Teach family the proper oral hygiene techniques and encourage them to perform oral hygiene.
NOC Self-Care Assistance: Bathing, Hygiene.

Self-care deficit *related to cognitive, neuromuscular, or musculoskeletal impairment; activity intoler-ance secondary to prolonged bed rest.*

Goals/Outcomes: The patient's physical needs are met by the patient, nursing staff, and/or significant others while the patient is being encouraged to participate as much as possible.
NOC Self-Care: Activities of Daily Living.

Self-Care Assistance: Bathing/Hygiene, Feeding, and Toileting
1. Assess the patient's ability to perform self-care on the basis of functional status (e.g., comatose state, hemi-plegia, sensory or motor deficit, alterations in vision).
   - Use assessment criteria for activity tolerance: If the patient experiences a decrease in BP of more than 20 mm Hg, an increase in HR of more than 20 bpm above resting HR, or a HR above 120 bpm in a patient receiving beta-adrenergic drugs, the patient is not fully tolerating the activity.
2. If the patient is comatose, meet all the patient's physical needs: bathing, oral hygiene, feeding, and elimination.
3. Explain all procedures to the patient and significant others before performing them.
   - Involve significant others in the plan of care.
   - Invite family and/or significant other in care as feasible.
   - Collaborate with the patient and/or significant other to develop the plan of care.
4. For the patient who is not comatose:
   - Promote as much self-care as the patient is capable of providing.
   - Schedule care activities around the periods of time the patient has the most energy.
   - Question the patient about activity intolerance when assessment findings reveal the activity may exceed the patient's tolerance.

5. If the patient is alert, keep toiletries and other necessary items within reach.
6. Do not rush the patient; allow adequate time for performance of self-care activities and try to schedule activities at a point in the work shift to allow the patient to have the time needed.
7. Encourage the patient; reinforce the value of progress that is made.
8. Provide assistive devices. Consult with the occupational therapy department regarding use of devices such as large handle utensils for eating.
9. If visual impairment exists, place all objects within the patient's field of vision. If diplopia is present, apply an eye patch and alternate it between the patient's eyes every 2 to 3 hours as prescribed.

NIC Energy Management; Self-Care Assistance: Dressing/Grooming.

Ineffective peripheral tissue perfusion *related to interrupted arterial and venous flow secondary to prolonged immobility.*

Goals/Outcomes: By discharge from ICU, the patient has adequate peripheral circulation, as evidenced by normal skin color and temperature, and adequate distal pulses (more than 21 on a 0 to 41 scale) in peripheral extremities. (Distal pulse scales may vary with facility.)
NOC Circulation Status.

Circulatory Care: Venous Insufficiency
1. Identify patients at highest risk for tissue impairment including those with altered LOC, extreme immobility/inability to assist with ADLs, hypothermia, hyperthermia, cachexia, hypoalbuminemia, and advanced age.
2. Identify patients at risk for DVT: chronic infection, malignancy, peripheral vascular disease, history of smoking, obesity, anemia, prolonged bed rest, and advanced age.
3. DVT/VTE prophylaxis should be initiated according to institutional guidelines (see Pulmonary Embolus, Chapter 4).

 Safety Alert *Note: All patients who are in bed greater than 50% of the time, including at night, should have deep vein thrombosis prophylaxis, either medical (heparin, enoxaparin) or mechanical.*

Embolus Precautions
The following measures are generally a part of a DVT prevention program.
1. Assess for a positive Homan sign. The Homan sign is not very sensitive or specific for DVT but can be elicited by flexing the knee 30 degrees and dorsiflexing the foot. Pain elicited with the dorsiflexion may indicate DVT and may warrant further evaluation by the physician.
2. Assess laboratory values and vital signs for risk of DVT.
   - Fever.
   - Tachycardia.
   - Elevated sedimentation rate.
   - CRP is a nonspecific marker of inflammation and may be elevated with DVT.
   - Patients who are "hypercoagulable" are at higher risk for DVT.
   - In patients prone to DVT:
     - Acquire bilateral baseline measurements of the midcalf, knee, and midthigh.
     - Record these measurements on the patient's initial assessment.
     - Monitor these measurements daily.
     - Compare measurements with the baseline measurements to rule out extremity enlargement that could be caused by DVT.
3. Teach the patient and family the signs of DVT.
   - Pain.
   - Swelling and warmth in the involved area.
   - Coolness, unnatural color or pallor in involved area.
   - Superficial venous dilation distal to the involved area.
   - Report signs to a staff member, physician, or midlevel practitioner promptly if they occur.
4. Advise the patient and family to perform only the exercises prescribed by the healthcare team. Discourage practices such as massaging the legs when swelling and discomfort are noted.

5. Exercises for DVT prevention.
   - Teach patient calf-pumping (ankle dorsiflexion-plantar flexion).
   - Teach patient ankle-circling exercises.
   - Unless symptomatic, instruct the patient to repeat each movement 10 times hourly during extended periods of immobility.
   - Help promote circulation by performing passive ROM or encouraging active ROM exercises.
   - Encourage deep breathing, which increases negative pressure in the lungs and thorax to promote emptying of large veins.
6. Provide mechanical venous compression for patients on bed rest.
   - When not contraindicated by peripheral vascular disease, ensure that the patient wears antiembolic hose or pneumatic sequential compression stockings.
   - Remove mechanical venous compression device for 10 to 20 minutes every 8 hours.
   - Inspect underlying skin for evidence of irritation or breakdown.
   - Reapply hose after elevating the patient's legs at least 10 degrees for 10 minutes.
7. Position for maximal venous circulation. Instruct the patient not to cross the feet at the ankles or knees while in bed because doing so may cause venous stasis. If the patient is at risk for DVT, elevate the foot of the bed 10 degrees to increase venous return.
8. Reduce the potential for thrombus formation and embolization.
   - Medications that inhibit blood clotting:
     - Heparin
     - Low-molecular-weight heparin
     - Aspirin
     - Platelet inhibitors
     - Sodium warfarin
9. Administer medication as prescribed, and monitor appropriate laboratory values:
   - Prothrombin time
   - International normalized ratio
   - Partial thromboplastin time
   - Heparin level
10. Educate patient to self-monitor for and report bleeding:
    - Epistaxis
    - Bleeding gums
    - Hematemesis
    - Hemoptysis
    - Melena
    - Hematuria
    - Ecchymoses

Safety Alert   *Note: High-risk patients may have an inferior vena cava filter placed to protect against pulmonary embolism.*

NIC Circulatory Precautions.

Altered cerebral tissue perfusion (orthostatic hypotension) *related to interrupted arterial flow to the brain secondary to prolonged bed rest.*

Goals/Outcomes: When getting out of bed, the patient has adequate cerebral perfusion, as evidenced by HR less than 120 bpm and BP $\geq$90/60 mm Hg immediately after position change (or within 20 mm Hg of the patient's normal range), nondiaphoretic skin, normal skin color, denial of vertigo, no syncope, and HR and BP to resting levels within 3 minutes of position change.
NOC Neurologic Status; Neurologic Status: Consciousness.

Cerebral Perfusion Promotion
1. Assess the patient for factors that increase the risk of orthostatic hypotension.
   - Fluid volume changes
     - Recent diuresis

- Diaphoresis
- Change in vasodilator therapy
- Altered autonomic control
  - Diabetic cardiac neuropathy
  - Denervation after heart transplant
  - Advanced age
  - Severe LV dysfunction

2. Educate the patient. Explain cause of orthostatic hypotension and measures for prevention.
3. Apply elastic stockings to help prevent orthostatic hypotension. For patients who continue to have difficulty with orthostatic hypotension, it may be necessary to supplement the hose with elastic wraps to the groin when the patient is out of bed. Ensure that these wraps encompass the entire surface of the legs.
4. Prepare the patient for getting out of bed. Encourage position changes within necessary confines. Consider using a tilt table to reacclimate the patient to upright positions.
5. Follow these guidelines for mobilization:
   - Closely monitor the BP of any high-risk patient for whom this will be the first time out of bed.
   - Dangle the patient's legs at the bedside. Be alert to indicators of orthostatic hypotension:
     - Diaphoresis
     - Pallor
     - Tachycardia
     - Hypotension
     - Syncope
     - Feeling of lightheadedness or dizziness
   - Check vital signs for indicators of orthostatic hypotension and return the patient to a supine position with:
     - Drop in systolic BP of 20 mm Hg
     - Increased pulse rate
     - Feeling of vertigo
     - Impending syncope
   - Stand at bedside if leg dangling is tolerated. Have at least two staff members assisting the patient. Progress to ambulation if no adverse signs or symptoms occur.

NIC Energy Management; Surveillance.

Constipation *related to less-than-adequate fluid or dietary intake and bulk; immobility; lack of privacy; positional restrictions; use of opioid analgesics.*

Goals/Outcomes: Within 24 hours of this diagnosis, the patient verbalizes knowledge of measures that promote bowel elimination. The patient relates the return of his or her normal pattern and character of bowel elimination within 3 to 5 days of this diagnosis. Older adults often experience constipation.
NOC Bowel Elimination.

Bowel Management
1. Assess the patient's bowel history. Determine normal bowel habits and interventions that are used successfully at home.
2. Monitor and document the patient's bowel movements, diet, and I&O. Be alert to the following indications of constipation:
   - Fewer than patient's usual number of bowel movements.
   - Abdominal discomfort or distention.
   - Straining at stool.
   - Patient complaints of rectal pressure or fullness.
   - Fecal impaction, which may be manifested by oozing of liquid stool and confirmed via digital examination.
3. Auscultate each abdominal quadrant for at least 1 minute to determine the presence of bowel sounds. Normal sounds are clicks or gurgles occurring at a rate of 5 to 34 per minute.

Safety Alert *Bowel sounds are decreased or absent with paralytic ileus. High-pitched rushing sounds may be heard during abdominal cramping, indicating an intestinal obstruction.*

4. Remove rectal fecal impaction. Use a gloved, lubricated finger to remove stool from the rectum. Digital stimulation alone may prompt a bowel movement. Oil-retention enemas may soften impacted stool.
5. Encourage a high-fiber/high-fluid diet. Unless contraindicated, a high-roughage diet and a fluid intake of at least 2 to 3 L/day help to promote regular bowel movements. Individualize fluid intake according to physiologic state for patients with renal, hepatic, or cardiac disorders.
6. Promote bowel regularity.
   - Offer the bedpan at intervals and allow for use of bedside commode when safe.
   - Ensure privacy.
   - Time laxatives, enemas, or suppositories to take effect at the time of day the patient normally has a bowel movement.
   - Provide warm fluids before breakfast.
   - Encourage toileting to gain advantage of gastrocolic or duodenocolic reflexes.
7. Promote peristalsis. Encourage as much activity as tolerated.
8. Consult the physician for pharmacologic interventions as necessary. To help prevent rebound constipation, make a priority list of interventions to ensure minimal disruption of the patient's normal bowel habits. The following is a suggested hierarchy of interventions:
   - Bulk-building additives (e.g., psyllium)
   - Mild laxatives (e.g., apple or prune juice, Milk of Magnesia)
   - Stool softeners (e.g., docusate sodium or docusate calcium)
   - Potent laxatives and cathartics (e.g., bisacodyl, cascara sagrada)
   - Medicated suppositories
   - Enemas
9. Discuss, with the patient, the role narcotics and other medications have in constipation. Consider alternative methods of pain control (see Box 1-15) in an attempt to reduce narcotic dosage.

NIC Constipation/Impaction Management.

Deficient diversional activity *related to prolonged illness and hospitalization*

Goals/Outcomes: Within 24 hours of intervention, the patient engages in diversional activities and relates the absence of boredom.
NOC Motivation.

Self-Responsibility Facilitation
1. Prevent boredom. Provide the patient with something to read or do. Explore activities the patient enjoys. Assess the patient's activity tolerance using the criteria listed in the Activity Intolerance nursing diagnosis on the first care plan in this section.
2. Personalize the patient's environment with favorite objects and photographs. Suggest that significant others bring in a radio or a television, if not part of the standard room furnishings.
3. Tailor activities to attention span. Initiate activities that require little concentration, and proceed to more complicated tasks as the patient's condition allows. For example, if reading requires more energy or concentration than the patient is capable of, suggest that significant others read to the patient or bring in audiotapes of books, such as those marketed for the visually impaired.
4. Remember the pleasant past. Encourage discussion of past activities or reminiscence as a substitute for performing favorite activities during convalescence.
5. Progress activities as the patient's endurance improves. Move from reading to other diversions, such as puzzles, model kits, handicrafts, and computerized games and activities.
6. Encourage visitation by significant others within limits of the patient's endurance. Involve significant others in patient activities, such as playing cards or backgammon. Encourage significant others to stagger their visits throughout the day.
7. Provide social interaction time. Spend time talking with the patient. Arrange for hospital volunteers to visit, play cards, read books, or play board games as appropriate. Consider relocation to a room in an area of high traffic if the patient desires more social interaction.
8. Remember the outdoors to promote normalcy. As the patient's condition improves, assist him or her with sitting in a chair near a window. When able, provide opportunities to sit in a solarium so that patients can interact together. If physical condition and weather permit, take the patient outside for brief periods. Natural sunlight helps to promote a more normal sleep-wake cycle.

9. Support spiritual, mental, and emotional health. Request consultation for interventions as appropriate from social services, occupational therapy, pastoral services, and psychiatric nursing.

NIC Energy Management; Activity Therapy; Art Therapy; Recreation Therapy; Spiritual Support; Family Support; Emotional Support.

Risk of injury *related to falls*

Goals/Outcomes: The patient will remain free from falls throughout stay in ICU.
NOC Cognitive Orientation, Distorted Thought Self-Control, Information Processing.

NIC: Self Responsibility Facilitation
1. Identify those patients at moderate or high risk for falls:
   - History of falls.
   - Needs assistance with ambulation.
   - Sensory impairment.
   - Confused or disoriented.
   - Needs assistance with elimination (bowel or bladder).
   - Vital signs are unstable (bradycardia, tachycardia, hypotension, fever, etc.).
   - Receiving cardiovascular or neurologic medications.
2. Use any or all of the following to notify those coming in contact with the patient that this patient is at risk for falls:
   - Place an armband on the patient's wrist.
   - Place hospital identification on door.
   - Place hospital identification on chart.
   - Share with the patient's family or significant others education related to the hospital's fall prevention program.
3. Universal fall prevention:
   - Instruct the patient to call for help before getting out of bed.
   - Provide the patient with non-skid footwear.
   - Familiarize the patient and family with the environment.
   - Keep the call light within the patient's reach.
   - Have the patient demonstrate use of the call light.
   - Have the patient's personal belongings within reach.
   - Maintain bed in the low position and wheels locked and turn on the bed alarm if needed.
   - Keep side rails up.
   - Use subdued lighting at night.
   - Maintain uncluttered environment at bedside.
   - Keep the floor clean and dry.
   - Have handrails in the patient's room, bathroom, and halls.
   - Consult pharmacy for medication review.
4. Hourly rounds by nursing staff (registered nurses, nurse assistants, nurse technicians [using the 5 Ps]): Hourly rounds proactively address the patient's needs and potentially prevent falls. Before leaving the room ask, "Is there anything I can help you with before I leave the room?" Remind the patient that a member of the nursing staff will return in 1 hour.
   - Pain: Assess the patient's pain level and offer pain medication.
   - Position: Assess the patient comfort and assist the patient to a more comfortable position as requested. For patients who are immobile, turn patients every 2 hours.
   - Personal needs: Assess and assist the patient to the toilet, offer snack or fluids.
   - Placement: Place the call light or button, phone, magazines or books, TV control, etc. within easy reach of the patient.

NIC Footwear.

ADDITIONAL NURSING DIAGNOSES

Also see nursing diagnoses and interventions under Nutritional Support, Sedation and Neuromuscular Blockade, and Risk for Disuse Syndrome, in Traumatic Brain Injury (Ch 3).

SEDATION AND NEUROMUSCULAR BLOCKADE

With the 2013 update of the SCCM guidelines for pain, agitation, and delirium, practice changes evolved. The term *analgosedation* refers to the use of analgesic medications, most commonly opiates, as first-line therapy for agitation, when another definitive treatable source of the agitation is not apparent (Box 1-17). Agitation is defined as nonpurposeful movement or motor restlessness. Inadequate pain control may manifest as agitation, and can result in decreased participation in ICU care (slower vent weaning and mobilization), chronic pain, and posttraumatic stress disorder. Clinically, undertreated or untreated pain can lead to serious consequences including hyperglycemia, embolic events, hemodynamic abnormalities, muscle breakdown, persistent catabolism, and impaired wound healing.

Many patients who are critically ill also experience anxiety, restlessness, and/or agitation, which may require the use of sedation. Unrelieved stress, manifested in the form of anxiety or agitation, retards healing and can increase mortality. Optimally, causes of agitation are identified and managed using nonpharmacologic methods (see Emotional and Spiritual Support of the Patient and Significant Others, Chapter 2). When nonpharmacologic methods fail, analgosedation is the recommended first-line drug therapy. Pain control is discussed in this chapter.

Following optimizing the analgesic agents, sedating or anxiolytic agents can be added to promote comfort and decrease anxiety. Anxiety and agitation in patients who are severely ill may be prompted by emotional factors, including fear, loss of physical control, life-threatening illness, inability to communicate (e.g., mechanical ventilation), and feelings of helplessness. Environmental factors such as noise, temperature extremes, and sleep deprivation add to anxiety and agitation. The influence of environmental factors is sometimes more pronounced in those with altered LOC (see Alterations in Consciousness). Common pathophysiologic factors that contribute to agitation include hypoxemia, impaired cerebral perfusion, infection, alcohol withdrawal, and encephalopathy (Box 1-17). These causes must be ruled out before initiating sedation because the use of sedative medications may mask a treatable problem. Litigation resulting from patient harm induced by use of sedation to manage hypoxia-induced agitation is not rare in the United States.

Box 1-17   PATHOLOGIC CONDITIONS CONTRIBUTING TO AGITATION

Addisonian crisis	Hyponatremia
Alzheimer disease	Hypophosphatemia
Anxiety disorder	Hypoxemia
Delirium	Impaired cerebral perfusion
Delirium tremens	Cerebral thrombosis
Developmental disability	Subarachnoid hemorrhage
Diabetes	Intracranial bleeding
Drugs	Cerebral vasospasm
Subtherapeutic	Cerebral edema
Supratherapeutic (toxic)	Increased intracranial pressure
Withdrawal syndromes	Tumor
Idiosyncratic reactions	Cerebrovascular accident
Drug interactions	Hydrocephalus
Steroids	Infection
Encephalopathy	Meningitis
Hepatic	Encephalitis
Metabolic	Brain abscess
Uremic	Sepsis syndrome
Fear	Pain, inadequately controlled
Fluid/electrolyte abnormalities	Sleep deprivation
Hypercarbia	Stress
Hyperthyroidism	Tachyphylaxis to drugs (drug resistance)
Hypoglycemia	Thyroid disease

DELIRIUM

Consideration of the possibility of delirium is imperative when beginning the management of agitation. Many of the clinical factors associated with agitation (see Box 1-17) are also causative for delirium, occurring in up to 50% of patients in ICU and up to 80% of patients who are mechanically ventilated. Causes are multifactorial and include the presence of invasive devices, use of benzodiazepines, sleep deprivation, and prolonged immobility. Following ruling out of other causes for agitation, the recommendation of the SCCM is to deliver light sedation to the patient using a validated agitation assessment scale, either the RASS or the Sedation-Agitation Scale (SAS) (see Appendices 1 and 2). A fluctuation in the patient's RASS or SAS score can be the first indication that delirium may be present. It is recommended that assessments be done on all patients in ICU every 12 hours, given that fluctuation in mental status is common. The diagnosis is made using one of two validated scales: the Confusion Assessment Method for the ICU (CAM-ICU) or the Intensive Care Delirium Screening Checklist (ICDSC). Delirium can be hyperactive (previously known as ICU-psychosis), but is much more commonly hypoactive or a mixture between the two. Hypoactive delirium may be manifested as a flat affect, withdrawal, lethargy, apathy, or an otherwise relatively unremarkable change in mental status. The unfortunate term "pleasantly confused" is sometimes used for these patients, but the outcome is often worse than for the hyperactive patient because it is so easy to ignore or undertreat. Delirium is associated with increased ICU and hospital length of stay, increased ventilator time, increased mortality, and some degree of permanent cognitive impairment in up to one third of patients. Studies have calculated that delirium may increase hospital costs by an average of almost $15,000. Treatment involves discontinuing medications that can be deliriogenic, identifying and modifying preexisting or precipitating risk factors if possible, nondrug treatment strategies (Box 1-18), and finally haloperidol or atypical antipsychotic medications. There is insufficient evidence to support the use of antipsychotics for prophylaxis in patients who are at high risk for delirium.

ADMINISTERING SEDATION

Assuming that pain and delirium are addressed, the goal of further pharmacologic sedation is to reduce anxiety and produce a calm but communicative state, if possible. This is best accomplished by administering frequent, incremental doses of sedatives only until the desired effects are achieved. For a majority of patients, the goal of therapy is light sedation, or 0 to −1 on the RASS, 3 to 4 on the SAS. Light sedation, as opposed to deeper levels, has been associated with decreased time on the ventilator, decreased hospital and ICU length of stay, and decreased incidence of delirium. Deeper levels of sedation may be appropriate for certain clinical conditions including elevated intracranial pressures, alcohol or other drug withdrawal, seizures, ARDS, hemodynamic instability, ventilator dyssynchrony, concomitant therapy with neuromuscular blocking agents (NMBAs), or comfort care.

If intermittent boluses of sedatives fail, it may be necessary to use a continuous infusion. SCCM guidelines recommend fentanyl as the initial infusion, followed by propofol or dexmedetomidine. If large amounts of medication are necessary, careful consideration should be

Box 1-18	NONDRUG TREATMENT STRATEGIES FOR DELIRIUM AND CONFUSION

Repeated reorientation of the patient
Repeated provision of cognitively stimulating activities
Nonpharmacologic sleep protocols; minimizing unnecessary noise and stimulation
Early mobilization/range-of-motion exercises
Timely removal of catheters and other invasive devices
Timely removal of physical restraints
Use of eyeglasses/magnifying lenses/hearing aids. Earwax disimpaction
Adequate hydration
Adequate pain control

given for consultation with a physician or midlevel practitioner who specializes in the management of patients who are critically ill using sedation, analgesia, and, if necessary, neuromuscular blockade. Major organ dysfunction, multiple medications, tissue catabolism, and other factors render patients who are critically ill especially vulnerable to the toxic effects of many sedatives.

Oversedation and toxicity should be carefully avoided through close monitoring, individualized dosing, and titration to desired effect. Excessive sedation has been associated with delayed recognition of neurologic events, muscle wasting, and nosocomial complications such as DVT, compression injury, and pneumonia. The literature supports performing daily wake up assessments on patients with continuous drips to assure that there has been no underlying neurologic changes and that the drips are at the lowest effective dose, if indeed they are still required at all.

When providing sedation, if anxiolytic or other adjunctive agents fail to help stabilize ventilation and perfusion in patients who are mechanically ventilated, NMBAs may need to be added. Neuromuscular blockade results in total paralysis of the striated muscle at the neuromuscular junction. Neither the nondepolarizing paralytic agents (see Table 1-36) nor succinylcholine possess anxiolytic nor analgesic properties. The patient may be terrified, given that they are fully aware that they have no ability to move, communicate, or breathe. Paralysis is always done in conjunction with sedation and analgesia to ensure that the patient is not overwhelmed with fear. If not done, the patient undergoes extreme stress, which can be further exacerbated if they also have unrelieved pain. The pain should be addressed with either scheduled (not PRN) opiates or a continuous opiate drip, usually fentanyl, and potential anxiety with a sedative drip such as propofol.

Patients may not tolerate or may inadvertently "fight" necessary treatments. Those with severe respiratory dysfunction may require use of specialized ventilator settings (ventilator dyssynchrony) such as reversing the inspiration to expiration time (reverse I:E ratios), or the use of oscillatory ventilation. Successful ventilation may not be possible without use of NMBAs to stop the patient from tensing in response to the treatment. Tensing reduces tidal volume and requires increased energy expenditure. Care providers must create an anticipatory plan for pain management and anxiolysis when the patient is no longer able to voice his or her needs.

RESEARCH BRIEF BOX 1-5

Delirium evaluation in patients in the intensive care unit (ICU) requires the use of an arousal/sedation assessment tool before assessing consciousness. The Richmond Agitation-Sedation Scale (RASS) and the Riker Sedation-Agitation Scale (SAS) are well-validated arousal/sedation tools. The concordance of RASS and SAS assessments in determining eligibility of patients in ICU for delirium screening using the confusion assessment method for ICU (CAM-ICU) was assessed. A prospective cohort study was performed in the adult medical, surgical, and progressive (step-down) ICUs of a tertiary care, university-affiliated, urban hospital in Indianapolis, Indiana. The cohort included 975 admissions to ICU between January and October 2009. In total, 2469 RASS and SAS paired screens were performed and the conclusion was that both SAS and RASS led to similar rates of delirium assessment using CAM-ICU.

From Khan BA: Comparison and agreement between the Richmond Agitation-Sedation Scale and the Riker Sedation-Agitation Scale in evaluating patients' eligibility for delirium assessment in the ICU. *Chest* 142(1):48-54, 2012.

NEUROMUSCULAR BLOCKADE

Monitoring paralytic agents: When a patient is paralyzed using NMBA therapy, it is of paramount importance to be able to evaluate whether the levels of sedation, analgesia, and paralysis are appropriate. The previously mentioned means of monitoring pain and agitation do not apply in the patient who is paralyzed, hence the need for continuous infusions or

Table 1-34	NERVE STIMULATION IN RELATIONSHIP TO PERCENT BLOCKAGE
Number of Twitches	**Percent Blockage**
4	0-50
3	60-70
2	70-80
1	80-90
None	>90

around-the-clock boluses of each for the duration of paralysis, without decreasing the doses. The "gold standard" for monitoring paralytics is the use of a peripheral nerve stimulator to deliver four (train of four or TO4) tiny, sequential stimulating shocks to nerves on the wrist, foot, or face. The muscle response is measured to evaluate how many of the four signals are blocked by the NMBA compared with the number perceived. In the absence of neuromuscular blockade, the muscle should move four times equally in response to four signals. As receptors are saturated with NMBAs, fewer muscle contractions are seen (Table 1-34). Nerve stimulators are the best monitoring option, with bispectral index (BIS) monitoring and drug holidays largely falling from favor, but can be uncomfortable for the patient being evaluated on an hourly basis. To avoid this, a baseline setting should be established before the paralytic is started. Termed the "supramaximal stimulation point," it is the electrical setting on the nerve stimulator after which no increased muscle movement is noted. Once the drip is started, under no circumstances should this electrical setting be increased. Also, it is very important to recognize that the purpose of the nerve stimulator is to avoid overexposure to these exceptionally dangerous drugs, in other words the nurse should attempt to decrease the drip rate if one or fewer twitches are present. Increasing the drip should only be done based on clinical necessity, never TO4 results, even if all four twitches are present.

COLLABORATIVE MANAGEMENT
CARE PRIORITIES
1. Ensure agitation is not caused by pathophysiology
All agitated patients should be evaluated for the presence of hypoxia, impending shock, hypoglycemia, sepsis, electrolyte imbalance, acid-base imbalance, drug reactions, and other common causes of abnormal behavior. History of mental illness and substance abuse should be evaluated, as psychiatric disorders and substance withdrawal often manifest with agitation. Ensure those with psychopathology are receiving appropriate prehospitalization medications, and those withdrawing from substances are placed on the appropriate management plan.

2. Attempt to manage pain and anxiety simultaneously, using an opiate analgesic with sedative effects
Opiates reliably relieve pain, are easily titrated, and have significant sedative effects. *Morphine* is widely administered using intermittent bolus dosing and as a continuous infusion. Morphine may be helpful in relieving hypoxia as it acts as a venodilator to reduce preload to help promote better circulation in patients with heart failure, as well as dilating the pulmonary vasculature to assist with gas exchange. In renal failure, dosing should be reduced by 50% as a result of the accumulation of an active metabolite of morphine. Other opiates commonly used include hydromorphone (Dilaudid) and fentanyl citrate (Sublimaze). Fentanyl and hydromorphone are rapidly absorbed by the CNS and therefore are more potent than morphine. Fentanyl is the shortest acting opiate and is best used as a continuous infusion. The SCCM recommends that fentanyl be used for rapid onset of analgesia and in patients who are hemodynamically unstable. Meperidine (Demerol) is not recommended as a primary analgesic, particularly in older adults and those with renal failure. Patients often report inadequate pain control, while experiencing euphoria. Meperidine accumulates with repeated doses and causes an increased risk of neurotoxicity (see Table 1-32).

3. Sedatives and antipsychotics options

After analgosedation is maximized, generally propofol or dexmedetomidine can be added for further sedation of ongoing agitation, followed by a benzodiazepine. Antipsychotics can be used if delirium is present. Patients who experience adverse reactions are sometimes given larger doses to correct the agitation associated with what is actually drug intolerance. Constant assessment of the patient's response to sedation is needed so that appropriate revisions can be made to drug dosage and selection. When patients are placed on sedation, the care team must keep in mind that the goal is not solely effective sedation but rather to manage the problem causing the agitation so that the patient can be weaned off the sedation.

Propofol (Diprivan): A lipid-based emulsion administered as a titratable, continuous infusion for short-term (several hours to 5 days) sedation for patients who are mechanically ventilated. Propofol contains significant fat calories, 1.1 kcal/mL, and this should be taken into account when patients are receiving TPN in addition to propofol. When discontinued, patients usually awaken readily with prompt return to baseline mental function. Downward titration by 5 μg/kg/min increments every 10 minutes is preferable to abrupt discontinuation, in that rebound agitation may occur. Hemodynamic changes (e.g., vasodilation, decreased MAP) can be minimized by adequate hydration and similarly slow increases in the infusion rate. Propofol is particularly useful for patients with neurologic impairment, because the short action facilitates daily awakening during the sedation vacation to evaluate underlying mental status. The drug is not an analgesic, thus pain medication should be prescribed. Effectiveness of pain management should be assessed during daily awakening. Scheduled doses or a continuous infusion of opiate analgesics provide effective pain control when used in combination with propofol. Doses in ventilated ICU patients should rarely exceed 50 μg/kg/min (or 3 mg/kg/h) because the agent is considered an anesthetic at higher doses. It is metabolized and eliminated largely independent of renal and hepatic function. The lipophilic drug accumulates more readily in patients who are obese, and dosing should be based on either IBW or adjusted body weight (ABW), (ABW $-$ IBW) $\times$ 0.4 $+$ IBW, in patients who are obese. These patients may also be at increased risk for a more prolonged recovery time after the infusion is discontinued. Prolonged recovery time may occur with any patient when the infusion is continued for more than 3 days at high doses.

- Propofol-related infusion syndrome: Propofol-related infusion syndrome (PRIS) is a rare, often fatal syndrome observed in patients who are critically ill receiving propofol for sedation. PRIS is characterized by acute bradycardia that progresses to asystole, associated with severe unexplained metabolic acidosis, acute renal failure, rhabdomyolysis, hyperkalemia, and cardiovascular collapse. The exact pathophysiology of PRIS has not been determined. Impaired tissue metabolism caused by propofol infusion has emerged as an important mechanism leading to complete cardiovascular collapse. Known risk factors include sepsis, severe cerebral injury, and high propofol doses. Early recognition is the key to successful management. If symptoms of PRIS are noted, propofol should be discontinued and an alternative sedative agent initiated. Measures to support cardiac and renal function should be promptly initiated.

Dexmedetomidine (Precedex): A novel agent with a mechanism of action similar to clonidine. The drug blocks sympathetic outflow through a central alpha stimulation to produce sedation when used as a continuous infusion. Although not an analgesic, dexmedetomidine has been shown to have opiate-sparing properties. Level of awareness may be assessed without downward titration of the drip. The drug is effective in managing alcohol withdrawal syndrome, delirium, and failed extubation. Dexmedetomidine is not associated with respiratory depression but can cause hypotension and bradycardia. The drug should be initiated in well-hydrated patients to avoid hypotension. The recommended initial bolus dose may be omitted in borderline hypovolemic patients. The SCCM has positioned the drug, as well as propofol, ahead of benzodiazepines in the treatment of agitation after analgosedation has been adequately attempted. Although the labeling gives a maximum duration of 24 hours, there are sufficient data that support extended use of the drug, up to 72 hours or more. The maximum dose is 1 μg/kg/h, although safety has been established at up to 1.5 μg/kg/h. It can also be used in nonintubated patients, unlike propofol.

Benzodiazepines: Benzodiazepines may be used to relieve anxiety, promote sleep, and produce sedation via nonspecific CNS depression or via a specific depressant effect on gamma-aminobutyric acid (GABA). Benzodiazepines produce muscle relaxation, which facilitates using a lesser dose of NMBAs if the patient requires paralysis. Dose-related effects on mental status range from relief of anxiety to sedation and coma. All benzodiazepines promote amnesia, an effect that is particularly useful in patients undergoing unpleasant procedures. Midazolam (Versed) is considered superior to other benzodiazepines in preventing recall. Ease of use, a general lack of paradoxic agitation, and lack of recall are advantages of benzodiazepines, but these are offset by a higher incidence of delirium and some pharmacokinetic disadvantages (see later). They are the primary drugs used to alleviate symptoms of acute alcohol withdrawal, which commonly contribute to agitation in the critically ill. However, benzodiazepines do not have analgesic properties present in opiates, thus pain should always be ruled out as a cause of agitation before using benzodiazepines solely. If present, pain should be treated with analgesics before these drugs are initiated. Table 1-35 describes specific characteristics of the widely used benzodiazepines.

- Lorazepam (Ativan): Commonly given as an intermittent IV or IM bolus and is sometimes used as a continuous infusion, particularly with alcohol withdrawal syndrome. Lorazepam has the slowest onset and the longest duration of action of all benzodiazepines. An advantage of lorazepam is that it is metabolized by glucuronidation, as opposed to oxidation as with the other benzodiazepines, thus liver impairment does not significantly affect drug metabolism. Lorazepam has no active metabolites, thus it is safer for use in patients who are renally impaired. However, at high doses for prolonged periods of time, hyperosmolality, acidosis, and ATN can occur resulting from the propylene glycol diluent in which the drug is delivered. Caution should be used when administering lorazepam to older adults, those who are severely ill, and those with limited pulmonary reserve. Despite possible complications, it is the benzodiazepine of choice for prolonged sedation. Patients who are lightly sedated should awaken within 30 minutes during the daily wake up assessment (sedation vacation). When patients have difficulty awakening during these assessments, the dosage should be decreased.
- Diazepam (Valium): An older benzodiazepine with a long half-life, which may result in prolonged sedation attributable to an active metabolite (up to 200 hours after a given dose). Diazepam should be avoided in patients with liver dysfunction or severe heart failure because of reduced hepatic clearance. Limited solubility in water restricts use of standard formulation to intermittent IV bolus injections.
- Midazolam (Versed): Short-acting and rapidly metabolized, the drug is particularly useful for short invasive procedures (e.g., bronchoscopy or endoscopy). Because of its short half-life, continuous infusions are required to maintain sedation for longer periods. Delayed drug metabolism in some patients who are critically ill may lead to extended sedation, particularly with sepsis or hepatic impairment. Midazolam is used with caution in patients with renal failure, because some of the active metabolites are renally secreted.

Table 1-35	BENZODIAZEPINE CHARACTERISTICS		
Benzodiazepines	**Lorazepam (Ativan)**	**Diazepam (Valium)**	**Midazolam (Versed)**
Intermittent	0.5 to 1 mg every 1 to 2 hours	2.5 to 5 mg every 3 to 4 hours	0.01 to 0.05 mg/kg every 15 minutes to 1 hour
Continuous	0.25 to 6 mg/h	Not applicable	0.02 to 0.2 mg/kg/h 0.5 to 4 µg/kg/min
Metabolism	Hepatic (glucuronidation)	Hepatic (oxidation)	Hepatic (oxidation)
Active metabolites	No	Yes	Yes
Excretion	Renal	Renal	Renal

Antipsychotics: These agents can be used to reduce agitation in disoriented and delirious or CAM-ICU positive patients. A component of delirium or psychosis should be identified before use of these agents is initiated. Patients should be well hydrated to avoid hypotension if given parenterally. Antipsychotics may be used as part of management of alcohol withdrawal syndrome.

- Haloperidol lactate (Haldol): A butyrophenone antipsychotic that is especially helpful in managing psychosis and during withdrawal of sedatives. Incremental IV or IM bolus doses are used, although the IV route is unlabeled on the package insert. The IV route has been widely used in patients who are critically ill because onset of action is rapid and extrapyramidal side effects occur less frequently than with the IM route. Haldol should be given cautiously to patients with severe cardiovascular disorders because of the possibility of transient hypotension and QT prolongation. There is a general lack of evidence proving the drug is useful in the treatment of delirium, although the benefit probably outweighs the risk of low-dose (less than 8 mg/day) PRN therapy.

Atypical Antipsychotics: The newer generation of antipsychotics used to reduce agitation when delirium has been established. These medications are associated with fewer extrapyramidal side effects than haloperidol.

- Aripiprazole (Abilify): Provides sedation via partial agonist activity at dopamine and serotonin ($5\text{-}HT_{1A}$) receptors and antagonist activity at serotonin ($5\text{-}HT_{1B}$) receptors. Also used to manage patients with schizophrenia and bipolar disorders. It is given in a dose of 9.75 mg IM at most every 2 hours to a maximum of 30 mg/day. Although it has the cleanest side effect profile of the injectable atypical antipsychotics, it is also less sedating, which can be a disadvantage.

- Ziprasidone (Geodon): A piperazine derivative that antagonizes alpha-adrenergic, dopamine, histamine, and serotonin receptors and inhibits reuptake of serotonin and norepinephrine. It is given as 10 mg IM every 2 hours or 20 mg every 4 hours to a maximum of 40 mg/day to diminish delirium, mania associated with bipolar disorders, and the symptoms associated with schizophrenia. It can have significant QT interval prolongation and should be monitored for this.

- Olanzapine (Zyprexa): A thienobenzodiazepine derivative that antagonizes $alpha_1$-adrenergic, dopamine, histamine, muscarinic, and serotonin receptors. It is given as 10 mg IM every 2 to 4 hours to a maximum of 30 mg/day to prompt CNS sedation and to decrease symptoms associated with delirium, schizophrenia, and bipolar mania. It generally has more anticholinergic side effects than the previously mentioned agents.

- Quetiapine (Seroquel): Although not available as a parenteral dosage form, this is a good option for PO or NG administration when that route is available. It has a mechanism of action similar to previous agents, with a fairly predictable sedative effect when used in patients who are delirious. It can be started at 25 mg every 8 to 12 hours and increased to 300 mg or more daily if needed. QT prolongation and orthostatic hypotension can occur with quetiapine.

- Risperidone (Risperdal): Another option for PO or NG administration, given as 1 to 2 mg every 12 to 24 hours for agitation associated with delirium, up to 6 mg/day. Its side effect profile is similar to quetiapine, with possibly more extrapyramidal side effects.

Neuromuscular Blocking Agents: NMBAs are used when longer periods of complete paralysis are necessary in patients who are mechanically ventilated. All possible causes of agitation (e.g., pain, fear, suctioning, hypoxemia) must be investigated thoroughly before neuromuscular blockade is initiated. Outside the operating room and other invasive procedural areas, paralysis should be used as "a last resort" to control energy expenditure in patients who are unstable, only when all methods of sedation have failed. NMBAs generally are used in the following situations: (1) to decrease O_2 consumption in patients who otherwise cannot obtain satisfactory O_2 saturation; (2) to alleviate specific medical conditions (e.g., status asthmaticus, tetanus, malignant hyperthermia, status epilepticus, ARDS); (3) to immobilize patients for surgical and invasive procedures; and (4) to manage increased ICP. NMBA therapy also provides effective management of shivering when deleterious effects occur during therapeutic hypothermia, a therapy used to facilitate neurologic recovery in patients postcardiac arrest.

- Depolarizing NMBAs: Succinylcholine (Anectine) is the only depolarizing NMBA with widespread clinical use. It is used to produce rapid, brief paralysis, most often during emergent intubation. Long-term blockade is not practical because of rapid tachyphylaxis and desensitization of receptors to blocking effects.

- Nondepolarizing NMBAs: The class of NMBAs most commonly used for paralysis in patients who are critically ill. The most common agents used are pancuronium (Pavulon), vecuronium (Norcuron), rocuronium (Zemuron), and cisatracurium (Nimbex). Pharmacokinetic and pharmacodynamic properties of the three agents are listed in Table 1-36. Cisatracurium is the most expensive of the three agents, but its cost is justified by decreased incidence of prolonged paralysis and weakness in patients with severe hepatic and/or renal impairment. The drug is beneficial in patients who require steroids, because it lacks the steroidal structure of other nondepolarizing agents. Steroid-induced myopathy associated with concomitant use of NMBAs and steroids is considered less likely with cisatracurium and will be less severe if it occurs. Numerous medications and several disease states augment or antagonize neuromuscular blockade (Box 1-19). The patient should be monitored throughout therapy for conditions affecting neuromuscular blockade.

Clinicians should determine a therapeutic end point or goal for paralysis and titrate neuromuscular blockade to achieve that goal. Examples of therapeutic end points are decreases in PIP or decreases in O_2 consumption. Negative end points include development of extreme weakness or inability to move. Monitoring the degree of neuromuscular blockade is essential. It cannot be overemphasized that NMBAs provide no analgesia or anxiolysis. All patients receiving NMBAs must also have therapy with continuously dosed opiates and anxiolytics.

Table 1-36	NEUROMUSCULAR BLOCKING AGENT CHARACTERISTICS				
	Neuromuscular Blocking Agents	Pancuronium (Pavulon)	Vecuronium (Norcuron)	Cisatracurium (Nimbex)	Rocuronium (Zemuron)
Dosage	Intermittent	0.04 to 0.1 mg/kg every 1 hour PRN	0.01 to 0.015 mg/kg every 15 minutes	0.03 mg/kg every 15 minutes	0.45 to 1.2 mg/kg, then 0.1 to 0.2 mg/kg every 15 to 30 minutes
	Continuous	1 to 1.6 μg/kg/min	0.8 to 1.2 μg/kg/min	0.5 to 10 μg/kg/min	6 to 12 μg/kg/min
Pharmacokinetics	Metabolism Excretion	Renal > hepatic renal	Hepatic > renal Renal (15%) Biliary (30% to 50%)	Hoffman (organ-independent) Elimination	Minimal hepatic metabolism; drug elimination primarily via bile; up to 30% renally eliminated
	Metabolites (active or toxic)	Yes	Yes	No	No
	Half-life (elimination)	132 to 257 minutes (2 to 4 hours)	80 to 97 minutes	22 to 29 minutes	84 to 131 minutes
Cardiovascular effects		Moderate ↑HR, ↑BP, CO	Minimal <1% ↑HR, ↑BP	None on HR and MAP	Minimal (2%)

BP, Blood pressure; CO, cardiac output; HR, heart rate; MAP, mean airway pressure; PRN, pro re nata (when necessary).

| Box 1-19 | DRUGS AND PHYSIOLOGIC CONDITIONS THAT AFFECT NEUROMUSCULAR BLOCKADE |

Drugs that augment neuromuscular blockade
Aminoglycoside antibiotics
Bacitracin
Calcium channel blockers
Clindamycin
Colistimethate
Cyclosporine
Inhaled anesthetics
Lidocaine
Piperacillin
Procainamide
Propranolol
Quinidine
Vancomycin

Drugs that antagonize neuromuscular blockade
Anticholinesterase agents
Azathioprine
Carbamazepine
Corticosteroids

Phenytoin
Ranitidine
Theophylline

Physiologic conditions that increase neuromuscular blockade
Acidosis
Dehydration
Hypercalcemia
Hypermagnesemia
Hypocalcemia
Hypokalemia
Hyponatremia
Hypothermia
Myasthenia gravis

Physiologic conditions that decrease neuromuscular blockade
Alkalosis
Decreased peripheral perfusion
Hyperkalemia
Hypernatremia

CARE PLANS FOR SEDATION AND NEUROMUSCULAR BLOCKADE

Anxiety   *related to actual or perceived threat of death; change in health status; threat to self-concept or role; unfamiliar people or environment; the unknown.*

Goals/Outcomes: Within 4 to 6 hours of initiating therapy, the patient's anxiety is diminished, as evidenced by verbalization of same, HR less than 100 bpm, RR less than 20 breaths/min, and decrease in restlessness and extraneous motor movement.
NOC Anxiety Self-Control.

Anxiety Reduction
1. Carefully assess for and correct factors contributing to anxiety (see Box 1-17).
2. Ensure pathophysiology is not overlooked as the cause of anxiety or agitation.
3. Provide emotional and spiritual support for the patient and family, especially if the patient requires neuromuscular blockade (see Emotional and Spiritual Support of the Patient and Significant Others, Chapter 2).
4. Evaluate adequacy of pain control. Administer opiate or other analgesics in appropriate doses on a schedule or through a continuous infusion (see Pain).
5. Initiate nonpharmacologic measures to reduce anxiety (see Box 1-15).
6. Assess the patient using a recognized agitation assessment tool (see Alterations in Consciousness).
7. If administering a short-acting benzodiazepine in small doses at frequent intervals, monitor carefully for excessive sedation and respiratory depression. Have flumazenil (Romazicon) immediately available for reversal of drug effects.
8. If anxiety is profound and associated with sensory/perceptual alterations (e.g., hallucinations), consider use of an antipsychotic agent. Perform a valid delirium assessment before using antipsychotics. Ensure adequate hydration before use and monitor closely for hypotension.
9. For patients undergoing neuromuscular blockade, provide careful monitoring of level of blockade with a peripheral nerve stimulator on the train of four settings, coupled with fixed, effective dosing of sedatives and analgesics.

Table 1-37	ASSESSMENT OF HEALING OF WOUNDS CLOSED BY PRIMARY INTENTION	
Expected Findings	**Abnormal Findings**
Edges well approximated	Edges not well approximated
Inflammatory response (redness, warmth, induration, pain) lasting 3 to 5 days	Decreased inflammatory response or inflammatory response that lasts more than 5 days after injury
No drainage (without drain present) 2 days after closure	Drainage continues more than 2 days after injury
Healing ridge present by postsurgical days 5 to 9	Absence of healing ridge by day 9
	Hypertrophic scar or keloid present

Risk for injury *related to impaired gas exchange resulting from hypoventilation associated with sedative induced respiratory depression.*

Goals/Outcomes: Within 1 hour of intervention, the patient has adequate gas exchange, as evidenced by orientation to time, place, and person; PaO_2 greater than 80 mm Hg; $PacO_2$ 24 to 30 mm Hg; SpO_2 greater than 90; and RR 12 to 20 breaths/min with normal depth and pattern. Achieving the patient's "healthy" baseline is generally the goal for improvement. Decreased O_2 supply secondary to decreased ventilatory drive occurring with sedative use and CNS depression or secondary to decreased chest wall movement occurring with residual neuromuscular blockade are resolved.
NOC Respiratory Status: Gas Exchange.

Ventilation Assistance
1. Assess the patient's respiratory rate, depth, and rhythm at least hourly when heavily sedated. Patients who are fully sedated require continuous direct monitoring until vital signs are stable and protective reflexes (e.g., gag reflexes) are present.
2. Propofol should only be used as part of sedation on patients who are mechanically ventilated to avoid the risk of apnea.
3. Provide appropriate care related to mechanical ventilation (see Mechanical Ventilation).
4. If NMBAs are used, assess depth of paralysis using peripheral nerve stimulator. Titrate dose to maintain desired level of paralysis (see Table 1-34). Only increase paralytic drip for clinical reasons, not in response to train of four results.
5. Provide a daily sedation vacation and/or drug holiday to assess LOC, ability to initiate spontaneous breaths, and ability to remain stable off sedation and/or neuromuscular blockade.
6. Continuously monitor SpO_2 via pulse oximetry and end tidal CO_2.
7. Alternatively, monitor chest wall movement via apnea monitor.
8. Have appropriate antidote (e.g., naloxone for opiates, flumazenil for benzodiazepines) and airway management equipment immediately available.
9. Position the patient to promote full lung expansion, and turn the patient to mobilize sputum.

Deficient knowledge *related to lack of recall, related to interrupted memory consolidation secondary to benzodiazepine use.*

Goals/Outcomes: Within 12 hours of cessation of benzodiazepine therapy, the patient recalls information essential to self-protection and self-care.
NOC Knowledge: Treatment Procedures.

Teaching: Procedure/Treatment
1. Remind the patient and family that recall of unpleasant procedures (e.g., cardioversion, endoscopy) will be diminished and that this is a desired effect of the medication.
2. Reinforce necessary information (e.g., NPO instructions, need to call for assistance when changing positions, need for deep breathing) with the patient and family at frequent intervals until comprehension is demonstrated.
3. Review outcome or findings of procedure with the patient as necessary until the patient expresses satisfactory understanding.

ADDITIONAL NURSING DIAGNOSIS

Additional nursing care plans are available in sections on Alterations in Consciousness, Pain, and Emotional and Spiritual Support of the Patient and Significant Others, Chapter 2).

WOUND AND SKIN CARE

A wound is a disruption of tissue integrity caused by trauma, surgery, or an underlying medical disorder. Wound management is designed to promote healing, prevent infection, and/or reduce deterioration in wound status. Principles of wound management are used to move a wound toward healing and should be integrated into the plan of care for the patient with a wound.

Renewed emphasis on the role of nurses in the prevention of pressure ulcers is evident in the Centers for Medicare and Medicaid Services (CMS) standards of care.

Noting that hospital-acquired conditions could be reasonably prevented with evidence-based guidelines, CMS discontinued additional payment to hospitals for pressure ulcers that were not present on admission. CMS will no longer pay for the treatment of hospital-acquired stage 3 and stage 4 pressure ulcers. Pressure ulcers are considered by some to be "avoidable" problems within the healthcare system. If a pressure ulcer is "present on admission" documented by a clinician who diagnoses and treats, the hospital will be entitled to reimbursement of treatment for stage 3 and stage 4 pressure ulcers. Pressure ulcer prevention programs should be in every healthcare facility and address issues such as skin and risk assessment, the use of products to both reduce risk and treat wound and skin issues, as well as patient and family education.

There are reliable and valid risk assessment tools to be used to identify risk factors that contribute to the development of pressure ulcers. The Braden Scale and Norton Scale have been extensively studied and found to be valid for the prediction of pressure ulcer risk. As a result of the emphasis on prevention of avoidable pressure ulcers and the accompanying economic impact of fiscal restraints, more effort is being placed on prevention. Norton scores of 14 are indicative of mild risk; a score of 12 indicates "high risk." Braden scores of 18 to 15 indicate mild risk, and 12 is high risk. A risk assessment tool should be used in acute care on admission and reassessment should be done at least every 24 to 48 hours or when the patient's condition changes or deteriorates.

WOUNDS CLOSED BY PRIMARY INTENTION

Clean surgical or traumatic wounds with edges that are closed with sutures, staples, sterile tape strips, or wound glue are referred to as wounds closed by *primary intention*. Impairment of healing most frequently manifests as dehiscence, evisceration, infection, or delayed healing. Individuals at high risk for disruption of wound healing include those who are obese, diabetic, older, malnourished, receiving steroids, immunosuppressed, undergoing chemotherapy or radiation therapy, or receiving vasopressors. Coexistent infections at another body site and colonization with microorganisms such as methicillin-resistant *Staphylococcus aureus* (MRSA) are factors that may contribute to the development of infection. The continuum of contamination of wounds ranges from colonized to critically colonized to infection. Once microorganisms adhere to the surface of the wound, a biofilm develops. Biofilms on the base of the wound inhibit efficacy of antibiotics and are suspected to delay wound healing. Proper wound management will decrease the risk of biofilm development, wound infections, and facilitate wound healing.

ASSESSMENT

OPTIMAL WOUND HEALING

Immediately after a surgical injury, the incision is warm, red, indurated, and tender. Inflammation normally subsides in 3 to 5 days. A healing ridge can be palpated just under the intact suture line by days 5 to 9. It is produced by the newly formed connective tissue (see Table 1-37).

IMPAIRED HEALING

Impaired healing is recognized by the lack of an adequate inflammatory response surrounding a wound, continued drainage from an incision line 2 days after injury (when no drain is present), absence of a healing ridge by day 9 after injury, and/or presence of purulent drainage (see Table 1-37). A chronic wound is one that fails to proceed to healing within a reasonable time, to progress through a normal repair process, and is usually associated with pathology (i.e., diabetes or pressure damage). Wound assessment should be done on an ongoing basis to determine the progress or deterioration of the wound. Assessment includes anatomic location, dimensions (length, width depth), percent of tissue type (granulation, slough, necrotic), exudate (amount, color, odor), and condition of the periwound skin. The wound should be cleansed before assessment to allow for visualization of the wound base.

Diagnostic Tests During Wound Healing

Test	Rationale	Abnormal Findings
Complete blood count (CBC) with differential	Assess for discrepancies in red blood cells, white blood cells, and hemoglobin, platelet count	Low red blood cells and hemoglobin may impair oxygen delivery. Platelet count: High will increase risk of clot. Low platelets will add to the risk of abnormal bleeding. An increase in the white blood cell count can indicate infection. Low white blood cells will reduce the body's ability to fight microorganisms.
Plasma protein levels: transferrin, albumin, and prealbumin	Protein levels assist with the regulation of fluid in the body and are necessary to make collagen, which is essential for wound healing	Transferrin less than 100 mg/dL, albumin less than 3.5 g/dL, and/or prealbumin less than 19.5 mg/dL indicate malnutrition. Request a nutrition consultation.
Wound culture and sensitivity	Determine the presence of microbes and susceptibility infection	Culture will identify the specific aerobic and anaerobic organisms and their susceptibility to antibiotics. Preliminary culture results in 24 hours, final in 48 hours.

COLLABORATIVE MANAGEMENT

CARE PRIORITIES FOR SURGICAL WOUNDS HEALING BY PRIMARY INTENTION

1. Application of a sterile dressing in surgery or at the time of injury: Protects wound from external contamination, trauma, or pressure injury. Usually, the surgeon or advanced practice nurse changes the initial dressing.
2. Nutrition (oral diet, enteral nutrition, PN): Provides sufficient nutrients for wound healing. Wounds require specific nutrients and adequate nutrition is key to meet healing needs.
3. Multivitamins (all but especially vitamin C) and minerals (especially zinc and iron): Corrects any deficits and supports healing.
4. Pain control: Maximizes subcutaneous blood flow to the wound to support healing.
5. Insulin: Necessary to control glucose levels in individuals with diabetes mellitus or hyperglycemia from other causes (e.g., steroid therapy, TPN, enteral nutrition). Hyperglycemia is associated with abnormal and prolonged inflammation, reduced collagen synthesis, and impaired epithelial migration. Patients who are critically ill often develop insulin resistance, resulting in hyperglycemia. Evidence-based hyperglycemia management protocols are available from many sources, including the SCCM and the American Association of Critical-Care Nurses. Choice of protocol is based on the ability of each nurse to comply with the recommended insulin dosage regime and associated monitoring. Protocols vary with number of steps, frequency of monitoring blood glucose, and need for available technology, such as access to computers, the Internet, point-of-care blood glucose meters, and other variables. Control of blood glucose has been consistently associated with more timely and effective would healing. Glucose stabilization must be done with a protocol that given the available resources, nurses are able to appropriately monitor blood glucose and manage hypoglycemia to maintain patient safety.

6. Topical or systemic antibiotics: Given when infection is present and can be used prophy-lactically for a limited period of time. CMS recommend that prophylactic antibiotics are discontinued within 24 hours after surgery is complete to decrease the occurrence of re-sistant microbes. Specific orders must be written for continuation to comply with the recommendation.

7. Antiseptics: Dakin solution at 0.25% may be used for a limited time to clean slough from a wound bed. Dressings that provide an antimicrobial affect against bacteria may have an active ingredient, that is, silver or cadexomer iodine, and can be used in treating a wound infection.

8. Incision and drainage: Removes wound exudate when infection is present and localized. Healing occurs by secondary intention. The wound may be irrigated to flush out organisms.

CARE PLANS FOR WOUND HEALING BY PRIMARY INTENTION

Impaired tissue integrity: wound *related to altered circulation; metabolic disorders (e.g., diabetes mellitus); alterations in fluid volume and nutrition; and medical therapy (chemotherapy, radiation therapy, steroid administration).*

Goals/Outcomes: The patient exhibits the following signs of wound healing: well-approximated wound edges, good initial postinjury inflammatory response (erythema, warmth, induration, pain), no inflammatory response after the fifth day postinjury, no drainage (without drain present) 48 hours after closure, and healing ridge present by postoperative days 5 to 9. Tissue integrity is restored.

NOC Tissue Integrity: Skin and Mucous Membranes.

Wound Care

1. Assess, document, and report impaired wound healing, including absence of a healing ridge, presence of drain-age or purulent exudate, and delayed or prolonged inflammatory response. Monitor vital signs and laboratory work for signs of infection, including elevated temperature, HR, and WBCs.

2. Use standard (universal) precautions and follow proper infection-control techniques when changing dressings. If a drain is present, assess patency and handle gently to prevent the drain from moving out of position, or being accidentally removed.

3. Provide wound care teaching and need for continued postdischarge care. Demonstrate care for the patient or caregiver and provide "teach back" time to validate knowledge and skills. Coordinate care with home healthcare agency, if appropriate.
   - For persons with hyperglycemia, maintain blood glucose within ordered range.
   - Explain to the patient that deep breathing promotes oxygenation, which enhances wound healing. Stress the importance of position changes and activity as tolerated to promote ventilation. Use an incentive spirometer to promote deep inspiration and expiration. Evaluate the patient for smoking, and if present, encourage smoking cessation because smoking increases vasoconstriction, which compromises perfusion impacting negatively on wound healing.
   - For nonrestricted patients, ensure a fluid intake of at least 1.5 L/24 h.
   - Provide nutrients for healing: a diet with adequate protein, calories, vitamins, and minerals. Encourage between-meal supplements and give frequent small feedings as needed/tolerated. (See Nutritional Support.)

SURGICAL OR TRAUMATIC WOUNDS HEALING BY SECONDARY INTENTION

Wounds healing by secondary intention are those with tissue loss or heavy contamination, not closed at the surface, and left open to fill with granulation tissue, contract, and reepithelize. Impaired healing is frequently caused by heavy contamination and impaired perfusion, oxy-genation, and/or nutrition, which delays the healing process. Individuals at risk for impaired healing include those who are obese, diabetic, malnourished, older, receiving steroids, immu-nosuppressed, undergoing radiation therapy or chemotherapy, or receiving vasopressors.

ASSESSMENT
OPTIMAL HEALING

Initially, the wound edges are inflamed, indurated, and tender. Pale granulation tissue on the wound floor and wound wall proliferates and progresses to a deeper pink and then red; the tissue should be moist. As the wound fills with granulation tissue, epithelial cells from the surrounding tissue migrate across the granulation tissue, fill the defect, and contraction occurs simultaneously to close the wound. As healing continues, the wound edges approximate and the newly resurfaced epithelium is pink and dry. If present, a wound tract or sinus gradually decreases in size. The time frame for healing depends on the size and location of the wound, as well as the patient's physical and psychological status (Table 1-38).

IMPAIRED HEALING

Exudate, slough, and necrotic material appear on the base and walls of the wound, indicating that healing has not progressed. The percentage of nonviable tissue in the wound must be assessed for distribution, color, presence of odor, and presence of wound exudate (color, amount, and consistency). Assess the periwound skin for signs of tissue damage, including disruption, moisture-related skin damage, discoloration, and increasing pain. Volume, color, and odor of drainage are assessed and measured if possible (see Table 1-38).

DIAGNOSTIC TESTS

See discussion on Wounds Closed by Primary Intention.

Test	Purpose	Abnormal Findings
Culture	Test for the presence of infection	Culture will identify the specific aerobic and anaerobic organisms and their susceptibility to antibiotics. Preliminary culture results in 24 hours, final in 48 hours.
Biopsy	To rule out the presence of cancer or dermatologic diagnosis	Consult appropriate treating specialty as needed (e.g., oncology or dermatology). Incorrect diagnosis of wound etiology can have untoward delay in treatment.

COLLABORATIVE MANAGEMENT

CARE PRIORITIES

1. Débride slough and necrotic tissue: To remove nonviable tissue, use surgical or sharp débridement (done by provider certified to perform débridement) for rapid removal and enzymatic (e.g., Santyl) or autolytic (e.g., hydrocolloid dressing) for slower removal.
2. Infection: Use systemic antibiotics specific to the pathogen. Each time wound care is provided, wound cleansing should be performed. This is to remove waste products and to dislodge and remove bacteria, necrotic tissue, foreign bodies, and exudate.
3. Moisture: Wound healing must take place in a moist environment. Dressing choices need to meet this need; excessive or inadequate moisture will delay wound healing.

Table 1-38	ASSESSMENT OF HEALING OF WOUNDS CLOSING BY SECONDARY INTENTION	
Expected Findings	**Abnormal Findings**	
Granulation tissue initially pale and moist and then becomes pink and red over time	Granulation tissue remains pale or is excessively dry	
No odor	Abnormal odor	
No slough (moist yellow avascular tissue) or necrotic (dead) tissue	Slough or necrotic tissue	
No tunneling (dead space caused by tissue destruction) or undermining, or decrease in size of tunnels or undermining areas	Tunneling or undermining that is not decreasing in size or length	
	Pain	
	Wound increases in size, tissue type changes from granulation tissue and becomes slough or necrotic	

4. Edges: Wound edges that are thickened and rolled downward may indicate premature closure of a chronic wound called epibole; cautery using silver nitrate may be needed to open the wound edges to move toward healing.
5. Fluids (oral/IV): Ensure adequate intravascular volume to support healing.
6. Topical or systemic vitamin A: When indicated, used to reverse adverse effects of steroids on healing.
7. Drain(s): Removes excess tissue fluid or purulent drainage. Closed drains are preferable to open drains because of infection control.
8. Negative pressure wound therapy: Reduces edema and wound exudate, promotes wound contraction, reduces bacterial bioburden, and stimulates granulation tissue formation.
9. Skin graft/cultured keratinocytes/cultured skin substitute: Provides coverage of wound if necessary.
10. Tissue flap: Fills tissue defect and provides wound closure with its own blood supply. Requires pressure redistribution bed surface to minimize pressure on operative flap.
11. Growth factors: These are naturally occurring proteins that stimulate new cell formation and have been approved for use in the treatment of diabetic foot ulcers. (e.g., platelet-derived growth factor).
12. Hyperbaric O_2: Used with difficult wounds to improve oxygen-carrying capacity and improve local tissue oxygenation.
13. Diet: Designed to maintain weight at optimal BMI with controlled blood glucose, includes multivitamins and minerals. See discussion on Wounds Closed by Primary Intention.

CARE PLANS FOR WOUNDS HEALING BY SECONDARY INTENTION

Impaired tissue integrity: *wound, related to presence of contaminants; metabolic disorders; medical therapy; altered perfusion; immunosuppression; and malnutrition.*

Goals/Outcomes: The patient's wound exhibits the following signs of healing: initially, postsurgical wound edges are inflamed, indurated, and tender; epithelialization begins, granulation tissue develops, and there is no odor or necrotic tissue. Exudate is minimal. The wound begins to contract and the base starts to fill with granulation tissue.

NOC Wound Healing: Secondary Intention.

Wound Care
1. Impaired wound healing: Assess and document wound condition daily. Report and manage decreased inflammatory response or inflammatory response lasting more than 5 days; epithelialization slowed or mechanically disrupted; granulation tissue remains pale or becomes dry; presence of odor, exudate, necrotic tissue, pain, wound breakdown, or if the wound edges close prematurely (epibole).
2. Pack wounds lightly: Apply prescribed dressings (Table 1-39). Lightly pack dressing into all tracts to promote gradual closure. Do not overpack wounds with dressings; fill wound without pressure. Thoroughly wash hands before and after dressing changes. Use clean gloves; dispose of contaminated dressings appropriately.
3. Manage wound drains: Maintain patency, prevent kinking, and secure drain/tubing to prevent accidentally moving or removing the drain. Medical device related pressure ulcers occur beneath drains; report and manage edema under drains.
4. Prevent contamination: Cleanse the skin surrounding the wound with normal saline. Use minimal friction if skin is friable.
5. Wound cleansing: Provide pressure irrigation using a 35-mL syringe with a 19-gauge Angiocath attached to provide a powerful irrigation stream. Commercial wound cleansers have the necessary pressure between 4 and 15 psi built into the spray nozzle. If the tissue is friable or the wound is over a major organ or blood vessel, use extreme caution with irrigation pressure. To remove contaminants effectively, use a large volume of irrigant (e.g., 100 to 150 mL).
6. Topical enzymes: If prescribed to assist in debridement, follow package directions carefully to help ensure efficacy. Certain other topical agents, such as povidone-iodine, deactivate enzymes. Protect undamaged skin with zinc oxide or liquid skin barrier.
7. Wound care teaching: Demonstrate, then have the patient or caregiver "teach back" to validate understanding and skills.

Table 1-39	DRESSINGS USED FOR WOUND CARE	
Dressing	**Advantages**	**Disadvantages**
Transparent dressing (e.g., Op-Site, Tegaderm, Bioclusive)	Provides moist environment and protects wound base. Transparent so can view wound; prevents loss of wound fluid; protects from friction and shear. Can use as secondary dressing and for securement.	Cannot absorb excessive moisture, may result in maceration of periwound tissue.
Hydrocolloid (e.g., DuoDerm, Restore, Exuderm)	Maintains moist wound environment; facilitates autolytic debridement; easy to apply, reduces pain.	Do not use with heavily draining wounds; opaque; exudate present on removal may be confused with infection; dressing can roll.
Hydrogel (e.g., Skintegrity, Elasto-gel, Replicare)	Nonadherent; provides moisture to wound, minimizes pain; can be used with infected wounds.	Cannot be used with heavily draining wounds; may macerate periwound skin.
Foam (e.g., Biatain, PolyMem)	Absorptive; nontraumatic; easy to apply and remove.	Not intended for dry wounds; may require tape or secondary dressing to secure.
Calcium Alginate (e.g., SeaSorb, Algisite)	Dressing is seaweed and is highly absorptive, used for heavily exudative wounds, appearance is gel-like upon removal.	Cannot be used for dry wounds; requires secondary dressing; may have foul odor when removed.
Gauze (e.g., 2×2, 4×4, rolled gauze)	Inexpensive; easy to use; ideal for packing wound.	May result in tissue maceration if inserted too moist; may result in tissue disruption if allowed to dry.
Composites (e.g., Alldress, Covaderm Plus)	Use for partial- to full-thickness wounds.	Adhesive borders may disrupt surrounding skin. Composite dressings come in a variety of sizes, may be difficult to carry a large supply.
Silver dressings: foam, alginates, gels	Antiseptic capability while in the wound. Different manufacturers will identify the length of time their dressing has in continuing to shed silver.	Silver sensitivity or allergy. Rare cases of issues of tattooing have been noted. Silver ions will be deactivated by some solutions.

PRESSURE ULCERS

The National Pressure Ulcer Advisory Panel (NPUAP) defines a pressure ulcer as localized injury to the skin and/or underlying tissue usually over a bony prominence, as a result of pressure, or pressure in combination with shear. High-risk patients include patients with impaired sensory perception, advanced age, skin moisture (incontinence, excessive sweating), decreased activity and mobility levels, poor nutritional intake, and exposure to friction and shear.

ASSESSMENT: PRESSURE ULCER RISK AND STAGING ULCERS

High-risk individuals should be assessed for risk on admission, with daily assessments during hospitalization, using a standard pressure ulcer assessment tool. Daily (or in some cases more often according to facility policy) use of the Braden Scale or Norton Scale will assist in identifying patients at risk for skin breakdown and help the nurse make decisions on when to use preventative interventions. A daily skin assessment should be done to assess for any alterations in skin integrity.

When pressure ulcers are present, staging of the tissue layers is an important evaluation of the level of tissue damage. A pressure ulcer can be staged on a scale of 1 to 4 if the base of the wound can be visualized. If the wound base cannot be seen, the wound is considered "unstageable." The following staging criteria are endorsed by the NPUAP and are widely used in healthcare settings.

Stage I: Nonblanchable erythema
Intact skin with nonblanchable redness of a localized area usually over a bony prominence. Darkly pigmented skin may not have visible blanching; its color may differ from the surrounding area. The area may be painful, firm, soft, warmer, or cooler compared with adjacent tissue. Stage I may be difficult to detect in individuals with dark skin tones. When seen under normal pressure conditions, may indicate "at-risk" persons.

Stage II: Partial thickness
A partial thickness loss of dermis, presents as a shallow, open ulcer with a red pink wound bed, without slough; can present as closed or a ruptured serum-filled or serosanguineous fluid-filled blister; may also be a shiny or dry shallow ulcer without slough or bruising*. This stage should not be used to describe nonpressure-related skin tears, tape burns, incontinence-associated dermatitis, maceration, or excoriation.
*Note: Bruising indicates deep tissue injury.

Stage III: Full thickness skin loss
Full thickness tissue loss. Subcutaneous fat may be visible. Bone, tendon, or muscle is not exposed nor directly palpable. Slough may be present, but does not obscure the depth of tissue loss. Wound undermining and tunneling may be present. The depth of a stage III pressure ulcer varies by anatomic location. The bridge of the nose, ear, occiput, and malleolus do not have (adipose) subcutaneous tissue and stage III ulcers can be shallow. Areas of significant adiposity can develop extremely deep stage III pressure ulcers.

Stage IV: Full thickness tissue loss
Full thickness tissue loss with exposed and/or directly palpable bone, tendon, or muscle. Slough or eschar may be present. Often includes undermining and tunneling. The depth of a stage IV pressure ulcer varies by anatomic location. The bridge of the nose, ear, occiput, and malleolus do not have (adipose) subcutaneous tissue and these ulcers can be shallow. Stage IV ulcers can extend into muscle and/or supporting structures (e.g., fascia, tendon, or joint capsule) making osteomyelitis or osteitis likely to occur.

Unstageable: Full thickness skin or tissue loss, depth unknown
Full thickness tissue loss in which actual depth of the ulcer is completely obscured by slough (yellow, tan, gray, green, or brown) and/or eschar (tan, brown, or black) in the wound bed. Until enough slough and/or eschar are removed to expose the base of the wound, the true depth cannot be determined. These wounds are either stage III or stage IV. Stable (dry, adherent, intact without erythema or fluctuance) eschar on the heels serves as "the body's natural (biological) cover" and should not be removed.

Suspected deep tissue injury, depth unknown
Purple or maroon localized area of discolored intact skin or blood-filled blister resulting from damage of underlying soft tissue from pressure and/or shear. The area may be preceded by tissue that is painful, firm, mushy, boggy, warmer, or cooler compared with adjacent tissue. Deep tissue injury may be difficult to detect in individuals with dark skin tones. Evolution may include a thin blister over a dark wound bed. The wound may further evolve and become covered by thin eschar. Evolution may be rapid exposing additional layers of tissue even with optimal treatment.

DIAGNOSTIC TESTS
See Diagnostic Tests.

COLLABORATIVE MANAGEMENT
See Collaborative Management in Surgical Wounds Healing by Primary Intention and Collaborative Management in Surgical or Traumatic Wounds Healing by Secondary Intention.

CARE PLANS FOR PREVENTION AND MANAGEMENT OF PRESSURE ULCERS

Risk for impaired tissue integrity related to excessive tissue pressure, shearing forces, friction, and altered circulation. Presence of pressure ulcer with increased risk for breakdown, related to altered circulation; presence of contaminants or irritants (chemical, thermal, mechanical).

Goals/Outcomes: High risk: skin integrity of the patient remains intact. After intervention/instructions, the patient/caregiver verbalizes causes and preventive measures for pressure ulcers and successfully participates in the plan of care to promote healing and prevent further breakdown if a pressure ulcer is present. Ulcers present have granulation tissue and are moving toward healing. There is a reduction in or no slough or necrotic tissue, or odor present.
NOC Tissue Integrity: Skin and Mucous Membranes.

Pressure ulcer prevention
1. Risk assessment: Identify individuals at risk daily with a reliable/valid risk assessment tool; systematically document skin condition from head to toe according to institutional policy.
2. Turning/Positioning: Turn or reposition the patient on a turning schedule.
   - Assist the patient with turning every 1 to 2 hours or as the patient's condition allows. Use pillows or foam wedges to prevent direct pressure on bony prominences.
   - Patients with a history of previous tissue injury will require pressure redistribution measures more frequently.
   - A high-Fowler position results in increased shearing. Use a low-Fowler position and alternate supine position with prone and 30-degree elevated side-lying positions.

 Safety Alert   *The Centers for Medicare and Medicaid Services has addressed the problem of ventilator-acquired pneumonia as an avoidable condition. The plan of care to avoid pneumonia incorporates the positioning of the patient with elevation of the head of the bed at 30 degrees or above. The clinician must perform a risk/benefit analysis for the individual patient regarding height of the head of the bed, weighing pressure ulcer prevention against ventilator-acquired pneumonia prevention.*

3. Heels: Float the heels using pillows placed under the length of the calf.
4. Sacrum: Consider the use of soft silicone border foam dressings over the sacrococcygeal area to prevent skin breakdown in high-risk patients. Several studies have provided evidence that pressure ulcer incidence is reduced when used.
5. Medical devices: To prevent medical device–related pressure ulcer, cushion skin with dressings in high-risk areas such as the nose; confirm that devices are not placed directly under a patient who has reduced sensation or is immobile.
6. Minimize friction on tissue during activity: Lift rather than drag the patient during position changes and transferring; use a draw sheet to facilitate patient movement. Ideally, the patient should be moved using lift equipment to prevent injury from friction and shearing as friable skin "drags" over the sheets. Do not massage bony prominences.
7. Minimize skin exposure to moisture: Cleanse at the time of soiling and at routine intervals. Use moisture barriers and moisture wicking underpads with minimization of disposable briefs. Consider use of bowel management systems if the patient has intractable fecal incontinence.
8. Pressure redistribution surfaces: Use an overlay or mattress that redistributes pressure, such as low air loss, alternating air, or gel. Choice of the most appropriate surface is based on the weight of the patient, ability to be turned, stage and location of the ulcer(s), and the overall goals of care for the patient.

Pressure ulcer care
1. Staging: Evaluate stage of pressure ulcer. See *Assessment*.
2. Maintain vigilant skin care: Research supports use of commercially available skin care products. Keep the patient's skin clean with regular bathing, and be especially conscientious about washing urine and feces from the skin. Commercial no-rinse cleansers are available. If soap must be used, then thoroughly rinse from the skin.
3. Moisture management: If the patient has excessive perspiration, ensure frequent cleansing and change bedding as needed.
4. Information sharing: Teach the patient and caregivers the importance of and measures for preventing and redistributing pressure as a means of treating pressure ulcers.

NIC Skin Surveillance; Incision Site Care; Wound Care; Pressure Ulcer Care; Pressure Ulcer Prevention; Wound Irrigation.

ADDITIONAL NURSING DIAGNOSES

For additional information on specific conditions, refer to the following:

Impaired Tissue Integrity under Surgical or Traumatic Wounds Healing by Secondary Intention.

Pain management; Pain decreasing with cutaneous stimulation.

Deficient knowledge related to care of wound/pressure ulcer.

Imbalanced Nutrition, less than body requirements for wound healing.

SELECTED REFERENCES

Ahlers SJ, van der Veen AM, van Dijk M, et al: The use of the Behavioral Pain Scale to assess pain in conscious sedated patients, *Anesth Analg* 110(1):127–133, 2010.

American Association of Critical-Care Nurses: *Prevention of aspiration.* http://www.aacn.org/WD/practice/docs/practicealerts/aacn-aspiration-practice-alert.pdf.

American Association of Critical-Care Nurses: *Verification of feeding tube placement.* http://www.aacn.org/WD/Practice/Docs/PracticeAlerts/Verification_of_Feeding_Tube_Placement_05-2005.pdf.

American College of Cardiology Foundation/American Heart Association: *ACCF/AHA guideline for coronary artery bypass surgery: a report of the ACCF/AHA task force on practice guidelines,* 2011. http://www.guideline.gov/search/search.aspx?term=accf%2faha+2011.

American College of Cardiology Foundation/American Heart Association: *ACCF/AHA guideline for the management of heart failure: a report of the ACCF/AHA task force on practice guidelines,* 2013. http://www.guideline.gov/search/search.aspx?term=accf%2faha+2011.

American College of Radiology: *ACR practice guideline for adult sedation/analgesia.* http://www.acr.org/SecondaryMainMenuCategories/quality_safety/guidelines/iv/adult_sedation.aspx.

American College of Radiology/Society of Interventional Radiology: *ACR/SIR practice guideline for adult sedation/analgesia: revision 2010 (Resolution 45).* http://www.acr.org/~/media/ACR/Documents/PGTS/guidelines/Adult_Sedation.pdf.

American Nurses Association (ANA): *Safe patient handling interprofessional standards across the care continuum,* Silver Springs, 2013, American Nurses Association.

American Society of Anesthesiologists Task Force on Pulmonary Artery Catheterization: Practice guidelines for pulmonary artery catheterization: an updated report by the American Society of Anesthesiologists Task Force on Pulmonary Artery Catheterization, *Anesthesiology* 99(4):988–1014, 2003.

American Society of Anesthesiology: Practice guidelines for sedation and analgesia by non-anesthesiologists, *Anesthesiology* 96(4):1004–1017, 2002.

American Society of Parenteral and Enteral Nutrition: *Parenteral nutrition trace element product shortage considerations,* December 2013. http://www.nutritioncare.org/Professional_Resources/Drug_Shortages/Parenteral_Nutrition_Trace_Element_Product_Shortage_Considerations/.

American Thoracic Society and Infectious Disease Society of America: Guidelines for prevention of adults with hospital acquired, ventilator associated and healthcare associated pneumonia, *Am J Respir Crit Care Med* 171:388–416, 2005.

Amorosa JK, Bramwit MP, Mohammed TL, et al: *ACR appropriateness criteria routine chest radiographs in ICU patients,* Reston, 2011, American College of Radiology.

Anand KJS, Craig KD: New perspectives on the definition of pain, *Pain* 67(1):3–6, 1996.

Anion Gap Calculator. http://www.mdcalc.com/anion-gap/.

Appel SJ, Downs CA: Understanding acid base balance, *Nursing* 38:9–11, 2008.

Arbour C, Gélinas C, Michaud C: Impact of the implementation of the Critical-Care Pain Observation Tool (CPOT) on pain management and clinical outcomes in mechanically ventilated trauma intensive care unit patients: a pilot study, *J Trauma Nurs* 18(1):52–60, 2011.

Arnold HM, Hollands JM, Skrupky LP, et al: Optimizing sustained use of sedation in mechanically ventilated patients: focus on safety, *Curr Drug Saf* 5(1):6–12, 2010.

Arroyo-Novoa CM, Figueroa-Ramos MI, Puntillo KA, et al: Pain related to tracheal suctioning in awake acutely and critically ill adults: a descriptive study, *Intensive Crit Care Nurs* 24(1):20–27, 2008.

Ayello EA, Sibbald RG: Preventing pressure ulcers and skin tears. In Capezuti E, Zwicker D, Mezey M, Fulmer T, editors: *Evidence-based geriatric nursing protocols for best practice,* ed 3, New York, 2008, Springer, pp 403–429.

Baranoski S, Ayello EA: *Wound care essentials: practice principles,* ed 3, Philadelphia, Lippincott, Williams and Wilkins.

Barr J, Fraser GL, Puntillo K, et al: Clinical practice guidelines for the management of pain, agitation, and delirium in adult patients in the intensive care unit, *Crit Care Med* 41(1):263-306, 2013.

Bednash G, Ferrell BR: *End-of-life nursing education consortium (ELNEC) faculty guide*, Duarte, 2007, American Association of Colleges of Nursing and City of Hope National Medical Center.

Bergeron N, Dubois M-J, Dumont M, et al: Intensive care delirium screening checklist: evaluation of a new screening tool, *Intensive Care Med* 27(5):859-864, 2001.

Bergstrom N, Braden B, Kemp M, et al: Predicting pressure ulcer risk: a multisite study of the predictive validity of the Braden Scale, *Nurs Res* 47(5):261-269, 1998.

Bergstrom N, Braden BJ: Predictive validity of the Braden Scale among black and white subjects, *Nurs Res* 51(6):398-403, 2002.

Besselink MG, van Santvoort HC, Buskins E, et al: Probiotic prophylaxis in predicted severe acute pancreatitis: a randomised, double-blind, placebo-controlled trial, *Lancet* 371(9613):6521-6529, 2008.

Biehl M, Kashiouris MG, Gajic O: Ventilator-induced lung injury: minimizing its impact in patients with or at risk for ARDS, *Respir Care* 58(6):927-937, 2013.

Birrer K: Pain agitation and delirium in the ICU. In Murphy JE, Lee MW, editors: *Pharmacotherapy self-assessment program 2014 book 1: critical and urgent care*, Lenexa, 2014, American College of Clinical Pharmacy, pp 177-191.

Black JM, Edsberg LE, Baharestani MM, et al: Pressure ulcer: avoidable or unavoidable, results of the national ulcer advisory panel consensus conference, *Ostomy Wound Manag* 57(2):24-27, 2011.

Bolton L: Which pressure ulcer risk assessment scales are valid for use in the clinical setting? *J Wound Ostomy Continence Nurs* 34(4):368-381, 2007.

Borg GA: Psychophysical basis of perceived exertion, *Med Sci Sports Exerc* 14(5):377-381, 1982.

Bridges E: *AACN practice alert pulmonary artery/central venous pressure measurement*, Revised December 2009, Aliso Viejo, 2009, American Association of Critical-Care Nurses (AACN). http://www.aacn.org/wd/practice/content/practicealerts.pcms?menu=practice.

Brindle CT, Wegelin JA: Prophylactic dressing application to reduce pressure ulcer formation in cardiac surgery patients, *J Wound Ostomy Continence Nurs* 39(2):133-142, 2012.

Bryant R, Nix D: *Acute and chronic wounds: current management concepts*, ed 4, St Louis, 2012, Mosby.

Bulechek GB, Butcher HK, Dochterman JM, editors: *Nursing interventions classification (NIC)*, ed 5, St Louis, 2008, Mosby.

Bulechek GB, Butcher HK, Dochterman JM, editors: *Nursing interventions classification (NIC)*, ed 6, St Louis, 2013, Mosby.

Bunn F, Trivedi D, Ashraf S: Colloid solutions for fluid resuscitation, *Cochrane Database Syst Rev* 1:CD001319, 2011.

Burns SM, Fisher C, Tribble S, et al: Multifactor clinical score and outcome of mechanical ventilation weaning trials: Burns Wean Assessment Program, *Am J Crit Care* 19(5):431-439, 2010.

Burns SM, Fisher C, Tribble SS, et al: The relationship between 26 clinical factors to weaning outcome, *Am J Crit Care* 21(1):52-59, 2012.

Cain S: Necrotizing fasciitis: recognition and care, *Practice Nurs* 21(6):297-302, 2010.

Callahan C, Unverzagt F, Hui S, et al: Six-item screener to identify cognitive impairment among potential subjects for clinical research, *Med Care* 40(9):771-781, 2002.

Cambron JA, Dexheimer J, Coe P: Changes in blood pressure after various forms of therapeutic massage: a preliminary study, *J Alternat Complement Med* 12(1):65-70, 2006.

Centers for Disease Control and Prevention: Guidelines for the prevention of intravascular catheter-related infections, *MMWR Recomm Rep* 51(RR-10):1-29, 2002.

Centers for Medicare and Medicaid Services: Changes to the hospital inpatient prospective payment systems and fiscal year 2008 rates, *Federal Register* 72(162):47201-47205, 2007.

Chaiken N: Reduction of sacral pressure ulcers in the intensive care unit using a silicone dressing, *J Wound Ostomy Continence Nurs* 39(2):143-145, 2012.

Chan LN: Drug-nutrient interactions, *JPEN J Parenter Enteral Nutr* 37(4):450-459, 2013.

Chanques G, Jaber S, Barbotte E, et al: Impact of systematic evaluation of pain and agitation in an intensive care unit, *Crit Care Med* 34(6):1691-1699, 2006.

Chanques G, Sebbane M, Barbotte E, et al: A prospective study of pain at rest: incidence and characteristics of an unrecognized symptom in surgical and trauma versus medical intensive care unit patients, *Anesthesiology* 107(5):858-860, 2007.

Chanques G, Viel E, Constantin JM, et al: The measurement of pain in intensive care unit: comparison of 5 self-report intensity scales, *Pain* 151(3):711-721, 2010.

Choban P, Dickerson R, Malone A, et al: A.S.P.E.N. clinical guidelines nutrition support of hospitalized adult patients with obesity, *JPEN J Parenter Enteral Nutr* 37(6):414-444, 2013.

Clark SF: Vitamins and trace elements. In Mueller CM, editor: *The A.S.P.E.N. adult nutrition support core curriculum*, ed 2, Silver Spring, 2012, American Society for Parenteral and Enteral Nutrition.

Cooper KL: Evidence based prevention of pressure ulcers in the intensive care unit, *Crit Care Nurse* 33(6):57–67, 2013.

Corkins MR, Guenter P, Dimaria-Ghalili RA, et al: Malnutrition diagnoses in hospitalized patients: United States, 2010, *JPEN J Parenter Enteral Nutr* 38(2):186–195, 2014.

Cox J: Predictors of pressure ulcers in adult critical care patients, *Am J Crit Care* 20(5):365–374, 2011.

Cresci G, Lefton J, Esper DH: Enteral formulations. In Mueller CM, editor: *The A.S.P.E.N. adult nutrition support core curriculum*, ed 2, Silver Spring, 2012, American Society for Parenteral and Enteral Nutrition.

Culleiton AL, Simko LC: Keeping fluids and electrolytes in balance (part 1), *Nursing* 6(2):30–35, 2011.

Daily E, Schroeder J: *Techniques in bedside hemodynamic monitoring*, ed 4, St Louis, 1989, Mosby.

Darovic G: *Hemodynamic monitoring, invasive and noninvasive clinical application*, Philadelphia, 2002, Saunders.

Department of Veterans Affairs: *Safe patient handling and movement algorithms*, Tampa, 2006, VISN 8 Patient Safety Center of Inquiry.

Devlin JW, Fraser GL, Ely EW, et al: Pharmacologic management of sedation and delirium in mechanically ventilated ICU patient: remaining evidence gaps and controversies, *Semin Respir Crit Care Med* 34(2):201–215, 2013.

Devlin JW, Roberts RJ, Fong JJ, et al: Efficacy and safety of quetiapine in critically ill patients with delirium: a prospective, multicenter, randomized, double-blind, placebo-controlled pilot study, *Crit Care Med* 38(2):419–427, 2010.

Dhaliwal R, Cahill N, Lemieux M, Heyland DK: The Canadian critical care nutrition guidelines in 2013: an update on current recommendations and implementation strategies, *Nutr Clin Pract* 29(1):29–43, 2014.

Diedrich DA, Brown DR: Analytic reviews: propofol infusion syndrome in the ICU, *J Intensive Care Med* 26(2):59–72, 2011.

Diehl T, Ambrose M, Goldgerg K, et al, editors: Fluid and electrolyte in medical surgical nursing made incredibly easy, Philadelphia, 2004, Lippincott.

Doherty M, Buggy DJ: Intraoperative fluids: how much is too much? *Br J Anaesth* 109(1):69–79, 2012.

Dorner B, Posthauer ME, Thomas D: The role of nutrition in pressure ulcer prevention and treatment: National Pressure Ulcer Advisory Panel white paper, *Adv Skin Wound Care* 22(5):212–221, 2009.

Elke G, Wang M, Weiler N, et al: Close to recommended caloric and protein intake by enteral nutrition is associated with better clinical outcome of critically ill septic patients: secondary analysis of a large international nutrition database, *Crit Care* 18(1):R29, 2014.

Epstein LJ, Kristo D, Strollo PJ, et al: Clinical guideline for the evaluation, management and long-term care of obstructive sleep apnea in adults, *J Clin Sleep Med* 5(3):263–276, 2009.

Erlich ML: *Urgent: propofol update (healthcare provider letter)*, June 19, 2012, APP Pharmaceuticals.

Esperanza ML, Estilo AA, Perez T, et al: Pressure ulcers in the intensive care unit: new perspectives on an old problem, *Crit Care Nurse* 32(3):65–70, 2012.

Ethier C, Burry L, Martinez-Motta C, et al: Recall of intensive care unit stay in patients managed with a sedation protocol or a sedation protocol with daily sedative interruption: a pilot study, *J Crit Care* 26(2):127–132, 2011.

European Pressure Ulcer Advisory Panel and National Pressure Ulcer Advisory Panel: *Prevention and treatment of pressure ulcers: clinical practice guidelines*, Washington, 2009, National Pressure Ulcer Advisory Panel.

Faigeles B, Howie-Esquive J, Miaskowski C, et al: Predictors and use of nonpharmacologic interventions for procedural pain associated with turning among hospitalized adults, *Pain Manag Nurs* 14(2):85–93, 2013.

Fleisher L, Beckman JA, Brown KA, et al: ACC/AHA 2007 guidelines on perioperative cardiovascular evaluation and care for noncardiac surgery, *J Am Coll Cardiol* 50(17):e159–e241, 2007.

Fontana CJ, Pittiglio LI: Sleep deprivation among critical care patients, *Crit Care Nurs Q* 33(1):75–81, 2010.

Fortin J, Habenbacher W, Heller A, et al: Non-invasive beat-to-beat cardiac output monitoring by an improved method of transthoracic bioimpedance measurement, *Comput Biol Med* 36(11):1185–1203, 2006.

Francis J Jr, Young G: Diagnosis of delirium and confusional states. In Aminoff M, Schmader K, editors: *UpToDate*, Waltham, 2014, Wolters Kluwer Health. http://www.uptodate.com.

Frankenfield D, Roth-Yousey L, Compher C: Comparison of predictive equations for resting metabolic rate in healthy nonobese and obese adults: a systematic review, *J Am Diet Assoc* 105(5):775–789, 2005.

Fukagawa M, Kurokawa K, Papadakis M: Fluid and electrolyte disorders. In Tierney L, McPhee S, Papadakis M, editors: *Current medical diagnosis and treatment*, ed 43, New York, 2004, Lange Medical Books/McGraw-Hill.

Gacouin A, Camus C, Le Tulzo Y, et al: Assessment of peri-extubation pain by visual analogue scale in the adult intensive care unit: a prospective observational study, *Intensive Care Med* 30(7): 1340-1347, 2004.

Gattinoni L, Caironi P, Cressoni M, Chiumello D, Ranieri VM, Quintel M, Russo S, Patroniti N, Cornejo R, Bugedo G. Lung Recruitment in Patients with the Acute Respiratory Distress Syndrome. *N Engl J Med* 354:1775-1786, 2006.

Garcia Lizana F, Peres Bota D, De Cubber M, Vincent JL: Long-term outcome in ICU patients: what about quality of life? *Intensive Care Med* 29(8):1286-1293, 2003.

Geerts WH, Bergqvist D, Pineo GF, et al: Prevention of venous thromboembolism: American College of Chest Physicians Evidence-Based Clinical Practice Guidelines (8th Edition), *Chest* 133(Suppl 6):S381-S453, 2008.

Gelinas C: Management of pain in cardiac surgery intensive care unit patients: have we improved over time? *Intensive Crit Care Nurs* 23(5):298-303, 2007.

Gelinas C, Arbour C: Behavioral and physiologic indicators during a nociceptive procedure in conscious and unconscious mechanically ventilated adults: similar or different? *J Crit Care* 24(4):628. e7-628.e17, 2009.

Gelinas C, Arbour C, Michaud C, et al: Patients and ICU nurses' perspectives of non-pharmacological interventions for pain management, *Nurs Crit Care* 18(6):307-318, 2013.

Gelinas C, Arbour C, Michaud C, et al: Implementation of the critical-care pain observation tool on pain assessment/management nursing practices in an intensive care unit with nonverbal critically ill adults: a before and after study, *Int J Nurs Stud* 48(12):1495-1504, 2011.

Gelinas C, Fillion L, Puntillo KA, et al: Validation of the critical-care pain observation tool in adult patients, *Am J Crit Care* 15(4):420-427, 2006.

Gelinas C, Puntillo KA, Joffe AM, Barr J: A validated approach to evaluating psychometric properties of pain assessment tools for use in nonverbal critically ill adults, *Semin Respir Crit Care Med* 34(2):153-168, 2013.

Girard TD, Pandharipande PP, Carson SS, et al: Feasibility, efficacy, and safety of antipsychotics for intensive care unit delirium: the MIND randomized, placebo-controlled trial, *Crit Care Med* 38(2):428-437, 2010.

Gordon DB, Dahl JL, Miaskowski C, et al: American Pain Society recommendations for improving the quality of acute and cancer pain management – American Pain Society Quality of Care Task Force, *Arch Intern Med* 165(14):1574-1580, 2005.

Gorji HM, Nesami BM, Ayyasi M, et al: Comparison of ice packs application and relaxation therapy in pain reduction during chest tube removal following cardiac surgery, *N Am J Med Sci* 6(1): 19-24, 2014.

Gregori JA, Nunez JM: Handling of water and electrolytes in the healthy old, *Rev Clin Gerontol* 19(1):1-12, 2009.

Grogano's Acid Based Tutorial. http://www.acid-base.com/.

Grossbach I, Chlan L, Tracy MF: Overview of mechanical ventilatory support and management of patient- and ventilator-related responses, *Crit Care Nurse* 31(3):30-45, 2011.

Gusmao-Flores D, Figueira Salluh JI, Chalhub RA, et al: The Confusion Assessment Method for the Intensive Care Unit (CAM-ICU) and Intensive Care Delirium Screening Checklist (ICDSC) for the diagnosis of delirium: a systematic review and meta-analysis of clinical studies, *Crit Care* 16(4):R115, 2012.

Hadjistavropoulos T, Craig KD: A theoretical framework for understanding self-report and observational measures of pain: a communications model, *Behav Res Ther* 40(5):551-570, 2002.

Harvey S, Jordan S: Diuretic therapy: implications for nursing practice, *Nurs Stand* 24(43):40-49, 2010.

Herr KA, Mobily PR: Comparison of selected pain assessment tools for use with the elderly, *Appl Nurs Res* 6(1):39-46, 1993.

Herr K, Coyne PJ, McCaffery M, et al: Pain assessment in the patient unable to self-report: position statement with clinical practice recommendations, *Pain Manag Nurs* 12(4):230-250, 2011.

Hess DR: Approaches to conventional mechanical ventilation of the patient with acute respiratory distress syndrome, *Respir Care* 56(10):1555-1572, 2011.

Hess DR: Noninvasive ventilation for acute respiratory failure, *Respir Care* 58(6):950-972, 2013.

Hill N: *Non-invasive ventilation in critical care, Critical Connections Newsletter*, February 2008, Society of Critical Care Medicine. http://www.sccm.org/Publications/Critical_Connections/Archives/February_2008/Pages/NoninvasiveVentilation.aspx.

Honiden S, McArdle JR: Obesity in the intensive care unit, *Clin Chest Med* 30(3):581–599, 2009.

Hospira Inc: *FDA package insert for dexmedetomidine.* http://www.precedex.com/wp-content/uploads.

Huff J: Evaluation of abnormal behavior in the emergency department. In Hockberger R, editor: *UpToDate*, Waltham, 2014, Wolters Kluwer Health. http://May 23, 2014, from www.uptodate.com.

Huff J, Farace E, Brady W, et al: The Quick Confusion Scale in the emergency department: comparison with the Mini-Mental State Examination, *Am J Emerg Med* 19(6):461–464, 2001.

Hughes F, Bryan K, Robbins I: Relatives' experiences of critical care, *Nurs Crit Care* 10(1):23–30, 2005.

Iglesias C, Nixon J, Cranny G, et al: Pressure relieving support surfaces. Trial: cost-effectiveness analysis, *BMJ* 332(7555):1416, 2006.

Iglesias C, Nixon J, Cranny G, et al: Pain: the fifth vital sign. In Ignatavicius DD, Workman ML, editors: *Medical-surgical nursing patient-centered collaborative care*, ed 6, Philadelphia, 2010, Saunders.

Inouye S: Delirium in older persons, *N Engl J Med* 354:1157–1165, 2006.

Institute for Healthcare Improvement: *Protecting 5 million lives from harm.* http://www.ihi.org/IHI/Programs/Campaign.

International Association for the Study of Pain (IASP): *Pain terminology*, 2011. http://www.iasp-pain.org/AM/Template.cfm?Section=Pain_Defi...isplay.cfm&ContentID=1728.

Jakob SM, Ruokonen E, Grounds RM, et al: Dexmedetomidine vs midazolam or propofol for sedation during prolonged mechanical ventilation: two randomized controlled trials, *JAMA* 307(11):1151–1160, 2012.

Jarzyna D, Jungquist CR, Pasero C, et al: American Society for Pain Management Nursing guidelines on monitoring for opioid-induced sedation and respiratory depression, *Pain Manag Nurs* 12(3):118–145, 2011.

Jensen GL, Binkley J: Clinical manifestations of nutrient deficiency, *JPEN J Parenter Enteral Nutr* 26(Suppl 5):S29–S33, 2002.

Johnson M, Maas M, editors: *Nursing outcomes classification (NOC)*, St Louis, 1997, Mosby.

Joshi GP, Ogunnaike BO: Consequences of inadequate postoperative pain relief and chronic persistent postoperative pain, *Anesthesiol Clin North Am* 23(1):21–36, 2005.

Kaarlola A, Pettila V, Kekki P: Quality of life six years after intensive care, *Intensive Care Med* 29(8):1294–1299, 2003.

Kalisvaart K, de Jonghe J, Bogaards M, et al: Haloperidol prophylaxis for elderly hip-surgery patients at risk for delirium: a randomized placebo-controlled study, *J Am Geriatr Soc* 53(10):1658–1666, 2005.

Kaye AD, Kaye AJ, Swinford J, et al: The effect of deep-tissue massage therapy on blood pressure and heart rate, *J Alternat Complement Med* 14(2):125–128, 2008.

Keckeisen M: Monitoring pulmonary artery pressure, *Crit Care Nurse* 24(3):67–70, 2004.

Keenan SP, Sinuff T, Burns KEA, et al: Clinical practice guidelines for the use of noninvasive positive-pressure ventilation and noninvasive continuous positive airway pressure in the acute care setting, *CMAJ* 183(3):E195–E214, 2011.

Kehlet H, Jensen TS, Woolf CJ: Persistent postsurgical pain: risk factors and prevention, *Lancet* 367(9522):1618–1625, 2006.

Khan BA: Comparison and agreement between the Richmond Agitation-Sedation Scale and the Riker Sedation-Agitation Scale in evaluating patients' eligibility for delirium assessment in the ICU, *Chest* 142(1):48–54, 2012.

Knape JTA, Adriaensen H, van Aken H, et al: Guidelines for sedation and/or analgesia by non-anaesthesiology doctors. Section and Board of Anaesthesiology, European Union of Medical Specialists, *Eur J Anaesthesiol* 24(7):563–567, 2007.

Kress JP, Pohlman AS, O'Connor MF, Hall JB: Daily interruption of sedative infusions in critically ill patients undergoing mechanical ventilation, *N Engl J Med* 342(20):1471–1477, 2000.

Kshettry VR, Carole LF, Henly SJ, et al: Complementary alternative medical therapies for heart surgery patients: safety, feasibility, and impact, *Ann Thorac Surg* 81(1):201–205, 2006.

Kumpf VJ, Gervasio J: Complications of parenteral nutrition. In Mueller CM, editor: *The A.S.P.E.N. adult nutrition support core curriculum*, ed 2, Silver Spring, 2012, American Society for Parenteral and Enteral Nutrition.

Larson C, Cavuto NJ, Flockhart DA, et al: Bioavailability and efficacy of omeprazole given orally and by nasogastric tube, *Dig Dis Sci* 41(3):475–479, 1996.

Lawson N, Thompson K, Saunders G, et al: Sound intensity and noise evaluation in a critical care unit, *Am J Crit Care* 19(6):e88–e98, quiz e99, 2010.

Lee K, Hong SB, Lim CM, Koh Y: Sequential organ failure assessment score and comorbidity: valuable prognostic indicators in chronically critically ill patients, *Anaesth Intensive Care* 36(4):528–534, 2008.

Lewis JL: *Hormonal and metabolic disorders: electrolyte balance. In The Merck manual, home edition.* http://www.merckmanuals.com/home/hormonal_and_metabolic_disorders/electrolyte_balance/electrolytes.html.

Lewis JL: *Overview of acid base balance. In The Merck manual, home edition.* http://www.merckmanuals.com/home/hormonal_and_metabolic_disorders/acid-base_balance/overview_of_acid-base_balance.html.

Lindberg JO, Engstrom A: Critical care nurses' experiences: "a good relationship with the patient is a prerequisite for successful pain relief management", *Pain Manag Nurs* 12(3):163–172, 2011.

Lobo DN, Lewington AJP, Allison SP: *Basic concepts of fluid and electrolyte therapy*, Melsungen, 2013, Bibliomed.

Loeser JD, Treede RD: The Kyoto protocol of IASP basic pain terminology, *Pain* 137(3):473–477, 2008.

Lonergan E, Britton A, Luxenberg J, Wyller T: Antipsychotics for delirium, *Cochrane Database Syst Rev* 2:CD005594, 2007.

Luetz A, Heymann A, Radtke FM, et al: Different assessment tools for intensive care unit delirium: which score to use? *Crit Care Med* 38(2):409–418, 2010.

Maccioli GA, Dorman T, Brown BR, et al: Clinical practice guidelines for the maintenance of patient physical safety in the intensive care unit: use of restraining therapies. American College of Critical Care Medicine Task Force 2001-2002, *Crit Care Med* 31(11):2665–2676, 2003.

Marcantonio E, Flaker J, Wright R, Resnick N: Reducing delirium after hip fracture: a randomized trial, *J Am Geriatr Soc* 49(5):516–522, 2001.

Marmo L, Fowler S: Pain assessment tool in the critically ill post-open heart surgery patient population, *Pain Manag Nurs* 11(3):134–140, 2010.

Marquis F, Ouimet S, Riker R, et al: Individual delirium symptoms: do they matter? *Crit Care Med* 35(11):2533–2537, 2007.

Martin B: *AACN practice alert non-invasive blood pressure monitoring*, Revised April 2010. Aliso Viejo, 2010, American Association of Critical-Care Nurses (AACN). http://www.aacn.org/wd/practice/content/practicealerts.pcms?menu=practice.

McClave S, Martindale RG, Vanek V, et al: Guidelines for the provision and assessment of nutrition support therapy in the adult critically ill patient. Society of Critical Care Medicine (SCCM) and American Society of Parenteral and Enteral Nutrition (A.S.P.E.N.), *JPEN J Parent Enteral Nutr* 33(3):277–316, 2009.

McMahon MM, Nystrom E, Braunschweig C: A.S.P.E.N. clinical guidelines: nutrition support of adult patients with hyperglycemia, *JPEN J Parenter Enteral Nutr* 37(1):23–36, 2013.

Moore ZE, Cowman S: Wound cleansing for pressure ulcers, *Cochrane Collaboration* 1:1–16, 2007.

Munoz P, Bouza E, Cuenca-Estrella M, et al: Saccharomyces cerevisiae fungemia: an emerging infectious disease, *Clin Infect Disease* 40(11):1625–1634, 2005.

Nassisi D, Korc B, Hahn S, et al: The evaluation and management of the acutely agitated elderly patient, *Mt Sinai Med J* 73(7):978–984, 2006.

National Guideline Clearinghouse (NGC): *Guideline synthesis: pressure ulcer prevention*, 2006 (revised 2008). http://www.guideline.gov.

National Pressure Ulcer Advisory Panel: *Support surface standards initiative.* http://www.npuap.org/NPUAP_S31_TD.pdf.

National Pressure Ulcer Advisory Panel: *Pressure ulcer staging.* http://www.npuap.org/resources/educational-and-clinical-resources/npuap-pressure-ulcer-stagescategories.

National Pressure Ulcer Advisory Panel: *Best practices for prevention of medical device-related pressure ulcer in critical care*, 2013. http://www.npuap.org/wp-content/uploads/2013/04/BestPractices-CriticalCare1.pdf.

Needham DM, Wozniak AW, Hough CL, et al: National Institutes of Health NHLBI ARDS network, *Am J Respir Crit Care Med* 189:1214–1224, 2014.

Nerbass FB, Feltrim MI, Souza SA, et al: Effects of massage therapy on sleep quality after coronary artery bypass graft surgery, *Clinics (Sao Paulo)* 65(11):1105–1110, 2010.

Neto AS, Nassar AP Jr, Cardoso SO, et al: Delirium screening in critically ill patients: a systematic review and meta-analysis, *Crit Care Med* 40(6):1946–1951, 2012.

O'Connor M, Bucknall T, Manias E: International variations in outcomes from sedation protocol research: where are we at and where do we go from here? *Intensive Crit Care Nurs* 26(4):189–195, 2010.

O'Donnell ML, Creamer M, Holmes ACN, et al: Posttraumatic stress disorder after injury: does admission to intensive care unit increase risk? *J Trauma* 69(3):627–632, 2010.

O'Mahony R, Murthy L, Akunne A, et al: Synopsis of the National Institute for Health and Clinical Excellence guideline for prevention of delirium, *Ann Intern Med* 154(11):746–751, 2011.

Owens D, Flom J: Integrating palliative and neurological critical care, *AACN Clin Issues* 16(4):542–550, 2005.

Pasero C, McCaffery M: *Pain assessment and pharmacologic management*, St Louis, 2011, Mosby Elsevier.

Pasero C, Puntillo K, Li D, et al: Structured approaches to pain management in the ICU, *Chest* 135(6):1665–1672, 2009.

Patton RM: Is diagnosis of pressure ulcers within an RN's scope of practice? *Am Nurse* 5(1):20, 2010.

Payen JF, Chanques G, Mantz J, et al: Current practices in sedation and analgesia for mechanically ventilated critically ill patients, *Anesthesiology* 106(4):687–695, 2007.

Payen JF, Bru O, Bosson JL, et al: Assessing pain in critically ill sedated patients by using a behavioral pain scale, *Crit Care Med* 29(12):2258–2263, 2001.

Pittman J, Beeson T, Terry C, et al: Methods of bowel management in critical care: a randomized controlled trial, *J Wound Ostomy Continence Nurs* 39(6):633–639, 2012.

Pittman RN: *Regulation of tissue oxygenation*, San Rafael, 2011, Morgan and Claypool Life Sciences.

Plank LD, Connolly AB, Hill GL: Sequential changes in the metabolic response in severely septic patients during the first 23 days after onset of peritonitis, *Ann Surg* 228(2):146–158, 1998.

Plank LD, Hill GL: Sequential metabolic changes following induction of inflammatory response in patients with severe sepsis or major blunt trauma, *World J Surg* 24(6):630–638, 2000.

Porter R, editor: Fluid and electrolyte metabolism. In *The Merck manual*, Whitehouse Station, 2006, Merck Research Laboratories.

Puntillo K, Arai SR, Cooper BA, et al: A randomized clinical trial of an intervention to relieve thirst and dry mouth in intensive care unit patients, *Intensive Care Med* 40(9):1295–1302, 2014.

Puntillo KA, White C, Morris AB, et al: Patients' perceptions and responses to procedural pain: results from Thunder Project II, *Am J Crit Care* 10(4):238–251, 2001.

Rajaram SS, Desai NK, Kalro A, et al: Pulmonary artery catheter for adult patients in intensive care, *Cochrane Database Syst Rev* 2:CD003408, 2013.

Rees J, Sharpe A: The use of bowel management systems in the high dependency setting, *Br J Nurs* 18(7):S19–S20, S22, S24, 2009.

Registered Nurses Association of Ontario (RNAO): *Risk assessment and prevention of pressure ulcers*, Toronto, 2005, Registered Nurses Association of Ontario.

Reilly EF, Karakousis GC, Schrag SP, et al: Pressure ulcers in the intensive care unit: the "forgotten" enemy, *OPUS 12 Scientist* 1(2):17–30, 2007.

Rice TW, The National Heart, Lung and Blood Institute Acute Respiratory Distress Syndrome (ARDS) Clinical Trials Network: Initial trophic versus full enteral feeding in patients with acute lung injury. The EDEN randomized trial, *JAMA* 307(8):795–803, 2012.

Rice TW, Wheeler AP, Thompson BT, et al: Enteral omega-3 fatty acid, gamma-linolenic acid, and antioxidant supplementation in acute lung injury, *JAMA* 306(14):1574–1581, 2011.

Richards KC, Gibson R, Overton-McCoy AL: Effects of massage in acute and critical care, *AACN Clin Issues* 11(1):77–96, 2000.

Riker RR, Fraser GL: Altering intensive care sedation paradigms to improve patient outcomes, *Anesthesiol Clin* 29(4):663–674, 2011.

Rock R: Get positive results from negative pressure wound therapy, *Wound Care Advisor* 1(2):15–19, 2012.

Rose L, Nokoyama N, Rezai S, et al: Psychological wellbeing, health related quality of life and memories of intensive care and a specialised weaning centre reported by survivors of prolonged mechanical ventilation, *Intensive Crit Care Nurs* 30(3):145–151, 2013.

Rose L, Smith O, Gelinas C, et al: Critical care nurses' pain assessment and management practices: a survey in Canada, *Am J Crit Care* 21(4):251–259, 2012.

Russo CA, Elixhauser A: *Hospitalizations related to pressure sores*, 2003. Healthcare cost and utilization project, Rockville, 2006, Agency for Healthcare Research and Quality. http://www.hcup_us.ahrq.gov/reprts/statbriefs/sb3.pdf.

Sauls J: The use of ice for pain associated with chest tube removal, *Pain Manag Nurs* 3(2):44–52, 2002.

Schier JG, Howland MA, Hoffman RS, Nelson LS: Fatality from administration of labetalol and crushed extended-release nifedipine, *Ann Pharmacother* 37(10):1420–1423, 2003.

Schlein KM, Coulter SP: Best practices for determining resting energy expenditure in critically ill adults, *Nutr Clin Pract* 29(1):44–55, 2014.

Sessler CN, Gosnell M, Grap MJ, et al: The Richmond Agitation-Sedation Scale: validity and reliability in adult intensive care patients, *Am J Respir Crit Care Med* 166(10):1338–1344, 2002.

Shehabi Y, Bellomo R, Reade MC, et al: Early intensive care sedation predicts long-term mortality in ventilated critically ill patients, *Am J Respir Crit Care Med* 186(8):724–731, 2012.

Siddiqi N, Stockdale R, Britton A, Holmes J: Interventions for preventing delirium in hospitalized patients, *Cochrane Database Syst Rev* 2:CD005563, 2007.

Siffleet J, Young J, Nikoletti S, Shaw T: Patients' self-report of procedural pain in the intensive care unit, *J Clin Nurs* 16(11):2142–2148, 2007.

Smith BS, Yogaratnam D, Levasseur-Franklin KE, et al: Introduction to drug pharmacokinetics in the critically ill patient, *Chest* 141(5):1327–1336, 2012.

Society of Critical Care Medicine and American Society of Health-System Pharmacists: Sedation, analgesia, and neuromuscular blockade of the critically ill adult: revised clinical practice guidelines for 2002, *Am J Health Syst Pharm* 59(2):147–149, 2002.

Stevens R, Nyquist P: Coma, delirium, and cognitive dysfunction in critical illness, *Crit Care Clin* 22(4):787–804, 2007.

Stotts NA, Puntillo K, Morris AB, et al: Wound care pain in hospitalized adult patients, *Heart Lung* 33(5):321–332, 2004.

Strom T, Martinussen T, Toft P: A protocol of no sedation for critically ill patients receiving mechanical ventilation: a randomised trial, *Lancet* 375(9713):475–480, 2010.

Tablan OC, Anderson LJ, Besser R, et al: Guidelines for preventing health care-associated pneumonia, 2003: recommendations of CDC and the Healthcare Infection Control Practices Advisory Committee, *MMWR Recomm Rep* 53(RR-3):1–36, 2004.

The Joint Commission: Sentinel event alert: *Preventing ventilator-related deaths and injuries*, February 26, 2005. http://www.jointcommission.org/SentinelEvents/SentinelEventAlert.

Tomasi CD, Grandi C, Salluh J, et al: Comparison of CAM-ICU and ICDSC for the detection of delirium in critically ill patients focusing on relevant clinical outcomes, *J Crit Care* 27(2):212–217, 2012.

Tracy MF, Lindquist R, Savik K, et al: Use of complementary and alternative therapies: a national survey of critical care nurses, *Am J Crit Care* 14(5):404–414, quiz 415–416, 2005.

Trompeo AC, Vidi Y, Locane MD, et al: Sleep disturbances in the critically ill patients: role of delirium and sedative agents, *Minerva Anestesiol* 77(6):604–612, 2011.

Tufano R, Piazza O, De Robertis E: Guidelines and the medical "art", *Intensive Care Med* 36(9):1612–1613, 2010.

van den Boogaard M, Schoonhoven L, van der Hoeven J, et al: Incidence and short-term consequences of delirium in critically ill patients: a prospective, observational, cohort study, *Int J Nurs Stud* 49(7):775–783, 2012.

van den Boogaard M, Schoonhoven L, van Achterberg T, et al: Haloperidol prophylaxis in critically ill patients with a high risk for delirium, *Crit Care* 17(R9):1–11, 2013.

van Eijk MM, Roes KC, Honing ML, et al: Effect of rivastigmine as an adjunct to usual care with haloperidol on duration of delirium and mortality in critically ill patients: a multicentre, double-blind, placebo-controlled randomised trial, *Lancet* 376(9755):1829–1837, 2010.

Vanek VW, Borum P, Buchman A, et al: A.S.P.E.N. position paper recommendations for changes in commercially available parenteral multivitamin and multi-trace element products, *Nutr Clin Pract* 27(4):440–491, 2012.

Vasilevskis EE, Ely EW, Speroff T, et al: Reducing iatrogenic risks: ICU-acquired delirium and weakness – crossing the quality chasm, *Chest* 138(5):1224–1233, 2010.

Verhaeghe S, Defloor T, Grypdonck M: Stress and coping among families of patients with traumatic brain injury: a review of the literature, *J Clin Nurs* 14(8):1004–1012, 2005.

Walsh NS, Blanck AW, Smith I, et al: Use of a sacral silicone border foam dressing as one component of a pressure ulcer prevention program in an intensive care unit setting, *J Wound Ostomy Continence Nurs* 39(2):146–149, 2012.

White JV, Guenter P, Jensen G, et al: Consensus statement: Academy of Nutrition and Dietetics and American Society for Parenteral and Enteral Nutrition: characteristics recommended for the identification and documentation of adult malnutrition (undernutrition), *JPEN J Parenter Enteral Nutr* 36(3):275–283, 2012.

Williams NT: Medication administration through enteral feeding tubes, *Am J Health Syst Pharm* 65(24):2347–2357, 2008.

Woolf CJ, Salter MW: Neuroscience-neuronal plasticity: increasing the gain in pain, *Science* 288(5472):1765–1768, 2000.

World Union of Wound Healing Societies: *Principles of best practice: minimizing pain at wound dressing-related procedures, a consensus document*, 2008. http://www.wuwhs.org.

Wound Ostomy and Continence Nurses (WOCN) Society: *Guideline for prevention and management of pressure ulcers*, Mount Laurel, 2010, Wound Ostomy and Continence Nurses (WOCN) Society.

Managing the Critical Care Environment

BIOTERRORISM

Bioterrorism is the intentional release of a biological agent, generally aimed at causing as great a number of people as possible to suffer illness and death. A bioterrorism event should be suspected when there is an unusual and unexplained increase in an illness.

The Centers for Disease Control and Prevention (CDC) identified six biological agents as Category A, of highest concern for use in terrorism: anthrax, botulism, hemorrhagic fever viruses, plague, smallpox, and tularemia. Several factors explain why these agents are more likely to be used:

1. Most people are susceptible to these organisms.
2. Most can be aerosolized, but not all are transmitted in the air.
3. They are fairly stable in aerosolized form.
4. Because of reason 3, agents transmitted through the air can cause disease in a large group of individuals without direct contact. Agents recognized as Category A transmitted by contact are exceptionally virulent and, when not recognized early, can spread rapidly and become an epidemic.
5. Resultant diseases are difficult to diagnose and treat.
6. They have high morbidity and/or mortality rates.
7. Despite prevention and surveillance efforts to date, the international community remains underprepared to fully address the threat. As of 2012, more than 80% of nations failed to meet the international requirements of the World Health Organization (WHO) to ensure they are prepared to manage pandemics or bioterrorism.

BIOTERRORISM ASSESSMENT: SURVEILLANCE

GOAL OF SURVEILLANCE
The goal is to detect a biological event as early as possible to limit the spread of the infection.

KEY SIGNS
Bioterrorism should be suspected when the following situations are seen:
- An outbreak of an illness within a short period of time, similar to one that happens in a healthy population, without a link to explain the transmission such as a similar food source.
- An outbreak of an illness that occurs at an unusual time of year.
- An outbreak with an unusual age distribution.
- A large cluster of patients are affected by an uncommon disease, which results in a higher than expected death rate.
- The severity of the disease is increased with patients having unusual routes of exposure.
- Strains of organisms seen have unusual antibiotic resistance.
- Those indoors are not as affected as or "as are those" who have been outdoors.
- With some strains, an increased number of dead animals is noted.
- Those presenting within 48 to 72 hours of exposure have likely been exposed to a biological agent, as opposed to those exposed to a toxin, who present within a few hours.

In 2003, the U.S. Department of Homeland Security introduced BioWatch; a federally supported environmental monitoring system designed to speed detection of specific bioterrorism agents released in aerosolized form during an attack. BioWatch air sampling devices have been deployed primarily outdoors, in more than 30 major urban areas. Samples are screened in designated laboratories every 24 hours for genetic material from specified pathogens.

In 2007, Homeland Security Presidential Directive 21 "Public Health and Medical Preparedness" (HSPD-21) recognized the health-related security threats to the nation. HSPD-21 was established a as federal advisory committee including "representatives from state and local government, public health authorities, and appropriate private sector health care entities, to ensure that the federal government is meeting the goal of enabling state and local government public health surveillance capabilities."

The U.S. Department of Health and Human Services received and subsequently delegated implementation of the mandate to the CDC. On May 1, 2008, the CDC established the National Biosurveillance Advisory Subcommittee (NBAS), a group of well-recognized experts from public health, health care providers, academics, the U.S. Department of Homeland Security, the U.S. Department of Defense, and the private sector to advise the federal government. The Advisory Committee of the Director is informed by the NBAS of issues that impact development and implementation of a nationwide biosurveillance strategy to promote human health.

MONITOR

- Observe for an unusual or unexplained increase in an illness, especially with the characteristics listed in Key Signs.

U.S. President Barack Obama developed a Global Health Security Agenda in 2014. The United States and several international partners are leading the global community to ensure appropriate steps are taken to increase worldwide security against infectious diseases.

The proposed strategy for international security against bioterrorism is as follows:

1. Prevent outbreaks by mitigating risks. Well-developed laboratory systems are needed in all countries to identify pathogens and facilitate "right care at the right time": right drug and right dosage at the right time. Protocols to protect and defend key laboratories from terrorists attempting to acquire biological weapons are needed, along with routine, universal immunizations for the worldwide population.
2. Detect disease threats immediately in all countries. Improved specialized biosurveillance systems require trained participants to monitor incidence of diseases, identify cases, determine the cause, and contain outbreaks before they become epidemics.
3. Respond more quickly to occurrences. All nations require well-developed emergency management systems with a unified response. Improved strategies are needed to mobilize international resources, including strengthening the ability of global health organizations to respond more quickly and comprehensively to crises.

As part of the 2014 Global Health Security Agenda, the United States pledged to assist more than 30 countries to meet these targets and has challenged the international community to assist in dedicating the resources needed to implement the proposed strategies.

REPORT

- All occurrences of the six Category A diseases must be reported to the CDC.
- The CDC also monitors Category B organisms (includes Brucellosis [*Brucella* sp.], epsilon toxin of *Clostridium perfringens*, food safety threats [e.g., *Salmonella* sp., *Escherichia coli* O157:H7, *Shigella*], glanders [*Burkholderia mallei*], melioidosis [*Burkholderia pseudomallei*], psittacosis [*Chlamydia psittaci*], Q fever [*Coxiella burnetii*], ricin toxin from *Ricinus communis* [castor beans], staphylococcal enterotoxin B, typhus fever [*Rickettsia prowazekii*], viral encephalitis [alphaviruses, e.g., Venezuelan equine encephalitis, Eastern equine encephalitis, Western equine encephalitis], and water safety threats [e.g., *Vibrio cholerae, Cryptosporidium parvum*]). These organisms are the second highest priority.
  - Category C organisms are the third highest priority agents and include emerging pathogens that could be engineered for mass dissemination in the future because of availability, ease of production and dissemination, and potential for high morbidity and mortality rates, and major health impact. The agents include emerging infectious diseases such as Nipah virus and hantavirus.

CONTAIN (PREVENT THE SPREAD OF THE DISEASE)

- Appropriate personal protective equipment (PPE) and isolation precautions need to be taken to inhibit the spread of the infectious agent.

LABWORK

* Appropriate laboratory studies should be done to confirm the presence of the suspected biological agent. Many of these diseases require testing at specialty laboratories because these are uncommon bacteria and most hospital laboratories are not set up to test for these agents.

ANTHRAX
PATHOPHYSIOLOGY

Anthrax is a serious disease caused by *Bacillus anthracis*, a spore-forming bacterium. A spore is a dormant (inactive) cell that activates under the right conditions. Anthrax spores, once inside the human body, are able to germinate. Once germinated, the replicating bacteria release endotoxins leading to hemorrhage, edema, and necrosis.

There are three types of anthrax: skin (cutaneous), lung (inhalation), and digestive (gastrointestinal). Hemorrhagic mediastinitis is present with the inhalation form, and bloody diarrhea is seen with the intestinal form. When enough endotoxin is released into the bloodstream, the disease can be fatal even if antibiotics eradicate the bacteria. Anthrax infections are usually very rare because it takes thousands of spores to cause an infection. Inhalation anthrax is usually fatal even with treatment. Gastrointestinal anthrax has a mortality rate of 25% to 60%, whereas 20% of those with untreated cutaneous anthrax die. Cutaneous anthrax is rarely fatal unless untreated.

TRANSMISSION

Anthrax has not been known to spread from one person to another. Humans may acquire anthrax by handling products from infected animals or inhaling anthrax spores from infected animal products (e.g., wool). People acquire gastrointestinal anthrax by eating undercooked meat from infected animals. Anthrax in soil may enter the body through open skin. The organism is easy to obtain, produce, and store.

ASSESSMENT

The symptoms (warning signs) of anthrax differ depending on the type of disease:

* Inhalation: The most serious form with the highest mortality rate, this begins 1 to 6 days after exposure with cold or influenza (flu)-like symptoms, with sore throat, mild fever, and muscle aches. Later symptoms include cough, chest discomfort, shortness of breath, fatigue, and muscle aches. Inhalation anthrax quickly progresses to respiratory failure and shock. Chest radiograph reveals a widened mediastinum and pleural effusions.
* Cutaneous: The first symptom is a raised, itchy bump that develops into a blister, seen 1 to 7 days after exposure. The blister progresses to a skin ulcer with a blackened center. The sore, the blister, and the ulcer are painless. Fever, headache, and swollen glands may occur.
* Gastrointestinal: At 2 to 5 days after exposure, the person exhibits nausea, loss of appetite, bloody diarrhea, and fever, followed by severe stomach pain. If untreated, it can progress to generalized toxemia and sepsis.

DIAGNOSTIC TESTS

Diagnostic tests to isolate anthrax antigen are not widely available. Confirmation of the diagnosis is made by sending a specimen to a national reference laboratory after the treatment begins. Clinicians should begin treatment based on clinical signs and symptoms, because early treatment is imperative to enhance chances of survival from inhalation anthrax. Standard blood culture may be useful if the laboratory is told to look for bacillus species. A Gram stain, enzyme-linked immunosorbent assay (ELISA), and nasal swab check for spores may also be useful.

COLLABORATIVE MANAGEMENT
CARE PRIORITIES
1. Antibiotics

Used to treat all three types of anthrax. Ideally, the antibiotic should be based on culture and sensitivity results. If those are not available, the antibiotics of choice are doxycycline and ciprofloxacin. Additionally, levofloxacin is recommended for adults. Occasionally, rifampin may also be used. Early identification and treatment are crucial to minimize the amount of endotoxin released.

2. Intubation and mechanical ventilation (inhalation)
To support gas exchange and help maintain acid-base balance.

3. Intravenous fluids (inhalation and gastrointestinal)
To prevent dehydration and maintain adequate circulatory volume.

4. Prevention after exposure
Treatment differs when a person exposed to anthrax is not yet having symptoms. Health care providers use antibiotics (e.g., ciprofloxacin, doxycycline, penicillin) combined with anthrax vaccine to prevent anthrax infection and, for contact anthrax, instruct the exposed person to immediately scrub hands and arms or take a shower (if available) and remove and place their clothes in a plastic bag when apprised of an exposure.

5. Treatment after infection
Treatment is usually a 60-day course of antibiotics. Success depends on the type of anthrax, the general health of the individual, and how early treatment begins. A 60-day course is necessary so that the antibiotic is in the person's system when the spores activate. Inactive spores are not susceptible to antibiotics.

6. Vaccination
A vaccine to prevent anthrax exists, but it is not yet available to the general public. Anyone at risk for anthrax exposure, including certain members of the U.S. Armed Forces, laboratory workers, and workers who may enter or reenter contaminated areas, may be vaccinated. If anthrax is used as a weapon, a vaccination program will be initiated to vaccinate as many exposed people as possible.

CARE PLANS: ANTHRAX

Gas exchange, impaired *related to respiratory insufficiency from respiratory tract infection secondary to inhalation of anthrax.*

Goals/Outcomes: Within 12 to 24 hours of treatment, the patient has adequate gas exchange, as evidenced by Pao_2 at least 80 mm Hg, $Paco_2$ 35 to 45 mm Hg, pH 7.35 to 7.45, presence of normal breath sounds, and absence of adventitious breath sounds. The respiratory rate (RR) is 12 to 20 breaths/min with normal pattern and depth.

NOC Respiratory Status: Gas Exchange.

Respiratory Monitoring
1. Monitor rate, rhythm, and depth of respirations.
2. Note chest movement for symmetry of chest expansion and signs of increased work of breathing such as use of accessory muscles or retraction of intercostal or supraclavicular muscles.
3. Monitor for diaphragmatic muscle fatigue.
4. Ensure airway is not obstructed by tongue (snoring or choking-type respirations) and monitor breathing patterns. New patterns that impair ventilation should be managed as appropriate for setting.
5. Auscultate breath sounds noting areas of decrease/absent ventilation and presence of adventitious sounds.
6. Note changes in oxygen saturation from arterial blood gases (Sao_2), pulse oximetry (Spo_2), and end-tidal CO_2 ($ETCO_2$) as appropriate.
7. Monitor for increased restlessness or anxiety.
8. If increased restlessness or unusual somnolence occurs, evaluate the patient for hypoxemia and hypercapnia as appropriate.
9. Monitor chest x-ray reports as new films become available.

Oxygen Therapy
1. Administer supplemental oxygen using liter flow and device as ordered. Add humidity as appropriate.
2. Restrict the patient and visitors from smoking while oxygen is in use.

3. Document pulse oximetry with oxygen liter flow in place at time of reading as ordered. Oxygen is a drug; the dose of the drug must be associated with the oxygen saturation reading or the reading is meaningless.
4. Obtain arterial blood gases (ABGs) if the patient experiences behavioral changes or respiratory distress, to check for hypoxemia or hypercapnia.
5. Monitor for changes in chest radiograph and breath sounds indicative of oxygen toxicity and absorption atelectasis in patients receiving higher concentrations of oxygen (greater than Fio$_2$ 45%) for longer than 24 hours. The higher the oxygen concentration, the greater the chance of toxicity.
6. Monitor for skin breakdown where oxygen devices are in contact with skin, such as nares and around edges of mask devices.
7. Provide oxygen therapy during transportation and when the patient gets out of bed.

Mechanical Ventilation
1. Monitor for conditions indicating a need for ventilation support.
2. Monitor for impending respiratory failure.
3. Consult with other health care providers to select the ventilatory mode.
4. Administer muscle-paralyzing agents, sedatives, and narcotic analgesics as appropriate.
5. Monitor the effectiveness of mechanical ventilation on the physiologic and psychological status of the patient.
6. Provide the patient with means of communication.
7. Monitor adverse effects of mechanical ventilation.
8. Perform routine mouth care.
9. Elevate the head of the bed (HOB) up to 45 degrees as tolerated.

BOTULISM
PATHOPHYSIOLOGY

Botulism is a muscle-paralyzing disease associated with respiratory dysfunction caused by a toxin produced from *Clostridium botulinum* bacteria. The toxin is the most potent lethal substance known to humans. Man-made inhalational botulism is brought into being when aerosolized botulinum toxin is inhaled. The bacterium naturally lives for weeks in nonmoving water and food. There are three naturally acquired types of botulism:

* Foodborne: A person ingests toxin that leads to illness in a few hours to days.
* Infant: Occurs in a small number of susceptible infants each year who harbor *C. botulinum* in their intestinal tracts.
* Wound: Occurs when a wound is infected with *C. botulinum*.

Botulinum toxin, once absorbed into the bloodstream, is transported to the peripheral cholinergic synapses, where it binds irreversibly. The toxin then blocks the release of acetylcholine in the neuromuscular junctions, causing paralysis of the muscles.

TRANSMISSION

Botulism is not spread from person to person. Botulinum toxin is absorbed through lung or intestinal mucosa and nonintact skin. Foodborne botulism occurs in all age groups.

ASSESSMENT

* Foodborne: Double vision, drooping eyelids, slurred speech, dysphagia, dry mouth, and descending muscle weakness are symptoms. Weakness starts in the shoulders and upper arms, descends to the lower arms and upper thighs, and eventually spreads down to the lower legs and feet. Paralysis of the respiratory muscles leads to respiratory failure unless ventilation is supported with mechanical ventilation. Patients are generally afebrile and alert.
* Respiratory assessment: Patients who are not intubated should have their respiratory status monitored closely to detect deterioration in respiratory muscle strength. One of the best assessment tools is periodic measurement of negative inspiratory force (NIF). If the NIF falls below 20 cm H_2O, the patient is likely to require intubation and mechanical ventilation.

DIAGNOSTIC TESTS

Currently, the CDC and fewer than 25 public health laboratories perform the diagnostic test for botulism. Diagnosis is made clinically, after ruling out other causes of paralysis. Classic botulism paralysis is descending in nature and involves the cranial nerves.

Bioterrorism

COLLABORATIVE MANAGEMENT
CARE PRIORITIES
1. Antitoxin
Botulinum antitoxin is available in two forms from the CDC. Because both are equine derivatives, it is important to perform a skin test as directed in the package insert to check for hypersensitivity before administering. Antitoxin helps prevent further nerve damage from the botulinum toxin but cannot reverse the existing paralysis. It is most effective if given within the first 24 hours. The antitoxin is not effective in infant botulism. For infant botulism, botulism immune globulin-intravenous (BIG-IV) is administered.

2. Antibiotic
Antibiotics are given to treat wounds infected with *C. botulinum* and secondary infections. Antibiotics have no effect on botulinum toxin.

3. Supportive care
Includes mechanical ventilation, nutrition support, care for immobility, and treatment for secondary infections.

CARE PLANS: BOTULISM
Breathing pattern, ineffective *related to respiratory tract infection*

Goals/Outcomes: The patient demonstrates effective air exchange, as evidenced by RR 12 to 20 breaths/min, $Pao_2 \geq 80$ mm Hg, $Paco_2$ 35 to 45 mm Hg, pH 7.35 to 7.45, Sao_2 greater than 95%, Svo_2 greater than 60%, and $Ecto_2$ 5% to 6% (35 to 45 mm Hg).
NOC Respiratory Status: Ventilation.

Respiratory Monitoring
1. Monitor rate, rhythm, depth, and effort of respirations.
2. Monitor for diaphragmatic muscle fatigue.
3. Auscultate breath sounds, noting areas of decreased/absent ventilation, and presence of adventitious sounds.
4. Assess for breathing effectiveness by monitoring Sao_2, Svo_2, $Ecto_2$, and changes in ABG values, as appropriate.
5. Insert oral or nasopharyngeal airway if the patient cannot maintain patent airway; if severely distressed, the patient may require endotracheal intubation.

Ventilation Assistance
1. Position the patient to alleviate dyspnea and insure maximal ventilation, generally in a sitting upright position unless severe hypotension is present.
2. Assist with incentive spirometer, as appropriate.
3. Clear secretions from airway by having the patient cough, or provide nasotracheal, oropharyngeal, or endotracheal tube suctioning as needed.
4. Have the patient breathe slowly or manually ventilate with an Ambu (manual resuscitation) bag slowly and deeply between coughing or suctioning attempts.
5. Turn the patient every 2 hours if immobile. Encourage the patient to turn self or get out of bed as much as tolerated if able to do so.

HEMORRHAGIC FEVER VIRUSES
PATHOPHYSIOLOGY
Hemorrhagic fever viruses (HFVs) include many diseases separated into four families of viruses; not all are viewed as risks for bioterrorism. Those thought to or that have posed a significant risk include Ebola virus disease, Marburg virus disease, Lassa fever, New World Arenaviridae, Rift Valley fever, yellow fever, Omsk hemorrhagic fever, and Kyasanur forest disease. In 2014, the largest, most devastating outbreak of Ebola virus occurred in West Africa, affecting thousands of African people and international aid workers including health care professionals. The pathophysiology of these diseases is not well understood. Outbreaks are sporadic and have occurred in areas with very limited health care. Infection with these viruses

leads to thrombocytopenia and possibly platelet dysfunction. The effects of these viruses vary, but all lead to coagulation problems, hemorrhage, and shock. Mortality ranges from less than 1% with Rift Valley fever to 50% to 90% with Ebola virus. Only one of the Arenaviridae viruses has been identified in the United States. Other HFVs have not emerged.

TRANSMISSION

HFVs reside in many animal hosts and arthropod vectors. Humans become infected when bitten by an infected arthropod, by inhaling aerosolized virus from infected rodent excreta, from direct contact with infected animal carcasses, and from other human beings. Humans infected with Ebola, Marburg, Lassa fever, and arenaviruses can spread the disease through contact with body fluids.

ISOLATION

Strict droplet and contact precautions are required if a patient is suspected of infection. The recommendations for management of Ebola patients has evolved worldwide. It was recognized that a large number of secondary infections from Ebola virus disease during the 2014 outbreak occurred in health care workers exposed during care of infected patients. Leading U.S. special contagious disease centers have used full-body Tyvek suits and powered air purifying respirator (PAPR) hoods as part of the contact and droplet precautions protocol.

ASSESSMENT

Clinical scenarios vary depending on the virus. The most common symptom is a fever.
- Ebola and Marburg: Maculopapular rash, bleeding, disseminated intravascular coagulation (DIC), jaundice, nausea, vomiting, diarrhea, and headache.
- Lassa fever and New World arenaviruses: Gradual onset of fever, nausea, abdominal pain, conjunctivitis, and jaundice. Severe exudative pharyngitis in Lassa fever.
- Rift Valley fever: Fever, headache, photophobia, and jaundice.

DIAGNOSTIC TESTS

Only the CDC and U.S. Army Research Institute of Infectious Diseases laboratories have testing available.

COLLABORATIVE MANAGEMENT

CARE PRIORITIES

1. Supportive care

Maintain fluid and electrolyte balances, and treat hypotension with early use of vasopressors if fluid therapy is not effective, mechanical ventilation, renal dialysis, and anticonvulsive therapy. Administration of clotting factor concentrates, platelets, fresh-frozen plasma, and heparin in patients with DIC.

2. Antivirals

These agents are not effective against these diseases.

3. Ribavirin

Institute a 10-day course if Lassa fever or New World arenavirus is confirmed.

4. Control risk for bleeding

Intramuscular injections, aspirin, nonsteroidal antiinflammatory drugs, steroids, and anticoagulant therapies are contraindicated.

5. Vaccine

A vaccine is available for yellow fever, which is only recommended for travelers going to South America or Africa where yellow fever is endemic and for laboratory personnel who are exposed to yellow fever samples. The vaccine is not helpful postexposure because the short incubation period does not allow immunity to develop if the vaccine is administered following exposure.

Bioterrorism

PLAGUE

PATHOPHYSIOLOGY

Plague is an infectious disease caused by the bacterium *Yersinia pestis* that is found in rodents and their fleas. Several forms of plague can occur individually or in combination: bubonic, pneumonic, and septicemic plague. Bubonic plague is the most common, occurring when an infected flea bites a human or when infectious materials enter through a break in the skin. Pneumonic plague occurs when *Y. pestis* infects the lungs through direct or close contact with a person who has pneumonic plague or in untreated patients with bubonic or septicemic plague, allowing bacterial spread to the lungs. Septicemic plague can occur as a complication of either of the previous types of plague or alone. The bacteria enter the bloodstream and multiply, prompting the systemic effects of sepsis.

The *Y. pestis* bacteria travel to lymph nodes, where they resist defense mechanisms and rapidly multiply, causing destruction of lymph nodes. Bacteria enter the bloodstream and prompt sepsis, septic shock, DIC, and coma. Without treatment, mortality approaches 100%; with treatment, the mortality can be as low as 5%.

TRANSMISSION

Pneumonic plague is spread through direct contact with an infected person. Neither bubonic nor septicemic plagues are transmitted by person-to-person contact.
- Pneumonic plague: Droplet precautions until the patient receives antibiotics for 72 hours.
- Bubonic or septicemic plague: Standard precautions.

ASSESSMENT

- Pneumonic plague: Fever, headache, weakness, and rapidly developing pneumonia with shortness of breath, chest pain, cough, and sometimes bloody or watery sputum. The pneumonia progresses and in 2 to 4 days can cause respiratory failure and shock. Without treatment, patients with pneumonic plague will die.
- Bubonic plague: Swollen, tender lymph glands (called buboes), fever, headache, chills, and weakness.
- Septicemic plague: Fever and chills, abdominal pain, and shock with bleeding (caused by DIC).

DIAGNOSTIC TESTS

- Gram stain of sputum or blood: Reveals gram-negative bacilli. A laboratory may misidentify the bacteria unless notified that *Y. pestis* is suspected.

COLLABORATIVE MANAGEMENT

CARE PRIORITIES

1. Antibiotics

Given within the first 24 hours of symptoms. Streptomycin, gentamicin, tetracyclines, and chloramphenicol are all effective in treating pneumonic plague. The preferred choice in adults is streptomycin 1 g intramuscularly (IM) twice a day for 10 days or gentamicin 5 mg/kg either IM or IV once a day or 2 mg/kg loading dose followed by 1.7 mg/kg administered IM or IV three times a day for 10 days. In children, the drug of choice is streptomycin 15 mg/kg IM twice a day with maximum dose of 2 g or gentamicin 2.5 mg/kg IM or IV three times a day for 10 days.

2. Vaccine

There currently is no vaccine available in the United States. Work is currently under way to develop a vaccine.

3. Supportive care

Ventilatory support, pain management, and treatment for shock, DIC, and multiorgan dysfunction syndrome, as appropriate.

SMALLPOX (VARIOLA)
PATHOPHYSIOLOGY

Smallpox is a serious, contagious, and sometimes fatal infectious disease. It is a member of the orthopoxvirus family, along with monkeypox, vaccinia, and cowpox. Although all of these can cause skin lesions, only smallpox is readily transmitted from person to person. There are two main clinical forms of smallpox: Variola major and Variola minor, with several additional strains. Variola major is the severe and most common form of smallpox, with a more extensive rash and higher fever. Historically, Variola major had a 30% mortality rate. Variola minor was less common and much less severe. Smallpox was eradicated after a successful worldwide vaccination program. The last case of smallpox in the United States was in 1949. The last naturally occurring case in the world was in Somalia in 1977. There is currently questionable access to the virus since the separation of the Soviet Union, because Moscow and the United States housed the only two storage laboratories at that time.

Smallpox virus enters the body through the mucosa in the oropharyngeal and respiratory tracts. The virus multiplies in the lymph nodes, the spleen, and the bone marrow. Eventually the virus, contained in lymphocytes, localizes in small blood vessels of the dermis and infects adjacent cells, causing the pustules to form.

Smallpox is an excellent agent for bioterrorism because it is easy to both transport and store, and because it is very stable and markedly virulent when aerosolized.

TRANSMISSION

Smallpox is transmitted via droplet nuclei or aerosols expelled from the oropharynx of an infected person. Usually direct and fairly prolonged face-to-face contact was required to spread smallpox from person to person. Smallpox can be spread through direct contact with infected bodily fluids or contaminated objects (e.g., bedding or clothing). Rarely, the virus spreads through the air in enclosed settings (e.g., buildings, buses, trains). Humans are the only natural hosts of variola (there is no recorded transmissions from animals or insects).

A person with smallpox is sometimes contagious with onset of fever (prodrome phase). Most infected persons become contagious with the onset of rash. At this stage, the person is usually very sick, unable to move around in the community. The person remains contagious until the last smallpox scab falls off.

ASSESSMENT

- Clinical case definition: An illness with acute onset of fever $\geq$101° F (38.3° C), followed by a rash characterized by firm, deep-seated vesicles or pustules in the same stage of development without any other apparent cause. These characteristics help differentiate the smallpox from chickenpox. Smallpox may be easily missed in the early stage by health care providers.
- Incubation period: Usually 12 to 14 days but can range from 7 to 17 days. During this time, the patient feels fine and is not contagious.
- Prodromal period: Begins with a high fever (101° F to 104° F), malaise, headache, and backache. The patient may exhibit severe abdominal pains, vomiting, and delirium. This period lasts for 2 to 4 days before a rash develops. The rash begins with small red spots on the tongue and mouth. During this phase, the person is most contagious.
- Rash development: Progresses in the mouth and develops on the skin, starting on the face and moving to the arms and legs and then to the feet and hands. It usually spreads to all parts within 24 hours. When the rash appears, the patient's fever subsides and the patient starts to feel better. On day 3, the rash consists of raised bumps. On day 4, the bumps fill with thick, cloudy fluid with a possible indent in the center. Indentation is the classic sign of smallpox rash. The bumps become pustules and eventually scab over. During the pustule stage, the patient is again febrile. After 2 weeks, most of the sores have scabs, which begin to fall off, leaving marks that will become pitted scars on the skin.

DIAGNOSTIC TESTS

Laboratory diagnostic testing for variola should be done by a CDC Laboratory Response Network (LRN) laboratory using LRN-approved polymerase chain reaction (PCR) tests and protocols for variola virus. Laboratory testing should be reserved for cases that meet the clinical case definition, thus classified as being a potential high risk for smallpox.

Safety Alert   *Initial confirmation of a smallpox outbreak requires additional testing at the Centers for Disease Control and Prevention.*

LABORATORY CRITERIA FOR CONFIRMATION OF SMALLPOX
- PCR identification of variola DNA in a clinical specimen.
- Isolation of smallpox (variola) virus from a clinical specimen (WHO Smallpox Reference Laboratory or laboratory with appropriate reference capabilities) with variola PCR confirmation.

COLLABORATIVE MANAGEMENT
There are no approved treatments for smallpox. Currently, treatment consists of supportive care. However, cidofovir, an antiviral, is currently being studied to see if it is effective against the smallpox virus.

CARE PRIORITIES
1. Vaccine
A key is to identify smallpox exposure and administer vaccine within 3 days, to prevent or significantly lessen the severity of the disease process. Vaccine administered within 4 to 7 days after exposure may provide some protection and lessen the disease severity.

2. Isolation
Patients presenting with symptoms should be isolated immediately in a negative-pressure room. The door should be kept closed at all times. All health care workers entering the room should wear an N-95 respirator mask. Because smallpox is also transmitted via body fluids (contaminating the bedding), health care workers should use contact precautions (i.e., gown, gloves, and shoe covers) when entering the room. Other infection control practices, such as limiting patient transport, designating patient care equipment, and so forth, should follow the institution's policies. Linen should be autoclaved and corpses cremated.

3. Supportive management
- Provide hydration: Intravenous fluids to prevent dehydration.
- Provide nutrition: To help strengthen the immune system.
- Initiate mechanical ventilation: If the patient experiences respiratory failure.
- Hemodynamic monitoring: If management of fluid balance and blood pressure is difficult.
- Control fever: Antipyretics to reduce body temperature if greater than 103° F.
- Reduce pain and anxiety: Analgesics and sedatives as indicated.

CARE PLANS: SMALLPOX
Body image, disturbed   *related to numerous skin lesions resulting from infection with smallpox.*

Goals/Outcomes: The patient will acknowledge change in physical appearance and express a positive self-worth. **NOC** Body Image, Self-Esteem.

Body Image Enhancement
1. Use anticipatory guidance to prepare the patient for predictable changes in body image.
2. Assist the patient to discuss changes caused by illness.
3. Assist the patient to separate physical appearance from feelings of personal self-worth.
4. Identify the effects of the patient's culture, religion, race, sex, and age in terms of body image.

Emotional Support
1. Discuss with the patient the emotional experience.
2. Make supportive or empathetic statements.
3. Support the use of appropriate defense mechanisms.
4. Encourage the patient to express feelings of anxiety, anger, or sadness.

5. Listen to and encourage expressions of feelings and beliefs.
6. Refer for counseling as appropriate.

TULAREMIA

PATHOPHYSIOLOGY

Tularemia is caused by a bacterial zoonosis called *Francisella tularensis*. One of the most infectious pathogenic bacteria known, it is found in infected water, soil, vegetation, small mammals, ticks, fleas, and mosquitoes. *F. tularensis* is a small, nonmotile, aerobic, gram-negative coccobacillus that targets the lymph nodes, lungs, pleura, spleen, liver, and kidneys. Bacteria enter through skin, mucous membranes, gastrointestinal tract, and lungs to invade cells, causing inflammation and permanent damage if untreated.

TRANSMISSION

Tularemia is transmitted by bites from infected arthropods; handling infectious animal tissues or fluids; direct contact with or ingestion of contaminated water, food, or soil; and inhaling infected aerosols. There is no evidence of person-to-person transmission. Patients should be placed on standard precautions.

ASSESSMENT

- Disease presentation: May vary depending on the infecting organism, dose, and site of inoculation. It usually starts abruptly with a fever of 100.1° F to 104° F (38° C to 40° C), headache, chills, generalized body aches, rhinitis, and a sore throat. Some patients have a dry cough, substernal pain, skin or mouth ulcers, swollen painful lymph glands, and swollen and painful eyes.
- Illness progression: Progressive weakness, malaise, anorexia, and weight loss. If untreated, symptoms may persist for several weeks to months. Secondary sepsis, pleuropneumonia, and, rarely, meningitis may develop.

DIAGNOSTIC TESTS

Rapid diagnostic testing for *F. tularensis* is not widely available. If tularemia is suspected, specimens of respiratory secretions and blood should be collected and sent to a designated laboratory for microscopic identification using fluorescent-labeled antibodies.

COLLABORATIVE MANAGEMENT

CARE PRIORITIES

1. Antibiotics

Several types of antibiotics have been effective. Oral tetracyclines (i.e., doxycycline) or fluoroquinolones (i.e., ciprofloxacin) can be used. IV streptomycin and gentamicin are effective. Bacterial cultures and sensitivity data are used to determine the most appropriate treatment. The patient may be placed on a 10-day course.

EMERGING INFECTIONS

Infectious diseases pose a serious health care threat. Although medicine has been able to develop strategies to successfully prevent and treat infections, both familiar and lesser known organisms continue to present treatment challenges. Emerging infections are complex, and their evolution has been challenging for health care personnel to recognize, understand, and treat. Many infections, such as H1N1, H5N1, hantavirus, and "mad cow" disease, originate from different species of animals and spread to humans. Other infectious diseases are acquired from exposure to specific environments such as health care settings, or are transmitted from person to person. Regardless of how infections and infectious diseases are transmitted, prevention and control are challenging.

INFECTION PREVENTION AND INFECTION CONTROL

For several decades, infection prevention and control programs have focused on breaking the chain or cycle of infection. The single most important way to prevent the spread of infection is through the use of appropriate hand hygiene. Hand hygiene should be used before and after all contact with a patient or the patient's environment. The WHO identifies "Five Moments of Hand Hygiene." These include (1) before touching a patient, (2) before clean or aseptic procedures, (3) after body fluid exposure or risk, (4) after touching a patient, and (5) after touching patient surroundings. The use of hand hygiene is crucial in infection prevention and control.

Standard precautions are infection prevention practices that are designed to prevent and control the spread of infections. Standard precautions include the use of barriers or PPE (e.g., gloves, masks, and gowns) to interrupt transmission of organisms between patients and health care providers. Health care personnel should use and be familiar with the appropriate PPE depending on the risk of transmission during the activity being performed.

A tiered subset of standard precautions is transmission-based precautions. Universal precautions and other infection prevention methods are the long-standing strategies used in hospitals commonly referred to as *isolation precautions*. The most recent revision (2007) by the CDC and the Healthcare Infection Control Practices Advisory Committee reflects evidence-based practices and the knowledge base of 2007. These techniques and procedures are transmission-based, interrupting the transmission of infectious agents and adhere to five basic principles:

1. To provide infection control recommendations for the entire health care system, including hospitals, long-term care facilities, ambulatory care, home care, and hospices.
2. To reaffirm standard precautions as the foundation for preventing transmission of organism during patient care in all settings.
3. To reaffirm the importance of implementing transmission-based precautions based on the clinical presentation of the syndrome and likely pathogens until the infectious etiology is known.
4. To provide epidemiologically sound and, whenever possible, evidence-based recommendations.
5. To provide a unified infection control approach to multidrug-resistant organisms (MDROs).

The 2007 guideline contains two tiers of precautions:

1. *Standard precautions:* Designed for the care of all patients in the health care setting, regardless of diagnosis or infection status.
2. *Transmission-based precautions:* Used for patients known to be infected or colonized with epidemiologically important pathogens that can be transmitted by airborne or droplet or contact with dry skin or contaminated surfaces. Isolation techniques that prevent transmission are the following:
   a. Airborne infection isolation: For patients known or suspected to be infected with microorganisms transmitted person to person by airborne droplet nuclei that remain suspended in the air and that can be dispersed widely by air currents.
   b. Droplet: For patients known or suspected to be infected with microorganisms transmitted by respiratory droplets (more than 5 μm in size), generated by the patient coughing, sneezing, or talking or during performance of cough-inducing procedures.
   c. Contact: For patients with known or suspected infections or evidence of syndromes that represent increased risk for contact transmission, including colonization or infection with MDROs according to recommendations in the CDC guidelines (2007).
   d. Protective environment: To minimize fungal spore counts in the air for patients undergoing allogeneic, hematopoietic stem cell transplantation. Specific requirements for the protective environment were defined by the CDC in 2000.

Humans can be vulnerable, with inadequate natural defenses to control all possible infections. Our inborn defenses must be augmented to enhance infection protection. Researchers are hard pressed to develop vaccines, medications, and treatments. Regardless of sex, age, socioeconomic status, or ethnic background, infectious disease can strike at any time and may lead to significant morbidity and mortality.

MULTIDRUG-RESISTANT ORGANISMS

MDROs pose a serious health risk to the patient who is hospitalized. These organisms are resistant to one or more classes of antimicrobial agents and thus are difficult to successfully manage. Prolonged treatment leads to increased length of stay, increased health care costs, and increased morbidity and mortality. Methicillin-resistant *Staphylococcus aureus* (MRSA) and vancomycin-resistant *Enterococci* (VRE) are the most common MDROs. Several gram-negative bacilli, including Carbapenem-resistant *Enterobacteriaceae* (CRE), are developing increased resistance to treatment. MDROs are spread by person-to-person contact and by contact with contaminated environmental surfaces. Treatment is prescribed based on the sensitivity of the causative organism to the available antimicrobial agents.

Many individuals are colonized with MDROs rather than having active infections. The organism is present within the body without signs or symptoms of infection. These patients are carriers. Patients are placed on contact precautions to prevent the spread of the MDRO to others. Hand hygiene remains the most important infection control measure for the prevention of MDROs.

METHICILLIN-RESISTANT *Staphylococcus aureus* (MRSA)

MRSA is the most common organism seen in community and health care settings. MRSA most commonly occurs in skin infections but can also occur as a bloodstream infection or pneumonia where it can become life threatening. The CDC reports that invasive MRSA infections have decreased 54% from 2006 to 2011 but still pose a serious health care risk in patients who are hospitalized. Vancomycin-intermediate *Staphylococcus aureus* (VISA) and vancomycin-resistant *Staphylococcus aureus* (VRSA) are also resistant strains of *Staphylococcus aureus*. These organisms pose treatment challenges, given their resistance to the commonly appropriate antimicrobial agents.

VANCOMYCIN-RESISTANT *Enterococcus* (VRE)

VRE developed from the *enterococci* normally present in the intestines, female genitalia, and the environment, which most often cause urinary tract, bloodstream, and surgical wound infections. Enterococcal infections have often been treated with vancomycin. After many years of managing these infections with vancomycin, various strains of *enterococci* developed resistance to eradication by vancomycin. Patients most likely to develop VRE infections include those previously treated with a prolonged regimen of vancomycin or other antibiotics; patients who are hospitalized and receiving antibiotics for an extended period of time; patients who are immunosuppressed, including critically ill, oncology, and patients who have had a transplant procedure; patients who have undergone abdominal and chest surgical procedures; those with the need for prolonged management using a urinary catheter or central IV catheter; and those already colonized with VRE.

CARBAPENEM-RESISTANT *Enterobacteriaceae* (CRE)

CRE is a serious health threat with a high mortality rate. CRE is not only resistant to the carbapenem class of antibiotics but is also resistant to most other classes of antimicrobials, thus leaving very limited treatment options. The most commonly seen *Enterobacteriaceae* are *E. coli* and *Klebsiella pneumoniae*. Others include KPC (*K. pneumoniae* carbapenemase) and NDM (New Delhi metallo-beta-lactamase). News agencies have shared disturbing comments from the CDC about new "dangerous bacteria," also called "superbug 2013," and "nightmare bacteria." The number of outbreaks of CRE remains small, is confined to hospitals and long-term care facilities, but has the potential to increase. When infected, the death rate is 50%, despite aggressive antibiotic treatment and supportive measures. With few drug companies developing new antibiotics, survival advantage may be in favor of the resistant organisms, rather than those who acquired the infection.

EBOLA VIRUS DISEASE

Ebola virus disease (EVD) or Ebola hemorrhagic fever is a rare and most often fatal disease caused by a virus from the family *Filoviridae*, genus *Ebolavirus*. There are five *Ebolavirus* species but only four are known to cause disease in humans, *Zaire ebolavirus*, *Sudan ebolavirus*, *Tai Forest ebolavirus*, and *Bundibugyo ebolavirus*. EVD was first identified in 1976 near the Ebola River in the Democratic Republic of the Congo. Since first identified, there have been sporadic outbreaks in Africa.

The 2014 Ebola outbreak is the largest in world history. The first cases reported occurred in Guinea in March of 2014 and is the first outbreak in West Africa. The 2014 West Africa outbreak has affected several countries with the majority of the cases occurring in Sierra Leone, Liberia, Guinea, and more recently, Mali. As of March 2015, there have been over 25,000 cases reported with over 10,000 confirmed deaths.

The natural reservoir remains unknown; however, researchers believe the virus is animal-borne with bats being the most likely reservoir. Ebola is also considered an agent of bioterrorism. Of the five subtypes listed earlier, four occur in an animal host that is native to Africa.

TRANSMISSION

Ebola is spread through direct contact to mucous membranes or broken skin with blood and body fluids, including but not limited to blood, sweat, vomit, feces, saliva, breast milk, and semen. It is not spread through the air or by water.

Screening tools should be used in all health care settings to establish risk factors for EVD. These include recent travel to areas that have active EVD and a fever of greater than 38.6° C or 101.5° F. Additional symptoms are severe headache, muscle pain, vomiting, diarrhea, unexplained hemorrhage, or abdominal pain. Health care providers should also include malaria as a working diagnosis because it is also the most common febrile illness in people who have recently travelled to the affected countries.

CASE DEFINITIONS

Early recognition and detection is crucial, and health care providers need to be alert and evaluate any patients suspected with EVD. The following categories have been defined by the CDC.

Person Under Investigation (PUI): A person who has both risk factors and symptoms as follows:
- Clinical criteria: Fever greater than 38.6° C or 101.5° F with severe headache, muscle pain, vomiting, diarrhea, abdominal pain, or unexplained hemorrhage;
  AND
- Risk factors within the past 21 days: Contact with blood/body fluids or human remains of a person with known or suspected EVD, residence in or travel to and area where there is active EVD, or direct handling of bats or nonhuman primates in areas with active EVD.

Probable Case: A PUI with risk factors of low-risk or high-risk exposure.
Low-risk exposure includes:
- Household contact with a person who has EVD.
- Close contact with a person who has EVD, such as being within 3 feet of a patient with EVD, in the room or in the care area of the person who is ill for a prolonged period of time.
- Direct contact without PPE.

High-risk exposure includes:
- Percutaneous or mucous membrane exposure to blood or body fluids of a patient with EVD.
- Direct unprotected skin contact with blood or body fluids of a patient with EVD.
- Direct contact with a dead body in a country with an EVD outbreak with PPE.

Confirmed Case: A person with a confirmed laboratory test for EVD.

No Known Exposure: A person who has been in a country where there is an EVD outbreak in the past 21 days but does not report a high-risk or low-risk exposure.

SIGNS AND SYMPTOMS

Symptoms of EVD usually appear from 2 to 21 days after an exposure and averages from 8 to 10 days. Symptoms include: fever greater than 38.6° C or 101.5° F, severe headache, muscle pain, weakness, diarrhea, vomiting, abdominal pain, and unexplained hemorrhage, which includes bleeding or bruising.

PREVENTION AND INFECTION CONTROL

All health care workers who enter rooms with patients who are PUI (probable, or known) should wear PPE including masks, gloves, gowns, and eye protection. Shoe covers and leg covers should be used as needed. It has been recognized that a large number of secondary infections from Ebola Virus Disease during the 2014 outbreak occurred in health care workers exposed during care of infected patients. Leading U.S centers addressing serious contagious diseases have used full-body Tyvek suits and powered air purifying respirator (PAPR) hoods as part of the contact and droplet precautions protocol when caring for patients with confirmed EVD. Patients should be isolated in private rooms with private bathrooms if possible or cohort patients with EVD in the same ward. Health care workers who handle dead bodies should also wear appropriate PPE.

Restrict visitors with the exception of individuals who may be essential to the well-being of the patient. This should be determined on a case-by-case basis. A logbook should be kept to document all persons entering the patient's room, including health care personnel. As of March, 2015, U.S centers managing patients with a confirmed diagnosis of EVD have not allowed visitors, outside of essential health care providers, into the room.

Aerosol-generating procedures should be avoided. If the patient's condition warrants these procedures, PPE including respiratory protection such as N-95 respirators or a higher level of respiratory protection should be used along with a negative-pressure environment or airborne isolation room. Powered air purifying respirator (PAPR) hoods have been used to provide additional protection with enhanced comfort.

Diligent environmental cleaning and disinfection measures should be used along with safe handling of potentially contaminated materials. Use of Environmental Protection Agency-registered hospital disinfectants with a label claim for nonenveloped viruses should be used to disinfect environmental surfaces in the patient's room with suspected or confirmed EVD. Patients with EVD should not be placed in rooms with carpet, upholstered furniture, or curtains. Mattresses or pillows should have a nonporous covering that fluids cannot penetrate. Any cloth products or textiles should not be laundered. These items should be disposed of into the waste stream. Any disposable single-use items should be placed in leak-proof containment. Any plastic waste bags should be placed in a rigid waste receptacle. U.S. centers have used more extensive environmental protection measures including autoclaving trash prior to placing it in rigid waste receptacles, treating toilet water with disinfectants when waste is deposited, and extensive terminal cleaning measures, based on lessons learned from care providers managing the EVD outbreak in West Africa.

DIAGNOSIS

Diagnosis is made by recent travel to areas where EVD is endemic and by symptoms. This can be difficult in the early stages but health care providers can follow the case definitions previously listed.

Laboratory tests include:

Timeline of Infection	Diagnostic Tests Available
Within a few days after symptoms begin	Antigen-capture enzyme-linked immunosorbent assay (ELISA) testing • Immunoglobulin M (IgM) ELISA • Polymerase chain reaction (PCR) • Virus isolation
Later in disease course or after recovery	• IgM and IgG antibodies
Retrospectively in deceased patients	• Immunohistochemistry testing • PCR • Virus isolation

TREATMENT

Treatment is dependent on symptoms and patients are provided supportive care. Early treatment and interventions increase the chance of survival. Managing fluid and electrolytes by providing IV fluids, maintaining oxygen levels and blood pressure are all essential to survival. Patients may produce 10 liters of diarrhea daily.

There are currently no U.S. Food and Drug Administration (FDA)-approved vaccines or medications available for EVD. There have been some experimental vaccines and treatments but they have not been fully tested for effectiveness and safety.

Recovery depends on good supportive care and the patient's immune response. Patients who recover develop antibodies that last for at least 10 years. At present, it is not known if they are immune for life or can become infected with different species of EVD. Long-term complications have occurred in patients who have recovered from EVD, such as joint and vision problems.

SEVERE ACUTE RESPIRATORY SYNDROME

Severe acute respiratory syndrome (SARS) is a febrile lower respiratory tract infection that mimics many other respiratory illnesses. To date, there are no specific clinical or laboratory findings that distinguish with certainty SARS-associated coronavirus (CoV) disease from other respiratory illnesses rapidly enough to facilitate management decisions that must be made soon after the patient presents to the health care system. Therefore, early recognition of this disease still relies on a combination of clinical and epidemiologic features.

The virus may have originated from animals and spread to humans. SARS first emerged in the Guangdong Province in China during November 2002 through June 2003, where approximately 15,000 probable cases were identified. A worldwide epidemic occurred when a SARS-infected physician contaminated several guests at a hotel in Hong Kong.

A novel CoV has been identified as the cause of SARS and is now labeled SARS-CoV. Research in China has detected several CoVs closely related to SARS-CoV in two animal species (masked palm civet cat and raccoon dog). Both are considered delicacies in China and are consumed by humans. One theory states that this CoV had mutated and was transmitted to humans through handling of these animals or contact with their saliva and feces.

PATHOPHYSIOLOGY

SARS begins much like the common flu, progressing to pneumonia, and potentially to acute respiratory distress syndrome (ARDS) and death. Lymphopenia, thrombocytopenia, and leucopenia are noted. SARS-CoV may infect blood cells and/or induce autoantibodies to damage these cells, leading to immunologic dysregulation in response to SARS-CoV.

TRANSMISSION

The most common mode of transmission for SARS is close person-to-person contact: kissing, sharing eating or drinking utensils, close conversation (less than 3 feet), physical examination, and any other direct physical contact. Respiratory droplets are expelled by the infected person by a cough or sneeze into the air. Droplets then reach the mucosal membrane of the nose, mouth, or eyes of a nearby person, infecting him or her.

Surfaces contaminated with SARS droplets may serve as a reservoir for the virus. SARS droplets can remain viable up to several days depending on the type of surface.

ASSESSMENT

GOAL OF ASSESSMENT

Evaluate for early clinical and epidemiologic features of SARS.

HISTORY AND RISK FACTORS

Evaluation of SARS-CoV disease among persons presenting with community-acquired illness

The CDC recommends the following approach for the evaluation of SARS-CoV disease among persons presenting with community-acquired illness. The suspicion of SARS-CoV disease is raised if, within 10 days of symptom onset, the patient:

- Has a history of recent travel to mainland China, Hong Kong, or Taiwan or close contact with ill persons with a history of recent travel to such areas,

OR

- Is employed in an occupation at particular risk for SARS-CoV exposure, including a health care worker with direct patient contact or a worker in a laboratory that contains live SARS-CoV,

OR

- Is part of a cluster of cases of atypical pneumonia without an alternative diagnosis.
- In addition, all patients with fever or lower respiratory symptoms (e.g., cough, shortness of breath, difficulty breathing) should be questioned about whether within 10 days of symptom onset they have had:
  - Close contact with someone suspected of having SARS-CoV disease,

  OR

- A history of foreign travel (or close contact with an ill person with a history of travel) to a location with documented or suspected SARS-CoV,

OR

- Exposure to a domestic location with documented or suspected SARS-CoV (including a laboratory that contains live SARS-CoV) or close contact with an ill person with such an exposure history.

SIGNS AND SYMPTOMS

The initial presentation of SARS is similar to that of other lower respiratory tract infections. No specific clinical or laboratory findings are available to rapidly distinguish SARS from any other respiratory illness. Early recognition of SARS requires assessment of clinical and epidemiologic features. The incubation period is 2 to 10 days. Early clinical manifestations include fever, myalgia, headache, and rhinorrhea. Fever is a key component. On the second day of the fever, a dry, nonproductive cough may develop, progressing to shortness of breath, hypoxemia, and ARDS. The CDC has delineated three different levels of how patients may clinically present with SARS:

Early illness
- Presence of two or more of the following: fever, chills, rigors, myalgia, headache, diarrhea, sore throat, rhinorrhea.

Mild-to-moderate respiratory illness
- Temperature of greater than 100.4° F (38° C), and
- One or more of the clinical findings of lower respiratory illness (e.g., cough, shortness of breath, difficulty breathing).

Severe respiratory illness
- Meets clinical criteria for mild-to-moderate respiratory illness including one or more of the following:
  - Chest radiograph illustrating pneumonia,
  - ARDS (see Acute Lung Injury and Acute Respiratory Distress Syndrome, Chapter 4), or
  - Autopsy findings of pneumonia or ARDS without an identifiable cause.

SCREENING LABWORK

Laboratory studies such as bacterial cultures and respiratory viral panels can be used to rule out other potential causes of respiratory tract infection. SARS-CoV reverse transcription (RT)-PCR and enzyme immunoassay (EIA) tests are not typically ordered until after a high index of suspicion by the physician and notification of public health officials.

Diagnostic Tests for Severe Acute Respiratory Syndrome Coronavirus (SARS-CoV)		
Test	**Purpose**	**Abnormal Findings**
Laboratory Studies		
SARS-CoV reverse-transcription–polymerase chain reaction (RT-PCR) test: A signed consent should be completed before collection of a sample. The sample should be forwarded to a state or local public health laboratory for processing.	Detects SARS-CoV viral RNA in respiratory samples, stool, and blood. The likelihood of detecting infection is increased if multiple specimens are collected at several times during the course of the illness.	A positive SARS-CoV RT-PCR test should be considered presumptive until confirmatory testing by a second reference laboratory is performed. A negative test result for SARs-CoV may not rule out SARS-CoV disease and should not affect patient management or infection control decisions.

Continued

Emerging Infections

Diagnostic Tests for Severe Acute Respiratory Syndrome Coronavirus (SARS-CoV) — cont'd

Test	Purpose	Abnormal Findings
SARS-CoV enzyme immunoassay (EIA) test: A signed consent should be completed before collection of the sample. The sample should be forwarded to a state or local public health laboratory for processing.	Detects SARS-CoV antibodies in blood samples. The Centers for Disease Control and Prevention considers detection of SARS-CoV antibody to be the most reliable indicator of infection. Has not been licensed by the U.S. Food and Drug Administration.	Detectable antibodies
SARS-CoV immunofluorescence assay (IFA) for antibody	Gives results identical to SARS-CoV EIA for antibody.	Detectable antibodies
Specimen culture for SARS-CoV	Isolation of SARS-CoV from a clinical specimen to confirm the virus.	SARS-CoV identified in specimen
Sputum and blood cultures	Test can aid in ruling out bacterial infection.	Positive for bacterial pathogen
Respiratory viral panels for influenza A and B, respiratory syncytial viruses, and specimens for *Legionella* and pneumococcal and urinary antigen.	These tests aid in ruling out other potential sources of infection.	Positive for pathogen
Complete blood count and clotting profile	Monitoring white blood cell counts to assist in evaluation of other bacterial infection.	Evaluation for lymphopenia, thrombocytopenia, and leucopenia
Radiology		
Chest radiograph	Assists in identifying the progression of disease and anatomic involvement.	Infiltrates suggestive of pneumonia
Respiratory Tests		
Arterial blood gases (ABGs)	Determination of patient oxygen saturation of arterial blood.	Alkalosis, acidosis (see Acid-Base Imbalances, p. 1)
Pulse oximetry	Measure patient oxygen saturation of arterial blood.	Values of <90%

COLLABORATIVE MANAGEMENT

The Centers for Disease Control and Prevention provides guidance on the clinical evaluation and management of patients who have presenting symptoms of fever and/or respiratory illness. These guidelines focus on identification of cases and infection control management. At present, treatment for severe acute respiratory syndrome is primarily supportive.

Management	Goal
Notify facility infection prevention leadership and the public health department.	Communicate suspected community health threat to comply with public health regulation and facilitate collaboration on the control and diagnosis of severe acute respiratory syndrome coronavirus (SARS-CoV).

At initial suspicion, place a mask on the patient and arrange for isolation. Place patient in an airborne infection isolation room/negative-pressure room and wear personal protective equipment, including gowns, gloves, N-95 respirators, and facial protection upon entry to the room. Removal of protective equipment in a manner that prevents contamination of skin and clothing is a priority.	To prevent the transmission of SARS-CoV to other patients and to yourself.
Oxygen therapy	To support gas exchange and circumvent development of hypoxemia. Maintain pulse oximetry of <90%.
Intubation and mechanical ventilation	To support gas exchange and help maintain acid-base balance.
Intravenous fluids	To prevent dehydration and maintain adequate circulatory volume.
Antibiotics	To prevent secondary infections. Empirical antibiotic therapy should be prescribed for typical and atypical community-acquired pneumonia. Therapy may include a fluoroquinolone or macrolide.
Antiviral	Ribavirin is the antiviral of choice, but has had mixed results. Adverse side effects include hemolytic anemia and electrolyte imbalances (i.e., hypokalemia and hypomagnesemia). Patients must be monitored closely for significant side effects.
Corticosteroids	May be beneficial in patients with pulmonary infiltrates and hypoxemia. Methylprednisolone dosage ranges from 40 mg twice daily to 2 mg/kg daily.

CARE PRIORITIES FOR SARS-CoV
(see Care Priorities for MERS-CoV)

MIDDLE EASTERN RESPIRATORY SYNDROME CORONAVIRUS (MERS-CoV)

Middle Eastern respiratory syndrome (MERS-CoV) is a viral respiratory illness caused by a coronavirus. It was first reported in Saudi Arabia in September 2012. Camels have been found to be the primary source of the virus. As of April 2014, there have been 536 laboratory-confirmed cases of MERS-CoV reported primarily in the Middle East; however, with international travel MERS-CoV has been seen in Europe, Asia, and the United States. All documented cases have had recent travel to the Middle East or are in close contact with individuals who are ill. Close contact is identified as those individuals who live or care for the ill, and there has been no evidence to support widespread spreading of MERS-CoV in the community setting.

PATHOPHYSIOLOGY

The clinical signs and symptoms of MERS-CoV include fever, cough, dyspnea, chills, rigor, headache, myalgia, and malaise. Other reported symptoms included nausea, vomiting, diarrhea, abdominal pain, and sore throat. Patients present with acute respiratory illness and can rapidly progress to pneumonitis, respiratory failure, septic shock, and multiorgan failure, which may result in death.

The incubation period ranges from 2 to 13 days with a median incubation period of 5 days. Most patients present to the hospital on day 4. The median time of onset of illness to death in the patient who is critically ill is 12 days.

TRANSMISSION

MERS-CoV can spread from a person who is ill to others through close contact. Close contact means individuals who care for the individual who is ill or those living with the person who is infected. There has been transmission to health care providers by patients who are infected. There have been no reported community outbreaks at this time, although this is being closely monitored. All cases that have been reported have been linked to countries in or near the Arabian Peninsula, and most people who have become ill have lived or recently traveled to the area.

ASSESSMENT

GOAL OF ASSESSMENT
Evaluate for early clinical and epidemiologic features of MERS-CoV.

HISTORY AND RISK FACTORS
Health care providers should consider MERS-CoV for any patient who has traveled to the Arabian Peninsula in the past 14 days and developed symptoms of acute respiratory illness such as fever, cough, or shortness of breath. Others at risk include individuals who have had close contact with anyone who has traveled to the Arabian Peninsula, anyone who has had close contact with someone with suspected or confirmed MERS-CoV, and any health care worker exposed to MERS-CoV and has not used the appropriate infection control measures. Individuals with other comorbidities appear to be at a higher risk as well as individuals who are immunosuppressed.

SIGNS AND SYMPTOMS
Most individuals come to the health care setting with symptoms of a severe acute respiratory illness. These symptoms include a fever, cough, and shortness of breath. There have also been reports of gastrointestinal symptoms that include nausea, vomiting, and diarrhea. MERS-CoV rapidly progresses to pneumonitis, severe respiratory distress syndrome, sepsis, and multisystem organ failure.

Diagnostic Tests for Middle Eastern Respiratory Syndrome Coronavirus (MERS-CoV)		
Test	**Purpose**	**Abnormal Findings**
Laboratory Studies		
MERS-CoV real-time reverse polymerase chain reaction assay (rRT-PCR)	Detects RNA expression levels in real time. This test quantifies the number of copies of viral RNA per given volume of specimen. rRT-PCR is considered the most optimal for detecting MERS-CoV.	A positive MERS-CoV rRT-PCR test should be considered presumptive until confirmatory testing by the Centers for Disease Control and Prevention (CDC) is performed. A negative test result should be reported through the CDC Laboratory Response Network (LRN) within 24 hours and an equivocal test result must be reported to the CDC immediately.
MERS-CoV antibodies	Detects MERS-CoV antibodies in blood samples.	Detectable antibodies
Sputum and blood cultures	Test can aid in ruling out bacterial infection.	Positive for bacterial pathogen
Respiratory viral panels for influenza A and B, respiratory syncytial viruses, and specimens for *Legionella* and pneumococcal and urinary antigen.	These tests aid in ruling out other potential sources of infection.	Positive for pathogen

Diagnostic Tests for Middle Eastern Respiratory Syndrome Coronavirus (MERS-CoV)—cont'd

Test	Purpose	Abnormal Findings
Complete blood count and clotting profile	Monitoring white blood cell counts to assist in evaluation of other bacterial infection.	Evaluation for lymphopenia, thrombocytopenia, and leukopenia.
Serum chemistries	Lactate dehydrogenase (LDH) is used to measure tissue damage. The protein LDH is found in many body tissues, especially the heart, liver, kidney, muscles, brain, blood cells, and lungs.	Elevated LDH levels
Radiology		
Chest radiograph	Assists in identifying the progression of disease and anatomic involvement.	Unilateral or bilateral patchy densities or opacities, interstitial infiltrates, consolidation, and pleural effusions.
Respiratory Tests		
Arterial blood gases (ABGs)	Determination of patient oxygen saturation of arterial blood.	Alkalosis, acidosis (see Acid-Base Imbalances, p. 1)
Pulse oximetry	Measure patient oxygen saturation of arterial blood.	Values of <90%

CARE PRIORITIES FOR MERS-CoV AND SARS-CoV

1. Treating the patient with supportive measures

As outlined earlier, this is recommended. There are no vaccines or specific management for MERS-CoV or SARS-CoV.

2. Infection control

Patients are to be placed in a negative-pressure room under airborne, contact, and standard precautions. Anyone who enters the patient's room must wear gowns, gloves, an N-95 respirator, and eye protection. Hand hygiene should be performed after contact with a patient on precaution. If there is a lack of negative-pressure rooms and/or there is a need to concentrate infection control efforts and resources, patients may be cohorted on a floor or nursing unit designated for the care of patients with MERS only if air-handling systems can be modified to allow these areas to operate under negative pressure relative to surrounding areas.

- Designate "clean" and "dirty" areas for isolation materials. Maintain a stock of clean patient care and PPE supplies outside the patient's room. Decide where contaminated linen and waste will be placed. Locate receptacles close to the point of use and separate from clean supplies.
- Limit the amount of patient-care equipment brought into the room to that which is medically necessary. Provide each patient with patient-dedicated equipment (e.g., blood pressure cuff, thermometer).
- Limit patient movement and transport out of the negative-pressure room. Whenever possible, use portable equipment to perform radiographs and other procedures in the patient room. Limit visits to patients to persons who are necessary for the patient's emotional well-being and care.
- Health care workers who perform aerosol-generating procedures should be alert to the fact that there may be an increased risk of SARS-CoV and MERS-CoV transmission when these procedures are performed. PPE should fit properly and protect all skin surfaces and clothing. A fluid-repellant gown or full-body suit, eye protection, N-95 respirator, and gloves that fit snuggly over the gown cuff should be worn. After an aerosol-generating procedure (e.g., intubation, bronchoscopy), clean and disinfect horizontal surfaces around the patient as soon as possible.

ADDITIONAL NURSING DIAGNOSES FOR MERS-CoV AND SARS-CoV

See nursing diagnoses for Acute Lung Injury and Acute Respiratory Distress Syndrome (Chapter 4), Acute Pneumonia (Chapter 4), Acute Respiratory Failure (Chapter 4), Mechanical Ventilation (Chapter 1), Fluid and Electrolyte Disturbances (Chapter 1), and Emotional and Spiritual Support of the Patient and Significant Others (Chapter 2).

CREUTZFELDT-JAKOB DISEASE

PATHOPHYSIOLOGY

Creutzfeldt-Jakob disease (CJD) is a rare, fatal, neurodegenerative disorder, believed to be caused by an abnormal isoform of a glycoprotein known as a prion, a proteinaceous infectious particle. The most common disorder is bovine spongiform encephalopathy, or "mad cow" disease. A new form of CJD has emerged, called new variant CJD (vCJD or nvCJD). This form of CJD is linked to consumption of cattle with "mad cow" disease. Clinical and epidemiologic evidence supporting this link between "mad cow" disease and vCJD has become stronger. vCJD generally affects younger people with a mean age of 29 years, whereas CJD occurs in those aged 65 to 69 years.

CJD is classified as a transmissible spongiform encephalopathy. *Prion disease* occurs in animals, particularly cattle, sheep, and goats. CJD is endemic around the world and its estimated incidence report is 1 case per 1 million population. Three forms of "classic" CJD have been identified. Sporadic CJD affects older adults with rapid-onset dementia and neurologic symptoms of unknown cause. Familial CJD is an inherited disease and generally strikes younger individuals. It has a longer course in comparison to sporadic CJD. Iatrogenic CJD occurs through contact with infected tissue via medical procedures or treatments.

Prion proteins are normal proteins in the body and brain. In CJD, these proteins become abnormally shaped, as a result either of genetics or of contamination from an outside source. This leads to surrounding normal prion proteins taking on the abnormal shape. Central nervous system (CNS) function is disrupted, leading to cognitive impairment and cerebellar dysfunction. As the process continues, the abnormal prions accumulate in the brain, causing neuronal dysfunction, neuron death, gliosis (proliferation of neuroglial tissue in the CNS), and ultimately death.

TRANSMISSION

CJD can spread via infectious or hereditary means. Prion infections are transmitted via the peripheral route, either orally or transcutaneously. They may be introduced to lymphatic organs, particularly the spleen and lymph nodes, where initial replication of the infected prions occurs. Infections can either enter the circulatory system and be hematogenously spread to the brain, or infected prions may travel via the vagus nerve to the brain. Genetic mutation of the human prion gene *PrP* on chromosome 20 leads to the dysfunction of the prion protein. More than 20 reported mutations of this chromosome have been reported. All mutations influence the onset and duration of CJD. vCJD is theorized to be caused by the consumption of meat from cattle that is infected. Once ingested, the infected prions follow the same neuro-invasion route of CJD.

ASSESSMENT: CREUTZFELDT-JAKOB DISEASE

GOAL OF ASSESSMENT

Evaluate for clinical signs of CJD.

RISK FACTORS AND HISTORY

- Family history of CJD.
- Exposure to contaminated tissue. People who have received human growth hormone derived from human pituitary glands or who have had dura mater grafts.

Sporadic CJD

- Reported as having "come out of the blue."

- Early symptoms are memory loss, loss of interest, and mood changes that progress quickly (within a few weeks) to confusion and memory problems. Complaints of clumsiness, with jerky and stiff limbs, are also seen.
- Median age at death is 68 years in patients who are initially seen with dementia and neurologic deterioration.
- Course of illness is often 4 months.
- Blurred eyesight and incontinence follow.
- At end stage, patients are unable to move or speak and need 24-hour care.
- Death occurs approximately 6 months after the onset of the disease.

Familial CJD
- Symptoms vary between different people, depending in part on the type of gene mutation responsible.
- In some cases, the illness is similar to sporadic CJD in type, duration, and progression, whereas in others, it is a more slowly developing dementia that progresses over a few years.

vCJD
- The incubation period is unknown and may take up to several years before manifesting.
- vCJD affects younger people, with a mean age of 29 years.
- Initial symptoms are more psychiatric than neurologic.
- Patients are anxious and depressed and display withdrawal or other behavioral changes.
- Persistent pain and odd sensations in the face and extremities are common. As disease progresses, the patient develops ataxia, sudden erratic movements, and progressive dementia with marked memory loss.
- Ultimately, the patient will lose the ability to move or speak and will require 24-hour care. Death soon follows.

DIAGNOSTIC TESTS
CJD is diagnosed based on typical signs, symptoms, and progression of disease.

Diagnostic Tests for Creutzfeldt-Jakob Disease (CJD)		
Test	**Purpose**	**Abnormal Findings**
Radiology		
Magnetic resonance imaging (MRI): T1-, T2-, and diffusion-weighted and FLAIR (fluid-attenuated inversion recovery) sequences should be ordered with MRI.	Identify abnormalities of the brain consistent with CJD.	Images will show abnormalities (hyperintensities and cortical ribboning) in specific areas of the brain (e.g., basal ganglia and medial and pons).
Neurophysiology		
Electroencephalogram (EEG)	For sporadic CJD cases. Identify alteration in brain waves.	Consistent slowing of brain waves and/or presence of periodic sharp wave complexes, generally late in the course of the disease.
Laboratory Studies		
Lumbar puncture: cerebrospinal fluid (CSF) examination	Assess for protein levels consistent with CJD.	Elevated CSF protein levels. A 14-3-3 CSF protein test should be highly sensitive and specific to CJD.
Brain biopsy	Assess region of brain that appears abnormal on MRI. Only means of confirming CJD besides autopsy.	Deposits or plaques of abnormal bundles of prion protein, spongiform encephalopathy.

Emerging Infections

COLLABORATIVE MANAGEMENT

There is no known treatment or cure for CJD. Management of these patients is supportive and palliative in nature. There is no vaccine for CJD.

CARE PRIORITIES

1. Supportive care

Ventilatory support, pain management, patient safety, intensive skin care, assessment, nutrition support, care for immobility, and treatment for secondary infections.

2. Infection control

Standard precautions are used to care for patients with CJD. If a brain biopsy or other procedure is performed on a patient with CJD or suspected CJD, inform the central sterile department so that stringent chemical and autoclave sterilization methods can be used to reprocess instruments.

ADDITIONAL NURSING DIAGNOSES

See nursing diagnoses and interventions in Nutrition Support, Mechanical Ventilation, Alterations in Consciousness, Wound and Skin Care, Prolonged Immobility (Chapter 1), Emotional and Spiritual Support for the Patient and Significant Others, and Ethical Considerations in Critical Care (Chapter 2).

WEST NILE VIRUS

PATHOPHYSIOLOGY

West Nile virus (WNV) is a single-stranded positive RNA virus from the Japanese encephalitis virus serogroup of the genus *Flavivirus*, family Flaviviridae, which is known for Japanese encephalitis and St. Louis encephalitis. In rare cases, WNV may lead to encephalitis or meningitis and death. WNV has an incubation period of 2 to 14 days. It can also be divided into two lineages. Lineage I strains are more widely distributed and linked to human infections.

TRANSMISSION

WNV is a disease that has spread worldwide. Initially, WNV was a disease that only occurred in bird species. Approximately 146 different species of birds have been reported to acquire this disease. This disease is spread among the bird population by 29 different species of mosquitoes (vectors). The natural cycle is from bird 1 to mosquito 1 to bird 2 to mosquito 2, and so forth. Because of a complex intensification of this natural cycle, bridge vectors (mosquitoes that bite both birds and humans) became infected with the WNV and spread the disease to humans. Only birds and humans in the United States and Israel have been known to die from WNV.

ASSESSMENT: WEST NILE VIRUS

GOAL OF ASSESSMENT

Evaluate for signs and symptoms of WNV.

HISTORY AND RISK FACTORS

Exposure to mosquitoes where WNV exists increases risk. WNV is common in areas such as Africa, West Asia, and the Middle East. It first appeared in the United States in the summer of 1999 and since then has been found in all 48 contiguous states. Older age is associated with a higher risk for developing more serious CNS disease.

INCUBATION PERIOD

- Generally 2 to 14 days, although longer incubation periods have been documented in persons who are immunosuppressed.

MILD INFECTION/WEST NILE FEVER

- Symptoms last 3 to 6 days.
- Sudden onset of a fever with malaise, anorexia, nausea, vomiting, eye pain, headache, myalgia, rash, and lymphadenopathy.

SEVERE INFECTION/WNV MENINGITIS, WNV ENCEPHALITIS, AND WNV POLIOMYELITIS

- When the CNS is affected, clinical syndromes ranging from febrile headache to aseptic meningitis to encephalitis may occur, and these are usually indistinguishable from similar syndromes caused by other viruses.
- WNV encephalitis or meningoencephalitis is characterized by altered mental status or focal neurologic findings.
- WNV meningitis involves fever, headache, and nuchal rigidity (stiff neck). Pleocytosis (abnormal increase in white blood cell [WBC] count in cerebrospinal fluid [CSF]) is present. Changes in consciousness are not usually seen and are mild when present.
- WNV encephalitis also involves fever and headache and more global symptoms. There is typically an alteration of consciousness, which may be mild and result in lethargy but may progress to confusion or coma. Focal neurologic deficits, including limb paralysis and cranial nerve palsies, may be observed. Tremor and movement disorders have also been identified.
- WNV poliomyelitis is characterized by the acute onset of asymmetric limb weakness or paralysis in the absence of sensory loss. Pain sometimes precedes the paralysis. The paralysis can occur in the absence of fever, headache, or other common symptoms associated with WNV infections. Involvement of the respiratory muscles, leading to acute respiratory failure, can occur.

Clinical features

- Fever
- Gastrointestinal (GI) disturbances
- Change in mental status
- Development of a maculopapular or morbilliform rash (infrequent) involving the neck, trunk, arms, or legs
- Seizures
- Myelitis
- Polyradiculitis
- Optic neuritis
- Cranial nerve abnormalities
- Severe weakness
- Flaccid paralysis sometimes
- Ataxia/extrapyramidal signs
- Myocarditis, pancreatitis, and fulminant hepatitis have been noted in outbreaks before 1990.

LABWORK

Certain findings are seen in patients with severe disease.

- Total leukocyte count is mostly normal but can be elevated with lymphocytopenia and anemia.
- Hyponatremia is sometimes present, particularly among patients with encephalitis.
- CSF examination shows pleocytosis, usually with a predominance of lymphocytes. Protein is universally elevated. Glucose is normal.

Diagnostic Tests for West Nile Virus (WNV)

Test	Purpose	Abnormal Findings
Laboratory Studies		
WNV immunoglobulin M (IgM) antibody capture enzyme-linked immunosorbent assay (MAC ELISA) of serum or CSF.	To diagnose WNV. Most efficient diagnostic test. Best to collect 8 to 21 days after the onset of symptoms.	Positive MAC ELISA. Patients who have been vaccinated or infected with other flaviviruses (e.g., Japanese encephalitis) may have positive results.

Continued

Diagnostic Tests for West Nile Virus (WNV) — cont'd

Test	Purpose	Abnormal Findings
Complete blood count (CBC)	Identify abnormalities associated with WNV.	Elevated leukocyte counts with lymphocytopenia and anemia. CBC can be normal with WNV.
Serum chemistry	To assess for hyponatremia, which can be seen in WNV.	Hyponatremia
Radiology		
Magnetic resonance imaging (MRI)	Identify possible abnormalities associated with WNV.	One third of patients show enhancements of the leptomeninges and the periventricular areas.

Testing for WNV can be obtained through local or state health departments. WNV is on the list of designated nationally notifiable arboviral encephalitides, and the proper authorities should be informed. Check your local or state health department for guidance.

COLLABORATIVE MANAGEMENT

Treatment of WNV infection is supportive. High-dose ribavirin and interferon alfa-2b have some activity against WNV in vitro. There is no specific antibiotic or antidote for the viral infection. Also, there is no vaccine.

CARE PRIORITIES
Supportive care
Includes IV fluids to prevent dehydration, antipyretics for fever management, oxygen therapy and ventilatory support, patient safety, nutrition support, and treatment for secondary infections. Standard precautions should be taken at all times; follow organization's policy for appropriate personal protection category.

ADDITIONAL NURSING DIAGNOSES

See nursing diagnoses and interventions in Nutrition Support (Chapter 1), Mechanical Ventilation (Chapter 1), Altered Mental Status/Alterations in Consciousness (Chapter 1), Wound and Skin Care (Chapter 1), Prolonged Immobility (Chapter 1), Emotional and Spiritual Support for the Patient and Significant Others (Chapter 2), and Ethical Considerations in Critical Care (Chapter 2).

PANDEMIC FLU

An epidemic occurs when there are an unusually high number of people affected by a disease. A pandemic is an international epidemic. An influenza pandemic may occur when a new influenza virus is detected and the human population has no immunity. With the increase in global travel and transportation, and urban development with areas of overcrowding, epidemics that result from a new influenza virus are likely to be disseminated around the world and rapidly become a pandemic. The WHO has defined the phases of a pandemic to create a global framework to aid countries in pandemic preparedness and response planning. Pandemics can be either mild or severe in the illness and death they cause. The severity of a pandemic can change during the time the illness continues to spread.

The WHO has developed a global influenza preparedness plan that outlines the responsibilities of WHO and national authorities in the event of an influenza pandemic. The WHO also offers guidance tools and training to assist in the development of national pandemic preparedness plans (www.who.int/csr/disease/influenza/A58_13-en.pdf).

AVIAN INFLUENZA ("BIRD FLU")
PATHOPHYSIOLOGY
Avian influenza is an infection caused by avian (bird) flu viruses, type A strains. These viruses occur naturally among birds. Wild birds carry the viruses in their intestines but usually do not

get sick from them. However, domesticated birds such as poultry can become very ill and die from avian influenza viruses.

It is theorized that certain subgroups of avian influenza mutated, crossed species, and infected humans. The subgroups of avian influenza linked to human infections include but are not limited to H5N1, H7N7, H9N2, H7N3, and H7N9. The H5N1 subgroup is of particular concern to humans because of its ability to mutate and its tendency to acquire genes from viruses from other animal species. It has demonstrated high pathogenicity and causes severe disease in humans. The H7N9 is a new subgroup first reported in March 2013, characterized by rapid development of serious pneumonia, which leads to sepsis, ARDS, and multisystem organ failure.

TRANSMISSION

Avian influenza is most commonly spread from infected birds to humans. The virus is harbored in birds (in the intestine), which shed the virus through their saliva, nasal secretions, and feces. The most common means of transmission among birds is fecal to oral. Humans who come in direct contact with infected poultry are susceptible to infection. Avian influenza survives on inanimate objects. Items contaminated with secretions/excretions of infected birds can be a vector for transmission to humans. The spread of avian influenza from one person who is ill to another has been reported very rarely, and transmission has not been observed to continue beyond one person.

ASSESSMENT

HISTORY AND RISK FACTORS
- Direct or close contact with infected poultry or contaminated surfaces. In outbreaks, most cases have occurred in previously healthy children and young adults.
- A Health Safety Alert will be sent out by the CDC to all hospitals if there are avian influenza outbreaks that lead this federal organization to recommend heightened surveillance and diagnostic testing of targeted patients. In this situation, the CDC will outline triage guidelines, which will likely include travel to the outbreak location within the past 10 days and hospitalization with a severe respiratory illness.

SIGNS AND SYMPTOMS
- Similar to the "common flu": fever, cough, sore throat, muscle aches, and eye infections.
- In more severe cases of avian influenza, when assessed, the patient may display signs and symptoms of viral pneumonia (see Acute Pneumonia, p. 373) and ARDS (see Acute Lung Injury and Acute Respiratory Distress Syndrome, p. 365).
- These symptoms can be accompanied by nausea, diarrhea, vomiting, and neurologic changes.

DIAGNOSTIC TESTS

Diagnostic Tests for Avian Influenza		
Test	**Purpose**	**Abnormal Findings**
Laboratory Studies		
Complete blood count	Assess for changes suggestive of other bacterial infections.	Elevated white blood cell count
Influenza A/H5 (Asian lineage) virus real-time reverse transcription–polymerase chain reaction (RT-PCR) assay: Must consult with and have authorization from local or state health departments. Test is conducted only in designated laboratories.	To identify causative agent.	Positive
Rapid bedside tests: Available but results are not confirmatory.	Conduct for rapid screening for virus.	Positive. Confirmatory tests should be performed.

Continued

Diagnostic Tests for Avian Influenza—cont'd		
Test	**Purpose**	**Abnormal Findings**
Viral culture: Must be conducted in biosafety Level 3 laboratory.	Identify causative agent.	Positive for pathogen
Radiology		
Chest radiograph	Identify progression of lung disease and anatomic involvement.	Infiltrates, atelectasis
Respiratory Tests		
Arterial blood gas (if patient is in respiratory distress)	Determination of oxygen saturation and blood gases.	Acidosis, alkalosis
Pulse oximetry	Measure oxygen saturation.	<90%

COLLABORATIVE MANAGEMENT

At present, the primary medication therapy option is oseltamivir (Tamiflu) and zanamivir (Relenza); however, there is concern that viruses may become resistant to both of these drugs. Treatment is supportive in accordance to the clinical status of the patient.

CARE PRIORITIES
1. Supportive management
Includes IV fluids to prevent dehydration, antipyretics for fever management, oxygen therapy and ventilatory support, patient safety, nutrition support, and treatment for secondary infections.

2. Infection control
Place patients in a negative-pressure room under airborne, contact, and standard precautions. An N-95 respirator should be worn by everyone who enters the room. Gowns and gloves are to be worn for all patient contact, and eye protection should be worn when within 3 feet of the patient. Good hand hygiene should be practiced. Precautions should be continued for 14 days after onset of symptoms or until either an alternative diagnosis is established or diagnostic test results indicate that the patient is not infected. Restricted visitation should be implemented and an ongoing log kept of all people entering the patient's room. Minimize the number of health care personnel caring for the patient. All equipment and other items should remain in the patient's room and should not be used with other patients or outside the isolation room.

3. Vaccination of health care workers
Health care workers caring for patients with documented or suspected avian influenza should be vaccinated with the most recent seasonal influenza vaccine. This allows for protection against the predominant circulating strain and reduces the likelihood of health care workers becoming coinfected with human and avian strains, which could lead to the emergence of a pandemic strain. At present, there is no vaccine for avian influenza.

ADDITIONAL NURSING DIAGNOSES
See nursing diagnoses for Acute Lung Injury and Acute Respiratory Distress Syndrome, Acute Pneumonia, Acute Respiratory Failure (Chapter 4), Mechanical Ventilation (Chapter 1), and Emotional and Spiritual Support of the Patient and Significant Others (Chapter 2).

EMOTIONAL AND SPIRITUAL SUPPORT OF THE PATIENT AND SIGNIFICANT OTHERS

Similar to all health care professionals, nurses must remain mindful of the need to remain objective and nonjudgmental; therefore, imposing one's own personal views upon others must be avoided. Instead, a patient's significant others may feel that they are in the best position to assign significance to an event, or to decide the most appropriate response. To facilitate therapeutic interactions when faced with challenging situations, nurses must assess both the patient's and significant others' understanding and perception of the situation before implementing a plan of care. Assessment of patient and significant others' needs requires that nurses employ active listening, are fully present during interactions, and invest as much high-quality time as possible during the process. An interdisciplinary team may be employed to assist with assessment and subsequent problem-solving. Given resource limitations, possible inconsistency of nurse assignment, and the amount of coverage available by other disciplines, time constraints may lead to dysfunctional situations that are not handled in the best manner to produce a sustainable solution or, in worst-case scenarios, to not being noticed at all.

It is of paramount importance that nurses are familiar with how to provide both emotional and spiritual support to patients and significant others, and to help guide them through the challenges posed by critical illness and hospitalization. Complex support system issues may include identification of high-risk dependent relationships among older adults, family members, domestic partners, children, or religious leaders. Actions required may include steps to prevent infliction of physical, emotional, or sexual harm, exploitation, or neglect of basic life necessities.

Effective exchange of information is foundational for collaboration among the health care team, patients, and their significant others. Accurate and timely information should be shared throughout the hospitalization to ensure the delivery of holistic patient care. In our current fast-paced, dynamic health care environment, relationships among health care professionals and their clients vary, and can evolve over time.

With less opportunity to establish relationships, trusting the clinical knowledge, decisions, and judgment of unknown providers may be difficult. In large teaching hospitals, the problem is compounded as the monthly rotation of multiple levels of physician house staff ensues. Nursing care is often delivered on a dynamic schedule and includes increasing numbers of contract and per diem clinical staff. Therefore, stabilizing the team and taking the time needed to provide effective communication can be challenging. The larger the number of health care team members or family/significant others involved, the greater the challenge of adequate communication. In addition, emotionally charged events are common in the critical care environment. To help provide care of the whole patient and family system, emotional support can be of assistance to promote healthy coping.

Occasionally, however, providers are also in need of emotional support to cope with difficult situations. Emotional support is defined as support for emotions that will help provide the best outcomes. Key elements of holistic care include providing encouragement, reassurance, and acceptance during times of stress. Mental, emotional, and spiritual interventions are often needed to help with coping and decision-making during critical illness. Emotional responses may be closely associated with mental processes; in other words, thoughts or perceptions drive feelings about life events. Knowledge affects perception, so keeping patients and families informed and up to date is of paramount importance to their emotional well-being. Knowledge will promote them having more perceived control of the situation. Frequent, repetitive, simple explanations are often needed. During emotional upset, the ability to recall and retain information is often impaired.

Nurses can facilitate adaptation to perceived stressors, changes, or threats that interfere with meeting the demands present in the lives of patients and their significant others. Coping techniques that are used vary with individuals, including health care providers, and are often affected by culture. Counseling or family-centered care team conferences may be provided, using an interactive, helpful approach, and may focus on the needs, problems, or feelings of the patient, significant others, and health care team members. Actions are designed to enhance or support coping, crisis management, problem-solving, and interpersonal relationships. Emotionally charged ethical issues frequently arise in the critical care environment. Care providers are prompted to address end-of-life decision-making, including "Do Not Resuscitate" issues, withdrawal of care, and whether or not the family desires to be present if resuscitation is needed. Involvement of the interdisciplinary team (which may include members such as pastoral care, mental health professionals, social work, palliative care, and an ethics professional) may be warranted on admission to the critical care unit and throughout the stay if complex end-of-life issues arise.

RESEARCH BRIEF 2-1

A large percentage of the U.S. general public has stated they would like to have loved ones present during resuscitation. Despite the countless benefits reported, family presence during resuscitation is still a controversial, highly debated issue among health professionals in adult critical care units. Baumhover and Hughes (2009) designed an exploratory, descriptive, and correlational study to determine the relationship between the spirituality of health care professionals and support for family presence during invasive procedures and resuscitation. The holistic Spirituality Assessment Scale (SAS) developed by Howden (1992) was used to obtain information regarding a more comprehensive meaning of spirituality; not focused exclusively on religious beliefs and feelings of patients but also including the feelings of health care providers. Data were collected from 73 nurses, 31 physicians, and 4 physician assistants. Results suggested a link between a holistic perspective and support for family presence. The higher the scores of spirituality for health care providers, the greater the likelihood that they supported family presence as a patient's right and essential part of holistic care. This study helps to fill the gap in the current literature regarding certain demographic characteristics affecting whether or not health care providers are willing to allow families to be present during invasive procedures and resuscitation. Further analysis of extraneous variables is needed before the results of this study can be generalized.

From Baumhover N, Hughes L: Spirituality and support for family presence during invasive procedures and resuscitations in adults. *Am J Crit Care* 18:357-367, 2009.

Promoting psychological peace in the final phase of life is of paramount importance to the patient and their significant others and involves exploration of the spiritual beliefs of all those involved in making decisions. Disagreement on the appropriate course of action stems from many factors. For example, confusion among significant others regarding the wishes of the patient, their own views on death and dying, or vacillating patient views may create a dysfunctional care environment. The problem is compounded when various subgroups of decision-makers share perspectives in isolation, rather than discussing them openly in a group composed of all key decision-makers.

In extreme cases, anger and confusion may result in violent behavior, and the lines of communication may deteriorate if appropriate avenues are not initiated to repair damages. The American College of Critical Care Medicine has developed patient and family guidelines that help widen perspectives, open new options, and suggest different ideas for health care providers to help abate situations before they escalate to the point of physical violence.

Spiritual support is regarded as a part of providing holistic care. Spirituality is not to be confused with religion. Although the vast majority of nurses believe spiritual care is a part of providing patient-centered, holistic care, over half feel inadequate to perform spiritual care interventions. Spirituality has been described as the values, beliefs, and behaviors of an individual related to purpose and meaning in life; connectedness to self, others, and life and universal dimensions; innerness or inner resources and capacity for transcendence. Using these characteristics, Howden developed the Spirituality Assessment Scale or SAS (Box 2-1). The 28 items on the SAS provide a strong operational framework for evaluating the ability of all involved with patient care and decision-making to connect or to be sensitive to the spiritual dimensions of others, and possibly frame the approach on addressing the emotional needs of others. If a health care provider has not developed the capacity to connect with others, providing care that requires embracing a viewpoint outside of his or her personal sphere of perception is extremely difficult. Behavior modification of the patient, significant others, or health care team members may be necessary as part of facilitating adaptation to life changes for the patient and significant others resulting from hospitalization. Values may collide, based on past

Box 2-1	ELEMENTS OF THE HOWDEN SPIRITUAL ASSESSMENT SCALE (SAS)*

Has a sense of belongingness	Feels part of the community lived in
Has capacity to forgive	Feels reconciling relationships is important
Can rise above or go beyond mental and physical problems	Can rise above or go beyond body changes or body losses
Is concerned about environmental destruction	Feels responsible for preserving the planet
Can find peace during a devastating event	Has inner resources for dealing with uncertainty
Has a sense of kinship to others	Has found inner strength during past struggles
Has a connection to all of life	Possesses life goals and aims
Relies on inner strength when struggling	Possesses inner strength
Enjoys serving others	Feels a sense of fulfillment in life
Has a sense of inner spiritual guidance	Trusts life is good despite discouraging events
Perceives ability for self-healing	Feels good about themselves
Perceives meaning of life provides peace	Has the sense life has meaning and purpose
Feels a sense of balance within life	Feels inner harmony and peace
Boundaries of personal universe extend beyond space and time	Inner strength is related to belief in a higher power or supreme being

From Howden JW: Development and psychometric characteristics of the Spirituality Assessment Scale. *Dissert Abstr Int* 54:166B, 1992. Abstract reproduced with permission from ProQuest LLC. © 2007 ProQuest LLC; all rights reserved. Further reproduction is prohibited without permission.
*Items are rated 1 (Strongly disagree) through 6 (Strongly agree) on a Likert scale after reading statements about the elements listed here.

experiences of all involved; therefore, staying focused on the present can assist all involved in remaining objective when approaching the situation.

ASSESSMENT OF NEED FOR EMOTIONAL AND SPIRITUAL SUPPORT

GOAL OF ASSESSMENT

The goal of assessment is to determine the ability of the patient and significant others to demonstrate a healthy response to changes brought forth by critical illness. In addition, a comprehensive assessment can ensure that appropriate emotional and spiritual support can be provided to facilitate appropriate decision-making as part of patient and family-centered care. True family-centered care requires the creation of mutually beneficial partnerships among patients, families, and health care providers. A concerted effort may be required to create one unified voice for the right course of action in every situation that arises.

HISTORY AND RISK FACTORS

Innumerable variables can affect coping and decision-making abilities. The factors listed in Box 2-1 have been demonstrated by various studies to affect how decisions are made and how they may adversely affect coping because of a difference in beliefs related to spirituality. The following characteristics in any member of a decision-making team may be associated with ineffective coping: poor self-image, a lack of fulfillment, significant financial problems, existing unhealthy and/or unrepaired relationships, resistance to change, a lack of meaning or purpose in life, difficulty in learning, a poor sense of belonging or connectedness, a lack of inner peace or strength, the inability to forgive others, difficulty relating to others, and/or unclear life goals.

CARE PLANS: EMOTIONAL AND SPIRITUAL SUPPORT OF THE PATIENT, FAMILY, AND SIGNIFICANT OTHERS

Anxiety *related to actual or perceived threat of death; change in health status; threat to self-concept or role; unfamiliar people and environment; the unknown.*

Goals/Outcomes: After intervention, anxiety is absent or reduced, as evidenced by the patient's verbalization of same, vital signs at the patient's baseline, and an absence of or decrease in irritability and restlessness. Family members appear calmer.

NOC Anxiety Level, Anxiety: Self-Control, Concentration, Coping.

Anxiety Reduction

1. Engage in honest communication with the patient and family; empathize. Actively listen and establish an atmosphere that enables free expression. Express to the patient that you care about his or her health.
2. Assess level of anxiety with the patient and family. Be alert to verbal and nonverbal cues:
   a. Mild: Restless.
   b. Moderate: Inattentive, expresses concern, narrowed perceptions, disturbed sleep pattern, altered vital signs.
   c. Severe: Expressing feelings of doom; rapid speech; tremors; poor eye contact; preoccupation with the past; inability to understand the present; possible presence of tachycardia, palpitations, nausea, and hyperventilation.
   d. Panic: Cannot concentrate or communicate, distorting reality, increased motor activity, vomiting, tachypnea.
3. For severe anxiety or panic state, refer to appropriate psychiatric health care team member.
4. If hyperventilation occurs, encourage slow, deep breaths and have the patient or significant other mimic your own breathing pattern.
5. Validate the nursing assessment of anxiety with the patient or significant other. ("You seem distressed; are you feeling anxious or overwhelmed?")
6. After an episode of anxiety, review and discuss the thoughts and feelings that led to the episode.
7. Identify coping behaviors currently being used (e.g., denial, anger, repression, withdrawal, daydreaming, drug or alcohol dependence). Review coping behaviors used in the past. Assist in using adaptive coping to manage anxiety.
8. Encourage expression of fears, concerns, and questions. ("This room may look like a maze of wires and tubes; please let me know when you have any questions.")
9. Reduce sensory overload by providing an organized, quiet environment. (See Alterations in Consciousness, Chapter 1).
10. Introduce one self and other health care team members; explain each individual's role as it relates to the plan of care or care map.
11. Teach relaxation and imagery techniques. See Sample Relaxation Technique in Appendix 7.
12. Enable significant others to be in attendance whenever possible.
13. Consult palliative care services if available and appropriate.
14. Engage in and promote awareness of touch to significant others when appropriate. Types of touch are described in Box 2-2.

NIC Coping Enhancement; Calming Technique, Active Listening, Presence.

| **Box 2-2** | **TYPES OF TOUCH** |

Instrumental touch
- Task- or procedure-related
- May be negatively perceived but accepted as impersonal

Affective touch
- Expressive, personal
- Caring
- Comforting
- May be positively or negatively perceived
- Influenced by cultural patterns

Therapeutic touch
- Deliberate intervention to accomplish a purpose
- Acupressure
- Use of space around the individual to mobilize energy fields

Social isolation   *related to altered health status; inability to engage in satisfying personal relationships; altered mental status; altered physical appearance.*

Goals/Outcomes: Within 24 hours after diagnosis, the patient demonstrates interaction and communication with others.

NOC Loneliness Severity, Mood Equilibrium, Personal Well-Being.

Socialization Enhancement
1. Assess factors contributing to social isolation.
   - Restricted visiting hours.
   - Absence of or inadequate support system.
   - Inability to communicate (e.g., presence of endotracheal tube/tracheostomy).
   - Physical changes that affect self-concept.
   - Denial or withdrawal.
   - Critical care environment.
2. Recognize patients at higher risk for social isolation: the older adult, disabled, chronically ill, socioeconomically disadvantaged.
3. Assist the patient with identification of feelings associated with loneliness and isolation. ("You seem very sad when your family leaves the room. Can you tell me more about your feelings?")
4. Determine the need for socialization and identify available and potential support systems. Explore methods for increasing social contact (e.g., recordings of loved ones, more frequent visitations/hospital volunteers, scheduled interaction with nurse or support staff).
5. Provide positive reinforcement for socialization that lessens feelings of isolation and loneliness. ("Please continue to call me when you need to talk to someone. Talking will help both of us to better understand your feelings.")
6. Facilitate the patient's ability to communicate with others (see Alterations in Consciousness, Chapter 1).

NIC Support System Enhancement, Mood Management.

Compromised family coping   *related to situational crisis (patient's illness)*

Goals/Outcomes: After intervention, family/significant others demonstrate effective adaptation to change/traumatic situation, as evidenced by seeking external support when necessary and sharing concerns.

NOC Family Coping, Family Normalization.

Coping Enhancement
1. Assess character of family/significant others: social, environmental, ethnic, and cultural factors; relationships; and role patterns. Identify developmental stage. Be aware that other situational or maturational crises may be ongoing, such as an older parent or teenager with a learning disability.
2. Assess previous adaptive behaviors. ("How do you deal with stressful situations?") Discuss observed conflicts and communication breakdown. ("I noticed that your brother has not visited your mother today. Has there been a problem we should be aware of? Knowing about it may help us better care for your mother.")
3. Acknowledge the family's or significant others' involvement in patient care and promote strengths. ("You were able to encourage your wife to turn and cough. That is very important to her recovery.") Encourage participation in patient care conferences. Promote frequent, regular patient visits as appropriate for the patient's situation.
4. Provide information and guidance related to the patient. Discuss the stresses of hospitalization and encourage discussions of feelings, such as anger, guilt, hostility, depression, fear, or sorrow. ("You seem to be upset since having been told that your husband is not leaving the hospital today.") Refer to clergy, case manager, clinical nurse specialist, social services, or palliative care specialist as appropriate.
5. Evaluate interactions among patient and family/significant others. Encourage reorganization of roles and priority setting as appropriate. ("It appears as though your husband is concerned about his insurance policy and seems to expect you to investigate it. I'll ask the financial counselor to talk with you.")
6. Encourage family/significant others to schedule periods of rest and activity and to seek support when necessary. ("Your neighbor volunteered to stay in the waiting room this afternoon. Would you like to rest at home? I'll call you if anything changes.")

NIC Family Support; Family Process Maintenance; Normalization Promotion, Financial Resource Assistance.

Emotional and Spiritual Support

Fear *related to patient's life-threatening condition; lack of information*

Goals/Outcomes: After the intervention, the patient and family/significant others relate that fear has been lessened or is manageable.

NOC Fear Level, Fear Self-Control.

Security Enhancement

1. Assess fears and understanding related to the patient's clinical situation. Evaluate verbal and nonverbal responses.

2. Acknowledge the fears. ("I understand these tubes may frighten you, but they are necessary to help nourish your son.")

3. Assess history of coping behavior. ("How do you cope with difficult situations?") Determine resources and significant others available for support. ("Who/what usually helps during stressful times?")

4. Provide opportunities for expression of fears and concerns, while setting boundaries of appropriate behavior. Recognize that anger, denial, withdrawal, and demanding behavior may be adaptive coping responses during the initial period of crisis.

5. Provide information at frequent intervals about the patient's status, and the therapies and equipment used. Demonstrate a caring attitude.

6. Encourage use of positive coping behaviors by identifying fear(s), developing goals, identifying supportive resources, facilitating realistic perceptions, and promoting problem-solving.

7. Be alert to maladaptive responses to fear: potential for violence, withdrawal, severe depression, hostility, and unrealistic expectations of staff or of patient's recovery. Provide referrals to psychiatric service or palliative care specialist as appropriate (see Box 2-3 for ways to reduce the risk of violence).

8. Assess your own feelings about the patient's life-threatening illness. Acknowledge that your attitude and fear may be reflected to the family/significant others.

NIC Coping Enhancement; Calming Technique; Support System Enhancement.

Box 2-3 SAFETY PRECAUTIONS IN THE EVENT OF VIOLENT BEHAVIOR

Patient safety

- Remove harmful objects from the environment, such as heavy objects, scissors, tubing.
- Apply padding to side rails according to agency protocol if the patient is acting out.
- If available, use bed alarms. Ensure all unit staff members are aware of potential for violence.
- Use physical or chemical restraints as necessary and prescribed. Monitor the patient's neurovascular status at frequent intervals.
- Set limits on the patient's behavior, using clear and simple commands.
- As prescribed, consider chemical sedation when unable to control the patient's behavior with other means.
- Explain safety precautions to the patient and family/significant others.

Caregiver safety

- Place the patient in bed closest to nursing station. Maintain visibility at all times by keeping door open.
- Alert hospital security department when risk of violence is present from the patient or family.
- Do not approach a violent patient or family member without adequate assistance from others.
- Never turn your back on a violent patient or family member.
- Maintain a calm, matter-of-fact tone of voice. Set limits on family's behavior.
- Monitor security measures at frequent intervals.
- Remain alert.

From Bureau of Labor Statistics (BLS), U.S. Department of Labor, for the National Institute for Occupational Safety and Health (NIOSH), Centers for Disease Control and Prevention: *Survey of workplace violence prevention*, Washington, 2005, U.S. Department of Labor. Retrieved from www.bls.gov/iif/osh_wpvs.htm.

Grieving *related to perceived potential loss of physiologic well-being (e.g., expected loss of body function or body part, changes in self-concept or body image, terminal illness).*

Goals/Outcomes: After interventions, patient and significant others/family express grief, participate in decisions about the future, and communicate concerns to health care team members and to one another.
NOC Adaptation to Physical Disability, Body Image Enhancement.

Acceptance Health Status
1. Assess the source of perception of loss.
2. Assess factors contributing to anticipated loss.
3. Assess patient and family's behavioral response. Expect reactions such as disbelief, denial, guilt, anger, and depression. Determine stage of grieving as described in Table 2-1.
4. Assess spiritual, religious, and sociocultural expectations related to loss. ("Is religion/spirituality an important part of your life? How do you and your family/significant others usually deal with serious health problems?") Refer to the clergy or community support groups as appropriate.

Emotional Support
1. Encourage the patient and family/significant others to share their concerns. ("Is there anything you'd like to talk about today?") Also, respect their desire not to speak or actively listen.
2. Demonstrate empathy. ("This must be a very difficult time for you and your family.") Touch when appropriate (see Box 2-2).
3. In selected circumstances, provide an explanation of the grieving process. This approach may assist in better understanding and acknowledging feelings.
4. Assess grief reactions of the patient and family/significant others, and identify a potential for dysfunctional grieving reactions (e.g., absence of emotion, hostility, avoidance). If the potential for dysfunctional grieving is present, refer to case manager, psychiatric service, clergy, or palliative care specialist as appropriate.
5. When appropriate, recruit tissue donation professionals to discuss donation. Assess the patient's wishes about tissue donation.

NIC Active Listening; Dying Care; Grief Work Facilitation.

Spiritual distress *related to separation from spiritual/religious/cultural supports; challenged belief and value system.*

Table 2-1	STAGES OF GRIEVING
Protest stage	Denial: "No, not me" Disbelief: "But I just saw her this morning" Anger Hostility Resentment Bargaining to postpone loss Appeal for help to recover loss Loud complaints Altered sleep and appetite
Disorganization	Depression Withdrawal Social isolation Psychomotor retardation Silence
Reorganization	Acceptance of loss Development of new interests and attachments Restructuring of lifestyle Return to preloss level of functioning

Emotional and Spiritual Support

Goals/Outcomes: After diagnosis, the patient and family verbalize spiritual or religious beliefs and express hope for the future, the attainment of spiritual or religious support, and the availability of what is required to resolve conflicts.
NOC Spiritual Health, Dignified Life Closure.

Spiritual Support
1. Assess spiritual or religious beliefs, values, and practices. ("Do you have a religious preference? How important is it to you? Are there any religious or spiritual practices you wish to participate in while in the hospital?")
2. Inform the patient and family/significant others of the availability of spiritual aids, such as a chapel, religious services, or pastoral care service. Discuss advance directives.
3. Present a nonjudgmental attitude toward religious or spiritual beliefs and values. Create an environment conducive to free expression and invite sharing of beliefs. Identify available support systems that may assist in meeting the patient's religious or spiritual needs (e.g., clergy, the patient's fellow church members, support groups).
4. Be sensitive to comments related to spiritual concerns or conflicts. ("I don't know why God is doing this to me." "I'm being punished for my sins.")
5. Use active listening and open-ended questioning to assist in resolving conflicts related to spiritual issues. ("I understand that you want to be baptized. We can arrange to do that here.")
6. Provide privacy and opportunities for religious practices, such as prayer and meditation.
7. If spiritual beliefs and therapeutic regimens are in conflict, provide honest, concrete information to encourage informed decision-making. ("I understand that your religion discourages receiving blood transfusions. Have the implications of not receiving blood transfusions been discussed with you?")

NIC Coping Enhancement, Conflict Mediation, Presence.

Ineffective individual coping and ineffective denial *related to health crisis; sense of vulnerability; inadequate support systems.*

Goals/Outcomes: After diagnosis, the patient verbalizes feelings, identifies strengths, and begins using positive coping behaviors.
NOC Coping, Acceptance Health Status, Personal Well-Being, Adaptation to Physical Disability.

Coping Enhancement
1. Assess the patient's perceptions and ability to understand current health status.
2. Establish honest communication. ("Please tell me what I can do to help you.") Assist with identifying strengths, stressors, inappropriate behaviors, and personal needs.
3. Support positive coping behaviors. ("I see that easy listening music seems to help you relax.")
4. Provide opportunities for expression of concerns; gather information from nurses and other support systems. Provide explanations about prescribed routine, therapies, and equipment. Acknowledge feelings and assessment of current health status and environment.
5. Identify factors that inhibit the ability to cope (e.g., unsatisfactory support system, knowledge deficit, grief, fear).
6. Recognize defensive and maladaptive coping behaviors (e.g., severe depression, drug or alcohol dependence, hostility, violence, suicidal ideations). Address these behaviors. ("You seem to be requiring more pain medication. How does the pain medication help you?") Refer the patient to case manager, psychiatric liaison, clergy, or palliative care specialist as appropriate (see Box 2-3 for ways to reduce the risk of violence).

Support System Enhancement
1. Encourage regular visits by significant others as appropriate. Encourage them to engage in conversation with the patient to help minimize the patient's emotional and social isolation.
2. Assess significant others' interactions with the patient. Attempt to mobilize support systems by involving them in patient care whenever possible.
3. As appropriate, explain to significant others that increased dependency, anger, and denial may be adaptive coping behaviors used by the patient in early stages of crisis until effective coping behaviors are learned.

NIC Socialization Enhancement; Resiliency Promotion, Self-Awareness Enhancement.

Disabled family coping *related to inadequate or incorrect information or misunderstanding; temporary family disorganization and role change; exhausted support systems; unrealistic expectations; fear; anxiety.*

Goals/Outcomes: After interventions, family/significant others verbalize feelings, identify ineffective coping patterns, identify strengths and positive coping behaviors, and seek information and support from the nurse or other support systems.

NOC Caregiver-Patient Relationship, Caregiver Performance: Direct Care, Caregiver Performance: Indirect Care.

Caregiver Support

1. Have the family designate one member as the primary point of contact. Explain how this will allow the nurse to spend more time taking care of the patient and less time on the telephone explaining the patient's status to each family member separately.
2. Establish open, honest communication. Assist in identifying strengths, stressors, inappropriate behaviors, and personal needs. ("I understand your mother was very ill last year. How did you manage the situation?" "I hear that your loved one is very ill. How can I help you?")
3. Assess for ineffective coping (e.g., depression, substance abuse, violence, withdrawal) and identify factors that inhibit effective coping (e.g., inadequate support system, grief, fear of disapproval by others, knowledge deficit). ("You seem to be unable to talk about your husband's illness. Is there anyone with whom you can talk about it?") (See Box 2-3 for ways to reduce the risk of violence.)
4. Assess knowledge regarding the patient's current health status and therapies. Provide information frequently, and allow sufficient time for questions. Reassess understanding at frequent intervals.
5. Provide opportunities in a private setting for both patients and significant others to talk and share concerns with nurses or other health care providers. If appropriate, refer to psychiatric clinical nurse specialist for therapy.
6. Offer realistic hope. Help family/significant others develop realistic expectations for the future and identify support systems that will assist them with planning for the future.
7. Reduce anxiety in significant others by encouraging diversionary activities (e.g., period of time outside of hospital) and interaction with outside support systems. ("I know you want to be near your son, but if you would like to go home to rest, I will call you if any changes occur.")
8. Establish open, honest communication and rapport. ("I am here to care for your mother and to help you, as well.")
9. Identify ineffective coping behaviors (e.g., violence, depression, substance abuse, withdrawal). ("You seem to be angry. Would you like to talk to me about your feelings?") Refer to psychiatric liaison, clergy, or support group as appropriate.
10. Identify perceived or actual conflicts. ("Are you able to talk openly among yourselves?" "Are your brothers and sisters able to help and support you during this time?")
11. Encourage healthy functioning. For example, facilitate open communication and encourage behaviors that support cohesiveness. ("Your mother seemed to enjoy your last visit. Would you like to see her now?")
12. Assess knowledge about the patient's current health status. Provide opportunities for questions; reassess understanding at frequent intervals.
13. Assist with developing realistic goals, plans, and actions. Refer to clergy, case manager, psychiatric nurse, social services, financial counseling, and family therapy as appropriate.
14. Encourage family/significant others to spend time outside of the hospital and to interact with/support individuals.
15. Include the family/significant others in the patient's plan of care. Offer them opportunities to become involved in patient care, for example, range-of-motion (ROM) exercises, patient hygiene, and comfort measures (e.g., backrub).

NIC Family Involvement Promotion; Family Mobilization; Family Support.

Powerlessness *related to health care environment; treatment regimen*

Goals/Outcomes: After diagnosis, assess the patient's and family's preferences, needs, values, and attitudes. The patient makes decisions about self-care and therapies and relates an attitude of realistic hope and a sense of self-control and the family accepts decisions.

NOC Depression Self-Control, Family Participation in Professional Care, Health Beliefs: Perceived Control.

Self-Responsibility Facilitation

1. Explain the Patient and Family Rights and Responsibilities information the hospital provides. Help the patient and significant others understand their rights and responsibilities, and responsibilities of the hospital with regard to patient care.
2. Ensure the patient and family know who is taking care of the patient. Tell the patient and family if a staff member does not have an identification badge visible, it is alright to ask for their name and their role in patient care.

3. Before providing information, ensure the patient's privacy is maintained, and assess the patient's and family's understanding of health condition, prognosis, and plan of care.
4. Recognize expressions of fear, lack of response to events, and lack of interest in information, any of which may signal a sense of powerlessness.
5. Evaluate medical and nursing interventions, and adjust them, as appropriate, to support the patient's and/or caregiver's sense of control. For example, if the patient always bathes in the evening to promote relaxation before bedtime, modify the care plan or map to include an evening bath rather than follow the hospital routine of giving a morning bath.
6. Assist the patient to identify and demonstrate activities that can be performed independently.
7. Encourage the patient and/or family to keep a notebook with them at all times, which can serve as a helpful tool to remember questions or write down information that will be shared with other family members during this stressful time.
8. Whenever possible, offer alternatives related to routine hygiene, diet, diversion activities, visiting hours, or treatment times.
9. Encourage the patient and family to ask to speak with the charge nurse, nurse manager, nurse supervisor, or patient advocate/patient representative if there is a problem with any member of the health care team.
10. Ensure privacy and preserve territorial rights whenever possible. For example, when distant relatives and casual acquaintances request information about the patient's status, refer them to the patient or a family member who can provide acceptable amounts of information.
11. Avoid paternal or parental behaviors with patients and families.
12. Assess support systems; enable significant others to be involved in care whenever possible.
13. Offer realistic hope for the future. If appropriate, encourage direction of thoughts beyond the present.
14. Provide referrals to clergy, palliative care specialists, and other support systems as appropriate.

NIC Emotional Support; Family Involvement Promotion, Support Group.

Sleep pattern, disturbed *related to environmental changes; illness; therapeutic regimen; pain; immobility; psychological stress.*

Goals/Outcomes: After discussion, the patient identifies factors that promote sleep. Within 8 hours of intervention, the patient attains adequate periods of uninterrupted sleep and verbalizes satisfaction with the ability to rest.
NOC Personal Well-Being, Sleep.

Sleep Enhancement
1. Assess usual sleeping patterns (e.g., bedtime routine, hours of sleep per night, sleeping position, use of pillows and blankets, napping during the day, nocturia).
2. Explore relaxation techniques that promote rest/sleep (e.g., imagining relaxing scenes, listening to soothing music or taped stories, using muscle relaxation exercises).
3. Identify causative factors and activities that contribute to sleep pattern disturbance, adversely affect sleep patterns, or awaken the patient. Examples include pain, anxiety, depression, hallucinations, medications, underlying illness, sleep apnea, respiratory disorder, caffeine, fear, and medical and nursing interventions.
4. Organize procedures and activities to allow for 90-minute periods of uninterrupted rest/sleep. Limit visiting during these periods.
5. Whenever possible, maintain a quiet environment by providing ear plugs or decreasing alarm levels. The use of "white noise" (e.g., low-pitched, monotonous sounds; electric fan; soft music) may facilitate sleep. Dim the lights for a period of time every 24 hours by drawing the drapes (if safe to do so) or providing blindfolds.
6. If appropriate, limit daytime sleeping. Attempt to establish regularly scheduled daytime activity (e.g., ambulation, sitting in chair, active ROM), which may promote nighttime sleep.
7. Investigate and provide nonpharmacologic comfort measures that are known to promote sleep (Table 2-2).

NIC Environmental Management; Environmental Management: Comfort.

Body image disturbance *related to loss of or change in body parts or function; physical trauma.*

Goals/Outcomes: Before hospital discharge, the patient acknowledges body changes and demonstrates movement toward incorporating changes into self-concept. Maladaptive responses, such as severe depression, are absent.
NOC Body Image, Adaptation to Physical Disability, Self-Esteem, Psychosocial Adjustment: Life Change.

Table 2-2	NONPHARMACOLOGIC MEASURES TO PROMOTE SLEEP
Activity	**Example(s)**
Mask or eliminate environmental stimuli	Use eye shields, ear plugs Play soothing music Dim lights at bedtime Mask odors from dressings/drainage; change dressing or drainage container as indicated
Promote muscle relaxation	Encourage ambulation as tolerated throughout the day Teach and encourage in-bed exercises and position change Perform back massage at bedtime If not contraindicated, use a heating pad
Reduce anxiety	Ensure adequate pain control Keep the patient informed of his or her progress and treatment measures Avoid overstimulation by visitors or other activities immediately before bedtime Avoid stimulant drugs (e.g., caffeine)
Promote comfort	Encourage the patient to use own pillows, bedclothes if not contraindicated Adjust bed; rearrange linens Regulate room temperature
Promote usual presleep routine	Offer oral hygiene at bedtime Provide warm beverage at bedtime Encourage reading or other quiet activity
Minimize sleep disruption	Maintain quiet environment throughout the night Plan nursing activities to allow long periods (at least 90 minutes) of undisturbed sleep Use dim lights when checking on the patient during the night

Emotional and Spiritual Support

Body Image Enhancement
1. Establish open, honest communication. Promote an environment that is conducive to free expression. ("Please feel free to talk to me whenever you have any questions.") Assess indicators suggesting body image disturbance, as listed in Box 2-4.
2. When planning care, be aware of interventions that may influence body image (e.g., medications, procedures, monitoring).
3. Assess knowledge of the patient's pathophysiologic process and current health status. Clarify any misconceptions.

Box 2-4	INDICATORS SUGGESTING BODY IMAGE DISTURBANCE
Nonverbal indicators	**Verbal indicators**
• Missing body part: internal or external (e.g., splenectomy, amputated extremity) • Change in structure (e.g., open, draining wound) • Change in function (e.g., colostomy) • Avoiding looking at or touching body part • Hiding or exposing body part	• Expression of negative feelings about body • Expression of feelings of helplessness, hopelessness, or powerlessness • Personalization or depersonalization of missing or mutilated part • Refusal to acknowledge change in structure or function of body part

4. Discuss the loss or change with the patient. Recognize that what may seem to be a small change may be of great significance to the patient (e.g., arm immobilizer, catheter, hair loss, ecchymoses, facial abrasions).
5. Explore expressions of concern, fear, and guilt. ("I understand that you are frightened." "What is your understanding of how your condition will change over time?")
6. Encourage the patient and family/significant others to interact with one another. Help family/significant others to support the patient's feelings related to the changed body part or function. ("It seems as though your son looks very different to you now, but it would help if you speak to him and touch him as you would normally.")
7. Encourage gradual participation in self-care activities as the patient becomes physically and emotionally able. Allow for some initial withdrawal and denial behaviors. For example, when changing dressings over traumatized part, explain what you are doing but do not expect the patient to watch or participate initially.
8. Discuss the potential for reconstruction of the loss or change (i.e., surgery, prosthesis, grafting, physical therapy, cosmetic therapies, organ transplant). ("What is your understanding of the potential for reconstruction?")
9. Recognize manifestations of severe depression (e.g., sleep disturbances, change in affect, change in communication pattern). As appropriate, refer to case manager, psychiatric liaison, clergy, or support group.
10. Help the patient attain a sense of autonomy and control by offering choices and alternatives whenever possible. Emphasize strengths and encourage activities that interest the patient.
11. Offer realistic hope for the future.

NIC Self-Esteem Enhancement; Emotional Support; Grief Work Facilitation, Suicide Prevention.

Complicated grieving *related to loss of physiologic well-being; fatal illness.*

Goals/Outcomes: After diagnosis, the patient and family express grief, explain the meaning of the loss, and talk with each other. The patient assumes necessary self-care activities.
NOC Mood Equilibrium, Grief Resolution, Depression Self-Control.

Grief Work Facilitation
1. Assess grief stage (see Table 2-1) and previous coping abilities. Discuss feelings of the patient and family, the meaning of loss, and goals. ("How do you feel about your condition/illness or your loved one's condition? What do you hope to accomplish in these next few days/weeks? Are you afraid your family will not be taken care of if you pass away?")
2. Acknowledge and permit anger; set limits on the expression of anger to discourage destructive behavior. ("I understand that you must feel very angry, but for the safety of others, you may not throw equipment.")
3. Identify suicidal behavior (e.g., severe depression, statements of intent, suicide plan, previous history of suicide attempt). Ensure safety and refer to case manager, psychiatric service, psychiatrist, clergy, or palliative care specialist.
4. Encourage the patient and family/significant others to participate in activities of daily living and diversion activities. Identify physiologic problems related to loss (e.g., eating or sleeping disorders) and intervene accordingly.
5. Collaborate with the care team about a visit by another individual with the same disorder, if appropriate.

Hope Instillation
1. Provide opportunities for the patient to feel cared for, needed, and valued by others. For example, emphasize the importance of relationships. ("Tell me about your grandchildren." "It seems that your family loves you very much.")
2. Support significant others who seem to spark or maintain the patient's feelings of hope. ("Your husband's mood seemed to improve after your visit.")
3. Recognize factors that promote sense of hope (e.g., discussions about family members, reminiscing about better times).
4. Promote anticipation of positive events (e.g., mealtime, grandchildren's visits, bathtime, extubation, removal of traction).
5. Help the patient recognize that although there may be no hope for returning to original lifestyle, there is hope for a new but different life.
6. Avoid insisting that the patient assume a positive attitude. Encourage hope for the future, even if it is the hope for a peaceful death.
7. Set realistic, attainable goals, and reward achievement.

NIC Suicide Prevention, Family Integrity Promotion.

Risk for self-directed violence or risk for other-directed violence by patient or family *related to sensory overload; suicidal behavior; rage reactions; neurologic disease; perceived threats; toxic reaction to medications; substance withdrawal.*

Goals/Outcomes: The patient or family does not harm themselves or others.
NOC Aggression Self-Control, Abusive Behavior Self-Restraint, Abuse Cessation.

Environmental Management: Violence Prevention

1. Assess factors that may contribute to or precipitate violent behavior (e.g., medication reactions, inability to cope, suicidal behavior, confusion, hypoxia, substance withdrawal, preictal and postictal states), or dysfunctional family behaviors such as arguing, pushing, and shoving.
2. Attempt to eliminate or treat causative factors. For example, provide patient teaching, assess the family for homicidal behavior, reorient the patient, and reduce sensory overload (see Alterations in Consciousness, p. 24). Facilitate mental health consults as appropriate.
3. Approach the patient and family in a positive manner, and encourage verbalization of feelings and concerns. ("You appear upset and frightened. I will be here from 3 pm to 11 pm to care for you, or for your family member.")
4. Help the patient distinguish reality from altered perceptions, including hallucinations, delusions, and illusions. Orient to time, place, and person. Alter the environment to promote reality-based thought processes (e.g., provide clocks, calendars, pictures of loved ones, familiar objects).
5. For acute confusion that becomes aggressive, do not attempt to reorient patient and avoid arguing. Instead, provide support by stating, "I believe that you (see, hear) that; however, I do not (see, hear) that." Use non-threatening mannerisms, facial expressions, and tone of voice.
6. Initiate measures that prevent or reduce excessive agitation for the patient or family:
   - Reduce environmental stimuli (e.g., alarms, loud or unnecessary talking).
   - Before touching the patient/family, ask for permission. Provide concise explanations.
   - Speak quietly (but firmly, as necessary), and project a caring attitude. ("We are very concerned for your comfort and safety. Can we do anything to help you feel more relaxed?")
   - Avoid crowding (e.g., of equipment, visitors, health care personnel) in the patient's personal environment.
   - Avoid direct confrontation.
7. Explain and discuss the patient's behavior with family/significant others. Acknowledge frustration, concerns, fears, and questions. Review safety precautions with family/significant others (see Box 2-3).

Abuse Protection Support

1. Assess for history of physical aggression, family violence, extreme dependence in relationships (including religious leaders), and substance abuse as maladaptive coping behaviors (see Box 2-3).
2. Discuss the need for Adult Protective Services involvement to protect the patient or family caregiver(s) with the medical team, case manager, and social worker if pathologic relationships are identified.
3. Monitor for early signs of increasing anxiety and agitation (e.g., restlessness, verbal aggressiveness, inability to concentrate). Assess for body language that is indicative of violent behavior: clenched fists, rigid posture, increased motor activity.

NIC Delusion Management, Anger Control Assistance, Anxiety Reduction, Surveillance: Safety, Crisis Intervention.

Readiness for enhanced family coping: potential for growth *related to use of support systems and referrals; choosing experiences that optimize wellness.*

Goals/Outcomes: At the time of the patient's diagnosis, family/significant others express their intent to use support systems and resources and identify alternative behaviors that promote communication and strengths. Family/significant others express realistic expectations and decrease use of ineffective coping behaviors.
NOC Family Functioning, Family Normalization, Respite Care.

Normalization Promotion

1. Assess relationships, interactions, support systems, and individual coping behaviors. Permit movement through stages of adaptation. Encourage further positive coping.
2. Acknowledge expressions of hope, future plans, and growth among family members/significant others.
3. Encourage development of open, honest communication. Provide opportunities in a private setting for interactions, discussions, and questions. ("I know the waiting room is very crowded. Would you like some private time together?")

Emotional and Spiritual Support

4. Refer the family/significant others to community or support groups (e.g., ostomy support group, head injury rehabilitation group).
5. Encourage exploration of outlets that foster positive feelings for significant others, for example, periods of time outside the hospital area, meaningful communication with the patient or support individuals, and relaxing activities (e.g., showering, eating, exercising).

NIC Support Group, Resiliency Promotion, Anticipatory Guidance.

Deficient knowledge *related to disease process, diet, medication, prescribed activity, fall prevention, infection control, health resources, treatment procedures, treatment regimen, substance use control, personal safety.*

Goals/Outcomes: The patient and family/significant others verbalize understanding of current diet, disease process, health resources, medication, prescribed activity, treatment procedures, and treatment regimen before discharge from the critical care unit.

NOC Knowledge: Disease Process, Diet, Fall Prevention, Health Behavior, Illness Care, Infection Control, Medication, Personal Safety, Substance Use Control.

Teaching Individual and Family Support

1. Assess current level of knowledge about all aspects of disease process and illness management, including health resources, medication, prescribed activity, treatment procedures, and treatment regimen.
2. Assess cognitive and emotional readiness to learn.
3. Recognize barriers to learning, such as impaired verbal communication, altered thought processes, confusion, impaired memory, sensory alterations, fear, anxiety, and lack of motivation.
4. Assess learning needs and establish short- and long-term goals.
5. Use individualized verbal or written information to promote learning and enhance understanding. Give simple, direct instructions. If indicated, use audiovisual tools to supplement information.
6. Encourage significant others to reinforce correct information rendered by health care providers.
7. Encourage interest about health care information by involving the patient in planning care. Explain rationale for care.
8. Interact frequently with the patient to evaluate comprehension of information given. Ask the patient and family to repeat what has been explained. Individuals in crisis often need repeated explanations before information can be understood. Also be aware that many individuals may not understand seemingly simple medical terms (e.g., "terminal," "malignant," "constipation").
9. As appropriate, assess understanding of informed consent. Assist the patient to use information received to make informed health care decisions (e.g., about invasive procedures, surgery, resuscitation).
10. Assess understanding of right to self-determination; provide information as indicated. If requested, assist the patient with mechanism for executing an advance directive for health care.
11. At frequent intervals, inform the family/significant others about the patient's current health status, therapies, and prognosis. Use individualized verbal, written, and audiovisual strategies to promote understanding.
12. Evaluate the family/significant others at frequent intervals for understanding of information that has been provided. Adjust teaching as appropriate. Some individuals in crisis need repeated explanations before comprehension can be assured. ("I have explained many things to you today. Would you mind summarizing what I've told you so that I can be sure you understand your husband's status and what we are doing to care for him?")
13. Encourage the family/significant others to relay correct information to the patient. This also reinforces comprehension for the family/significant others and the patient.
14. Ask if needs for information are being met. ("Do you have any questions about the care your mother is receiving or about her condition?")
15. Help the family/significant others use the information they receive to guide health care decisions (e.g., regarding the patient's surgery, resuscitation, organ donation).
16. Promote active participation in patient care when appropriate. Encourage the family/significant others to seek information and express feelings, concerns, and questions.

NIC Teaching: Disease Process, Prescribed Medication, Procedure/Treatment, Health System Guidance, Fall Prevention; Health Education; Patient Rights Protection; Infection Protection, Learning Facilitation; Learning Readiness Enhancement.

Impaired verbal communication *related to neurologic or anatomic deficit (e.g., hearing impairment, visual impairment); psychological or physical barriers (e.g., tracheostomy, intubation); cultural or developmental differences.*

Goals/Outcomes: At the time of intervention, the patient communicates needs and feelings, and relates decrease in or absence of frustration over communication barriers.
NOC Communication: Expressive, Communication: Receptive, Information Processing.

Communication Enhancement: Speech, Hearing, and/or Visual Deficit

1. Assess etiology of impaired communication (e.g., tracheostomy, stroke, cerebral tumor, Guillain-Barré syndrome).
2. With the patient and significant others, assess the patient's ability to hear, see, speak, read, write, and comprehend English. If the patient speaks a language other than English, collaborate with an English-speaking family member or interpreter to establish effective communication.
3. When communicating, use eye contact; speak in a clear, normal tone of voice; and face the patient.
4. If the patient cannot speak because of a physical barrier (e.g., tracheostomy, wired mandibles), provide reassurance and acknowledge frustration. ("This may be frustrating for you, but please do not give up. I want to understand you.")
5. Provide slate, word cards, pencil and paper, alphabet board, pictures, or other communication device to assist the patient. Adapt the call system to meet the patient's needs. Document the meaning of the patient's signals in response to questions.
6. Explain to significant others the source of the communication impairment; demonstrate effective communication alternatives (see preceding intervention).
7. Be alert to nonverbal messages, such as facial expressions, hand movements, and nodding of the head. Validate meanings of nonverbal cues with the patient.
8. Recognize that the inability to speak may foster maladaptive behaviors. Encourage the patient to communicate needs; reinforce independent behaviors.
9. Be honest; do not relate understanding if you cannot interpret the patient's communication.

NIC Active Listening; Communication Enhancement: Hearing Deficit, Speech Deficit, Visual Deficit.

Disturbed sensory perception *related to therapeutically or socially restricted environment; psychological stress; altered sensory reception, transmission, or integration; chemical alteration.*

Goals/Outcomes: At the time of intervention, the patient verbalizes orientation to time, place, and person; relates the ability to concentrate; and expresses satisfaction with the degree and type of sensory stimulation being received.
NOC Distorted Thought Self-Control, Neurologic Status: Cranial/Sensory Motor Function, Vision Compensation Behavior.

Environmental Management

1. Assess factors contributing to the sensory/perceptual alteration.
   - Environmental: Excessive noise in the environment; constant, monotonous noise; restricted environment (immobility, traction, isolation); social isolation (restricted visitors, impaired communication); therapies.
   - Physiologic: Altered organ function; sleep or rest pattern disturbance; medication; history of altered sensory perception.
2. Determine the appropriate sensory stimulation needed; plan care accordingly.
3. Control factors that contribute to environmental overload. For example, avoid constant lighting (maintain day/night patterns); reduce noise whenever possible (e.g., set alarms appropriately, avoid loud talking, keep room door closed [if safe for the patient], provide ear plugs).
4. Provide meaningful sensory stimulation:
   - Display clocks, large calendars, and meaningful photographs and objects from home.
   - Depending on the patient's preferences, provide a radio, music, reading materials, and tape recordings of family and significant others. Earphones help block out external stimuli.
   - Position the patient toward window when possible.
   - Discuss current events, time of day, holidays, and topics of interest during patient care activities.
   - As needed, orient the patient to surroundings. Direct the patient to reality as necessary.
   - Establish personal contact by touch to help promote and maintain contact with the real environment.
   - Encourage significant others to communicate with the patient frequently, using a normal tone of voice.
   - Convey concern and respect. Introduce yourself, and call the patient by name.

Emotional and Spiritual Support

- Stimulate vision with mirrors, colored decorations, and pictures.
- Stimulate sense of taste with sweet, salty, and sour substances if appropriate.
- Encourage use of appropriate eyeglasses and hearing aids.
5. Inform the patient before initiating interventions and using equipment.
6. Encourage participation in health care planning and decision-making whenever possible by asking the patient first.
7. Provide patient with choices when possible.
8. Assess sleep-rest pattern to evaluate its contribution to the sensory/perceptual disorder. Ensure that the patient attains at least 90 minutes of uninterrupted sleep as frequently as possible.

NIC Environmental Management; Cognitive Restructuring; Cognitive Stimulation.

ETHICAL CONSIDERATIONS IN CRITICAL CARE

Perhaps more attention is paid to health care decisions in critical care than in any other health care area. Because of the sudden onset of life and death scenarios, interprofessional team members in intensive care areas seem to discuss and notice ethical dilemmas more frequently than other areas of the hospital. These decisions have been debated vigorously in the literature, and although some of these issues have had reasonable and workable solutions, others continue to be argued. A brief overview of common ethical considerations in critical care will be presented.

Health care providers must develop a clear understanding of ethical issues to ensure that the care provided is morally and legally acceptable. Ethical reasoning enables the health care professional to examine the moral principles involved in decision-making and identify appropriate options. Although there are many ethical principles, the following four principles are probably the most widely referenced: (1) respect for autonomy (recognizing that each patient has a right to make decisions for himself/herself), (2) nonmaleficence (not harming a patient), (3) beneficence (helping a patient), and (4) justice (treating patients equally).

INFORMED CONSENT

Without adequate knowledge, patients and their significant others cannot make good decisions. Part of a nurse's obligation is to inform patients and families, in a caring manner, what is to be expected from different treatment options. Informed consent serves not only to protect the health care provider from liability but its primary purpose is to support the ethical principle of respect for autonomy. Informed consent is instrumental to a patient's right to accept, continue, or reject all or part of health care interventions. The elements of informed consent should be used as a guide but are not absolutely necessary for all nursing or medical interventions (Box 2-5).

If a patient is unsure, does not understand, or feels pressured about consenting to the treatment plan, nurses are responsible for advocating for the patient and communicating this to the physician, other health care professionals, and administration if necessary.

| **Box 2-5** | **ELEMENTS OF INFORMED CONSENT** |

Threshold elements (preconditions)
1. Competence (to understand and decide)
2. Voluntaries (in deciding)

Information elements
3. Disclosure (of material information)
4. Recommendation (of a plan)

5. Understanding (of items 3 and 4)

Consent elements
6. Decision (in favor of a plan)
7. Authorization (of the chosen plan)

From Beauchamp TL, Childress JF: *Principles of biomedical ethics*, ed 6, New York, 2009, Oxford University Press.

DECISION-MAKING CAPACITY

A patient's ability to make a decision is fundamental to informed consent. The four components of decision-making capacity are the ability to: (1) express a choice, either verbally or via another means, (2) understand the relevant information, (3) appreciate the importance of the information to one's own situation, including risks and benefits of options, and (4) reason about options consistently with one's beliefs, values, etc.

Patients are presumed to have decision-making capacity. Lack of orientation to person and place, medications, psychological disorders, and cognitive decline may be reasons to question a patient's capacity, but they are not sufficient reasons to declare that a patient cannot make a decision. Health care professionals should try to maximize the patients' capacity, such as removing or adding medications, having discussions during a certain part of the day, or discussing in the presence of family members.

Decision-making capacity is decision-specific. The more critical and complex the decision, the higher level of decision-making capacity required. Capacity should be assessed on an ongoing basis as decisions need to be made. All health care providers must be familiar with individual state laws regarding who can legally assess a patient's capacity and how it should be documented.

ADVANCE DIRECTIVES

Advance directives refer to a patient's directions on how to provide care in the event that the patient becomes unable to make decisions or verbalize them on his or her own behalf. An advance directive can be written or verbal and can be in the form of a living will or a durable power of attorney for health care (DPAHC).

A living will specifies what treatment a patient wants or does not want in the event that the condition is terminal and the patient cannot make health care decisions. A DPAHC appoints a person to make decisions for a patient when the patient cannot make decisions.

A surrogate decision-maker is someone named in the DPAHC. When no DPAHC exists, the legal next of kin becomes the surrogate decision-maker for the patient. If the patient does not have family or a DPAHC, a court-appointed guardian becomes the surrogate decision-maker. This person is obligated to make choices that the patient would make if able. If those choices are unknown, the surrogate decision-maker must try to determine, based on the patient's values, what the patient would want.

Interpretation of advance directives can be problematic. Although many patients express a desire for no "extraordinary measures," the meaning of this term can vary. For example, a ventilator can be considered "extraordinary," but it is also part of very common temporary treatments regularly used in critical care. Despite problems with interpretation, caregivers must responsibly deal with these ambiguities and seek to honor the patient's wishes.

Many states are adopting Physician Orders for Life Sustaining Treatment (POLST, also known as MOST and POST) to clarify patient choices. POLST forms differ from a living will insofar as the form becomes a physician order as soon as it is signed. Therefore, there should be careful deliberation regarding when it is appropriate for a patient to complete a POLST form.

CONFIDENTIALITY

Confidentiality in a relationship between a health care provider and a patient means that one does not identify or expose information that is not relevant to care. Also, one does not communicate information gained from a patient except with providers and decision-maker identified by the patient. Health care provider codes of ethics generally include provisions for keeping all information about a patient confidential. Any disclosure of patient information should be considered very carefully.

The Health Insurance Portability and Accountability Act of 1996 (HIPAA) was mandated by the U.S. Congress to establish a federal standard regarding confidentiality of specific electronic medical information. Individual states may have stricter privacy laws. HIPAA sets the lowest acceptable standard for privacy. State laws apply over HIPAA.

There are situations in which one is legally obligated to breach patient confidentiality. These situations include public welfare risks, sexually transmitted diseases, gunshot wounds, and suspected abuse and/or neglect of children, older adults, or developmentally disabled individuals. HIPAA supports the disclosure of protected health information when required by law.

QUALITY OF LIFE

A person's quality of life is based on physical, intellectual, emotional, and social components. Although improving quality of life is a primary focus of health care, assessing quality of life is difficult at best. Numerous studies have demonstrated that health care providers consistently rate patients' quality of life lower than the patients do themselves. Studies also reveal that such judgments by health care providers do affect care. A life of dependence on medications, treatments, and care rendered by others is generally viewed as "not desirable" by many people, including health care providers, until they are actually faced with the choice between a dependent life versus death involving a family member or themselves. Nurses and care team members in critical care should be aware of all the dynamics underlying choices of patients and families, because hospitalization reflects a minuscule part of a patient's entire life.

A patient's assessment of quality of life may be compromised when that patient becomes depressed or newly disabled (e.g., stroke, paraplegia, quadriplegia). Although critical care nurses care for many patients in such situations, it is usually the first time that this patient or family has faced such life-altering circumstances. The stress of the situation makes evaluation of quality of life difficult for them. It is important to provide the patient and family with support and time before making critical decisions.

Studies indicate that health care providers not only base quality of life on the patient's medical condition but also have social prejudices that affect care. These include biases against older adults, people with alternative lifestyles, those with alcohol and/or other substance abuse, and patients with a history of criminal activity. Comments about perceived flawed decision-making by patients and families may be passed on to others during nursing reports and hand-off communications between other team members. Rather than viewing care with objectivity, the team is at risk of developing the plan of care with biases shared in conversation. The team must regularly evaluate the plan of care and patterns of communication with the patient and family. Poor communication may undermine the relationship between the health care team with patients/significant others and overall success of the interdisciplinary plan of care.

TRUTH TELLING

Respect for patient autonomy and the principles of informed consent require that patients are told the truth about their medical condition. There are times when family members or treating professionals believe that telling patients the truth about their condition may negatively affect their outcomes. Sometimes called the therapeutic exception to truth telling, it should be used very rarely, and only with confirming evidence that telling the truth would truly harm the patient. Sometimes requests from family members to withhold medical information from a patient entail religious and/or cultural considerations. These requests should be addressed on a case-by-case basis.

WITHHOLDING AND WITHDRAWING TREATMENT

The acts of withholding (not starting) and withdrawing (stopping) treatment are considered to have no moral or legal difference. However, health care providers and patients' family members often feel more comfortable withholding than withdrawing treatment. Once a treatment has been started and is determined to be of no benefit to the patient, the reasons used to justify withholding treatment can be used when stopping or withdrawing supportive measures. One question to ask about withdrawing treatment is, "If the patient was not already receiving the treatment, would it be morally acceptable not to initiate it?"

It has been noted that when decisions to withhold resuscitation (do not resuscitate [DNR] or allow natural death [AND]) have been made, it seems unclear what other care should be provided. DNR and AND should not be interpreted as "do not treat." Many patients with DNR orders receive critical care interventions, surgery, and other treatments and then survive to discharge. Once a decision has been made to withhold resuscitation, it is important to clearly define treatments to be withheld or provided.

ASSISTED SUICIDE AND EUTHANASIA

Euthanasia refers to one person killing another person for a "compassionate" reason, and without causing pain. Assisted suicide occurs when someone provides a means for a patient to commit suicide (such as deliberately providing enough medicine for an overdose) but the patient actually performs the act that results in death. Although controversy surrounds assisted suicide, the American Nurses Association (ANA), the American Association of Critical-Care

Nurses (AACN), the American Medical Association (AMA), and the National Hospice Organization (NHO) explicitly oppose it. As of 2014, assisted suicide is legal in the states of Oregon, Montana, Vermont, Washington, and New Mexico, and is being debated in New Jersey. A ballot that explored legalizing physician-assisted suicide failed to be accepted by voters in Massachusetts in 2012. A Gallup Poll conducted in May 2013 revealed that 70% of respondents agreed that when patients and their families requested assisted suicide, physicians should be allowed to "end the patient's life by some painless means."

COMFORT CARE

Patients who are chronically ill, debilitated, or dying are generally isolated from and by society, as well as by health care providers. Health care providers now recognize that pain and depression may be undertreated in the routine care of patients and while caring for those who are chronically ill or dying. Health care professionals express fears of causing dependence, unresponsiveness, and even death resulting from use of sedatives and narcotic analgesics. When faced with a patient who is dying, it is unreasonable to worry about potential dependence on medication. The benefits of analgesics far outweigh the risks of dependence. Health care providers should try to provide the maximal pain relief possible while preserving responsiveness. When that is not possible, many patients and families choose to accept a decreased responsiveness to ensure that adequate pain relief is provided for the patient who is dying.

Many health care providers voice concerns that giving potent opioids or opiates to a patient who is dying may actually kill the patient. This concern is magnified when decisions to withdraw and withhold treatments have been made simultaneously. Opioid and opiate analgesics afford a broad therapeutic index and have a long history of safe use in patients who are medically frail. Many patients can tolerate increasing doses of these drugs without adverse respiratory or cardiovascular effects. Doses must be individualized or titrated based on pain relief using a pain scale. It is nearly impossible to predict a "perfect dose" of medication, given that not everyone responds to opioid analgesics the same way.

Even though it is very difficult to determine what amount of opioid or opiate will cause a person's death, such medicines can still be given by applying the principle of double effect. Simplified, this principle explains that giving narcotics to relieve pain is morally acceptable, even while knowing that it may also cause the patient to die sooner. However, growing evidence suggests that opiates, even at high doses, when given according to the latest palliative care guidelines, do not hasten death while meeting the patient's needs for comfort. The principle of double effect rarely needs to be used to justify the administration of opioids.

ETHICAL REASONING

When nurses find themselves in a situation in which they think something is "wrong," they should first consider the situation logically and systematically. By doing this, nurses can defend their positions rationally and provide ethically as well as medically sound care.

1. Determine the relevant facts of the case: These facts include the patient's medical, mental, and emotional condition, as well as the current plan of care.
2. Evaluate personal biases: The nurse must consider his or her personal values and ethical position regarding the situation as it may affect care. Nurses should consider the values and ethical positions of all the decision-makers involved.
3. Identify the problem: Do the facts support your view of the problem? Would others view the problem differently? If so, how?
4. Consider what ethical values and principles are at stake: Think about patient autonomy, patient harm (maleficence and beneficence), justice, and other considerations.
5. Explore options and their consequences: Consider identified values and principles; explore all plausible options for resolving the dilemma.

If direct communication with those involved does not resolve the issue, the bedside nurse should then involve the charge nurse or unit manager. The medical director's involvement may also be beneficial. If assistance is still needed in resolving the dilemma, The Joint Commission (TJC) requires that health care providers have access to institutional means for resolving ethical dilemmas (such as an ethics consultant or committee).

PREVENTIVE ETHICS

Just as it is easier to prevent heart disease than it is to cure it, it is easier to prevent an ethical conflict than it is to resolve one. When evaluating actions taken to resolve a dilemma, nurses should consider how those actions can provide guidance in future situations. When the bedside nurse first detects a problem, strategies used in previous, similar situations can be employed to prevent this situation from developing into a conflict. Many problems may be resolved after the first few steps of an ethical inquiry; gathering information and coordinating a patient care conference involving all relevant people. The interdisciplinary team should refrain from speculation or gossip and instead openly communicate with the patient, family, and other members of the care team about the plan of care. The nurse should promote discussions regarding the possible patient outcomes, ensuring that significant others have considered that they could be facing the patient's lifelong debility, the possibility of death, and are aware of the extent of time that may be needed to achieve a reasonable recovery. Lastly and most importantly, nurses should respect each patient as a person and treat that patient accordingly. The local ethics committee or team may be consulted for assistance with any ethical questions or concerns.

CARE PLANS FOR ETHICAL CONSIDERATIONS

Deficient knowledge *related to medical/nursing interventions related to end-of-life care.*

Goals/Outcomes: Before any medical or nursing intervention, the patient and significant others will verbalize understanding of explanations and agree to or refuse the intervention.
NOC Knowledge: Treatment Procedure(s).

Teaching: Procedure/Treatment
1. Have the patient identify appropriate decision-maker. If the patient has not executed an advance directive before becoming unable to speak for themselves, state law dictates the appropriate chain of decision-makers within the support system.
2. Assess decision-making capacity.
3. Determine that the patient has not been coerced into making decisions that are not in harmony with their wishes.
4. Accept the patient's/significant others' permission for or refusal of the intervention.

NIC Teaching: Procedure/Treatment; Teaching: Disease Process; Learning Facilitation.

Deficient knowledge *related to end-of-life decisions related to available documents.*

Goals/Outcomes: The patient will verbalize understanding of the options available regarding advance directives (living wills and DPAHC).
NOC Knowledge: Disease Process

Decision-Making Support
1. Provide the patient with information regarding living wills and DPAHC.
2. Assess understanding of living wills/DPAHC; provide information as indicated.
3. Identify who is legally empowered as a surrogate decision-maker.

NIC Health System Guidance; Patient Rights Protection.

Grieving *related to withholding/withdrawal of treatment; anticipation of loss.*

Goals/Outcomes: After intervention, the patient and significant others communicate feelings and participate in decisions regarding death and dying.
NOC Grief Resolution.

Anticipatory Guidance
1. Assess the patient's/significant others' understanding of medical prognosis and planned interventions.
2. Provide specific information regarding what to expect, what care/interventions will be given, and what will be withheld/discontinued; answer questions openly.
3. Allow for significant others to be with the patient during the dying process if they desire to be present.
4. Provide comfort measures for the patient/significant others.

NIC Grief Work Facilitation; Support System Enhancement; Active Listening; Family Support; Environmental Management: Comfort; Spiritual Support; Decision-Making Support.

PATIENT SAFETY

In 1999, the Institute of Medicine (IOM) released the report, To Err Is Human: Building a Safer Health Care System, which focused national attention on patient safety. The IOM estimated that between 44,000 and 98,000 persons die annually as a result of health care errors and that more than 1 million patients sustain injury as a result of health care errors. Since its release over 10 years ago, regulatory agencies, health care facilities, and consumers have joined together to enhance patient safety with minimal improvement. The report emphasized that individual clinicians' competency, hard work, and good intentions were not the cause of these errors but that the complex health care system with complicated processes were leading to these errors.

Shifting the goal from eliminating individual errors to reducing or eliminating the potential for patients to be harmed is significant. A proactive approach generally yields more globally successful outcomes. Nurses can contribute significantly to keeping patients safe by focusing on system-wide improvements, rather than reacting to adverse events. Nurses spend extensive periods of time with patients and are placed in roles that require interdisciplinary care coordination. The coordinative role prompts familiarity with a variety of hospital processes that may place the patient at risk for harm. Although it is not an easy journey, health care facilities now focus attention on designing systems where errors are prevented, and when they occur, practitioners can easily recognize and recover from actual and potential errors.

PATIENT SAFETY STANDARDS

Patient safety standards are set by a variety of organizations, including The Joint Commision (TJC), Centers for Medicare and Medicaid Services (CMS), Agency for Health care Research and Quality (AHRQ), National Quality Forum (NQF), Institute for Healthcare Improvement (IHI), and National Patient Safety Foundation (NPSF). All agencies have completed extensive research related to health care quality and provide extensive materials to support health care providers in performance improvement efforts to improve patient safety. The descriptions for these agencies are as follows:

AHRQ

The mission of the AHRQ (www.AHRQ.gov) is to improve the quality, safety, efficiency, and effectiveness of health care for all Americans. The agency's research assists both consumers and professionals in making more informed decisions about health care and facilitate quality improvement in health care services. The AHRQ was formerly known as the Agency for Health Care Policy and Research.

CMS

The Medicare and Medicaid programs were signed into law on July 30, 1965. The CMS (www.cms.gov) administers the Medicare program and jointly with state governments administers the Medicaid program. The CMS activities are focused to ensure access to safe and quality health care for beneficiaries.

IHI

The IHI (www.ihi.org) is an independent, nonprofit organization that strives to lead the improvement of worldwide health care. The IHI facilitates improvement by augmenting the desire or will for change, developing concepts for improving patient care, and helping health care systems put those ideas into action.
- Transforming Care at the Bedside (TCAB) was a national initiative developed by the Robert Wood Johnson Foundation (RWJF) in partnership with the IHI to improve hospital patient care and the hospital work environment by empowering front-line nurses to implement innovative new practices on their units.
  - TCAB emphasized a "bottom-up" approach to change; unlike the majority of quality programs, which use a "top-down" strategy.

Patient Safety

- The goal was to make the hospital experience safer and more pleasant for patients and to create time for nurses to spend more time in direct patient care.
- Nurse job satisfaction, retention, and quality of care were all expected to improve.
- TCAB was a three-phase program lasting from 2003 to 2008. The initial two phases were targeted at development and pilot testing of the TCAB approach in 13 select hospitals; the third phase continued the pilot projects and more broadly disseminated the model.

NQF

The NQF (www.qualityforum.org) is a not-for-profit organization focused on improving the quality of health care for all Americans. Their three-part mission includes setting priorities for performance improvement, supporting national consensus standards for performance measurement and public reporting of this information, and facilitating attainment of national goals by offering education and outreach programs.

NPSF

The NPSF (www.npsf.org) is an independent, not-for-profit organization founded in 1997, with a mission to improve safety of patients and families within the health care system. The NPSF is committed to a collaborative, interprofessional approach including key stakeholders. The goal of the group is to unite professional disciplines with organizational leaders across the continuum of care.

TJC

The mission of TJC (www.jointcommission.org) is to continuously improve the safety and quality of care provided to patients through the provision of health care accreditation. The organization has set standards that include National Patient Safety Goals and Sentinel Event Alerts. The 2007 Joint Commission Annual Report on Quality and Safety revealed inadequate communication between health care providers, or between providers and the patient and family members, as the main or root cause of at least half the serious adverse events in hospitals. Other causes included inadequate assessment of the patient's condition and poor leadership or training. TJC has launched several patient safety initiatives including the "Do Not Use Abbreviation" list, Infection Control, "Speak Up," and Universal Protocol ("Time Out"). Many of these initiatives have risen as a result of sentinel events that have occurred across the United States. TJC was formerly known as the Joint Commission on Accreditation of Health care Organizations (JCAHO).

Websites for additional resources are listed in Table 2-3.

Sentinel Event Alerts

In 1996, TJC established the sentinel event policy, which called for the identification, reporting, evaluation, and prevention of sentinel events, defined as any unexpected occurrence

Table 2-3	RESOURCES ON PATIENT SAFETY
Agency for Healthcare Research and Quality	www.ahrq.gov
American Hospital Association	www.aha.org
Centers for Medicare and Medicaid Services	www.cms.hhs.gov
Emergency Care Research Institute	www.ecri.org
Institute for Safe Medication Practices	www.ismp.org
National Patient Safety Foundation	www.npsf.org
National Priorities Partnership	www.nationalprioritiespartnership.org
The Institute for Health Care Improvement	www.ihi.org
The Joint Commission	www.jointcommission.org
Outcome Engenuity Just Culture Community	www.justculture.org
WHO Collaborating Centre for Patient Safety Solutions	www.ccforpatientsafety.org

involving death or serious physical or psychological injury or risk thereof (Boxes 2-6 and 2-7). One of the fundamental aspects of the sentinel event policy is the publication of sentinel event alerts by TJC. Sentinel event alerts consolidate experiences and "lessons learned" by accredited health care organizations with the goal of preventing health care errors in the future. Accredited organizations are expected to analyze current practices in order to recommend practices outlined by sentinel event alerts and close any inconsistencies that may exist in practice.

National patient safety goals

In July 2002, TJC launched the National Patient Safety Goal (NPSG) program in all accredited facilities. NPSGs are identified and prioritized by the Patient Safety Advisory Group, which consists of physicians, nurses, pharmacists, and other clinicians with expertise in patient safety for all accredited bodies (i.e., acute care facilities, ambulatory health care, behavioral health, etc.). The Patient Safety Advisory Group uses data from sentinel events and other authoritative sources to define NPSGs from year to year. NPSGs are evaluated each year, and a decision is made to continue current goals, add to the goal, delete the goal, move the goal to

---

Box 2-6 | SENTINEL EVENT POLICY

A sentinel event is an unexpected occurrence involving death or serious physical or psychological injury, or the risk thereof. The terms "Sentinel Event" and "Health Care Error" are not synonymous. Not all sentinel events are caused by a health care error, nor do all health care errors result in a sentinel event. All accredited organizations are required to define "sentinel event" for its own purpose and establish how all sentinel events will be identified and managed. Accredited organizations' response to a "sentinel event" includes conducting a timely, thorough, and credible root cause analysis, and development of an action plan.

From The Joint Commission. Retrieved from www.jointcommission.org.

Box 2-7 | OCCURRENCES THAT ARE SUBJECT TO REVIEW BY THE JOINT COMMISSION UNDER THE SENTINEL EVENT POLICY

- Event has resulted in an unanticipated death or major permanent loss of function, not related to the natural course of the patient's illness or underlying condition OR
- Suicide of any patient receiving care, treatment, and services in a staffed around-the-clock care setting or within 72 hours of discharge
- Unanticipated death of a full-term infant
- Abduction of any patient receiving care, treatment, and services
- Discharge of an infant to the wrong family
- Rape, assault (leading to death or permanent loss of function), or homicide of any patient receiving care, treatment, and services
- Rape, assault (leading to death or permanent loss of function), or homicide of a staff member, licensed independent practitioner, visitor, or vendor while on site at the health care organization
- Hemolytic transfusion reaction involving administration of blood or blood products having major blood group incompatibilities
- Invasive procedure, including surgery, on the wrong patient, wrong site, or wrong procedure
- Unintended retention of a foreign object in a patient after surgery or other procedure
- Severe neonatal hyperbilirubinemia (bilirubin >30 mg/dL)
- Prolonged fluoroscopy with cumulative dose >1500 rad to a single field or any delivery of radiotherapy to the wrong body region or >25% above the planned radiotherapy dose

Box 2-8	THE 2014 JOINT COMMISSION NATIONAL PATIENT SAFETY GOALS

For Acute Care Hospitals
- Identify patients correctly
- Improve staff communication
- Use medicines safely

- Use alarms safely
- Prevent infections
- Identify patient safety risks
- Prevent mistakes in surgery

Box 2-9	"SERIOUS REPORTABLE EVENTS" (previously known as "Never Events")

Seven Categories
1. Surgical or invasive procedure events
2. Product or device events
3. Patient protections events

4. Care management events
5. Environmental events
6. Radiologic events
7. Potential criminal events

the accreditations standards, and/or add additional goals (Box 2-8). Some of the patient safety goals may be moved from the NPSG chapter to the main body of standards in the TJC standards manual over time. Patient safety goals evolve into the standard of care.

"Serious Reportable Events" (SRE) or "Never Events"

In 2001, Ken Kizer, MD, the former CEO of the NQF, introduced a list of 21 adverse events that were serious and should never occur. Over the years, the list has expanded and as of 2011 encompasses 29 events in 7 categories (Box 2-9). Effective October 2008, health care facilities no longer receive payment from the CMS for any patient who suffers a "Never Event" while in the care of the facility. The condition lists included on the CMS "Never Events" and the NQF "Never Events" overlap but are not identical. Refer to the CMS website (www.cms.hhs.gov) for current regulations surrounding payment structure for "Never Events."

"Patient Safety Organizations"

Recognizing the need to capture information from adverse events, Congress passed the Patient Safety and Quality Improvement Act of 2005 (Patient Safety Act). The act authorized the creation of Patient Safety Organizations (PSOs) to collect and analyze data from patient safety events. PSOs include public and private entities demonstrating the goal to collect, aggregate, and analyze data for the improvement of patient safety.

CULTURE OF SAFETY

Health care organizations have identified that 95% of health care errors are directly related to system flaws, whereas only 5% of health care errors are caused by incompetent or poorly intended care (Sexton and Thomas, 2004). System flaws are largely related to flawed communication, which may lead to disjointed or uncoordinated care. Not all members of the team are consistently aware of key information that, if omitted, may cause harm to the patient. Therefore, to improve patient safety and address health care errors, health care organizational culture must value communication and team collaboration. Focus on these two factors will result in improved clinical effectiveness and job satisfaction among health care professionals (Box 2-10).

COMMUNICATION

Despite years of training, coaching, and experience, communication among health care professionals remains a challenge and a leading root cause of sentinel events in many facilities. In a metaanalysis of research studies, Seago (2008) found that the evidence remains mixed on a preferred format for communication strategies. In the AACN Standards for Establishing and Sustaining a Healthy Work Environment, Skilled Communication is the first standard addressed and is the one standard that weaves its way into the five other standards. The emphasis by the AACN on healthy work environment standards is a testimony to the importance of excellent communication skills in acute and critical care (Table 2-4).

Box 2-10	COMPONENTS OF SUCCESSFUL TEAMWORK

- Trust
- Respect
- Collaboration
- Open communication
- Nonpunitive environment
- Clear direction
- Methods to evaluate outcomes and amend processes as needed

- Defined roles and responsibilities of team members
- Atmosphere of respect
- Flattening of caregiver hierarchy
- Methodologies to resolve conflict
- Defined decision-making procedures

From O'Daniel M, Rosenstein AH: Professional communication and team collaboration. In Hughes RG, editor: *Patient safety and quality: an evidence-based handbook for nurses,* Rockville, 2008, Agency for Health care Research and Quality.

Table 2-4	AMERICAN ASSOCIATION OF CRITICAL-CARE NURSES STANDARDS FOR ESTABLISHING AND SUSTAINING HEALTHY WORK ENVIRONMENTS
Skilled communication	Nurses must be as proficient in communication skills as they are in clinical skills
True collaboration	Nurses must be relentless in pursuing and fostering true collaboration
Effective decision-making	Nurses must be valued and committed partners in making policy, directing and evaluating clinical care, and leading organizational operations
Appropriate staffing	Staffing must ensure effective match between patient needs and nurse competencies
Meaningful recognition	Nurses must be recognized and must recognize others for the value each brings to the work of the organization
Authentic leadership	Nurse leaders must fully embrace the imperative of a healthy work environment, authentically live it, and engage others in its achievement

From American Association of Critical-Care Nurses: *AACN Advanced critical care nursing,* Aliso Viejo, 2008, American Association of Critical-Care Nurses, p 7.

Patient Safety

Nurses and physicians are trained to deliver and receive communication using different strategies that often lead to a communication gap between these highly skilled health care professionals. Nurses tend to communicate in a lengthier manner, unfolding patient conditions in a narrative and highly descriptive style (e.g., a patient has an alteration in comfort versus a patient is in pain). Physicians are taught in medical school to present "highlights" to their attending physician, giving them only the needed data to make a clinical decision. Therefore, when a nurse communicates with a physician or midlevel practitioner and does not provide a focused report, key patient care data may not be communicated effectively.

The power of structured communication methods has been successfully used in many industries including the airline industry, nuclear power, and the U.S. Department of Defense. One such method of structured communications is the Situation-Background-Assessment-Recommendation (SBAR) documentation format. Using SBAR is helpful to those who have difficulty with focused, concise communications. The AHRQ and others across the United States have advocated for SBAR as a form of standardized communication among complex health care teams (Table 2-5).

TJC recognizes the importance of communication and has woven communication throughout many of the NPSGs. In particular, TJC calls for each accredited facility to define a methodology for which staff communicates information about patient care in a consistent manner when moving a patient from one practitioner to the care of a different practitioner. A report at the time of transition of caregivers is called "hand-off communication" (Box 2-11).

Table 2-5	**STRUCTURED COMMUNICATION: SITUATION-BACKGROUND-ASSESSMENT-RECOMMENDATION (SBAR)**	
Before initiating an SBAR conversation, nurses should assess the patient; review the health care record for appropriate physician or other care provider to call; know the patient's diagnoses, procedures, and medical history; read all recent physician progress notes (especially from the past 12 hours); have available the following clinical data (chart, allergies, medications recently given, recent diagnostic tests, and patient code status); and, last, take a moment to organize all data, thoughts, and requests.		
S Situation	Give your name and unit you are calling from, the patient's full name, room number, and attending physician name if calling the on-call physician. If the problem is urgent, please notify the provider at the beginning of the call. The patient's code status if appropriate.	"Dr. James, I'm Susie, a critical care RN. Mr. Smith is a 42-year-old currently in radiology for a computed tomography (CT) of the head after a motor vehicle crash (MVC). I am the rapid response nurse and was called to see him for anxiety and shortness of breath."
B Background	The patient's admission diagnosis, admission date, and pertinent medical history. Provide a brief synopsis of the treatments and plan of care thus far.	"Mr. Smith was the driver and sustained blunt chest trauma during the MVC approximately 3 hours ago. There is no significant medical history."
A Assessment	Provide a brief description of the problem or primary concern. If uncertain of the problem, acknowledge the uncertainty. Provide clinical data such as most recent vital signs, physical assessment findings, and clinical changes specific to the problem you are calling about. Provide update of all pertinent therapies (IVs, O_2, etc.).	"I think Mr. Smith has a pneumothorax on the right. Breath sounds are absent in the right middle and lower lobes. He is short of breath, anxious, and tachypneic with an oxygen saturation of 88% on 4 liters of oxygen."
R Recommendation	Express what you think the patient needs to address the problem. If unclear on what interventions are needed, acknowledge uncertainty. If requesting the practitioner to come and assess the patient, clarify with the practitioner the exact time frame to expect their arrival.	"I think Mr. Smith needs more oxygen and a chest tube right away. I have asked the radiology technician to obtain the supplies for chest tube placement. Can you come to radiology to assess the patient for chest tube placement, or is there someone else we should call?"

Several national programs have been developed to enhance both intradisciplinary and interdisciplinary communication among health care providers:

TeamSTEPPS

The AHRQ and the U.S. Department of Defense have partnered together to develop an evidence-based curriculum and training program with the goal of promoting patient safety through improving communication and teamwork skills among health care professionals (Table 2-6).

The focus of TeamSTEPPS is to develop competency in four primary trainable teamwork skills. These skills are leadership, communication, situation monitoring, and mutual support. When all individuals of a team possess competency in these skills, research has demonstrated that the team can enhance three types of teamwork outcomes: performance, knowledge, and attitudes.

"JUST CULTURE"

The creation of a "Just Culture" has been advocated as a means to enhance the patient safety culture of an organization. A culture of learning must exist that encourages the reporting of

Box 2-11 HAND-OFF COMMUNICATION

Elements of Hand-Off Communication
- Standardized to the situation to which it applies
- When to use certain techniques (i.e., read-back or repeat-back)
- Interactive: Allow for questioning between giver and receiver of the patient information.
- Contain the most recent information regarding patient care, treatment, services, condition, and any recent or anticipated changes.
- Interruptions during hand-offs are limited.

Strategies to Improve Hand-Off Communication
- Use clear language and avoid all abbreviations or terms that can be misinterpreted.
- Use effective communication techniques.
- Limit interruptions and distractions.
- Provide adequate time for interaction.
- Standardize use of tools to facilitate the interaction, especially during high-volume, high-distraction times, such as shift-to-shift, unit-to-unit.
- Use technology to enhance communications—electronic health care records, portable computers, handheld devices, etc.

Table 2-6	THREE PHASES OF THE TeamSTEPPS IMPLEMENTATION
Phase 1 Assess the Need	Determine the organizational readiness for undertaking a TeamSTEPPS-based initiative. • Establish an organizational change team. • Conduct a site assessment. • Define the problem, challenge, or opportunity for improvement. • Define the goal of the intervention.
Phase 2 Planning, Training, and Implementation	TeamSTEPPS is designed to be customized to the organization. Implementation options include use of all tools and strategies across the entire organization or a phased-in approach that targets specific units or departments, or selected individual tools can be introduced at specific intervals. • Define the intervention. • Develop a plan for determining the interventions and effectiveness. • Develop an implementation plan. • Gain leadership commitment to the plan. • Develop a communication plan. • Prepare the facility. • Implement training.
Phase 3 Sustainment	Sustain and spread improvements in teamwork performance, clinical processes, and outcomes. Continual learning and reinforcement of skills on the unit or within the facility: • Provide opportunities for clinicians to practice skills. • Ensure leaders emphasize new skills. • Provide regular feedback and coaching. • Celebrate and measure successes. • Update the plan.

adverse events and near misses without the fear of retribution. The practitioner must be offered protection from disciplinary action when they report injuries, errors, and near misses when personally involved. This implies that errors are most often not intentional, nor are they caused by human failures alone. Most are often a series of system failures that come together at an intersection involving the patient.

The creation of a "Just Culture" does acknowledge that there are exceptions where health care workers do not have protection. Protection should not be granted for risky and/or criminal behavior, for active malfeasance, or in cases in which an injury is not reported in a timely manner (Box 2-12).

PATIENT/FAMILY INVOLVEMENT

Patient and family involvement in the plan of care can be a crucial element of patient safety, because both are familiar with key information that, if known, may prevent harm. Understanding of medications, the health history, and proposed plan of care is vital to a safe patient care experience. Patients and families may feel reluctant to challenge, remind, or question their health care providers. There has been a recent shift within all patient safety organizations as well as professional organizations to include the patient in daily rounds, to provide time for daily goal setting, and to ensure all parts of the treatment plan have been communicated and are understood. Several national programs have been developed and promoted to facilitate the involvement of patients and families in the plan of care (Box 2-13).

SPEAK UP

TJC supports a national campaign urging patients to partner with their health care provider to prevent health care errors by becoming involved in their care. The campaign offers a variety of tools (videos, brochures, artwork, etc.) to educate patients on steps they can take to partner with health care workers to enhance safe care delivery. Topics include but are not limited to "Help Avoid Mistakes with Your Medication," "Five Things You Can Do to Prevent Infection," and "What You Should Know about Pain Management" (Box 2-14).

NOTHING ABOUT ME, WITHOUT ME

In 2001, the NPSF established a Patient and Family Advisory Council to provide guidance and expertise on all NSPF's activities. One of the fundamental principles advocated by this

---

Box 2-12	**"JUST CULTURE"**

Creation of a culture where clinicians are willing to report errors so that the process can be analyzed and solutions found, but clinician responsibility for events is maintained. The culture is not "blame-free" but blame-appropriate.

From Marx D: *Patient safety and the "just culture": a primer for health care executives,* New York, 2001, Columbia University. Retrieved from www.psnet.ah rq.gov/resource.aspx?resourceID-1582.

Box 2-13	**STEPS TO INVOLVING PATIENTS IN PATIENT SAFETY**

Obtain patient feedback through a variety of sources such as patient satisfaction, focus groups, community groups, hotlines, etc.

Review patient plan of care and daily goals with patients and their families.

Never separate a patient from their family unless that is desired; allow patient access 24 hours per day.

Never deny a patient information; a variety of tools can be used to enhance communication and sharing of information such as reviewing the health care record; orientation to the unit, equipment, and team members; wipe boards; sharing clinical pathways; patient conferences with interdisciplinary team; and customized discharge instructions.

Encourage patient's and family's involvement in care by inviting them to participate through creative campaigns; staff wearing buttons asking "Ask me if I've washed my hands"; tent cards in patient rooms; brochures and pamphlets educating patients on how to be involved in their care.

From Roizen M, Oz M, The Joint Commission: *You: the smart patient,* New York, 2006, Simon & Schuster Inc. Retrieved from www.jointcommission.org/GeneralPublic/smart_patient.htm.

Box 2-14	SPEAK UP

Speak up if you have questions or concerns. If you still do not understand, ask again. It is your body and you have a right to know.

Pay attention to the care you get. Always make sure you are getting the right treatments and medicines by the right health care professionals. Do not assume anything.

Educate yourself about your illness. Learn about the medical tests you get and your treatment plan.

Ask a trusted family member or friend to be your advocate (advisor or supporter).

Know what medicines you take and why you take them. Health care errors are the most common health care mistakes.

Use a hospital, clinic, surgery center, or other type of health care organization that has been carefully checked out. For example, The Joint Commission visits hospitals to see if they are meeting The Joint Commission's quality standards.

Participate in all decisions about your treatment. You are the center of the health care team.

From The Joint Commission: *Speak Up: help prevent errors in your care, and speak up: know your rights.* Retrieved from www.jointcommission.org/assets/1/18/speakup_hc.pdf.

council is the philosophy of "Nothing about Me, without Me." This phrase was suggested in 1998 by an English midwife at a seminar advocating that patients should be involved in every step of their health care. This phrase has now been quoted by key patient safety leaders such as but not limited to Delbanco, Berwick, Tye, and IOM's Crossing the Quality Chasm report and is the title of a consumer book on health care safety. (Table 2-7 outlines the NPSF recommendations.)

HIGH-RELIABILITY ORGANIZATIONS

High-reliability organizations (HROs) are those that are known to be complex and risky yet maintain safety and effectiveness. Key characteristics of HROs include preoccupation with failure and safety, deference to expertise, sensitivity to operations, commitment to resilience, and reluctance to simplify. HROs are continually analyzing and asking questions to prevent failures within the systems and analyzing how to minimize effects from failures when and if they occur. The use of the prospective tool of a failure mode and effects analysis (FMEA) and the use of a retrospective tool such as a root cause analysis (RCA) have proven valuable to health care organizations (Table 2-8).

Table 2-7	NATIONAL AGENDA FOR ACTION: PATIENTS AND FAMILIES IN PATIENT SAFETY: ROAD MAP FOR ACTION
Education and Awareness	• Raise public awareness on the definition and frequency of health care error and patient safety. • Educate the public on how to aid in safeguarding their own care. • Educate health care professionals and leadership about the importance of the patient/family perspective. • Raise health care providers' awareness of the experiences of patients and their families. • Raise awareness in the behavioral health community on health care errors. • Educate the media. • Build patient safety and health care error prevention into all health care professional education curricula. • Build interactive, interdisciplinary education programs. • Develop a central clearinghouse and interactive resource center.

Continued

Table 2-7	NATIONAL AGENDA FOR ACTION: PATIENTS AND FAMILIES IN PATIENT SAFETY: ROAD MAP FOR ACTION—cont'd
Build a Culture of Patient- and Family-Centered Patient Safety	• Teach and encourage effective communication skills. • Engage leadership in promoting and training providers in open communication about health care error. • Empower hospital patient representatives to effectively advocate. • Establish patient and family advisory councils. • Represent patients' interests on boards and trustees. • Establish patient safety task forces. • Create a national forum for state coalitions.
Research	• "Bridging the gap." • Disclosure. • Short- and long-term effects of incorporating patients and families into the system. • Current patient safety information and resource landscape for patients and families. • Posttraumatic stress specific to health care error. • Team relationships.
Support Services	• National resource center and information line. • Emergency hotline. • Peer resource counseling. • Support groups for families and individuals who have suffered as a result of a health care error. • Disclosure and communication programs. • National training programs for hospitals implementing any of the above programs.

From National Patient Safety Foundation: *National agenda for action: patients and families in patient safety: Nothing about Me, without Me*, 2003. Retrieved from www.npsf.org/pdf/paf/AgendaFamilies.pdf.

Table 2-8	FAILURE MODE AND EFFECTS ANALYSIS VERSUS ROOT CAUSE ANALYSIS	
Failure Mode and Effects Analysis (FMEA)	**Root Cause Analysis (RCA)**	
Proactive analysis of a process or equipment to anticipate any potential process or product failure	Retrospective analysis of an event that has already occurred; actual failure	
Looks forward through a process to identify any potential failure points	Looks back chronologically after a process has failed	
Multidisciplinary team involvement is key to success	Multidisciplinary team involvement by all who were involved in the failure is key to success	
Three key questions are addressed: • How likely is the equipment or process to fail? • What is the significance of the failure? • How likely it is that someone will be able to detect this failure?	Three key questions are addressed: • What happened? • Why did it happen? • What can be done to prevent it from happening again?	
Analytical tools used: • Flow diagrams of all main and subprocesses • Brainstorm • Cause-and-effect diagrams	Analytical tools used: • Timeline • Cause-and-effect diagrams • Frequency plots • Scatterplots	

Patient safety is an ever-changing specialty within health care; new resources and knowledge are constantly being defined as research is completed. The provision of safe care delivery is demanded by regulators, payers, health care providers, and, most important, the patient. Therefore, it is crucial that every clinician accept accountability for the provision of a health care environment that both supports and provides a culture of safe care delivery.

SELECTED REFERENCES

Agency for Health Care Research and Quality: Team STEPPS™: national implementation, Rockville, February 2, 2009, Agency for Health Care Research and Quality. http://from teamstepps.ahrq.gov/index.htm. Accessed July 5, 2015.

American Academy of Microbiology (AAM) Bioinformatics and Biodefense: Keys to understanding natural and altered pathogens, Washington, 2009, American Academy of Microbiology.

American Association of Critical-Care Nurses: AACN standards for establishing and sustaining healthy work environments: a journey to excellence, Am J Crit Care 14:187–197, 2005.

Baumhover N, Hughes L: Spirituality and support for family presence during invasive procedures and resuscitations in adults, Am J Crit Care 18:357–367, 2009.

Beauchamp TL, Childress JF: Principles of biomedical ethics, ed 6, New York, 2009, Oxford University Press.

Berghs M, Dierckx D, Gastmans C: The complexity of nurses' attitudes toward euthanasia: a review of the literature, J Med Ethics 31:441–446, 2005.

Centers for Disease Control and Prevention [CDC]: Avian influenza A virus infections in humans, March 18, 2015. http://www.cdc.gov/flu/avianflu/avian-in-humans.htm. Access date July 5, 2015.

Centers for Disease Control and Prevention [CDC]: Bioterrorism. http://www.bt.cdc.gov/bioterrorism/.

Centers for Disease Control and Prevention [CDC]: Bioterrorism: anthrax. http://www.cdc.gov/anthrax/bioterrorism/.

Centers for Disease Control and Prevention [CDC]: Botulism, April 25, 2015. http://www.bt.cdc.gov/agent/botulism/. Access date July 5, 2015.

Centers for Disease Control and Prevention [CDC]: Clinical guidance on the identification and evaluation of possible SARS-CoV disease among persons presenting with community-acquired illness, May 3, 2005. http://www.cdc.gov/ncidod/sars/clinicalguidance.htm.

Centers for Disease Control and Prevention [CDC]: Consent form (SARS-CoV EIA laboratory testing), May 3, 2005. http://www.cdc.gov/ncidod/sars/lab/eia/consent.htm.

Centers for Disease Control and Prevention [CDC]: Creutzfeldt-Jakob disease, classic questions and answers, CJD infection control practices, June 2008. http://www.cdc.gov/ncidod/dvrd/cjd/qa_CJD_infection_control.htm.

Centers for Disease Control and Prevention [CDC]: Fact sheet: variant Creutzfeldt-Jakob disease, June 2008. http://www.cdc.gov/ncidod/dvrd/vcjd/factsheet_nvcjd.htm.

Centers for Disease Control and Prevention [CDC]: Guideline for isolation precautions: preventing transmission of infectious agents in health care settings, June 2007. http://www.cdc.gov/ncidod/dhqp/pdf/guidelines/Isolation2007.pdf.

Centers for Disease Control and Prevention [CDC]: Ebola (Ebola Virus Disease), July 2, 2015. http://www.cdc.gov/vhf/ebola/index.html. Access date July 5, 2015.

Centers for Disease Control and Prevention [CDC]: Health care Infection Control Practices Advisory Committee (HICPAC). http://www.cdc.gov/hicpac/pubs.html.

Centers for Disease Control and Prevention [CDC]: Infection control in health care facilities, Feb 12, 2013. http://www.cdc.gov/flu/professionals/infectioncontrol/.

Centers for Disease Control and Prevention [CDC]: Methicillin-resistant Staphylococcus aureus (MRSA) infections, April 3, 2014. http://www.cdc.gov/mrsa/health care/index.html#q3.

Centers for Disease Control and Prevention [CDC]: Middle Eastern respiratory syndrome (MERS), May 22, 2014. http://www.cdc.gov/coronavirus/mers/clinical-features.html.

Centers for Disease Control and Prevention [CDC]: Plague information, June 13, 2012. http://www.bt.cdc.gov/agent/plague/.

Centers for Disease Control and Prevention [CDC]: Severe acute respiratory syndrome (SARS), May 3 2005. http://www.cdc.gov/ncidod/sars/.

Centers for Disease Control and Prevention [CDC]: Severe acute respiratory syndrome (SARS); public health guidance for community-level preparedness and response to severe acute respiratory syndrome (SARS) version 2, Supplement F: laboratory guidance, January 2004. http://www.cdc.gov/ncidod/sars/absenceofsars.htm.

Centers for Disease Control and Prevention [CDC]: Supplement I: infection control in health care, home, and community settings, January 8 2004. http://www.cdc.gov/ncidod/sars/guidance/i/pdf/i.pdf.

Centers for Disease Control and Prevention [CDC]: *Smallpox.* http://www.bt.cdc.gov/agent/smallpox/.

Centers for Disease Control and Prevention [CDC]: *Tularemia.* http://www.bt.cdc.gov/agent/tularemia/.

Centers for Disease Control and Prevention [CDC]: *Viral hemorrhagic fevers* June 18, 2013. http://www.cdc.gov/vhf/virus-families.

Centers for Disease Control and Prevention [CDC]: *West Nile virus (WNV)* Feb 12, 2015. http://www.cdc.gov/westnile/index.htm.

Cheng VC, Lau SK, Woo PC, Yuen KY: Severe acute respiratory syndrome coronavirus as an agent of emerging and reemerging infection, *Clin Microbiol Rev* 20:660–694, 2007.

Davidson JE, Powers K, Hedayast KM, et al: Clinical practice guidelines for the support of the family in the patient centered intensive care unit. American College of Care Medicine Task Force 2004-2005, *Crit Care Med* 35:605–622, 2007.

Delgado C: Meeting clients' spiritual needs, *Nurs Clin North Am* 42:279–293, 2007.

Dreher H, Dean JL, Moriarty DM, et al: What you need to know about SARS now, *Nursing* 34: 58–64, 2004.

Edgman-Levitan S: Involving the patient in safety efforts. In Leonard A, Frankel A, Simmonds T, editors: *Achieving safe and reliable health care: strategies and solutions*, Chicago, 2004, ACHE Health Administration Press.

Engel JP, Lipkin WI: *Improving the nation's ability to detect and respond to 21st century urgent health threats: second report of the National Biosurveillance Advisory Subcommittee*, April 2011. http://www.cdc.gov/about/advisory/pdf/NBASFinalReport_April2011.pdf.

Frankel A: Accountability: defining the rules. In Leonard A, Frankel A, Simmonds T, editors: *Achieving safe and reliable health care: strategies and solutions*, Chicago, 2004, ACHE Health Administration Press.

Friesen MA, White SV, Byers JF: Handoffs: implications for nurses. In Hughes RG, editor: *Patient safety and quality: an evidence-based handbook for nurses*, Rockville, 2008, Agency for Health Care Research and Quality.

Fry ST, Johnstone M: *Ethics in nursing practice: a guide to ethical decision making*, ed 3, Chichester, 2008, Wiley-Blackwell.

Grace PJ: *Nursing ethics and professional responsibility in advanced practice*, Sudbury, 2009, Jones and Bartlett.

Grisso T, Appelbaum PS: *Assessing competence to consent to treatment: a guide for physicians and other health professionals*, Oxford, 1998, Oxford University Press.

Haggerty LA, Grace PJ: Clinical wisdom: the essential component of 'good' nursing care, *J Prof Nurs* 24:235–240, 2008.

Huhn GD, Sejvar JD, Montgomery SP, Dworkin MS: West Nile virus in the United States: an update on an emerging infectious disease, *Am Fam Physician* 68:653–660, 2003.

Institute of Medicine: *Keeping patients safe: transforming the work environment of nurses*, Washington, 2004, National Academies Press.

Institute of Medicine: *Patient safety: achieving a new standard for care*, Washington, 2004, National Academies Press.

Institute of Medicine: *To err is human: building a safer health system*, Washington, 2000, National Academies Press.

Institute of Medicine (US) and National Research Council (US) Committee on Effectiveness of National Biosurveillance Systems: *Biowatch and the public health system*, Washington, 2011, National Academies Press.

Jonsen AR, Siegler M, Winslade WJ: *Clinical ethics: a practical approach to ethical decisions in clinical medicine*, ed 6, New York, 2006, McGraw-Hill.

Karwa M, Currie B, Kvetan V: Bioterrorism: preparing for the impossible or the improbable, *Crit Care Med* 33:S75–S95, 2005.

Leonard M, Frankel A: Focusing on high reliability. In Leonard A, Frankel A, Simmonds T, editors: *Achieving safe and reliable health care: strategies and solutions*, Chicago, 2004, ACHE Health Administration Press.

Leonard M, Graham S, Taggart B: The human factor: effective teamwork and communication in patient strategy. In Leonard A, Frankel A, Simmonds T, editors: *Achieving safe and reliable health care: strategies and solutions*, Chicago, 2004, ACHE Health Administration Press.

Lipkin WI: The changing face of pathogen discovery and surveillance, *Nat Rev Microbiol* 11:133–141, 2013.

Marx D: *Patient safety and the "just culture": a primer for health care executives*, New York, 2001, Columbia University.

Maze CD: Registered nurses' personal rights vs. professional responsibility in caring for members of underserved and disenfranchised populations, *J Clin Nurse* 14:546–554, 2005.

Mazur MA, Cox LA, Capon JA: The public's attitude and perception concerning witnessed cardio-pulmonary resuscitation, *Crit Care Med* 4:2925–2928, 2006.

Meade C, Bursell A, Ketelsen L: Effects of nursing rounds on call light use, satisfaction and safety, *Am J Nursing* 106:58–70, 2006.

Medline Plus: *Lactate dehydrogenase test*, February 8, 2012. http://www.nlm.nih.gov/medlineplus/ency/article/003471.htm.

Nance JJ: *Why hospitals should fly: the ultimate flight plan to patient safety and quality care*, Bozeman, 2008, Second River Health care Press.

National Patient Safety Foundation: *National agenda for action: patients and families in patient safety: Nothing about Me, without Me*, 2003. http://www.npsf.org/pdf/paf/AgendaFamilies.pdf.

National Quality Forum: *National Quality Forum updates endorsement of serious reportable events in health care*, Oct 17, 2012. http://www.qualityforum.org/pdf/news/prSeriousReportableEvents10-15-06.pdf.

O'Daniel M, Rosenstein AH: Professional communication and team collaboration. In Hughes RG, editor: *Patient safety and quality: an evidence-based handbook for nurses*, Rockville, 2008, Agency for Health care Research and Quality.

Reason J, Hobbs A: *Managing maintenance error: a practical guide*, Burlington, 2003, Ashgate.

Rice SE: Susan Rice: prepare to fight tomorrow's Ebola. *USA Today*, September 26, 2014. http://www.usatoday.com/story/opinion/2014/09/26/ebola-west-africa-americans-treatment-help-aid-who-column/16233605/.

Rutherford P, Moen R, Taylor J: TCAB: the how and what, *Am J Nursing* 109:5–17, 2009.

Scholtes PR, Joiner BL, Streibel BJ: *The team handbook*, ed 3, Madison, 2003, Oriel.

Seago JA: Professional communication. In Hughes RG, editor: *Patient safety and quality: an evidence-based handbook for nurses*, Rockville, 2008, Agency for Health care Research and Quality.

Sexton B, Thomas E: Measurement: assessing a safety culture. In Leonard A, Frankel A, Simmonds T, editors: *Achieving safe and reliable health care: strategies and solutions*, Chicago, 2004, ACHE Health Administration Press.

Siegel JD, Rhinehart E, Jackson M, Chiarello L: Management of multidrug-resistant organisms in health care settings, *Am J Infect Control* 35:S165–S193, 2007.

Simmonds T, Whittington J: Analytical tools. In Leonard A, Frankel A, Simmonds T, editors: *Achieving safe and reliable health care: strategies and solutions*, Chicago, 2004, ACHE Health Administration Press.

The Bipartisan WMD Terrorism Research Center: *Bio-response report card*, October 2011. http://www.wmdcenter.org/wp-content/uploads/2011/10/bio-response-report-card-2011.pdf.

The Joint Commission: *Hand-off communications*. http://www.jointcommission.org/Accreditation-Programs/HomeCare/Standards/09_FAQs/NPSG/Communication/NPSG.02.05.01/hand_off_communications.htm.

The Joint Commission: *National patient safety goals*. http://www.jointcommission.org/assets/1/6/HAP_NPSG_Chapter_2014.pdf.

The Joint Commission: *Patient safety*. http://www.jointcommission.org/topics/patient_safety.aspx.

The Joint Commission: *Sentinel event policy*. http://www.jointcommission.org/Sentinel_Event_Policy_and_Procedures/.

The Joint Commission: *Speak Up initiatives*. http://www.jointcommission.org/speakup.aspx.

Wainwright P, Gallagher A: Ethical aspects of withdrawing and withholding treatment, *Nurs Stand* 21:46–50, 2007.

Watson J: *Nursing. The philosophy and science of caring*, Boulder, 2008, University Press of Colorado.

Weick KE, Sutcliffe KM: *Managing the unexpected: assuring high performance in an era of complexity*, San Francisco, 2001, Jossey-Bass.

Wheeler DJ: *Understanding variation: the key to managing chaos*, ed 2, Knoxville, 2000, SPC Press.

Willis DG, Grace PJ, Roy C: A central unifying focus for the discipline: facilitating humanization, meaning, choice, quality of life, and healing in living and dying, *Adv Nurs Sci* 31:E28–E40, 2008.

Wolf ZR, Hughes RG: Error reporting and disclosure. In Hughes RG, editor: *Patient safety and quality: an evidence-based handbook for nurses*, Rockville, 2008, Agency for Health Care Research and Quality.

World Health Organization: *Background and summary of human infection with avian influenza A (H7N9) virus*, January 31, 2014. http://www.who.int/influenza/human_animal_interface/20140131_background_and_summary_H7N9_v1.pdf?ua=1.

World Health Organization: *Middle Eastern respiratory syndrome coronavirus (MERS-CoV) summary and literature update*, May 9, 2014. http://www.who.int/csr/disease/coronavirus_infections/MERS_CoV_Update_09_May_2014.pdf?ua=1.

Patient Safety

3   Trauma

MAJOR TRAUMA

PATHOPHYSIOLOGY

Traumatic injuries account for over 5 million deaths worldwide. In the United States, traumatic injuries are the leading cause of death for patients between the ages of 1 and 44 years. Traumatic injuries also account for over 2.6 million hospitalizations each year. Major trauma occurs when energy is applied to body tissues in excess of what the tissues are able to absorb. The energy can be in the form of kinetic, thermal, chemical, electrical, and radiant energy. Trauma can also occur when the body is deprived of an essential element such as oxygen or heat. Kinetic energy is the most common cause of trauma and includes mechanisms such as motor vehicle collisions (MVCs), falls, and gunshot wounds. Thermal, chemical, electrical, and radiation energy cause burns. Lack of oxygen occurs in drowning and hanging injuries. The amount of damage to the tissue will depend on the amount of force applied, the length of time the force is applied, and the resiliency of the tissue. Hollow organs tend to absorb more energy and are injured less frequently than are solid organs because the organ tissue has more flexibility to withstand the forces.

The primary pathophysiologic process that occurs with major trauma is shock. Patients with major trauma are at risk for all types of shock, but the most common type is hypovolemic shock resulting from hemorrhage. Hypovolemic shock is usually broken into four stages that are used to describe the physiologic response to hemorrhage and are useful in estimating the amount of blood loss.

All body systems require both oxygen and glucose for cellular energy production. The classic signs of hypovolemic shock occur from activation of the central nervous system (CNS). Following major injury, the CNS triggers a series of reactions to increase delivery of oxygen and glucose to the cells. Catecholamines (epinephrine and norepinephrine) and glucocorticoids are released from the adrenal glands to preserve perfusion to vital organs, mobilize glycogen stores, increase available glucose and oxygen, suppress pancreatic insulin secretion, and enhance glucose uptake. Hyperglycemia is common following major trauma. Glycogen stores are rapidly depleted (within 24 hours). Without nutrition, energy is generated from the breakdown of the body or catabolism. Breakdown of muscle tissue, fat, and viscera creates a negative nitrogen balance. Subclinical adrenal insufficiency may become clinically apparent after severe injury.

The posterior pituitary release of antidiuretic hormone promotes water absorption in the distal renal tubules. Intravascular volume increases as urinary output decreases. Blood pressure (BP) is increased by the renin-angiotensin-aldosterone system. Aldosterone promotes sodium and water reabsorption to increase intravascular volume, and angiotensin II causes vasoconstriction.

Several factors can alter the patient's response to blood loss and must be considered in the resuscitation of these patients. These factors include the patient's age, location of injury, type and severity of the injury, the amount of time that has elapsed since the injury, prehospital interventions to address blood loss, and medications taken for chronic conditions, especially anticoagulants and beta-blockers. Because the patient has many other injuries, the classic signs of shock may be altered.

The source of the bleeding must be identified and stopped as soon as possible. The patient must be adequately resuscitated or the patient is at risk of developing acidosis, coagulopathy, and hypothermia, which are considered the deadly triad of trauma. Once these conditions occur, they tend to stimulate each other and become a vicious cycle that is difficult to break.

Acidosis occurs when the number of red blood cells is reduced from blood loss and cellular oxygen supply is reduced, resulting in end-organ hypoxia caused by inadequate tissue perfusion. Anaerobic metabolism may ensue if blood and volume replacement is inadequate to maintain perfusion. While anaerobic metabolism continues, lactic acid builds up, leading to an increase in the base deficit and decrease in the pH.

After initial restoration of circulating fluid volume, the body may develop a hyperdynamic circulatory state to help compensate for the cellular oxygen debt incurred. This phase should peak at 48 to 72 hours and diminish within 7 to 10 days. The hyperdynamic state is evidenced by an increased cardiac index (CI), oxygen delivery (DO_2), and oxygen consumption ($\dot{V}O_2$). Inability to achieve and maintain a hyperdynamic state is associated with higher mortality and shock-related organ failure.

Coagulopathy develops from both the consumption of clotting factors as the body forms clots in an attempt to stop the bleeding of injured tissues and the dilution of the blood from infusion of crystalloids and massive transfusion of packed red blood cells when clotting factors are not replaced. If coagulopathy is not reversed, disseminated intravascular coagulopathy (DIC) can occur. Factors contributing to development of DIC include hypotension, impaired tissue perfusion, and capillary dysfunction leading to stasis, hypoxemia, and hypothermia.

Multiple factors increase the likelihood of hypothermia in major trauma. Exposed body surface area or viscera may occur at the scene of injury or during the initial resuscitation. If blood and resuscitation fluids are infused without warming, the core body temperature can drop. Prolonged exposure to cool temperatures in resuscitation or operative areas can also lower the body temperature. When present, central thermoregulatory failure caused by CNS injury, intoxication, or hypoperfusion contributes to hypothermia. Mild hypothermia can help preserve the function and viability of major organs, particularly when tissue perfusion is diminished as a result of injury, shock, or surgical clamping of arteries. Severe hypothermia creates significant physiologic alterations, including CNS depression, dysrhythmias, acidosis, and substantial electrolyte imbalances. Catecholamine infusions are often ineffective until body temperature approaches 33.9 °C (93 °F).

In patients who sustain major trauma, a widespread inflammatory response known as systemic inflammatory response syndrome (SIRS) may be triggered by massive tissue injury and the presence of foreign bodies such as road dirt, shrapnel, and invasive medical devices. Inflammatory mediators activate the coagulation cascade, increased catecholamines stimulate the production and release of white blood cells, and endothelial dysfunction ensues. The hemodynamic response and clinical findings are similar to those with sepsis. (See Chapter 11 for information on SIRS.)

The overwhelming inflammation associated with SIRS may lead to multiple organ dysfunction syndrome (MODS). MODS is a leading cause of late mortality in patients with multitrauma, accounting for approximately 10% of trauma deaths. Inadequate initial resuscitation or inability to achieve and maintain a compensatory hyperdynamic state contributes to the development of organ failure in patients with trauma. Presence of endotoxin, tumor necrosis factor, interleukin-1, and other inflammatory mediators cause vasodilation, leading to hypotension. Capillary dysfunction results in poor cellular circulation and subsequent tissue destruction. Acidosis, pulmonary compromise, and circulatory collapse may result. Clinical trials are under way for therapies to help control inflammatory mediators.

PSYCHOLOGICAL RESPONSE

Victims of major trauma sustain life-threatening injuries. The patient often is aware of the situation and fears death. Even after the physical condition stabilizes, the patient may have a prolonged and severe psychological reaction triggered by the trauma called posttraumatic stress disorder.

MAJOR TRAUMA ASSESSMENT: PRIMARY

GOAL OF SYSTEM ASSESSMENT
Evaluate and treat life-threatening injuries.

AIRWAY ASSESSMENT
Determine airway patency.
- Is the airway open?
- Can the patient maintain the open airway?

- Is there potential for airway obstruction?
- Inspect the face and neck for signs of trauma.
- Look in the mouth for secretions, blood, vomitus, or loose teeth.
- Palpate the neck for crepitus.

BREATHING ASSESSMENT
- Is there adequate air exchange?
- Inspect the chest for signs of trauma that could interfere with chest excursion.
- Inspect the neck for tracheal deviation and jugular vein distention (JVD).
- Palpate the chest for crepitus, tenderness over the ribs or sternum.
- Auscultate breath sounds.
- What is the oxygen saturation?

CIRCULATORY ASSESSMENT
- Observe skin color.
- Is there any obvious bleeding?
- Palpate for pulses, and note strength and rate.
- Palpate skin for temperature.
- Auscultate heart sounds and BP.

DISABILITY ASSESSMENT
- Observe the patient's responsiveness.
- If not alert, does the patient respond to shout or pain?
- Determine the patient's Glasgow Coma Scale (GCS) score.
- Assess pupils for size, equality, and responsiveness.

EXPOSURE
- Expose the patient to observe for signs of trauma.
- Institute measures to keep the patient warm.

MAJOR TRAUMA ASSESSMENT: SECONDARY

GOAL OF SYSTEM ASSESSMENT
Identify all the injuries the patient has incurred.

VITAL SIGNS
- Pulse rate may be elevated if the patient has experienced blood loss or stimulation of the sympathetic nervous system (SNS) or be decreased in response to elevated intracranial pressure (ICP) from a severe head injury.
- Respiratory rate (RR) may also be increased as a result of SNS stimulation or hypoxia, or may be decreased secondary to decreased level of consciousness (LOC).
- BP will be elevated with SNS stimulation or increased ICP, or decreased as a result of hemorrhage.
- Temperature may be decreased from exposure to cold environment and development of hemorrhagic shock.

HISTORY
- AMPLE (Allergies, Medications, Past surgeries and pertinent medical conditions, Last meal, Events leading up to incident).
- Last menstrual period for women of child-bearing age.
- Determine the mechanism of the trauma.
    - Determine any injury modifiers.
    - Identify safety devices used.
- Determine the use of intoxicants.
- Tetanus status.

HEAD-TO-TOE ASSESSMENT
- Observe each area for signs of trauma including bruising, abrasions, lacerations, and contusions.
- Auscultate for lung sounds, heart sounds, bowel signs, and bruits.
- Palpate each area to feel for crepitus and swelling.

Head and neck
- Observe head for Battle signs (temporal bruising indicating a basilar skull fracture [BSF]) and raccoon eyes (periorbital bruising).
- Observe the neck for tracheal alignment, JVD, and expanding hematomas.

Chest
- Observe for symmetrical chest wall movement.
- Percuss chest for dullness or hyperresonance.
- Palpate over ribs and sternum for tenderness.
- Listen to breath sounds, noting equality and for any abnormal breath sounds.

Abdomen and pelvis
- Observe the abdomen for distention.
- Auscultate for bowel sounds.
- Palpate for tenderness and guarding.

Extremities
- Observe for deformities.
- Palpate for crepitus.
- Check neurovascular status of all four extremities.

Posterior surface
- Inspect the posterior surface; if the patient's spine has not been cleared, the patient must be logrolled, maintaining spinal precautions.
- Palpate along the vertebral column, accessing for tenderness, deformity, or crepitus.

LABORATORY WORK
Blood studies can reveal indications of hypoxia and/or continued bleeding and developing shock, as well as identify special circumstances such as pregnancy and intoxication.
- Blood typing and screening or cross-matching.
- Complete blood counts: hemoglobin (Hgb), increased white blood cell (WBC) count.
- Coagulation studies including platelets, prothrombin time (PT), partial thromboplastin time (PTT), and international normalized ratio (INR).
- Serial arterial blood gases (ABGs).
- Electrolytes.
- Urine or serum beta human chorionic gonadotropin for pregnancy.
- Blood alcohol levels and toxicology screens.

Diagnostic Tests for Major Trauma		
Test	**Purpose**	**Abnormal Findings**
Blood Studies		
Type and screen/type and cross-match	To have type-specific and cross-matched blood available for resuscitation	Inability to cross-match if specimen is collected after multiple units of blood are transfused.

Continued

Diagnostic Tests for Major Trauma — cont'd

Test	Purpose	Abnormal Findings
Arterial blood gas	Assess for adequacy of oxygenation and ventilation and to determine the level of anaerobic metabolism.	pH <7.35 with increased $Paco_2$ (>45 mm Hg) indicates respiratory acidosis. Serum bicarbonate <22 mEq/L with a pH <7.35 can indicate metabolic acidosis. Decreased Pao_2 indicates hypoxemia. Increased $Paco_2$ indicates inadequate ventilation. Base deficit >2.0 mEq/L indicates increased oxygen debt.
Complete blood count Hemoglobin (Hgb) Hematocrit (Hct)	Assess for blood loss.	Decreased Hgb and Hct indicate blood loss. Often Hgb and Hct are within normal range initially, especially if the patient has not received a significant amount of fluid to replace the blood loss. The Hgb and Hct should be repeated after the patient has a fluid challenge if there is any indication of significant bleeding.
Electrolytes Potassium (K^+) Glucose Creatinine	Provide a baseline and assess for possible alterations.	Potassium may be elevated with crush injuries. Glucose is usually elevated after injury. Decreased glucose indicates hypoglycemia and may cause decreased level of consciousness. Elevated creatinine indicates decreased renal functioning, and care should be taken when administering contrast for radiologic studies.
Coagulation profile Prothrombin time (PT) with international normalized ratio (INR) Partial thromboplastin time Fibrinogen D dimer	Assess for causes of bleeding, clotting, and disseminated intravascular coagulation indicative of abnormal clotting present in shock or ensuing shock.	Decreased PT with low INR promotes clotting; elevation promotes bleeding; elevated fibrinogen and D dimer reflect abnormal clotting is present.
Blood alcohol	To determine the level of alcohol in the patient's blood.	Greater than 10 mg/dL indicates the presence of alcohol in the patient's blood. The higher the level, the more chance the patient has of showing signs of intoxication, but an absolute value will depend on the patient's tolerance. This may interfere with neurologic assessment.
Carbohydrate-deficient transferrin	To identify patients who have had excessive drinking for the past few weeks and may be at risk for alcohol withdrawal	Greater than 20 units/L for males and >6 units/L for females indicate excessive drinking.
Drug screen	To identify the presence of drugs in the patient's system.	A positive value indicates recent use of the substance.

Diagnostic Tests for Major Trauma — cont'd

Test	Purpose	Abnormal Findings
Radiology		
Chest radiograph	Assess thoracic cage (for fractures), lungs (pneumothorax, hemothorax); size of mediastinum, size of heart.	Displaced lung margins will be present with pneumothoraces and hemothoraces. Cardiac enlargement may reflect cardiac tamponade.
Pelvic radiograph	Assess the integrity of the pelvic ring to identify fractures and determine the stability of the pelvis.	Fracture lines through any of the bones in the pelvis, widening of the symphysis pubis, and widening of the sacroiliac joint(s)
Computerized tomography: head, neck, chest, abdomen, and/or pelvis	Assess for internal injuries.	Any findings of skeletal fractures, misalignment, organ damage, or abnormal collections of blood indicate injury to the organ/tissue involved.
Ultrasound: Focused Assessment with Sonography for Trauma (FAST)	Assess for fluid around the heart, liver, spleen, and bladder.	Abnormal collection of fluid
Invasive Studies		
Diagnostic peritoneal lavage	Assess for blood or in the peritoneal cavity or abnormal substrates in the peritoneal lavage fluid.	The presence of red or white blood cells, bile, food fibers, amylase, or feces in the lavage fluid suggests injury to the abdominal organs. Lavage fluid coming from the Foley catheter indicates bladder rupture. Lavage fluid coming from the chest tube, if present, indicates diaphragm rupture.

COLLABORATIVE MANAGEMENT

The primary goals of initial assessment in major trauma are to identify life-threatening injuries, stop bleeding, and restore adequate oxygenation to the tissues. Once life-threatening injuries have been addressed, a secondary assessment is performed to identify all injuries the patient may have sustained; perform a thorough organized head-to-toe assessment to minimize the chance of missing injuries. The following treatments may be required.

CARE PRIORITIES

1. Secure a patent airway

A patent airway must be secured when a GCS score of 8 or less or potential for airway compromise is possible and/or the patient has respiratory failure requiring mechanical ventilation. The airway is secured by intubation using a rapid sequence intubation protocol to prevent patient movement and aspiration during the procedure. If the patient is unable to be intubated, a surgical airway must be performed. The surgical airway of choice in an emergency situation is a cricothyroidotomy. If the cervical spine has not been cleared, the spine must be stabilized during the procedure by maintaining constant in-line positioning with gentle traction.

2. Support ventilation

If the patient is not adequately ventilating to maintain oxygen saturations greater than 93%, the patient should be placed on supplemental oxygen. Most patients with major trauma will require supplemental oxygen. Blood loss creates reduced oxygen-carrying capacity, and tissue demand for oxygen is greatly increased during the hypermetabolic phase. High-flow oxygen by mask is indicated initially. Oxygen therapy can be titrated according to ABG and pulse oximetry values. Mechanical ventilation may be required if the patient is not ventilating well enough to remove CO_2. If the patient does not have equal breath sounds, a pneumothorax or hemothorax may have occurred and a tube thoracotomy may be indicated. Capnography should be considered for patients who are mechanically ventilated, because it is an early marker of hypoventilation and apnea.

3. Manage hemorrhage and hypovolemia

Stopping blood loss and restoring adequate circulating blood volume are imperative. Lack of resuscitation will lead to increasing oxygen debt and eventually to MODS and death. The goal of resuscitation in any patient with trauma should be to restore adequate tissue perfusion. Two or more large-bore ($\geq$16-gauge) short catheters should be placed to maximize delivery of fluids and blood. Use of intravenous (IV) tubing with an exceptionally large internal diameter (trauma tubing), absence of stopcocks, and use of external pressure are techniques used to promote rapid fluid volume therapy when indicated. In some cases, the patient may require large central venous access, such as an 8.5 Fr introducer. When rapid infusion of large amounts of fluid is required, all fluid should be warmed to body temperature to prevent hypothermia. Rapid warmer/infuser devices are available to facilitate rapid administration of blood products. Fluid resuscitation should be used more judiciously in pediatric and older patients, as well as patients with significant craniocerebral trauma, who have precise fluid requirements (see Traumatic Brain Injury).

- Crystalloids: Initial IV fluid used for resuscitation should be an isotonic electrolyte solution such as 0.9% normal saline (NS) or lactated Ringer (LR). Other balanced electrolyte solutions such as Normosol-R pH 7.4 (Hospira) or Plasmalyte-A 7.4 (Baxter) may be used after initial fluid resuscitation has been completed.
- Rapid bolus: Between 1 and 2 L of rapid IV fluid infusion for adults and 20 mL/kg for pediatric patients should be initiated in the prehospital setting. If the patient continues to show signs of shock after the bolus is complete, blood transfusions should be considered.
- Packed red blood cells (PRBCs): Typed and cross-matched blood is ideal, but in the immediate resuscitation period, if cross-matched blood is not available, type O blood may be used. Once the patient has been typed, type-specific blood can be used. Those patients requiring continuous blood transfusions need reassessment to identify the source of bleeding and definitive treatment to stop ongoing blood loss. A massive transfusion protocol may also need to be initiated.
- Massive transfusion is defined as replacement of one half of the patient's blood volume at one time or complete replacement of the patient's blood volume over 24 hours. A massive transfusion protocol ensures that the patient receives plasma, platelets, and cryoprecipitate in addition to PRBCs to prevent the complications related to coagulopathy. Another concern with massive transfusion is hypocalcemia caused by calcium binding with citrate in stored PRBCs, resulting in depressed myocardial contractility, particularly in patients with hypothermia or in those with impaired liver function. One ampule of 10% calcium chloride should be considered for administration after every 4 units of PRBCs.

> **Safety Alert**
> *Only O-negative packed cells should be transfused into prepubescent females and women in childbearing status to prevent sensitization and future complications during pregnancy.*

- Autotransfusion: Shed blood from the patient can be collected, filtered, and reinfused. Shed blood is captured from chest tube drainage or the operative field and reinfused immediately. Various techniques are used to capture and reinfuse the blood. Advantages of autotransfusion include reduced risk of disease transmission, absence of incompatibility problems, and availability. Disadvantages include risk of blood contamination and presence of naturally occurring factors that promote anticoagulation.
- Colloids: Resuscitation with colloids has not been shown to reduce mortality and is not used in the initial resuscitation of patients with trauma.
- Recombinant factor VIIa (rFVIIa): The standard use of rFVIIa in the resuscitation of patients with trauma is still controversial. Some studies have shown a decrease in the number of units of PRBCs required for patients in hemorrhagic shock but have not shown a decrease in mortality. More studies are needed to determine the appropriate indications, contraindications, dosage, and timing of rFVIIa administration in patients with trauma who experience hemorrhagic shock.

4. Identify, prevent, and/or manage hypothermia

Warmed blankets, forced warm air blankets, and warmers for IV fluids and blood should be used to prevent hypothermia. If the patient is already hypothermic, more aggressive measures to rewarm the patient may be necessary. Warming lights are useful for pediatric patients. Core rewarming measures can include irrigation of the peritoneal and/or thoracic cavities with warmed saline, use of heated humidified oxygen, and extracorporeal blood rewarming.

5. Provide gastric decompression

Gastric intubation permits gastric decompression, aids in removal of gastric contents, and helps to prevent vomiting or possible aspiration. The nasal route is contraindicated in patients with basilar skull fractures because of the need to prevent tubes entering the cranial vault via abnormal openings in the fractured skull. In patients with facial trauma or suspected or known BSF, gastric tubes should be placed orally.

6. Ensure urinary drainage

An indwelling catheter is inserted to obtain a specimen for urinalysis and to monitor hourly urine output. See Renal and Lower Urinary Tract Trauma for precautions.

7. Prevent infection with antibiotics

Broad-spectrum antibiotics are used initially to prevent infections if there are open wounds or compound fractures. More specific antimicrobial agents are used when results from culture and sensitivity tests are available.

8. Control pain and anxiety with analgesics and anxiolytics

Relief of pain and anxiety are accomplished using IV opiates and anxiolytics. All IV agents should be carefully titrated to desired effect, while avoiding respiratory depression, masking injury, or disguising changes in physiologic variables. Use of the World Health Organization ladder for pain management and a pain-rating scale are essential for the trauma population.

9. Provide tetanus prophylaxis

Tetanus immunoglobulin (TIG) and tetanus-toxoid (Tt) are considered on the basis of the Centers for Disease Control and Prevention recommendations (Table 3-1).

Table 3-1	GUIDE TO TETANUS PROPHYLAXIS IN ROUTINE WOUND MANAGEMENT			
	Clean Minor Wounds		**All Other Wounds***	
History of Adsorbed Tetanus Toxoid (Doses)	Tdap or Td[†]	TIG[‡]	Tdap or Td[†]	TIG[‡]
3 or unknown	Yes	No	Yes	Yes
≥3 doses[§]	No[‖]	No	No[¶]	No

From Centers for Disease Control and Prevention: *Manual for the surveillance of vaccine-preventable diseases,* Atlanta, 2008, Centers for Disease Control and Prevention.
*Such as (but not limited to) wounds contaminated with dirt, feces, soil, and saliva; puncture wounds; avulsions; and wounds resulting from missiles, crushing, burns, and frostbite.
[†]For children younger than 7 years, DTaP (Diphtheria, Tetanus, and Pertussis) is recommended; if pertussis vaccine is contraindicated, DT is given. For individuals 7 to 9 years of age or 65 years or older, Td is recommended. For individuals 10 to 64 years, Tdap is preferred to Td if the patient has never received Tdap and has no contraindication to pertussis vaccine. For individuals 7 years of age or older, if Tdap is not available or not indicated because of age, Td is preferred to TT.
[‡]TIG is human tetanus immunoglobulin. Equine tetanus antitoxin should be used when TIG is not available.
[§]If only three doses of fluid toxoid have been received, a fourth dose of toxoid, preferably an adsorbed toxoid, should be given. Although licensed, fluid tetanus toxoid is rarely used.
[‖]Yes, if it has been 10 years or longer since the last dose.
[¶]Yes, if it has been 5 years or longer since the last dose. More frequent boosters are not needed and can accentuate side effects.

10. Initiate nutrition support therapy

Infection and sepsis contribute to the negative nitrogen state and increased metabolic needs. Prompt initiation of nutrition therapy is essential for rapid healing and prevention of complications. Parenteral nutrition or postpyloric (jejunal) feedings may be used if postoperative ileus or injury to the gastrointestinal (GI) tract is present. For more information, see Nutrition Support.

11. Facilitate evaluation for surgery

Need for surgery depends on the type and extent of injuries. The surgical team is coordinated by the trauma surgeon. When several specialty surgeons are required for various injuries, the order of surgeries is coordinated carefully to preserve life and limit the potential for disability.

CARE PLANS: MAJOR TRAUMA

Ineffective tissue perfusion, cardiopulmonary *related to substantial loss of blood volume.*

Goals/Outcomes: Within 24 hours of this diagnosis, the patient exhibits adequate tissue perfusion, as evidenced by BP within normal limits for the patient, heart rate (HR) 60 to 100 beats per minute (bpm), normal sinus rhythm on electrocardiogram (ECG), peripheral pulses greater than 2+ on a 0-to-4+ scale, warm and dry skin, hourly urine output ≥0.5 mL/kg, base deficit between −2 and +2 mmol/L, serum lactate less than 2.2 mmol/L, measured cardiac output (CO) 4 to 7 L/min, central venous pressure (CVP) or pulmonary artery wedge pressure (PAWP) 6 to 12 mm Hg, and patient awake, alert, and oriented.

NOC Blood Loss Severity.

Shock Management: Volume
1. Monitor for sudden blood loss or persistent bleeding.
2. Prevent blood volume loss (e.g., apply pressure to site of bleeding).
3. Monitor for fall in systolic BP to less than 90 mm Hg or a fall of 30 mm Hg in patients who are hypertensive.
4. Monitor for signs/symptoms of hypovolemic shock (e.g., increased thirst, increased HR, increased systemic vascular resistance [SVR], decreased urinary output [urine output], decreased bowel sounds, decreased peripheral perfusion, altered mental status, or altered respirations).
5. Position the patient for optimal perfusion.
6. Insert and maintain large-bore IV access.
7. Administer warmed IV fluids, such as isotonic crystalloids, as indicated.
8. Administer blood products (e.g., PRBCs, platelets, plasma, and cryoprecipitate), as appropriate.
9. Administer oxygen and/or mechanical ventilation, as appropriate.
10. Draw ABGs and monitor tissue oxygenation.
11. Monitor Hgb/hematocrit (Hct) level.
12. Monitor coagulation studies, including INR, PT, PTT, fibrinogen, fibrin degradation/split products, and platelets.
13. Monitor laboratory studies (e.g., serum lactate, acid-base balance, metabolic profiles, and electrolytes).
14. Monitor fluid status, including intake and output, as appropriate.
15. Monitor for clinical signs and symptoms of overhydration/fluid excess.

Vital Signs Monitoring
1. Monitor BP, pulse, temperature, and respiratory status, as appropriate.
2. Note trends and wide fluctuations in BP.
3. Auscultate BPs in both arms and compare, as appropriate.
4. Initiate and maintain a continuous temperature monitoring device, as appropriate.
5. Monitor for and report signs and symptoms of hypothermia and hyperthermia.
6. Monitor the presence and quality of pulses.
7. Monitor cardiac rate and rhythm.

Acid-Base Monitoring
1. Examine the pH level in conjunction with the $PaCO_2$ and HCO_3 levels to determine whether the acidosis/alkalosis is compensated or uncompensated.
2. Monitor for an increase in the anion gap (greater than 14 mEq/L), signaling an increased production or decreased excretion of acid products.
3. Monitor base excess/base deficit levels.
4. Monitor arterial lactate levels.
5. Monitor for elevated chloride levels with large volumes of NS.

Impaired gas exchange *related to airway obstruction, inadequate oxygenation*

Goals/Outcomes: Within 12 to 24 hours of treatment, the patient has adequate gas exchange, as evidenced by $PaO_2 \geq 80$ mm Hg, $PaCO_2$ 35 to 45 mm Hg, pH 7.35 to 7.45, presence of normal breath sounds, and absence of adventitious breath sounds. RR is 12 to 20 breaths/min with normal pattern and depth.

NOC Respiratory Status: Gas Exchange; Respiratory Status: Ventilation.

Airway Management
1. Assess for patent airway; if snoring, crowing, or strained respirations are present, indicative of partial or full airway obstruction, open airway using chin-lift or jaw-thrust technique and maintain cervical spine alignment.
2. Insert oral or nasopharyngeal airway if the patient cannot maintain patent airway; if severely distressed, the patient may require endotracheal intubation.
3. When the spine is cleared, position the patient to alleviate dyspnea and ensure maximal ventilation, generally in a sitting inclined position unless severe hypotension is present.
4. Clear secretions from airway by having the patient cough vigorously, or provide nasotracheal, oropharyngeal, or endotracheal tube suctioning as needed.
5. Have the patient breathe slowly or manually ventilate with bag-valve-mask device slowly and deeply between coughing or suctioning attempts.
6. Assist with use of incentive spirometer, as appropriate.
7. Turn the patient every 2 hours if immobile. Encourage the patient to turn self, or get out of bed as much as tolerated if the patient is able.
8. Provide chest physical therapy as appropriate, if other methods of secretion removal are ineffective.

Oxygen Therapy
1. Provide humidity in oxygen.
2. Administer supplemental oxygen using liter flow and device as ordered.
3. Restrict the patient and visitors from smoking while oxygen is in use.
4. Document pulse oximetry with oxygen liter flow in place at time of reading as ordered. Oxygen is a drug; the dose of the drug must be associated with the oxygen saturation reading or the reading is meaningless.
5. Obtain ABGs if the patient experiences behavioral changes or respiratory distress to check for hypoxemia or hypercapnia.
6. Monitor for changes in chest radiograph and breath sounds indicative of oxygen toxicity and absorption atelectasis in patients receiving higher concentrations of oxygen (FIO_2 greater than 45%) for longer than 24 hours. The higher the oxygen concentration, the greater the chance of toxicity.
7. Monitor for skin breakdown where oxygen devices are in contact with skin, such as nares and around edges of mask devices.
8. Provide oxygen therapy during transportation and when the patient gets out of bed.

Respiratory Monitoring
1. Monitor rate, rhythm, and depth of respirations.
2. Note chest movement for symmetry of chest expansion and signs of increased work of breathing such as use of accessory muscles or retraction of intercostal or supraclavicular muscles.
3. Ensure airway is not obstructed by tongue (snoring or choking-type respirations) and monitor breathing patterns. New patterns that impair ventilation should be managed as appropriate for setting.
4. Note that trachea remains midline, because deviation may indicate that the patient has a tension pneumothorax.
5. Auscultate breath sounds following administration of respiratory medications to assess for improvement.
6. Note changes in oxygen saturation (SaO_2), pulse oximetry (SpO_2), end-tidal CO_2 ($ETCO_2$), and ABGs as appropriate.
7. Monitor for dyspnea and note causative activities/events.
8. If increased restlessness or unusual somnolence occurs, evaluate the patient for hypoxemia and hypercapnia as appropriate.
9. Monitor chest x-ray reports as new films become available.

Acute pain *related to physical injury*

Goals/Outcomes: Within 30 minutes of intervention, the patient's subjective evaluation of discomfort improves, as documented by a pain scale. Nonverbal indicators, such as grimacing, are absent. Vital signs return to baseline. ECG changes present during event resolve.

NOC Comfort Status: Physical, Pain Level.

Pain Management
1. Assess and document the location and intensity of the pain. Devise a pain scale with the patient, rating discomfort from 0 (no pain) to 10 or any system that assists in objectively reporting pain level. If intubated, use a physiologic scale such as adult nonverbal pain scale or the FLACC (Face, Legs, Activity, Cry, Consolability) scale.
2. Determine the needed frequency of making an assessment of patient comfort and implement monitoring plan.
3. Provide the patient with optimal pain relief with prescribed analgesics.
4. Ensure pretreatment analgesia and/or nonpharmacologic strategies before painful procedures.
5. Evaluate the effectiveness of the pain control measures used through ongoing assessment of the pain experience.

Hypothermia *related to altered temperature regulation*

Goals/Outcomes: The patient will maintain a normal body temperature greater than 36° C (96.8° F).
NOC Thermoregulation.

Temperature Regulation
1. Monitor temperature at least every 2 hours, as appropriate.
2. Institute a continuous core temperature monitoring device, as appropriate.
3. Monitor BP, pulse, and respirations, as appropriate.
4. Monitor skin color and temperature.

Treatment for Hypothermia
1. Cover with warmed blankets, as appropriate.
2. Administer warmed (37° C to 40° C) IV fluids, as appropriate.
3. Administer heated oxygen, as appropriate.
4. Infuse all whole blood and PRBCs through a warmer.
5. Institute active core rewarming techniques (e.g., colonic lavage, hemodialysis, peritoneal dialysis, and extracorporeal blood rewarming), as appropriate.
6. Minimize exposure of the patient.
7. Keep the room temperature comfortable for the patient.

Posttrauma syndrome *related to inadequate coping ability resulting from major physical and emotional stress.*

Goals/Outcomes: The patient exhibits appropriate coping mechanism and reduced anxiety, as evidenced by decreased restlessness, pulse rate 60 to 100 bpm, RR 12 to 20 breaths per minute, and decrease in the amount of pain medication requested.
NOC Anxiety Level; Coping.

Anxiety Reduction
1. Explain all procedures, including sensations likely to be experienced during the procedure.
2. Provide factual information concerning diagnosis, treatment, and prognosis.
3. Encourage the family to stay with the patient, as appropriate.
4. Create an atmosphere to facilitate trust.
5. Control stimuli, as appropriate for patient needs.
6. Determine the patient's decision-making ability.
7. Administer medications to reduce anxiety, as appropriate.
8. Assess for verbal and nonverbal signs of anxiety.
9. Support the use of appropriate defense mechanisms.

Coping Enhancement
1. Provide an atmosphere of acceptance.
2. Provide the patient with realistic choices about certain aspects of care.
3. Acknowledge the patient's spiritual/cultural background.
4. Encourage the use of spiritual resources, if desired.
5. Encourage verbalization of feelings, perceptions, and fears.
6. Assist the patient to identify available social supports.
7. Encourage family involvement, as appropriate.

Emotional Support
1. Make supportive and empathetic statements.
2. Encourage the patient to express feelings of anxiety, anger, or sadness.
3. Refer for counseling, as appropriate.

ADDITIONAL NURSING DIAGNOSES

Also see nursing diagnoses and interventions as appropriate in Nutrition Support, Mechanical Ventilation, Hemodynamic Monitoring, Prolonged Immobility, and Emotional and Spiritual Support of the Patient and Significant Others (Chapters 1 and 2).

ABDOMINAL TRAUMA
PATHOPHYSIOLOGY

The patient with abdominal injury can be the most challenging and difficult to manage. Forces may be blunt or penetrating and the organs are either solid (pancreas, kidneys, adrenal glands, liver, and spleen) or hollow (stomach, small bowel, and colon).This patient may have subtle signs of internal hemorrhage, which can be a major contributor to the increase in mortality and morbidity noted after the initial injury has been managed. The severity of abdominal injury is related to the type of force applied to the organs suspended inside the peritoneum. Motor vehicle collision (MVC), either auto-auto or auto-pedestrian, is the most common cause of blunt abdominal trauma worldwide.

BLUNT TRAUMA

There are three mechanisms of action with blunt trauma.
1. **Rapid deceleration:** On impact, the different organs that reside inside the abdominal cavity move at different speeds depending on their density. This creates what is known as shear force, that is, two different directions applied to the organ, usually at the point of attachment, causing injury to other organs such as the aorta.
2. **Crush of contents between the walls:** Solid viscera are exceptionally affected when compression occurs from the anterior abdominal wall and the spine or posterior cage.
3. **External compression force:** The force of external traumatic impact may increase the organ and abdominal pressures to such a degree that the hollow organs rupture.

MECHANISMS OF ACTION WITH PENETRATING INJURY

External penetration to the abdominal cavity can be caused by any missile or object that intrudes into the abdominal cavity. Penetrating forces injure the organ(s) in the direct path of the instrument or missile, and shock waves from high-velocity weapons (e.g., high-powered rifles) may also injure adjacent organs. Stab wounds are generally easier to manage than gunshot wounds but may be fatal if a major blood vessel (aorta) or highly vascular organ (liver) is penetrated. The three most common injuries associated with penetrating abdominal trauma are those to the small bowel, liver, and colon. With blunt trauma, injuries to the liver, spleen, and kidney are more common. Undetected mesenteric damage may cause compromised blood flow, with eventual bowel infarction. Perforations or contusions result in release of bacteria and intestinal contents into the abdominal cavity, causing serious infection.

The abdomen can be divided into four areas: (1) intrathoracic abdomen, (2) pelvic abdomen, (3) retroperitoneal abdomen, and (4) true abdomen.

Intrathoracic abdomen

The upper abdomen resides beneath the rib cage and includes the diaphragm, liver, spleen, and stomach.
- Diaphragm: Commonly injured at the left posterior portion after blunt trauma, the tear is best visualized by chest radiograph, which reveals an elevation of the left hemidiaphragm and air under the diaphragm.
- Spleen: The organ most frequently injured after blunt trauma. Massive hemorrhage from splenic injury is common. Damage to the spleen may occur with the most trivial of injuries, thus index of suspicion should be high. Splenic injury is often associated with

hepatic or pancreatic injury because of the close proximity of these organs. Splenectomy is the treatment of choice for major spleen injuries. Minor splenic injuries may be managed with direct suture techniques.

- Liver: Most frequently involved in penetrating trauma (80%) because of its large size and location, the liver is less often affected by blunt injury (20%). Control of bleeding and bile drainage is the priority with hepatic injury. Mortality from liver injuries is approximately 10%. In most patients, bleeding from a liver injury can be controlled, such as with perihepatic packing. Approximately 5% of injuries require packing for bleeds. Major arterial bleeding from the liver parenchyma will require further attention. Biliary tree injuries may require surgical repair and are associated with liver injury. The patient may be asymptomatic or have mild to moderate abdominal discomfort with biliary tree injury.

Pelvic abdomen

As defined by bony pelvis, this includes the urinary bladder, urethra, rectum, small intestine, and, in females, the ovaries, fallopian tubes, and uterus. Diagnosis is difficult because many of these injuries are extraperitoneal (outside the peritoneal cavity).

Retroperitoneal abdomen

This includes the kidneys, ureters, pancreas, aorta, and vena cava. Evaluation may require a computed tomography (CT) scan, angiography, and an IV pyelogram (IVP).

- Retroperitoneal vessels: Tears in retroperitoneal vessels associated with pelvic fractures or damage to retroperitoneal organs (pancreas, duodenum, and kidney) can cause bleeding into the retroperitoneum.
- Although the retroperitoneal space can accommodate up to 4 L of blood, detection of retroperitoneal hematomas is difficult and sophisticated diagnostic techniques may be required.

True abdomen

This includes the small and large intestines, uterus (when enlarged), and bladder (when distended). Perforation usually presents with peritonitis such as pain and tenderness.

- Colon: Injury is most frequently caused by penetrating forces, although lap belts, direct blows, and other blunt forces cause a small percentage of colonic injuries. Because of the high bacterial content, infection is even more a concern than it is with small bowel injury. Most patients with significant colon injuries require a temporary colostomy.
- Undetected mesenteric damage: May cause compromised blood flow, with eventual bowel infarction. Perforations or contusions result in release of bacteria and intestinal contents into the abdominal cavity, causing serious infection.
- Pelvis: See Renal and Lower Urinary Tract Trauma (Chapter 3).

Occasionally the lower portion of the esophagus is involved in penetrating trauma. The stomach is usually not injured with blunt trauma because it is flexible and readily displaced, but it may be injured by direct penetration. Injury to either the esophagus or stomach results in the escape of irritating gastric fluids as a result of gastric perforation and the release of free air below the level of the diaphragm. Esophageal injuries are often associated with thoracic injuries. Once hemorrhage has been controlled, attention is turned to prevention of further contamination by controlling spillage of gut contents.

Traumatic pancreatic or duodenal injury is uncommon but is associated with high morbidity and mortality. These injuries are difficult to detect and may be associated with massive injury to nearby organs, prompting spillage of irritating fluids, activated enzymes, and bile, which augments the inflammatory response. Pancreatic injury is rare; however, the pancreas can be contused or lacerated. Clinical indicators of injury to these retroperitoneal organs may not be obvious for several hours.

Injuries to major vessels such as the abdominal aorta and inferior vena cava most often are caused by penetrating trauma but also occur with deceleration injury. Hepatic vein injuries are frequently associated with juxtahepatic vena cava injury and result in rapid hemorrhage. Blood loss after major vascular injury is massive. Survival depends on rapid transport to a trauma center and immediate surgical intervention.

ASSESSMENT: ABDOMINAL TRAUMA

GOAL OF SYSTEM ASSESSMENT

Rapidly evaluate for significant primary and secondary injuries (for all systems) while performing basic and advanced trauma life support. Airway, breathing, circulation, disability, and exposure are the structural components of all trauma assessment.

Safety Alert	*In a patient who is unstable, immediate identification of free intraabdominal fluid by Focused Assessment with Sonography for Trauma (FAST) examination or a diagnostic peritoneal lavage (DPL) is imperative and supports decisions to move straight to the operating room.*

 In the traditional perspective of the "Golden Hour of Trauma" (period of time immediately after traumatic injury in which rapid intervention may prevent death), the American College of Surgeons guideline recommends that rapid assessment of hemorrhage includes aggressive volume resuscitation.

HISTORY AND RISK FACTORS

First and foremost, it is essential to establish how the injury occurred (Box 3-1). Details regarding circumstances of the accident and mechanism of injury are invaluable in detecting the presence of specific injuries. Second, allergies, medications, and last meal eaten will play an important role in the maintenance of good resuscitation. Other information, previous abdominal surgeries, and use of safety restraints (if appropriate) should be noted. Hollow viscous injury is often missed but is more likely to be present when a contusion is seen on the abdomen. Medical information including current medications and last Tt immunization should be obtained. The history is sometimes difficult to obtain because of alcohol or drug intoxication, head injury, breathing difficulties, or impaired cerebral perfusion. Family members and emergency personnel may be valuable sources of information.

VITAL SIGNS

Assess for impending hemorrhagic shock: Pulse greater than 100 bpm, decreased pulse pressure, oliguria: blood loss 750 to 1500 mL; pulse greater than 120 bpm, hypotension, oliguria, confusion: blood loss 1500 to 2000 mL; pulse greater than 140 bpm, severe oliguria, lethargy: blood loss greater than 2000 mL.

HIGH ALERT!   Persistent Tachycardia

Persistent tachycardia: Should always be considered a clue to tissue hypoxia. While the neuroendocrine response ensues, persistent tachycardia indicates a response to tissue hypermetabolism and inadequate resuscitation.

---

* Hypotension: Presence of hypotension is a sign of impending doom, but the absence of hypotension does not always accurately reflect an absence of hemorrhage. After an

Box 3-1	**INITIAL HISTORY TAKING OF PATIENTS IN MOTOR VEHICLE COLLISIONS (BYSTANDERS, PASSENGERS, AND RESCUE PERSONNEL)**

* Extent of damage to the vehicle
* Approximate speed
* Did the airbag deploy?
* Were they wearing a seat belt?
* Were they ejected?
* Was prolonged extrication required?

* Was there a "T-bone" type of occurrence (intrusion into the passenger/or driver side)?
* Alcohol or drugs?
* Possible psychiatric problems/suicide attempts?

All patients in motor vehicle collisions are suspected as having dual diagnosis of head and spine until cleared.

Abdominal Trauma

injury, a profound neuroendocrine response ensues to activate the beta receptors (sinus node and ventricular contractile tissue), the alpha receptors (smooth muscle in the arteries), and the renal tubules (promoting preservation of fluid), resulting in significant tachycardia, profound vasoconstriction, and progressive oliguria. These responses may mask the severity of hemorrhage. Patients on alpha- or beta-antagonists or those with acute spinal cord injuries (above C5) will not manifest these responses and therefore will have few compensatory mechanisms.

- Pulse pressure: This measure may be effectively used to determine the amount of volume in the arteries (systolic minus diastolic BP, normal greater than 40 mm Hg). Pulse pressure generally correlates with the volume ejected by the left ventricle and therefore is a valuable tool to evaluate the volume in the vascular bed. Presence of pulsus paradoxus (Box 3-2) may be visualized with either the invasive arterial pressure trace or the plethysmograph of the pulse oximeter and is an invaluable tool in evaluating arterial volume.

OBSERVATION AND SUBJECTIVE/OBJECTIVE SYMPTOMS

- Inspection of all surfaces of trunk, head, neck, and extremities, including anterior lateral and posterior exposure, with notation of all penetrating wounds, contusions, tenderness, ecchymosis, or other marks and indicators. Multiple wounds may represent entrance or exit wounds but do not eliminate the possibility of objects that may remain internally.
- Kehr sign (left shoulder pain caused by splenic bleeding) may also be noted, especially when the patient is recumbent.
- Nausea and vomiting may occur, and the conscious patient who has sustained blood loss often complains of thirst; an early sign of hemorrhagic shock.
- Preoperative pain is anticipated and is a vital diagnostic aid. The nature of postoperative pain can also be important. Incisional and some visceral pain can be anticipated, but intense or prolonged pain, especially when accompanied by other peritoneal signs, can signal bleeding, bowel infarction, infection, or other complications.

 Safety Alert *It is important to note that damage to retroperitoneal organs such as the pancreas and duodenum may not cause significant signs and symptoms for 6 to 12 hours or longer. Relatively slow bleeding from abdominal viscera may not be clinically apparent for 12 hours or longer after the initial injury. In addition, the nurse should be aware that complications such as bowel obstruction caused by adhesions or narrowing of the bowel wall from localized ischemia, inflammation, or hematoma may develop days or weeks after the traumatic event. The need for vigilant observation in the care of these patients cannot be overemphasized.*

INSPECTION

- Abrasions and ecchymoses may indicate underlying injury. The absence of ecchymosis does not exclude major abdominal trauma and massive internal bleeding. In the event of gunshot wounds, entrance and exit (if present) wounds should be identified.

Box 3-2   MEASURING PARADOXICAL PULSE

- After placing blood pressure (BP) cuff on the patient, inflate it above the known systolic BP. Instruct the patient to breathe normally.
- While slowly deflating the cuff, auscultate BP.
- Listen for the first Korotkoff sound, which will occur during expiration with cardiac tamponade.
- Note the manometer reading when the first sound occurs, and continue to deflate the cuff slowly until Korotkoff sounds are audible throughout inspiration and expiration.
- Record the difference in millimeters of mercury between the first and second sounds. This is the pulsus paradoxus.

- Ecchymosis over the left upper quadrant suggests splenic rupture, and erythema and ecchymosis across the lower portion of the abdomen suggest intestinal injury caused by lap belts.
- Grey-Turner sign, a bluish discoloration of the flank, may indicate retroperitoneal bleeding from the pancreas, duodenum, vena cava, aorta, or kidneys.
- Cullen sign, a bluish discoloration around the umbilicus, may be present with intraperitoneal bleeding from the liver or spleen. Ecchymosis may take hours to days to develop, depending on the rate of blood loss.

AUSCULTATION

It is important to auscultate before palpation and percussion, because these maneuvers can stimulate the bowel and confound assessment findings.

- Bowel sounds: These are likely to be decreased or absent with abdominal organ injury or intraperitoneal bleeding. The presence of bowel sounds, however, does not exclude substantial abdominal injury. Immediately after injury, bowel sounds may be present, even with major organ injury. Bowel sounds should be auscultated in each quadrant every 1 to 2 hours in patients with suspected abdominal injury. Absence of bowel sounds is expected immediately after surgery. Failure to auscultate bowel sounds within 24 to 48 hours after surgery suggests ileus, possibly caused by continued bleeding, peritonitis, or bowel infarction.

PALPATION

- Tenderness to light palpation suggests pain from superficial or abdominal wall lesions, such as that occurring with seat belt contusions.
- Deep palpation may reveal a mass, which may indicate a hematoma. Internal injury with bleeding or release of GI contents into the peritoneum results in peritoneal irritation and certain assessment findings. Box 3-3 describes signs and symptoms that suggest peritoneal irritation.
- Subcutaneous emphysema of the abdominal wall is usually caused by thoracic injury but also may be produced by bowel rupture.
- Measurements of abdominal girth may be helpful in identifying increases in girth attributable to gas, blood, or fluid. Visual evaluation of abdominal distention is a late and unreliable sign of bleeding.
- Peritoneal signs (pain, guarding, rebound tenderness) or abdominal distention in a patient who is unconscious requires immediate evaluation in either case.

HIGH ALERT! Flank (Grey-Turner sign) or umbilical (Cullen sign) ecchymosis may be delayed several hours to days in patients with retroperitoneal hemorrhage. Based on the index of suspicion, persistent hypotension is always investigated with ultrasound or radiography.

- Mild tenderness to severe abdominal pain may be present, with the pain either localized to the site of injury or diffuse.
- Blood or fluid collection within the peritoneum causes irritation that results in involuntary guarding, rigidity, and rebound tenderness.
- Fluid or air under the diaphragm may cause referred shoulder pain.

PERCUSSION

- Unusually large areas of dullness may be percussed over ruptured blood-filled organs. For example, a fixed area of dullness in the left upper quadrant suggests a ruptured spleen.

Box 3-3	SIGNS AND SYMPTOMS THAT SUGGEST PERITONEAL IRRITATION

- Generalized abdominal pain and tenderness.
- Involuntary guarding of the abdomen.
- Abdominal wall rigidity.
- Rebound tenderness.
- Abdominal pain with movement or coughing.
- Decreased or absent bowel sounds.

An absence (or decrease in the size) of liver dullness may be caused by free air below the diaphragm, a consequence of hollow viscous perforation, or, in unusual cases, displacement of the liver through a ruptured diaphragm.
- The presence of tympany suggests gas; dullness suggests that the enlargement is caused by blood or fluid.

HIGH ALERT! Massive intestinal edema is common following laparotomy and prolonged shock. Inflammatory response, neuroendocrine stimulation, aggressive crystalloid resuscitation, bowel handling, intraabdominal packing, and retroperitoneal hematomas may cause a delay in abdominal closure. If the abdomen is closed, the intraabdominal volume may compress arteries, capillaries, the bladder, and the ureters. This compartment hypertension (abdominal compartment syndrome) may cause significant hypotension, oliguria, and base deficit that will be difficult to combat. (See Abdominal Hypertension and Abdominal Compartment Syndrome, Chapter 10).

Diagnostic Evaluation of Abdominal Trauma

Test	Purpose	Abnormal Findings
FAST: Focused Assessment with Sonography for Trauma	Rapid, portable, noninvasive method to detect hemoperitoneum. Uses four views to evaluate.	Based on the assumption that all clinically significant abdominal injuries are associated with hemoperitoneum. If positive result for blood, may require CT. If negative result, but indicative, proceed to DPL.
DPL: Diagnostic Peritoneal Lavage	DPL is indicated for selected patients who are more likely to have abdominal injury in the setting of blunt trauma: • Spinal cord injury • Multiple injuries and unexplained shock • Obtunded patients • Intoxicated patients • Those who will undergo prolonged anesthesia for another procedure.	Based on the assumption that all clinically significant abdominal injuries are associated with hemoperitoneum. If positive result for blood, requires CT.
Computed tomography (CT) scan	Used to evaluate integrity of cavities and organs.	Wound tract outlined by hemorrhage, air, bullet, or bone fragments that clearly extend into the peritoneal cavity; the presence of intraperitoneal free air, free fluid, or bullet fragments; and obvious intraperitoneal organ injury.
Rectal examination	Evaluate for bony penetration.	Blood in the stool (gross or occult) and/or the presence of a high-riding prostate (indicates genitourinary or bowel injury).
Chest radiograph	Assess size and integrity of heart, thoracic cage, and lungs; rules out chest cavity penetration.	Hemothoraces or pneumothoraces; air under diaphragm indicates peritoneal penetration.

Diagnostic Evaluation of Abdominal Trauma — cont'd

Test	Purpose	Abnormal Findings
Blood Studies		
Complete blood count Hemoglobin (Hgb) Hematocrit (Hct) Red blood cell count White blood cell count	Assess for occult bleeding or effects of gross bleeding.	Decreased Hgb or Hct reflects blood loss, may be false-negative result when the patient has lost significant volume. Repeat after 2 L of isotonic fluid resuscitation.
Electrolytes Potassium (K+) Magnesium (Mg2+) Calcium (Ca2+) Sodium (Na+)	Assess for possible causes of dysrhythmias and/or heart failure.	Decrease in K^+, Mg^{2+}, or Ca^{2+} may cause dysrhythmias. Elevation of Na^+ may indicate dehydration.
Coagulation profile Prothrombin time (PT) with international normalized ratio (INR) Partial thromboplastin time Fibrinogen D dimer	Assess for causes of bleeding, clotting, and disseminated intravascular coagulation indicative of abnormal clotting present in shock or ensuing shock.	Decreased PT with low INR promotes clotting; elevation promotes bleeding; elevated fibrinogen and D dimer reflect abnormal clotting is present.

COLLABORATIVE MANAGEMENT

The initial focus should be stabilization and supporting hemodynamics, but the highest priority is to diagnose and repair causes of hemorrhage. Timely provision of needed surgery, preferably in a trauma center, is the crucial factor impacting survival. Prolonged hypovolemia and shock result in organ ischemia and ultimately failure. See Major Trauma (Chapter 3) Acute Respiratory Distress Syndrome (Chapter 4) Cardiogenic Shock (Chapter 5), Acute Renal Failure (Chapter 6), and Hepatic Failure (Chapter 9).

CARE PRIORITIES

1. Identify and manage hypothermia

Patients with trauma are often profoundly hypothermic on arrival in the emergency department as a result of inadequate protection, IV fluid administration, ongoing blood loss, and environmental exposure. Hemorrhagic shock leads to decreased cellular perfusion and oxygenation and impoverished heat production. Hypothermia interferes with coagulation and platelet aggregation, and therefore exacerbates hemorrhage.

- Remove all wet clothing and make sure the patient is dry. The patient should be actively warmed with blankets, air-warming devices, or possibly continuous arteriovenous warming techniques. A simple method is to cover all extremities and the abdomen with plastic (e.g., blue side of underpads or trash bags) to trap all heat produced.

2. Provide oxygen therapy to manage hypoxia

Abdominal injury may result in poor ventilatory efforts caused by pain or compression of thoracic structures. High-flow supplemental oxygen is indicated initially and then titrated according to ABG values. Mechanical ventilation may be necessary.

3. Manage hypovolemia and anemia

Because massive blood loss is associated with most abdominal injuries, immediate volume resuscitation is crucial. Initially, LR or a similar balanced salt solution is given. Colloid solutions may be helpful in the postoperative period if there are low filling pressures and evidence of decreased plasma oncotic pressure. Typed and cross-matched fresh blood is the optimal fluid for replacement of large blood losses. However, because fresh whole blood is rarely available, a combination of packed cells and fresh-frozen plasma is often used. Overaggressive use of colloids and PRBCs may increase third spacing and SIRS. (See Major Trauma for more information.)

- Indication for immediate blood transfusion: Ongoing blood loss indicates hemodynamic instability despite the administration of 2 L of fluid to adult patients.
- Acidosis: Hemorrhagic shock reduces perfusion, resulting in hypoxemia, anaerobic metabolism, and lactic acidosis. The compensatory vasoconstrictive response shunts blood to the heart, lungs, and brain from the skin, muscles, and abdominal organs. Base deficit or lactate levels should be used to guide fluid resuscitation, ventilation, and BP support.
- Coagulopathy: Hypothermia, acidosis, and massive blood transfusion all lead to coagulopathy. The top priority is to stop the bleeding. Coagulopathy is treated by the administration of fresh-frozen plasma, factor VII, cryoprecipitate, and platelets, and correcting hypothermia and acidosis. If bleeding persists, consider vasopressin infusion, which causes vasoconstriction and calcium chloride.

4. Consider surgery for penetrating abdominal injuries

- Indication for emergency laparotomy:
  - Signs of peritonitis.
  - Uncontrolled shock or hemorrhage.
  - Clinical deterioration during observation.
  - Positive hemoperitoneum findings with FAST (Focused Assessment with Sonography for Trauma) or DPL (diagnostic peritoneal lavage) examinations.
- Removing penetrating objects can result in additional injury; thus, attempts at removal should be made only under controlled situations with a surgeon and operating room immediately available.
- If evisceration occurs initially or develops later, do not reinsert tissue or organs. Place a saline-soaked gauze over the evisceration, and cover with a sterile towel until the evisceration can be evaluated by the surgeon.
- The issue of mandatory surgical exploration versus observation and selective surgery, especially with stab wounds, remains controversial. There is a trend toward observation of patients without obvious injury or peritoneal signs.
- Indications for laparotomy include one or more of the following: (1) penetrating injury indicative of invading the peritoneum (e.g., abdominal gunshot wound or abdominal stab wound with evisceration, hypotension, or peritonitis); (2) positive peritoneal signs (e.g., tenderness, rebound tenderness, involuntary guarding); (3) shock; (4) GI hemorrhage; (5) free air in the peritoneal cavity as seen on x-ray film; (6) evisceration; (7) massive hematuria; and (8) positive findings on DPL.

> **Safety Alert** *The patient should be evaluated for peritoneal signs at least hourly by the same examiner. Consult the surgeon immediately if the patient shows peritoneal signs, evidence of shock, gastric or rectal bleeding, or gross hematuria.*

5. Consider an appropriate surgical intervention based on type of injury

- Blunt, nonpenetrating abdominal injuries: Physical examination is important in determining the necessity for surgery in patients who are alert, cooperative, and nonintoxicated. Additional diagnostic tests such as abdominal ultrasound, DPL, or CT are necessary to evaluate the need for surgery in the patient who is intoxicated or unconscious or who has sustained head or spinal cord trauma.
  - Nonoperative management: In blunt abdominal trauma, including severe solid organ injuries, selective nonoperative management (closely monitoring vital signs and frequently repeating the physical examination) is considered the standard of care, and based on CT scan diagnosis and hemodynamic stability of the patient.
    - Pediatric patients can generally be resuscitated and treated without surgery; some pediatric surgeons often transfuse up to 40 mL/kg of blood products to stabilize a pediatric patient.
    - Hemodynamically stable adults with solid organ injuries, primarily liver and spleen, may be candidates.
  - Splenic artery embolotherapy may be used for adult blunt splenic injury.

- These patients should be evaluated in the same manner as that described in the section Surgical Considerations for Penetrating Abdominal Injuries.
- Immediate laparotomy for blunt abdominal trauma is indicated under the following circumstances: (1) clear signs of peritoneal irritation (see Box 3-3); (2) free air in the peritoneum; (3) hypotension caused by suspected abdominal injury, or persistent and unexplained hypotension; (4) positive DPL findings; (5) GI aspirate or rectal smear-positive result for blood; and (6) other positive findings in diagnostic tests such as CT or arteriogram.
- Need for immediate surgery versus triad of failure: Once in the operating room, it may become apparent that the patient cannot survive a long procedure, or that the triad of failure (acidosis, hypothermia, and coagulopathy) may cause death. At this point the surgeon may do limited repair and packing, choosing to delay major surgical repair.
  - Transfer the patient to the intensive care unit (ICU), where the triad may be corrected. Survival from abdominal trauma and surgery requires an integrated team effort.
  - Focus is to limit the effects of hemorrhage, acidosis, and coagulopathy and to promote perfusion of all organs.

6. Considerations regarding closure of the abdominal surgical incision

During closure after surgery, if the bowel (intestines) can be visualized with an abdominal horizontal view, the abdomen fascia should not be closed. If the abdomen has been closed, it may become necessary to open it again either in the ICU or the operating room. There are multiple methods discussed in the literature to supplement closure.

1. Silo bag closure: A 3-L sterile plastic irrigation bag is emptied and cut to lie flat. The edges are trimmed and sutured to the skin.
2. Vacuum pack: A 3-L sterile plastic irrigation bag is emptied and cut to lie flat, then placed into the abdomen, and the edges are placed under the sheath. Two suction drains are placed on top of the bag, and a large adherent Steri-Drape is then placed over the whole abdomen. The catheters are placed to suction, providing continuous drainage.
3. Vacuum-assisted closure: This consists of a sterile sponge dressing with an adherent dressing and a continuous negative pressure; it promotes closure, blood flow, and collagen formation.

HIGH ALERT!   Sudden release of abdominal pressure may lead to further injuries such as ischemia-reperfusion, acute vasodilatation, and cardiac dysfunction and arrest. The nurse should hydrate the patient with at least 2 L of intravenous fluids and vasopressors should be immediately available in case severe hypotension occurs.

7. Provide nutrition support

Patients with abdominal trauma have complex nutritional needs because of the hypermetabolic state associated with major trauma and traumatic or surgical disruption of normal GI function. Often, infection and sepsis contribute to a negative nitrogen state and increased metabolic needs. Prompt initiation of parenteral or postpyloric feedings, as appropriate, in patients unable to accept conventional enteric feedings and the administration of supplemental calories, proteins, vitamins, and minerals are essential for healing. For additional information, see Nutrition Support (Chapter 1).

8. Prevent infection with antibiotics

Abdominal trauma is associated with a high incidence of intraabdominal abscess, sepsis, and wound infection, particularly with injury to the terminal ileum and colon. Patients with penetrating or blunt trauma and suspected intestinal injury are started on parenteral antibiotic therapy immediately. Broad-spectrum antibiotics are continued postoperatively and stopped after approximately 72 hours unless there is evidence of infection.

9. Manage pain using analgesics

Because opiates alter the sensorium, frequent assessment of LOC is important. Analgesics are used in the immediate postoperative period to relieve pain and promote ventilatory excursion. Nonsteroidal antiinflammatory drugs (NSAIDs) can increase risk of bleeding and should be used cautiously.

CARE PLANS: ABDOMINAL TRAUMA

Deficient fluid volume *related to active loss of blood volumes or secondary to management of fluids.*

Goals/Outcomes: Within 12 hours of this diagnosis, the patient becomes normovolemic, as evidenced by mean arterial pressure (MAP) greater than 70 mm Hg, HR 60 to 100 bpm, normal sinus rhythm on ECG, CVP 2 to 6 mm Hg, PAWP 6 to 12 mm Hg, CI greater than 2.5 L/min/m^2, SVR 900 to 1200 dynes/s/cm^{-5}, urinary output greater than 0.5 mL/kg/h, warm extremities, brisk capillary refill (less than 2 seconds), and distal pulses greater than 2+ on a 0-to-4+ scale. Although hemodynamic measurements are helpful to determine adequacy of resuscitation, serum lactate and base deficit are essential to evaluate cellular perfusion.

NOC Fluid Balance; Electrolyte and Acid-Base Balance.

Fluid Management

1. Monitor BP every 15 minutes, or more frequently in the presence of obvious bleeding or unstable vital signs. Be alert to changes in MAP of greater than 10 mm Hg.

> **Safety Alert** *Even a small but sudden decrease in blood pressure signals the need to consult the advanced practice provider and/or surgeon, especially for the patient with trauma in whom the extent of injury is unknown.*

2. Monitor HR, ECG, and cardiovascular status every 15 minutes until volume is restored and vital signs are stable. Check ECG to note HR elevations and myocardial ischemic changes (i.e., ventricular dysrhythmias, ST segment changes), which can occur because of dilutional anemia in susceptible individuals.
3. In the patient with evidence of volume depletion or active blood loss, administer pressurized fluids rapidly through several large-caliber (16-gauge or larger) catheters. Use short, large-bore IV tubing (trauma tubing) to maximize flow rate. Avoid use of stopcocks, because they slow the infusion rate.
4. Fluids should be warmed to prevent hypothermia.

 HIGH ALERT!   Evaluate patency of intravenous catheters continuously during rapid volume resuscitation.

5. Measure central pressures and thermodilution CO every 1 to 2 hours or more frequently if blood loss is ongoing. Calculate SVR and pulmonary vascular resistance every 4 to 8 hours or more often in patients who are unstable. Be alert to low or decreasing CVP and PAWP.

HIGH ALERT!   An elevated heart rate (HR), along with decreased pulmonary artery wedge pressure, decreased cardiac output/cardiac index (CO/CI), and increased systemic vascular resistance suggest hypovolemia (see Table 5-10 for hemodynamic profile of hypovolemic shock). Anticipate slightly elevated HR and CO caused by hyperdynamic cardiovascular state in some patients who have undergone volume resuscitation, particularly during the preoperative phase. Also anticipate mild to moderate pulmonary hypertension, especially in patients with concurrent thoracic injury, such as pulmonary contusion, smoke inhalation, or early acute respiratory distress syndrome. Acute respiratory distress syndrome is a concern in patients who have sustained major abdominal injury, considering that there are many potential sources of infection and sepsis that make the development of acute respiratory distress syndrome more likely (see Acute Respiratory Distress Syndrome).

6. Measure urinary output every 1 to 2 hours. Be alert to output of less than 0.5 mL/kg/h for 2 consecutive hours. Low urine output usually reflects inadequate intravascular volume in the patient with abdominal trauma.
7. Monitor for physical indicators of arterial hypovolemia: (1) cool extremities, (2) capillary refill greater than 2 seconds, (3) absent or decreased amplitude of distal pulses, (4) elevated serum lactate, and (5) base deficit.
8. Estimate ongoing blood loss. Measure all bloody drainage from tubes or catheters, noting drainage color (e.g., coffee grounds, burgundy, bright red; Table 3-2). Note the frequency of dressing changes as a result of saturation with blood to estimate amount of blood loss by way of the wound site.

Table 3-2	CHARACTERISTICS OF GASTROINTESTINAL DRAINAGE*
Source	**Composition and Usual Characteristics**
Mouth and oropharynx	Saliva; thin, clear, watery; pH 7
Stomach	Hydrochloric acid, gastrin, pepsin, mucus; thin, brown to green, acidic
Pancreas	Enzymes and bicarbonate; thin, watery, yellowish brown; alkaline
Biliary tract	Bile, including bile salts and electrolytes; bright yellow to brownish green
Duodenum	Digestive enzymes, mucus, products of digestion; thin, bright yellow to light brown, may be green, alkaline
Jejunum	Enzymes, mucus, products of digestion; brown, watery with particles
Ileum	Enzymes, mucus, digestive products, greater amounts of bacteria; brown, liquid, feculent
Colon	Digestive products, mucus, large amounts of bacteria; brown to dark brown, semiformed to firm stool
Postoperative (gastrointestinal surgery)	Initially, drainage expected to contain small amounts of fresh blood appearing bright to dark; later, drainage mixed with old blood appearing dark brown ("coffee grounds"), and then approaches normal composition
Infection present	Drainage cloudy, may be thicker than usual; strong or unusual odor, drain site often erythematous and warm

*It is important to know the normal to recognize the abnormal.

NIC Electrolyte Management; Fluid Monitoring; Hypovolemia Management.

Acute pain *related to physical injury secondary to trauma or surgical intervention.*

Goals/Outcomes: The patient's subjective evaluation of discomfort improves, as assessed by use of a pain scale and/or assessed by nonverbal indicators of discomfort, such as grimacing, restlessness, and/or physiologic indicators. **NOC** Pain Control; Comfort Level.

Pain Management
1. Medicate appropriately for pain relief. It is important to note that opiate analgesics can decrease GI motility, causing nausea, vomiting, and delay of bowel activity. These factors are especially important if the patient has had a recent laparotomy.
2. Provide comfort measures, maintain proper positioning of affected extremities while turning the patient and supporting incisional areas.
3. Explain procedures to the patient and include education regarding pain relief measures.

Risk for infection *related to inadequate primary infection defenses secondary to physical trauma or surgery; inadequate secondary defenses caused by decreased Hgb or inadequate immune response; tissue destruction and environmental exposure (especially to intestinal contents); multiple invasive procedures.*

Goals/Outcomes: The patient is free of infection, as evidenced by core or rectal temperature less than 37.7° C (100° F); HR less than 100 bpm; CI less than 4 L/min/m²; SVR greater than 900 dynes/s/cm⁻⁵; orientation to time, place, and person; and absence of unusual redness, warmth, or drainage at surgical incisions and drain sites. **NOC** Risk Control.

Infection Protection
1. Note color, character, and odor of all drainage from any surgical site, orifice, drain, or site of invasive catheters.
2. Report the presence of foul-smelling or abnormal drainage. See Table 3-2 for a description of the usual characteristics of GI drainage.
3. Monitor temperature, hemodynamics, and vital signs closely.

Abdominal Trauma

Safety Alert *Administer pneumococcal vaccine to patients with total splenectomy to minimize the risk of postsplenectomy sepsis.*

4. For more interventions, see this diagnosis in the section on Major Trauma.

NIC Infection Control; Infection Protection.

Ineffective tissue perfusion: GI *related to interruption of arterial or venous blood flow or episodes of hypovolemia resulting in decreased perfusion to GI organs.*

Goals/Outcomes: The patient has adequate GI tract tissue perfusion, as evidenced by normoactive bowel sounds; soft, nondistended abdomen; and return of bowel elimination.
NOC Tissue Perfusion: Abdominal Organs.

Circulatory Precautions
1. Auscultate for bowel sounds hourly during the acute phase of abdominal trauma and every 4 to 8 hours during the recovery phase. Report prolonged or sudden absence of bowel sounds during the postoperative period, because these signs may signal bowel ischemia or mesenteric infarction.
2. Evaluate the patient for peritoneal signs (see Box 3-3), which may occur initially as a result of injury or may not develop until days or weeks later, if complications caused by slow bleeding or other mechanisms occur.
3. Ensure adequate intravascular volume (see Deficient Fluid Volume).
4. Evaluate laboratory data for evidence of bleeding (e.g., serial Hct) or organ ischemia (e.g., aspartate aminotransferase [AST], alanine aminotransferase [ALT], lactic dehydrogenase [LDH]). Desired values are as follows: Hct greater than 28% to 30%, AST 5 to 40 International Unit/L, ALT 5 to 35 International Unit/L, and LDH 90 to 200 U/L.
5. Document amount and characteristics of GI secretions, drainage, and excretions.
6. Assess and report any indicators of infection or bowel obstruction (e.g., fever, severe or unusual abdominal pain, nausea and vomiting, unusual drainage from wounds or incisions, change in bowel habits).

HIGH ALERT! Note changes that suggest bleeding (presence of frank or occult blood), infection (e.g., increased or purulent drainage), or obstruction (e.g., failure to eliminate flatus or stool within 3 to 4 days after surgery).

NIC Circulatory Care: Arterial Insufficiency; Bowel Management.

Impaired skin integrity *related to mechanical factors (including physical injury); increased metabolic needs secondary to trauma/stress response; altered circulation secondary to hemorrhage or direct vascular injury; exposure to irritants (gastric secretions).*

Goals/Outcomes: The patient has adequate tissue integrity by the time of hospital discharge, as evidenced by wound healing within an acceptable time frame (according to extent of injury) and absence of skin breakdown caused by GI drainage.
NOC Tissue Integrity: Skin and Mucous Membranes.

Skin Surveillance
1. Protect the skin surrounding tubes, drains, or fistulas, keeping the areas clean and free from drainage. Gastric and intestinal secretions and drainage are highly irritating and can lead to skin excoriation. If necessary, apply ointments, skin barriers, or drainage pouches to protect the surrounding skin. If available, consult the ostomy nurse for complex or involved cases.
2. For other interventions, see this diagnosis in the section on Major Trauma.

NIC Wound Care; Tube Care.

Imbalanced nutrition: less than body requirements *related to decreased intake secondary to disruption of GI tract integrity (traumatic or surgical); increased need secondary to hypermetabolic posttrauma state.*

Goals/Outcomes: The patient has adequate nutrition, as evidenced by maintenance of baseline body weight and state of nitrogen balance on nitrogen studies.
NOC Nutritional Status: Food and Fluid Intake; Nutritional Status.

Nutrition Management
1. Collaborate with advanced practice providers, dietician, and pharmacist to estimate the patient's metabolic needs on the basis of type of injury, activity level, and nutritional status before injury.
2. Consider the patient's specific injuries when planning nutrition. For example, expect patients with hepatic or pancreatic injury to have difficulty with blood glucose regulation.
3. Patients with trauma to the upper GI tract may be fed enterally, but feeding tube must be placed distal to the injury. Disruption of the GI tract may require a feeding gastrostomy or jejunostomy. Patients with major hepatic trauma may have difficulty with protein tolerance.
4. Ensure patency of gastric or intestinal tubes to maintain decompression and encourage healing and return of bowel function. Avoid occlusion of the vent side of sump suction tubes, because this may result in vacuum occlusion of the tube.

Safety Alert	*Use caution when irrigating gastric or other tubes that have been placed in or near recently sutured organs.*

- For additional information, see sections on Nutrition Support (Chapter 1) and Major Trauma.

NIC Electrolyte Management; Feeding; Nutrition Therapy; Tube Feeding.

Disturbed body image *related to creation of stoma (often without the patient's previous knowledge); as part of management of penetrating physical injury to internal organs.*

Goals/Outcomes: The patient is able to acknowledge body changes, views and touches affected body part, and demonstrates movement toward incorporating changes into self-concept and is able to verbalize some level of coping.
NOC Body Image; Self-Esteem.

Body Image Enhancement
1. Evaluate the patient's reaction to the stoma or missing/mutilated body part by observing and noting evidence of body image disturbance (see Box 2-4).
2. Anticipate feelings of shock and disbelief initially. Be aware that patients with trauma usually do not receive the emotional preparation for ostomy, amputation, and other disfiguring surgery that the patient undergoing elective surgery receives.
3. Anticipate and acknowledge normalcy of feelings of rejection and isolation (and uncleanliness in the case of fecal diversion).
4. Offer the patient an opportunity to view the stoma/altered body part. Use mirrors if necessary.
5. Encourage the patient and significant others to verbalize feelings regarding altered/missing body part.
6. Offer the patient an opportunity to participate in the care of the ostomy, wound, or incision.
7. Confer with the surgeon regarding advisability of a visit by an ostomate or a patient with similar alteration in body part.
8. Be aware that most colostomies are temporary in patients with colonic trauma. This fact can be reassuring to the patient, but it is important to verify the type of colostomy with the surgeon before explaining this to the patient.

NIC Ostomy Care.

ADDITIONAL NURSING DIAGNOSES

Also see Major Trauma for Hypothermia (Chapter 2) and Posttrauma Syndrome. For additional information, see other diagnoses under Major Trauma, as well as nursing diagnoses and

Abdominal Trauma

interventions in the following sections, as appropriate: Hemodynamic Monitoring (Chapter 1), Prolonged Immobility (Chapter 1), Emotional and Spiritual Support of the Patient and Significant Others, Peritonitis (Chapter 9), Enterocutaneous Fistula (Chapter 9), SIRS, Sepsis, and MODS (Chapter 10), and Acid-Base Imbalances (Chapter 1).

ACUTE CARDIAC TAMPONADE

PATHOPHYSIOLOGY

Cardiac tamponade is a condition that results in a low CO state caused by decreased filling of the chambers of the heart from pressure exerted by fluid, blood, purulent liquid, or gas in the pericardial space surrounding the heart. Cardiac tamponade is classified as acute, subacute, occult, or regional. Acute cardiac tamponade occurs when there is a rapid accumulation of fluid in the pericardial space that compresses the heart, resulting in sudden hemodynamic instability that can be life threatening.

Potential causes of cardiac tamponade include the following:

- Trauma: Blunt or penetrating cardiac trauma.
- Iatrogenic: Cardiac surgery, cardiac catheterization, pacemaker implant.
- Nontraumatic hemorrhage: Dissecting aortic aneurysm, anticoagulation therapy.
- Left ventricular rupture: Following extensive myocardial infarction.
- Infection: Viral, bacterial, or fungal.
- Neoplasms/carcinoma: Most commonly breast and lung.
- Other: Connective tissue disease, pleural effusions, radiation therapy, uremic states.

Acute cardiac tamponade is usually a result of trauma, iatrogenic causes, and hemorrhage resulting in inadequate CO, decreased tissue perfusion, and possibly death. *Subacute tamponade* causes are related to the slower accumulation of fluids seen with infections, neoplasms, and tissue disease. Occult or low pressure tamponade is seen in hypovolemic settings. Regional tamponade can occur with large pleural effusions or with fluid localized or loculated within one part of the pericardial space. Pericardial effusions can be described using the Horowitz classification system based on the echo-free space seen with echocardiograms (Box 3-4). Any nonacute tamponade may become acute when rapid deterioration in patient condition causes shock related to low CO.

Acute cardiac tamponade manifests when the heart is compressed within the pericardial sac to the point where the chambers of the heart cannot fill. The pressure within the sac must be relieved. The rapid detection and treatment of acute tamponade are key to patient survival. The pericardial sac contains 20 to 50 mL of fluid to protect and provide a friction-free surface for the beating heart. The pericardial sac has a fibroelastic quality, which allows limited stretching ability. A sudden addition of 50 to 100 mL of fluid can markedly increase intrapericardial pressure. Conversely, a slowly accumulating tamponade can result in 2000 mL of fluid collection without life-threatening cardiac compromise because the pericardial sac has an opportunity to stretch slowly, expanding to accommodate the slow accumulation of fluid volume within the pericardial sac.

When there is a rapid increase in intrapericardial pressure, the heart is compressed causing a decrease in intraventricular filling. The compliance of the right side of the heart is limited, because it is competing for the fixed volume within the pericardium. The right atrium (RA), as a low pressure heart chamber is the most susceptible to collapse, which decreases filling of the right ventricle. This decreased filling results in JVD. While the pressure continues to increase, the right ventricle has partial collapse during early diastole. The decreased right ventricle free wall compliance causes a right-to-left shift of the septum, which is pronounced during inspiration, causing the pulsus paradoxus seen with cardiac tamponade. An unresolved

---

Box 3-4	HOROWITZ CLASSIFICATION OF PERICARDIAL EFFUSIONS

Grade 1: Small: Echo-free space in diastole less than 10 mm.
Grade 2: Moderate: Echo-free space at least greater than 10 mm posteriorly.
Grade 3: Large: Echo-free space greater than 20 mm.
Grade 4: Very Large: Echo-free space greater than 20 mm and compression of heart is present.

tamponade puts pressure on all chambers of the heart, pulmonary vessels, and coronary arteries, causing hemodynamic instability. Hemodynamically, while pulmonary artery pressures (PAPs) increase, an equalization of pressures of the right and left atria are seen, and decreased ventricular filling occurs. This hemodynamic compromise results in decreased CO and hypotension with decreased tissue perfusion.

ASSESSMENT: ACUTE CARDIAC TAMPONADE

GOAL OF SYSTEM ASSESSMENT

Determine rapid diagnosis and treatment of acute cardiac tamponade to prevent cardiac collapse and irreversible shock.

> **HIGH ALERT!** Pulseless electrical activity may be the presenting sign of cardiac tamponade. Have a high suspicion of tamponade if presenting rhythm is narrow-complex tachycardia without a pulse. Cardiopulmonary resuscitation must be initiated immediately.

- IV insertion and advanced airway placement as soon as possible.
- Epinephrine 1 mg IVP or vasopressin 40 units IVP with ongoing cardiopulmonary resuscitation.
- Fluid administration: LR or NS bolus.
- Emergent pericardiocentesis.
- Prepare for emergent thoracotomy if qualified surgeon is present.

OBSERVATION

- Early signs and symptoms: Beck triad consisting of muffled or distant heart tones, distended neck veins, and hypotension; an unwillingness to lay flat/supine, high anxiety, dyspnea, a change in mental status and pulsus paradoxus. Pulsus paradoxus is a decrease of greater than 10 mm Hg in systolic BP that occurs during inspiration in the setting of increased intrathoracic pressure. Stroke volume is reduced by the increased intrathoracic pressure compressing the heart and blood vessels. The decrease in systolic BP during inspiration is heard when slowly auscultating the BP.
- Important bariatric considerations: Distended neck veins may be difficult or impossible to assess related to neck size and adipose distribution. Additionally, proper BP cuff size is essential to accurately assess for pulsus paradoxus in the absence of invasive arterial pressure monitoring. Without a large enough cuff, the subtle drop in the systolic BP heard during inspiration when auscultating the BP is almost impossible to recognize.
- Early hemodynamic changes: Decreased BP, increase in RA pressure (RAP) or CVP. Pulsus paradoxus of greater than 10 mm Hg (see Box 3-2); low CO.
- Late signs and symptoms: Signs of cardiogenic shock including decreased BP, weak or thready pulse, confusion, restlessness, cold clammy skin, pallor.
- Late-stage hemodynamic changes: Continued hypotension, low CO, right and left atrial pressures equalize, and PAP increases.

VITAL SIGNS

- Sinus tachycardia, commonly seen as compensatory response to decreased stroke volume.
- Monitor BP; assess for significant hypotension, narrow pulse pressure, systolic BP less than 90 mm Hg, and pulsus paradoxus.
- Exertional dyspnea early, progressing to dyspnea and orthopnea.
- Hoarseness and hiccups may be present resulting from laryngeal and phrenic nerve involvement.
- Low urine output is a result of low CO, and taken with other signs should be viewed as a signal for intervention in the absence of hemodynamic monitoring.

AUSCULTATION

- Beck triad, although described as classic, is seen in 10% to 33% of patients. Muffled heart tones may not be apparent with the patient sitting upright, depending on the volume of tamponade, and may be difficult to hear in a busy, noisy environment. JVD is not always present in acute tamponade, but is commonly seen in constrictive pericarditis. Differentiating constrictive pericarditis from cardiac tamponade is important. In the presence of hypovolemia, blood flowing toward the RA during inspiration makes the finding of JVD less likely with tamponade. Pericardial friction rub may be heard with pericarditis.

PERCUSSION

- Dullness to percussion under the left scapula posteriorly, related to compression of the left lower lobe. The Bamberger-Pins-Ewart sign is a localized pulmonary auscultation and percussion finding noted in the setting of large pericardial effusions. There is dullness to percussion, increased fremitus, and bronchial breathing between the vertebral column and the scapula. A blowing sound can be heard, generally on the left side, resulting from atelectasis caused by the enlarged pericardial sac.

HEMODYNAMIC MONITORING

If hemodynamic monitoring is not already in progress, do not delay other treatments, but prepare for appropriate monitoring, according to the hemodynamic system used. This may include insertion and monitoring of an arterial line and pulmonary artery catheter or another system capable of CO measurement.

- Decreased BP: Systolic BP less than 90 mm Hg requires intervention.
- Increased CVP: Greater than 12 mm Hg or increasing above base line. The CVP may also be decreased if significant hypovolemia is present.
- Pulsus paradoxus: Systolic arterial pressure decreases greater than 10 mm Hg during inspiration; easily seen in arterial waveform with lower systolic BP during inspiration. This may be less apparent with severe shock.
- Absence of Kussmaul sign: Kussmaul sign is a paradoxical increase in jugular venous (JV) pressure with noticeable external JV distention during inspiration seen with constrictive pericarditis, but rarely with cardiac tamponade. The right ventricle can accommodate increased volume with inspiration in the setting of tamponade, and thus a decline in JV pressure can be seen on the CVP waveform. With cardiac tamponade, jugular veins are distended with a prominent x descent and an absent y descent on the CVP waveform. The right atrial y descent is lost because no blood can enter the atrium. Patients with constrictive pericarditis have a prominent x and y descent. This is important in differentiating tamponade from constrictive pericarditis.
- Low CO: CI less than 2.2.
- PAP: Increased.
- Stroke volume variation (SVV): Increased. May be less apparent with severe shock, but is inaccurate in setting of dysrhythmias.
- CVP equalizes with left atrial pressure or pulmonary artery occlusive pressure.
- BP, CO, and CI continue to decrease, requiring fluid and vasopressor and inotropic support until definitive treatment is provided.
- If untreated, tamponade can lead to pulseless electrical activity (PEA) or total cardiac arrest.

Safety Alert   *Abnormally elevated central venous pressure, pulmonary artery pressure, and pulsus paradoxus may not be seen with the patient who is hypovolemic until fluid administration is begun.*

- Pulsus paradoxus related to hypovolemia will resolve with fluid administration.
- Pulsus paradoxus will not resolve in acute cardiac tamponade with fluid administration alone.

SCREENING DIAGNOSTIC TESTS

- Echocardiogram is indicated as a quick diagnostic tool for assessment.

Diagnostic Tests for Acute Cardiac Tamponade

Test	Purpose	Abnormal Findings
Noninvasive Cardiology		
Electrocardiogram (ECG): 12-lead	Assess for any ischemia or infarct, underlying rhythm disturbances, or pericarditis.	Electrical alternans is a beat-to-beat change in the QRS, from swinging of the heart within the pericardium. It is rare and seen with very large volume effusions. Presence of ST segment depression or T wave inversion (myocardial ischemia), ST elevation (acute myocardial infarction), new bundle branch block (especially left bundle branch block), or pathologic Q waves (resolving/resolved myocardial infarction) in two contiguous or related leads. Pericarditis shows ST segment and T wave changes, which are often confused with ischemic changes but are more diffuse and follow a four stage pattern (Table 5-9). Low voltage of QRS highly indicative of tamponade.
Radiology		
Chest radiograph	Assess for a widening mediastinum. Assess size of heart, thoracic cage (for fractures), thoracic aorta (for aneurysm), and lungs (pneumonia, pneumothorax); assists with differential diagnosis of chest pain.	Widening mediastinum is indicative of acute cardiac tamponade, especially important for trauma, postprocedural, and postsurgical patients. Cardiac silhouette enlargement with clear lung fields is indicative of pericardial effusion; but >200 mL of fluid must be present for this finding to be apparent.
Echocardiography (2D or Doppler ECHO)	It is the most definitive test for diagnosing early cardiac tamponade. Assessment of thoracic aneurysms that might have dissected into the valve or coronary arteries causing tamponade. Determine type of fluid within the pericardial space. Assess for mechanical abnormalities related to effective pumping of blood from both sides of the heart.	Pericardial effusions with and without tamponade. Aortic dissections and aneurysms. Abnormal ventricular wall movement or motion, low ejection fraction, incompetent or stenosed heart valves, and abnormal intracardiac chamber pressures.

Continued

Acute Cardiac Tamponade

Diagnostic Tests for Acute Cardiac Tamponade—cont'd

Test	Purpose	Abnormal Findings
Transesophageal ECHO (TEE)	Postcardiac surgery effusions often accumulate at the posterior wall with compression of right atrium. Useful for assessment of regional cardiac tamponade. Also can be done without delay while patient is being prepped in operating room for emergent thoracotomy or can be done in operating room. Assess for mechanical abnormalities related to ineffective pumping of blood from both sides of the heart using a transducer attached to an endoscope.	Same as above but can provide enhanced views, particularly of the posterior wall of the heart. Also, useful in determining pericardial thickness and filling dynamics associated with restrictive pericarditis.
Blood Studies		
Complete blood count Hemoglobin (Hgb) Hematocrit (Hct) Red blood cell (RBC) count White blood cell (WBC) count Erythrocyte sedimentation rate (ESR)	Assess for anemia, inflammation, and infection; assists with differential diagnosis of cause of tamponade.	Decreased RBCs, Hgb, or Hct reflects hemorrhage or anemia. Elevated WBC and or ESR indicative of infection or inflammatory pericarditis unless secondary to uremia.
Coagulation profile Prothrombin time (PT) with international normalized ratio (INR) Partial thromboplastin time (PTT) Fibrinogen D dimer Antifactor Xa assay (heparin level) Activated clotting time (ACT)	Assess for causes of bleeding, clotting, and disseminated intravascular coagulation indicative of abnormal clotting present in shock or ensuing shock. Patients who are anticoagulated are at higher risk for tamponade with procedures.	Elevated PTT, PT with high INR promotes bleeding; elevated fibrinogen and D dimer reflect abnormal clotting is present. Antifactor Xa assay reflects where heparin specifically affects the clotting cascade and indicates that further heparin reversal may be needed. ACT is often used in surgery and occasionally in the intensive care unit to determine clotting status.
Electrolytes Potassium (K^+) Magnesium (Mg^{2+}) Calcium (Ca^{2+}) Sodium (Na^+)	Assess for possible causes of dysrhythmias and/or heart failure.	Decrease in K^+, Mg^{2+}, or Ca^{2+} may cause dysrhythmias. Elevation of Na^+ may indicate dehydration (blood is more coagulable). Low Na^+ may indicate fluid retention and/or heart failure.
Other C-Reactive protein (CRP) Antistreptolysin O (ASO)	Assess for cause of pericarditis.	CRP can be indicative of inflammation unless the patient has uremia. ASO elevated with immunologic cause.

COLLABORATIVE MANAGEMENT

From www.acc.org/qualityandscience/clinical/statements.htm.

Guidelines on the Diagnosis and Management of Pericardial Disease from the Task Force on the Diagnosis and Management of Pericardial Diseases of the European Society of Cardiology

In 2004, findings were published from the Task Force on the Diagnosis and Management of Pericardial Diseases in the *European Heart Journal*. These findings included specific recommendations for various forms of pericardial disease to include cardiac tamponade. The treatment guidelines have been widely cited in the worldwide medical literature. The following are limited to the recommendations for the treatment of acute (surgical) cardiac tamponade.

Intervention	Rationale
The diagnostic tests as presented reflect these guidelines with the addition of computed tomography (CT), spin-echo, and cine magnetic resonance imaging (MRI).	To assess the size and extent of simple and complex pericardial effusions. These are also helpful to measure the size of very large effusions.
Pericardiocentesis (Class I)	Absolute indication for cardiac tamponade with hemodynamic instability, except in the presence of aortic dissection–associated tamponade.
Surgical drainage with bleeding suppression (Class I)	For wounds, ruptured ventricular aneurysm, or dissecting aorta aneurysm with hemorrhage or any tamponade in which needle clotting would make needle evacuation impossible.
Thoracoscopic drainage, subxiphoid window, or open surgery	Indicated for loculated tamponade.

In 2003, the American College of Cardiology, the American Heart Association, and the American Society of Echocardiography presented a task force recommendation for the use of echocardiography for all patients with pericardial disease. This recommendation would include the patient with cardiac tamponade unless an emergent surgical procedure was needed before evaluation.

> **Safety Alert** *Pericardiocentesis should be avoided when cardiac tamponade is associated with aortic dissection; immediate surgical intervention is indicated.*
> The American College of Cardiology Foundation (ACCF)/American Heart Association (AHA)/American Association for Thoracic Surgery (AATS)/American College of Radiology(ACR)/Society of Cardiovascular Anesthesiologists (SCA)/Society for Cardiovascular Angiography and Interventions (SCAI)/Society of Interventional Radiology (SIR)/Society of Thoracic Surgeons (STS)/Society for Vascular Medicine (SVM) issued Guidelines for the Diagnosis and Management of Patients With Thoracic Aortic Disease in 2010. This safety alert information was derived from that report.

CARE PRIORITIES

1. Stabilize ventilation with oxygen, intubation, and mechanical ventilation

Oxygen is administered using the equipment that most effectively corrects each patient's hypoxia. Devices used range from nasal cannula to 100% nonrebreather masks to mechanical ventilators. If the patient presented in cardiac arrest, chest compressions should be in progress while ventilation is being stabilized.

2. Facilitate providing pericardiocentesis

Needle aspiration of the pericardium can be performed using a subxiphoid or left parasternal approach to drain excess fluid from the pericardial space. The blood removed often will not clot, because the heart action can cause clotting factors within the pericardial sac to break down (defibrination). Pericardiocentesis alone may not suffice to manage acute pericardial tamponade. Surgical exploration with pericardial window is recommended because of the high incidence of recurrent bleeding if surgery is not performed. A drain may stay in place until fluid output decreases or ceases.

3. Anticipate the need to provide a surgical procedure

Subxiphoid pericardiostomy is a resection of the xiphoid process to drain the pericardial sac. It is performed using either local or general anesthesia. Other, more extensive surgical procedures, including a pericardiectomy, can be used for cardiac decompression. An immediate thoracotomy can be done in the ICU or emergency department if the patient becomes suddenly bradycardic (HR less than 50 bpm) or severely hypotensive (systolic BP less than 70 mm Hg) or has PEA or cardiac arrest. Thoracotomy allows for pericardial sac evacuation, hemorrhage control, and internal cardiac massage if needed.

4. Provide fluid resuscitation

IV fluid infusion is used to increase ventricular filling pressures during diastole and may result in increased CO and BP. Blood products, colloids, or crystalloids may be used.

5. Administer vasoconstrictors

Medications used to increase BP by stimulating vasoconstriction in the peripheral vasculature include neosynephrine or norepinephrine. These medications are less effective in a setting of hypovolemia.

6. Administer inotropic agents

Medications used to increase myocardial contractility and CO include dopamine, dobutamine, and milrinone (see Appendix 6).

7. Stabilize BP with ongoing titration of medications and fluids

This must be done with hemodynamic monitoring and goal-directed therapy derived at by the entire critical care team.

CARE PLANS: ACUTE CARDIAC TAMPONADE

Decreased CO related to decreased preload secondary to compression of ventricles by fluid in the pericardial sac.

Goals/Outcomes: Within 4 to 6 hours after fluid resuscitation or evacuation of tamponade, the patient has adequate CO, as evidenced by CVP 4 to 6 mm Hg, CO 4 to 7 L/min, CI $\geq$2.5 L/min, systolic BP at least 90 mm Hg (or within the patient's normal range), HR 60 to 100 bpm, normal sinus rhythm on ECG, SVV 13% or lower, and absence of new murmurs or gallops, distended neck veins, and pulsus paradoxus.

NOC Cardiac Pump Effectiveness.

Cardiac Care: Acute Hemodynamic Regulation

1. Assess cardiovascular function by evaluating heart sounds and neck veins hourly. Consult provider for muffled heart sounds, new murmurs, new gallops, irregularities in rate and rhythm, and distended neck veins.
2. Monitor all patients with blunt or penetrating trauma to the chest and abdomen for physical signs of acute cardiac tamponade, persistent hemodynamic instability, and shock symptoms more severe than expected for the blood loss.
3. Evaluate the patient for pulsus paradoxus (see Box 3-2).
4. Measure and record hemodynamic measurements. Consult the advanced practice provider for sudden abnormalities or changes in trend. Early signs of tamponade include elevated CVP with normal BP SVV greater than 13% and pulsus paradoxus. Later signs include equalization of CVP and left atrial pressure (pulmonary artery occlusive pressure) and elevated PAP in the presence of hypotension, SVV greater than 13% and not fluid responsive, low CO and CI (see Box 3-4).
5. Evaluate ECG for ST segment changes, T wave changes, rate, and rhythm. The optimum is sinus rhythm or sinus tachycardia. Maintain continuous cardiac monitoring.
6. For patients presenting with PEA and narrow complex tachycardia on ECG, suggest acute cardiac tamponade and follow ACLS (Advanced Cardiac Life Support) guidelines to treat and relieve cardiac tamponade.
7. Administer blood products, colloids, or crystalloids as prescribed. For patients with trauma, use large-bore IV lines in the periphery, if possible. Use pressure infusers and rapid volume/warmer infusers for patients who require massive fluid resuscitation.
8. Be prepared to administer vasoconstrictor agents (e.g., norepinephrine, phenylephrine, dopamine) if fluid resuscitation does not support the patient's BP. Positive inotropic agents (e.g., milrinone) may be used to support CO in short-term management. The underlying problem is decreased ventricular filling, thus these are temporizing measures for hemodynamic support until correction of the tamponade occurs.

9. Have emergency equipment available for immediate pulmonary artery catheterization, central line insertion, arterial line insertion, pericardiocentesis, or thoracotomy.

10. Assess heart rate and monitor ECG: sinus tachycardia, commonly seen as compensatory response to decreased stroke volume.

NIC Cardiac Care; Cardiac Care: Acute; Emergency Care; Hemodynamic Regulation; Invasive Hemodynamic Monitoring; Fluid Monitoring; Fluid Management; Blood Product Administration; Medication Administration; Oxygen Therapy; Resuscitation; Shock Management: Cardiac; Vital Signs Monitoring; Dysrhythmia Management.

Ineffective tissue perfusion: pulmonary, peripheral, and cerebral *related to interruption of arterial and venous flow secondary to compression of the myocardium, by the collection of fluid within the pericardial sac.*

Goals/Outcomes: Within 4 to 6 hours after management with fluids or evacuation of tamponade, the patient has adequate perfusion, as evidenced by orientation to time, place, and person; systolic BP at least 90 mm Hg (or within the patient's normal range); RR 12 to 20 breaths/min with normal depth and pattern (eupnea) and ease of respirations; Sao_2 at least 95%; peripheral pulses at least 2+ on a 0-to-4+ scale; equal and normoreactive pupils; warm and dry skin; brisk capillary refill (less than 2 seconds); and urine output at least 0.5 mL/kg/h.
NOC Circulation Status.

Shock Management: Cardiac

1. Assess tissue perfusion by evaluating the following at least hourly: LOC, BP, pulses, pupillary response, skin temperature, capillary refill, and hemodynamic monitoring measurements if available.

2. Evaluate urine output hourly to ensure that it is at least 0.5 mL/kg/h for patients with nonrenal failure.

3. Maintain tissue perfusion by delivering prescribed blood products, colloids, crystalloids, vasopressors, and positive inotropes.

4. If hypotension occurs, ensure that hypovolemia is treated, with fluid administration, before or simultaneously with vasopressors for treatment of hypotension. Administer vasopressors via the central line whenever possible. Frequently assess peripheral IV lines for evidence of infiltration. If vasopressor agents infiltrate subcutaneous tissues, necrosis occurs. Follow appropriate management protocol for your institution.

5. Have emergency oxygen and intubation and mechanical ventilation equipment available.

6. Anticipate and prepare for pericardiocentesis and/or emergent cardiac surgery (pericardial window, possible pericardiostomy or pericardiectomy). If needle aspiration of the pericardium is ineffective, surgical evacuation of the pericardium is immediately required if the patient is in shock.

7. Prepare for emergency open chest procedure in the postcardiac surgery patient exhibiting signs of tamponade.

Safety Alert *Vasoconstrictors (e.g., norepinephrine, phenylephrine, dopamine) should be infused through a central line.*

NIC Cardiac Care: Acute; Circulatory Care; Emergency Care; Invasive Hemodynamic Monitoring; Respiratory Monitoring; Shock Management; Vital Signs Monitoring; Cerebral Perfusion Promotion; Neurologic Monitoring; Medication Administration; Medication Management; Oxygen Therapy; IV Therapy; Fluid/Electrolyte Management.

ADDITIONAL NURSING DIAGNOSES

For other nursing diagnoses and interventions, see also Major Trauma, Chest Trauma, Hemodynamic Monitoring (Chapter 9), and Emotional and Spiritual Support of the Patient and Significant Others (Chapter 2).

ACUTE SPINAL CORD INJURY
PATHOPHYSIOLOGY

Injury to the spinal cord can be a devastating event initiating a cascade of physical and psychological changes that may last a lifetime. Spinal cord injury (SCI) affects approximately 12,000 people each year; this number depicts a continuing trend in injuries associated with

Acute Spinal Cord Injury

motor vehicle crashes (39.2%), falls (28.3%), and violent acts, primarily gunshot wounds (14.6%) but a decreasing trend in sports injuries (8.2%) with 9.7% classified as other. The average age at injury is increasing and is now 41.6 years; the rising trend may reflect referral patterns survival of older adults at the scene, or an increase in the number of injuries in those who are 60 years and older. Young white males continue to be injured most frequently but a mixed racial/ethnicity pattern has emerged since 2005 that may reflect the U.S. population trend; a decrease in white populations with an increase in African-American and Hispanic populations being injured. Cervical injuries occur most frequently at a rate of 56% over lumbar and thoracic injuries. There are estimated to be between 250,000 and 400,000 people living with an SCI, and approximately 85% of patients with SCI who survive the initial 24 hours live at least 10 years. Less than 1% of patients experience complete recovery at the time of discharge from the hospital.

The spinal cord is approximately 18 inches in length running from the base of the brain to the lumbar (L) spine area between L1 and L2 where the cord tapers to form the conus medullaris, a bulbous end that terminates into a collection of nerve roots known as the cauda equina (horse's tail). The spinal nerve roots exit the spinal cord at corresponding levels below the vertebral body of the spinal column and are the anatomic connection between the central and peripheral nervous system. Because the spinal cord ends at L1 and L2, the nerves descending from the conus medullaris making up the cauda equina are considered peripheral nerves. The brain and spinal cord communicate sensory and motor information along a complex system of tracts, some descending from the brain (motor) and others ascending from the periphery (sensory). Damage to pathways along this communication system results in unique but very distinguishable syndromes that include upper motor neurons (UMNs), which carry messages between the brain and the periphery along the spinal cord, and lower motor neurons (LMNs), those nerves that branch out from the vertebrae (peripheral nerves). Damage to UMNs results in muscle spasticity and hyperreflexia, whereas damage to LMNs results in muscle flaccidity and areflexia.

Mechanisms of injury to the spinal cord can be traumatic or nontraumatic. Traumatic injuries include MVCs, falls, sports injuries, or acts of violence (e.g., gunshot wounds or stabbings). These mechanical force injuries result in sudden flexion, hyperextension, vertebral fracture, compression of the cord, rotation of the cord, or direct injury to the cord such as in a stabbing or gunshot wound. Nontraumatic injuries may be a result of vascular injury (aortic disruption or spinal artery occlusion), degenerative diseases (spondylosis), inflammatory events, neoplasms, or autoimmune diseases (multiple sclerosis). Injuries to the spinal cord regardless of mechanism of injury include concussion, contusion, laceration, transsection, hemorrhage, ischemia, and avascularization. See SCI classifications and terminology in Table 3-3.

FRACTURES INVOLVING THE VERTEBRAL BODIES

Vertebral column fractures may or may not cause SCI. Severe SCI can occur without damage to the vertebrae but rather result from ischemia. With severe fractures, such as the "burst" fracture (fragmentation of a vertebral body with penetration of the spinal cord), paralysis almost always occurs. Penetration of the spinal cord with bony fragments may cause hemorrhage, infection, and leakage of cerebrospinal fluid (CSF).

SPINAL SHOCK

Spinal shock occurs following both complete and partial transsection of the cord. It is a temporary loss of reflex and sensorimotor function in all segments below the level of injury. Spinal shock does not involve the classic shock symptoms, including hypotension, tachycardia, and cardiovascular compensation to help support the BP. The "shock" manifests as temporarily "stunning" the function of the spinal cord. Spinal shock occurs immediately after SCI, lasting several hours to weeks and is a separate phenomenon from neurogenic shock. Sensorimotor function of the disrupted portion of the spinal cord can return once spinal shock resolves.

NEUROGENIC SHOCK

Neurogenic shock occurs in patients who injure the cervical or upper thoracic cord, disrupting sympathetic innervation to the vasculature and the heart. Cardiovascular compensatory mechanisms controlled by sympathetic nerves in the upper thoracic cord are lost. The loss of sympathetic innervation causes widespread vasodilation and venous pooling in the

Table 3-3	SPINAL CORD INJURY CLASSIFICATIONS AND TERMINOLOGY
Type	Closed (blunt)
	Open (gunshot wound or stabbing)
Cause	Motor vehicle collisions, falls, sports-related injury, acts of violence
Site	Level of injury involved (cervical thoracic, lumbar, sacral)
Mechanism	Flexion (deceleration injury, backward fall, diving injury)
	Extension (whiplash or fall with hyperextension of neck)
Stability	Integrity of supporting anatomy including vertebral bodies, ligaments, articulating processes, and facet joints
Complete	Tetraplegia (quadriplegia) or paraplegia (absence of motor, sensory, and vasomotor function below the level of injury)
	More frequently seen in cervical injuries
Incomplete	Sparing of some motor and sensory function below the level of the lesion
	More frequently seen in lumbar injuries

extremities and splanchnic vasculature. Loss of sympathetic innervation to the heart leads to bradycardia. The ensuing hypotension and bradycardia reduce CO as a result of decreased preload (decreased venous return) and inability to increase heart rate, putting patients at risk for secondary injury related to ischemia.

SPINAL SHOCK WITH NEUROGENIC SHOCK
Patients who injure the cervical or upper thoracic cord may experience neurogenic shock and spinal shock simultaneously.

Safety Alert *Although spinal shock is seen in spinal cord injuries (SCIs) at any level, the loss of central control of peripheral vascular tone (neurogenic shock) occurs most dramatically in high cervical spine injuries, with interruption of the sympathetic nervous system. Profound bradycardia and hypotension are possible. With SCIs lower than the midthoracic area, the patient will experience a phase of neurogenic shock, with loss of sympathetic innervation to vasculature below the level of the lesion; however, the effects of that loss are not as dramatic.*

SEPTIC SHOCK
Septic shock (see Septic Shock) may occur in patients with SCI as a result of infections related to pneumonia, urinary tract infections (UTIs), pressure sores, overuse of corticosteroids, and other causes.

HIGH ALERT! Autonomic Dysreflexia
 A life-threatening condition affecting victims with lesions at or above T6, stemming from stimulation of the SNS by relatively minor events. The resultant uncompensated cardiovascular response may cause seizures, subarachnoid hemorrhage, fatal cerebrovascular accident, and myocardial infarction if not immediately recognized and treated.
Once spinal shock resolves, autonomic dysreflexia may occur at any time from the acute phase to several years following the injury.

Causes
Most commonly, stimuli to the bladder, including distention, infection, calculi, cystoscopy; or from the bowel with fecal impaction, rectal examination, suppository insertion; or from the

skin, such as tight clothing or sheets, temperature extremes, sores, or areas of broken skin. Initiating a regular toileting program is of paramount importance as the patient recovers.

ACUTE PHASE ASSESSMENT

GOAL OF ASSESSMENT

There are two goals for spinal cord assessment: (1) identify and initiate management of fractures, spinal shock, and cord syndromes; and (2) prevent further injury.

CLINICAL ASSESSMENT

The clinical assessment of the patient with SCI begins with the trauma primary survey at the time of arrival to the emergency department (see sections on Major and Abdominal Trauma discussed earlier). Once stabilized the secondary trauma survey can be completed and an extensive neurologic and functional assessment can be performed.

Neurologic examination: Use of the American Spinal Injury Association Scale (ASIA) documents the motor and sensory impairment related to the injury (Table 3-4).

Functional Assessment: The Functional Independence Measure (FIM, an 18-item scale) provides measurement of disability based on the International Classification of Impairment, Disabilities, and Handicaps. The scale is useful in determining the ability of the patient with SCI to carry out activities of daily living.

INTERPRETATION OF PHYSICAL ASSESSMENT FINDINGS

Interpretation of physical assessment findings begins with vital signs, respiratory status, including oxygen saturation (pulse oximetry), vital capacity, and monitoring for ascending edema. Consideration for cardiac monitoring, placement of nasogastric (NG) tubes, or Foley catheters occurs as a result of cardiac, GI, and genitourinary assessment. Interpretation of laboratory values and diagnostic studies assist in the development of the plan of care.

TYPES OF INJURY

Complete SCI is total loss of motor and sensory function below the level of the lesion. Symptoms are a result of physiologic transsection of the cord either from bruising or compression of cord and blood vessels. Both sides of the body are affected equally. Approximately 50% of injuries are complete.

Incomplete SCI has preservation of some motor or sensory function below the level of the lesion. The pattern of injury may not be symmetrical. Several cord syndromes (anterior cord syndrome, central cord syndrome, lateral cord/Brown-Séquard syndrome, posterior cord syndrome, conus medullaris syndrome, and cauda equina syndrome) have been identified and will be discussed under Acute Phase Assessment.

LEVELS OF INJURY

Tetraplegia (quadriplegia): Injury to the cervical cord resulting in motor loss in all four extremities.

Table 3-4	AMERICAN SPINAL INJURY ASSOCIATION SCALE
Level	**Description of Impairment**
A	No motor or sensory function preserved below the level through the sacral segments (S4-S5). Complete injury.
B	Sensory but no motor function preserved below the level through the sacral segments (S4-S5).
C	Motor function is preserved below the level but the majority of muscle groups has muscle grade strength level of less than 3 (has no antigravity movement).
D	Motor function is preserved below the level but the majority of muscle groups has muscle grade strength level of 3 (has antigravity movement).
E	Normal motor and sensory functions (no cord injury).

Paraplegia: Injury to the thoracic and lumbar cord resulting in motor loss in the lower trunk and extremities.

The patient should be evaluated for the following SCI specific conditions:

Spinal shock initial symptoms:

- Flaccid paralysis below the level of injury of all skeletal muscles with absence of deep tendon reflexes.
- Loss of cutaneous sensation.
- Loss of temperature control with development of anhidrosis (absence of sweating).
- Loss of vasomotor tone.
- Loss of proprioception (position sense).
- Loss of visceral and somatic sensation, and loss of the penile reflex.
- GI shutdown resulting in paralytic ileus.
- Bowel and bladder paralysis resulting in urinary retention and fecal retention.

Recovery phase of spinal shock: As spinal shock subsides, the patient may experience:

- Flexor spasms evoked by cutaneous stimulation.
- Reflex emptying of the bowel and bladder.
- Extensor or flexor rigidity.
- Hyperreflexic deep tendon reflexes, and reflex priapism or ejaculation in the male, evoked by cutaneous stimulation.

Neurogenic shock symptoms include:

- Vasodilation.
- Hypotension.
- Bradycardia.

Septic shock symptoms include:

- Vasodilation.
- Hypotension.
- See Chapter 11.

Autonomic dysreflexia symptoms include:

- Pounding headache.
- Paroxysmal hypertension (up to 300 mm Hg systolic).
- Flushing of the skin with sweating above the level of the lesion.
- Nasal congestion.
- Blurred vision.
- Nausea.
- Bradycardia (30 to 40 bpm).
- Chest pain.
- Below the level of the lesion, pilomotor erection (goose bumps), pallor, chills, and vaso-constriction will be present (Table 3-5).

CORD SYNDROMES

Anterior cord syndrome: Injury to the anterior two thirds of the spinal cord supplied by the anterior spinal artery caused by an acute burst fracture, herniation of an intervertebral disk, a vascular injury or occlusion resulting from trauma, clot, or surgical procedure, such as aortic aneurysm repair.

The prognosis varies with each patient and depends on the degree of structural damage and edema.

Symptoms include:

- Loss of varying degrees of motor function below the level of injury.
- Loss of pain and temperature sensation below the level of injury.
- Position, pressure, and vibration sensations remain intact.

Central cord syndrome: Most common SCI affecting the central gray matter of the spinal cord. Primary causes of injury include compression of the cord, low-velocity injuries, fractures and dislocations, and interruption of blood supply to the central spinal cord. In older persons with underlying conditions such as cervical spondylosis, a hyperextension injury related to a fall may result in central cord injury. Vertebral injury may be noted on the radiograph. Motor and sensory deficits are less severe in the lower extremities than in the upper extremities because of the central arrangement of cervical fibers in the spinal cord. Incomplete injuries carry a relatively good prognosis. Many patients can ambulate with an assistive device and may

Table 3-5	LEVELS OF CORD INJURY
Level of Injury	**Manifestation**
C4 and above	Loss of muscle function, including respiratory function; fatal outcome unless ventilation is provided immediately.
C4-C5	Same as above; phrenic nerve may be spared; assisted ventilation; quadriplegia/tetraplegia.
C6-C8	Diaphragm and accessory muscles or respiration retained; movement of neck, shoulders, chest, and upper arms; quadriplegia.
T1-T3	Neck, chest, shoulder, arm, hand, and respiratory function retained; difficulty maintaining a sitting position; paraplegia.
T4-T10	More stability of trunk muscles; paraplegia.
T11-L2	Use of upper extremities, neck, and shoulders; some function of upper thigh; reflex emptying of bowel; males may have difficulty achieving and maintaining an erection; decreased seminal emission.
L3-S1	Reflex emptying of bowel/bladder; decreased/lack of ability to have an erection; decreased seminal emission; all muscle groups in upper body function; most muscles of lower extremities function.
S2-S4	Flaccid bowel and bladder; lower extremity weakness; all muscle groups function; no ability to have a reflex erection.

regain bowel and bladder function. There is a less favorable prognosis regarding regaining useful function in the hands.
Symptoms include the following:
- Motor and sensory deficits are usually severe in the upper extremities and profound in the hands and fingers.
- Sacral and some lumbar fibers are spared, therefore motor and sensory function in the perineum, genitalia, and lower extremities is present.
- Bladder dysfunction varies with each patient.

Lateral cord (Brown-Séquard) syndrome: Results from a horizontal hemisection of the spinal cord (e.g., from a gunshot or stab wound). Patients usually have bilateral motor and sensory impairment, with a relative difference in function from one side to the other. Prognosis is usually good for recovery of upper and lower extremity function.
Symptoms include:
- Ipsilateral weakness.
- Decrease in light touch, vibratory and position senses.
- Contralateral pain (hypalgesia) and temperature loss.
- Usually there are bilateral motor and sensory deficits, but motor activity will be better on the contralateral side and sensory activity will be better on the ipsilateral side.

Posterior cord syndrome: Although rare, posterior cord syndrome represents an incomplete injury to the posterior columns of the spinal cord.
Symptoms include:
- Loss of proprioception.
- Preserved motor function, pain, and light touch.

Conus medullaris syndrome: The conus medullaris is the tapered end of the spinal cord between the first and second lumbar disks. The conus medullaris consist of sacral spinal cord segments. Injury at this level is considered an UMN lesion. Injury is as a result of a lumbar burst fracture, lateral disk herniation, lumbar stenosis (multilevel), ankylosing spondylitis, neoplasm, infection (abscess), spinal anesthesia, congenital anomalies (tethered cord, arteriovenous malformations), spinal hemorrhage, and multiple sclerosis. Because the injury is at the junction of the conus medullaris and the cauda equina, the lower cord as well as individual peripheral nerves of the cauda equina may be injured, presenting a mixed clinical picture of UMN and LMN lesions.

Symptoms include:

* Motor strength: mixed UMN (symmetrical) and LMN paralysis (asymmetrical).
* Sensation (numbness) varies but tends to be symmetrical, bilateral, and in the perianal area.
* Bladder function is either preserved (UMN) or areflexic (LMN).
* Erectile dysfunction and impotence (UMN) or anesthesia to sacral dermatomes (LMN).
* May exhibit increased muscle tone (spasticity), especially if the lesion is isolated and primarily UMN.
* Deep tendon reflexes demonstrate hyperreflexia (UMN).

Differentiation from cauda equina may be difficult. Signs and symptoms are very similar except for the bilateral presentation in conus medullaris, sacral sparing with preservation of the bulbocavernosus reflex, and normal sphincter tone.

Cauda equina syndrome: The cauda equina (horse's tail) is a bundle of nerve roots at the end of the spinal cord representing the lumbar and sacral nerve roots. Injury at this level is an LMN. Injury to the cauda equina is associated with a central disk fracture or lumbar disk below the level of the *conus medullaris*.

Symptoms include:

* Pattern of LMN responses (flaccid paralysis, areflexia, and loss of muscle tone with muscle fasciculation).
* Diminished muscle strength in the lower extremities consistent with the involved nerve root.
* Greater involvement in the lower lumbar and sacral roots based on the muscle group distribution innervated by the spinal nerve involved.
* Sensation is diminished or lost to pinprick and light touch along the dermatome pattern of the nerve; often there is saddle anesthesia with diminished or absent sensation to the glans penis or clitoris.

HIGH ALERT! Requires immediate attention (decompression) to prevent permanent injury.

* Anal sphincter tone may or may not be present.
* There may be a history of urinary retention or loss of bladder tone and incontinence.
* Diminished or absent muscle strength in the muscles listed as follows assists in localizing the injury:
    * L2 iliopsoas (hip flexion).
    * L3 quadriceps (knee extension).
    * L4 tibialis anterior (ankle dorsiflexion).
    * L5 extensor hallucis longus (big toe extension).
    * S1 gastrocnemius/soleus (ankle plantar flexion).

HIGH ALERT! Vertebral artery injury (VAI): Recognizing the potential for VAI in patients with cervical spine injuries is important. These are occult injuries but may account for changes in mental status in a patient without a history of brain injury. Patients may be asymptomatic or complain of headache. Some go on to have posterior fossa infarcts. Magnetic resonance imaging should be part of the diagnostic workup for early detection of VAI. Patients with VAI may be placed on anticoagulants.

DIAGNOSTIC TESTS

Following trauma, the commonly used radiologic investigations do not rule out injury to the spinal cord, especially for children, particularly resulting from the elasticity of the cervical spine. There is a possibility of SCI without radiologic abnormality (SCIWORA). The changes may be identified using magnetic resonance imaging (MRI). SCIWORA may be present in patients who have experienced blunt trauma who report immediate or transient symptoms of neurologic deficit or who exhibit symptoms upon initial assessment. Treatment within 6 hours with high-dose methylprednisolone improves the outcome. It is possible to reduce the incidence of neurologic complications by increasing awareness and initiating early treatment with steroids and immobilization of the affected area, most often, the cervical spine.

SPINAL RADIOGRAPH

Plain radiographs provide information on the bony anatomy of the spine, thereby delineating fractures, dislocations, and subluxations of the vertebral bodies, as well as demonstrating narrowing of the spinal canal and level of hematomas, neoplasms, or abscesses. Additional views such as open mouth, bilateral oblique, or flexion-extension films also aid in diagnosis.

Cervical spine x-rays taken to rule out fracture on patients with traumatic brain injury or SCI include three views: anterior posterior (AP), lateral, and odontoid. Visualization from C1 to T1 is imperative but may be difficult in patients with large necks and shoulder muscles. If visualization is clear, CT or MRI must be done before removing cervical spine collars.

HIGH ALERT!   Films must be obtained with extreme caution in the evaluation of the patient with a possible spinal cord injury because any sudden or incorrect movement of the injured area could cause further trauma to the spinal cord or cause injury in a patient who is neurologically intact. Flexion-extension films should only be obtained when a patient is alert and able to describe pain on manipulation or under the supervision of a radiologist using fluoroscopy techniques.

CT SCANS

The CT scan provides detailed information on the bony structures of the vertebral bodies, especially related to encroachment on the spinal canal by bone fragments or vertebral body displacement. CT images are especially useful for evaluation of the cervical thoracic junction. Helical or spiral CT scans are used to reconstruct the sagittal and coronal planes. The entire spine should be imaged if there is an SCI to identify injuries at other levels.

SPINAL MRI SCANS

MRI identifies the extent of cord injury and provides information on the cause of cord compression, degree of compression, extent of contusion, degree of ligament involvement, and other related soft tissue injuries. MRI is also the best method to differentiate between swelling/edema and ischemia.

COLLABORATIVE MANAGEMENT

CARE PRIORITIES

1. Immobilize the injured site

Additional injury to the spinal cord as a result of inadequate stabilization after injury is sustained by 10% to 25% of patients with SCI. Immobilization continues until the spine is stable either by traction or surgical decompression and fixation. Remove the patient from the spine board as soon as possible to prevent skin breakdown. This is usually done after the primary survey is completed. There is new evidence to suggest that use of spine boards should be reserved only for those with obvious SCI during prehospital care.

Cervical spine injury

Cervical collar and/or head blocks and backboard: The initial treatment for a suspected cervical spine injury.

Cervical traction: Once the injury has been diagnosed, cervical traction to immobilize and reduce the fracture or dislocation can be achieved in several ways including application of a *cervicothoracic* orthotic, a halo device with a vest, or a traction system using Gardner-Wells, Vinke, or Crutchfield tongs. In traction therapy, the tongs are inserted through the outer table of the skull and attached to ropes and pulleys with weights to achieve bony reduction and proper alignment. Guidelines recommend 3 to 5 lb for each vertebral body fractured but not to exceed 70 lb total weight for all involved vertebrae. Use of muscle relaxants is also recommended. Cross-table lateral radiographs should be obtained until desired realignment of the vertebral bodies is achieved (this may take several hours and several trials with weights). Another alternative is special frames or beds (e.g., kinetic treatment table). The use of the *cervicothoracic* orthotic or halo device for skeletal fixation of the head and neck allows for earliest mobilization and rehabilitation if no surgery is needed. Closed reduction should be done with use of MRI if the patient has brain injury or has an altered LOC from other causes (alcohol intoxication).

Surgical intervention: During the immediate postinjury phase, surgery is controversial, and immediate or early surgery postinjury may have little effect on the neurologic outcome and the benefit-to-harm ratio is uncertain. Surgery may be performed (1) if the neurologic deficit is progressing—for example, if cord compression is imminent, in the presence of an expanding hematoma or neoplasm; (2) in the presence of compound fractures; (3) if there is a penetrating wound of the spine; (4) if bone fragments are localized in the spinal canal; or (5) if there is acute anterior spinal cord trauma. Surgeries may include decompression laminectomy, closed or open reduction of the fracture, or spinal fusion for stabilization. Anterior cervical decompression is advocated for significant disk herniation. Once stabilization of the spine occurs, the patient can be mobilized unless contraindicated for other reasons.

Thoracic and lumbar spine injuries: May require surgical stabilization with laminectomy with or without fusion. Bone grafts, pedicle screws, and rods are used for fusions. If the injury is stable, it may be treated with closed reduction using a thoracolumbosacral orthotic (turtle shell–like immobilizer). If the fracture is unstable and the patient is unable to go to surgery for repair because of medical instability, bed rest with the use of the thoracolumbosacral orthotic should be a priority.

2. Prevent secondary injury

Although administration of methylprednisolone within 8 hours of injury may still be used in some trauma centers, the use of steroids in the treatment of acute SCI is under scrutiny. As a result of methodological flaws in the original study that demonstrated improved neurologic outcomes with methylprednisolone and the increasing evidence of complications associated with steroid use, the standard of acute care for SCI management is changing and high-dose methylprednisolone is now one of several treatment options, not a standard of care. More recent studies are emphasizing arterial oxygenation and spinal cord perfusion. Modulating postinjury inflammation may arrest the secondary injury cascade. The more common secondary injuries include spasticity, pain, respiratory insufficiency leading to pneumonia, genitourinary problems that may prompt infection, pressure ulcers, and autonomic dysreflexia. Other promising therapies emerging include thyrotropin-releasing hormone, neuroprotection with minocycline (a semisynthetic second-generation tetracycline derivative), use of calcium channel blockers to aid in axonal conduction, use of Cethrin (a Rho antagonist) for neuroregeneration and neuroprotection, and the use of anti-Nogo monoclonal antibodies to augment plasticity and regeneration. Cell-mediated repair is being investigated using stem cells and bone marrow stromal cells. The use of GM1 gangliosides to improve spinal cord outcomes has not been supported.

Methylprednisolone protocol is as follows: Within 8 hours of injury, a loading dose (30 mg/kg) is administered by IV bolus over a 15-minute period. After a 45-minute wait, 5.4 mg/kg/h is then administered in a continuous IV infusion over a 23-hour period and then stopped. If the infusion is interrupted for any reason, it must be recalibrated so that the entire dose can be completed within the original 23-hour time frame.

HIGH ALERT! Use of this protocol and the 48-hour protocol is no longer the standard of care and is used only if benefit outweighs the risk.

3. Maintain hemodynamic stability

Hypotension: Maintain MAP between 85 and 90 mm Hg for the first 7 days after injury to reduce secondary SCI (e.g., ischemia and cord injury) and maximize recovery.

Orthostatic hypotension: This is a lifelong problem, especially in patients with cervical and high thoracic injuries. Caregivers should move the patient slowly into the upright position (slow elevation of the head of the bed before 90 degrees) to avoid a sudden drop in BP, prompting cerebral hypoxia and loss of consciousness. Abdominal binders and Ace bandages or thigh-high antiembolic stockings may also help prevent orthostatic hypotension. These interventions should be applied before mobilizing the patient.

Vasopressors (e.g., vasopressin, norepinephrine): To treat the hypotension during the immediate postinjury stage caused by loss of vasomotor control below the level of injury, with resultant vasodilation and a relative hypovolemia (see Appendix 6).

HIGH ALERT! Vasopressor support should be initiated only after fluid resuscitation has been done or in cases of refractory hypotension or low systemic vascular resistance.

Antihypertensives (e.g., hydralazine hydrochloride, methyldopa, nitroprusside sodium): To treat the severe hypertension that occurs in autonomic dysreflexia. There is some support for the use of enteral theophylline to treat bradycardia in cervical cord injury in an effort to avoid use of the long-term infusions of inotropic or chronotropic agents.

4. Manage vasodilation-induced hypovolemia
In patients with neurogenic or septic shock, blood volume is normal but the vascular space is enlarged, causing peripheral pooling, decreased venous return, and decreased CO. Careful fluid repletion, usually with crystalloids, is indicated. Vasopressor therapy is initiated for patients unresponsive to fluid volume replacement. (For fluid management in patients with multisystem trauma, see Major Trauma).

5. Support ventilation
Respiratory insufficiency is a hallmark in SCI, and the higher the level of injury, the more likely the injury will affect ventilation. The need for assisted ventilation is based on the level of injury, ABG values, pulse oximetry, capnography, and the results of pulmonary function tests, pulmonary fluoroscopy, and physical assessment data. The need for mechanical ventilation is likely with injuries at C4 and above, patients older than 40 years, smokers, and patients with associated chest trauma and immersion injuries. Initially, the patient may require intubation and, later, tracheotomy. Patients with low cervical or high thoracic injuries whose respiratory status is stable initially may need temporary intubation later if ascending edema develops. Patients with high cervical injury who survive the initial injury but have paralysis of the muscles of respiration may require permanent tracheotomy and mechanical ventilation.

6. Provide aggressive pulmonary care
Respiratory complications are the most common cause of morbidity and mortality in patients with cervical SCI accounting for up to 80% of deaths, with pneumonia accounting for 50% of deaths. Prevention, detection, and treatment of atelectasis, pulmonary infection, and respiratory failure must be priorities. Recognition of signs and symptoms of pulmonary embolism (PE) are crucial in patients with SCI who may have no complaints of chest pain. Chest physiotherapy and noninvasive positive-pressure ventilation using bilevel continuous positive airway pressure may provide support, but intubation with mechanical ventilation is sometimes required.

Bronchodilators (e.g., beta-2-agonists, methylxanthines): To dilate bronchioles and facilitate removal of secretions. Consider early treatment especially in patients who have a history of *chronic obstructive pulmonary disease* (COPD) or smoking and who show evidence of difficulty moving secretions.

Mucolytic agents (e.g., guaifenesin, acetylcysteine): To reduce tenacity and viscosity of purulent and nonpurulent secretions.

Antibiotics: As prescribed to treat pulmonary infections related to aspiration or ventilator-acquired pneumonia.

7. Prevent aspiration using gastric decompression
Gastric tube placement to decompress the stomach, prevent aspiration of gastric contents, and manage paralytic ileus is necessary (often seen within 72 hours of injury in patients with lesions higher than T6). Placement of an NG tube may be necessary before surgery to prevent development of ileus, which commonly occurs postoperatively.

8. Gastric ulcer prevention
Proton-pump inhibitors (PPIs; e.g., pantoprazole, omeprazole): PPIs are recommended over histamine blockers for stress ulcer (a Cushing ulcer) prophylaxis. Cushing ulcers are related to CNS trauma and occur more often in the stomach than the duodenum, and occasionally affect the esophagus. PPIs reduce the production of acid in the stomach by blocking gastric parietal cell hydrogen-potassium ATPase. Recommended therapy for PPIs is 4 weeks.

9. Relieve pain and anxiety

Analgesics (e.g., acetaminophen, NSAIDs, or opioids): Use of analgesics is necessary to minimize pain associated with injury or surgery in patients who are alert and unconscious. Sensory loss may be incomplete giving rise to pain in areas below the level of the lesion.

Sedatives (e.g., midazolam, lorazepam): Sedation should be used cautiously in patients with SCI who are not intubated. Thorough assessment of respiratory status should be performed if the patient is anxious, restless, or agitated. Rule out hypercapnia and hypoxia in these patients first. Capnography can provide information about declining effectiveness of respiration before pulse oximetry detects a change in oxygen saturation. If the respiratory status is stable, anxiolytics or benzodiazepines can be used to decrease anxiety caused by the injury, hospitalization, or fear of the prognosis. These agents may also be useful when the patient is being mechanically ventilated.

10. Prevent deep venous thrombosis and thromboembolism

Patients with SCI are at high risk for development of vascular complications because of immobility, loss of vasoconstriction capabilities below the level of injury, and loss of muscle innervation in the lower extremities that facilitates venous flow. Interventions to prevent or treat vascular complication should be put in place at the time of admission.

Early stabilization and mobilization: Once spinal stability is achieved either through orthotic devices or surgery, patients should be out of bed. A rehabilitation plan that includes physical and occupational therapy should be initiated.

Early detection of vascular complications: Use of Doppler ultrasonography or plethysmography for detection of deep venous thrombosis (DVT) is recommended. CT angiography has a greater specificity to diagnose PE than D dimer and ventilation-perfusion scan.

Anticoagulants (heparin or low–molecular-weight heparins such as dalteparin [Fragmin] or enoxaparin [Lovenox]): To prevent thrombophlebitis, DVT, and PE.

> **HIGH ALERT!** Patients who are not candidates for anticoagulation therapy may have an inferior vena cava filter inserted to trap emboli traveling from the lower extremities to the lungs.

11. Nutrition Support

As a result of the massive catabolic demand associated with CNS injuries, nutrition therapy should be started as early as possible. If the patient is not able to take oral nutrients, enteral feeding should be started. If there is a coexisting problem with the GI tract from injury, ileus, or surgery, total parenteral nutrition should be considered.

12. Skin care

Prevent pressure sores: Remove from spinal board as soon as possible after admission to the emergency department. Begin turn schedule either manually or using specialty beds. Monitor bony prominences (occiput of head, heels, elbows, sacrum, iliac rests) every shift for signs of pressure. Check beneath cervical spine collar if still in place. Early consult to wound therapy if the patient is vulnerable (prolonged hemodynamic instability, nutrition problems, ventilator dependence, inability to mobilize) for prevention strategies including specialty beds.

13. Bladder program

Once the stability of the patient is ensured, a bladder program using an intermittent straight catheterization procedure is recommended.

> **HIGH ALERT!** Early bladder decompression and drainage using a Foley catheter is necessary during the acute phase (3 to 4 days after injury). To prevent bladder infections, begin bladder training and remove the Foley catheter once the patient is stable. Bladder distention can be a trigger for onset of autonomic dysreflexia.

Bladder training: Begin intermittent straight catheterizations on a q3-4h (every 3 to 4 hours) schedule and advance to q6h. If urine output is greater than 300 mL, increase frequency of intermittent catheterizations; if less than 300 mL, increase time between catheterizations. Once oral feeding is initiated, monitor fluid intake to match catheterization output to prevent overdistension of the bladder. The goal is to maintain detrusor stretch and relaxation until spinal shock dissipates and reflexive bladder can be trained.

Prevent spinal shock by decompressing the bladder: Insert an indwelling or intermittent catheter to decompress an atonic bladder in the immediate postinjury phase (spinal shock). With the return of the reflex arc after spinal shock subsides, a reflex neurogenic bladder that fills and empties automatically will develop in patients with lesions above T12. Patients with lesions at or below T12 generally have an atonic, areflexic neurogenic bladder that overfills, distending the bladder, and causing overflow incontinence. Intermittent catheterization may be necessary.

14. Bowel management

Initiation of a bowel regimen at the time of admission assures GI function and prevents constipation and impaction. Liquid or oral stool softeners (e.g., docusate sodium), suppositories, and small-volume enemas are used.

Bowel training: Part of the rehabilitation plan commences with the return of spinal reflexes. Medication along with digital stimulation of the external sphincter is a common bowel training protocol. The aim is to begin training for bowel independence and to prevent fecal impaction and distention of the bowel, which could stimulate an episode of autonomic dysreflexia.

Hyperosmolar laxatives (e.g., glycerin suppository): To facilitate movement of the bowels on a regular basis and prevent fecal impaction.

Irritant or stimulant laxatives (e.g., senna bisacodyl): To stimulate bowel movements as part of a bowel training program.

15. Prevent infections

Pneumonia: Aggressive pulmonary hygiene.

UTI: Remove Foley catheter as soon as the patient is stable.

Skin: Avoid pressure sores and wound infections.

CARE PLANS: ACUTE SPINAL CORD INJURY

Impaired gas exchange related to altered oxygen supply associated with hypoventilation secondary to paresis or paralysis of the muscles of respiration (diaphragm, intercostal muscles) and/or inability to maintain clear airway occurring with high cervical spine injury or ascending cord edema.

Goals/Outcomes: The patient has adequate gas exchange, as evidenced by orientation to time, place, and person; $Pao_2 \geq 80$ mm Hg; and $Paco_2 \leq 45$ mm Hg. RR 12 to 20 breaths/min with normal depth and pattern, HR 60 to 100 bpm, BP stable and within the patient's normal range, and vital capacity (depth or volume of inspiration) is ≥ 1 L. Motor and sensory losses remain at the same spinal cord level as the initial findings.

HIGH ALERT! Patients with cervical injuries usually arrive in the intensive care unit (ICU) already intubated. However, with some high thoracic or low cervical lesions, patients who ventilate independently in the emergency department may arrive in the ICU without assisted ventilation. This patient is at risk for an increasingly higher level of cord damage because of hemorrhage and edema, which can result in a higher level of dysfunction and a change in respiratory status that requires assisted ventilation. Before attempting oral intubation with neck flexion, ensure that cervical x-ray studies have confirmed the absence of cervical involvement. Use either nasal intubation or orotracheal intubation with manual cervical spine immobilization if cervical spine injury is not ruled out. Fiber optic intubation may also be considered.

NOC **Respiratory Status:** Ventilation.

Respiratory Monitoring
1. Assess for signs of respiratory dysfunction: shallow, slow, or rapid respirations; poor cough; vital capacity; changes in sensorium; anxiety; restlessness; tachycardia; pallor; adventitious breath sounds (i.e., crackles, rhonchi); decreased or absent breath sounds (bronchial, bronchovesicular, vesicular); decreased tidal volume

(less than 75% to 85% of predicted value); or vital capacity (less than 1 L). Capnography can be used for early detection of elevations in pCO_2 levels, which may signal early respiratory insufficiency, which can lead to hypoxia if not promptly addressed.

2. Monitor ABG tests; report abnormalities. Be particularly alert to Pao_2 less than 60 mm Hg, $Paco_2$ greater than 50 mm Hg, and decreasing pH, considering that these findings indicate the need for assisted ventilation possibly caused by atelectasis, pneumonia, or respiratory fatigue.

3. Monitor vital capacity at least q8h. If it is less than 1 L, Pao_2/Pao_2 ratio is ≤ 0.75, or copious secretions are present, intubation is recommended.

4. Monitor for signs and symptoms of pulmonary embolism (PE). The patient may not have sensory symptoms (chest pain or tightness) based on the level of the lesions.

5. If the patient does not require intubation with mechanical ventilation, implement the following measures to improve airway clearance:
   - Place the patient in a semi-Fowler position unless it is contraindicated (e.g., the patient is in cervical tongs with traction or has unstable thoracic or lumbar fractures).
   - Turn the patient from side to side at least every 2 hours to help mobilize secretions.
   - Keep the room humidified to help loosen secretions.
   - Unless contraindicated, keep the patient hydrated with at least 2 to 3 L fluid/day.
   - Teach deep-breathing and coughing exercises, which should be performed at least every 2 hours.

6. Suction secretions as needed and hyperoxygenate before suctioning.

HIGH ALERT! Be alert for bradycardia associated with tracheal suctioning. If the patient's cough is ineffective, implement the following method, known as quad coughing: place palm of hand under the patient's diaphragm, and push up on the abdominal muscles as the patient exhales. Be aware that using the quad cough maneuver in patients with intracaval filters to prevent pulmonary emboli has been reported to have significant complications, including bowel perforation and filter migration and deformation.

---

7. Monitor the patient for evidence of ascending cord edema: increasing difficulty with swallowing secretions or coughing, presence of respiratory stridor with retraction of accessory muscles of respiration, bradycardia, fluctuating BP, and increased motor and sensory loss at a higher level than the initial findings.

8. If the patient has cranial tongs or traction with a halo apparatus in place, monitor the patient's respiratory status every 1 to 2 hours for the first 24 to 48 hours and then every 4 hours if patient's condition is stable. Be alert to absent or adventitious breath sounds, and inspect chest movement to ensure that the vest is not restricting diaphragmatic movement.

HIGH ALERT! Have a plan to remove the vest if cardiopulmonary resuscitation is needed.

---

9. If intubation via endotracheal tube or tracheotomy becomes necessary, explain the procedure to the patient and significant others.

NIC Airway Management; Oxygen Therapy; Respiratory Monitoring; Mechanical Ventilation.

Autonomic dysreflexia (or risk for same) *related to abnormal response of the autonomic nervous system to a stimulus.*

Goals/Outcomes: The patient has no symptoms of autonomic dysreflexia, as evidenced by dry skin above the level of injury, BP within the patient's normal range, HR ≥ 60 bpm, and absence of headache and other clinical indicators of autonomic dysreflexia. ECG demonstrates normal sinus rhythm.
NOC Risk Detection.

Dysreflexia Management

1. Assess for the classic triad of autonomic dysreflexia: throbbing headache, cutaneous vasodilation, and sweating above the level of injury. In addition, extremely elevated BP (e.g., ≥ 250 to $300/150$ mm Hg), nasal stuffiness, flushed skin (above the level of injury), blurred vision, nausea, bradycardia, and chest pain can occur. Be alert to the following signs of autonomic dysreflexia that occur below the level of injury: pilomotor erection, pallor, chills, and vasoconstriction.

2. Assess for cardiac dysrhythmias, via cardiac monitor during initial postinjury stage (2 weeks).
3. Implement measures to prevent factors that may precipitate autonomic dysreflexia: bladder stimuli (i.e., distention, calculi, infection, cystoscopy); bowel stimuli (i.e., fecal impaction, rectal examination, suppository insertion); and skin stimuli (i.e., pressure from tight clothing or sheets, temperature extremes, sores, areas of broken skin).
4. If indicators of autonomic dysreflexia are present, implement the following measures:
   - Elevate the head of the bed or place the patient in a sitting position. This will decrease BP by promoting cerebral venous return.
   - Monitor BP and HR every 3 to 5 minutes until the patient stabilizes.
   - Identify and remove offending stimulus. If the patient's bladder is distended, catheterize cautiously, using sufficient lubricant containing a local anesthetic. If the patient has an indwelling urinary catheter, check for obstruction, such as granulation in catheter or kinking of tubing; as indicated, irrigate catheter, using no more than 30 mL NS. If UTI is suspected, obtain a urine specimen for culture and sensitivity once the crisis stage has passed. Check for fecal impaction; perform the rectal examination gently, using an ointment containing a local anesthetic (e.g., Nupercainal). Check for sensory stimuli and loosen clothing, bed covers, or other constricting fabric as indicated.
5. Consult the physician for severe or prolonged hypertension or other symptoms that do not abate. Severe or prolonged elevations of BP may result in life-threatening consequences: seizures, subarachnoid or intracerebral hemorrhage, and fatal cerebrovascular accident.
6. As prescribed, administer an antihypertensive agent and monitor its effectiveness.
7. Remain calm and supportive of the patient and significant others during these episodes.
8. Upon resolution of the immediate crisis, answer the patient's and significant others' questions regarding the cause of autonomic dysreflexia. Provide the patient and family education regarding signs and symptoms and methods of treatment of autonomic dysreflexia. This is particularly crucial for the patient with SCI who has sustained injury above T6, because these patients are at risk for autonomic dysreflexia for life.

NIC Dysreflexia Management.

Decreased CO *related to relative hypovolemia secondary to enlarged vascular space occurring with neurogenic shock.*

Goals/Outcomes: The patient has adequate CO, as evidenced by orientation to time, place, and person; systolic BP ≥90 mm Hg (or within the patient's normal range); HR 60 to 100 bpm; RAP 4 to 6 mm Hg; PAP 20 to 30/8 to 15 mm Hg; PAWP 6 to 12 mm Hg; SVR 900 to 1200 dynes/s/cm^{-5}; normal amplitude of peripheral pulses (greater than 2+ on a 0-to-4+ scale); urinary output ≥0.5 mL/kg/h; and normal sinus rhythm on ECG.
NOC Circulation Status.

Hemodynamic Regulation
1. Monitor the patient for indicators of decreased CO: drop in systolic BP less than 20 mm Hg, systolic BP greater than 90 mm Hg, or a continuous drop of 5 to 10 mm Hg with each assessment; HR greater than 100 bpm, irregular HR, lightheadedness, fainting, confusion, dizziness, flushed skin; diminished amplitude of peripheral pulses; change in BP, HR, mental status, and color associated with a change in position. Monitor input and output; urine output less than 0.5 mL/kg/h for 2 consecutive hours should be reported. Assess hemodynamic measurements. In the presence of neurogenic shock, anticipate decreased RAP, PAP, PAWP, and SVR (see Table 1-13).
2. Continuously assess cardiac rate and rhythm; report changes in rate and rhythm.
3. Prevent episodes of decreased CO caused by orthostatic hypotension:
   - Change the patient's position slowly.
   - Perform range-of-motion (ROM) exercises every 2 hours to prevent venous pooling.
   - Apply elastic antiembolic hose as prescribed to promote venous return.
   - Avoid placing pillows under the patient's knees, "gatching" the bed, or allowing the patient to cross the legs or sit with legs in a dependent position.
   - Collaborate with physical therapy personnel in progressing the patient from a supine to upright position, using a tilt table.
4. As prescribed, administer fluids to control mild hypotension.
5. Administer and monitor therapeutic effects of vasopressor therapy (see Appendix 6).
6. Ensure adequate volume repletion before or concurrently with vasopressor therapy.

NIC Cardiac Care; Fluid Management.

Risk for injury: gastric *related to risk of development of gastric ulcer (a Cushing ulcer) or gastritis secondary to increased gastric acid production.*

Goals/Outcomes: The result of the patient's gastric pH test is greater than 5, and the patient has no symptoms of gastric ulcer, as evidenced by gastric aspirate and stool culture that are negative for blood; BP within the patient's normal range; HR ≤100 bpm; and absence of midepigastric or referred shoulder pain.

HIGH ALERT!   Patients sustaining major trauma are at high risk for development of gastritis/gastric ulcers caused by increased production of gastric acid. Although ulceration can occur at any time in the patient with spinal cord injury, it is most likely to occur within 3 weeks of the injury. Cushing ulcers develop in the stomach, duodenum, and rarely the esophagus in the setting of central nervous system trauma, whereas Curling ulcers are stress ulcers related to burns and other trauma that occur almost exclusively in the duodenum.

NOC Risk Control.

Bleeding Precautions
1. Assess for indicators of GI ulceration or hemorrhage: midepigastric pain (dull, gnawing, burning ache) if the patient has sensation; and hematemesis, melena, constipation, anemia, pallor, decreased BP, increased HR, and complaints of shoulder pain.
2. Test gastric aspirate and stools for blood q8h. Promptly consult the physician if blood is present.
3. Monitor complete blood count (CBC) for signs of anemia: decreases in Hct, Hgb, and red blood cells (RBCs). Monitor clotting factors PTT, PT/INR, and platelets.
4. As prescribed, implement measures to treat or prevent ulceration and hemorrhage:
   - Administer PPIs to suppress secretion of gastric acids, decrease irritating effects of gastric secretions, and facilitate healing.
   - Insert gastric tube and attach to low, intermittent suction to remove gastric contents.
   - Prepare the patient for surgery as indicated.
5. For the patient with GI ulceration and hemorrhage, bowel perforation is an added risk. Be alert to the following indicators: pallor, shock state, abdominal distention, may or may not have voluntary or involuntary guarding, vomiting of material that resembles coffee grounds, absent bowel sounds, elevated WBC count (greater than 11,000/mm^3), and presence of air on abdominal x-ray view. In some cases the only indicators are tachycardia and shoulder pain. Lack of pain is not a reliable indicator of bowel perforation in the patient with SCI. Bowel perforation is an emergency situation, requiring immediate surgical intervention.

NIC Surveillance; Medication Administration; Bleeding Precautions; Risk Identification.

Ineffective tissue perfusion (or risk for same): peripheral and cardiopulmonary *related to interruption of blood flow associated with thrombophlebitis, DVT, and PE secondary to venous stasis, vascular intimal injury, and hypercoagulability occurring as a result of decreased vasomotor tone and immobility.*

Goals/Outcomes: The patient is free of symptoms of thrombophlebitis, DVT, and PE, as evidenced by absence of heat, swelling, discomfort, and erythema in the calves and thighs; HR ≤100 bpm; RR ≤20 breaths/min with normal pattern and depth; BP within the patient's normal range; Pao$_2$ ≥80 mm Hg; oxygen saturation greater than 90%; and absence of chest or shoulder pain.
NOC Tissue Perfusion: Pulmonary.

Cardiac Care: Acute
1. The high-risk interval for this diagnosis is the 6- to 12-week period after injury. Assess for indicators of thrombophlebitis and DVT: unusual heat and erythema of calf or thigh, increased circumference of calf or thigh, unilateral tenderness or pain in extremity (depending on the patient's level of injury and whether injury is complete or incomplete). Pain in the calf area with dorsiflexion (positive reaction for Homan sign) is not a reliable sign and should be avoided. Recommend Doppler ultrasonography for definitive diagnosis of DVT.
2. Assess for indicators of PE: sudden chest or shoulder pain, tachycardia, dyspnea, tachypnea, hypotension, pallor, cyanosis, cough with hemoptysis, restlessness, increasing anxiety, and low Pao$_2$.

3. Implement measures to prevent development of thrombophlebitis, DVT, and PE:
   - Change the patient's position at least every 2 hours to prevent venous pooling.
   - Perform ROM exercises on all extremities every 1 to 2 hours to promote venous return and prevent stasis.
   - Avoid use of knee gatch or pillows under the knees, which can compromise circulation.
   - If the patient is out of bed and in a chair, do not allow the patient to cross legs at the knee or sit with legs dependent for longer than 0.5 to 1 hour. For the patient experiencing some return of spinal reflexes below the lesion with spasticity of lower extremities, instruct the patient to alert the nurse should legs become crossed.
   - Apply sequential compression devices or antiembolic hose as prescribed.
   - Maintain adequate hydration of at least 2 to 3 L/day, unless contraindicated, to prevent dehydration and concomitant increase in blood viscosity, which can promote thrombus formation.
   - Administer prophylactic low-dose, low–molecular-weight heparin as prescribed.
   - Begin transition from low–molecular-weight heparin to warfarin following PT/INR.

HIGH ALERT! Patients with spinal cord injury who are not candidates for anticoagulation because comorbidities may require surgical intervention (insertion of intracaval filter) to prevent pulmonary emboli as a result of thrombophlebitis or deep venous thrombosis.

NIC Circulatory Care: Arterial Insufficiency; Circulatory Care: Venous Insufficiency; Peripheral Sensation Management; Cardiac Care: Acute; Respiratory Monitoring; Shock Management: Cardiac.

Risk for impaired skin integrity *related to prolonged immobility secondary to immobilization device or paralysis.*

Goals/Outcomes: The patient's skin remains intact without areas of breakdown or irritation.
NOC Tissue Integrity: Skin and Mucous Membranes.

Pressure Management
1. Perform a complete skin assessment at least every 8 hours. Pay close attention to skin that is particularly susceptible to breakdown (i.e., skin over bony prominences and around halo vest edges, occiput of head, edges of C spine collar). Be alert to erythema, warmth, open or macerated tissue, and foul odors (indicative of infection with tissue necrosis).
2. Turn and reposition the patient and massage susceptible skin at least every 2 hours. Post a turning schedule and include the patient in the planning and initiating of the schedule.

HIGH ALERT! Do not turn the patient until the injury has been stabilized or a turning protocol has been ordered. If turning is allowed before immobilization with tongs, halo, or surgery, use the logrolling technique only, using at least three people to turn the patient: one to support the head and neck and keep them in alignment during the procedure, and two to turn the patient.

3. Keep skin clean and dry.
4. Pad halo vest edges (e.g., with sheepskin) to minimize irritation and friction.
5. Provide pressure relief mattress most appropriate for the patient's injury.
6. For more information related to the maintenance of skin and tissue integrity, see Wound and Skin Care, Chapter 1.

NIC Pressure Management; Pressure Ulcer Prevention; Skin Surveillance.

Imbalanced nutrition: less than body requirements *related to decreased oral intake secondary to anorexia, difficulty eating in prone position, fear of choking and aspiration, and inability to feed self because of paralysis of upper extremities; decreased GI motility secondary to autonomic nervous system dysfunction.*

Goals/Outcomes: The patient has adequate nutrition, as evidenced by balanced nitrogen state per nitrogen balance studies, serum albumin 3.5 to 5.5 g/dL, thyroxine-binding prealbumin 20 to 30 mg/dL, and retinol-binding protein 4 to 5 mg/dL.

NOC Nutritional Status.

Nutrition Management
1. Perform a complete baseline assessment of nutritional status.
2. Assess the patient's readiness for oral intake: presence of bowel sounds, passing of flatus, or bowel movement.
3. If unable to receive proper oral nutrition, prepare to insert a postpyloric enteral feeding tube or a peripherally inserted central catheter line for total parenteral nutrition.
4. When the patient begins an oral diet, progress slowly from liquids to solids as tolerated.
5. Monitor and record percentage of each meal eaten by the patient.
6. Implement measures to maintain or improve the patient's intake.
   - Obtain dietary consultation to provide the patient with his or her favorite foods, as well as those that are highly nutritious.
   - Provide oral hygiene before and after meals, and decrease external stimuli (which will also help the patient concentrate on chewing and swallowing and thus minimize the risk of aspiration).
   - Provide small, frequent feedings; feed the patient slowly, providing small, bite-size pieces, which facilitate digestion and help prevent choking; also less likely to cause abdominal distention, which may compromise respiratory movement; and less fatiguing.
   - Feed the patient in a position to minimize aspiration risk, and if the patient is in a halo device or has been stabilized, feed in high-Fowler position or get out of bed to chair.
7. Once the patient's condition has been stabilized, consult with occupational therapy personnel for selection of assistive devices that will enable the patient to learn independent feeding techniques.

NIC Fluid/Electrolyte Management; Swallowing Therapy; Self-Care Assistance: Feeding.

Urinary retention or reflex urinary incontinence *related to inhibition of the spinal reflex arc secondary to spinal shock after SCI or related to loss of reflex activity for micturition and bladder flaccidity secondary to cord lesion at or below T12.*

Goals/Outcomes: The patient has urinary output without incontinence.

HIGH ALERT! Urinary retention with stretching of the bladder muscle may trigger autonomic dysreflexia. Therefore, it is crucial to assess for retention and to treat it promptly.

NOC Urinary Elimination.

Urinary Retention Care
1. Assess for indicators of urinary retention: suprapubic distention and intake greater than output.
2. Assess for effects of medications that can cause urinary retention such as tricyclic antidepressants and anticholinergics.
3. Catheterize the patient as prescribed. Patients usually have an indwelling catheter for the first 3 to 4 days after injury. Then, intermittent catheterization is used to try to retrain the bladder. If intermittent catheterization is used and episodes of urinary incontinence occur, catheterize more frequently. If greater than 300 mL of urine is obtained, catheterize more often and space fluids to match output.
4. Measure the amount of residual urine and attempt to increase the length of time between catheterizations, as indicated by decreased amounts (i.e., less than 50 to 100 mL of urine).
5. Ensure continuous patency of the drainage system to prevent reflux of urine into the bladder or blockage of flow, which could lead to urinary retention or UTI, which may cause autonomic dysreflexia. Tape the catheter over the pubis to prevent traction on the catheter, which can lead to ulcer formation in the urethra and erosion of the urethral meatus.
6. Maintain a fluid intake of at least 2.5 to 3 L/day to prevent early stone formation caused by mobilization of calcium. Do not reduce fluids to accommodate bladder training; increase frequency of intermittent catheterization instead.

Acute Spinal Cord Injury

7. Teach the patient and significant others the procedure for intermittent catheterization. Alert them to the indicators of UTI (restlessness, incontinence, malaise, anorexia, fever, and cloudy or foul-smelling urine) and the importance of adequate fluid intake, regular urine cultures, good handwashing technique, and cleansing of the urinary catheter before catheterization.

 HIGH ALERT! Urinary tract infection (UTI) is one of the leading causes of morbidity and mortality in the patient with spinal cord injury. This patient may not be aware of the presence of UTI until he or she is severely ill as a result of pyelonephritis (calculi, infection, septicemia).

---

8. Monitor and record input and output. Distribute fluids evenly throughout the day to prevent overdistention, which can cause incontinence and increase the risk for autonomic dysreflexia.
9. Decrease fluid intake before bedtime to prevent nighttime incontinence.
10. For other treatment interventions, see Autonomic Dysreflexia (or risk for same).

NIC Urinary Catheterization; Urinary Retention Care.

Ineffective thermoregulation *related to inability of the body to adapt to environmental temperature changes secondary to poikilothermic reaction occurring with SCI.*

Goals/Outcome: Within 2 to 4 hours of this diagnosis, the patient becomes normothermic.

 HIGH ALERT! With spinal cord injury the patient is poikilothermic, that is, the patient has a decreased ability to regulate temperature below the level of the lesion through vasodilation or vasoconstriction (sweating and shivering). Because there is no autonomic control of core body temperature, the patient is susceptible to temperature variations in the environment. Attention to room temperature and use of external cooling or warming devices may be necessary.

NOC Thermoregulation.

Temperature Regulation
1. Monitor the patient's temperature at least every 4 hours and assess the patient for signs of ineffective thermoregulation: complaints of being too warm, excessive diaphoresis, warmth of skin above the level of injury, complaints of being too cold, pilomotor erection (goose bumps), or cool skin above the level of injury.
2. Implement measures to attain normothermia: regulate room temperature, provide extra blankets to prevent chills, protect the patient from drafts, provide warm food and drink if the patient is chilled; provide cool drinks if the patient is warm, remove excess bedding to facilitate heat loss, provide a tepid bath or cooling blanket to facilitate cooling.

NIC Temperature Regulation; Environmental Management.

Constipation *related to atonic bowel, paralytic ileus with concomitant autonomic dysreflexia or loss of anal sphincter control.*

Goals/Outcomes: The patient remains free of symptoms of constipation and/or paralytic ileus, as evidenced by auscultation of normal bowel sounds, and free of symptoms of autonomic dysreflexia, and the patient has bowel elimination of soft and formed stools.

 HIGH ALERT! Paralytic ileus occurs most often in patients with spinal cord injury at T6 and above and usually within the first 72 hours after injury.

NOC Bowel Elimination.

Constipation/Impaction Management

1. Obtain history of the patient's preinjury bowel elimination pattern.
2. Assess for indicators of paralytic ileus: decreased or absent bowel sounds, abdominal distention, anorexia, vomiting, and altered respirations as a result of pressure on the diaphragm. Report significant findings promptly.
3. Keep the patient NPO (nil per os) until evidence of return of bowel function (flatus or bowel movements are the most reliable signs).
4. If indicators of paralytic ileus appear, implement the following, as prescribed:
   - Discontinue oral or enteral intake.
   - Insert NG tube to decompress the stomach; attach to low intermittent suction.
   - Monitor NG tube output as large amount may result in dehydration or metabolic alkalosis.
   - Insert a rectal tube if prescribed.
5. Perform a gentle digital examination for fecal impaction and check for rectal reflexes. Before the return of rectal reflexes, manual removal of feces may be needed. If a fecal impaction is present in an atonic bowel, administration of a small-volume enema may be necessary.
6. Observe closely for signs of autonomic dysreflexia, which can be triggered by distention of the abdomen (for assessment and treatment of autonomic dysreflexia, see interventions with Autonomic Dysreflexia or risk for same).
7. Monitor the patient for indicators of constipation (nausea, abdominal distention, and malaise) and fecal impaction (nausea, vomiting, increasing abdominal distention, palpable colonic mass, or presence of hard fecal mass on digital examination).

HIGH ALERT!   Be aware that overdistention of the bowel or stimulation of the anal sphincter caused by impaction, rectal tube, rectal examination, or enema may precipitate autonomic dysreflexia. Use generous amounts of anesthetic lubricant when performing a rectal examination or administering an enema.

---

8. Monitor skin at rectal tube site for breakdown. Sensation to rectum may be spared in incomplete injuries and thus the patient may have complaints of discomfort with the rectal tube. Remove the tube as soon as possible to prevent injury to rectal mucosa and damage to the rectal sphincter.
9. Administer stool softeners (e.g., docusate sodium) daily.
10. If possible, avoid enemas for long-term bowel management, because the patient with SCI cannot retain the enema solution. However, if impaction occurs, a gentle, small-volume cleansing enema may be necessary, followed by manual removal of fecal material.
11. Assess the patient's readiness for a bowel retraining program, including neurologic status and current bowel patterns, noting frequency, amount, and consistency. Bowel retraining is initiated when the patient is neurologically stable.
12. Patients with upper extremity function should be engaged in learning how to perform digital rectal stimulation, insert suppository, and massage abdomen to facilitate bowel movements.

NIC Surveillance: Bowel Management; Dysreflexia Management; Tube Care; Constipation/Impaction Management.

Risk for infection *related to inadequate primary defenses (broken skin) secondary to presence of invasive immobilization devices.*

Goals/Outcomes: The patient is free of infection at insertion site for tongs or halo device, as evidenced by normothermia; negative culture results; and absence of erythema, swelling, warmth, purulent drainage, or tenderness at insertion site.
NOC Risk Control.

Infection Protection

1. Assess insertion sites every 8 hours for indicators of infection: erythema, swelling, warmth, purulent drainage, and increased or new tenderness. Note pin migration. If the pin appears to be loose, consult the advanced practice provider and instruct the patient to remain still until the pin can be secured.
2. Perform pin care as prescribed. Cleanse the site with soap and water or NS; the area may be left open to air. Monitor for drainage or infection.

NIC Infection Control; Infection Protection; Skin Surveillance.

Disturbed sensory perception visual *related to presence of immobilization device; use of therapeutic bed.*

Goals/Outcome: After intervention(s), the patient expresses satisfaction with visual capabilities.
NOC Vision Compensation Behavior.

Environmental Management
1. Assess for factors that limit the patient's visual capabilities: presence of tongs, cervical traction, halo device, and use of specialty beds.
2. Provide for increased visualization of the patient's surroundings:
   - Obtain prism glasses or hand mirror for patients who are supine or have restricted head movement because of halo traction devices.
   - Position mirrors to increase the amount of area that can be visualized from the patient's position.
   - Approach the patient and converse within the patient's visual field.
   - Keep clocks, calendars, and other personal objects within the patient's visual field.

NIC Positioning.

Sexual dysfunction or ineffective sexuality patterns *related to trauma-associated SCI.*

Goals/Outcomes: The patient verbalizes sexual concerns before discharge from ICU.
NOC Sexual Functioning.

Sexual Counseling
1. Assess the patient's level of sexual function or loss from a neurologic and psychological perspective. The general rule for men is that the higher the lesion, the greater is the chance of maintaining the ability to have an erection, but with less chance for ejaculation. For women, ovulation may stop for several months because of stress after the injury. Ovulation usually returns, however, and the woman can become pregnant and have a normal pregnancy. Both men and women with high lesions may experience feelings of excitement similar to a preinjury orgasm.
2. Allow the patient to speak about sexual concerns or consult with a counselor.
3. Check level of patient's knowledge, questions, and concerns about sexual function after the SCI.
4. It is normal for men to experience a reflex erection upon resolution of the spinal shock, particularly for individuals with lesions in the cervical and thoracic areas. Reassure the patient that this is normal and minimize embarrassment by providing coping skills.
5. Expect acting-out behavior related to the patient's sexuality. This is a normal response to the patient's concern regarding his or her sexual prognosis.
6. Provide accurate information regarding expected sexual function in an open, interested manner, based on your assessment of the patient's readiness for information.
7. Facilitate communication between the patient and his or her partner.
8. Refer the patient and partner for sexual counseling by a sex therapist, psychologist, or other knowledgeable rehabilitation professional upon resolution of the critical stages of SCI.
9. Provide the patient with information on the following organizations that can be accessed through the internet: National Spinal Cord Injury Association and Spinal Cord Injury Network International.

NIC Sexual Counseling; Anxiety Reduction; Body Image.

ADDITIONAL NURSING DIAGNOSES

Also see nursing diagnoses and interventions as appropriate under sections on Nutrition Support, Mechanical Ventilation, and Prolonged Immobility in Chapter 1, and Emotional and Spiritual Support of the Patient and Significant Others in Chapter 2.

BURns
■
PATHOPHYSIOLOGY

Burn injuries involve damage to the skin and underlying tissues, but other organ systems may be affected, especially with extensive (greater than 20% total body surface area [TBSA]) burn injuries. The cause of injury may be thermal (flame/flash; contact with hot liquids, semiliquids, hot objects), electrical, chemical, or radiation. Relative risk of injury differs by age, gender, occupation, and recreational activities. Estimates for the number of burn injuries in the United States range from 1.4 to 2 million injuries annually, and of those, approximately 450,000 seek medical treatment. Of these, it is estimated that 40,000, including 30,000 at hospital burn centers, require hospitalization. For those who survive their injury, the average hospital length of stay is slightly greater than 1 day per 1% TBSA burn. The number of deaths as a result of fire, burns, and/or smoke inhalation each year is approximately 3400. In the United States, the two most common reported etiologies are fire/flame (43%) and scalds (34%); electrical burn injuries account for 4% of all admissions to burn centers each year. The burning agent, intensity, and duration of exposure, location, and depth of burn, and the extent or size of injury, determine overall injury severity.

Burn injuries are categorized based on depth of injury. The longer and more intense the exposure to the burning agent, the greater is the depth of injury. A burn injury is described as either a partial-thickness or full-thickness injury, relative to the layer(s) of skin and tissues injured. A superficial injury, commonly referred to as "first-degree" burn (e.g., sunburn), damages only the epidermis. These burns typically heal within 3 to 5 days and without permanent scarring. Partial-thickness injury, called a "second-degree" burn, involves varying levels of the dermis, which contain structures essential to skin function (e.g., sweat and sebaceous glands, hair follicles, sensory nerves, capillary network). These burns typically heal within 14 to 21 days, depending on the depth. Full-thickness injury, a "third-degree" burn, destroys the epidermis and dermis and exposes the less vascularized fat layer, which contains adipose tissue, roots of sweat glands, and hair follicles. These wounds require surgical excision of the dead tissue and skin grafting to provide the best functional and cosmetic outcomes. In very small full-thickness wounds (e.g., size of a quarter or smaller), healing may occur by granulation and migration of healthy epithelium from the wound margins. When full-thickness injuries include destruction of tendon and bone, clinicians often describe these injuries as "fourth-degree" burns. These injuries are the deepest and require excision, possibly amputation of extremities, and skin grafting to heal. Refer to Table 3-6 for detailed burn wound classification and descriptions.

In patients admitted to burn centers, approximately 10% to 20% have an associated inhalation injury. Inhalation injury commonly occurs with flame injuries, particularly if the victim is trapped in an enclosed, smoke-filled space, and is an important determinant of survival (60% to 70% of patients who die in burn centers have inhalation injuries). The associated pathophysiology can be divided into three types of injury as follows.

- Inhalation of carbon monoxide and other noxious gases: Most fatalities occurring at the scene of a fire are as a result of asphyxiation and/or carbon monoxide inhalation (poisoning). Carbon monoxide binds to Hgb with an affinity that is 200 times greater than oxygen, resulting in tissue hypoxia.
- Injury above the glottis: Injury above the glottis (nasopharynx, oropharynx, and larynx) can be thermal or chemical in nature. The heat exchange capability of the respiratory tract is very efficient such that tissue damage from breathing in heated air occurs most often above the vocal cords. Heat damage to the pharynx can be severe enough to cause upper airway edema resulting in obstruction.
- Injury below the glottis: Injury below the glottis is almost always chemical in nature, causing direct damage to airway epithelium from inhalation of the noxious chemicals (e.g., aldehyde, sulfur oxide, phosgene) of smoke.

Overall, the age of the patient, concomitant injury, and preinjury health—in combination with injury severity—impact mortality, length of hospitalization, and ultimately rehabilitation outcomes in the patient with burn injuries.

Care for the patient with a major burn injury is based on the patient's stage of recovery from the pathophysiologic changes resulting from the cutaneous burn and inhalation injury. The initial resuscitative period lasts from the time of injury until capillary membrane integrity is restored, typically 48 to 72 hours after the burn occurs. Following resuscitation, the acute phase may last for days to months. It begins with resolution of the fluid shifts and continues until all or nearly all wounds are healed. The last stage, or rehabilitative stage, can continue for many months to years and is seldom a focus for critical care nurses. However, early rehabilitative efforts such as patient positioning, splinting, exercise, and patient and family education begin on admission to the hospital.

Burns

Table 3-6	BURN WOUND DESCRIPTION AND CHARACTERISTICS			
	Cause of Injury	Depth	Characteristics	Treatment and Recovery
First-degree burn	Prolonged ultraviolet light exposure (sun); brief exposure to hot liquids	Limited damage to epithelium; skin remains intact	Erythematous, hypersensitive, no blister formation	Complete healing within 3 to 5 days without scarring
Superficial partial-thickness (second-degree) burn	Brief exposure to flash, flame, or hot liquids	Epidermis destroyed; minimal damage to superficial layers of dermis; epidermal appendages intact	Moist and weepy, pink or red, blisters, blanching, hypersensitive	Complete healing within 21 days with minimal to no scarring
Deep partial-thickness (second-degree) burn	Intense radiant energy; scalding liquids, semiliquids (e.g., tar), or solids; flame	Epidermis destroyed; underlying dermis damaged; some epidermal appendages remain intact	Pale; decreased moisture; blanching absent or prolonged; intact sensation to deep pressure but not to pinprick	Prolonged healing (often longer than 21 days); may require skin graft to achieve complete healing with better functional outcome
Full-thickness (third-degree) burn	Prolonged contact with flame, scalding liquids; steam; hot objects; chemicals; electrical current	Epidermis, dermis, and epidermal appendages destroyed; injury through dermis	Dry, leatherlike; pale, mottled brown, or red; thrombosed vessels visible; insensate	Requires skin grafting
Full-thickness (fourth-degree) burn	High-voltage electrical injuries; prolonged contact with flame (often in a victim who is unconscious)	Epidermis, dermis, epidermal appendages, fat, muscle, and bone can be destroyed	Dry, leatherlike eschar; color variable; charring visible in deepest area; insensate; extremity movement limited	Requires skin grafting; may require amputation of extremities involved

Modified from Carrougher GJ, editor: *Burn care and therapy*, St Louis, 1998, Mosby.

INJURY SEVERITY ASSESSMENT

The American Burn Association (ABA) has developed an injury severity classification system that categorizes burn injuries as minor, moderate, and major. The ABA advocates that patients with major burns be treated in a burn center or a facility with expertise in burn care. Moderate burns usually require hospitalization, although not necessarily in a burn center, and minor burns are often treated on an outpatient basis. Box 3-5 outlines the ABA criteria for patients who should be referred to a recognized burn center.

HISTORY AND RISK FACTORS FOR A MAJOR BURN

Several factors affect survival after a major burn injury. The patient's age is a determining factor with those at the extremes of age (less than 2 years and greater than 65 years of age) being at highest risk of death. Preexisting cardiac or lung disease (e.g., COPD) or history of smoking increases susceptibility to respiratory distress. Patients who sustain a thermal injury in a confined area may have a concomitant inhalation injury and are also at increased risk. Patients with preexisting cardiac, vascular, renal, or respiratory conditions may not tolerate aggressive fluid resuscitation therapy and may experience complications. Conditions such as immunosuppression, diabetes, collagen vascular disease, history of cardiopulmonary or vascular disease, and invasive procedures contribute to the likelihood of infection, sepsis, and

Box 3-5	AMERICAN BURN ASSOCIATION BURN CENTER REFERRAL GUIDELINES

- Partial-thickness burns greater than 10% total body surface area (TBSA) burn in patients younger than 10 years or older than 50 years.
- Partial-thickness burns greater than 20% TBSA burn in patients 11 to 50 years of age.
- Burns that involve the face, hands, feet, genitalia, perineum, or major joints.
- Full-thickness burns in any age group.
- Electrical burns (to include lightning injuries).
- Chemical burns.
- Burn injuries with associated inhalation injury.
- Burn injury in patients with preexisting medical disorders that could complicate management, prolong recovery, or affect mortality.
- Any patient with burns and concomitant trauma in which the burn injury poses the greatest risk of morbidity/mortality.
- Burn injury in children at hospitals without qualified personnel or equipment for the care of children.
- Burn injury in patients who will require special social, emotional, or long-term rehabilitative interventions.

Excerpted from American Burn Association/American College of Surgeons Committee on Trauma: *Guidelines for the operation of burn centers. Resources for optimal care of the injured patient 2006*, Chicago, 2006, American Burn Association, pp. 79-86.

prolonged healing. Those patients with a history of drug and/or alcohol abuse have an increased mortality risk and often have longer hospital stays. Burn injury can be associated with a concomitant traumatic injury from a blast, motor vehicle crash, or fall. Careful evaluation for secondary injury is essential.

INITIAL ASSESSMENT

In the prehospital setting or emergency department, patients with a burn injury should be evaluated using a primary survey followed by a more thorough, secondary survey; the principles of which are taught in the Advanced Burn Life Support (ABLS) course. The primary patient survey includes the basic ABCs, with the addition of D and E: A: airway and cervical spine immobilization (based on mechanism of injury); B: breathing; C: circulation; D: disability or neurologic deficit; and E: exposure and evaluation. Once the primary survey is complete, a secondary survey should be performed and includes a detailed head-to-toe assessment, exploration of the circumstances of the injury, and the patient's medical history. Injury severity is assessed according to patient's age, potential for inhalation injury, TBSA burn, depth and location, past medical history, and concomitant trauma.

INITIAL SYSTEM ASSESSMENT
- Assess airway for obstruction.
- Assess breathing for distress.
- Assess for decreased tissue perfusion.
- Assess for TBSA burn and depth of burn injury.
- Trauma assessment to identify concomitant injury.
- Assess for pain and anxiety.

AIRWAY/BREATHING
- Observe for foreign objects in mouth, including a large tongue that may obstruct the airway.
- Observe for signs of accessory muscle use for respirations.
- If intubated, verify tube placement, work of breathing, and appropriate ventilator settings.

HEART RATE, HEART RHYTHM, BP TO EVALUATE CO AND PERFUSION

- Assess HR and rhythm, especially if the TBSA burn is greater than 20% because patients tend to be tachycardic (pain will also increase HR).
- Central line monitoring for hemodynamic status (e.g., CVP, PAP, PAWP, CO) is not commonly used unless the patient exhibits signs of hemodynamic instability.
- Take BP on uninjured extremity if possible. Arterial line may be necessary for BP monitoring if burn injury to bilateral extremities is extensive and/or patient exhibits hemodynamic instability. Compare cuff BP to arterial line BP if arterial line is in place; decide which pressure is deemed the most accurate.
- Evaluate for distal tissue perfusion, appearance of uninjured skin, color of nail beds, capillary refill, and temperature of extremities. Assess for the six "Ps":
  - Pain out of proportion to the injury.
  - Pallor.
  - Pulselessness.
  - Paresthesias.
  - Paralysis.
  - Poikilothermia (or "polar"/cold to touch).

BURN WOUND EXTENT (CALCULATION OF TBSA BURN)

The extent of the burn wound is reported as a percent of the TBSA injured. In adults, this is easily estimated by using the rule of nines (Figure 3-1). In children, this rule is altered slightly, reflecting the different body proportion in infants and children. The rule of nines technique is used in prehospital settings and emergency departments when a quick assessment is necessary. For very small and/or irregularly shaped or scattered burns, it helps to remember that the surface area of the patient's palm (palm plus fingers) equals 1% of the patient's TBSA. A more accurate assessment tool is the Lund-Browder chart (Figure 3-2), which is more detailed and accounts for changes in body areas according to age. This chart may be used for both children and adults and is frequently used in critical and acute care settings. More recent studies have called into question the use of these measures in the morbidly obese population and suggest that as the body mass index increases, the size of the palmer surface in relation to the percent TBSA burn decreases.

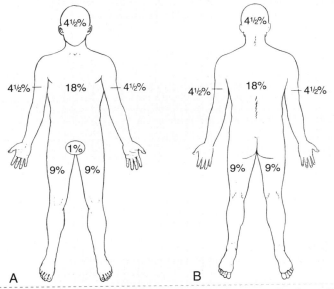

Figure 3-1 Estimation of adult burn injury: rule of nines. **A,** Anterior view. **B,** Posterior view. (From Thompson M, McFarland GK, Hirsch JE, et al: *Mosby's clinical nursing,* ed 4, St Louis, 1997, Mosby.)

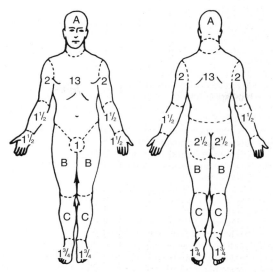

Relative percentages of areas affected by growth
(age in years)

	0	1	5	10	15	Adult
A: Half of head	9½	8½	6½	5½	4½	3½
B: Half of thigh	2¾	3¼	4	4¼	4½	4¾
C: Half of leg	2½	2½	2¾	3	3¼	3½

Second degree_____and
Third degree_____=
Total percent burned___

Figure 3-2 Estimation of burn injury: Lund and Browder chart. Areas represent percentages of body surface area that vary according to age. The accompanying table indicates the relative percentages of these areas in various stages of life. (From Sabeston DC Jr, editor: *Textbook of surgery: the biographical basis of modern surgical practice,* ed. 11, Philadelphia, 1977, Saunders.)

Safety Alert *Electrical burn injuries may reveal only cutaneous injuries on initial inspection, but extensive damage can occur to deep and underlying tissues, nerves, blood vessels, and muscles along the conduction path and at the electrical current contact sites.*

- Estimate wound size (percent TBSA burn) and assess depth (partial- or full-thickness burn injury).

PALPATION
- Pulse assessment to evaluate for decreased tissue perfusion of all extremities:
  - Pulse quality and regularity bilaterally (0-to 4+ scale);
  - Edema (0-to-4+ scale): unburned tissue of extremities.
- Turgor assessment of unburned extremities.
- Temperature of extremities (cool extremities may be indicative of poor distal perfusion of extremities).

AUSCULTATION

- Respiratory sounds to assess for adventitious breath sounds; confirm for bilateral breath sounds.
- Heart sounds to evaluate for contributors to decreased CO (note changes with body positioning and respirations):
  - S1 and S2: quality, intensity, pitch;
  - Extra sounds: S3 (after S2), S4 (before S1) indicative of heart failure.
- Bowel sounds: presence or absence; location.

RESPIRATORY SYSTEM

Respiratory compromise may occur as a result of upper airway swelling, inhalation injury, carbon monoxide poisoning, or respiratory tract infection. The upper airway is injured when hot air causes heat injury to the respiratory mucosa. The lower respiratory tract can be damaged by contact with products of combustion and inhalation of vaporized caustic substances, such as sulfur, hydrogen cyanide, ammonia, acrolein, aldehydes, and hydrochloric acid. These noxious gases are produced from the combustion of common household items, such as carpeting, furniture, and decorations. Airway injury, obstruction, or respiratory distress may not occur immediately following injury.

- Secure and protect airway; check for any cervical injuries and need to stabilize neck area for appropriate airway protection positioning.
- Progressive swelling of the upper airway (above the glottis) may lead to airway obstruction. Check for airway obstruction as a result of swelling caused by heat, smoke, or chemical injury to nasopharyngeal mucosa or by constriction around the neck or chest caused by eschar (burned, devitalized tissue) formation.
- Assess for singed nasal hairs, perioral burns, change in voice, or coughing, especially if productive for soot (mucus will have gray or black particles).
- Carbon monoxide, a byproduct of combustion, displaces oxygen from Hgb, resulting in hypoxia. Headache, decreased visual acuity, tinnitus, vertigo, confusion, unresponsiveness, and convulsions are signs of carbon monoxide poisoning. Refer to Table 3-7 for signs and symptoms of carbon monoxide poisoning.

Safety Alert *Unresponsiveness is not normally associated with burn injuries; patients who are difficult to arouse at the scene or in the emergency department should be evaluated for carbon monoxide exposure or other potential causes (i.e., traumatic brain injury, drugs/alcohol).*

- Epithelial or mucosal sloughing with bronchitis and respiratory distress may occur 6 to 72 hours after the burn occurs and may further contribute to airway obstruction. The top layer of the mucosal lining of the airway "peels" away; similar to the skin peeling after a sunburn.
- Stridor, severe hoarseness, hacking cough, labored breathing, dyspnea, tachypnea, and possible altered LOC caused by hypoxia.

Table 3-7	CARBON MONOXIDE POISONING
Carboxyhemoglobin Saturation (%)	**Signs and Symptoms**
≤10	Impaired vision
11-20	Headache, facial flushing
21-30	Nausea, trouble with dexterity
31-40	Nausea, vomiting, dizziness, syncope
41-50	Tachypnea, tachycardia, loss of consciousness
>50	Coma, death

- Pulmonary excursion is limited by circumferential full-thickness wounds of the neck and torso. Circumferential full-thickness burns of the torso often cause inadequate pulmonary excursion, leading to inadequate ventilation. When pronounced, a chest wall escharotomy may need to be performed.
- Assess for low blood oxygen content, respiratory distress, impaired chest wall excursion, increased peak pressures, decreased compliance, and abnormal ABG values.
- Patients with inhalation injury are at risk for pneumonia. On average, 50% of all burn patients with inhalation injury who require mechanical ventilation will develop pneumonia.
- Assess for bronchial breath sounds over areas of consolidation, crackles.

CARDIOVASCULAR SYSTEM

Circulatory compromise results from the fluid shifts that occur following a significant (typically greater than 20% TBSA) burn injury. Increased capillary permeability caused by the inflammatory response results in a shift of intravascular fluid into the interstitial spaces in the first 72 hours postburn. This causes a decrease in circulating volume and increased blood viscosity. Other systemic responses include increases in catecholamines, cortisol, renin-angiotensin, antidiuretic hormone, and aldosterone production as the body attempts to retain sodium and water to replenish intravascular fluid. Rapid fluid shifts can result in massive edema in unburned and burned areas, hemoconcentration, and thrombus formation.

- Signs of hypovolemic shock, such as thirst, pallor, dry mucous membranes, decreased LOC, and cool skin temperature; tachycardia, hypotension, and decreased filling pressures (CVP, PAP, PAWP); decreased or absent peripheral pulses and delayed capillary refill; and impaired peripheral perfusion with possible obstruction caused by vascular compression with circumferential full-thickness burns or thrombus formation.
- Cardiac dysrhythmias caused by direct cardiac damage (electrical burns).
- Electrolyte imbalance (e.g., hyperkalemia caused by cellular hemolysis).
- Peripheral edema as a result of fluid shifts and hypoproteinemia.

GASTROINTESTINAL SYSTEM

Initially, blood flow is shunted away from the GI tract and peristalsis is slowed or stopped completely, causing a gastric ileus (usually resolves within 72 hours after burn injury).

- Before the initiation of early enteral feedings, life-threatening stomach and intestinal ulcerations (Curling ulcers) and hemorrhage (associated with low gastric pH) often occur. Prophylaxis should be initiated with the use of PPIs or H_2-receptor antagonists and/or early enteral feeding.
- Large fluid resuscitation volumes pose a significant risk for abdominal compartment syndrome.
- Assess for diminished or absent bowel sounds; presence of nausea and vomiting; abdominal distention.

RENAL SYSTEM

Hemoconcentration and reduced circulatory volumes result in decreased renal blood flow and low urinary output. Dark concentrated urine in the presence of muscle injury implies myoglobinuria or hemoglobinuria. Continued poor renal perfusion results in acute tubular necrosis and renal failure. Urine output guides fluid resuscitation measures and recognition of renal compromise or poor CO is essential.

- Urine output less than 30 mL/h in adults and 0.5 mL/kg/h in children less than 30 kg; dark-colored, concentrated urine.

Safety Alert *Bladder pressures exceeding 20 mm Hg may constitute an emergency as it may indicate abdominal compartment syndrome. Thus it is important for the nurse to monitor any increases in trending of bladder pressures.*

- Consider bladder pressure monitoring every 4 hours during excessive fluid administration. During the resuscitation period, excessive fluid administration is usually defined as greater than 1.5 to 2 times the calculated fluid resuscitation estimates (see Collaborative Management).

INTEGUMENTARY SYSTEM

Loss of skin integrity results in increased fluid loss through evaporation, hypothermia, pain, and increased risk of infection. Evaporative fluid losses can be substantial, especially in patients with large surface area burns and in pediatric patients with burn injuries who have larger surface area per kilogram of body weight. Significant hypothermia can result in patients with large surface area burns, long transports to the hospital, and long surgeries and in those who require prolonged wound care.

Patients with burn injuries can experience three types of pain:

- Procedural pain is experienced during painful procedures (e.g., wound debridement, dressing changes, staple removal, active physical therapy) and is often described as pain that is of short duration and high intensity.
- Background pain, which is experienced at rest or while doing minimal physical activities, and is often described as constant and of low intensity.
- Breakthrough pain is experienced during activities or painful procedures despite the administration of procedural pain medication and is intense and of short duration.

 Circumferential full-thickness burns can cause constriction of underlying tissue, blood vessels, and muscles with circulatory compromise to underlying muscles and distal extremities. Healed skin may result in some scar formation, which can lead to contractures that limit joint ROM.

See Table 3-6 for a complete description of partial-thickness and full-thickness burn wound injuries.

WOUND INFECTION

Loss of skin integrity means that the body's first line of defense against infection is compromised. Ongoing evaluation for burn wound infection is imperative because a significant infection may lead to delayed healing, tissue loss, and sepsis. Typically, the larger the wound or delay in complete healing, the greater is the risk for wound infection. Early signs of wound infection include fever, increase or decrease in WBC count, erythema surrounding the burn wound, increased wound pain, change in exudate or wound appearance, and loss of previously healed skin grafts. Invasive wound infection is indicated by rapid eschar separation (invasive fungal infections); focal, dark red, brown, or black discolorations in the eschar; rapid conversion of an area of partial- to full-thickness injury; and hemorrhagic fat necrosis.

SYSTEMIC INFLAMMATORY RESPONSE SYNDROME/SEPTIC SHOCK

All patients who are severely burned display signs and symptoms of SIRS; therefore, this term is not used to describe the inflammatory processes in the patient with burn injuries. However, if more than three signs and symptoms of SIRS (modified slightly for the patient with burn injuries) are present along with a documented source of infection, sepsis is present.

Signs of burn sepsis include:

- Tachycardia: HR greater than 110 bpm (depending on baseline, age, and comorbidity).
- Tachypnea: RR greater than 25 breaths/min (age-dependent).
- Decreased BP with low SVR.
- Labile core body temperature (may fluctuate by more than 3° C, as low as 36.5° C).
- Low platelet count (thrombocytopenia).
- Changes in LOC (confusion, disorientation, agitation).
- Hyperglycemia or increasing insulin requirements.
- Feeding intolerance; increased enteral feeding residuals; loss of appetite.
- Gastric distention or gastric ileus.

Diagnostic Tests for Major Burn Injury

Test	Purpose	Abnormal Findings
Noninvasive Cardiology		
Electrocardiogram (ECG): 12-lead ECG on admission	To assess cardiac health. A baseline ECG should be completed on patients with a history of cardiac disease and those with a major burn injury (to include electrical injury).	Presence of ST segment depression or T wave inversion (myocardial ischemia), ST elevation (acute myocardial infarction), new bundle branch block (especially left BBB) or pathologic Q waves (resolving/resolved myocardial infarction), and arrhythmias.
Invasive Pulmonary		
Bronchoscopy: Technique of visualizing the inside of the airways for both diagnostic and therapeutic purposes	To assess for evidence of inhalation injury and/or to obtain fluid specimen (bronchoalveolar lavage).	Presence of carbonaceous particles, erythema, edema, and bronchial casts; presence of microorganisms $>10^5$
Noninvasive Metabolic Study		
Indirect calorimetry: Provides the most accurate measurement of energy expenditure	To measure resting energy expenditure. With these data, calories used during the testing period can be extrapolated as well as providing the respiratory quotient (RQ) — the ratio of carbon dioxide produced to oxygen consumed.	RQ values >1.0 may indicate overfeeding of total calories or excessive carbohydrate infusion. RQ values <0.6 may indicate ketosis.
Noninvasive Blood Study		
Pulse oximetry: Noninvasive method allowing cutaneous monitoring of the oxygenation of the patient's hemoglobin	To assess oxygenation. Not reliable in patients who are profoundly hypovolemic, in shock, or hypothermic or with baseline chronic obstructive pulmonary disease.	Less than 92% may indicate impaired oxygenation and need for oxygen therapy. Unreliable in the presence of carbon monoxide poisoning. False readings may occur when hemoglobin is bound to carbon monoxide that may delay the recognition of hypoxemia (low blood oxygen levels).
End-tidal CO_2: Noninvasive reflection of Pa_{CO_2}	To assess ventilation.	Levels greater than or less than normal (35 to 45 mm Hg) reflect ventilatory problems.
Blood Studies		
Complete blood count Hemoglobin (Hgb) Hematocrit (Hct) Red blood cell (RBC) count White blood cell (WBC) count Platelet count	To assess for polycythemia, anemia, inflammation, infection, sepsis, coagulation disorders, and dehydration.	Increased RBCs, Hgb, or Hct reflect concentration (secondary to under-resuscitation during the initial 24 hours postburn). Decreased levels may reflect anemia. Infection or inflammation may increase WBCs. Sepsis may increase or decrease WBCs. Thrombocytopenia (decreased platelet count) may reflect coagulation disorders or sepsis.

Continued

Burns

Diagnostic Tests for Major Burn Injury — cont'd

Test	Purpose	Abnormal Findings
Metabolic Panel		
Glucose	Determine whether glucose control is necessary; glucose levels in response to premorbid medical condition, concomitant injuries, or secondary conditions. To assess for changes resulting from large-volume fluid shifts or increasing needs.	Hyperglycemia may indicate premorbid medical condition (e.g., diabetes) or injury stress response. Hypoglycemia may indicate depletion of glycogen stores, especially in children. Hypoglycemia or hyperglycemia may indicate sepsis or adrenal insufficiency.
Potassium (K^+) Magnesium (Mg^{2+}) Calcium (Ca^{2+})		Decrease in K^+, Mg^{2+}, or Ca^{2+} may cause dysrhythmias.
Sodium (Na^+)		Elevation of Na^+ may indicate dehydration; low Na^+ may indicate fluid retention.
Lactate Base deficit		Increase in lactate and base deficit levels may indicate inadequate fluid resuscitation or shock state (first 12 to 24 hours postburn) or infection.
Coagulation profile Prothrombin time with international normalized ratio Partial thromboplastin time Fibrinogen D dimer	To assess for bleeding, clotting, and disseminated intravascular coagulation indicative of abnormal clotting present in shock or ensuing shock or coagulation disorder.	Severe burn injury results in a postburn hypercoagulation — characterized by the activation of coagulation, decreased fibrinolytic activity, and decreased natural anticoagulant activity.
Arterial Blood Gas (ABG) Analysis		
pH	To assess for acid-base disorders by measuring the concentration of gases (carbon dioxide and oxygen), bicarbonate, and pH of the blood. Early ABGs may be normal. Early acidemia may reflect inadequate fluid resuscitation. Later studies may reflect hypoxemia secondary to respiratory failure, with progressive metabolic acidosis in patients with impending shock or systemic inflammatory response syndrome.	pH range: 7.35–7.45. The pH indicates if a patient is acidemic (pH < 7.35) or alkalemic (pH > 7.45).
PO_2		PO_2: 80–100 mm Hg. A low O_2 indicates that the patient is not respiring properly and is hypoxemic.
pCO_2		pCO_2: 35–45 mm Hg. A high pCO_2 indicates underventilation; a low pCO_2 indicates hyperventilation or overventilation. pCO_2 levels can also become abnormal when the respiratory system is working to compensate for a metabolic issue.
HCO_3		HCO_3 range: 22 to 26 mmol/L. A low HCO_3 indicates metabolic acidosis; a high HCO_3 indicates metabolic alkalosis. HCO_3 levels can also become abnormal when the kidneys are working to compensate for a respiratory issue.

Diagnostic Tests for Major Burn Injury — cont'd		
Test	**Purpose**	**Abnormal Findings**
Carboxyhemoglobin analysis	To assess for carbon monoxide poisoning. Carbon monoxide, a byproduct of combustion, displaces oxygen from hemoglobin, resulting in hypoxia.	Carboxyhemoglobin levels above 5% to 10% in individuals not routinely exposed to carbon monoxide. Smokers and those routinely exposed to heavy traffic (truckers, taxi drivers) may routinely have nonsignificant carboxyhemoglobin levels of 5% to 15%.
Radiology		
Chest radiograph	To aid in the assessment of pulmonary status on admission and serially for any progression of lung involvement. Done serially.	Chest radiographs are often normal on admission and then progressively worsen within 24 to 48 hours with significant smoke inhalation and development of acute respiratory distress syndrome. Pneumonia exhibits a "white out" picture demonstrating pulmonary infiltrates.
Skeletal radiographs	To assess for potential injuries in at-risk patients. Patients with known high-voltage electrical contact should be evaluated for long bone or spinous process fractures resulting from prolonged muscle tetany.	Fractures, foreign objects.

DIAGNOSTIC TESTS

BRONCHOSCOPY

The ABA Consensus Conference on Burn Sepsis and Infection Group has determined that bronchoscopy is the best and most reliable test for diagnosis of smoke inhalation injury below the glottis. Signs of injury below the glottis that can be observed with bronchoscopy include carbonaceous material, edema, and ulceration. Therapeutic bronchoscopy facilitates removal of carbonaceous material and nonviable tissue.

FLUORESCEIN EXAMINATION

This procedure uses orange dye (fluorescein) and an ultraviolet light (Wood lamp) to detect foreign bodies in the eye and/or damage to the cornea. This examination should occur in all patients with possible eye injury and should be performed early (first 24 hours after burn injury), before swelling prevents a thorough examination.

CULTURE AND SENSITIVITY STUDIES

This diagnostic test evaluates sputum (pneumonia), blood (bacteremia or septicemia), urine (UTI), and wound tissue for evidence of colonization and infection.

Burn wound infection is defined as more than 10^5 microorganisms/g of burn wound tissue with active invasion of adjacent, viable, unburned skin. Gram-negative organisms include *Pseudomonas aeruginosa, Klebsiella, Serratia, Acinetobacter, Escherichia coli,* and *Enterobacter cloacae.* Gram-positive organisms (*Staphylococcus* and *Streptococcus*) and fungal pathogens (*Candida* and *Aspergillus*) may also be present. Colonization of burn wounds is common and not treated with systemic antimicrobial therapy. Topical agents are used to reduce microbes. Surveillance cultures may be collected on admission for screening of multidrug-resistant organisms and methicillin-resistant *Staphylococcus aureus.* An epidemiologic investigation may be needed to evaluate infection trends.

URINE COLLECTIONS

Perform urinalysis and culture and sensitivity early to detect UTI. A 24-hour urine collection to measure total nitrogen, urea nitrogen, creatinine, and amino acid nitrogen values may indicate return of capillary integrity (3 to 5 days after burn occurrence) and mobilization of third-spaced fluids, the degree of catabolism present, and the onset or resolution of acute renal failure. Myoglobinuria can result from muscle injury sustained from an electrical injury or deep full-thickness burn.

HEMATOLOGY

Elevated Hct resulting from hemoconcentration during initial resuscitation. Hgb will be decreased secondary to dilution, surgical burn wound excision, hemolysis, or multiple laboratory draws. During the first 24 hours postburn, neither the Hgb level nor the Hct is a reliable guide to fluid resuscitation. WBCs may be elevated resulting from systemic inflammatory response or sepsis. Patients with burn injuries will typically be leukopenic initially because WBCs migrate to areas of burned tissue.

ELECTROLYTE PANEL

Hyperglycemia is common in patients related to the normal stress response of injury. Hyperglycemia may also be seen in patients with sepsis and multiple organ failure. Sodium shifts occur during resuscitation; carefully monitor and adjust type of resuscitation fluid 24 hours postinjury. Vigilant monitoring of the ECG for T wave elevation indicative of hyperkalemia is of paramount importance. Early identification of hyperkalemia facilitates prompt treatment. Potassium may be elevated as a result of cell lysis, fluid shifts, or renal insufficiency. Blood urea nitrogen (BUN) is elevated because of hypovolemic state, increased protein catabolism, or possible acute renal failure. Persistent elevation of BUN and creatinine signals inadequate fluid intake or acute renal failure. Total protein and albumin are decreased secondary to leakage of plasma proteins into interstitial spaces. Creatine kinase (CK) is sometimes used as an index of muscle damage, but a burn injury that damages even a small quantity of muscle tissue will result in markedly elevated CK levels in the first 24 hours. Troponin levels are more indicative of cardiac damage. Increase in lactate may indicate inadequate fluid resuscitation (first 12 to 24 hours postburn), infection, or shock state from decreased tissue perfusion or sepsis.

ECG

Evaluate for tachycardia secondary to hypovolemia or pain. Tachycardia of 100 to 120 bpm is common in the adult patient who appears adequately resuscitated. Myocardial damage secondary to high-voltage electrical burn injury may be evident (e.g., dysrhythmias, prolonged QT interval). Dysrhythmias related to electrolyte imbalance may occur. Hyperkalemia is relatively common and, if extreme, requires immediate care to avoid a lethal dysrhythmia.

COLLABORATIVE MANAGEMENT

CARE PRIORITIES

1. Manage hypoxemia and protect the upper airways by using humidified oxygen therapy

Treats hypoxemia and prevents drying and sloughing of the mucosal lining of the tracheobronchial tree. If the patient is awake, oxygen administration by nonrebreather face mask may be sufficient; intubation may be required if the patient is stuporous, unconscious, or with significant burn injuries to the face or upper airway area. Any patient with suspected carbon monoxide poisoning/inhalation injury should receive humidified 100% oxygen by nonrebreather face mask until the carboxyhemoglobin level falls below 10%. Hyperbaric oxygen therapy (HBOT) is a treatment sometimes used to accelerate resolution of carbon monoxide poisoning in patients with burn injuries, as well as healing of gangrene, wounds, and infections in which tissues are unable to receive adequate oxygen. The purpose of HBOT in carbon monoxide poisoning is to reduce the amount of carbon monoxide in the blood by displacing carbon monoxide molecules bound to hemoglobin (carboxyhemoglobin), and replacing them with oxygen (O_2) molecules (oxyhemoglobin) to restore the oxygen level to normal quickly. The high pressure within the chamber increases blood oxygen level 10- to 15-fold. HBOT can break the cycle of swelling, tissue hypoxia, and tissue necrosis. HBOT is used consistently to resolve carbon monoxide poisoning, but on a case-by-case basis to manage tissue damage associated with thermal burn injuries.

2. Support ventilation by providing intubation and mechanical ventilation:

Endotracheal intubation is indicated if respiratory distress or failure is present, airway obstruction from laryngeal edema associated with the superheated gases is imminent (e.g., progressive hoarseness and/or stridor), or the patient cannot protect their airway (impaired LOC). Large burn injury (more than 40% TBSA) may result in generalized tissue edema even in the absence of inhalation injury, requiring prophylactic intubation for airway protection. Because laryngeal edema typically resolves in 3 to 5 days after the burn injury, tracheostomy is avoided for upper airway distress unless there is acute obstruction or prolonged need for ventilatory support.

For patients requiring intubation and mechanical ventilation, implementation of measures (e.g., Ventilator Bundle) to prevent ventilator-associated pneumonia are instituted. Ventilator-associated events are identified by using a combination of objective criteria: deterioration in respiratory status after a period of stability or improvement on the ventilator, evidence of infection or inflammation, and laboratory evidence of respiratory tract infection (www.cdc.gov/nhsn/pdfs/pscManual/10-VAE_FINAL.pdf). Ventilator-associated pneumonia is the leading cause of death among patients with hospital-acquired infections; it prolongs time spent on the ventilator, in the ICU, and the total hospital length of stay.

The key components of the Institute for Healthcare Improvement (IHI) Ventilator Bundle are noted as follows (*); other key preventative interventions are also suggested:

- Hand hygiene.
- Elevation of the head of the bed 30 to 45 degrees.*
- Mouth care and endotracheal tube care.
- Daily "sedative interruptions" and assessment of readiness for extubation.*
- Peptic ulcer disease prophylaxis.*
- DVT prophylaxis* (unless contraindicated).
- Lung protective ventilator strategies.
- Early mobilization.

> **Safety Alert**
> *The Institute for Healthcare Improvement (IHI) Ventilator Bundle is a set of key evidence-based interventions related to mechanical ventilator care that when implemented collectively and consistently lead to better patient outcomes.*

3. Thin secretions with bronchodilators and mucolytic agents

Aid in promoting gas exchange and in loosening of pulmonary secretions.

4. Relieve constriction of circumferential burns with escharotomy

An incision through eschar to relieve constriction caused by circumferential, full-thickness burns. Escharotomies of the chest wall relieve respiratory distress secondary to circumferential, full-thickness burns of the trunk. Escharotomies of the extremities lessen pressure created by underlying edema to restore adequate tissue perfusion. Escharotomies of the torso and/or extremities may be performed at the bedside or in the emergency department by trained personnel. Indicated when patients have burns of thorax, when respiratory excursion is restricted or exhibit cyanosis and cold temperature of distal unburned skin, prolonged capillary filling, decreased sensation and movement, or weak or absent peripheral pulses (mimics compartment syndrome).

5. Hydrate using large-bore IV access

Peripheral veins should be used to establish IV access using two large-bore IV catheters. Veins underlying unburned skin are preferred; however, veins beneath burned skin can be used if necessary. If peripheral IV access is not possible, obtain central venous line access (preferably through nonburned skin) for IV administration. Intraosseous infusion may be necessary if peripheral or central venous access is not possible.

> **Safety Alert** *Patients with less than 20% total body surface area burns may be candidates for oral fluid resuscitation. Oral resuscitation should be considered when the patient is able to tolerate oral intake (intact gastrointestinal tract) or when resources are limited (e.g., mass casualty situation).*

6. Fluid resuscitation

The goal of fluid resuscitation is to maintain tissue perfusion and organ function while avoiding the complications of inadequate or excessive fluid therapy (Advanced Burn Life Support). Fluid replacement protocols are based on body weight and percent of TBSA burned and provide an estimate for resuscitation. The ABA Consensus formula recommends administration of 2 to 4 mL fluid per kilogram body weight per percent TBSA burned (adult) and 3 to 4 mL fluid per kilogram body weight per percent TBSA burned (infants and young children weighing less than 30 kg) to provide the total estimate of fluids to be administered in the first 24 hours following the time the burn occurred. Give half in the first 8 hours and then the second half over the next 16 hours. The initial infusion rate is calculated using the Consensus formula and subsequent hourly titration is guided by urinary output (30 to 50 mL/h for adults and 1 mL/kg/h in children weighing less than 30 kg). LR solution is used in the first 24 hours, with small amounts of colloid fluids added during the second 24 hours after injury. Colloids are generally avoided during the first 12 to 24 hours after injury because increased capillary permeability allows leakage of protein into the interstitial tissues. The greater surface area–to–body mass ratio of children necessitates the administration of relatively greater amounts of resuscitation fluid. In addition, infants and young children should receive fluid with 5% dextrose (e.g., $D_5^{1/4}$ NS or $D_5^{1/2}$ NS) at a maintenance rate in addition to the LR resuscitation fluid. Maintenance fluids are provided at a constant rate and are based on the child's dry weight. A child weighing up to 10 kg should receive 4 mL/kg/h; those 11 to 20 kg should receive 2 mL/kg/h, and those 21 to 30 kg should receive 1 mL/kg/h during the first 24 hours following injury. Patients who are particularly sensitive to excessive fluid resuscitation include children, older adults, and those with preexisting cardiac disease.

> **Safety Alert** *Calculate fluid infusion from the time of injury, not the time of hospital admission. Fluid resuscitation and maintenance formulas should be modified based on individual patient responses and needs. Hourly urine output serves to guide infusion rates. Patients with electrical injuries, very deep burns, inhalation injury, prior dehydration, ethanol intoxication, and concomitant trauma (e.g., crushing injuries) may have greater fluid needs than suggested by their cutaneous burn injury alone.*

7. Maintain an accurate record of the fluid balance

Insertion of an indwelling urinary catheter may be essential for accurate hourly measurement of urine output and evaluation of renal status in patients with a major burn injury.

8. Facilitate core body temperature regulation

For patients with extensive burn injuries, the body's response to injury is to increase core and skin temperatures by 2° C above normal. Increasing the ambient room temperature to 33° C (91.4° F) helps to attenuate the hypermetabolic response. Limit body exposure during wound care and dressing changes.

9. Prevent aspiration of gastric contents by NG intubation

Permits gastric decompression, reducing risk of aspiration. Aids in the removal of gastric contents, which may be necessary during the resuscitative phase because of the potential for gastric ileus in patients with greater than 20% TBSA burn and in patients with intubated airway.

10. Provide proper patient positioning to decrease the potential for further injury

Burn injured extremities should be elevated to reduce dependent edema formation. Patients with burns of the head or ears should be positioned without a pillow (to prevent the incidence of neck flexion contractures and ear chondritis [can develop from pressure on injured, fragile ear cartilage]). Patients should be routinely positioned to reduce contracture formation with frequent position changes to reduce the incidence of pressure sores.

11. Provide aggressive nutrition support

High metabolic activity and increased protein catabolism related to burn injury result in dramatic increases in energy requirements and nutritional needs. Additional injury (e.g., long bone fractures) or poor nutritional status before the burn injury may further increase nutritional needs. This hypermetabolic response to injury typically continues beyond the acute phase of recovery and may last up to 1 year for those with extensive burn injuries (i.e., >40% TBSA burn). Energy requirements are estimated using one of several predictive formulas based on body size and extent of burn, with adjustment for age, and are calculated by nutritionists. Indirect calorimetry is also used to measure energy expenditure, thus providing a measure of calories needed. However, the equipment required for indirect calorimetry is expensive and requires trained personnel to administer the test.

Although nutrition practices vary, nutrition support should be initiated early in the recovery process. The appropriate mix of protein, fat, and carbohydrates to be provided is not standardized, but a positive nitrogen state can be achieved with patients who are administered high-protein, moderate-carbohydrate, and low-fat diets.

Oral, enteral, or parenteral methods of delivery are used, based on patient tolerance. Many critically ill patients with burn injuries are unable to meet their increased nutrition requirements with oral intake alone. Enteral feedings are preferred in these patients and have the added benefit of decreasing GI acidity and ulcer formation. Either gastric or postpyloric jejunal feedings may be used. Elemental jejunal feedings may be tolerated when conventional feedings are not. Total parenteral nutrition may be initiated for the patient with gastric ileus or inability to tolerate an adequate amount of enteral feedings.

For patients who are difficult to wean from the ventilator, it has been suggested that the use of higher-fat, lower-carbohydrate diets may be beneficial because excess carbohydrate increases CO_2 production.

- Support nutrition status with multivitamin and mineral supplements: Many vitamins and minerals affect immune function, protein synthesis, and wound healing. Vitamins A and C and zinc are especially important for promoting wound healing. Multivitamins are commonly prescribed for patients with burn injuries.

12. Perform wound care

Wound cleansing is accomplished with use of mild soap and water. Burns are débrided using manual, enzymatic, or surgical techniques. Topical antimicrobial agents, such as silver sulfadiazine and mafenide acetate, are used to control bacterial proliferation. Burn wounds may be covered and ultimately closed with various temporary and permanent coverings as in the following list. Care of the patient with these coverings depends on the type of wound closure technique used.

Wound coverage and closure techniques:
- Cutaneous autograft: includes split-thickness skin graft and cultured epithelial autograft; provides permanent wound coverage.
- Cutaneous allograft: fresh or preserved donated adult cadaver skin; provides temporary wound coverage until the wound bed is ready for autografting.
- Cutaneous xenograft: harvested adult porcine epidermis (pigskin); provides temporary wound coverage until the wound bed beneath is healed or is ready for permanent autografting.
- Biosynthetic coverings: artificial dermis (e.g., Integra); provides a permanent dermal tissue layer that requires a thin autograft for permanent coverage.
- Synthetic coverings: various dressings often used to cover partial-thickness burns and/or donor sites; provide temporary wound coverage until the wound bed beneath is healed or is ready for permanent autografting; often include an antimicrobial agent (e.g., silver) that is released over time. Use and care of wounds when treated using these specialized dressings are specific to the type of product used; follow directions by manufacturer for use based on burn depth (some dressings may only be appropriate for use in partial-thickness burn injuries), length of use (this is of particular importance in dressings providing time release of silver), and dressing removal procedure.

Burns

13. Prepare for surgery as needed

Need for surgery depends on the depth and extent of the burn injury. The burn surgeon coordinates the surgical team.

PHARMACOTHERAPY

1. Provide tetanus prophylaxis

Tetanus immunoglobulin (TIG) or tetanus-toxoid (Tt) should be provided based on the patient's previous immunization for tetanus prophylaxis. Obtain a history of tetanus immunization from the patient or medical records so that appropriate tetanus prophylaxis can be accomplished. Individuals with risk factors for inadequate tetanus immunization status should be treated as tetanus immunization—unknown. The tetanus prophylaxis administered should be consistent with the recommendations of the American College of Surgeons (see www.facs.org/trauma/publications/tetanus.pdf). Burn injuries are considered "tetanus-prone wounds." Tetanus prophylaxis is given intramuscularly.

2. Manage pain with IV analgesics and anxiolytics

Morphine sulfate and fentanyl are common agents used for pain management. They are administered in small, frequent IV doses, as needed for comfort and before painful procedures. Consider adjunctive treatment using benzodiazepines (e.g., lorazepam, diazepam, midazolam) to decrease anxiety. Anxiety increases the perception of pain.

 Safety Alert *During the resuscitative phase of care, all medications, except tetanus immunoglobulin or tetanus-toxoid, are administered intravenously to avoid sequestration of medication, which then would "flood" the vascular system with the return of capillary integrity and the diuresis of third-spaced (interstitial) fluids.*

3. Consider gastric acid suppression therapy

Maintain gastric pH greater than 5.0 to prevent development of gastric ulcers. Early initiation of enteral tube feedings or use of IV PPIs and an H_2-blocking agent assist with maintenance of gastric pH and the prevention of ulcers.

4. Administer antibiotics for known infections

Antibiotics are not routinely prescribed unless a known or suspected infection exists. Broad-spectrum antibiotics may be used initially to treat a suspected infection. More specific antimicrobial agents are used when results from culture and sensitivity tests are available. Burn wound colonization is treated with topical antimicrobial agents only.

5. Provide DVT prophylaxis

Prophylactic measures may include the selective use of sequential compression devices on unburned extremities, subcutaneous heparin, low–molecular-weight heparin, or IV heparin drip. The incidence of DVT in the burn population is unknown; however, it is logical to assume that this patient population is at high risk because of hypercoagulability, altered vascular integrity from the burn injury, imposed immobilization, and multiple operative procedures.

CARE PLANS: BURNS

Ineffective airway clearance (or risk for same) *related to increased pulmonary secretions and inflammation, swelling of nasopharyngeal mucous membranes secondary to smoke irritation or impaired cough; potential of constricting neck and thorax burns and decreased expansion of alveoli secondary to circumferential thorax burns, or pneumonia.*

Goals/Outcomes: The patient maintains a clear airway, as evidenced by auscultation of normal breath sounds over the lung fields and a state of eupnea.
NOC Respiratory Status: Airway Patency.

Airway Management

1. Assess and document respiratory status, noting breath sounds and rate and depth of respirations. Identify deteriorating respiratory status, as evidenced by crackles, rhonchi, stridor, labored breathing, dyspnea, tachypnea, restlessness, and decreasing LOC. Consult physician promptly for all significant findings.
2. Assess and document characteristics and amount of secretions after each deep-breathing and coughing exercise.
3. Reposition the patient from side to side every 1 to 2 hours to help mobilize secretions; position the head of the bed at a 30 degree elevation. Consider the use of a specialized rotation bed.
4. As prescribed, administer percussion and postural drainage to facilitate airway clearance (this is contraindicated with fresh skin grafts over thorax). Perform oropharyngeal or endotracheal suctioning, as indicated by the presence of adventitious breath sounds and the patient's inability to clear the airway effectively by coughing.
5. Administer bronchodilating medications, if prescribed.

NIC Airway Management; Airway Suctioning; Artificial Airway Management; Aspiration Precautions; Cough Enhancement; Mechanical Ventilation.

Impaired gas exchange (or risk for same) *related to inhalation injury with tracheobronchial swelling and carbonaceous debris; competition of carbon monoxide with oxygen for Hgb; hypoventilation associated with constricting circumferential burns to the thorax or large fluid volume resuscitation.*

Goals/Outcomes: The patient exhibits adequate gas exchange, as evidenced by $PaO_2 \geq 80$ mm Hg, oxygen saturation $\geq 95\%$, $PaCO_2$ 35 to 45 mm Hg, age-appropriate RR with a normal pattern and depth, and absence of adventitious breath sounds and other signs of respiratory dysfunction. These outcomes should be adjusted for patients with preinjury respiratory disease (e.g., COPD).
NOC Respiratory Status: Gas Exchange.

Respiratory Monitoring

1. Assess and document respiratory status, noting rate and depth, breath sounds, and LOC. Identify deteriorating respiratory status, as evidenced by indicators of upper airway distress (e.g., severe hoarseness, stridor, dyspnea) and lower airway distress (e.g., crackles, rhonchi, hacking cough, labored or rapid breathing). Consult the physician promptly for all significant findings.

> **Safety Alert** *Infants and young children have relatively smaller airways, thus placing them at greater risk for airway occlusion.*
> In the obese adult, common alterations in lung function include restrictive lung pattern (resulting from abnormally high diaphragmatic position and increase in chest wall mass) and obstructive sleep apnea. This combination results in increased work of breathing and predisposes patients to apneic episodes and/or oxygen desaturations.

2. Administer humidified oxygen therapy, mechanical ventilation, or bronchodilator treatment, as prescribed.
3. Unless contraindicated, place the patient at a minimum of 30 degrees head elevation to limit upper airway edema formation and to enhance respiratory excursion and prevent aspiration.
4. Monitor for hypoxemia and hypercapnia. Serial ABG values, pulse oximetry, and end-tidal CO_2 monitoring provide crucial information concerning arterial oxygen and CO_2 levels. Declining vital capacity, tidal volume, and/or inspiratory force indicates respiratory insufficiency (patients who are mechanically ventilated only).
5. Teach the patient who is not intubated the necessity of deep-breathing and coughing exercises every 2 hours, including use of incentive spirometry while awake.
6. Prepare equipment and the patient for intubation and mechanical ventilation, if needed. Note that the position of the patient's head is crucial for successful intubation.

NIC Airway Management; Respiratory Monitoring; Oxygen Therapy; Bedside Laboratory Testing; Cough Enhancement: Laboratory Data Interpretation.

Deficient fluid volume *related to active loss through the burn wound and leakage of fluid, plasma proteins, and other cellular elements into the interstitial space.*

Goals/Outcomes: The patient fluid volume status stabilizes, as evidenced by MAP greater than 60 mm Hg, peripheral pulses greater than 2+ on a 0-to-4+ scale, and urine output 30 to 50 mL/h (adult) or 1 mL/kg/h (child less than 30 kg dry body weight). Outcomes for urine output should be adjusted for those patients with preexisting renal failure/compromise. In the presence of myoglobinuria (red-pigmented urine indicative of myoglobin or red blood cells in the urine), a urinary output of 1 to 1.5 mL/kg/h (approximately 75 to 100 mL/h in the adult) is the desired outcome until the heme pigments clear from the urine (urine color returns to normal). **NOC** Fluid Balance.

Fluid Management

1. Monitor the patient for evidence of fluid volume deficit, including tachycardia, decreased MAP, decreased amplitude of peripheral pulses, urine output less than 30 mL/h (adult), urine output less than 1 mL/kg/h (child weighing less than 30 kg), thirst, and dry mucous membranes.
2. Establish two large-bore peripheral IV lines, preferably through nonburned skin. Establish central line if necessary.

 Safety Alert *Consider placement of intraosseous device if unable to achieve peripheral or central venous access.*

3. Monitor intake and output; administer fluid therapy using the ABA Consensus formula or as prescribed. Adjust infusion to maintain desired urine output at the desired resuscitation hourly rate. Do not exceed 50 mL/h urine output (adults) or 1 mL/kg/h in children during initial 48 hours of resuscitation (unless heme pigments are present in the urine). Avoid colloids during first 12 to 24 hours following the burn injury, if possible.

Safety Alert *Evaluate patency of intravenous catheters continuously during rapid volume resuscitation.*

4. Monitor weight daily during fluid resuscitation; report significant gains or losses. A significant weight gain will occur with large volume fluid resuscitation. A significant weight loss may also occur as a result of catabolism, an increased metabolic rate, and with extensive removal of burn tissue (e.g., large body fascial excisions).
5. Monitor serial Hct and Hgb values. During the first 24 hours postburn, neither the Hct nor Hgb levels are reliable guides to fluid resuscitation. While the circulating volume is restored, hemoconcentration is no longer present and Hct returns to within normal limits. Consult the physician for significant anemia.
6. Monitor the patient for signs and symptoms of large volume fluid administration (shortness of breath, tachypnea, excessive urine output). Central hemodynamic monitoring is recommended for patients who have preexisting heart or lung disease.
7. In the presence of myoglobinuria (associated with high-voltage electrical injuries or significant soft tissue injury from mechanical trauma), confer with the physician regarding the need to increase the rate of fluid administration and to consider urine alkalinization. On occasion, the use of mannitol to promote osmotic diuresis and prevent renal tubular sludging is considered. Other diuretics are avoided because they further deplete an already compromised intravascular volume. Administration of a diuretic precludes the subsequent use of hourly urine output as a guide to fluid resuscitation.
8. With the onset of spontaneous diuresis (48 to 72 hours postburn), decrease infusion rates as prescribed. Continue to reduce rates gradually according to intake/output ratio and clinical status.

NIC Fluid/Electrolyte Management; Fluid Monitoring; Hypovolemia Management; Shock Prevention; Venous Access Devices Maintenance.

Ineffective tissue perfusion: peripheral *related to thermal injury, circumferential burns, edema, hypovolemia.*

Goals/Outcomes: The patient maintains adequate tissue perfusion.
Note: Tissue perfusion in burned extremities is adequate when peripheral pulses are greater than 2+ on a 0-to-4+ scale, capillary refill is brisk (less than 2 seconds), and uninjured and healing skin is warm to the touch.
NOC Tissue Perfusion: Peripheral; Circulation Status.

Circulatory Precautions

1. Monitor tissue perfusion hourly in burned extremities during the resuscitation phase of care. Note capillary refill, temperature, and peripheral pulses. Report signs of impaired tissue perfusion to the advanced practice provider

immediately, including coolness of the extremity, weak or absent peripheral pulses, pain or paresthesias, and delayed capillary refill.
2. Elevate burned extremities at or above heart level to promote venous return, prevent excessive dependent edema formation, and reduce risk for compartment syndrome of the extremities.

Hypothermia *related to exposure at the scene of injury; large body surface area burns, administration of large volumes of unwarmed fluid.*

Goals/Outcomes: The patient's temperature returns to normal (smaller burn injuries) or is slightly elevated (38.5° C; extensive burn injuries) within 24 hours of this diagnosis. Complications of hypothermia have been avoided.
NOC Thermoregulation.

Temperature Management
1. Warm fluids administered during the initial resuscitation phase and until the patient approaches desired core temperature. Keep room temperature as warm as possible. Goal is 33° C (91.4° F) ambient room temperature.
2. Avoid unnecessary exposure of the body. Keep the patient covered with warmed or warming blanket.
3. Monitor core temperature via rectal or esophageal probe, urinary catheter attachment, or pulmonary artery catheter.
4. Be aware that vasodilation during rewarming can result in further intravascular fluid volume deficit.
5. Monitor for and promptly report serious dysrhythmias (i.e., atrial fibrillation with rapid ventricular response, ventricular dysrhythmias, atrial ventricular conduction block) associated with severe or prolonged hypothermia.
6. Monitor ABG values for evidence of hypoxemia. Hypothermia causes a shift to the left in the oxyhemoglobin dissociation curve and may impair oxygen unloading to peripheral tissue.

Risk for infection *related to inadequate primary and secondary defenses secondary to traumatized tissue, bacterial proliferation in burn wounds, presence of invasive IV lines or urinary catheter, and immunocompromised status.*

Goals/Outcomes: The patient is free of infection, as evidenced by core temperatures of 38.5° C (101.3° F) for those with extensive burn injuries, WBC count less than 11,000/mm³, negative culture results, and absence of purulent matter and other clinical indicators of burn wound infection.
NOC Risk Control.

Infection Prevention
1. Practice universal precautions to reduce the risk of transmission of microorganisms. Contact isolation measures as appropriate.
2. Recommend sequestration of patients with methicillin-resistant *Staphylococcus aureus*, vancomycin-resistant enterococci, or other multidrug-resistant organisms.
3. Administer TIG or Tt, as prescribed.
4. Assess burn wound daily for signs of infection.
5. Report to the physician if:
   - fever is greater than 39° C (102.2° F), or temperature is less than 35° C (95° F),
   - elevated or decreased WBC count,
   - change in color or odor of wound exudate and purulent material, and
   - signs of wound deterioration: loss of previously healed wounds, disappearance of a well-defined burn margin with edema formation, and hemorrhagic discoloration.
6. Wash burn wound with a mild soap and rinse thoroughly with water.
7. Except for eyebrows, shave all hair within burn wound to prevent wound contamination on a daily basis. Eyebrows are left in place because if shaved, may not grow back, or the new growth may appear distorted. This practice continues until wound closure.
8. Administer antipyretic and antimicrobial agents, as prescribed. Ensure aseptic technique when administering care to burned areas and performing invasive techniques.
9. Assess appearance of graft sites, including adherence to recipient bed, appearance, color, and odor. Be alert to erythema, hyperthermia, increasing tenderness, purulent drainage, and swelling around the grafted site.
10. Assess all invasive lines and devices (e.g., urinary catheters) daily. Review necessity with prompt removal of unnecessary lines and devices.
11. For patients with a central line, implement the IHI central line bundle:
    - Hand hygiene.

Burns

- Maximal barrier precautions upon insertion.
- Chlorhexidine skin antisepsis.
- Optimal catheter site selection, with avoidance of the femoral vein in adult patients.
- Daily review of line necessity with prompt removal of unnecessary lines.

12. Observe for clinical indicators of sepsis: tachypnea, hypothermia, hyperthermia, ileus, subtle disorientation, unexplained metabolic acidosis, low platelet count, feeding intolerance, and glucose intolerance. If sepsis is suspected, obtain wound, blood, sputum, and urine culture specimens as prescribed.

NIC Environmental Management; Infection Control; Infection Protection; Surveillance; Wound Care; Shock Management.

Acute pain *related to burn injury and treatment*

Goals/Outcomes: Within 30 minutes of treatment/intervention, the patient's subjective evaluation of discomfort improves and/or nonverbal indicators of discomfort are absent or diminished.
NOC Pain Control.

Pain Assessment and Management

1. Assess the patient's level of discomfort at frequent intervals. Patients with partial-thickness burns may experience severe pain because of damage and exposure of sensory nerve endings. Pain tolerance often decreases with prolonged hospitalization, multiple painful procedures, and sleep deprivation.
2. Monitor the patient for clinical indicators of pain: increased BP/MAP, tachypnea, shivering, rigid muscle tone, or guarded position. Pain assessment using observational tools may be required for preverbal children or those requiring intubation and sedation.
3. For verbal children (generally children older than 3 years), adolescents, and adults, use age-appropriate self-reporting pain assessment tools.
4. Assess preinjury coping abilities.
5. Administer opioid analgesia and anxiolytics, as prescribed. Time dosage for optimal effectiveness before painful procedures.
6. Provide simple explanations of all procedures.
7. Employ adjunctive nonpharmacologic interventions, as indicated (relaxation breathing, guided imagery, distraction, and music therapy).
8. If possible, avoid wound care procedures during sleeping hours.
9. Ensure that the patient receives periods of uninterrupted sleep by grouping care procedures when possible.

NIC Analgesic Administration; Anxiety Reduction; Environmental Management: Comfort; Pain Assessment and Management.

Impaired tissue integrity *related to burn injury; edema*

Goals/Outcomes: The patient's wound exhibits evidence of healing. Wound healing occurs without hypertrophic scarring (late outcome finding).
Note: Healing time varies with the extent and depth of injury.
NOC Tissue Integrity: Skin and Mucous Membranes.

Healing

1. Assess and document extent and depth of burn wound (see Table 3-6).
2. Cleanse and débride the wound, as prescribed.
3. Apply topical antimicrobial treatments, as prescribed, using aseptic technique.
4. Elevate burned extremities at or above heart level to facilitate venous return and reduce edema formation and risk for compartment syndrome.

For patients with skin grafts:

5. Help prevent graft loss if fluid collection beneath graft occurs. Notify the burn surgeon. Small fluid collections should be removed; if caught early and removed, will allow for graft readherence.
6. Monitor type and amount of drainage from wounds. Promptly report the presence of bright red bleeding, which would inhibit graft take, or purulent exudate, which indicates infection.
7. Maintain immobility of grafted site for 3 to 5 days or as prescribed. This is achieved with a combination of positioning, splinting, or light pressure and sedation. In some instances, bulky or occlusive dressings may be required to maintain immobilization and promote hemostasis of graft.

8. Apply elastic wraps, as prescribed, to legs that have grafts and/or donor sites to promote venous return and to promote graft adherence when out of bed.
9. Provide donor site care, as prescribed, and be alert to signs of donor site infection.
10. Teach the patient about need for compression to prevent bleeding and to promote graft adherence.

NIC Infection Protection; Positioning; Wound Care.

Ineffective tissue perfusion: gastrointestinal *related to hypovolemia and interruption in blood flow associated with splanchnic vasoconstriction secondary to fluid shifts and catecholamine release.*

Goals/Outcomes: The patient has adequate GI tissue perfusion, as evidenced by auscultation of bowel sounds within 48 to 72 hours after burn injury; bowel elimination and appetite within the patient's normal pattern; and absence of nausea and vomiting.

| **Safety Alert** | *Be aware that prolonged impaired perfusion to gastrointestinal organs increases the likelihood of complications such as impaired gastric motility, adynamic ileus, gastritis, and gastric ulcer development.* |

NOC Tissue Perfusion: Abdominal Organs.

Gastrointestinal Intubation
1. Assess bowel function every 2 to 4 hours. Identify abdominal distention and decreasing or absent bowel sounds, which occur with adynamic ileus or abdominal compartment syndrome. Consider bladder pressure monitoring; notify the physician if pressures reach 20 mm Hg.
2. During period of absent bowel sounds, maintain gastric tube to intermittent low suction as prescribed. Check at intervals to ensure patency and position of the tube. Before removing tube, clamp for several hours to be certain that the patient has sufficient GI motility. Abdominal distention, nausea, vomiting, or return of a large volume of gastric contents when tube is reconnected indicates insufficient motility to tolerate tube removal.
3. Maintain NPO status until return of bowel sounds. Provide mouth care for comfort and hygiene.
4. Administer PPIs, H$_2$-receptor antagonists, and other agents prescribed to reduce formation of gastric acids. If prescribed, start enteral feedings.
5. Test gastric aspirate for occult blood, as indicated, and report to the physician.

NIC Gastrointestinal Intubation; Hemodynamic Regulation; Nutrition Management; Tube Care: Gastrointestinal.

Imbalanced nutrition: less than body requirements of protein, vitamins, and calories *related to hypermetabolic state.*

Goals/Outcomes: The patient has adequate nutrition, as evidenced by stable weight (following resuscitation period), balanced nitrogen state per nitrogen tests, serum albumin 3.5 g/dL, thyroxine-binding prealbumin 20 to 30 mg/dL, retinol-binding protein 4 to 5 mg/dL, and evidence of continued burn wound healing and graft take.
NOC Nutritional Status.

Nutrition Management
1. Collaborate with the physician and dietitian to estimate the patient's metabolic needs on the basis of injury extent, dry weight, and nutritional status before injury.
2. Consider the patient's specific injuries, ability to consume diet, and preexisting medical condition when planning nutrition.
3. Provide diet as prescribed. When the patient can take foods orally, promote supplemental feedings/snacks between meals.
4. Consider placement of a soft Silastic feeding tube for provision of enteral tube feedings for those who are unable to meet their caloric and protein requirements orally.
5. Recognize that opioids decrease GI motility and may cause nausea and vomiting.
6. Administer medications to prevent/treat opioid-associated GI complications (constipation, decrease in GI motility).
7. Recognize that patients with an ileus that persists for longer than 4 days or those unable to meet caloric needs enterally may require total parenteral nutrition.

Burns

8. Record all intake for daily calorie counts.
9. Monitor the patient's weight. Minimize error by weighing the patient without dressings or splints, if possible.
10. Monitor markers of nutritional status: serum albumin, thyroxine-binding prealbumin, retinol-binding protein, and urine nitrogen measurements. Long periods of catabolism cause these serum values to decrease. Be alert to measures of protein deficiencies, weight loss, and poor wound healing, all of which are signals that nutritional needs are not being met.

NIC Nutrition Management; Nutrition Therapy; Nutrition Monitoring.

Fear *related to potentially threatening situation (e.g., serious injury, hospitalization) and supported by presence of pain, unfamiliarity, and noxious environmental stimuli present in critical care area; communication barrier (e.g., intubation); sensory impairment from direct injuries.*

Goals/Outcomes: The patient exhibits decreased symptoms of fear: apprehension, tension, nervousness, tachycardia, aggressiveness, and withdrawal.
NOC Fear Control.

Anxiety Reduction
1. Assess level of fear and understanding of present condition.
2. Plan care to provide as restful an environment as possible.
3. Provide information regarding nursing care, treatment plan, and progress. It is often necessary to repeat information because injury, stress, and fear can interfere with comprehension.
4. Promote visits by family members and significant others.
5. Offer to consult hospital spiritual care or the patient's clergy as desired by the patient.
6. Assess and promote the patient's usual coping strategies. Consult with a psychologist for assistance.
7. Provide referral to burn survivor support groups.

NIC Coping Enhancement; Security Enhancement; Support System Enhancement.

Disturbed sensory perception: tactile and visual *related to altered reception secondary to medications, sleep pattern disturbance, pain, swollen eyelids, and full-thickness burn wound.*

Goals/Outcomes: The patient verbalizes orientation to time, place, and person and describes rationale (age-appropriate understanding) for necessary treatments.
NOC Vision Compensation Behavior: Cognitive Orientation.

Sensory Perception Management
1. Assess the patient's orientation to time, place, and person using age-appropriate questions.
2. Answer the patient's questions simply and succinctly, providing information regarding immediate surroundings, procedures, and treatments. Anticipate the necessity of having to repeat information at frequent intervals.
3. For the patient with cutaneous burn injury, explain why tactile sensation is decreased or absent. If the patient's eyelids are swollen shut because of facial edema, reassure the patient that he or she is not blind and that swelling will resolve within 3 to 5 days. Apply eye lubricant, as prescribed, for those patients with excessive swelling and/or inhibited blink.
4. Touch the patient on unburned skin to provide nonpainful tactile stimulation.
5. Explain that alterations in perception can be related to opioids and other medications commonly prescribed during the acute phase of burn recovery.

NIC Peripheral Sensation Management; Surveillance: Safety; Communication Enhancement: Visual Deficit; Environmental Management.

Risk for disuse syndrome *related to immobilization from pain, splints, or scar formation.*

Goals/Outcomes: The patient displays complete ROM without verbal or nonverbal indicators of discomfort.
NOC Risk Control.

Positioning
1. Provide ROM exercises every 4 hours while awake. When possible, combine when medicated with analgesics for other procedures and during activities of daily living.
2. Apply splints, as prescribed, to maintain extremities in functional position and to prevent contracture formation.
3. For the patient with grafts, institute ROM exercises and ambulation on prescribed postgrafting day (often 3 to 7 days postgrafting). Premedicate with analgesic to aid in mobility and reduce discomfort.

NIC Exercise Therapy: Ambulation; Exercise Therapy: Joint Mobility; Exercise Promotion; Nutrition Management.

Disturbed body image *related to biophysical changes secondary to burn injury.*

Goals/Outcomes: The patient begins to acknowledge body changes and demonstrates movement toward incorporating changes into self-concept.
NOC Body Image.

Body Image Enhancement
1. Assess the patient's perceptions and feelings about the burn injury and changes in lifestyle and relationships, especially those with significant others.
2. Involve significant others in as much care as possible to maintain bond with the patient.
3. Respect the patient's need to express anger over body changes.
4. Consider consultation with a rehabilitation psychologist and/or child life therapy.
5. Provide information concerning eventual appearance of grafts and donor sites.
6. Provide names and telephone numbers of local and national support groups for burn survivors: the American Burn Association, National Headquarters Office, website: www.ameriburn.org, phone: (312) 642-9260; the Phoenix Society for Burn Survivors, Inc., National Headquarters Office, website: www.phoenix-society.org, phone: (800) 888-2876.

NIC Anxiety Reduction; Coping Enhancement; Grief Work Facilitation; Self-Esteem Enhancement; Support System Enhancement.

Deficient knowledge *related to lack of knowledge regarding ability for self-care management and/or use of resources for supportive care.*

Goals/Outcomes: Within 24 hours of initiation of acute care, the patient and significant others verbalize knowledge about prescribed medications and techniques that facilitate continued wound healing and limb mobility.
NOC Knowledge: Medication; Knowledge: Treatment Regimen.

Teaching: Disease Process
1. Review the splinting and exercise program for contracture prevention, as directed by the physical therapist.
2. Teach the patient and significant others to monitor for pain or pressure caused by improperly applied splint and to assess splinted extremity for coolness, pallor, cyanosis, decreased pulses, and impaired function.
3. Discuss current skin and wound care plan.
4. Explain indicators of wound infection.
5. Review nutritional needs.
6. Review current pain and anxiolytic medications.

NIC Learning Facilitation; Learning Readiness Enhancement; *Teaching:* Individual.

ADDITIONAL NURSING DIAGNOSES

For other nursing diagnoses and interventions, see the following, as appropriate: Nutrition Support, (Chapter 1); Mechanical Ventilation, (Chapter 1); Prolonged Immobility, (Chapter 1); Compartment Syndrome/Ischemic Myositis, (Chapter 3); Emotional and Spiritual Support of the Patient and Significant Others, (Chapter 2).

Burns

COMPARTMENT SYNDROME/ISCHEMIC MYOSITIS

PATHOPHYSIOLOGY

Compartment syndrome is caused by pathologic elevation of intercompartmental pressures within nonexpansible tissue envelopes. The pressure increase may come from either an increase in volume within a tissue compartment or externally applied pressure compressing a tissue compartment. While pressure within the anatomic space increases, local perfusion is compromised, leading, if untreated, to irreversible damage of the tissues within the compartment. Compartment syndrome is a surgical emergency that requires rapid intervention to prevent permanent cosmetic or functional deformity or loss of limb. Compartment syndrome may be acute or chronic (exercise-related forms); this section focuses on the acute peripheral type.

Most compartment syndromes are associated with trauma, but the condition may also occur from multiple other etiologies including reperfusion injuries, ischemia, burns, prolonged limb compression, drug abuse, or poor positioning during prolonged surgical procedures (Table 3-8). The incidence of compartment syndrome in those younger than 35 years is increased probably secondary to the larger muscle mass contained within the osteofascial space.

Any muscle may be affected as long as the pressure within a muscle is sustained for a prolonged period of time. Most often the muscles affected are those that are contained within an osteofascial space in the upper or lower extremity. The most common site in the upper arm is the forearm. The forearm contains two compartments: the volar and dorsal. The volar compartment contains the flexors of the wrist and fingers and the dorsal compartment contains the extensors. The lower extremity contains a total of seven compartments: three in the thigh and four in the calf. The three compartments of the thigh are the anterior, posterior, and medial. The calf compartments are the anterior, lateral/peroneal, deep posterior, and superficial posterior. The tibial nerve lies within the posterior compartment and provides sensation to the plantar surface of the foot and flexion of the toes. The anterior compartment contains the peroneal nerve providing sensation to the first web space and motor function of the extensors of the calf and foot. The anterior compartment of the calf is the most common site of compartment syndrome.

Increased and sustained pressure within a muscle compartment can develop because of increased volume in the compartment from a hematoma or edema. A second etiology is

Table 3-8	CAUSES OF COMPARTMENT SYNDROME		
Localized Compartmental Trauma	**Tissue Reaction/Edema Formation**	**Coagulation Defects**	**Other**
Fractures Surgery Hematoma Venomous bites (snake, spider) Vascular injury Postischemic swelling Crush injuries Electrical injuries	Prolonged use of operative tourniquets Arterial or venous obstruction Limb reimplantation Burns (especially when circumferential) Excessive exercise (e.g., march gangrene) Nephrotic syndrome	Hemophilia Anticoagulant therapy	Compression during obtundation (anesthesia, drug overdose) Infiltrated IV therapy Constrictive dressings, inflatable splints or casts Closure of fascial defects Hypothermia or hyperthermia *Clostridium perfringens* infections Rocky Mountain spotted fever Use of pneumatic antishock garment Hypovolemia Hypotension

Modified from Callahan J: Compartment syndrome. *Orthop Nurs* 4:11-15, 1985.

prolonged ischemia, which may be as a result of external compression or arterial compromise. Finally, compartment syndrome may be caused by decreased overall size of the muscle compartment from scar formation, especially following circumferential burns (see Table 3-8).

Regardless of the etiology or location, ischemia begins when the metabolic demands of the tissues cannot be met. The normal pressure in muscle compartments is less than 10 to 12 mm Hg. Whitesides' theory states that the development of compartment syndrome depends on both the intracompartmental pressure and the systemic BP. The diastolic BP minus the compartmental pressure should be greater than 30 mm Hg to avoid ischemia in the tissues. Thus, increasing the compartmental pressure or decreasing the perfusion pressure can each lead to a compartment syndrome.

When injury occurs, the depletion of intracellular energy stores causes cellular swelling and increasing venous pressures, allowing edema to develop and local blood flow to decrease. Lymphatic drainage initially increases and then decreases as a result of congestion from the growing tissue edema. Compartmental tissue pressure increases, compromising capillary blood flow. Histamine is released, producing vasodilation and increased capillary permeability. Rising compartmental pressure further increases venous congestion and results in reduction in the arteriovenous pressure gradient, reducing local tissue perfusion and further increasing capillary pressure. Fluids and proteins escape from the capillaries and contribute to even higher tissue pressures. The higher tissue pressures eventually exceed both capillary and venous pressures, stopping nutrient blood flow and promoting further ischemia. Local blood flow to muscles is severely compromised when the interstitial tissue pressure equals or exceeds the diastolic pressure. As a result of impaired venous return, anaerobic metabolism creates more lactic acid, which stimulates vasodilation further, decreasing BP and elevating tissue pressure. The pressure within the compartment continues to increase, equaling or exceeding the capillary pressure and leading to arteriolar compression, causing further ischemia of the muscle and nerves.

Sustained hypotension and shock are associated with greater incidence of compartment syndrome resulting from the lowered pressure gradient. Less compartmental pressure is needed to result in arteriolar spasm and ischemic changes in the muscles.

The earliest signs of compartment syndrome are often subtle but are primarily neurologic as a result of the susceptibility to hypoxia of the nonmyelinated sensory fibers. Sensory changes in the extremity begin with paresthesias or hyperesthesias within 30 minutes of the onset of ischemia and may become functionally irreversible after 12 to 24 hours. The average interval between the initial injury to the compartment and the beginning symptoms of compartment syndrome is 2 hours. Compartmental tissue ischemia that lasts longer than 6 hours results in muscle necrosis and irreversible tissue changes.

Late-onset compartment syndrome is seen in patients who are comatose or confused and who are unable to communicate symptoms. Late-onset compartment syndrome is often more difficult to recognize and manage, sometimes worsening following treatment with fasciotomy. The late syndrome may occur in compartments already treated with fasciotomy. Healthy granulation tissue may cover necrotic muscle within partially opened compartments. With sufficient muscle tissue injury (e.g., after crush injuries) or undiagnosed compartment syndrome, rhabdomyolysis may develop with the release of metabolic toxin and intracellular components, especially myoglobin. The release of toxins can result in secondary myoglobinemia, leading to acute tubular necrosis, which may progress to acute kidney injury and multisystem failure.

COMPARTMENT SYNDROME ASSESSMENT
GOAL OF ASSESSMENT
The goals are to prevent ischemia and reduce long-term sequelae by earlier diagnosis and treatment through reduction in internal or external pressure.

HISTORY AND RISK FACTORS
* Any patient with a peripheral injury listed in Table 3-8 is at risk for compartment syndrome.
* Patients admitted for acute renal failure after treatment for crush injuries or compartment syndrome should be suspected of having late-onset or continuing compartment syndrome.

- Patients with profound shock who receive aggressive fluid resuscitation are at risk for acute compartment syndrome.

VITAL SIGNS
- Hypotension potentiates compartment syndrome.

OBSERVATION AND SUBJECTIVE SYMPTOMS

Early indicators
- Unusually severe pain for an injury is a cardinal symptom. Passive stretch of an involved muscle group significantly increases the pain.

Late-onset syndrome indicators
- Persistent peripheral edema or continued elevation of tissue pressures even after fasciotomy.
- If compartment syndrome is not treated, the necrosing muscles become fibrotic and contract and can no longer function (e.g., Volkmann ischemic contracture).
- Late decompression fasciotomy seldom restores lost myoneural function. Early recognition is the key to successful management and preservation of function.
- Extreme pain is out of proportion to the injury.
- Increased pain occurs on passive ROM (stretch) of the affected extremity.

Late findings
- Paresthesias (early loss of vibratory sensation).
- Pallor of the extremity.
- Paralysis.

PALPATION
- Feel for temperature of affected area; polar (coolness) of affected area is a late sign.
- Palpation of the compartment reveals tension and slowed capillary refill.
- Assess pulses in all extremities; pulselessness is a late sign.

Diagnostic Tests for Compartment Syndrome		
Test	**Purpose**	**Abnormal Findings**
Blood Chemistry: Creatine phosphokinase	Elevation is caused by the release of the enzyme by the injured muscle tissue.	Continued elevation in the course of treatment may indicate late-onset compartment syndrome. Extensive muscle necrosis may lead to myoglobinemia and myoglobinuria, and may lead to rhabdomyolysis. Blood urea nitrogen and creatinine levels will be elevated if acute renal failure results from rhabdomyolysis.
Serum creatine kinase (CK)-MM	CK-MM isoenzyme is most specific for skeletal muscle damage. Serum CK levels begin increasing 2 to 12 hours after the onset of muscle injury. They peak within 1 to 3 days and decrease 3 to 5 days after muscle injury ceases.	In compartment syndrome, CK levels may rise as high as 100,000 units/L. Levels greater than 2000 units/L raise the possibility of muscle damage. CK values greater than 2000 units/L after surgery can be a warning sign of acute compartment syndrome in patients who are ventilated and sedated.

Diagnostic Tests for Compartment Syndrome — cont'd

Test	Purpose	Abnormal Findings
Intracompartmental pressure monitoring	Compartment pressure and associated critical values may be monitored intermittently by inserting needles (pressure within 10 to 30 mm Hg of diastolic blood pressure), which get obstructed by muscle tissue. Continuous infusion catheters (pressure >45 mm Hg) and wick or slit catheters (>30 to 35 mm Hg) monitor continuously via fluid-filled catheters and pressure monitors. In patients who are hypotensive and at higher risk for compartment syndrome, the delta pressure should be calculated. Delta pressure equals mean arterial pressure minus compartmental pressure.	Delta pressures of ≤30 mm Hg for 6 hours or ≤40 mm Hg for 8 hours require prompt consultation with the physician. Pressures warranting fasciotomy vary with clinical indicators, the patient's systemic condition, and measurement technique.
Near-infrared spectroscopy (NIRS)	Based on the different light absorption properties, NIRS can measure the local changes in concentration of oxygenated and deoxygenated hemoglobin and perfusion in different tissues including muscle.	More studies are needed, but NIRS may provide the benefit of a rapid, continuous, noninvasive, sensitive, and specific tool for early detection of acute compartment syndrome.
Ultrasound: pulsed phase–locked loop (PPLL)	More investigation is needed to determine effectiveness. The PPLL ultrasound locks on to a characteristic reflection that comes from a specific tissue and can detect the very subtle movements of fascia that correspond to local arterial pulsation.	Increased intracompartmental pressure during compartment syndrome causes a reduction in normal fascial displacements in response to arterial pulsation.
Scintigraphy	Radionuclide imaging that shows the physiologic function of the system being investigated as opposed to its anatomy.	Can study all compartments of an extremity at once but limited usefulness because of inability to study over time.
Pulse oximetry	Assesses perfusion of distal tissues. Readings should be compared with readings from a contralateral, uninvolved extremity.	Decreased perfusion will result in lower pulse oximetry measurements but may not be decreased until significant time and injury has occurred. Pulse oximetry cannot measure intracompartmental tissue oxygen saturation and requires adequate pulsatile flow.
Magnetic resonance imaging (MRI)	MRI is useful in detecting soft tissue edema on T1 images.	MRI cannot differentiate the edema from trauma with edema from a compartment syndrome in the acute phases and thus is of limited value in diagnosis in the acute phase. MRI is useful in identifying the tissue changes in an established compartment syndrome in a very late stage.

Continued

Diagnostic Tests for Compartment Syndrome—cont'd		
Test	**Purpose**	**Abnormal Findings**
Arteriograms and venograms	Radiologic examination of blood vessels may be performed when embolus, thrombus, or other vascular injury is indicated.	

COMPARTMENTAL PRESSURE MONITORING

Compartmental pressure monitoring continues to be the preferred method of definitive diagnosis of acute compartment syndrome. Several methods of direct compartment measurement exist including the needle manometer, the wick catheter, and the slit catheter. Continuous readings are not possible with the needle manometer method and may result in falsely high levels caused by the injection of saline into the muscle. Pressures within compartments may be continuously monitored with either the wick method or the slit catheter method by attaching a pressure transducer to an implanted catheter within a muscle compartment. Indications for continuous or intermittent pressure monitoring are in the patient who is unconscious, children or other patients difficult to assess, patients with nerve injury, and those with multiple orthopedic traumas. Regardless of technique, compartmental pressures greater than 30 mm Hg above the systemic diastolic pressure indicate the need for a compartment fasciotomy.

Early indicators
- Palpation of the compartment reveals tension and slowed capillary refill.
- Tissue pressures vary with the method of measurement. Generally, normal tissue pressures vary from 10 to 12 mm Hg, and sustained pressures greater than 30 mm Hg above the systemic diastolic pressure result in tissue necrosis.
- The thin-walled lower extremity veins may collapse at lower pressures, further contributing to the pathogenesis.

COLLABORATIVE MANAGEMENT

CARE PRIORITIES
1. Eliminate external pressure on the affected compartment
Identify and relieve circumferential constriction: Loosen or remove circumferential casts and padding or dressings; escharotomy for circumferential burns or frostbite.

2. Manage pain
Analgesia: Parenteral opiates often with sedative adjuncts.

3. Reduce internal compartmental pressure
IV hypertonic mannitol: Used as a preventive measure to reduce compartmental pressure via systemic diuresis and to help the kidneys excrete the large molecules of myoglobin if extensive tissue necrosis is present. This diuresis may potentiate more ischemia if the patient is hypovolemic.

4. Provide surgical intervention
Fasciotomy of myofascial compartment: The goal of treatment of acute compartment syndrome is to decrease tissue pressure, restore blood flow, and minimize tissue damage.
- Treatment of choice to accomplish these goals is a surgical fasciotomy to allow unrestricted swelling. The affected compartment alone may be opened but, more commonly, adjacent or all tissue compartments in the area are prophylactically incised. In the forearm, a volar aspect fasciotomy is most common. In the thigh, a lateral incision can decompress at three compartments, and in the calf, a lateral fasciotomy expansible to release all compartments or medial and lateral incisions is generally adequate.
- Persistent peripheral edema with elevated creatine phosphokinase, or the presence of acute renal failure, may justify reexploration and wide excision of all necrotic muscle in involved and adjacent compartments.

- Complications of fasciotomy include wound infection, the potential for osteomyelitis, and large scars.
- Secondary wound closure may be accomplished after 3 to 4 days once the compartmental pressure has returned to normal. Multiple methods of wound closure have been used, including mechanical closure devices, dynamic skin sutures, vacuum-assisted closure, and healing by secondary intention.
- Skin grafting may be needed to ensure complete coverage of the exposed compartments.

5. Provide vascular surgical intervention if blood vessel injury caused the compartment syndrome

Treat vascular injury: The involved blood vessel is explored and treated.
- Papaverine, a vasodilating drug that relaxes smooth muscle, can be injected in a bolus of fluid to reestablish normal internal artery dynamics.
- Blood vessel lacerations can be repaired or severely damaged vessels can be resected.

6. Renal protection

- Ischemia that persists for at least 4 hours causes significant myoglobinuria, which peaks approximately 3 hours following restoration of the circulation. Myoglobinuria can persist for up to 12 hours. When rhabdomyolysis is apparent, aggressive IV fluid administration and, possibly, bicarbonate may be administered to maintain urine output at 1 to 2 mL/kg/h.
- A combination of myoglobinemia, hypovolemia, and acidemia may lead to acute renal failure. Alkalization of the urine coupled with diuresis may be renal protective because hemoglobin and myoglobin are more soluble in an alkaline solution. Patients with trauma who generally survive recover renal function, including patients who require extended support using hemodialysis. Current recommendations include:
  - Manage hypovolemia with crystalloid solution.
  - Administer 500 mL/h IV crystalloid solution and 22.4 mEq bicarbonate (total 12 L/day, prompting diuresis of approximately 8 L/day).
  - If urine output is less than 300 mL/h, one dose of mannitol 1 g/kg IV is given.
  - For a pH greater than 7.45, acetazolamide, 250 mg, is administered IV.
  - Vital signs, urine pH level, and volume are monitored hourly.
  - Osmolarity, electrolytes, and ABG values are evaluated every 6 hours.

CARE PLANS: COMPARTMENT SYNDROME

Ineffective tissue perfusion (or risk for same): peripheral (compartment) *related to interruption of capillary blood flow secondary to increased pressure within the anatomic compartment.*

Goals/Outcomes: Throughout the hospitalization, the patient has adequate perfusion to compartment tissues, as evidenced by brisk (less than 2 seconds) capillary refill, peripheral pulses greater than 2+ on a 0-to-4+ scale, normal tissue pressures (0 to 10 mm Hg), and absence of edema or tautness. Within 2 hours of admission, the patient verbalizes understanding of reporting symptoms of impaired neurovascular status.

NOC Circulation Status.

Circulatory Precautions
1. Monitor neurovascular status of injured extremity at least every 2 hours.
2. Assess for increased pain on passive extension or flexion of the digits.
3. Monitor for sluggish capillary refill, decrease in or loss of two-point discrimination, increasing limb edema, and tautness over individual compartments.
4. Use pulse oximetry to help assess distal tissue perfusion and report significant differences from oximetry readings taken from the uninvolved contralateral extremity.
5. Assess for the six "Ps":
   - Pain (especially on passive digital movement and with pressure over the compartment).
   - Pallor.
   - Polar (coolness).
   - Pulselessness.
   - Paresthesia.
   - Paralysis.

6. Report deficits in neurovascular status promptly.
7. Loosen circumferential dressings as indicated.
8. Educate the patient about the symptoms to be promptly reported: severe, unrelieved pain; paresthesias (diminished sensation, hyperesthesia, or anesthesia); paralysis; coolness; or pulselessness.
9. Monitor tissue pressures continuously, with an intracompartmental pressure device if needed.
10. Consult the advanced practice provider if pressures exceed normal or preestablished levels or if the patient manifests brown urine indicative of myoglobinuria.

HIGH ALERT! Pressures greater than 10 mm Hg may reflect significant elevation. Myoglobinuria may indicate that rhabdomyolysis has ensued, which if not immediately managed may lead to acute renal failure.

11. Monitor closely for additional tissue injury if the patient becomes hypotensive.

NIC Cast Care: Maintenance; Heat/Cold Application; Peripheral Sensation Management; Shock Management; Skin Surveillance; Teaching: Disease Process.

Acute pain *related to physical factors (tissue ischemia) secondary to compartment syndrome.*

Goals/Outcomes: Throughout the hospitalization, the patient's pain is controlled, as reflected by a pain scale. Nonverbal indicators of discomfort (e.g., grimacing) are reduced or absent. Within 2 hours of admission, the patient verbalizes understanding of the need to report uncontrolled or increasing pain.
NOC Pain Control; Comfort Level.

Pain Management
1. Assess for pain: onset, duration, progression, and intensity. Devise a pain scale with the patient, rating discomfort "0" for no pain to "10" for unbearable pain. Patients who are noncommunicative or of low-level intellect may require a simpler or different pain scale.
2. Determine if passive stretching of digits and pressure over limb compartments increases the pain. Both may indicate early compartment syndrome.
3. Adjust the medication regimen to the patient's needs; document medication effectiveness.
4. Promptly report uncontrolled pain.
5. Prevent pressure from being applied on involved compartment and neurovascular structures.
6. Following a fasciotomy, pain that remains unrelieved may indicate that the fasciotomy is incomplete.
7. Pain that increases several days after a fasciotomy may signal compartmental infection.
8. Continue to monitor neurovascular function with each vital sign check to assess for recurring compartment syndrome or infection.

NIC Analgesic Administration; Anxiety Reduction; Coping Enhancement; Progressive Muscle Relaxation; Simple Guided Imagery.

Risk for infection *related to inadequate primary defenses secondary to necrotic tissue, wide excision fasciotomy, and open wound.*

Goals/Outcomes: Throughout the hospitalization the patient is free of infection, as evidenced by normothermia, WBC count less than 11,000/mm³, and absence of wound erythema and other clinical indicators of infection. Within 24 hours of admission, the patient verbalizes understanding of the need to promptly report any indicators of infection.
NOC Risk Control; Wound Healing: Primary Intention.

Infection Protection
1. Monitor the patient for fever, increasing pain, and laboratory data indicative of infection (e.g., increased WBC count or erythrocyte sedimentation rate).
2. Assess exposed wounds for erythema, increasing wound drainage, purulent wound drainage, increasing wound circumference, edema, and localized tenderness.
3. Assess neurovascular deficits, which may signal infection or pressure in adjacent inflamed tissues.
4. After primary closure or grafting of wound, assess for signs of infection beneath the closure.
5. Assess for chronic infection and osteomyelitis; key complications of compartment syndrome.

6. Instruct the patient to report the following indicators of infection: fever, localized warmth, increasing pain, increasing wound drainage (especially if purulent), swelling, and redness.
7. Consult with the advanced practice provider promptly regarding significant findings.

NIC Environmental Management; Medication Management; Surveillance; Vital Signs Monitoring; Wound Care; Wound Care: Closed Drainage.

Disturbed body image *related to physical changes secondary to large, irregular fasciotomy wound and skin-grafted scar; loss of function in or change in appearance of an extremity; or amputation.*

Goals/Outcomes: Within the 24-hour period before discharge from ICU, the patient acknowledges body changes and demonstrates movement toward incorporating changes into self-concept. The patient does not exhibit maladaptive response (e.g., severe depression) to wound or functional loss.
NOC Body Image; Self-Esteem.

Body Image Enhancement
1. Discuss compartment syndrome, therapeutic interventions, and long-term effects.
2. Provide time for the patient to share feelings about his or her changed appearance and function. Encourage questions and discussion of these feelings with the patient's significant others.
3. Help the patient set realistic goals for recovery.
4. Facilitate progression through the grieving process, as appropriate.
5. Recognize when patient is ready to view or discuss the injury. Adjustment time varies.
6. Encourage self-care. Provide necessary adjunctive aids (e.g., built-up utensils, button hooks, orthotics) to facilitate independence in activities of daily living.
7. Collaborate with the advanced practice provider for patients with functional loss or amputation, introduce use of orthotics and adjunctive devices to facilitate self-care.

NIC Active Listening; Amputation Care; Anxiety Reduction; Coping Enhancement; Emotional Support; Self-Care Assistance; Wound Care.

DROWNING

INCIDENCE
Drowning accounts for over 4000 deaths annually in the United States according to the Centers for Disease Control and Prevention and 388,000 deaths worldwide according to the World Health Organization, making drowning the third leading cause of unintentional deaths worldwide. The highest mortality rates are in children younger than 5 years of age; drowning occurs more frequently among males than females.

PATHOPHYSIOLOGY
Drowning is defined as a process of experiencing respiratory impairment from submersion/immersion in a liquid by the World Health Organization. The terms *drowning* and *near-drowning* are often used to distinguish between individuals who die within 24 hours of the drowning incident and those who live 24 hours or longer following the incident (termed "near-drowning"). Individuals classified as "near-drowning" may eventually die from the submersion/immersion. Healthcare providers cannot always determine who will die within the first 24 hours. Both populations receive the same treatment. The 2010 American Heart Association guidelines support these definitions to maintain consistency in the reporting of data related to drowning. A current term used to describe patients who survive a submersion is *nonfatal drowning*.

The main effects of drowning are decreased lung compliance, ventilator-perfusion mismatch, and intrapulmonary shunting leading to hypoxemia and decreased oxygen delivery to the tissues, which can lead to failure of multiple organs, most importantly, the CNS. Hypotension, pulmonary edema, hypothermia, and respiratory and metabolic acidosis occur after nonfatal drowning, compounding the detrimental effects of the hypoxemia. In addition to the neurologic deficits from cerebral anoxia, acute lung injury or acute respiratory distress syndrome, pneumonia, acute renal failure secondary to acute tubular necrosis, and DIC can occur. Cervical SCI is not common in nonfatal drowning. Any aspirated contaminants (e.g., algae, chemicals, sand) may cause or contribute to obstruction and lead to asphyxiation. Bacterial pneumonia can develop, depending on the type of contaminant in the aspirant, and chemical pneumonitis can occur if gastric contents were aspirated.

Drowning was formerly categorized by the type of water (freshwater versus saltwater) and whether the person aspirated fluid into the lungs (wet versus dry drowning). These distinctions are thought to be irrelevant in providing care to patients following nonfatal drowning.

WET VERSUS DRY DROWNING

An individual experiencing the drowning process will initially attempt to hold their breath. During breath holding there is some degree of laryngospasm that is followed by falling oxygen levels and increasing carbon dioxide levels in the blood. Eventually, the drive to breathe takes over and the individual begins to aspirate fluid into the lung (wet drowning). In individuals with prolonged laryngospasms, oxygen tension drops and the laryngospasm eventually subsides, prompting aspiration of water before cardiac arrest. Other causes of cardiac arrest are possible in individuals found in water without water in their lungs (dry drowning).

FRESHWATER VERSUS SALTWATER DROWNING

Literature previously reported a difference in freshwater drowning versus saltwater drowning. The prevailing thought was that the hypertonic nature of saltwater would cause water to be pulled into the lungs leading to massive pulmonary edema, whereas the hypotonic freshwater entering the lungs would be rapidly absorbed into the circulatory system, causing dilution of electrolytes and volume overload. An individual must aspirate over 11 mL/kg before these effects occur and most victims of drowning aspirate far less. Given how rarely massive aspiration occurs, this distinction is now thought to be unimportant. Both types of drowning result in loss of surfactant leading to noncardiogenic pulmonary edema.

Hypothermia, defined as a drop in core temperature to 33° C (91.4° F) or below, may also occur. Its progression can cause muscle activity and vital functions to cease, resulting in ventricular fibrillation (occurs at approximately 28° C [82.4° F]). These patients must be handled carefully to avoid prompting ventricular dysrhythmias. Hypothermia may protect the brain from permanent anoxic damage by decreasing cerebral metabolism by as much as 50%. The hypothermic protection is dependent on the temperature dropping to the point of slowing cerebral metabolism before the ischemic injury occurring in the brain. This occurs most often with drowning in icy waters or where the victim has been able to stay afloat for a period of time while the temperature drops before being submersed. Because these factors are not often known about the victim, all victims of drowning should receive aggressive initial resuscitation. Resuscitation should be continued until the victim is rewarmed to at least 32° C (89.6° F), because the heart may start beating at that temperature. The adage, "a patient is not dead until warm and dead," describes the need to ensure that proper rewarming has occurred in all patients who are hypothermic before pronouncing them dead. Many medications used during resuscitation are ineffective until the patient is warmed. Resuscitation remains possible after 30 minutes of submersion. Resuscitation efforts frequently should be continued for at least 1 hour.

ASSESSMENT: DROWNING
GOAL OF SYSTEM ASSESSMENT

Evaluate for respiratory and neurologic functioning, as well as determining if concurrent injuries were sustained such as head and/or spinal trauma.

HISTORY AND RISK FACTORS

Age of the victim, inability to swim, submersion time, temperature of the water, degree of water contamination, use of alcohol and/or drugs, associated injuries such as head and spine injuries, underlying medical conditions, and prehospital resuscitation received should all be considered.

VITAL SIGNS

- Temperature may be low if drowning occurred in cold water.
- RR may be elevated or absent if the patient is in arrest.

- Hypotension.
- HR may be increased or decreased depending on the temperature and respiratory status. The patient may also have presenting symptoms including atrial fibrillation, asystole, or ventricular tachycardia/fibrillation.
- RR may be increased with dyspnea or may be absent if arrest has occurred. Absent respiratory effort may indicate a high cervical spinal cord injury (SCI).

OBSERVATION

Evaluate for signs of trauma to head and neck, skin coloring as an indication of hypoxia, signs of neurologic functioning including pupil size and equality and response to stimuli.
- Pink, frothy sputum may indicate pulmonary edema.

PALPATION

- Evaluate skin for temperature, neck for deformities, and head for signs of trauma including swelling.

AUSCULTATION

Evaluate lung fields to identify abnormal breath sounds.
- Decreased breath sounds may indicate a pneumothorax or hemothorax.
- Sucking sound on inspiration may indicate an open pneumothorax.
- Crackles, rhonchi, wheezing.

Diagnostic Tests for Drowning

Test	Purpose	Abnormal Findings
Noninvasive		
Pulse oximetry	Continuous monitoring of oxygen saturation.	$SaO_2 < 95\%$.
Capnometry	Continuous monitoring of ventilation.	Increased.
Blood Studies		
Arterial blood gas analysis	Assess for adequacy of oxygenation and ventilation.	pH <7.35 with increased $PaCO_2$ (>45 mm Hg) indicates respiratory acidosis. Serum bicarbonate <22 mEq/L with a pH <7.35 can indicate metabolic acidosis. Decreased PaO_2 indicates hypoxemia.
Complete blood count White blood cell (WBC) count	Assess for inflammation and infection.	WBCs may be elevated as a result of the inflammatory process that occurs following injury to the tissues and/or infection from exposure to dirty water.
Electrolytes, glucose	Assess for abnormalities resulting from water aspiration.	Electrolyte changes are unusual, will depend on amount of water aspiration. Glucose level may be low.
Blood urea nitrogen (BUN) and creatinine	Assess for renal function.	Increased BUN and creatinine can indicate acute tubular necrosis from the severe hypoxemia that can accompany near-drowning.
Toxicology screen	Determine the degree of alcohol and/or drug usage that can interfere with an accurate neurologic assessment.	Presence of high alcohol level or drug/substance abuse.

Continued

Drowning

Diagnostic Tests for Drowning — cont'd		
Test	Purpose	Abnormal Findings
Radiology		
Chest radiograph	Assess lung fields.	Presence of infiltrates, atelectasis, and pulmonary edema.
Skull radiograph	Assess for fractures.	Linear skull fracture, depressed skull fracture.
Spinal radiographs	Assess for fractures.	Fracture in any bony structure or misalignment of the spinal column.
Computed tomography: head	Assess for head injury.	Presence of blood in the brain matter or dural spaces indicates a head injury. Blurring of the gray and white matter indicates anoxic brain injury.

COLLABORATIVE MANAGEMENT

CARE PRIORITIES

The primary goal of treatment is to restore ventilation and correct hypoxemia and acidosis. Once ventilation is normal, hypoxemia and acidosis may resolve without further treatment; however, many patients, especially those submerged for more than a few minutes may require additional measures. The following treatments may be required:

1. Provide oxygen therapy

Oxygen (100%) is initiated immediately to treat hypoxia and is continued. All patients, including those who are alert with spontaneous ventilation, are at risk for hypoxia and acidosis. Warmed oxygen 40° C to 43° C (104° F to 109.4° F) may be used as part of the rewarming process for patients with hypothermia.

2. Correct hypothermia with rewarming

Warm, moist oxygen 40° C to 43° C (104° F to 109.4° F) may be used to elevate core temperature. Peritoneal and gastric lavage are used for rewarming. Fluid for lavage is warmed to 37° C (98.6° F). The goal is to rewarm as safely and quickly as possible to achieve a normal core temperature. Care must be taken not to rewarm too quickly because blood can pool in the extremities, especially with external rewarming strategies, prompting hypotension. IV fluids should also be warmed to prevent further exacerbation of the hypothermia. Rewarming cannot be safely accomplished as quickly as cooling.

3. Manage ventilation and acid-base balance

Profound metabolic acidosis is treated with sodium bicarbonate, aggressive ventilation, and careful monitoring of arterial pH. If bronchospasm is present, aerosolized bronchodilators such as epinephrine, albuterol, or isoproterenol HCl may be used.

4. Assess for need for endotracheal intubation and mechanical ventilation

Intubation provides a patent airway for patients who are unable to manage secretions. Mechanical ventilation is used to manage respiratory failure resulting from reduced lung compliance, or if for any reason the patient is unable to maintain effective respiratory effort. Patients may require 1.5 to 2 times normal tidal volume at slower rates to allow optimal lung expansion and ventilation of alveoli.

5. Initiate positive end-expiratory pressure

If the patient is unresponsive to high levels of oxygen ($FIO_2 \geq 0.50$ to maintain a $PaO_2 \geq 60$ mm Hg), positive end-expiratory pressure improves oxygenation by preventing the collapse of alveoli during expiration. The pressure keeps alveoli open despite inadequate surfactant. Positive end-expiratory pressure should be removed cautiously, because levels of surfactant can remain low for 48 to 72 hours after a nonfatal drowning.

6. Consider bronchoscopy
To remove aspirated contaminants, if necessary.

7. Assess for the need of extracorporeal membrane oxygenation
Extracorporeal membrane oxygenation (ECMO), if available, may be useful when the patient is unable to maintain good oxygenation despite intubation and mechanical ventilation.

8. Promote neurologic/brain recovery
Depends on the severity of the neurologic impairment. Severe impairment may require ICP monitoring, steroids, osmotic diuretics (e.g., mannitol), and mechanical ventilation. Recent studies have not supported the use of barbiturate coma or therapeutic hypothermia. Avoid hyperthermia resulting from the increase in metabolic demand and potential of further neurologic damage.

9. Manage fluid and electrolyte imbalance
Although uncommon, fluid and electrolyte abnormalities may occur. Usually, no specific therapy is required for minor disturbances. Fluid volume may be replaced with crystalloid solutions (LR or NS).

10. Prevent and/or control infection
Temperature elevation up to 38° C (100.4° F) during the first 24 hours can be a normal response to injury. Antibiotics may be prescribed if fever greater than 38° C (100.4° F) persists for longer than 24 hours after the submersion or the patient develops pneumonia. Use of steroids and prophylactic antibiotics is not recommended.

11. Identify and manage the event that precipitated the drowning
Conditions such as substance abuse, seizure, myocardial infarction, or cervical spine fracture. Cervical spine injuries are uncommon in the victim of nonfatal drowning. Unless the mechanism of injury suggests the possibility of a cervical spine injury, routine cervical spine immobilization is not recommended because of the chance of interfering with airway management.

CARE PLANS: DROWNING
Impaired gas exchange *related to asphyxiation and aspiration*

Goals/Outcomes: Within 12 hours of initiation of treatment, the patient has adequate gas exchange, as evidenced by the following ABG values: PaO_2 greater than 80 mm Hg and $PaCO_2$ less than 45 mm Hg. Within 3 days of treatment, RR is less than 20 breaths/min with normal depth and pattern; breath sounds are clear and bilaterally equal; and the patient is oriented to time, place, and person (depending on degree of permanent neurologic impairment).
NOC Respiratory Status: Gas Exchange.

Respiratory Monitoring
1. Monitor rate, rhythm, and depth of respirations.
2. Note chest movement for symmetry of chest expansion and signs of increased work of breathing such as use of accessory muscles or retraction of intercostal or supraclavicular muscles.
3. Auscultate breath sounds, noting decrease/absent ventilation and presence of adventitious sounds.
4. Determine the need for suctioning by auscultating for crackles and rhonchi over major airways.
5. Monitor the patient's respiratory secretions.
6. Note changes in oxygen saturation (SaO_2), pulse oximetry (SpO_2), end-tidal CO_2 ($ETCO_2$), and ABGs as appropriate.
7. Monitor for increased restlessness or anxiety.
8. If the patient is restless or has unusual somnolence, evaluate for hypoxemia and hypercapnia as appropriate.
9. Monitor chest x-ray results while new films become available.

Oxygen Therapy
1. Administer supplemental oxygen using liter flow and device as ordered.
2. Add humidity as appropriate.

3. Restrict the patient and visitors from smoking while oxygen is in use.
4. Document pulse oximetry with oxygen liter flow in place at time of reading as ordered. Oxygen is a drug; the dose of the drug must be associated with the oxygen saturation reading or the reading is meaningless.
5. Obtain ABGs if the patient experiences behavioral changes or respiratory distress to check for hypoxemia or hypercapnia.
6. Monitor for changes in chest radiograph and breath sounds indicative of oxygen toxicity and absorption atelectasis in patients receiving higher concentrations of oxygen (greater than FIO_2 45%) for longer than 24 hours. The higher the oxygen concentration, the greater is the chance of toxicity. The rapid movement of oxygen molecules across the alveolar capillary membranes can damage the membranes, prompting a syndrome that mimics acute lung injury.
7. Monitor for skin breakdown where oxygen devices are in contact with skin, such as nares and around edges of mask devices.
8. Provide oxygen therapy during transportation and when the patient gets out of bed.

Mechanical Ventilation
1. Monitor for conditions indicating a need for ventilation support.
2. Monitor for impending respiratory failure or signs of pneumonia.
3. Consult with other healthcare personnel in selection of the ventilatory mode.
4. Administer muscle paralyzing agents, sedatives, and narcotics analgesics as appropriate.
5. Monitor for activities that increase oxygen consumption (fever, shivering, seizures, pain, or basic nursing activities) that; may supersede ventilator support settings and cause O_2 desaturation.
6. Monitor the effectiveness of mechanical ventilation on the patient's physiologic and psychological status.
7. Provide the patient with means of communication, if he or she is alert.
8. Monitor adverse effects of mechanical ventilation.
9. Perform routine mouth care.
10. Elevate the head of the bed minimally at 30 degrees.

Hypothermia *related to immersion in cold water*
- -

Goals/Outcomes: Within 24 hours of initiating therapy, the patient's core temperature increases to 35° C to 37° C (95° F to 98.6° F). BP, RR, and HR are normalizing for the patient.
NOC Thermoregulation.

Hypothermia Treatment
1. Monitor the patient's temperature using a low-recording thermometer, if necessary.
2. Institute a continuous core temperature–monitoring device, as appropriate.
3. Monitor for and treat ventricular fibrillation.
4. Minimize stimulation of the patient to avoid precipitating ventricular fibrillation.
5. Institute active external rewarming measures (e.g., warming lights, warmed baths, warmed blankets, forced air warming blankets), as appropriate. Do not attempt surface or external warming until core temperature is within acceptable limits (i.e., 35° C to 37° C [95° F to 98.6° F]). Premature surface rewarming can lead to the return of cold blood to the heart and precipitate an "after drop" in core temperature.
6. Institute active core rewarming techniques (e.g., colonic lavage, hemodialysis, peritoneal dialysis, and extracorporeal blood rewarming), as appropriate.
7. Monitor for rewarming shock.

Risk for infection *related to aspiration*
- -

Goals/Outcomes: The patient is free of infection, as evidenced by body temperature less than 37.5° C (99.5° F) after the first 24 hours, WBC count within normal limits for the patient, clear sputum, and negative culture results.
NOC Infection Severity.

Infection Protection
1. Monitor for signs and symptoms of infection (fever, changes in sputum).
2. Monitor absolute granulocyte count, WBC, and differential results.
3. Obtain cultures, as needed.
4. Encourage deep breathing and coughing, as appropriate.
5. Use aseptic technique when suctioning the secretions.

ADDITIONAL NURSING DIAGNOSES

Also see Posttrauma Syndrome in Major Trauma, see other nursing diagnoses and interventions and Emotional and Spiritual Support of the Patient and Significant Others, Chapter 2.

PELVIC FRACTURES

PATHOPHYSIOLOGY

The pelvis is composed of three bones: two innominate bones and the sacrum. The innominate bones are each composed of three bones (ilium, pubis, and ischium) that fuse after childhood. The two innominate bones are joined by the symphysis pubis, a fibrous cartilage joint that connects the two pubic bones anteriorly; they are attached posteriorly to a third bone, the sacrum, by a system of ligaments termed the *posterior osseous ligamentous* structures. Many blood vessels run through the pelvis and join to form the large venous plexus.

MVCs and auto-pedestrian trauma cause approximately two thirds of all pelvic fractures, which have a mortality rate of up to 50% in some studies. A large force is needed for a pelvic fracture to occur, because these bones are stabilized by a strong network of ligaments. Pelvic fractures have been classified by several systems, but perhaps the most helpful are the systems that classify fractures by their stability and the mechanism of injury (Table 3-9). Pelvic fractures are considered stable fractures when the posterior osseous ligamentous structures are intact. An unstable pelvic fracture occurs when the osseous ligamentous structures are disrupted posteriorly and portions of the pelvis can move in any direction.

The most serious complications from a pelvic fracture are hemorrhage and exsanguination, which cause up to 60% of deaths. The pelvis receives a rich supply of blood from a complex system of interconnected collateral arteries and the venous plexus of the iliac system, often called the vascular sink. The aorta and internal iliac artery are close to the pelvis. This vascular network can easily be damaged or disrupted by the same forces that injure the pelvis. Pelvic fragments can damage vascular structures. The retroperitoneal space can hold as much as 4 L of blood before spontaneous tamponade occurs. Acute blood loss is difficult to identify until systemic symptoms, such as those occurring with shock, appear. In addition, damage to the sciatic and sacral nerves may occur with sacral and sacroiliac disruption.

The most common cause of pelvic fractures in older adults is falls, as opposed to MVCs in younger people. Older adults with a pelvic fracture have a 20% mortality rate. Older adults have more problems related to preexisting conditions. Cardiovascular disease often causes insufficient compensatory function to manage the stress of injury. Despite a less severe mechanism of injury, rates of sepsis and death are higher in older adults than in patients with trauma who are younger than 65 years with similar injuries.

ASSESSMENT: PELVIC FRACTURES

GOAL OF SYSTEM ASSESSMENT

Evaluate for stability of the pelvis and the probability of substantial blood loss.

HISTORY AND RISK FACTORS

The most common mechanisms of injuries are MVCs, motorcycle collisions, pedestrians struck by motor vehicles, and falls. Up to 15% of patients with a pelvic fracture have associated renal and lower urinary tract (LUT) injuries. Fifty percent of patients with both pelvic fractures and urologic injuries also have abdominal injuries.

Risk factors include:

- Age.
- Smoking.
- History of bone disease including osteoporosis.
- Previous hysterectomy.
- Use of anticoagulants.
- Concomitant injuries including intraabdominal organ injuries and bladder and urethral injuries.

Stable pelvic fracture

- Can withstand normal physiologic forces without abnormal deformation.

Table 3-9	**CLASSIFICATION OF PELVIC FRACTURES**

Pelvic fractures are most commonly classified using one of two systems: the Tile Classification System and the Young Classification System.

1. **Tile Classification System:** Focuses on whether the posterior sacroiliac complex is intact:
   - Type A Injuries: The sacroiliac complex is intact with a pelvic ring stable fracture that can be managed without surgery.
   - Type B Injuries: The posterior sacroiliac complex is partially disrupted, are often unstable, and result from internal rotational forces.
   - Type C Injuries: The posterior sacroiliac complex is completely disrupted, have both rotational and vertical instability, and result from motor vehicle collisions, a fall from great heights, or severe compression.

2. **Young Classification System:** Focuses on mechanism of injury including lateral compression, antero-posterior compression, vertical shear, or a combination of forces. Lateral compression fractures include transverse fractures of the pubic rami, located ipsilateral or contralateral to a posterior injury.
   - Grade I: Associated sacral compression on side of impact.
   - Grade II: Associated posterior iliac ("crescent") fracture on side of impact.
   - Grade III: Associated contralateral sacroiliac joint injury.

Classification of Injury	*Mechanism of Injury*	*Description*
Anteroposterior compression	External rotation is caused by a crushing force on the posterior superior iliac spines.	"Open book injury"; the force causes the symphysis pubis to spring open. Rupture of anterior sacroiliac and sacrospinous ligaments occurs, but posterior ligaments are intact. Stable vertically but can rotate externally. May be associated with ruptured bladder (intraperitoneal) if injury occurs when bladder is full.
Lateral compression	Internal rotation from a high-energy injury that causes direct pressure to crush anterior sacrum. Pressure on the greater trochanter causes the femoral head to displace the anterior pubic rami.	Most common type of injury. Often does not affect posterior ligamentous complex. Partially unstable fracture that is rotationally unstable but vertically stable. May have extensive soft tissue injury. May be associated with ruptured bladder (extraperitoneal).
Vertical shear (Malgaigne fracture)	Excessive force from trauma such as falls and crush injuries in a vertical plane leads to unstable disruption of the anterior and posterior ring.	Most severe injury with the highest mortality rates. Very unstable. Complete disruption of the posterior osseous ligamentous system. Often accompanied by injuries of the skin and subcutaneous tissues or injuries to the gastrointestinal, genitourinary, vascular, and neurologic systems.
Complex fracture	Excessive and powerful forces from many directions.	Pelvic ring disruptions resulting in bizarre fractures or dislocations in a combination of injury patterns. Usually very unstable.

Unstable pelvic fracture
- Fracture of the pelvic ring in more than one place that results in displacement.

VITAL SIGNS
- Temperature may be low if the patient is developing shock.
- RR may be elevated as a compensatory mechanism in hypovolemic shock.
- BP may be decreased in response to substantial blood loss.
- HR will be increased with substantial blood loss.

OBSERVATION

Evaluate for signs of trauma to the abdominal and pelvic regions.
* Lower extremity shortening and abnormal external rotation of the leg.
* Pelvic instability and/or pain with palpation.
* Lacerations of the vagina, peritoneum, groin, or anus may indicate an open pelvic fracture.
* Groin, genitalia, and suprapubic swelling may be present.
* Blood at the meatus, signifying urethral trauma, which often accompanies pelvic fractures.
* Evidence of hypovolemic shock.

PALPATION

The pelvis is palpated by placing inward and posterior compression on the iliac crests.
* Assess for pain with palpation.
* Feeling of movement of the pelvic bones upon palpation.
* Neurovascular status of the lower extremities should be checked.
* Palpate for pulses in lower extremities, femoral.
* Check for sensation bilaterally.

Diagnostic Tests for Pelvic Fractures		
Test	**Purpose**	**Abnormal Findings**
Blood Studies		
Complete blood count Hemoglobin (Hgb) Hematocrit (Hct)	Assess for blood loss.	Decreased Hgb and Hct indicate blood loss. Often Hgb and Hct are within normal range initially, especially if the patient has not received a significant amount of fluid to replace the blood loss. Hgb and Hct testing should be repeated after the patient has a fluid challenge if there is any indication of significant bleeding.
Coagulation profile Prothrombin time (PT) with international normalized ratio (INR) Partial thromboplastin time Fibrinogen D dimer	Assess for causes of bleeding, clotting, and disseminated intravascular coagulation indicative of abnormal clotting present in shock or ensuing shock.	Decreased PT with low INR promotes clotting; elevation promotes bleeding; elevated fibrinogen and D dimer reflect abnormal clotting.
Radiology		
Pelvic radiograph	Assess bony integrity of the pelvis.	Fractures that disrupt the pelvic ring.
Pelvic computed tomography (CT) scan	Assess bony integrity of the pelvis and presence of retroperitoneal hemorrhage.	Fractures within the pelvic ring, retroperitoneal bleeding.

Continued

Diagnostic Tests for Pelvic Fractures—cont'd		
Test	**Purpose**	**Abnormal Findings**
Interventional Radiology		
Angiography	Indicated when the patient has evidence of hemodynamic instability with an ongoing need for blood transfusion where there is no evidence of any other bleeding source besides the pelvic fracture. If contrast extravasation or a false aneurysm is identified, then embolization can be done. Angiography is currently the gold standard for diagnosis of arterial bleeding secondary to pelvic fracture.	Extravasation of dye from torn blood vessels.

COLLABORATIVE MANAGEMENT

CARE PRIORITIES

1. Stabilize the pelvis

External immobilization: Defined as any device that is applied to immobilize the pelvis either externally or percutaneously through the skin into the bone. Noninvasive external fixation can be accomplished in several ways and can be applied at the scene of injury to preserve function and prevent further orthopedic and neurovascular injury. When an unstable pelvis is identified, the pelvis should be stabilized. Stabilization can be achieved with several methods including:

- A sheet wrapped around the pelvis and secured with towel clips.
- Commercially available devices such as the T-POD, SAM Sling, and Pelvic Binder.
- Internal rotation and taping the lower extremities, which is referred to as IRTOTLE.

With external immobilization, care should be taken to limit the amount of pressure and time the pressure is applied to prevent skin damage. Most of these devices/techniques should not be used for longer than 24 hours. These are temporary measures to limit the amount of hemorrhaging until more definite treatment can be initiated.

An invasive emergency external fixation device, consisting of one pin in each iliac wing connected by a bar, can be inserted to provide pelvic stability. If an emergency laparotomy is performed, more complex fixation devices may be applied.

If abnormal shortening or rotation has occurred with the injury, the lower extremities should be supported and stabilized in the position in which they were found. A backboard supported by pillows, towels, or blankets taped in place with cloth tape are used until a traction splint can be applied.

Safety Alert Use of an external fixation device is not sufficient for maintaining reduction in the posterior pelvis or for stabilizing the pelvic posterior elements. As long as the patient is on bed rest or in traction, however, it can be used to manage the acute phase of the fracture.

Internal immobilization: Surgical open reduction and immobilization of unstable pelvic ring disruptions with surgically implanted plates, screws, or other devices. Permanent fixation requires closed reduction for final pelvic stabilization.

2. Initiate surgical exploration

Done to identify blood vessels in need of ligation or repair for ongoing hemorrhage. Inflow of blood to the pelvic circulation can be limited by ligation of the internal iliac artery to control bleeding. Because many collateral vessels exist in the pelvic circulation, infarction rarely occurs with this procedure. Surgical exploration is not always recommended. When the peritoneal space is entered, the tamponade is released and bleeding can increase. The extensive vascular sink makes identification of bleeding vessels difficult. Some patients may undergo angiography and selective embolization of bleeding points with either an autologous blood clot or particulate gel foam instead of surgery.

3. Replace blood loss with massive transfusion

Patients who continue to exhibit signs of shock after receiving 2 L of crystalloid IV fluid should receive blood transfusions. Blood replacement is best given according to established massive transfusion protocols, which have been shown to decrease mortality by eliminating the deadly triad of acidosis, hypothermia, and coagulopathy. See Major Trauma for further discussion of massive transfusion protocols. Some studies have supported withholding aggressive fluid resuscitation until after operative or embolic repair because an increase in MAP will increase intravascular hydrostatic pressure and may increase bleeding from torn vessels.

4. Initiate pharmacotherapy for the following

Manage pain with analgesics: IV morphine sulfate usually relieves pain and can be readily reversed with naloxone if hypotension or respiratory insufficiency is noted.

Control BP with vasopressors: For hypotension only after sufficient volume replacement has occurred (see Appendix 6).

Provide protection from disease with tetanus immunization: Booster is given if history is unknown or if a booster is needed (see Table 3-1).

Manage infection with antibiotics: Initial use for prophylaxis against infection is controversial in patients with open fractures. Used later for positive cultures of wounds, blood, or urine.

CARE PLANS: PELVIC FRACTURES

Decreased CO *related to blood loss from severity of fracture(s) and/or concomitant injuries.*

Goals/Outcomes: Within 24 hours of injury, the patient demonstrates adequate perfusion, as evidenced by the following ABG values: pH between 7.35 and 7.45 and base deficit level greater than 2.0 mmol/L, regular HR ≤100 bpm, bilaterally strong and equal peripheral pulses, warm and dry extremities, brisk (less than 2 seconds) capillary refill, systolic BP ≥90 mm Hg (or within 10% of patient's normal range), and urine output ≥0.5 mL/kg/h. If hemodynamic monitoring is present, PAWP is ≥6 mm Hg and CI is ≥2.5 L/min/m². The patient is awake, alert, and oriented to time, place, and person without restlessness or confusion.

NOC Tissue Perfusion: Peripheral; Blood Loss Severity.

Hemorrhage Control

1. Apply compression device or sheet to pelvic area or tape feet in an internal rotation position to align broken pelvis and decrease bleeding.
2. Note Hgb/Hct levels before and after blood loss.
3. Monitor trends in BP and hemodynamic measurements, if available (e.g., CVP and pulmonary capillary/artery wedge pressure).

Hypovolemia Management

1. Monitor the patient for evidence of fluid volume deficit, including tachycardia, decreased MAP, decreased amplitude of peripheral pulses, urine output less than 30 mL/hr (adult), urine output less than 1 mL/kg/hr (child weighing less than 30 kg), thirst, and dry mucous membranes.
2. Establish two large-bore peripheral IV lines. Establish central line if necessary.
3. Monitor intake and output; administer fluid therapy as prescribed. Adjust infusion to maintain desired urine output at the desired resuscitation hourly rate. Do not exceed 50 mL/hr urine output.
4. Monitor weight daily during fluid resuscitation; report significant gains or losses. A significant weight gain will occur with large-volume fluid resuscitation.
5. Monitor serial Hct and Hgb values. While the circulating volume is restored, hemoconcentration is no longer present and Hct returns to within normal limits (WNL).
6. Monitor the patient for signs and symptoms of large-volume fluid administration (shortness of breath, tachypnea, excessive urine output).

Risk for infection *related to impaired wound healing*

Goals/Outcomes: The patient is free of infection, as evidenced by normothermia, WBC count 11,000/mm³, negative culture results, HR 100 bpm, BP within the patient's normal range, and absence of agitation, purulent drainage, and other clinical indicators of infection.

NOC Risk Identification.

Incision Site Care
1. Inspect the incision for redness, swelling, or signs of dehiscence.
2. Note the characteristics of any drainage.
3. Monitor the healing process at the incision site.
4. Change the dressing at appropriate intervals.
5. Perform pin care as prescribed. Current evidence does not support any one method of pin care.

Infection Prevention
1. Monitor for systemic and localized signs and symptoms of infection.
2. Monitor vulnerability to infection.
3. Monitor absolute granulocyte count, WBC, and differential results.
4. Promote sufficient nutrition intake.
5. Encourage rest.
6. Obtain cultures as needed.

Impaired physical mobility *related to limitation in movement of pelvis needed to stabilize fracture with fixation device and other loss of joint movement or ability to ambulate independently.*

Goals/Outcomes: The patient will not develop complications of impaired mobility such as skin breakdown on any dependent areas or areas involved with fracture stabilization; venous thromboembolism; or constipation.

NOC Immobility Consequences: Physiologic.

Bed Rest Care
1. Place on appropriate therapeutic mattress/bed.
2. Keep bed linen clean, dry, and wrinkle-free.
3. Apply devices to prevent foot drop, as needed.
4. Attach a trapeze bar to the bed, as appropriate.
5. Turn immobilized patients every 2 hours, according to a specific schedule.
6. Perform passive and active ROM exercises.
7. Apply antiembolism devices (e.g., stocking, sequential compression devices, foot pump).
8. Monitor for constipation, urinary function, and pulmonary status.

Positioning
1. Premedicate the patient before turning as appropriate.
2. Position in proper body alignment.
3. Support the legs during turning to minimize movement of the pelvis.
4. Monitor fixation/traction devices for proper setup, and maintain position and integrity of traction when repositioning the patient.
5. Minimize friction and shearing forces when positioning and turning the patient.
6. Place call light within reach.
7. Place frequently used items within reach.

RENAL AND LOWER URINARY TRACT TRAUMA

PATHOPHYSIOLOGY

Injuries to the genitourinary tract represent a small proportion of patients severe enough for admission to a trauma service. The majority of patients experience blunt trauma caused by MVCs, falls from heights, and blows to the torso or external genitalia. Genitourinary tract injury is rarely life threatening. However, shattered kidney, major renal vascular laceration with hemorrhage, renal artery dissection, or pedicle avulsion can be a result of a significant deceleration injury that may be life threatening or a threat to the kidney itself. These can be seen as a result of a high-speed MVC or a fall from a substantial height.

Pelvic fractures are most commonly associated with injury to the female genital tract. Injuries to the external genitalia, urethra, and bladder are often overlooked in the initial trauma assessment because they frequently accompany life-threatening injuries that require aggressive and immediate management. Urethral disruption is seen with pelvic fracture in approximately 5% of women and 25% of men. In males, penile injury results from rupture of the tunica albuginea, with concomitant urethral injury in approximately 20% of patients.

The genitourinary tract is divided into upper and lower tracts. The upper tract consists of the kidney and the ureters, and the LUT involves the external genitalia, urethra, and bladder. Renal and LUT trauma can also occur with penetrating injuries (stab and gunshot wounds). Other mechanisms of injury include physical or sexual assault and rough consensual sexual intercourse. Injury to the vulva or penis is uncommon and should alert one for prompt screening for interpersonal violence. Pathophysiology for renal and LUT trauma is shown in Table 3-10.

Table 3-10	PATHOPHYSIOLOGY FOR RENAL AND LOWER URINARY TRACT TRAUMA		
Type of Injury	**Anatomic Considerations**	**Pathophysiology and Mechanism of Injury**	**Result of Injury**
Renal trauma	Kidneys are well protected from injury posteriorly by muscles of the back, anteriorly by organs of the gastrointestinal tract, and by a tough outer capsule and adipose tissue. Kidneys are fixed in retroperitoneal space only by renal pedicle (vascular system in renal helium) and ureters. Blunt renal injury is often caused by compression of the kidney by the twelfth rib, which rotates inwardly and squeezes the kidney into the lumbar spine.	Renal trauma can be divided into three classifications: Minor trauma: Incidence 85%. Bruising of renal parenchyma; superficial lacerations of renal cortex without rupture of renal capsule. Major trauma: Incidence 10% to 15%. Major lacerations through cortex and medulla; continuation of laceration through renal capsule. Critical trauma: Incidence is less than 5%. Renal vascular trauma in which kidney is shattered and renal pedicle is injured; fragmentation (renal fracture).	Minor trauma: Hematuria and flank tenderness that will usually result in a full recovery with rest and observation. Major trauma: Hematuria, flank pain, and possible hypotension that may require surgical intervention. Critical injury: Severe blood loss and shock requiring immediate surgical intervention.
Ureteral trauma	Injury to the upper part of the ureter is uncommon because of its location deep in the retroperitoneum. Ureteral lacerations are most common at the ureteropelvic junction, where the upper ureter joins the renal pelvis.	Ureteral injury is most commonly associated with iatrogenic injuries during gynecologic, colonic, and vascular surgery. Blunt injury may occur when the ureter becomes crushed against the spinal column. When ureteral injury is not associated with iatrogenic injury, it usually occurs in the setting of severe abdominal compression or significant penetrating abdominal injury.	Extravasation of urine or blood may lead to infection, abscess formation, hemorrhage, or shock; late complications include prolonged voiding time, ureteral strictures, and fistula formation.

Continued

Table 3-10	PATHOPHYSIOLOGY FOR RENAL AND LOWER URINARY TRACT TRAUMA—cont'd		
Type of Injury	**Anatomic Considerations**	**Pathophysiology and Mechanism of Injury**	**Result of Injury**
Bladder trauma	When the bladder is distended, it extends above the umbilicus and has less protection from trauma; the bladder ruptures at its point of least resistance (the dome), and blood and urine extravasate into the peritoneal cavity (intraperitoneal rupture). Extraperitoneal rupture occurs most often in conjunction with pelvic fractures; sharp bone fragments perforate the bladder at its base, leading to extravasation of blood and urine into the space surrounding the bladder base.	Motor vehicle collisions are the most common cause of bladder rupture; bladder contusion often results from a direct blow or the cavitational effect of missiles (outward tissue acceleration away from the tract of the bullet); bladder rupture does not require extensive force, which may be a blunt blow to the lower abdomen.	Bladder lacerations or rupture can lead to blood or urine extravasation outside of the peritoneal cavity (80%) and into the peritoneal cavity (20%); infection or hemorrhage can follow.
Urethral trauma	Urethral injury is more common in males than in females because the male urethra is five times longer; the male urethra is also rigidly fixed at the urogenital diaphragm (bulbous urethra), whereas the female urethra is short and mobile.	Perineal trauma, straddle injuries, and pelvic fractures are often the causes of urethral injury; motor vehicle collisions with deceleration and shearing may also lead to injury of the posterior urethra.	Urethral injury may lead to extravasation of blood and/or urine within the penis; if disruption to Buck fascia occurs, extravasation into the upper thighs and peritoneum follows; hemorrhage or infection may also occur.

Urethral injury may cause males long-term problems with sexual intercourse and voiding. Sexual dysfunction may be a result of damage to neural and vascular structures. Incontinence may result from damage to the sphincters or their innervations. In patients with complete urethral disruption, approximately 20% have voiding dysfunction and 25% have sexual dysfunction.

RENAL AND LOWER URINARY TRACT ASSESSMENT

GOAL OF SYSTEM ASSESSMENT
Identify specific location of physical injuries and presence of signs and symptoms indicating injury to organs affected by the renal system or surrounding organs.

HISTORY AND RISK FACTORS
- Ask about allergies, current medications, preexisting medical conditions, and factors surrounding the injury.
- Patients with preexisting renal diseases such as polycystic kidney disease and pyelonephritis are at higher risk for renal injury.
- Ask about any suprapubic tenderness.

- Ask about inability to void spontaneously or any past bloody urine.
- Ask about flank pain, pain at the costovertebral angle, back tenderness, and colicky pain with the passage of blood clots.

OBSERVATION AND SUBJECTIVE SYMPTOMS

- Renal trauma: Abdominal or flank pain, back tenderness, colicky pain with passage of blood clots, pallor, diaphoresis, gross hematuria, restlessness, confusion, obvious wounds, contusions, or abrasions in the flank or abdomen; abdominal distention; Grey Turner sign (bruising over the lower portion of the back and the flank caused by a retroperitoneal hemorrhage); pain at the costovertebral angle.

> **HIGH ALERT!** Gross hematuria is present in only slightly more than half of patients with renal trauma and is considered an unreliable diagnostic sign.

- Ureter trauma: Gross hematuria may be present; if the ureter is transected, normal urine from the unaffected kidney may still be voided. Late signs may include fever and flank or abdominal discomfort. Urine may be found at the entrance or exit sites of penetrating abdominal wounds or wounds of the middle to lower back areas.
- Bladder trauma: Inability to void spontaneously, gross hematuria (present in approximately 95% of patients), and abdominal discomfort. Perineal or scrotal edema and hematoma, abnormal position of prostate, abdominal distention, palpable suprapubic mass, and palpable and overdistended bladder.
- Urethral trauma: Blood at the meatus, inability to void spontaneously, urethral bleeding, prostate tenderness, microscopic or gross hematuria, pain and tenderness of genitalia, and perineal hematoma. Tracking of urine into tissues of the thighs or abdominal wall, bruised to discolored genitalia.

> **HIGH ALERT!** Physical signs may be masked because the kidneys are located beneath abdominal organs, back muscles, and bony structures.

VITAL SIGNS

- Hypotension.
- Tachycardia.
- Flank or abdominal mass.
- Bladder trauma: Late signs may include fever.

PALPATION

- Bladder trauma: Suprapubic tenderness.
- Renal trauma: Hematoma over the flank of the eleventh or twelfth ribs.
- Ureter trauma: Enlarging retroperitoneal mass.

INSPECTION

- Digital rectal examination to check for rectal tone, gross blood, and the position of the prostate. Posterior urethral disruption may result in a "high riding" prostate in males, which moves away from the examiner during the procedure. The finding indicates rupture of the urethra, which requires surgical repair or "railroading" as soon as the patient's general condition permits. Diminished rectal tone may indicate SCI or imply that the patient engages in anal intercourse.
- A meticulous vaginal examination should be performed in all women with pelvic fractures to assess for bone fragments or lacerations that could result in hemorrhage and infection.

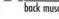

Renal and Lower Urinary Tract Trauma

Diagnostic Tests for Renal and Lower Urinary Tract Trauma

Test	Purpose	Abnormal Findings
Urinalysis	To rule out blood in urine; cloudiness, odor.	Hematuria; sediment, malodor.
Urine culture and sensitivity	Rule out infection or injury.	Urethral injury: microscopic (>3 to 5 red blood cells/high power field); presence of microorganisms.

Imaging

Check the patient's history for allergy to iodine, iodine-containing foods, or contrast material. Hydration and sometimes diuretics are needed to facilitate excretion of contrast material after testing. Evaluate blood urea nitrogen/creatinine level before use of dye to determine renal functioning.

Test	Purpose	Abnormal Findings
Computed tomography (CT) scan	CT is the method of choice to assess patients with severe renal trauma.	May reveal hematomas, renal lacerations, renal infarcts, or extravasation of urine. Contrast-enhanced CT detects kidney laceration and arterial occlusion. Delay images are necessary to assess for extravasation of contrast and determination of injury. Triple phase contrast examinations can help evaluate collecting duct injuries.
Retrograde urethrogram	Diagnose urethral tears or rupture. A small urinary catheter is inserted, and the balloon is inflated in the distal anterior urethra. Contrast material is injected, and a single radiograph film is taken to outline the inner size and shape of the urethra.	Used to evaluate urethral injuries. In urethral rupture, extravasation of the contrast material occurs. With a partial disruption, extravasation is accompanied by contrast appearing in the bladder. Contrast does not appear in the bladder with complete disruption. This procedure is deferred, however, if there is an indication for pelvic angiography.
Cystogram	If no urethral tear is found on retrograde urethrogram, a catheter is inserted into the bladder. The bladder is filled with 400 mL of contrast material. It is important to fill the bladder to the point of contraction and then forcefully instill another 50 mL of contrast. It is necessary to distend the bladder adequately to ensure extravasation and a meaningful test.	If intraperitoneal or extraperitoneal extravasation of contrast material occurs, the bladder is drained and repeat radiographs are taken to check for small posterior ruptures.
CT cystography	Assess for bladder injuries.	Abnormal filling of bladder.
Excretory urogram/intravenous pyelogram	Visualize the normal or injured structures of the kidneys, ureters, or bladder. This test has been supplanted with the use of CT imaging. It may, however, be used and is useful in instances when there is a suspected urethral injury and delayed CT images prove nondiagnostic.	Abnormal passage of contrast through the structures of the urinary system.

Diagnostic Tests for Renal and Lower Urinary Tract Trauma — cont'd

Test	Purpose	Abnormal Findings
Renal ultrasound	This test is rarely used for early identification of injury because it is too imprecise. The ultrasound is not sensitive enough for diagnosis and exclusion of a significant renal injury.	
Radionuclide imaging	Evaluates for injured lower urinary tract structures and alterations in renal blood flow. After intravenous injection of a radionuclide, a radioactivity-detecting device scans and records the radioactive uptake. The substance is excreted in 6 to 24 hours following the test.	Injury to structures of the urinary tract.
Kidney-ureter-bladder radiography	Evaluates position, size, structure, and defects of the urinary tract.	May reveal foreign bodies, retroperitoneal hematoma, fracture of the lower ribs or pelvis, organ displacement, or fluid accumulation.
Renal angiography	Arterial injection of a contrast medium, permitting identification on radiograph film of renal vasculature and functional tissue. Identification of any renal injury.	Renal pedicle injury, renal infarct, intrarenal hematoma, lacerations, and shattered kidney.
Magnetic resonance imaging	Used to identify the best surgical approach for more difficult injuries, such as traumatic posterior urethral injury. Identifies severity of injury and may help estimate time needed for recovery.	Localized injury to specific organ or surrounding structures.

Blood Studies

 HIGH ALERT! If an intraperitoneal bladder rupture has occurred, hyperkalemia, hypernatremia, uremia, and acidosis may occur as a result of reabsorption of urine from the peritoneal cavity.

Hemoglobin, hematocrit	Evaluate for low level or trend.	Below normal level may indicate bleeding, hemorrhage, and should lead to further examination for hematuria or other areas of potential internal hemorrhage.
Blood urea nitrogen (BUN)	Evaluate for elevation denoting level of effect.	Renal dysfunction causes insufficient excretion of urea, elevating nitrogenous wastes in the blood. In renal trauma, BUN level may increase because of body catabolism, dehydration, or from absorption of peritoneal extravasation of urine. When the BUN is elevated as a result of urine absorption, the serum creatinine levels remain normal. Normal BUN is 10 to 20 mg/dL.

Continued

Diagnostic Tests for Renal and Lower Urinary Tract Trauma—cont'd

Test	Purpose	Abnormal Findings
Serum creatinine	Assessment of renal function. Damage from trauma may result in decreased renal function with increased creatinine.	Renal impairment is virtually the only cause of elevated serum creatinine. Creatinine production is fairly constant because production is proportional to muscle mass. Creatinine is freely filtered at the glomerulus and minimally re-sorbed, thus creatinine excretion is proportional to glomerular filtration rate. Normal value is 0.7 to 1.5 mg/dL.
Clearance tests	Clearance is the volume of plasma that can be cleared of a specific substance during a specified period of time. Clearance tests evaluate the extent of injury by assessing renal filtration, reabsorption, secretion, and renal plasma flow. Creatinine, inulin (a plant starch), and urea may be tested.	Currently, most laboratories will provide an estimated glomerular filtration rate determination in addition to other renal function measurements. This provides a more practical estimation of clearance for the clinician.

COLLABORATIVE MANAGEMENT

CARE PRIORITIES

1. Identify and manage bleeding complications, including hypovolemic or hemorrhagic shock
- Hemorrhagic shock: Volume resuscitation with crystalloids, colloids, or blood products as indicated.

2. Manage pain
- Analgesics: IV narcotics may be used as a first line to relieve pain.
- Phenazopyridine (Pyridium) is a urinary antispasmodic agent that helps to relieve burning and frequency.
- Both of these strategies provide symptom relief only. Managing the cause of the pain treats the injury.

3. Prevent and/or manage infection
- Source control: Avoid urinary catheterization when possible to prevent catheter-associated UTI. Remove the catheter when no longer needed, according to the Centers for Disease Control and Prevention guidelines for prevention of catheter-associated UTI and/or nurse-driven Foley catheter removal protocol.
- Infections: As indicated, obtain blood and urine cultures and initiate appropriate antibiotics and other infection control measures.
- Antibiotics: Consider initiating for positive urine culture results, penetrating injuries, or peritonitis.

4. Support renal function
- Renal dysfunction: Fluids need to be carefully managed with goal-directed therapy; fluids may be administered or restricted depending on the phase of renal dysfunction; renal replacement therapies may be indicated for fluid and electrolyte management if the degree of dysfunction is severe enough. See Acute Renal Failure, Chapter 5, for more information.

5. Manage urinary elimination without causing further injury

Catheterization

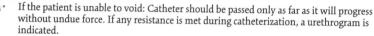

- If the patient is unable to void: Catheter should be passed only as far as it will progress without undue force. If any resistance is met during catheterization, a urethrogram is indicated.
- If blood is present at the urethral meatus: The patient should not be catheterized until diagnostic tests are completed, because the blood may signal urethral injury. In the presence of urethral injury, an improperly placed catheter can result in an incomplete injury progressing to a complete disruption.
- Urethral trauma: A suprapubic catheter may be used to manage severe urethral lacerations and urethral disruption.
- Renal trauma: In addition to direct surgical intervention, diversion of urine may be required by nephrostomy tube, depending on location of injury or in cases of coexisting pancreatic and duodenal injury.
- Ureteral trauma: Internal ureteral catheters (ureteral stents) may be indicated for ureteral trauma, particularly for gunshot wounds, to maintain ureteral alignment, ensure urinary drainage, and provide support during anastomosis.

6. Facilitate a timely surgical intervention

- Surgical intervention is required in a minority of patients who sustain renal trauma. The majority of patients who undergo surgical intervention have sustained penetrating trauma.
- Surgical correction: Surgical correction may be performed open or with minimally invasive technology, such as in interventional radiology. Surgical correction may be indicated for transected ureter, partial ureteral tears of more than one third of the circumference of the ureter, bladder perforation with associated abdominal injuries or intraperitoneal rupture, and injuries accompanied by rapidly expanding, pulsating hematomas. See Table 3-11 for examples of procedures for the various types of renal and LUT injuries.
- In the incidence of multiple trauma: The collaboration of the trauma surgeon and the urologist is paramount in the effort to decrease morbidity and mortality.
- Organ Injury Scale: The American Association for the Surgery of Trauma Organ Injury has developed an Organ Injury Scale of solid organs including the kidney. This scale was designed to provide a system to describe injuries by a common nomenclature and severity of injury. The severity score for the kidney is described in Table 3-12.

Table 3-11	SURGICAL PROCEDURES FOR RENAL AND LOWER URINARY TRACT TRAUMA
Type of Injury	**Surgical Indications/Surgical Management**
Minor renal trauma	Conservative management. Rest and observation with careful follow-up to prevent progressive deformity and to evaluate blood pressure.
Major renal trauma	Surgical intervention if hypotension and hemodynamic instability occur.
Critical renal trauma	Immediate surgical exploration; low rates of renal salvage.
Proximal ureteral injury	Primary ureterostomy with end-to-end anastomosis.
Distal ureteral injury	Ureteral stenting or percutaneous nephrostomy, depending on location and extent of injury.
Bladder injury	Use of urinary or suprapubic drainage. Surgical repair may be indicated.
Urethral injury	Urinary or suprapubic catheterization is used for long-term management.

Table 3-12		AMERICAN ASSOCIATION FOR THE SURGERY OF TRAUMA ORGAN INJURY SEVERITY SCORE FOR THE KIDNEY
Grade	Type	Injury Definition
1	Parenchyma	Subcapsular hematoma and/or contusion
	Collecting system	No injury
2	Parenchyma	Laceration less than 2 cm in depth and into the cortex, small hematoma contained within Gerota fascia
	Collecting system	No injury
3	Parenchyma	Laceration greater than 1 cm in depth and into the medulla, hematoma contained within Gerota fascia
	Collecting system	No injury
4	Parenchyma	Laceration through the parenchyma into the urinary collecting system
	Collecting system	Vascular segmental vein or artery injury
		Laceration, one or more in the collecting system with urinary extravasation
		Renal pelvis laceration and/or complete ureteral pelvic disruption
5	Vascular	Main renal artery or vein laceration or avulsion main renal artery or vein thrombosis

From Buckley JC, McAninch JW: Revision of the current American Association for the Surgery of Trauma Renal Injury Grading System. *J Trauma* 70:35-37, 2011.

CARE PLANS: RENAL AND LOWER URINARY TRACT TRAUMA

Impaired urinary elimination *related to mechanical trauma secondary to injury to the kidney and LUT structures.*

Goals/Outcomes: Within 6 hours after immediate trauma management, the patient has a urinary output of ≥0.5 mL/kg/h with no evidence of bladder distention.

NOC Urinary Elimination.

Urinary Elimination Management

1. Monitor urinary outflow. Encourage the patient to void. If patient is unable to void, assess for full bladder. Urinary catheterization or suprapubic drainage may be needed. Report findings to the physician. Monitor for the following signs of kidney or LUT trauma:
   - Urge but inability to void spontaneously despite adequate volume replacement.
   - Blood at the urethral meatus.
   - Difficult or unsuccessful urinary catheterization.
   - Anuria after urinary catheterization.
   - Hematuria.
2. Do not catheterize the patient if there is blood at the urethral meatus. Call the advanced practice provider for consultation for a possible urethral injury.
3. Monitor serum BUN and creatinine.
4. Document input and output hourly. Consult the advanced practice provider if urine output is less than 0.5 mL/kg/h.
5. Assess whether clots may be occluding the drainage system. If indicated, obtain order for catheter irrigation or call the advanced practice provider to irrigate the catheter. Sudden cessation of urine flow through the collection system (particularly if past output was greater than 50 mL/h) indicates possible catheter obstruction. If catheter irrigation does not resume urine drainage, consider changing the urinary catheter after discussion with the physician.
6. Ensure that nephrostomy tubes are not occluded by the patient's weight or external pressure. Irrigate the nephrostomy tube only if prescribed with ≤5 mL of fluid. The renal pelvis holds less than 10 mL of fluid.
7. Assess entrance site of the nephrostomy tube for bleeding or leakage of urine. Catheter blockage or dislodging causes a sudden decrease in urine output. Inspect urine color and for blood clots. Hematuria is normal for 24 to 48 hours after nephrostomy tube insertion. Consult the physician if gross bleeding (with or without clots) occurs.
8. Hydrate to allow for clearing of contrast material from the patient's system after diagnostic testing.

NIC Urinary Catheterization; Fluid Management; Fluid Monitoring; Tube Care: Urinary.

Risk for infection *related to inadequate primary defenses and tissue destruction secondary to bacterial contamination of the urinary tract system occurring with penetrating trauma, rupture of the bladder into the perineum, or instrumentation.*

Goals/Outcomes: The patient is free of infection, as evidenced by normothermia, WBC count ≤11,000/mm³, and negative results of urine and wound drainage testing for infective organisms.
NOC Immune Status; Risk Control.

Infection Protection

1. Use aseptic technique when caring for drainage systems. Keep catheters and collection container at a level lower than the bladder to prevent reflux; ensure that drainage tubing is not kinked.
2. Record the color and odor of urine each shift. Culture urine specimen when signs or symptoms of infection are present.
3. Monitor the patient's WBC count daily and temperature every 4 hours for elevations.
4. Assess for signs of peritonitis: abdominal pain, abdominal distention with rigidity, nausea, vomiting, fever, malaise, and weakness.
5. Assess catheter exit site each shift for the presence of erythema, swelling, or drainage.
6. Assess thigh, groin, and lower portion of abdomen for indicators of urinary extravasation: swelling, pain, mass(es), erythema, and tracking of urine along fascial planes.
7. Assess surgical incision for approximation of suture line and evidence of wound healing, noting presence of erythema, swelling, and drainage. Note color, odor, and consistency of drainage. Notify the physician of purulent or foul-smelling drainage. Consider obtaining a culture.
8. Assess skin at invasive sites for indicators of irritation: erythema, drainage, and swelling.
9. Cleanse catheter insertion sites with antimicrobial solution or per hospital policy. Manage catheter exit sites per protocol.
10. Consider dressing changes every 24 hours or as soon as noted they are wet. If skin is irritated from contact with urine, consider use of a pectin wafer skin barrier for extra protection.

NIC Incision Site Care; Wound Care; Infection Control; Surveillance; Tube Care: Urinary.

Acute pain (acute tenderness in lower abdomen) *related to physical injury associated with LUT structural injury, procedures for urinary diversion, or surgical incisions.*

Goals/Outcomes: Within 2 hours after giving analgesic agent, the patient's subjective evaluation of discomfort improves, as documented by an approved pain scale. Nonverbal indicators of discomfort, such as grimacing, are absent.
NOC Pain Control; Comfort Level.

Pain Management

1. Assess the patient for pain at least every 4 hours.
2. Be alert to shallow breathing in the presence of abdominal pain, which can cause inadequate pulmonary excursion. Medicate promptly, and document the patient's response to analgesic agent, using the appropriate pain scale. IV narcotics may be indicated if the injury is severe.
3. Explain the cause of the pain to the patient.
4. Assist the patient into a position of comfort. Often knee flexion will relax lower abdominal muscles and help reduce discomfort.
5. Implement nonpharmacologic measures for coping with pain: diversion, touch, and conversation.

NIC Analgesic Administration; Positioning; Presence.

THORACIC TRAUMA
PATHOPHYSIOLOGY
Thoracic trauma may be caused by blunt or penetrating injuries to the chest, back, flanks, and upper abdomen region. Thoracic trauma accounts for up to 60% of all trauma-related deaths in the United States. Careful assessment is needed to quickly identify life-threatening

injuries to the heart, lungs, and great vessels. Close monitoring is required to prevent complications secondary to injuries that develop over the first 24 hours, such as pulmonary contusions.

Thoracic injuries can result from both direct and indirect forces. Direct force such as direct impact involving an object can result in bony fractures, tissue bruising, and ruptured organs. Indirect forces can cause tissues to stretch beyond their limits and can result in tears leading to rupture of blood vessels and disruption of organs, such as the bronchus and esophagus. Thoracic injuries often lead to problems with ventilation, oxygenation, and perfusion, causing a decrease in the delivery of oxygen and nutrients to the tissues.

The lungs are often affected by space-occupying injuries, such as hemothoraces, pneumothoraces, and hemopneumothoraces, which compress lung tissue, interfering with lung expansion, thereby limiting the amount of ventilation and decreasing oxygen exchange at the alveoli level. The most serious of these injuries is a tension pneumothorax where the pressure in the chest is so high that not only is oxygenation impaired but also venous return to the heart is diminished, leading to decreased CO and shock.

One of the most common thoracic injuries is contusions to the lungs. When the lung tissue is bruised, alveolar hemorrhage and parenchymal destruction occur, leading to both local and systemic consequences. The reduced compliance impairs ventilation and causes an increase in shunting with decreased pulmonary blood flow. Hypoxemia and hypercarbia develop and usually worsen over the following 72 hours.

Blunt thoracic trauma can cause injury to the heart muscle by one or more of the following four mechanisms: compression of the heart between the sternum and vertebrae, bruising of heart tissue by bony structures, rupture or compression of coronary arteries by the blow, or cardiac rupture caused by intrathoracic or intraabdominal pressure. Causes of blunt cardiac injury are MVCs, direct blows to the chest, falls from great heights, sporting and industrial injuries, and kicks from animals. There are no reliable diagnostic tests to identify blunt cardiac injury. Cardiac injury is considered significant when the patient has new findings, such as new dysrhythmias, abnormal cardiac wall motion, or injury to the heart.

Penetrating thoracic trauma is caused by gunshot wounds, stab wounds, or foreign bodies entering the chest or upper abdomen. Open chest injuries can result in an open pneumothorax or lacerations to the lung tissue or the airways, heart, great vessels, and/or the esophagus. Penetrating injuries to the heart are the most common cause of intrapericardial hemorrhage.

ASSESSMENT: THORACIC TRAUMA

GOAL OF SYSTEM ASSESSMENT
Evaluate for traumatic injuries of the heart, lung, great vessels, and bony thorax.

HISTORY AND RISK FACTORS
Age, smoking history, mechanism of injury, chronic lung disease.

VITAL SIGNS
- RR may be increased if hypoxia is present.
- BP may be decreased.
- HR may increase as a result of hypoxia or hemorrhage.

OBSERVATION
Check chest for signs of trauma and chest excursion.
- Bruising, abrasions, contusions, and lacerations indicate that the thoracic area of the body received some of the force.
- Carefully observe chest wall for signs of penetrating injuries because the skin may close up, masking the entry, especially with low-velocity injuries such as stabbings.
- Logroll the patient to inspect the back of the chest.
- Observe position of the trachea.
- Observe for neck vein distention.

PERCUSSION
* Percuss over the lung fields to identify areas of hyperresonance, indicating a collection of air in the pleural space. Dullness may indicate atelectasis or a collection of blood in the pleural space.

PALPATION
* Over the ribs, sternum, and scapula to identify areas of tenderness and step-offs.
* Feel chest for crepitus or subcutaneous emphysema.

AUSCULTATION
* Lung fields to identify abnormal breath sounds.
* Decreased breath sounds may indicate a pneumothorax or hemothorax.
* Sucking sound on inspiration may indicate an open pneumothorax.
* Heart to identify abnormal heart sounds.
* Muffled heart sounds may indicate a pericardial tamponade.

ASSESSMENT
The nurse and interdisciplinary team assess for the following common injuries.

Pneumothorax/tension pneumothorax
* Chest pain.
* Respiratory distress.
* Decreased chest wall excursion.
* Hypoxia.
* Decreased breath sounds on the affected side.
* Tachycardia.
* Additionally, with a tension pneumothorax, tracheal deviation, JVD, hypotension, and cyanosis (late sign) may be present.

Hemothorax
* Chest pain.
* Respiratory distress.
* Decreased breath sounds on the affected side.
* Signs/symptoms of blood loss up to and including shock.

Flail chest
* Paradoxical chest wall movement.
* Pain over affected chest wall on palpation.
* Hypoxia.
* Decreased chest excursion resulting from pain.
* Decreased breath sounds.

Pulmonary contusion
* Hypoxia.
* Respiratory distress.

Blunt cardiac injury
* Arrhythmias.
* Chest wall contusions.
* Chest pain.

Aortic trauma
* Hypotension/hypertension.
* Tachycardia.
* Unequal pulses, absent pulses below the level of injury.
* Mottling below the level of injury.

Diagnostic Tests for Thoracic Trauma

Test	Purpose	Abnormal Findings
Noninvasive		
Pulse oximetry	Continuous monitoring of oxygen saturation.	Sao_2 <95%.
Capnography	Continuous monitoring of ventilation.	Increased.
Electrocardiogram	Assess for dysrhythmias, which can occur from blunt cardiac injury.	The most common findings with blunt cardiac injury are: Multiple premature ventricular contractions Unexplained sinus tachycardia Atrial fibrillation Bundle branch block, usually on the right ST segment changes.
Blood Studies		
Arterial blood gas analysis	Assess for adequacy of oxygenation and ventilation.	pH <7.35 with increased $Paco_2$ indicates respiratory acidosis. Decreased Pao_2 indicates hypoxemia. Increasing base deficit indicates inadequate delivery of oxygen to the tissues and an increase in anaerobic metabolism.
Serial cardiac enzymes Myoglobin Creatine kinase (CK)-MB isoform CK-MB Troponin I Troponin T	Assess for enzyme changes indicative of myocardial tissue damage.	Elevated enzymes reflect muscle damage; if CK-MB and troponins are elevated, the patient may have suffered an acute myocardial infarction. Not useful in diagnosing blunt cardiac injury.
Complete blood count Hemoglobin (Hgb) Hematocrit (Hct) White blood cell (WBC) count	Assess for blood loss, inflammation, and infection.	Decreased Hgb and Hct reflect amount of blood loss. WBCs will be elevated as a result of the inflammatory process that occurs following injury to the tissues.
Radiology		
Chest radiograph	Assess thoracic cage for fractures, pleural space for the presence of air or fluids, size of heart, thoracic aorta and diaphragm, or displacement of organs and structures.	Displaced lung margins indicate a pneumothorax or hemothorax. Cardiac enlargement reflects possible cardiac tamponade. Widened mediastinum and blurring of the aortic knob indicate possible aortic injury. Deviation of the trachea could indicate tension pneumothorax or aortic injury. Intestinal gas pattern in chest may indicate a ruptured diaphragm. Irregular, nonlobular opacifications in the pulmonary parenchyma indicate pulmonary contusions but are not usually seen on chest radiograph for the first 24 hours.

Diagnostic Tests for Thoracic Trauma—cont'd

Test	Purpose	Abnormal Findings
Computed tomography (CT) Thoracic CT scan CT angiography (CTA)	Assess pulmonary and vascular structures for damage.	Air or blood in the pleural space (pneumothorax or hemothorax). Mediastinal hematoma on CTA can indicate an aortic injury.
Ultrasound echocardiography (ECHO)	Assess for mechanical abnormalities related to effective pumping of blood and for collection of fluid in the pericardial sac.	Abnormal ventricular wall movement or motion, low ejection fraction, damaged valves, collection of fluid in the pericardial sac.
Transesophageal ECHO (TEE)	Assess for mechanical abnormalities related to effective pumping of blood from both sides of the heart using a transducer attached to the endoscope.	Same as above but can provide enhanced views, particularly of the posterior wall of the heart.
Aortogram	Useful as an adjunct to spiral CT in diagnosing thoracic aorta injuries; may be able to delineate the exact location and extent of the injury.	Hematoma formation and extravasation of fluid around the aorta indicate injury.
Flexible or rigid esophagoscopy	To identify esophageal injuries.	Laceration or bruising to the esophageal wall.
Flexible or rigid bronchoscopy	To identify tracheobronchial injuries.	Tear in the wall of the trachea or bronchus

COLLABORATIVE MANAGEMENT

Collaborative management should start with addressing the ABCs as outlined in the section on Major Trauma, including oxygen, IV fluids, and blood as indicated. During the initial assessment, several conditions involving injuries to the thoracic organs may warrant immediate intervention. These include the following:

- Open pneumothorax.
- Tension pneumothorax.
- Massive hemothorax.
- Flail chest.
- Cardiac tamponade.
- Torn aorta or great vessels.

CARE PRIORITIES

With pulmonary injuries, interventions are directed toward managing acute respiratory compromise while correcting the underlying injuries that may cause deterioration in the patient's condition. Intervention should be aimed at correcting and preventing hypoxia. With cardiac and great vessel injuries, the care priorities are focused on stopping hemorrhage, restoring perfusion, and supporting cardiac function.

1. Ensure patent airway

- When the patient is unable to maintain a patent airway either as a result of trauma or a decreased LOC, an artificial airway is inserted through oral intubation or via emergent tracheostomy.
- Intubation: Maintains patent airway, decreases airway resistance and respiratory effort, provides route for easy removal of airway secretions, and allows for manual or mechanical ventilation, as necessary.

2. Restore intrathoracic negative pressure

- Interventions are aimed at restoring the negative pressure in the thoracic cavity to allow for adequate ventilation.

- Pleural decompression: Relieves life-threatening tension pneumothorax. A 14-gauge needle or IV catheter is inserted into the second intercostal space at the midclavicular line to relieve the pressure in the chest cavity.

> **Safety Alert** *If a tension pneumothorax is suspected, pleural decompression should not be delayed for a confirmation chest radiograph.*

- Tube thoracostomy: Chest tubes are used to remove fluid or trapped air from the chest cavity as in a hemothorax or pneumothorax. A thoracic catheter is inserted, usually through the second intercostal space, the midclavicular line, or the fifth lateral intercostal space, midaxillary line. Placement depends on the location and extent of the hemothorax, effusion, or pneumothorax. The catheter can be connected to a one-way flutter valve (for air evacuation only) or to a closed chest drainage system. Tension pneumothorax is a life-threatening emergency requiring pleural decompression.

3. Enhance oxygenation and ventilation
- Oxygen therapy: Device is determined by the patient's response to therapy and may range from nasal cannula to 100% nonrebreathing mask, depending on extent of hypoxemia.
- Pulmonary toileting: Use of incentive spirometer, chest percussion, and suctioning to prevent atelectasis.
- Analgesia: Manages pain to minimize splinting and improve breathing. Opioid analgesics are used cautiously to avoid respiratory depression. An epidural patient-controlled analgesia pump or an intercostal nerve block may help to relieve local rib pain.
- Mechanical ventilation: Must be implemented for extreme respiratory distress or ventilatory collapse.
- Stabilization and fixation of flail chest: Most flail chest injuries stabilize within 10 to 14 days without surgical intervention. Stabilization of fractures is achieved using a volume-cycled ventilator. During surgery, a flail segment can be externally fixated by wiring or otherwise attaching the segment to the intact bony structures.

4. Restore perfusion and oxygen-carrying capacity
- Volume replacement: A high priority in the victim of trauma. Blood loss is replaced with PRBCs or whole fresh blood, if available. Blood replacement via autotransfusion may also be used. Use of colloid versus crystalloid fluids for volume replacement remains controversial. Volume is more often replaced with crystalloid fluids (e.g., NS, LR) rather than colloidal IV fluids (e.g., plasma, albumin). Colloids increase the risk of developing acute respiratory distress syndrome and acute renal failure, and are more expensive; furthermore, research has failed to demonstrate a significant benefit.
- Thoracotomy: Consider in patients with penetrating injuries to the chest who arrive in PEA or develop PEA shortly after arrival. This procedure should only be performed if a qualified surgeon is present. Opening the chest allows the surgeon to gain control over bleeding and restore intravascular volume to get the patient to the operating room for more definitive care.
- Repair of thoracic aortic injuries: If the patient is stable, repair should be delayed until the other injuries have been addressed and the patient is over the critical period. Repair may even occur on an elective basis after the patient is discharged from the hospital. Repair using endovascular stenting has been shown to decrease patient morbidity.

5. Support cardiac function
- Monitoring of hemodynamic status: If there is major cardiac or pulmonary involvement, use pulmonary artery monitoring and CO determinations with direct arterial pressure monitoring if indicated.
- Treatment of dysrhythmias: Use the ACLS protocols of the American Heart Association. If rhythm disturbances do not appear in the first 5 days after trauma, they rarely occur later.
- Immediate corrective surgical repair: Indicated for ruptured valve, torn papillary muscle, or torn intraventricular septum accompanied by hemodynamic instability.

- Treatment of shock: Initially, shock should be treated with fluid resuscitation to ensure adequate intravascular volume. Once intravascular volume has been restored and the patient remains hypotensive, vasopressor drugs (i.e., norepinephrine, epinephrine, vasopressin) may be necessary to enhance BP.
- Treatment of myocardial failure: Oxygen, diuretics, positive inotropic agents, and monitoring with a pulmonary artery catheter for right-sided and left-sided heart pressures.

> **Safety Alert** *Because of the potential for hemorrhage, never remove a penetrating object until the surgeon is present and studies have been completed to determine what the object has penetrated.*

CARE PLANS: THORACIC TRAUMA

Ineffective breathing pattern *related to pulmonary and/or cardiac injury*

Goals/Outcomes: Within 24 hours of this diagnosis, RR stabilizes to 12 to 20 breaths/min with normal work of breathing; lung injuries are managed to provide expanded lungs with minimal fluid and/or blood accumulation in the thoracic cavity; sources of bleeding are identified and managed to provide adequate Hgb level for adequate oxygenation; lost intravascular volume is replaced to reflect a CVP of 6 to 12 mm Hg; oxygen saturation is at least 95%, with Pao_2 at least 80 mm Hg with oxygen and $Paco_2$ less than 45 mm Hg with (or without) mechanical ventilation; and HR is 60 to 100 bpm with BP stable (at least 100 mm Hg systolic and 60 mm Hg diastolic).
NOC Respiratory Status: Ventilation.

 Airway Management
1. Monitor for sudden blood loss or persistent bleeding.
2. Prevent blood volume loss (e.g., apply pressure to site of bleeding).
3. Administer oxygen and/or mechanical ventilation, as appropriate.
4. Draw ABGs and monitor tissue oxygenation.

Ventilation Assistance
1. Monitor fluid status, including intake and output, as appropriate.
2. Maintain patent IV access.

Respiratory Monitoring
1. Monitor BP, pulse, temperature, and respiratory status.
2. Note trends and wide fluctuations in BP and auscultate BPs in both arms and compare.
3. Initiate and maintain a continuous temperature-monitoring device.

Decreased CO *related to cardiac injury or ineffective cardiac compensatory response to oxygenation or perfusion deficits.*

Goals/Outcomes: Within 24 hours of this diagnosis, the patient exhibits adequate CO, as evidenced by BP within normal limits for the patient; HR 60 to 100 bpm; normal sinus rhythm on ECG; peripheral pulses at least 2+ on a 0-to-4+ scale; warm and dry skin; hourly urine output at least 0.5 mL/kg; measured CO 4 to 7 L/min; CVP 2 to 6 mm Hg; PAP 20 to 30/8 to 15 mm Hg; PAWP 6 to 12 mm Hg; and patient awake, alert, oriented, and free from angina pain.
NOC Blood Loss Severity, Cardiac Pump Effectiveness.

 Hemorrhage Control
1. Apply manual pressure and/or pressure dressing as indicated.
2. Identify the cause of the bleeding.
3. Monitor the amount and nature of the blood loss.
4. Monitor Hgb and Hct levels.
5. Monitor clotting status via PT/PTT and INR values.

Shock Management
1. Monitor vital signs, mental status, and urinary output.
2. Use arterial line monitoring to improve accuracy of BP readings, as appropriate.
3. Monitor ABG results and tissue oxygenation.
4. Monitor trends in hemodynamic measurements (e.g., CVP, MAP, pulmonary capillary/artery wedge pressure).

5. Monitor determinants of tissue oxygen delivery (e.g., PaO_2, SaO_2, Hgb levels, CO), if available.
6. Insert and maintain large-bore IV access.
7. Administer crystalloids, as appropriate.
8. Administer blood and blood products, as appropriate.
9. Monitor fluid status, including daily weights and hourly urine output.
10. Administer inotropes, as appropriate.
11. Administer DVT and stress ulcer prophylaxis, as appropriate.

ADDITIONAL NURSING DIAGNOSES

For other nursing diagnoses and interventions, see sections on Major Trauma (Chapter 3), Acute Cardiac Tamponade (Chapter 1), Pain (Chapter 3), and Emotional and Spiritual Support of the Patient and Significant Others (Chapter 2).

TRAUMATIC BRAIN INJURY

PATHOPHYSIOLOGY

Traumatic brain injury (TBI), also known as acquired brain injury, occurs as a result of either blunt or penetrating forces to the head. Approximately 1.5 million TBIs occur each year with 52,000 resulting in death. Males are twice as likely to suffer a TBI as are females. Peak ages in the very young (until 1 year of age), young adults (15 to 24 years), and older adults (older than 65 years). Blunt injuries to the head are caused by acceleration, deceleration, and rotational forces (e.g., vehicular collisions, falls, high-impact sports). Penetrating injuries occur from piercing forces that traverse the skull and damage underlying brain tissue and support structures.

The initial impact (force) results in widespread injury resulting from tissue stresses and strain, which activate biomolecular processes within the cells. Injury results from structural and neuronal damage, vascular insufficiency, and inflammation. The cerebral vasculature and skull are often damaged. Tissue stresses result in contusions, diffuse axonal injuries, and compression injuries. Biomolecular processes cause neuroexcitation and deafferentation of the neurons. The neuroexcitatory injury activates excitatory neurotransmitters (glutamate and aspartate), which depolarize neurons. This neurotransmitter surge causes aberrant cell signaling, leading to long-lasting or permanent neuronal dysfunction. Deafferentation destroys the neurofilament of the axon, and the axon swells and retracts. Reduced blood flow, through cerebral edema or vasoconstrictive mechanisms, causes ischemia and augments cell death.

Outcome after TBI can be predicted to some extent based on the type of lesion, severity of injury, and length of coma. Age, preinjury medical status, mechanism of injury, ICP, and brainstem integrity are important factors influencing outcome.

CHANGES IN INTRACRANIAL PRESSURE DYNAMICS

Intracranial pressure dynamics is based on the volume-pressure relationship within the cranium (Monro-Kellie hypothesis). Three volumes exist within the fixed, rigid cranial vault: the brain, the blood, and the cerebrospinal fluid (CSF). Under normal conditions these volumes exert a pressure that is less than 15 mm Hg. The brain requires a constant blood supply to maintain normal function and when volume increases, pressure increases and compensatory mechanisms (shunting of CSF into the intrathecal space or vasoconstriction to reduce blood volume) are activated to reduce the volume. In brain injury, when the intrinsic compensatory mechanisms are damaged or overwhelmed, the functions that serve to maintain cerebral perfusion are compromised. Extrinsic measures are necessary to maintain the normal pressure-volume relationship and preserve cerebral perfusion pressure (CPP). Box 7-1 lists indicators of increased ICP (IICP). Treatment of derangements in ICP dynamics is based on the relationship between ICP and CPP and is stated simply: CPP = MAP − ICP.

MAP is calculated using the following equation:

$$MAP = (2 \times Diastolic + Systolic) \div 3.$$

The goal of treatment is to maintain CPP greater than 50 to 70 mm Hg and reduce ICP to less than 20 mm Hg.

PRIMARY BRAIN INJURIES

When the skull and brain are subjected to mechanical forces, a host of injuries in the cerebral cortex, brainstem, or cerebellum may change CPP. Severity of brain injuries is classified using the GCS: mild (GCS score = 13 to 15), moderate (GCS score = 9 to 12), and severe (GCS score ≤8). The FOUR score (Full Outline of UnResponsiveness) has been used with increasing frequency as a predictor of outcomes in patients with TBI. Verbal assessment is not possible with intubated patients using the GCS, which also lacks testing of brainstem reflexes. The FOUR score features four elements: eye, motor, brainstem, and respiration with a maximum score of 4 points for each element. The FOUR score provides additional details lacking in the GCS, can recognize locked-in syndrome, assesses brainstem reflexes, breathing patterns, and can recognize the different stages of herniation. Specific injuries arising from the mechanical forces are as follows:

- Contusion: Bruising that occurs as a result of mechanical forces to the head typically from the brain striking the skull or the dural folds. Cerebral contusions are seen as scattered areas of bleeding on the surface of the brain or the undersurface of the frontal and temporal poles. Coup (brain injury is directly beneath the site of impact) or contrecoup (brain injury is opposite the site of impact) injuries, herniation contusions (parahippocampal structures and cerebellar tonsils forced against the tentorium), and gliding contusions (from rotational forces in the parasagittal areas) can result in focal hemorrhage of the cortex and adjacent white matter. Surface (scalp) contusions are focal bruises, lacerations, and capillary hemorrhages found with contact forces. Surface or brain contusions may or may not be associated with fractures.
- Diffuse axonal injuries: Mild to severe injuries that occur when diffuse areas of white matter have been torn or sheared or when axons have been stretched. Injury evolves and generally worsens over time. The initial CT scan may not demonstrate a pathologic condition and does not reflect the severity that will manifest over time.
- Concussion: Neuroexcitatory injury sometimes associated with diffuse, axonal brain injuries. Classified as mild (no loss of consciousness, possible brief episodes of confusion or disorientation); moderate (brief loss of consciousness, transient focal neurologic deficits); or severe (prolonged loss of consciousness with sustained neurologic deficits lasting less than 24 hours). No changes are seen on CT scan, but patients with neurologic deficits require observation.
- Extra axial: Injuries are located outside the brain and are attributable to forces that disrupt the superficial layers of the brain resulting in bleeding (see Hematomas discussed later).

SECONDARY BRAIN INJURIES

Secondary injuries such as inflammation, edema, and changes in blood flow occur after the primary processes and further contribute to brain damage. They may be intrinsic or extrinsic. Secondary injury, despite the underlying cause, compromises the supply-demand ratio for cerebral oxygenation. Failure to manage secondary injury can result in irreversible neuronal damage superimposed on the already compromised injured brain.

- Intrinsic: Injuries that result from primary brain injury including intracranial hypertension, hypotension, hypovolemia, impaired autoregulation (causes reduced cerebral blood flow), reperfusion injury, brain edema, hemorrhage, herniation, cerebral vasospasm, hypoxia, inflammation, seizures, shivering, agitation, electrolyte imbalances, and hyperthermia.
- Extrinsic: Injuries unrelated to primary brain injury resulting from inadequate resuscitation, poor oxygenation, extreme hyperventilation, substance abuse, or hospital-acquired factors such as infections (meningitis), pneumonia, atelectasis, pulmonary edema, respiratory insufficiency, ventilatory-associated lung injury, or anesthetic agents used for surgical repair of injuries (see Meningitis, Chapter 7).

ASSOCIATED SKULL FRACTURES

Skull fractures occur as a result of blunt or penetrating impact force. Primary and secondary brain injuries are usually present.

- Linear skull fractures: Nondisplaced, associated with low-velocity impact.
- Basilar skull fractures: Linear fracture, involving the base of the anterior, middle, and posterior fossae of the cranium.
- Depressed skull fractures: Depression of the skull over the point of impact; may be comminuted (usually closed without direct brain penetration), compressed, or compound (open).

VASCULAR INJURIES

Vascular injuries are intrinsic brain injuries resulting from impact force that causes bleeding of cerebral arteries or veins. These injuries usually accompany moderate and severe primary injuries.

- Epidural hematomas: Commonly occur after a temporal linear skull fracture that lacerates the middle meningeal artery below it or from fractures of the sagittal and transverse sinuses. The hematoma develops rapidly in the space between the skull and dura and represents a life-threatening emergency.
- Subdural hematomas: Bleeding from veins between the dura and the arachnoid spaces; may be acute, subacute, or chronic. With the increased use of therapeutic anticoagulation for cardiac, stroke, and vascular problems, an increase in spontaneous and injury (falls) related subdural hematomas are being seen in the older population and alcoholics.
- Subarachnoid hemorrhage: Bleeding in the subarachnoid space seen over convexities of the brain or in the basal cisterns.
- Intracranial hematomas: Blood collection from injury to the small arteries and veins within the subcortical white matter of the temporal and frontal lobes; usually associated with petechiae, contusions, and edema.

NEUROLOGIC COMPLICATIONS
Herniation syndromes

Displacement of a portion of the brain through openings within the intracranial cavity that result from increased ICP. Herniation occurs when there is a pressure difference between the supratentorial and infratentorial compartments within the skull. When herniation occurs, significant portions of the cerebral vasculature are compressed, destroyed, or lacerated, resulting in ischemia, necrosis, and ultimately death.

- Cingulate herniation: Occurs with IICP or swelling in one brain hemisphere (left shift or right shift on CT). The affected high-pressure side shifts toward the low-pressure side causing compression of the anterior cerebral artery and internal cerebral vein. Reduced blood flow results in development of cerebral ischemia, edema, and IICP. Neurologic deficits include decreased LOC, with unilateral or bilateral lower extremity weakness or paralysis.
- Uncal herniation: Life-threatening, emergent situation that occurs when an expanding lesion (blood, edema, tumor) of the middle or temporal fossa forces the tip (uncus) of the temporal lobe toward the midline. The uncus protrudes over the edge of the tentorium cerebelli and compresses the oculomotor (third cranial) nerve and posterior cerebral artery. The uncus may be lacerated in the process and the midbrain is compressed against the tentorial edge. The patient manifests with an irregularly shaped pupil that may become fixed and dilated on the side of herniation, a change in respiratory pattern, marked deterioration in LOC, further elevation in ICP or decrease in ICP as the herniation progresses.
- Central (transtentorial) herniation: Life-threatening, emergent situation that occurs with expanding lesions of the frontal, parietal, or occipital lobes or with severe, generalized cerebral edema. Often, cingulate and uncal herniation precede this life-threatening process. Table 3-13 describes the clinical features of uncal and central herniation syndromes. Subcortical structures, including the basal ganglia and diencephalon (thalamus and hypothalamus), herniate through the tentorium cerebelli, causing compression of the midbrain and posterior cerebral arteries bilaterally. Symptoms of increased ICP often occur too rapidly to be observed. Changes in respiratory patterns may not be seen in patients who are critically ill and mechanically ventilated, depending on mode of ventilation (e.g., controlled or intermittent mandatory ventilation).
- Transcranial (extracranial) herniation: Occurs when intracranial contents under pressure are forced through an open wound, surgical site, or cranial vault fracture. Although the resultant loss of brain volume lowers ICP and may prevent intracranial herniation, this is an ominous sign and the patient is at risk for infection, further brain injury, and death.

ASSESSMENT: TRAUMATIC BRAIN INJURY

Neuroimaging is performed on all patients indicative of brain injury (see list as follows). CT scans demonstrate fractures, hematomas, and cerebral edema. Baseline physical examination data should include assessment of:

- Mental status
- Cranial nerves
- Motor status

Table 3-13	ASSESSMENT OF CENTRAL AND UNCAL HERNIATIONS			
	Diencephalic		Midbrain/ Upper Pons	Lower Pons/ Upper Medulla
Criteria	**Early**	**Late**		
Central Herniation				
Respiratory pattern	Deep sighs, yawning	Cheyne-Stokes pattern of respiratory rate increases, followed by decreases, then apnea, which repeats	Hyperventilation that is sustained and regular	Shallow, rapid, irregular
Pupils: size/ reaction	Small; react to bright light; small range of contraction	Small; react to bright light; small range of contraction	Midpositioned; irregularly shaped; fixed reaction to light	Midpositioned; fixed
Oculocephalic/ oculovestibular responses (doll's eyes phenomenon/ ice water caloric)	Full conjugate or slightly roving eye movements; full conjugate lateral; ipsilateral response to ice water ear irrigation	Same as early; nystagmus absent	Impaired; may be disconjugate	No response
Motor Responses				
At rest	Contralateral paresis, which may worsen	Motionlessness	Abnormal extension posturing	Flaccidity
To stimulus	Bilateral Babinski sign	Abnormal flexion posturing	Rigidity	Bilateral Babinski sign
	Early third nerve		Late third nerve	
Uncal Herniation				
Respiratory pattern	Normal		Hyperventilation that is regular and sustained	
Pupils: size/ reaction	Moderate dilation; ipsilateral to primary lesion; sluggish constriction; brisk contralateral papillary reaction		Widely dilated and fixed ipsilateral pupil	
Oculocephalic/ oculovestibular responses (doll's eyes phenomenon/ ice water caloric)	Present or disconjugate, full conjugate, slow ipsilateral eye movement or disconjugate caused by contralateral eye not moving medially		Impaired or absent Full lateral movement with contralateral eye; absence of medial movement with ipsilateral eye	
Motor response to stimulus	Contralateral extensor plantar reflex		Ipsilateral hemiplegia; abnormal posturing; absence of all responses	

Modified from Plum F, Posner J: *Diagnostic of stupor and coma*, ed 3, Philadelphia, 1980, Davis.

- Sensory status
- Reflexes

Thereafter, ongoing neurologic assessment should be based on the clinical status of the patient. Ideally, a complete neurologic assessment should be performed. However, many components of the examination require patients to follow commands. For patients unable to follow commands, the neurologic assessment should be tailored individually to the patient's abilities and redesigned as necessary. The Glasgow Coma Scale (see Appendix 2) is applicable for use in the acute phase, and the Rancho Los Amigos Cognitive Functioning Scale (see Cognitive Rehabilitation Goals, Table 1-6) can be used for recovery/rehabilitation assessment and should be part of the neurologic assessment.

The following are assessment findings related to specific types of brain injuries.

EPIDURAL HEMATOMA/LINEAR SKULL FRACTURE

- Scalp lacerations, swelling, tenderness, and ecchymosis of the head and scalp are associated injuries.
- Classic epidural signs are loss of consciousness, followed by a lucid interval and then rapid deterioration.
- Ipsilateral pupil dilation and contralateral weakness, followed by brainstem compression, occur if treatment is not initiated emergently.

BASILAR SKULL FRACTURE

- Dural tears resulting in rhinorrhea and otorrhea are common.
- Anterior fossa injuries are associated with periorbital ecchymosis (raccoon eyes), epistaxis, damage to cranial nerves I and II, and meningitis.
- Middle and posterior fossa injuries may damage cranial nerves VII and VIII and are associated with tinnitus, hemotympanum, and destruction of the cochlear vestibular apparatus.
- Ecchymosis of the mastoid process (Battle sign) is common.

COMPOUND DEPRESSED SKULL FRACTURE

- Changes in LOC, pupillary changes
- Headache
- Increased ICP (if measured invasively)
- CSF leaks if the dura has been torn, tympanum rupture
- Comminuted fractures are open wounds with or without dural tears, CSF leak, and transcalvarial herniation.

CONCUSSION

- Headache, although there are no overt signs of injury
- Dizziness
- Vomiting
- Memory loss
- Decreased attention and concentration skills

 HIGH ALERT! Moderate and severe injuries require close observation because cerebral edema and increased intracranial pressure can develop. Changes in behavior, level of consciousness, or refractory intracranial pressure require an immediate computed tomography scan.

CONTUSION

- Loss of consciousness is common. May have surface bruising of face or scalp along with hematoma.
- Neurologic deficits may be generalized or focal, depending on the site and severity of injury.

DIFFUSE AXONAL INJURY

- May occur with other injuries and is characterized by an immediate loss of consciousness. Duration of coma varies, depending on the severity of the injury, but often coma is prolonged and recovery of function is minimal to moderate.
- Edema and unstable ICP dynamics are common.

SUBDURAL HEMATOMA

- With acute subdural hematoma, neurologic deterioration is seen within 24 to 72 hours (or earlier), changing LOC, ipsilateral dilated pupil, and contralateral extremity weakness.
- Subacute hematoma may present within 48 hours to days after injury and manifests initially as a headache as LOC begins to deteriorate and focal neurologic deficits ensue.
- Chronic subdural are associated with progression of elusive, fluctuating deficits, such as personality changes, memory loss, headache, extremity weakness, and incontinence, especially in high-risk groups such as older adults and chronic alcohol users. The insidious nature of the bleed and hematoma formation delays critical signs and symptoms weeks to months after the injury occurs.

HIGH ALERT! Neurologic signs associated with a chronic subdural hematoma may occur weeks or months after injury.

SUBARACHNOID HEMORRHAGE

- Severe headache often reported as "the worst headache of my life."
- Changes in LOC.
- Meningeal signs: nuchal rigidity, elevated temperature, and positive Kernig sign and Brudzinski sign (loss of ability to extend leg when thigh is flexed on abdomen).
- Noncommunicating hydrocephalus is a delayed complication that requires placement of an external ventricular shunt to drain CSF.

INTRACRANIAL HEMATOMA

- Neurologic deficits are based on the site and severity of injury.

Diagnostic Tests for Traumatic Brain Injury

Test	Purpose	Abnormal Findings
Skull radiograph	Detect structural deficits.	Skull fractures, facial bone destruction, air-fluid level in sinuses, unusual intracranial calcification, pineal gland location (normally midline), and radiopaque foreign bodies.
Cervical spine radiograph	Evaluate for structural deficits of the spine. Cervical spine immobilization is mandated in all patients with trauma until the cervical spine (C1-T1) is visualized completely and fractures are ruled out.	Cervical spine injuries, including fractures, dislocations, and subluxations.
Computed tomography (CT) without contrast Spiral CT can be used for angiographic imaging	Fast diagnostic tool to evaluate for primary and secondary brain injuries and structural changes secondary to injury.	Gray and white matter, blood, and cerebrospinal fluid (CSF) are identified by their different radiologic densities. CT is used to diagnose cerebral hemorrhage, infarction, hydrocephalus, cerebral edema, and structural changes.
Magnetic resonance imaging (MRI)	Identify type, location, and extent of injury.	Spatial resolution can follow metabolic processes and detect tissue and structural changes.

Continued

| **Diagnostic Tests for Traumatic Brain Injury—cont'd** | | |
Test	Purpose	Abnormal Findings
Cerebral angiography	Examine the cerebral vasculature.	Abnormalities in cerebral circulation, filling defects, diminished blood flow.
Electroencephalography (EEG)	Measure spontaneous brain electrical activity via surface electrodes. Drug therapy, especially with narcotics, sedatives, and anticonvulsants, alters brain activity. Use of these drugs should be documented if the drug cannot be withheld 24 to 48 hours before performing EEG.	Abnormal brain activity (irritability) associated with seizures and generalized brain activity related to drug overdose, coma, or suspected brain death.
Evoked responses	Evaluates the electrical potentials (responses) of the brain to an external stimulus (i.e., auditory, visual, somatosensory). Evoked potentials are used to determine the extent of injury in patients who are uncooperative, confused, or comatose.	Abnormal or delayed expected response levels indicating lesions of the cortex or ascending pathways of the spinal cord, brainstem, or thalamus
CSF analysis	Evaluate for infection and bleeding	Abnormal color, turbidity/cloudiness, red blood cell (RBC) and white blood cell (WBC) counts, protein, glucose, electrolytes, gram stain, culture, and sensitivity.
Laboratory work WBCs Hemoglobin Hematocrit Partial thromboplastin time, prothrombin time/international normalized ratio Electrolyte panel Glucose Osmolality Alcohol and urine drug screen (admission)	Evaluate for metabolic imbalances, infection, coagulation status, bleeding, and drug use.	Can indicate infection, anemia, nutritional deficiencies, electrolyte imbalances, and drug use. All need to be monitored closely during emergency and acute phases.

COLLABORATIVE MANAGEMENT

CARE PRIORITIES

1. Surgical intervention

- Performed to evacuate mass lesions (epidural, subdural, and intracranial hematomas), place an ICP monitoring system (often placed in the emergency department or at the bedside), elevate depressed skull fractures, debride open wounds and brain tissue, and repair dural tears or scalp lacerations. Decompressive craniectomies and frontal and/or temporal lobectomies may be necessary to control severe increases in ICP.

2. Preoperative and postoperative management of coagulopathies

- Home medication history is imperative along with preoperative PT/INR and PTT evaluation in all patients with TBI.
- Subdural hematomas or intracerebral hemorrhage are more common in patients on clopidogrel (Plavix), aspirin, warfarin, or other anticoagulants.

Safety Alert *Stop all anticoagulation medication including heparin. If the patient is to have an emergent craniotomy for evacuation of a subdural hematoma or other injury, prothrombin time/international normalized ratio, partial thromboplastin time, and platelets must be normalized.*

- For patients on warfarin with INR greater than 1.2, infuse fresh-frozen plasma, or factor VII, and administer vitamin K until INR is in nontherapeutic range (less than 1.2). Monitor PT/INR daily and continue infusion of fresh-frozen plasma and administration of vitamin K based on results.
- For patients on Plavix (clopidogrel) or other antiplatelet medications, infuse platelets to achieve homeostasis. Platelet counts will appear normal, but their coagulation function has been altered by the clopidogrel or aspirin. Daily regimen of platelet replacement should continue for up to 5 postoperative days.

HIGH ALERT! There are no evidence-based studies for reversing coagulopathies because patients' response to medication is very individual. These strategies are aimed at monitoring the coagulopathy while they wax and wane over the postoperative course.

3. Management of ICP dynamics
- ICP monitoring is performed by a variety of techniques (Table 3-14). All monitoring systems provide a digital display of ICP, but CPP must be calculated (see Chapter 3).
- The goal is to maintain CPP greater than 50 to 70 mm Hg. Intraventricular catheters and parenchymal catheters are recommended for monitoring ICP over subarachnoid and epidural monitoring systems.

RESEARCH BRIEF 3-1

Intracranial pressure (ICP) monitoring is indicated for patients with a Glasgow Coma Scale (GCS) score ≤8 after resuscitation and an abnormal admission computed tomography (CT) scan. Placement of an ICP monitor is also suggested in patients who have a GCS ≤8 with a normal CT scan and if two or more of the following are noted on admission: (1) the patient is older than 40 years, (2) the patient has unilateral or bilateral abnormal posturing, or (3) the patient's systolic blood pressure is less than 90 mm Hg. Physician discretion may also determine the use of ICP monitoring.

Adapted from Brain Trauma Foundation: Guidelines for the management of severe head injury. *J Neurotrauma* 24(Suppl 1):S1-S106, 2007.

---

4. Reduction of ICP by CSF drainage
- Performed using intraventricular or ventriculostomy systems.
- To prevent overdraining, the drainage collection bags must be maintained at the level of the tragus of the ear or higher, thereby preventing excessive CSF flow caused by a higher-to-lower pressure gradient.

5. Hyperventilation via mechanical ventilation

Safety Alert *Hyperventilation is no longer recommended as a first-line treatment and should be used only with cerebral oxygen monitoring to reduce intracranial pressure. Hyperventilation should be avoided during the first 24 hours after injury.*

- Prophylactic hyperventilation ($Paco_2$ greater than 25 Hg) is recommended for short periods until more definitive therapies are initiated or increased ICP is reduced to avoid

Traumatic Brain Injury

Table 3-14		TYPES OF INTRACRANIAL MONITORING		
System	Type	Placement	Advantages/ Uses	Disadvantages
Fluid-filled or fiber optic	Intraventricular cannula	Lateral ventricle in nondominant hemisphere through burr hole	CSF measurement CSF drainage Drug administration Volume-pressure response testing	Rapid CSF drainage can result in collapsed ventricles or subdural hematoma Cannula tip may catch on ventricular wall Risk of intracerebral bleeding and infection May become plugged with debris Possible difficult insertion because of shifting or collapse of ventricle
Fluid-filled	Subarachnoid screw	Subarachnoid space through twist drill hole	Pressure monitoring Less risk of infection than with cannula Useful with small ventricles Does not penetrate brain	Compliance testing may be unreliable No CSF drainage Some risk of infection Risk of hemorrhage or hematoma during insertion Brain may be herniated into bolt, making recording unreliable
Electrical sensor	Epidural sensor	Epidural space Burr hole Fiber optic sensor	Lowest risk of infection Easy to insert Dura not penetrated	No direct measurement of CSF No CSF drainage Inability to recalibrate to zero Cannot measure volume-pressure response
Fiber optic	Intraparenchymal	Intraparenchymal via twist drill Fiber optic sensor	Easy to insert Direct pressure Compliance testing One-time zero and calibration before insertion	Risk of intracerebral bleeding and infection No CSF drainage

CSF, Cerebrospinal fluid.

herniation. Maintaining $Paco_2$ within a normal range is now considered optimal ventilation. Recent evidence suggests that hyperventilation may cause neurologic dysfunction as a result of decreased cerebral perfusion.

6. Monitoring jugular venous oxygen saturation (SjO_2)

- Used to measure cerebral oxygenation by determining oxygen content of cerebral venous blood as a global measurement of oxygen supply and demand. Three types of blood flow can be discriminated:
  - Normal (SjO_2 = 55% to 70%).
  - Oligemic (SjO_2 less than 55%).
  - Hyperemia (SjO_2 greater than 70%).
  - Treatment should be aimed at maintaining normal range.

7. Monitoring brain tissue oxygenation (PbTO₂)

- Used to monitor the partial pressure of regional brain tissue oxygenation at catheter tip to detect cerebral ischemia and hypoxia. Cerebral hypoxia, a secondary brain injury event, has been associated with poor patient outcomes.
- PbTO₂ levels greater than 20 are recommended.

> **HIGH ALERT!** Optimal management of a severe traumatic brain injury should include monitoring of cerebral perfusion pressure (CPP), intracranial pressure (ICP), and PbTO₂, as well as ventilation management. ICP threshold should be less than 20 mm Hg, optimal CPP is 50 to 70 mm Hg, and optimal PbTO₂ is greater than 20 mm Hg. While ICP rises and PbTO₂ falls, it may be necessary to adjust the FiO_2 to keep PbTO₂ greater than 20. It is not uncommon for FiO_2 to be 0.1 or 100% to maintain adequate cerebral oxygenation. PaO_2 less than 60 mm Hg should be avoided.

- Other ways to improve PbTO₂ include raising BP, treating anemia, and adjusting pCO_2.

8. Hyperosmolar therapy

- Reduces cerebral brain volume by removing fluid from the extracellular compartment of the brain.
- Mannitol, an osmotic diuretic, and hypertonic saline are generally used. Mannitol may be given in 0.25 to 1.0 g/kg body weight doses as needed to reduce ICP or may be given as a scheduled dose every 4 to 6 hours. Although there is no level 1 evidence supporting the use of hypertonic saline, patients with TBI who received hypertonic saline in a small study of patients with polytrauma had improved survival and restoration of hemodynamic stability. It may be useful as an adjunct therapy in refractory IICP.
- Dehydration is a major complication with the continued use of hyperosmolar therapies. Serum electrolyte and osmolality values should be closely monitored.
- Fluid balance is maintained with fluid therapy (75 to 100 mL/h). Replacement of urine losses may be prescribed based on the volume of urine collected 1 hour after giving hyperosmolar agents. Given either milliliter for milliliter or 0.5 mL for milliliter over a 3- to 4-hour period.

9. Maintenance of blood pressure to maintain CPP

- Hypotension and hypertension both contribute to cerebral edema, which compresses blood vessels. Hypotension can result in decreased oxygen delivery to brain cells. Elevated $PaCO_2$ reduces pH causing cerebral vessels to vasodilate. Hypotension reduces MAP and thus CPP. Glucose solutions are not used for fluid resuscitation in TBI.
- Vasoconstrictive medications (phenylephrine, norepinephrine) or inotropic medications (dobutamine) may be used. The aim is to avoid systolic BP less than 90 mm Hg.
- Effects of hypertension (elevated CPP and increased cerebral edema) are unclear, but increased capillary permeability and petechial hemorrhage are seen. Antihypertensive medications, such as labetalol HCl (Normodyne) or nitroprusside sodium (Nipride), may be required.

10. Reduction of metabolic demand

- Important strategy when treating ICP problems, because cerebral blood supply must match demand to maintain cerebral function.
- Sedating agents: Use of individual or combined continuous infusions of sedatives, analgesics, and paralytic drugs to reduce metabolic demand. Midazolam HCl (Versed), opiate analgesics such as fentanyl citrate (Sublimaze), sufentanil, or morphine sulfate, and anesthetic agents such as propofol (Diprivan) are used. Propofol may be preferred for its short half-life. Watch for "propofol infusion syndrome" (metabolic acidosis, rhabdomyolysis, hyperkalemia, and renal failure). Recommendations of doses are given in Table 3-15. Nondepolarizing neuromuscular blocking agents, including vecuronium bromide (Norcuron) or atracurium, are used but must be used with sedation and can mask seizure activity. (See also Sedation and Neuromuscular Blockade, Chapter 1.)
- Seizure control: Seizure activity increases the metabolic demand of the brain. Anticonvulsants are recommended to prevent early posttraumatic seizures (7-day course) despite

Table 3-15	ANALGESICS AND SEDATIVES RECOMMENDATIONS FOR USE IN TRAUMATIC BRAIN INJURY	
Agent	**Dose**	**Comments**
Morphine sulfate	4 mg/h continuous infusion	Titrate PRN Reverse with Narcan
Midazolam	2 mg test dose; then 2 to 4 mg/h continuous infusion	Reverse with flumazenil
Fentanyl	2 μg/kg test dose; then 2 to 5 μg/kg/h continuous infusion	
Sufentanil	10 to 30 μg test dose; then 0.05 to 2 μg/kg continuous bolus	
Propofol	0.5 mg/kg test bolus; then 20 to 75 μg/kg/min continuous infusion	Do not exceed 5 mg/kg/h Monitor closely, especially young adults

From Brain Trauma Foundation: Guidelines for the management of severe brain trauma. *J Neurotrauma* 24(Suppl 1):S1-S73, 2007.

- the fact that early posttraumatic seizure is not associated with worse outcomes. Posttraumatic seizure may occur with all TBIs but there is a higher incidence in patients with focal brain injuries such as depressed, comminuted, or compound skull fractures, contusions, lacerations, and penetrating injuries.
- Seizure prophylaxis with anticonvulsant agents such as phenytoin sodium (Dilantin) or, less often, levetiracetam (Keppra) or valproic acid is often prescribed. When using phenytoin, a weight-based loading dose of 15 to 20 mg/kg is given slowly at 50 mg/min, followed by a daily dose of 100 mg three times daily. Phenytoin cannot be administered with a dextrose solution because it will precipitate. Therapeutic levels are reported to be between 10 and 20 mg/mL. Doses should be scheduled to maintain free Dilantin levels between 1 and 2 mg/mL. Doses should be patient-specific (higher levels may be necessary to prevent breakthrough seizures, whereas lower levels may be acceptable if seizures are controlled).

Safety Alert   *In a patient with normal albumin levels, the free level correlates closely with the therapeutic level, but in patients who are hypoalbuminemic, such as patients with acute traumatic brain injury, the free level can be significantly higher and more accurately represents the patient's "true" phenytoin (Dilantin) level.*

- Barbiturate coma: A less-often used method of reducing metabolic demand, barbiturate administration, is recommended to control ICP refractory to standard medical and surgical treatment.
  - High doses of barbiturates should not be used without continuous ICP and hemodynamic monitoring and controlled mechanical ventilation. Barbiturates may induce profound cardiac and cerebral depression. Pentobarbital sodium (Nembutal) is the drug of choice.
  - A loading dose between 5 and 10 mg/kg is given (discontinue if MAP falls to less than 70 mm Hg), followed by a maintenance dose of 1 to 3 mg/kg/h.
  - Clinically significant hypotension is usually seen with barbiturate coma. It is not responsive to fluid resuscitation and requires the use of vasopressors such as dopamine or phenylephrine.
  - Barbiturates are withdrawn gradually while the patient improves. Patients with barbiturate coma require intensive physical care and physiologic monitoring.
  - Assessment of brain death criteria, if appropriate, cannot be initiated until barbiturate levels return to zero.

- Maintaining body temperature: For every 1° C in temperature elevation, there is a 10% to 13% increase in metabolic rate. Body temperature should be normal to control metabolic demand.

> **HIGH ALERT!** Normal temperatures range from 35.8° C to 37.5° C (96.4° F to 99.5° F) with a diurnal variation of 1° C. Rectal temperatures are 0.2° C to 0.6° C higher than oral and can be 0.8° C higher than right atrial, esophageal, and oral temperatures. Evaluation of the etiology of fever is important with brain injury, because it influences treatment choice.

- Fever may be caused by brain injury (central fever), an infectious process (peripheral fever), or drugs (drug fever). Central fever reflects disturbance in the hypothalamic thermoregulatory mechanism. It is characterized by lack of sweating, no diurnal variation, plateau-like elevation patterns, elevations up to 41° C (105.8° F), absence of tachycardia, persistence for days or weeks, and temperature reduction with external cooling rather than with antipyretic agents.
- Peripheral fever is associated with wound infections, meningitis, sepsis, pneumonia, and other bacterial invasion. Sweating, diurnal variation, response to antipyretic agents, and tachycardia are present.
- Drug fever occurs in response to certain medications including antibiotics.

External cooling with a hypothermia blanket may cause shivering, the body's mechanism to increase heat production.

> **HIGH ALERT!** Shivering increases metabolic demand and may increase intracranial pressure. Shivering may be controlled by wrapping distal extremities in bath towels before initiating hypothermia or using chlorpromazine (Thorazine), which must be used with caution because it may cause hypotension. Research on use of hypothermia in treatment of acute brain injury is evolving. If used, follow a strict hypothermia protocol. Currently, there is no support for prophylactic hypothermia.

11. Modifying nursing care activities that raise ICP

- Transient brief and rapid elevations in ICP, which cannot always be avoided, are commonly seen during position changes or other nursing care activities. Generally, ICP returns to resting baseline within a few minutes.

> **HIGH ALERT!** All nursing care activities that increase intracranial pressure (ICP) should be spaced to enable a return of ICP to baseline and maximizing of cerebral perfusion pressure. Clustering nursing care such as bathing, turning, and suctioning creates a stair-step rise in ICP. Sustained increases (longer than 5 minutes) should be avoided.

- Suctioning: Causes a significant rise in ICP. To minimize adverse effects associated with suctioning, implement the guidelines outlined in Box 3-6.
- Neck positioning: Flexion, extension, and lateral movements of the neck can significantly raise ICP. Maintaining the neck in a neutral position at all times is important. In patients with poor neck control, stabilize the neck with towel rolls or sandbags.
- Elevating head of bed: Although head of bed elevation at 30 degrees is believed to improve venous drainage and contribute to ICP reduction, ICP may be improved at higher or lower elevations. Adjust head of bed elevation to optimize the patient's CPP and $PbTO_2$ and minimize ICP.
- Turning: Turning is necessary to prevent pressure ulcer formation and is not contraindicated. Individual patient responses to turning should be evaluated. Initially, turning from side to side will elevate pressure, but ICP should return to resting baseline after a few minutes. If ICP does not return to resting baseline within 5 minutes, CPP may be compromised and the patient should be returned to a position that reduces ICP and

Box 3-6	GUIDELINES FOR SUCTIONING SECRETIONS FROM PATIENTS AT RISK FOR INCREASED INTRACRANIAL PRESSURE

- Suction only if the clinical status of the patient warrants.
- Precede suctioning with preoxygenation using 100% oxygen.
- Limit each suctioning pass to ≤10 seconds.
- Limit suction passes to two.
- Follow each pass with 60 seconds of hyperventilation using 100% oxygen.
- Use negative suction pressure less than 120 mm Hg.
- Keep the patient's head in a neutral position.
- Use a suction catheter with an outer-to-inner diameter ratio of 2:1.

maximizes CPP. Hip flexion also increases ICP. If independent nursing activities do not decrease ICP, then medical protocols must be used.

- Bathing: Although bathing itself has not been documented as raising ICP, the rapid turning from side to side associated with linen changes raises ICP. These "turn procedures" are actually clustered activities because the length of the procedure does not allow sufficient time for ICP to return to baseline. Evaluation of the patient's response may necessitate performing the linen change in stages or allowing adequate time for ICP to return to resting baseline.
- Sensory stimulation: A sensory stimulation program may be implemented safely in patients who are comatose early after injury when ICP is stable. This rehabilitative technique may be an important adjunct to traditional care and improve admission to an active rehabilitation program (Table 3-16).

12. Nutrition support: Feeding should be initiated as early as possible to achieve full caloric replacement within 7 days of injury

- Enteral nutrition helps to maintain the integrity of the gut mucosa and should be initiated as early as possible after injury.
- When postpyloric (duodenum or jejunum) feeding tubes are used, enteral feedings can be initiated before bowel sounds return to normal.
- In some cases, gastric tubes for decompression are used simultaneously with the postpyloric tubes. See Nutrition Support (Chapter 1) for documentation of proper placement and checking of residual volumes. If enteral feedings are contraindicated or not tolerated by the patient, total parenteral nutrition must be started.

13. Prevention of aspiration

- Prevalent complication after brain injury.
- Aspiration may occur at the time of injury or as an iatrogenic complication of intubation, enteral feedings, or prolonged use of artificial airways.
- Tracheobronchial secretions should be checked for glucose (a sign that tube feedings have been aspirated).
- Follow enteral feeding protocols initiated.
- Initial and ongoing swallowing assessments can be done at the bedside or under fluoroscopy.

14. DVT prophylaxis

- Patients with TBI are at risk for developing DVT as well as PE as a result of prolonged bed rest. There is concern for the use of anticoagulation therapies because there is risk for expansion of intracranial hemorrhage. There is level III support for the prophylactic use of low–molecular-weight heparin or unfractionated heparin along with mechanical measures to prevent DVT (sequential compression devices); however, there is no evidence to support optimum doses or time when to begin therapy. Clinical practice guidelines for TBI also support the use of graduated compression stockings, unless the lower extremity injuries prevent their use. However, there are no recommendations for the therapeutic treatment of DVT or PE. DVT management is determined by the attending physician based on risk-benefit ratios.

Table 3-16	**MANAGEMENT OF SEVERE BRAIN INJURY**	
Treatment	**Level of Evidence***	**Recommendation**
Blood pressure	Level II†	Avoid early postinjury episodes of hypotension <90 mm Hg.
Oxygenation	Level III	Avoid Pao_2 <60 mm Hg and O_2 saturation <90%.
ICP treatment threshold	Level II	Treatment to lower ICP should be initiated at 20 mm Hg.
CPP treatment	Level III	CPP should be maintained at ≥50 mm Hg. Maintain MAP >90 mm Hg.
Cerebral oxygenation	Level III	Keep $PbTO_2$ >20.
Hyperventilation	Level II	Avoid prophylactic hyperventilation; hyperventilate for short duration for refractory increased ICP >25 mm Hg.
	Level III	Avoid hyperventilation in the first 24 hours postinjury.
Hyperosmolar therapy	Level II	Mannitol: use intermittent boluses of 0.25 to 1 mg/kg.
	Option	Hypertonic saline (3%). No recommended dose.
Barbiturates	Level II	May be considered in patients with hemodynamic stability refractory to other methods to reduce ICP.
Propofol	Level II	Use for control of ICP.
Glucocorticoids	Standard	Use is not recommended.
Nutrition	Level II	Full caloric replacement by postinjury day 7
Seizure prophylaxis	Level II	Anticonvulsants can be considered an option for high-risk patients early after injury. Not recommended for preventing late posttraumatic seizures.

Data from Brain Trauma Foundation: Guidelines for the management of severe head injury.
J Neurotrauma 24(Suppl 1):S1-S106, 2007.
*Level of evidence denotes the degree that the recommendation represents clinical certainty.
†*Level II,* Moderate clinical certainty; *Level III/Option,* unclear clinical certainty; *Standard,* high level of certainty. Level of evidence is based on scientific literature where the highest degree of certainty is drawn from prospective randomized clinical trials.
CCP, Cerebral perfusion pressure; *ICP,* intracranial pressure; *MAP,* mean arterial pressure.

15. Management of cardiac dysrhythmias
- Commonly seen in patients with brain injuries and probably related to autonomic (sympathetic and parasympathetic) derangement or compression of midbrain and brainstem structures.
- ECG changes seen with elevated ICP are prominent U waves, ST segment changes, notched T waves, and prolongation of the QT interval.
- Bradycardia, supraventricular, tachycardia, and ventricular dysrhythmias are common.

16. Glucose management
- Keep serum glucose ranges within normal limits. Avoid levels greater than 170 mg/dL and less than 50 mg/dL to avoid worsening the brain injury. Insulin therapy may be required to control hyperglycemia.

17. Glucocorticoid
- Use of glucocorticoids (dexamethasone) is not indicated for brain injury and may result in worse outcomes.

18. Rehabilitation
- Brain injury often results in physical (paralysis, spasticity, and contractures) and cognitive impairments.

- Consult with physical, occupational, and speech therapists early to minimize deficits and prepare the patient for an acute rehabilitative program.
- National Institutes of Health (NIH) Consensus Development Conference Recommendations on Rehabilitation of Persons with Brain Injury are available. Support also is available through the Brain Injury Association of America (www.biausa.org).

19. Neuroprotective strategies
- Ongoing brain injury research is targeting neuroprotective strategies that include hypothermia, IV progesterone, and use of magnesium, cyclosporine, erythropoietin, and hyperbaric therapies.

CARE PLANS: TRAUMATIC BRAIN INJURY

Impaired gas exchange *related to decreased oxygen supply and increased CO_2 production secondary to decreased ventilatory drive occurring with pressure on respiratory center, imposed inactivity, pneumonia, acute respiratory distress syndrome, and possible neurologic pulmonary edema.*

Goals/Outcomes: Keep $Paco_2$ values in normal range greater than 35 mm Hg and Pao_2 greater than 60 mm Hg. By the time of discharge from ICU or transfer to rehabilitation unit, the patient has adequate gas exchange, as evidenced by appropriate mental status and orientation; $Pao_2 \geq 60$ mm Hg; RR 12 to 20 breaths/min with normal depth and pattern; and absence of adventitious breath sounds.

NOC *Respiratory Status:* Gas Exchange.

Respiratory Monitoring
1. Assess the patient's RR, depth, and rhythm. Auscultate lung fields for breath sounds every 1 to 2 hours and as needed. Monitor for respiratory patterns described in Table 3-13. Be alert to IICP (see Box 7-1).
2. Assess the patient for signs of hypoxia, including confusion, agitation, restlessness, and irritability. Remember that cyanosis is a late indicator of hypoxia.
3. Ensure a patent airway via proper positioning of neck and frequent assessment of the need for suctioning. Ensure hyperoxygenation of the patient before and after each suction attempt to prevent dangerous, suction-induced hypoxia or $PbTO_2$ less than 20. Do not overventilate. Keep $Paco_2$ between 35 and 45 mm Hg.
4. Monitor ABG values; consult the physician for significant findings or changes. Be alert to levels indicative of hypoxemia (Pao_2 less than 80 mm Hg) and to $Paco_2$ less than 35 mm Hg, considering that levels higher than this range may increase cerebral blood flow and thus increase ICP.
5. Ensure that oxygen is delivered within prescribed limits.
6. Assist with turning every 2 hours, within limits of the patient's injury, to promote lung drainage and expansion and alveolar perfusion. Unless contraindicated, raise the head of the bed 30 degrees to enhance gas exchange.
7. Encourage deep breathing at frequent intervals to promote oxygenation. Avoid coughing exercises for patients at risk for IICP.
8. Evaluate the need for an artificial airway in patients unable to maintain airway patency or adequate ventilatory effort.

NIC Airway Management; Oxygen Therapy; Respiratory Monitoring.

Risk for infection: CNS *related to inadequate primary defenses secondary to direct access to the brain in the presence of skull fracture, penetrating wounds, craniotomy, intracranial monitoring, or bacterial invasion caused by pneumonia or iatrogenic causes.*

Goals/Outcomes: The patient is free of infection, as evidenced by normothermia, WBC count $\leq 11,000/mm^3$, negative culture results, HR ≤ 100 bpm, BP within the patient's normal range, and absence of agitation, purulent drainage, and other clinical indicators of infection.

NOC Risk Identification.

Infection Protection
1. Assess vital signs at frequent intervals for indicators of CNS infection. Be alert to elevated temperature and increased HR and BP.
2. Monitor the patient for signs of systemic infection, including discomfort, malaise, agitation, and restlessness.
3. Inspect cranial wounds for the presence of erythema, tenderness, swelling, and purulent drainage. Obtain prescription for culture as indicated.

4. Monitor CSF from intraventricular catheter for cloudy appearance or blood. Analysis of CSF should be done on a routine basis.
5. Other infection sites: Monitor for signs of UTI if the patient has an indwelling Foley catheter. Monitor other injury and surgical sites.
6. Apply a loose sterile dressing (sling) to collect CSF drainage from nose. Do not pack the nose or ears if there is CSF drainage. Record amount, color, and characteristics of drainage.
7. Caution the patient against coughing, sneezing, nose blowing, or Valsalva or similar maneuvers, because these activities can further damage the dura. Use orogastric tubes if BSFs or severe frontal sinus fractures are present.
8. Ensure timely administration of prescribed antibiotics.
9. Apply basic principles for care of any invasive device used with ICP monitoring:
   - Use good handwashing technique before caring for the patient.
   - Discourage the patient from touching devices if awake; apply restraints only if necessary to keep the patient from harm. Restraints can increase ICP by causing straining and agitation.
   - Maintain aseptic technique during care of device, following agency protocol for infection control.

Decreased intracranial adaptive capacity *related to decreased CPP or infections that can occur with secondary head injury.*

Goals/Outcomes: Within 12 to 24 hours of treatment/interventions, the patient has adequate intracranial adaptive capacity, as evidenced by equal and normoreactive pupils; RR 12 to 20 breaths/min with normal depth and pattern (eupnea); HR 60 to 100 bpm; ICP up to 15 mm Hg; CPP greater than 50 mm Hg; and absence of headache, vomiting, and other clinical indicators of IICP. Optimally, by the time of discharge from ICU or transfer to rehabilitation unit, the patient is oriented to time, place, and person and has bilaterally equal strength and tone in the extremities.
NOC Neurologic Status.

Neurologic Monitoring
1. Assess neurologic status at least hourly (GCS and FOUR score are commonly used). Monitor pupils, LOC, and motor activity; also perform cranial nerve assessments (see Appendix 3). A decrease in LOC is an early indicator of IICP. Changes in the size and reaction of the pupils, a decrease in motor function (e.g., hemiplegia, abnormal flexion posturing), and cranial nerve palsies.
2. Monitor vital signs at frequent intervals. Be alert to changes in respiratory pattern, fluctuations in BP and pulse, widening pulse pressure, and slow HR.
3. Monitor the patient for indicators of IICP (see Box 7-1).
4. Monitor hemodynamic status to evaluate CPP and ensure that it is greater than 50 mm Hg. Be alert to decreases in mean systolic arterial BP (less than 80 mm Hg) or increases in MAP. Perform ongoing assessment of ICP, CPP, and PbTO$_2$ recording levels hourly until stable. Consult the physician if pressure changes significantly (e.g., ICP greater than 20 mm Hg; PbTO$_2$ less than 20 or other preestablished ranges for PbTO$_2$). Perform ongoing calibration and zeroing of transducer to ensure accuracy of readings.
5. Maintain a patent airway and ensure precise delivery of oxygen to promote optimal cerebral perfusion.
6. Facilitate cerebral venous drainage by maintaining the neck in a neutral position avoiding hyperflexion.
7. To help prevent fluid volume excess, which could add to cerebral edema, ensure precise delivery of IV fluids at consistent rates.
8. Ensure timely administration of medications that are prescribed for the prevention of sudden increase or decrease in BP, HR, or RR.
9. Treat elevations in ICP immediately (Box 3-7).

NIC Cerebral Edema Management; Cerebral Perfusion Management; Intracranial Pressure Monitoring; Neurologic Monitoring.

Ineffective thermoregulation *related to trauma associated with injury to or pressure on the hypothalamus.*

Goals/Outcomes: The patient becomes normothermic within 24 hours of the diagnosis.
NOC Thermoregulation.

Temperature Regulation
1. Monitor for signs of hyperthermia: temperature greater than 38.3° C (101° F), pallor, absence of perspiration, torso that is warm to the touch.

Box 3-7 NURSING INTERVENTIONS FOR PATIENTS WITH INCREASED INTRACRANIAL PRESSURE

- Maintain head of bed elevation at level that keeps intracranial pressure (ICP) less than 20 mm Hg and cerebral perfusion pressure (CPP) greater than 50 mm Hg.
- Loosen constrictive objects around the neck to facilitate venous blood flow from the head.
- With position changes, ensure ICP and CPP return to baseline or stay within acceptable measurements within 5 minutes of turn.
- Maintain head in neutral position.
- Correct factors that may increase ICP such as hypoxia, pain, anxiety, fear, and abdominal or bladder distention.
- Evaluate activities that increase ICP (e.g., suctioning, bathing, dressing changes) and reorganize care to minimize elevations and hip flexion.

---

2. As prescribed, obtain blood, urine, and sputum specimens for culture to rule out underlying infection.
3. Be alert to signs of meningitis: fever, chills, nuchal rigidity, Kernig sign, Brudzinski sign (see Meningitis, Chapter 7).
4. Assess wounds for evidence of infection, including erythema, tenderness, and purulent drainage.
5. If the patient has hyperthermia, remove excess clothing and administer tepid baths, hypothermic blanket, or ice bags to axilla or groin, but avoid inducing shivering.
6. As prescribed, administer antipyretics such as acetaminophen.
7. As prescribed, administer chlorpromazine to treat or prevent shivering, which can cause further increases in ICP.
8. Keep environmental temperature at optimal range.
9. Assess for possible drug fever reaction, which can occur with antimicrobial therapy.

NIC Fever Treatment.

Risk for disuse syndrome *related to immobilization and prolonged inactivity secondary to brain injury, spasticity, or altered LOC.*

Goals/Outcomes: The patient has baseline/optimal ROM without verbal or nonverbal indicators of pain.
NOC Mobility Level: Muscle Function.

Positioning
1. Begin performing passive ROM exercises every 4 hours on all extremities as soon as the patient's acute condition stabilizes. Monitor ICP during exercise, being alert to dangerous elevations outside of the established measurements. Consult with the physical therapist accordingly.
2. Teach passive ROM exercises to significant others. Encourage their participation in patient exercise as often as they are able.
3. Reposition the patient every 2 hours within restrictions of the head and other injuries, using the logrolling technique as indicated.
4. Ensure proper anatomic position and alignment. Support alignment with pillows, trochanter rolls, and wrapped sandbags.
5. For the patient with spasticity, use foot cradles to keep linens off the feet. To maintain dorsiflexion, provide the patient with shoes that are cut off at the toes, with the shoes ending just proximal to the head of the patient's metatarsal joints. Because there is no contact of the balls of the feet with a hard surface, the risk of spasticity will be minimized. Consult the occupational therapist for use of splints or other supportive device.
6. For the patient without spasticity, use foot supports to prevent plantar flexion and avoid external hip rotation.
7. To maintain anatomic position of the hands, provide the patient with spasticity with a splint or a cone that is secured with an elastic band. Either device will limit spasticity by pressing on the muscles, whereas the elastic band will stimulate the extensor muscles, thereby promoting finger extension.

NIC Exercise Therapy: Joint Mobility.

Impaired tissue integrity: corneal (or risk for same) related to irritation associated with corneal drying and reduced lacrimal production secondary to altered consciousness or cranial nerve damage.

- -

Goals/Outcomes: The patient's corneas are moist and intact.

NOC Tissue Integrity: Skin and Mucous Membranes.

Risk Identification

1. Assess for indicators of corneal irritation: red and itching eyes, ocular pain, sensation of a foreign object in the eye, scleral edema, and blurred vision.
2. Avoid exposing the patient's eyes to irritants such as baby powder or talc.
3. Lubricate the patient's eyes every 2 hours with isotonic eye drops or ointment.
4. Facilitate an ophthalmology consultation as indicated.

NIC Medication Administration: Eye.

ADDITIONAL NURSING DIAGNOSES

Also see Decreased Adaptive Capacity: Intracranial in Cerebral Aneurysm and Subarachnoid Hemorrhage (Chapter 7). As appropriate, see nursing diagnoses and interventions under Alterations in Consciousness (Chapter 1), Care of the Patient after Intracranial Surgery (Chapter 7), and Meningitis (Chapter 7). See Risk for Trauma in Status Epilepticus (Chapter 7). Also see nursing diagnoses and interventions under Nutrition Support (Chapter 1), Mechanical Ventilation (Chapter 1), Hemodynamic Monitoring (Chapter 1), Prolonged Immobility (Chapter 1), Emotional and Spiritual Support of the Patient and Significant Others (Chapter 2). The patient with craniocerebral trauma is at risk for diabetes insipidus and syndrome of inappropriate antidiuretic hormone. See Diabetes Insipidus (Chapter 8) and Syndrome of Inappropriate Antidiuretic Hormone (Chapter 8).

SELECTED REFERENCES

Alsikafe NF, McAninch JW, Elliott SP, Garcia M: Nonoperative management outcomes of isolated urinary extravasation following renal lacerations due to external trauma, *J Urol* 176:2494-2497, 2006.

American Burn Association, Burn incidence fact sheet. September 9, 2014. http://www.ameriburn.org/resources_factsheet.php.

American Burn Association Consensus Conference on Burn Sepsis and Infection Group: American Burn Association Consensus Conference to define sepsis and infection in burns, *J Burn Care Res* 28:776-790, 2007.

American College of Cardiology Foundation (ACCF)/American Heart Association (AHA)/American Association for Thoracic Surgery (AATS) American College of Radiology(ACR), Society of Cardiovascular Anesthesiologists (SCA)/Society for Cardiovascular Angiography and Interventions (SCAI)/Society of Interventional Radiology (SIR)/Society of Thoracic Surgeons (STS)/Society for Vascular Medicine (SVM): Guidelines for the diagnosis and management of patients with thoracic aortic disease, *Circulation* 121:e266-e369, 2010.

American College of Surgery Committee on Trauma: *Textbook on advanced trauma life support for doctors: ATLS student course manual*, Chicago, 2008, American College of Surgeons.

American Heart Association: *ACLS: Principles and practice*, Dallas, 2011, American Heart Association.

American Heart Association: *Handbook of emergency cardiovascular care for healthcare providers*, Dallas, 2011, American Heart Association.

American Spinal Injury Association: *International standards for neurological classification of spinal cord patients*, Chicago, 2002, American Spinal Injury Association.

Bailey JR, Stinner DJ, Blackbourne LH, et al Combat-related pelvis fractures in nonsurvivors, *J Trauma* 71(Suppl 1):S58-S61, 2011.

Baptiste D, Fehlings M: Update on the treatment of spinal cord injury, *Prog Brain Res* 161:217-233, 2007.

Baptiste D, Fehlings M: Emerging drugs for spinal cord injury, *Expert Opin Emerg Drugs* 13:63-80, 2008.

Bartal CA, Yitzhak AB: The role of thromboelastometry and recombinant factor VIIa in trauma, *Curr Opin Anaesthesiol* 22:281-288, 2009.

Bodden J: Treatment options in the hemodynamically unstable patient with a pelvic fracture, *Orthop Nurs* 28:109–116, 2009.

Bongiovanni MS, Bradley SL, Kelley DM: Orthopaedic trauma: critical care nursing issues, *Crit Care Nurs* 28:60–71, 2005.

Brain Trauma Foundation: Guidelines for the management of severe head injury, *J Neurotrauma* 24(Suppl 1):1–106, 2007.

Brain Trauma Foundation, American Association of Neurological Surgeons, Congress of Neurological Surgeons: Guidelines for the management of severe traumatic brain injury. V. Deep vein thrombosis prophylaxis, *J Neurotrauma* 24(Suppl 1):S32–S36, 2007.

Brain Trauma Foundation, American Association of Neurological Surgeons, Congress of Neurological Surgeons: Guidelines for the management of severe traumatic brain injury. VI. Indications for intracranial pressure monitoring, *J Neurotrauma* 24(Suppl 1):S37–S44, 2007.

Brasel KJ, Pham K, Yang H, et al: Significance of contrast extravasation in patients with pelvic fracture, *J Trauma* 62:1149–1152, 2007.

Broering B, Campbell M, Galvin A, Holleran R: For the Emergency Nurses Association. (2007) TNCC Trauma Nurse Core Course Provider Manual (6th ed, revised printing.) Des Plaines, IL: Emergency Nurses Association: Brain and Cranial Trauma 91-112; Thoracic Trauma 133-147; Abdominal Trauma 149-164; Spinal Cord and Vertebral Column Trauma 165-182; Musculoskeletal Trauma 183-195.

Carr JA, Phillips BD, Bowling WM: The utility of bronchoscopy after inhalation injury complicated by pneumonia in burn patients: results from the National Burn Repository, *J Burn Care Res* 30:967–974, 2009.

Carrougher GJ: Burn wound assessment and topical treatment, In *Burn care and therapy*, 104–132, St Louis, 1998, Mosby.

Carrougher GJ, Ptacek JT, Honari S, et al: Self-reports of anxiety in burn injured hospitalized adults during routine wound care, *J Burn Care Res* 27:676–681, 2006.

Caviness AC: Spinal cord injury without radiographic abnormality (SCIWORA) in children. In Bachur RG, editor: *UpToDate*, Waltham, 2014, Wolters Kluwer. http://www.uptodate.com/contents/spinal-cord-injury-without-radiographic-abnormality-sciwora-in-children.

Chandy D, Weinhouse GL: Drowning (submersion injuries). In Danzl DF, editor: *UpToDate*, Waltham, 2010, Wolters Kluwer. http://www.uptodate.com/contents/drowning-submersion-injuries.

Cheatham ML, Malbrain ML, Kirkpatrick A, et al: Results from the International Conference of experts on intra-abdominal hypertension and abdominal compartment syndrome. II. Recommendations, *Intensive Care Med* 33:951–962, 2007.

Cheatham ML, White MW, Sagraves SG, et al: Abdominal perfusion pressure: a superior parameter in the assessment of intra-abdominal hypertension, *J Trauma* 49:621–627, 2000.

Cheitlin MD, Armstrong WF, Aurigemma GP, et al: *ACC/AHA/ASE 2003 guideline for the clinical application of echocardiography.* http://circ.ahajournals.org/content/108/9/1146.full.

Cirocchi R, Abraha I, Montedori A, et al: Damage control surgery for abdominal trauma, *Cochrane Database Syst Rev* 20:CD007438, 2010.

Como JJ, Bokhari F, Chiu WC, et al: Practice management guidelines for selective nonoperative management of penetrating abdominal trauma, *J Trauma* 68:721–733, 2010.

Cothren CC, Osborn PM, Moore EE, et al: Preperitoneal pelvic packing for hemodynamically unstable pelvic fractures: a paradigm shift, *J Trauma* 62:834–842, 2007.

Criddle LM: Recombinant factor VIIa and the trauma patient, *J Emerg Nurs* 32:404–408, 2006.

Davis JW, Moore FA, McIntyre RC Jr, et al: Western trauma association critical decisions in trauma: management of pelvic fracture with hemodynamic instability, *J Trauma* 65:1012–1015, 2008.

Dechert TA, Duane TM, Frykberg BP, et al: Elderly patients with pelvic fracture: interventions and outcomes, *Am Surg* 75:291–295, 2009.

Demetriades D, Velmahos GC, Scalea TM, et al: Blunt traumatic thoracic aortic injuries: early or delayed repair – results of an American Association for the Surgery of Trauma prospective study, *J Trauma* 66(4):967–973, 2009.

Demetriades K, Hadjizacharia P, Constantinou C, et al: Selective nonoperative management of penetrating abdominal solid organ injuries, *Ann Surg* 244:620–628, 2006.

Dente CJ, Shaz BH, Nicholas JM, et al: Improvements in early mortality and coagulopathy are sustained better in patients with blunt trauma after institution of a massive transfusion protocol in a civilian level I trauma center, *J Trauma* 66:1616–1624, 2009.

Dorsey DP, Bowman SM, Klein MB, et al: Perioperative use of cuffed endotracheal tubes is advantageous in young pediatric burn patients, *Burns* 36:856–860, 2010.

Dries DJ: Management of burn injuries – recent developments in resuscitation, infection control and outcomes research, *Scand J Trauma Resusc Emerg Med* 17:14, 2009.

Elie MC: Blunt cardiac injury, *Mount Sinai J Med* 73:542–552, 2006.

Emergency Nurses Association: *Textbook of trauma nursing core course*, Des Plaines, 2007, Emergency Nurses Association.

Emergency Nurses Association: *Trauma nursing core course provider manual*, ed 7, Des Plaines, 2014, Emergency Nurses Association.

Faucher LD, Conton KM: Practice guidelines for deep venous thrombosis prophylaxis in burns, *J Burn Care Res* 28:661–663, 2007.

Faucher L, Furukawa K: Practice guidelines for the management of pain, *J Burn Care Res* 27:659–668, 2006.

Fox CJ, Mehta SG, Cox ED, et al: Effect of recombinant factor VIIa as an adjunctive therapy in damage control for wartime vascular injuries: a case control study, *J Trauma* 66:S112–S119, 2009.

Furey AJ, O'Toole RV, Nascone JW, et al: Classification of pelvic fractures: analysis of inter- and intraobserver variability using the Young-Burgess and Tile classification systems, *Orthopedics* 32:401, 2009.

Gardner MJ, Parada S, Chip Routt ML Jr: Internal rotation and taping of the lower extremities for closed pelvic reduction, *J Orthop Trauma* 23:361–364, 2009.

Gonzales EA: Fluid resuscitation in the trauma patient, *J Trauma Nurs* 15:149–151, 2008.

Gordon MD, Gottschlich MM, Helvig EI, et al: Review of evidence-based practice for the prevention of pressure sores in burn patients, *J Burn Care Res* 25:388–410, 2004.

Gourgiotis S, Villias C, Germanos S, et al: Compartment syndrome: a review, *J Surg Educ* 64:178–186, 2007.

Gourlay D, Hoffer E, Routt M, Bulger E: Pelvic angiography for recurrent traumatic pelvic arterial hemorrhage, *J Trauma* 59:1168–1174, 2005.

Goutos I, Sadideen H, Pandya AA, et al: Obesity and burns, *J Burn Care Res* 33:471–482, 2012.

Greenhalgh DG, Saffle JR, Holmes JH, et al: American Burn Association consensus conference to define sepsis and infection in burns, *J Burn Care Res* 28:776–790, 2007.

Hadley M, Walters B, Grabb P, et al: Guidelines for the management of acute cervical spine and spinal cord injuries, *Neurosurgery* 50(Suppl 3):S1–S199, 2002.

Hadley M, Walters B: Introduction to the guidelines for the management of acute cervical spine and spinal cord injuries, *Neurosurgery* 72:5–16, 2013.

Harvey CA: Complications, *Orthop Nurs* 26:410–412, 2006.

Heetveld MJ, Harris I, Schlaphoff G, et al: Hemodynamically unstable pelvic fractures: recent care and new guidelines, *World J Surg* 28:904–909, 2004.

Hemmila MR, Wahl WL: Management of the injured patient. In Doherty GM, Way LW, editors: *Current surgical diagnosis and treatment*, New York, 2006, Lange.

Hemphill J, Phan N: Management of acute severe traumatic brain injury. In Aminoff M, Moreira M, editors: *UpToDate*, Waltham, 2013, Wolters Kluwer. http://www.uptodate.com/contents/management-of-acute-severe-traumatic-brain-injury.

Hemphill J, Phan N: Traumatic brain injury: epidemiology, classification, and pathophysiology. In Aminoff M, editor: *UpToDate*, Waltham, 2013, Wolters Kluwer. http://www.uptodate.com/contents/traumatic-brain-injury-epidemiology-classification-and-pathophysiology.

Honari S: Topical therapies and antimicrobials in the management of burn wounds, *Crit Care Nurs Clin North Am* 16:1–11, 2004.

Hurlbert R: Strategies of medical intervention in the management of acute spinal cord injury, *Spine* 32:S16–S21, 2006.

Husain FA: Serum lactate and base deficit as predictors of mortality and morbidity, *Am J Surg* 185:485–491, 2003.

Ibsen LM, Koch T: Submersion and asphyxial injury, *Crit Care Med* 30:S402–S408, 2002.

Jeschke MG, Finnerty CC, Emdad F, et al: Mild obesity is protective after severe burn injury, *Ann Surg* 258:1119–1129, 2013.

Kaplan LJ: Critical care considerations in trauma. In *Medscape*, New York, 2008, WebMD. http://emedicine.medscape.com/article/434445-overview.

Kobziff L: Traumatic pelvic fractures, *Orthop Nursing* 25:235–241, 2006.

Konstantakos EK, Dalstrom DJ, Nelles ME, et al: Diagnosis and management of extremity compartment syndromes: an orthopaedic perspective, *Am Surg* 73:1199–1210, 2007.

Kosir R, Moore FA, Selby JH, et al: Acute lower extremity compartment syndrome (ALECS): screening protocol in critically ill trauma patients, *J Trauma* 63:268–275, 2007.

Köstler W, Strohm PC, Südkamp NP: Acute compartment syndrome of the limb, *Injury* 36:992–998, 2005.

Kramer G: Pathophysiology of burn shock and burn edema. In Herndon DN, editor: *Total burn care*, ed 3, London, 2007, Saunders.

LaBorde P: Burn epidemiology: the patient, the nation, the statistics, and the data resources, *Crit Care Nursing Clin North Am* 16:13–25, 2004.

Layton AJ, Modell JH: Drowning update 2009, *Anesthesiology* 110:1390–1401, 2009.

Lettieri CJ: Nonsurgical management of thoracic trauma, *Medscape Pulmon Med* 10:2, 2006.

Littlejohns L, Bader M, March K: Brain tissue oxygen monitoring in severe brain injury. I. Research and usefulness in critical care, *Crit Care Nurse* 23:17–27, 2003.

Maisch B, Seferovic PM, Ristic AD, et al: Guidelines on the diagnosis and management of pericardial diseases, *Eur Heart J* 25:1–28, 2004.

Malbrain ML: Abdominal perfusion pressure as a prognostic marker in intra-abdominal hypertension. In Vincent JL, editor: *Yearbook of intensive care and emergency medicine*, Berlin, 2002, Springer-Verlag, pp. 792–814.

Malbrain ML, Deeren D, De Potter TJ: Intra-abdominal hypertension in the critically ill: it is time to pay attention, *Curr Opin Crit Care* 11:156–171, 2005.

McCall JE, Cahill TJ: Respiratory care of the burn patient, *J Burn Care Res* 26:200–206, 2005.

McGahan PJ, Richards JR, Bair AE, Rose JS: Ultrasound detection of blunt urological trauma: a 6-year study, *Injury Int J Care Injured* 36:762–770, 2005.

Meecham CC, Kulkami R: Pelvic fracture in emergency medicine. In *Medscape*, New York, 2013, WebMD. http://www.emedicine.medscape.com/article/825869-overview#showall.

Michetti CP, Sakran JV, Grabowski JG, et al: Physical examination is a poor screening test for abdominal pelvic injury in adult blunt trauma patients, *J Surg Res* 159:456–461, 2010.

Moeller MS: Indications for use of recombinant factor VII: a case study with implications for research, *J Trauma Nurs* 13:190–192, 2006.

Moltzan CJ, Anderson DA, Callum J, et al: The evidence for the use of recombinant factor VIIa in massive bleeding: development of a transfusion policy framework, *Transfus Med* 18:112–120, 2008.

Moore KM: Controversies in fluid resuscitation, *J Trauma Nurs* 13:168–172, 2006.

Mosier MJ, Pham TN: American Burn Association practice guidelines for prevention, diagnosis, and treatment of ventilator-associated pneumonia (VAP) in burn patients, *J Burn Care Res* 30:910–928, 2009.

Papa L, Hoelle R, Idris A: A systematic review of definitions for drowning incidents, *Resuscitation* 65:255–264, 2005.

Patanwala AE: Factor VIIa (recombinant) for acute traumatic hemorrhage, *Am J Health Syst Pharm* 65:1616–1623, 2008.

Patterson DR, Hoffman HG, Weichman SA, et al: Optimizing control of pain from severe burns: a literature review, *Am J Clin Hypn* 47:43–54, 2004.

Perel P, Roberts I: Colloids versus crystalloids for fluid resuscitation in critically ill patients, *Cochrane Database Syst Rev* 17:CD000567, 2007.

Pham TN, Cancio LC, Gibran NS: American Burn Association practice guidelines: burn shock resuscitation, *J Burn Care Res* 29:257–266, 2008.

Phoenix Society for Burn Survivors, Inc., Professional Resources: Bring SOAR to your hospital, 2014, The Phoenix Society National Headquarters Office: http://www.phoenix-society.org/resources/professionals.

Rasul AT, Lorenzo CT: Acute compartment syndrome treatment and management. In Lorenzo CT, editor: *Medscape*, New York, 2014, WebMD. http://www.emedicine.medscape.com/article/307668-treatment#showall.

Raza A, Byrne D, Townell N: Lower limb compartment syndrome after urological pelvic surgery, *J Urol* 171:5–11, 2004.

Sadaka F, Naydenov S, Ponzillo J: Theophylline for bradycardia secondary to cervical spinal cord injury, *Neurocrit Care* 13:389–392, 2010.

Sagrista-Sauleda J, Angel J, Sambola A, et al: Low-pressure cardiac tamponade: clinical and hemodynamic profile, *Circulation* 114:945–952, 2006.

Salcido R, Lepre SJ: Compartment syndrome: wound care considerations, *Adv Skin Wound Care* 20:559–565, 2007.

Sathy AK, Starr AJ, Smith WR, et al: The effect of pelvic fracture on mortality after trauma: an analysis of 63,000 trauma patients, *J Bone Joint Surg Am* 91:2803–2810, 2009.

Schecter SC, Schecter WP, McAninch JW: Penetrating bilateral renal injuries: principles of management, *J Trauma* 67:E25–E28, 2009.

Seiler JG, Casey PJ, Binford SH: Compartment syndrome of the upper extremity, *J South Orthop Assoc* 9:4, 2000.

Shadgan B, Menon M, O'Brien PJ, Reid WD: Diagnostic techniques in acute compartment syndrome of the leg, *J Orthop Trauma* 22:581–587, 2008.

Shariat SF, Roehrborn CG, Karakiewicz PI, Dhami C: Evidence-based validation of the predictive value of the American Association for the Surgery of Trauma Kidney Injury Scale, *J Trauma* 62:933–939, 2007.

Shepherd SM: Drowning. In *Medscape*, New York, 2014, WebMD. http://www.emedicine.com/emerg/TOPIC744.htm.

Simon B, Ebert J, Bokhari F, et al: Pulmonary contusion and flail chest: practice management guideline, Chicago, 2006, *Eastern Association for the Surgery of Trauma*. http://www.east.org/tpg/pulmcontflailchest.pdf.

Singisetti K: Postoperative acute compartment syndrome in the nonoperated "well leg": implications to orthopaedic nursing, *Orthop Nurs* 28:91–93, 2009.

Spahn DR, Bouillon B, Cerny V, et al: Management of bleeding and coagulopathy following major trauma: an updated European guideline, *Crit Care* 17:R76, 2013.

Spahn DR, Cerny V, Coats TJ, et al; Task Force for Advanced Bleeding Care in Trauma: Management of bleeding following major trauma: a European guideline, *Crit Care* 11:R17, 2007.

Spaniol JR: Fluid resuscitation therapy for hemorrhagic shock, *J Trauma Nurs* 14:152–160, 2007.

Spodick DH: Acute cardiac tamponade, *N Engl J Med* 349:648, 2003.

Styl J: *Compartment syndromes: diagnosis, treatment and complications*, Boca Raton, 2004, CRC Press.

Thalmann M, Trampitsch E, Haberfellner N, et al: Resuscitation in near drowning with extracorporeal membrane oxygenation, *Ann Thorac Surg* 72:607–608, 2001.

Tinkoff G, Esposito TJ, Reed J, et al: American Association for the Surgery of Trauma Organ Injury Scale, I: spleen, liver, and kidney, validation based on the National Trauma Data Bank, *J Am Coll Surg* 207:646–655, 2008.

Tisherman SA, Barie P, Bokhari F, et al: Clinical practice guideline: endpoints of resuscitation, *J Trauma* 57:898–912, 2004.

Tremblay LN, Feliciano DV, Schmidt J, et al: Skin only or silo closure in the critically ill patient with an open abdomen, *Am J Surg* 182:670, 2001.

Vanden Hoek TL, Morrison LJ, Shuster M, et al: Part 12: cardiac arrest in special situations: 2010 American Heart Association Guidelines for Cardiopulmonary Resuscitation and Emergency Cardiovascular Care, *Circulation* 122(18 Suppl 3):S829–S861.

Cantwell GP, Verive M, Shoff WH: Near drowning. In *Medscape*, New York, 2014. http://emedicine.medscape.com/article/772753-clinical.

Wallen MA, Morrison AL, Gillies D, et al: Mediastinal chest drain clearance for cardiac surgery, *Cochrane Database Syst Rev* 4:CD003042, 2002.

Ward RS: Physical rehabilitation. In Carrougher GJ, editor: *Burn care and therapy*, St Louis, 1998, Mosby.

Weber JM: Epidemiology of infections and strategies for control. In Carrougher GJ, editor: *Burn care and therapy*, St Louis, 1998, Mosby.

Wijdicks EF, Bamlet WR, Maramattom BV, et al: Validation of a new coma scale: the FOUR score, *Ann Neurol* 58:585–593, 2005.

Wilensky E, Bloom S, Leichter D, et al: Brain tissue oxygenation practice guidelines using the LICOX® CMP monitoring system, *J Neurosci Nurs* 37:278–288, 2005.

Williams FN, Jeschke MG, Chinkes DL, et al: Modulation of the hypermetabolic response to trauma: temperature, nutrition, and drugs, *J Am Coll Surg* 208:489–502, 2009.

Wing P: Early acute management in adults with spinal cord injury, *J Spinal Cord Med* 31:360, 2008.

World Society on Abdominal Compartment Syndrome: *Consensus definitions and recommendations*. http://www.wsacs.org/.

Yan S, Tsurumi A, Que Y, et al: Prediction of multiple infections after severe burn trauma: a prospective cohort study, *Ann Surg* Jun 19, 2014 (Epub ahead of print).

Yarlagadda C: Cardiac tamponade. In Lange RA, editor: *Medscape*, New York, 2008, WebMD. http://emedicine.medscape.com/article/152083-overview.

Yu JS, Habib P: MR imaging of urgent inflammatory and infectious conditions affecting the soft tissues of the musculoskeletal system, *Emerg Radiol* 16:267–276, 2009.

Zimmer M, Nantwi K, Goshgarian H: Effect of spinal cord injury on the respiratory system: basic research and current clinical treatment options, *J Spinal Cord Med* 30:319–330, 2007.

RESPIRATORY ASSESSMENT: GENERAL

GOAL OF SYSTEM ASSESSMENT

Evaluate for ineffective breathing patterns, impaired gas exchange, and airway obstruction.
- Considerations for the bariatric patient: The majority of bariatric patients admitted for diagnoses other than weight loss surgery are women 20 to 30 years of age with respiratory diagnoses.

VITAL SIGN ASSESSMENT

- Respiratory rate (RR) and depth to evaluate for tachypnea, bradypnea, and work of breathing.
- Pulse oximetry to help identify low readings reflective of impaired gas exchange.
- Heart rate (HR) to evaluate for tachycardia or bradycardia; generally associated with RR changes.
- Considerations for the bariatric patient: Tachypnea is more common with this population.

CONTINUOUS PULSE OXIMETRY (Spo$_2$ MONITORING)

- Evaluate for changes over time and/or since the last recorded reading. Results should be correlated with the arterial oxygen saturation (Sao$_2$) readings derived from arterial blood gases (ABGs).
- Pulse oximetry accuracy is dependent on the presence of an adequate pulse in the area in which the measurement probe has been applied.
- Ensure readings are done using an appropriate probe placed on the anatomic location with the best pulse and least interference. Probes are available for the finger, forehead, and ear lobe.
- Readings must be correlated with physical assessment findings and can remain normal despite signs of impending deterioration. Physical assessment findings such as use of accessory muscles or presence of tachypnea are indicative of respiratory distress but may not be reflected in a change in Spo$_2$. If an increasing amount of oxygen (O$_2$) is needed to maintain Spo$_2$, this is also indicative of impending deterioration of the patient.

Considerations for the bariatric patient: Patients who are extremely obese are at higher risk of hypoxemia than people of average size, which, combined with problems positioning patients for intubation and difficult anatomy, makes securing an airway challenging.

OBSERVATION

- Evaluate for use of accessory muscles, shortness of breath, and air hunger.
- Ensure that the patient is evaluated for the presence of chronic obstructive pulmonary disease (COPD) before applying O$_2$ therapy so that appropriate liter flow is determined to prevent respiratory impairment.
- Evaluate facial and lip color for pallor or cyanosis indicative of hypoxemia.

CONSIDERATIONS FOR THE BARIATRIC PATIENT

- Persons of size have an increased probability of lung derecruitment resulting from the increased weight of the chest wall, protuberant abdomen encroaching on the diaphragm in the recumbent position, and provider reticence to extubate an extremely obese patient at high risk for having a difficult airway.

• Assess for obstructive sleep apnea (OSA), which is very common in the bariatric population.

AUSCULTATION

- Listen to breath sounds to evaluate for presence of adventitious sounds that reflect factors contributing to respiratory distress, including those related to both airway obstruction and impaired gas exchange.
- Adventitious sounds: Crackles (rales) indicative of fluid in alveoli, bubbles (rhonchi) indicative of secretions in bronchioles, wheezing (inflammation), inspiratory stridor (narrowing of airways as a result of massive inflammation or obstruction by secretions or foreign body), or pleural friction rub (inflammation).
- Lungs must be auscultated anteriorly and posteriorly in all three lobes of the right lung, the two lobes of the left lung, over the right and left main bronchi, and over the trachea.
- Considerations for the bariatric patient: Breath sounds may be distant resulting from the layers of adipose tissue between the skin and chest wall.

SCREENING LABWORK

- ABG analysis can reveal increases or decreases in pH; levels of O_2, O_2 saturation, CO_2, and bicarbonate; base excess or base deficit indicative of impending respiratory failure; hyperpnea/tachypnea; and metabolic derangements affecting breathing patterns. Blood gas analysis may be done using either arterial blood or mixed venous blood samples. Mixed venous blood samples are available only using a pulmonary artery catheter and can be used to calculate efficacy of both O_2 delivery and O_2 consumption. ABGs cannot be used to calculate O_2 consumption.

Considerations for the bariatric patient: Obesity creates values similar to those seen in restrictive lung disease. Increased pulmonary blood volume and increased chest wall mass from adipose tissue restrict normal chest wall movements. Abnormal diaphragm position, upper airway resistance, and increased daily CO_2 production further increase the work of breathing. The restrictive pattern results in decreased functional residual capacity, vital capacity, total lung capacity, inspiratory capacity, minute ventilator volume, and expiratory reserve volume.

CARE PLANS: GENERAL APPROACHES TO RESPIRATORY DISORDERS
IMPAIRED SPONTANEOUS VENTILATION WITH OR WITHOUT IMPAIRED GAS EXCHANGE

Goals/Outcomes: Within 12 to 24 hours of treatment, the patient has adequate gas exchange, reflected by Pao_2 greater than 80 mm Hg, $Paco_2$ 35 to 45 mm Hg, pH 7.35 to 7.45, presence of normal breath sounds, and absence of adventitious breath sounds. RR is 12 to 20 breaths/min with normal pattern and depth or back to normal baseline. **NOC** Respiratory Status: Ventilation, Vital Signs Status, Respiratory Status: Gas Exchange, Symptom Control Behavior, Comfort Level, Endurance.

Ventilation Assistance

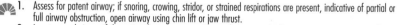

1. Assess for patent airway; if snoring, crowing, stridor, or strained respirations are present, indicative of partial or full airway obstruction, open airway using chin lift or jaw thrust.
2. Insert an oral airway if the patient becomes unconscious and cannot maintain patent airway; use a nasopharyngeal airway if the patient is conscious to avoid provoking vomiting. If severely distressed, the patient may require endotracheal intubation.
3. Position the patient to alleviate dyspnea and ensure maximal ventilation; generally, sitting in an upright position unless severe hypotension is present.
4. Monitor changes in oxygenation following position change: Spo_2, Svo_2, $Scvo_2$, end-tidal CO_2 ($ETCO_2$), $A\text{-}aDo_2$ levels, and ABGs.
5. Clear secretions from airway by having the patient cough vigorously, or provide nasotracheal, oropharyngeal, or endotracheal tube suctioning, as needed.
6. Have the patient breathe slowly or manually ventilate with manual resuscitator or bag-valve-mask device slowly and deeply between coughing or suctioning attempts.
7. Assist with use of incentive spirometer as appropriate.
8. Turn the patient every 2 hours if immobile. Encourage the patient to turn self, or get out of bed as much as tolerated if he or she is able.

9. Provide mucolytic and bronchodilating medications orally, intravenously, or by inhaler, aerosol, or nebulizer as ordered to assist with thinning secretions and relaxing muscles in lower airways.
10. Provide chest physical therapy as appropriate, if other methods of secretion removal are ineffective.
11. Considerations for the bariatric patient: The prevalence of OSA syndrome in bariatric surgical patients is 39% to 71%. Sleep studies (polysomnography) are recommended as part of preoperative evaluation. Continuous positive airway pressure (CPAP) via mask (10 cm H_2O) is begun if patients are unable to complete sleep studies before surgery. OSA is characterized by repetitive, partial, or complete obstruction of the upper airway, which prompts arterial blood oxygen desaturations and awakenings from sleep. Frequent decreases in RR with periods of apnea occur, resulting in instances of severe hypoxia. Patients manifest snoring, systemic and pulmonary hypertension, nocturnal angina, sleep-related cardiac dysrhythmias, gastroesophageal reflux disease (GERD), insomnia, polycythemia, and daytime somnolence.

Oxygen Therapy
1. Ensure humidity is provided when using O_2 or bilevel positive airway pressure (BiPAP) device for more than 12 hours to help thin secretions.
2. Administer supplemental O_2 using liter flow and device as ordered.
3. Restrict the patient and visitors from smoking while O_2 is in use.
4. Document pulse oximetry with O_2 liter flow in place at time of reading as ordered. Oxygen is a drug; the dose of the drug must be associated with the O_2 saturation or the reading is meaningless.
5. Obtain ABGs if the patient experiences behavioral changes or respiratory distress to check for hypoxia or hypercapnia.
6. Monitor for hypoventilation, especially in patients with COPD.
7. Monitor for changes indicative of O_2 toxicity in patients receiving higher concentrations of O_2 (greater than 45% FiO_2) for longer than 24 hours. Changes will be apparent in chest radiograph and breath sounds. Absorption atelectasis may be present. The higher the O_2 concentration, the greater is the chance of toxicity.
8. Monitor for skin breakdown where O_2 devices are in contact with the skin, such as nares, around the ears, and around edges of mask devices.
9. Provide O_2 therapy during transportation and when the patient gets out of bed.
10. If the patient is unable to maintain SpO_2 reading of more than 88% off O_2, consult with the respiratory care practitioner/therapist and the physician about the need for home O_2 therapy.

Respiratory Monitoring
1. Monitor rate, rhythm, and depth of respirations.
2. Note chest movement for symmetry of chest expansion and signs of increased work of breathing such as use of accessory muscles or retraction of intercostal or supraclavicular muscles. Consider use of noninvasive positive-pressure ventilation (NPPV or NiPPV) for impending respiratory failure.
3. Monitor for snoring, coughing, and possibly choking-type respirations when patient has a decreased level of consciousness to assess if airway is obstructed by tongue.
4. Monitor for new breathing patterns that impair ventilation, which may need aggressive management in a specialized, highly skilled setting.
5. Note that trachea remains midline, because deviation may indicate that the patient has a tension pneumothorax.
6. Auscultate breath sounds before and after administration of respiratory medications to assess for improvement.
7. Evaluate changes in SaO_2, SpO_2, $ETcO_2$, $ScvO_2$, and ABGs as appropriate.
8. Monitor for dyspnea and note causative activities/events.
9. If increased restlessness or unusual somnolence occurs, evaluate the patient for hypoxemia and hypercapnia as appropriate.
10. Monitor chest radiograph reports when new images become available.
11. Considerations for the bariatric patient: Mechanical ventilation for the obese patient with respiratory failure is challenging. Delivered tidal volume should be calculated based on ideal body weight (IBW) rather than actual body weight to avoid high airway pressures and barotrauma. End-tidal CO_2 monitors are unreliable because of widened alveolar-arterial gradients present in most obese patients. The reverse Trendelenburg position at 45 degrees facilitates liberation from the ventilator 24 hours of mechanical ventilation postoperatively.

NIC Cough Enhancement; Acid-Base Management; Mechanical Ventilation; Artificial Airway Management; Oral Health Maintenance.

ACUTE ASTHMA EXACERBATION

PATHOPHYSIOLOGY

The incidence of asthma is growing steadily by 2.9% each year in the United States. The number of people with asthma has increased from 20.3 million in 2001 to 25.7 million in 2010. Asthma manifests variable, recurrent symptoms related to airflow limitation stemming from chronic airway inflammation. Bronchiolar smooth muscles manifest overactive bronchoconstriction and are hyperresponsive to internal and environmental stimuli. Airflow obstruction is fully or partially reversible, but as the disease progresses, chronic airway inflammation creates edema, mucus, and eventually mucus plugging, which further decreases airflow. Eventually, irreversible changes in airway structure occur, including fibrosis, smooth muscle hypertrophy, mucus hypersecretion, injury to epithelial cells, and angiogenesis. Persons with asthma eventually develop air trapping, increased functional residual capacity, and decreased forced vital capacity. Several types of cells and cellular elements are affected including mast cells, epithelial cells, T lymphocytes, macrophages, eosinophils, and neutrophils, which when triggered can sometimes prompt sudden, fatal exacerbations of coughing, wheezing, chest tightness, and breathlessness.

Life-threatening asthma exacerbation results from bronchial smooth muscle contraction (bronchospasm), bronchial inflammation leading to airway edema, and mucus plugging. When an episode of bronchospasm (critical airway narrowing) is not reversed after 24 hours of maximal doses of traditional inhaled short-acting beta$_2$-adrenergic agonists (SABAs) such as albuterol or levalbuterol, injected systemic beta$_2$-agonists such as epinephrine, inhaled anticholinergics such as ipratropium, and systemic steroid therapy with prednisone, prednisolone, or methylprednisolone, the refractory patient may be diagnosed with status asthmaticus. Common triggers for asthma exacerbations include respiratory tract infections, allergens (airborne or ingested), air pollutants, smoke, and physical irritants (e.g., cold air, exercise). Anxiety or "panic" attacks and use of beta-adrenergic blocking agents and nonsteroidal antiinflammatory drugs (NSAIDs) may predispose patients to development or exacerbation of severe asthma. Activities that prompt deeper inhalation, such as vigorous laugher or physical exertion, can trigger an episode. Exercise-induced asthma or exercise-induced bronchospasms are well recognized in the literature.

Several clinical patterns for development of an asthma exacerbation are recognized. An "attack" can happen suddenly (over several hours) or it may take several days to reach critical airway obstruction. The more common gradual presentation manifests with increasing symptoms of sputum production, coughing, wheezing, and dyspnea. As air trapping increases, lung hyperinflation prompts increased work of breathing. Rapid exhalations increase insensible water loss through exhaled water vapor and diaphoresis. Oral intake may be decreased, contributing to hypovolemia. Without adequate oral intake to promote hydration, mucus becomes thick and begins to plug the airways. Terminal bronchioles can become occluded completely from mucosal edema and tenacious secretions. Ventilation-perfusion mismatch or shunting occurs as poorly ventilated alveoli continue to be perfused, which leads to hypoxemia. Tachycardia is an early compensatory mechanism to increase O_2 delivery to the body cells, but it increases myocardial O_2 demand. Oxygen requirements and work of breathing increase, leading to respiratory failure, hypercapnia, and respiratory arrest if not managed promptly and appropriately.

ASSESSMENT

GOAL OF SYSTEM ASSESSMENT

- Evaluate for ineffective breathing patterns, impaired gas exchange, and airway obstruction.
- Determine the patient's previous treatment regimen; classify which "step" of treatment has been needed to control symptoms; the patient may need to move to the next step of treatment to maintain control.
- Classify severity of exacerbation: should be determined following initial assessment and diagnostic testing.

HISTORY AND RISK FACTORS

For asthma

- Asthma symptoms: Cough (especially if worse at night), wheezing, recurrent difficulty breathing, and recurrent chest tightness.

- Family history: Patients with either family history or atopic disease are at higher risk of asthma.
- Common triggers: Symptoms worsen with viral respiratory infections, environmental airborne allergens, irritants in the home (mold, mildew, wood-burning stove, cockroaches, dust mites, animal dander, carpeting laid over concrete), recent emotional upset, aggressive exercise or physical exertion, fear, anxiety, frustration, food, new medications, changes in weather (especially exposure to cold air), occupational chemicals or allergens, and hormonal changes (menstrual cycle).
- Comorbid conditions: Sinusitis, rhinitis, GERD, OSA, and allergic bronchopulmonary aspergillosis.

For asthma exacerbation
- Classify asthma severity: Intermittent (step 1 treatment) or persistent: mild, moderate, severe (steps 2, 3, 4, 5, and 6 treatments); steps differ for children younger than 5 years old, children between 5 and 12 years old, and adults.
- Classify severity of exacerbation: Mild to severe or life threatening.
- Assess control: Determine if pattern of previous exacerbations is inherent to the current episode.
- Compliance/ability to control: Assess the patient's knowledge and skills for self-management.
- Identify precipitating factors: Situation: exposure at home, work, daycare, or school to inhalant allergens or irritants; time of day, season or time of year, relationship of symptoms to meals, deterioration in other health conditions, or menses.
- Identify comorbid conditions that may impair asthma management (e.g., sinusitis, rhinitis, GERD, OSA, obesity, stress, or depression).
- Surgery: Patients with asthma are at high risk for exacerbations following endotracheal intubation, general anesthesia, and ventilation provided during surgical or other invasive procedures. Impaired cough, hypoxemia, and hypercapnia may trigger exacerbation.

SPIROMETRY OR PEAK EXPIRATORY FLOW
- Peak expiratory flow (PEF): Measurement of rate or force of exhalation; those with easier breathing will have higher values than those in distress. A peak flow meter is used by patients at home to assess asthma control. Those with more severe asthma may have difficulty discerning worsening of symptoms and may use PEF several times daily to assess for declining rate of exhalation.
- Assesses degree of obstruction and reversibility in patients older than 5 years.
- Spirometry is essential for establishing the diagnosis of asthma. Patients' perceptions of airflow obstruction are highly variable. Spirometry or PEF provides an objective measurement to help classify severity of exacerbation.
- Decreased to less than 40% of predicted value indicates severe exacerbation; less than 25% of predicted value for life threatening.

VITAL SIGNS (SEVERE TO LIFE-THREATENING ASTHMA EXACERBATION)
- Presence of fever: Temperature elevation helps discern whether the patient's condition is related to a microbe (fever) versus an allergen (afebrile).
- Pulse oximetry: Oxygen saturation is decreased from the patient's baseline value.
- Tachycardia (HR greater than 140 beats/min [bpm]) and tachypnea (RR greater than 40 breaths/min).
- Hypotension may be present; hypotension is exacerbated by underlying dehydration often present in patients with severe asthma.

OBSERVATION
- Severe attacks render patients unable to speak resulting from breathlessness.
- Use of accessory muscles; fatigued, with or without diaphoresis.
- Ashen, pale, or gray/blue facial color, lip color, or nail beds.
- Chest expansion may be decreased or restricted.
- Altered level of consciousness (confusion, disorientation, agitation).
- Agitation is more commonly associated with hypoxemia, whereas somnolence is associated with hypercapnia (elevated CO_2 level).

- Frequent nonproductive coughing unless associated with superimposed infection.
- Increased nasal secretions, mucosal swelling, and nasal polyps.
- Prolonged phase of forced expiration.

AUSCULTATION
- Wheezing bronchial breath sounds; wheezing on inspiration is more indicative of acute airway narrowing, versus wheezing on expiration, which is more common.
- Wheezing during normal breathing is common.
- Chest may be nearly silent if airflow is severely obstructed. During an asthma attack, if wheezing stops, the patient may either have resolution of symptoms or complete airway occlusion.

PALPATION
- Palpate to assess for chest expansion; chest may be hyperinflated or may be asymmetrical; chest expansion during inspiration may be decreased.
- Decreased tactile fremitus may be present.

PERCUSSION
- May reveal hyperresonance (pneumothorax), a complication of asthma.

SCREENING LABWORK
- Complete blood count (CBC) with white blood cell (WBC) differential: Evaluates for elevated WBCs indicative of chronic inflammation as a result of allergic response and infection including presence of eosinophils, neutrophils, and mononuclear cells.
- ABG analysis: Evaluates for hypoxemia and hypercapnia.

RESEARCH BRIEF 4-1

Important changes in prescribing practices resulting from recent studies are occurring in primary care. The Asthma Clinical Research Network is reporting evidence that improvement in FEV_1 (forced expiratory volume in 1 second) in response to albuterol is a reliable predictor of improved asthma control using tiotropium, a long-acting muscarinic antagonist. This holds particular promise for long-term control in patients with severe asthma. There is evidence supporting improvement in lung function with tiotropium as an add-on therapy to inhaled corticosteroids and long-acting beta-agonists. These practical studies are examples of what is commonly referred to as real-world research, an effort to investigate the patient's disease course at the interface of their daily life and activities. Patient-reported outcome measures (PROMs) are guiding investigators toward a better appreciation of the relevance of investigational end points. Improvements in PROMs include morning peak expiratory flow and asthma control days among other outcomes.

From Peter SP, Bleecker ER, Kunselman SJ, et al: Predictors of response to tiotropium versus salmeterol in asthmatic adults. *J Allergy Clin Immunol* 132:1068-1074, 2013.

Diagnostic Tests for Acute Asthma Exacerbation

Test	Purpose	Abnormal Findings
Arterial blood gas (ABG) analysis	Assess for abnormal gas exchange or compensation for metabolic derangements. Initially PaO_2 is normal and then decreases as the ventilation-perfusion mismatch becomes more severe. A normal PCO_2 in a distressed patient with asthma receiving aggressive treatment may indicate respiratory fatigue, which causes a progressively ineffective breathing pattern, which can also lead to respiratory arrest. Oxygenation assessment differs from acid-base balance assessment, wherein the PCO_2 value is used as the hallmark sign for respiratory failure induced acidosis.	*pH changes:* Acidosis may reflect respiratory failure; alkalosis may reflect tachypnea. *Carbon dioxide:* Elevated CO_2 reflects respiratory failure; decreased CO_2 reflects tachypnea; rising PCO_2 is ominous, because it signals severe hypoventilation, which can lead to respiratory arrest. *Hypoxemia:* PaO_2 less than 80 mm Hg. *Oxygen saturation:* SaO_2 less than 92%. *Bicarbonate:* HCO_3 less than 22 mEq/L. *Base deficit:* less than -2.
Complete blood count (CBC) with white blood cell (WBC) differential	WBC differential evaluates the strength of the response of the immune system to the trigger of exacerbation and for the presence of infection.	*Eosinophils:* Increased in patients not receiving corticosteroids; indicative of magnitude of inflammatory response. *Increased WBC count:* More than 11,000/mm^3 is seen with bacterial pneumonias. WBCs may be increased by asthma in the absence of infection. *Hematocrit (Hct):* May be increased from hypovolemia and hemoconcentration.
Pulmonary function tests/ spirometry	The hallmark sign of asthma is a decreased FEV_1 (forced expiratory volume in 1 second)/FVC (forced vital capacity). If peak expiratory flow (PEF) rate does not improve with initial aggressive inhaled bronchodilator treatments, morbidity increases.	*Forced expiratory volume (FEV):* Decreased during acute episodes; if less than 0.7, narrowed airways prevent forceful exhalation of inspired volume (Table 4-1). *PEF rate:* Less than 100 to 125 L/min in a normal-sized adult indicates severe obstruction to air flow.
Pulse oximetry (SpO_2)	Noninvasive technology that measures the oxygen saturation of arterial blood intermittently or continuously using a probe placed on the patient's finger or ear. When using pulse oximetry, it is helpful to obtain ABG values to compare the oxygen saturation and evaluate the PaO_2, $PaCO_2$, and pH.	*Normal SpO_2:* Greater than 95%. Correlation of SpO_2 with SaO_2 (arterial saturation) is within 2% when SaO_2 is greater than 50%. Temperature, pH, $PaCO_2$, anemia, and hemodynamic status may reduce the accuracy of pulse oximetry measurements. Presence of other forms of hemoglobin in the blood (carboxyhemoglobin or methemoglobin) can produce falsely high readings.
Serologic studies	Acute and convalescent titers are drawn to diagnose a viral infection.	*Increased antibody titers:* A positive sign for viral infection.
Chest radiograph	Evaluates the severity of air trapping; also useful in ruling out other causes of respiratory failure (e.g., foreign body aspiration, pulmonary edema, pulmonary embolism, pneumonia).	*Lung hyperinflation:* Caused by air trapping *Flat diaphragm:* Related to increased intrathoracic volume.
12-Lead ECG (electrocardiogram)	Evaluates for dysrhythmias associated with stress response and asthma medications.	*Sinus tachycardia:* Important baseline indicator; use of some bronchodilators (e.g., metaproterenol) may produce cardiac stimulant effects and dysrhythmias.

Diagnostic Tests for Acute Asthma Exacerbation—cont'd		
Test	**Purpose**	**Abnormal Findings**
Sputum Gram stain, culture, and sensitivity	Culture and sensitivity may show microorganisms if infection is the precipitating event. The most reliable specimens are obtained via bronchoalveolar lavage (BAL) during bronchoscopy, or using a protected telescoping catheter (mini-BAL or using BAL) to decrease the risk of contamination from oral flora.	Gross examination may show increased viscosity or actual mucous plugs. *Gram stain positive:* Indicates organism is present. *Culture:* Identifies organism. *Sensitivity:* Reflects effectiveness of drugs on identified organism.
Diagnostic fiber optic bronchoscopy using a PSB (protected specimen brush) and BAL	Obtains specimens during simple bronchoscopy without contaminating the aspirate; modified technique (mini-BAL) is also effective without the need of full bronchoscopy.	*Gram stain positive:* Indicates organism is present. *Culture:* Identifies organism. *Sensitivity:* Reflects effectiveness of drugs on identified organism.
Serum theophylline level	Important baseline indicator for patients who take theophylline regularly; therapeutic level is close to toxic level. If additional theophylline is given, serial levels should be measured within the first 12 to 24 hours of treatment and daily thereafter. Patients are monitored for side effects (e.g., nausea, nervousness, dysrhythmias).	Acceptable therapeutic range is 10 to 20 μg/mL. There is little evidence to support clinical benefit for adding theophylline to inhaled beta-adrenergic blocking agents and steroids for patients with acute, severe asthma who were not already using theophylline regularly.

COLLABORATIVE MANAGEMENT

CARE PRIORITIES

The goal of asthma management is to control the disease using a stepwise approach to therapies. Ideal control is attained when patients are free of daytime symptoms, do not awaken breathless or coughing at night, have few or no limitations on activities, do not regularly use rescue medications, have no exacerbations, and maintain a forced expiratory volume in 1 second (FEV_1) and/or peak expiratory flow rate (PEFR) greater than 80% of the predicted value. When prevention fails, the potential for life-threatening respiratory failure is high during exacerbations unresponsive to treatment within the first hour. Management is directed toward decreasing bronchospasm and increasing ventilation. Other interventions are directed toward treatment of complications (Table 4-1).

1. Determine severity of asthma exacerbation

    a. Acute severe: PEFR is less than 40% of predicted or personal best in a patient who is unable to speak a complete sentence in one breath, with RR greater than 25 breaths/min and HR greater than 110 bpm.

    b. Life threatening: In a patient with severe asthma, the PEFR is less than 25% of predicted or personal best, SpO_2 less than 90%, PaO_2 less than 80 mm Hg; PCO_2 35 to 45 mm Hg, silent chest, weak respiratory effort, exhaustion, cyanosis, bradycardia, hypotension, dysrhythmias, confusion, and coma.

    c. Near fatal: PCO_2 greater than 45 mm Hg and/or requiring mechanical ventilation using increased positive pressure to overcome inspiratory pressures; the patient also has other findings of life-threatening exacerbation.

2. Oxygen therapy

Patients have profound hypoxia and can tolerate high doses of O_2 (FIO_2) unless they retain CO_2 and breathe by hypoxic drive. Most patients with asthma are able to tolerate high flow O_2, versus those with other obstructive lung disease who cannot. Oxygen dosage must be limited in nonintubated, mechanically ventilated patients who breathe via hypoxic drive to avoid hypoventilation and respiratory arrest. Humidified O_2 therapy is begun immediately to correct hypoxemia and thin secretions. PaO_2 is maintained slightly above normal unless the

Table 4-1	PULMONARY FUNCTION TESTS IN ASTHMA EXACERBATION		
Test	**Description**	**Normal Values**	**Exacerbation Values**
FEV₁ Forced expiratory volume (1 second)	Volume of gas exhaled over first second of full exhalation measured by FVC	≥75% of predicted normal	Severe: Less than 40% of predicted or personal best. Life threatening: Less than 25% of predicted or personal best. Decreased as a result of narrowed airways, which are resistant to airflow during exhalation.
FVC Forced vital capacity	Total amount of gas exhaled as forcefully and rapidly as possible after maximal inspiration	≥80% of predicted normal	With severe or life-threatening exacerbation: Decreased because of air trapping.
FEF Forced expiratory flow	Average rate of flow during middle half of FEV; an accurate estimate of airway resistance	≥80% of predicted normal	Decreased because of small airway obstruction; may return to normal after inhalation of aerosolized bronchodilator.
PEFR or PEF Peak expiratory flow rate	Maximal rate of air flow throughout FVC	>100-125 L/min in a normal-sized adult indicates severe obstruction to air flow	Decreased because of small airway obstruction; may return to normal after inhalation of aerosolized bronchodilator.

patient retains CO_2 to compensate for the increased O_2 demands imposed by the increased work of breathing. The degree of hypoxemia and patient response determines the method of O_2 delivery. A high-flow device (e.g., 100% nonrebreather mask) delivers more precise and higher FIO_2. Management of anxiety must be considered, especially if the patient will not wear a mask because of feelings of suffocation.

3. Heliox therapy

A blended mixture of helium and O_2, available in mixtures of 60:40, 70:30, and 80:20, which is delivered either through a tight-fitting face mask or through a mechanical ventilator circuit. Heliox reduces the turbulent flow of air in narrowed airways. Helium is not as dense as nitrogen, which accounts for the decreased turbulence, therefore reducing the work of breathing and improving gas exchange. Findings of upper airway sounds in the bronchopulmonary system are inconsistent with the diagnosis of asthma. The advanced practice provider should be consulted for further actions should auscultation reveal this finding.

4. Intubation and mechanical ventilation

Strongly considered when the patient has severe hypoxemia or hypercapnia indicative of impending respiratory failure: confusion, somnolence, agitation, or central cyanosis; or if the patient experiences intolerable respiratory distress. There are varying practices and no consensus guideline regarding the criteria for intubation and mechanical ventilation for the patient with asthma. These interventions can create significant complications for the patient related to intubation and concomitant bronchial reactivity. Intubation and mechanical ventilation should be considered cautiously. Hypoventilation with low minute ventilation, low tidal volume (6 mL/kg), and long exhalation time are necessary to prevent barotrauma, increased intrathoracic pressures, and cardiac compromise. Plateau pressure should not exceed 30 cm H_2O and auto-positive end-expiratory pressure (auto-PEEP) should be maintained at less than 10 cm H_2O. In exceptionally severe cases, neuromuscular blockade may be warranted in addition to sedation and analgesia.

5. Pharmacotherapy to manage acute asthma exacerbation

Vigorous therapy is initiated to decrease bronchospasms, help reduce airway inflammation, and help remove secretions. Treatment is continued until wheezing is eliminated and pulmonary function tests return to baseline (Table 4-2).

Table 4-2	MEDICATIONS USED FOR ASTHMA EXACERBATION*		
Drug Type	**Medication and Dosage**	**Action**	**Side Effects**
Short-acting inhaled beta$_2$-adrenergic agonist (SABA)	Albuterol: Nebulized 2.5 to 5 mg every 20 minutes for three doses, then 2.5 to 10 mg every 1 to 4 hours as needed, or 10 to 15 mg/h continuously. Levalbuterol [(R)-albuterol]: Nebulizer solution (0.63 mg/3 mL, 1.25 mg/0.5 mL, 1.25 mg/3 mL) given 1.25 to 2.5 mg every 20 minutes for three doses, then 1.25 to 5 mg every 1-4 hours as needed.	Immediate adrenergic stimulant effects; activates beta$_2$-adrenergic receptors; relaxes smooth muscle to relieve bronchospasm.	The adverse effects of SABAs are important to consider. They can be very unpleasant and are fairly common. They include tachycardia, tremor, anxiety, or irritation following their use. These side effects can be effectively minimized by rinsing the mouth out after use.
Nonselective beta-agonist therapy	Epinephrine: 0.3 to 0.5 mg every 20 minutes for three doses subcutaneously (SC). Terbutaline: 0.25 mg every 20 minutes for three doses SC; also available orally as 5 mg per os (PO) three times a day (maximum dose 15 mg daily). There is no proven advantage of systemic therapy over aerosolized therapy.	Stimulates both alpha- and beta-adrenergic receptors; relaxes bronchial smooth muscle; epinephrine may cause peripheral vasoconstriction; terbutaline is the drug of choice in pregnant women.	Increased heart rate (>120 bpm), nervousness, tremor, palpitations, nausea, vomiting, headache, and paradoxical bronchospasm.
Corticosteroids	Prednisone, methylprednisolone, or prednisolone: 40 to 80 mg/day in 1 or 2 divided doses until peak expiratory flow rate reaches 70% of predicted or personal best.	Antiinflammatory effects help to decrease both swelling and reactivity of airways.	Mood swings, insomnia, agitation, osteoporosis, gastrointestinal upset, nausea, heartburn; if tapered improperly, the patient may experience adrenal insufficiency.
Anticholinergics	Ipratropium bromide nebulizer solution 0.25 mg/mL (*Atrovent*): 0.5 mg every 20 minutes for three doses, then as needed; generally used in conjunction with beta-agonist therapy. May mix in same nebulizer with albuterol. Should not be used as first-line therapy; should be added to SABA therapy for severe exacerbations. The addition of ipratropium has not been shown to provide further benefit once the patient is hospitalized. Ipratropium with albuterol nebulizer solution (each 3 mL vial contains 0.5 mg ipratropium bromide and 2.5 mg albuterol): 3 mL every 20 minutes for three doses, then as needed. May be used for up to 3 hours in the initial management of severe exacerbations.	Blocks action of acetylcholine at parasympathetic sites of bronchial smooth muscle to cause inhibition of nasal secretions and bronchodilation.	Dry mouth, dizziness, transient increased bronchospasm; may cause narrow-angle glaucoma if eyes are contaminated in susceptible patients. Use of mouthpiece nebulizer is safer than face mask.

*Recommendations originate from the National Institutes of Health (NIH) Expert Panel on the Diagnosis and Management of Asthma (2007). Intravenous theophylline and magnesium are not recommended for general use in a hospitalized patient with acute asthma by the NIH guidelines. A 20-minute intravenous magnesium sulfate infusion for poorly responding patients is recommended by the British Thoracic Society guidelines. All patients receiving theophylline before hospitalization should have a theophylline level determined before a loading dose is given.

- **Bronchodilators:** Dilate smooth muscles of the airways to help relieve bronchospasms, resulting in increased diameter of functional airways. SABAs are the mainstay of asthma exacerbation management, whereas long-acting beta-adrenergic agonists (LABAs) are used for long-term control of asthma. Theophylline and aminophylline are no longer recommended for management of acute bronchospasms.
- **Corticosteroids:** Given intravenously during the acute phase of the exacerbation to decrease the inflammatory response, which causes edema in upper airways. Administration should decrease reactivity and swelling of the airways. Dosage varies according to severity of episode and whether or not the patient is currently taking steroids. The patient may be converted to inhaled corticosteroids once the acute phase has been resolved. Acute adrenal insufficiency can develop in patients who take steroids routinely at home, if these drugs are not given to the patient during hospitalization.
- **Anticholinergics:** Inhaled medications used to reduce vagal tone of the airways, thus helping to reduce bronchospasms. Ipratropium (Atrovent) is used in combination with inhaled SABAs for severe, acute asthma.
- **Magnesium sulfate:** Magnesium sulfate has been shown to inhibit smooth muscle contraction, inhibit acetylcholine release, and decrease histamine release from mast cells. The American Thoracic Society asthma management guidelines (2008) recommend consideration of a single dose of magnesium sulfate 1.2 to 2 g over 20 minutes for patients with severe, life-threatening, or fatal exacerbation who have an inadequate or ineffective response to inhaled bronchodilators. Recent metaanalyses and high-quality random control trials have identified intravenous (IV) magnesium sulfate as an effective adjunct to standard therapy in the context of severe or life-threatening exacerbation. However, the use of nebulized $MgSO_4$ is not supported by adequate evidence.
- **Sedatives and analgesics:** Used in more limited doses in patients who are not intubated or mechanically ventilated, unless the patient is extremely anxious, agitated, and unable to cooperate with therapy. These agents depress the central nervous system (CNS) response to hypoxia and hypercapnia. Once mechanical ventilation is in place, the dosage is titrated until the patient is comfortable and/or hypoxemia or hypercapnia begins to resolve.
- **Buffers:** Sodium bicarbonate may be given to correct severe acidosis not corrected by intubation and mechanical ventilation. Generally, this is only a temporizing measure to help relieve lactic acidosis. The physiologic response to bronchodilators improves with correction of metabolic acidosis.
- **Antibiotics:** Given if a respiratory infection is indicated, as evidenced by fever, purulent sputum, or leukocytosis.

6. Fluid replacement

To liquefy secretions and replace insensible losses. Generally, crystalloid fluids (e.g., 5% dextrose in water [D_5W], 5% dextrose in normal saline [D_5NS]) are used.

7. Chest physiotherapy

Generally contraindicated in acute phases of exacerbation because of acute respiratory decompensation and hyperreactive airways. Once the crisis is over, the patient may benefit from percussion and postural drainage every 2 to 4 hours to help mobilize secretions.

CARE PLANS: ACUTE ASTHMA EXACERBATION

IMPAIRED GAS EXCHANGE *related to ineffective breathing patterns secondary to narrowed airways.*

- -

Goals/Outcomes: Within 2 to 4 hours of initiation of treatment, the patient has adequate gas exchange reflected by Pao_2 greater than 80 mm Hg, $Paco_2$ 35 to 45 mm Hg, and pH 7.35 to 7.45 (or ABG values within 10% of the patient's baseline), with mechanical ventilation, if necessary. Within 24 to 48 hours of initiation of treatment, the patient is weaning or weaned from mechanical ventilation, and RR is approaching baseline rate, depth, and pattern.

NOC Respiratory Status: Ventilation, Vital Signs Status; Respiratory Status: Gas Exchange, Symptom Control Behavior, Comfort Level, Endurance.

Ventilation Assistance

1. Monitor for signs of increasing hypoxia at frequent intervals: Restlessness, agitation, and personality changes are indicative of severe exacerbation. Cyanosis of the lips (central) and of the nail beds (peripheral) are late indicators of hypoxia.
2. Monitor for signs of hypercapnia at frequent intervals: Confusion, listlessness, and somnolence are indicative of respiratory failure and near-fatal asthma exacerbation.
3. Monitor ABGs when continuous pulse oximetry values or patient assessment reflects progressive hypoxemia: ABGs will also identify the pH and level of CO_2, alerting the provider to impending hypoxemic and/or hypercapnic respiratory failure. Be alert to decreasing Pao_2 and increasing $Paco_2$ or decreasing O_2 saturation levels, indicative of impending respiratory failure.
4. Monitor for decreased breath sounds or changes in wheezing at frequent intervals: Absent breath sounds in a distressed patient with asthma may indicate impending respiratory arrest.
5. Position the patient for comfort and to promote optimal gas exchange: High-Fowler position, with the patient leaning forward and elbows propped on the over-the-bed table to promote maximal chest excursion, may reduce use of accessory muscles and diaphoresis resulting from work of breathing. The use of a portable electric fan is sometimes reported by the patient as greatly improving comfort and stamina.
6. Monitor Fio_2 to ensure that O_2 is within prescribed concentrations: If the patient does not retain CO_2, a 100% nonrebreather mask may be used to provide maximal O_2 support. If the patient retains CO_2 and is unrelieved by positioning, lower-dose O_2, bronchodilators, steroids, intubation, and mechanical ventilation may be necessary sooner than in patients who are able to receive higher doses of O_2 by mask.

Mechanical Ventilation

1. Monitor patients who are intubated and mechanically ventilated for increased intrathoracic pressure (auto-PEEP) as a result of "breath stacking," wherein the next breath is delivered before complete emptying of the first breath. Each subsequent breath failing to completely empty lung volume and predisposes the patient to barotrauma, pneumothorax, and decreased cardiac output resulting from dynamic hyperinflation (DHI) causing pressure increases inside the thorax, which impede venous return to the heart.
2. Monitor for hypotension: Decreased venous return can lead to hypotension. DHI should be suspected in an intubated patient with asthma who is hypotensive following intubation and initiation of mechanical ventilation, when there is no other obvious cause (e.g., tension pneumothorax). Current evidence and outcome data support judicious fluid administration in response to hypotension in patients who are mechanically ventilated. Fluid boluses should be done cautiously, based on objective indicators including an assessment of stroke volume variation. A fluid bolus may be attempted for differential diagnosis of ventilation versus intravascular volume changes affecting the blood pressure (BP). If DHI is suspected, consult with the respiratory therapist and the advanced practice provider to modify ventilator settings.

INEFFECTIVE AIRWAY CLEARANCE *related to increased tracheobronchial secretions and bronchoconstriction; decreased ability to expectorate secretions secondary to fatigue.*

Goals/Outcomes: Within 24 hours of initiating treatment, the patient's airway has reduced secretions, as evidenced by return to baseline RR (12 to 20 breaths/min) and absence of excessive coughing. Within 24 to 48 hours of resolution of severe, refractory asthma, the patient reports an increased energy level with decreased fatigue and associated symptoms.

NOC Respiratory Status: Airway Patency.

Cough Enhancement

1. Monitor the patient's ability to clear tracheobronchial secretions frequently. Set up suction equipment at the bedside.
2. Encourage oral fluid intake or administer IV fluids within the patient's prescribed limits to help decrease viscosity of the secretions.
3. Encourage coughing to clear secretions and deep breathing unless the patient is already coughing uncontrollably or going into respiratory failure. If the patient can manage to take deep breaths, respiratory failure is manageable.
4. Provide humidified O_2 to help liquefy tracheobronchial secretions.
5. Evaluate whether or not the patient may benefit from chest physiotherapy, after crisis phase of exacerbation has been resolved. Discuss with the advanced practice provider. If appropriate, teach significant others to perform chest physiotherapy.
6. Teach the patient proper coughing technique for effective management of secretions.
7. Instruct the patient to take several deep breaths. Instruct significant others in coaching this technique.

8. After the last inhalation, teach the patient to perform a succession of coughs (usually three or four) on the same exhalation until most of the air has been expelled.
9. Explain that the patient may need to repeat this technique several times before the cough becomes productive.

Asthma Management
1. Determine the patient's previous asthma control status, including which "step" of therapy was implemented (Table 4-3).
2. Compare current status to past exacerbation responses to determine respiratory status.
3. Ensure spirometry measurements (FEV_1, FVC, FEV_1/FVC ratio) or PEFR readings are obtained before and after use of a short-acting bronchodilator.
4. Educate the patient about use of a PEFR meter at home.

Table 4-3	STEPPED MEDICATION MANAGEMENT FOR ASTHMA CONTROL				
Intermittent Asthma	**Persistent Asthma***				
Step 1	**Step 2**	**Step 3**	**Step 4**	**Step 5**	**Step 6**
SABA as needed	Preferred Low-dose ICS	Preferred Low-dose ICS + LABA or Medium-dose ICS	Preferred Medium-dose ICS + LABA	Preferred High-dose ICS + LABA	Preferred High-dose ICS + LABA + oral corticosteroid
	Alternative Cromolyn, LTRA, nedocromil, theophylline	Alternative Low-dose ICS + either LTRA, nedocromil, theophylline, or zileuton	Alternative Medium-dose ICS + either LTRA, nedocromil, theophylline, or zileuton	Alternative Consider omalizumab for patients with allergies	Alternative Consider omalizumab for patients with allergies
			Asthma specialist should manage the patient		
	Consider subcutaneous allergen immunotherapy for patients with allergic asthma				

Long-term Asthma Control Medications: Adults

Medications	Dosage	Side Effects
ICS		
Beclomethasone HFA	80 to 480 μg daily	Cough, dysphonia, oral thrush. Cytochrome P-450 metabolism: Drugs that inhibit isoenzyme CYP3A4 may increase systemic concentration of ICS. Systemic adverse effects may be seen. Should be used following bronchodilators after washing out the mouth.
Budesonide DPI	160 to 1200 μg daily	
Flunisolide	500 to 2000 μg daily	
Flunisolide HFA	320 to 640 μg daily	
Fluticasone HFA/MDI	88 to 440 μg daily	
Fluticasone DPI	100 to 500 μg daily	
Mometasone DPI	200 to 400 μg daily	
Triamcinolone acetonide	300 to 1500 μg daily	
Systemic Oral Corticosteroids		
Methylprednisolone	7.5 to 60 mg daily; short course "burst" 40 to 60 mg daily as single or divided doses for 3 to 10 days to gain control	Hyperglycemia, increased appetite, fluid retention, weight gain, peptic ulcer, aseptic necrosis. Long term: Cushing syndrome, adrenal axis suppression, growth suppression, muscle weakness, cataracts, rarely immunosuppression.
Prednisolone		
Prednisone		

Table 4-3	STEPPED MEDICATION MANAGEMENT FOR ASTHMA CONTROL—cont'd

Long-term Asthma Control Medications: Adults

Medications	Dosage	Side Effects
Inhaled LABAs		
Salmeterol DPI Formoterol DPI	One blister every 12 hours One capsule every 12 hours	Tachycardia, tremors, hypokalemia, QTc interval prolongation. Not used as a rescue inhaler for acute distress.
Combined Medications		
Fluticasone/Salmeterol Budesonide/Formoterol	One inhalation two times a day Two puffs two times a day	See LABA and ICS; dose depends on level of control.
Cromolyn/Nedocromil		
Cromolyn MDI Cromolyn nebulizer Nedocromil MDI	Two puffs four times a day One ampule four times a day Two puffs four times a day	Cough and irritation; 15% to 20% of patients have bad taste from nedocromil.
Immunomodulators		
Omalizumab (anti-IgE)	150 to 375 mg subcutaneously every 2 to 4 weeks	Pain, burning at injection site; possible anaphylaxis.
Leukotriene Modulators		
LTRAs		
Montelukast Zafirlukast	10 mg at bedtime 40 mg daily	No specific adverse effects.
5-Lipoxygenase Inhibitor		
Zileuton	2400 mg daily	Liver enzyme elevation.
Methylxanthines		
Theophylline	Starting dose 10 mg/kg daily up to 300 mg; maximum dose 800 mg daily	Tachycardia, nausea, vomiting, SVT, CNS stimulation, headache, seizures, hyperglycemia, hypokalemia, insomnia, gastric upset, increased reflux and PUD, difficulty voiding in older adult men, increased hyperactivity in children.

*Information based on National Institutes of Health Asthma Management Guidelines (2007). Retrieved from www.nhlbi.nih.gov/health-pro/guidelines/current/asthma-guidelines. Accessed February 6, 2014. *CNS*, Central nervous system; *DPI*, dry powder inhaler; *HFA*, hydrofluoroalkanes (ozone-benign propellant for inhalation); *ICS*, inhaled corticosteroid; *IgE*, immunoglobulin E; *LABA*, long-acting beta2-agonist; *LTRA*, leukotriene receptor antagonist; *MDI*, metered dose inhaler; *PUD*, peptic ulcer disease; *SABA*, short-acting beta2-agonist; *SVT*, supraventricular tachycardia.

5. Determine the patient's compliance with treatments.
6. Note onset, frequency, and duration of coughing and advise the patient to avoid triggers of coughing if identified.
7. Coach in breathing or relaxation exercises.
8. Encourage the patient to breathe slowly and deeply. Teach pursed-lip breathing technique to assist the patient with controlling respirations as appropriate:
   - Inhale through the nose.
   - Form lips in an O shape as if whistling.
   - Exhale slowly through pursed lips.
   - Record the patient's response to the breathing technique. Educate significant others in coaching.

9. Teach the patient and family how to decrease metabolic demands for O_2 by limiting or pacing the patient's activities and procedures.

10. Schedule rest times after meals to avoid competition for O_2 supply during digestion.

11. Monitor Spo_2 by pulse oximetry during activity to evaluate limits of activity, set future activity goals, and recommend optimal positions for oxygenation.

12. Assess for fever every 2 to 4 hours. Consult the advanced practice provider and provide treatment as prescribed to decrease temperature and thus O_2 demands.

Anxiety Reduction

1. Ascertain and alleviate the cause of restlessness to decrease metabolic demands (e.g., if restlessness is related to anxiety, help reduce anxiety by providing reassurance, enabling family members to stay with the patient, and offering distractions such as soft music or television).

   • Restlessness may be an early sign of hypoxemia.

2. Explain all procedures and offer support to minimize fear and anxiety, which can increase O_2 demands.

NIC Acid-Base Management; Acid-Base Monitoring; Airway Management; Bedside Laboratory Testing; Cough Enhancement; Emotional Support; Energy Management; Fluid Management; Fluid Monitoring; Laboratory Data Interpretation; Mechanical Ventilation; Oxygen Therapy; Positioning; Respiratory Monitoring; Vital Signs Monitoring.

ADDITIONAL NURSING DIAGNOSES

Also see the section on Acute Respiratory Failure for information about support of breathing. For other nursing diagnoses and interventions, see Emotional and Spiritual Support of the Patient and Significant Others (Chapter 2).

ACUTE RESPIRATORY DISTRESS SYNDROME

PATHOPHYSIOLOGY

The primary goal of the pulmonary system is to promote an appropriate and reasonable gas exchange at the alveolar-capillary surface, generally measured by pulse oximetry and ABGs. Acute respiratory failure is a general term that identifies a primary lung dysfunction. Mild to severe symptoms of acute respiratory distress syndrome (ARDS) are potentially lethal complications of critical illness that are unfortunately common in some intensive care units (ICUs). This dysfunction ultimately results in failure to promote appropriate and proportionate O_2 uptake at the alveolar-capillary interface. Type I (hypoxemic) is oxygenation failure, whereas type II (hypercapnic) is ventilation failure. Many patients manifest respiratory failure of types I and II simultaneously. Clinically, type I failure exists when Pao_2 is less than 50 mm Hg with the patient at rest and breathing room air ($Fio_2 = 0.21$ or 21% of the atmospheric pressure, which is 760 mm Hg at sea level). Ultimately there will also be failure to remove CO_2 (known as hypoventilation), and/or $Paco_2$ greater than 50 mm Hg (type II) is significant for acute ventilation failure or hypercapnia. A wide variety of disease states create a single or mixed respiratory failure. One of the simplest methods of evaluating patients relates to the understanding of basic gas exchange. Oxygenation occurs primarily during inspiration and the removal of CO_2 occurs during exhalation. The basic concepts applied here include compliance and recoil. Lung compliance is the measure of expansion of the alveoli (the gas-exchanging surface), which occurs on inspiration, whereas elasticity refers to the ability of the alveoli to recoil, as they do on exhalation. Restrictive airway diseases generally present with significant hypoxemia, whereas obstructive disorders are more likely to develop a persistent and chronic hypercapnia. See Box 4-1 for a description of some of the disease processes that can lead to acute respiratory failure.

The terms acute lung injury (ALI) and ARDS were historically used to differentiate and describe a continuum of lung dysfunction. ARDS was defined in 1994 by the American-European Consensus Conference. Many concerns regarding the evaluation methods and categorization of lung dysfunction and interventions have evolved since that time. In 2011, the Berlin definition equalized the diagnosis and divided the disorder by levels of hypoxemia, as well as Fio_2 and PEEP requirements (Table 4-4).

The term *ALI* no longer exists. Under the Berlin definition, patients with Pao_2/Fio_2 200 to 300 are diagnosed with "mild ARDS." The onset of ARDS (diagnosis) must be acute, defined

Box 4-1	DISEASE PROCESSES LEADING TO THE DEVELOPMENT OF RESPIRATORY FAILURE

Obstructive disease states, impaired exhalation, impaired minute ventilation, CO_2 retention
- Chronic obstructive pulmonary disease (emphysema, bronchitis, asthma, cystic fibrosis)
- Neuromuscular defects (Guillain-Barré syndrome, myasthenia gravis, multiple sclerosis, muscular dystrophy, polio, brain/spinal injury)
- Depression of respiratory control centers (drug-induced cerebral infarction, inappropriate use of high-dose oxygen therapy, drug/toxic agents)

Restrictive disease states, impaired inspiration, impaired alveolar recruitment: Hypoxemia, refractory hypoxemia
- Restrictive pulmonary disease (interstitial fibrosis, pleural effusion, pneumothorax, kyphoscoliosis, obesity, diaphragmatic paralysis)
- Pulmonary emboli
- Atelectasis
- Pneumonia
- Bronchiolitis
- Acute respiratory distress syndrome
- Chest trauma (rib fractures)
- Chest wall issues

Diffusion disturbances
- Pulmonary/interstitial fibrosis
- Pulmonary edema
- Acute respiratory distress syndrome
- Anatomic loss of functioning lung tissue (pneumonectomy)

Table 4-4	STAGING ACUTE RESPIRATORY DISTRESS SYNDROME BASED ON BERLIN DEFINITIONS	
Mild	$Pao_2/Fio_2 < 200$ mm Hg	$Pao_2/Fio_2 < 300$ mm Hg with PEEP or CPAP ≥ 5 cm H_2O
Moderate	$Pao_2/Fio_2 < 100$ mm Hg	$Pao_2/Fio_2 < 200$ mm Hg with PEEP or CPAP ≥ 5 cm H_2O
Severe	$Pao_2/Fio_2 < 100$ mm Hg with PEEP or CPAP ≥ 5 cm H_2O	

CPAP, Continuous positive airway pressure; *PEEP,* positive end-expiratory pressure.

as occurring within 7 days of a particular event, such as sepsis, pneumonia, or simply a patient's recognition of worsening respiratory symptoms. Bilateral opacities consistent with pulmonary edema must be present and can be detected on computed tomography or chest x-ray. Heart failure is not excluded from the current definition because patients with high pulmonary capillary wedge pressures or known congestive heart failure with left atrial hypertension can still have ARDS.

There may be a primary (intrapulmonary) or secondary (extrapulmonary) insult to both the lung endothelium and the epithelium. The associated release of mediators, increasing vascular and alveolar permeability (leak), eventually perpetuates alveolar collapse and supports the accumulation of fluids in the pulmonary interstitium. While the capillary permeability and alveolar epithelial damage continue to worsen, surfactant activity is reduced, protein production increases, and therefore gas exchange decreases as a result of widened diffusion distance and intrapulmonary shunting. The alveoli tend to collapse, communicating the loss of opening pressure to other alveoli in the sac. All resist reexpansion in the absence of surfactant and the presence of significant infiltration and collapsing fluid pressure. Initially, acute hypoxemia develops, worsens, and ultimately progresses into hypercapnic respiratory failure. The shunt fraction (blood flow past derecruited alveoli rejoins in the pulmonary venous circulation without adequate O_2 exposure) as well as alveolar (physiologic) dead space (overventilation of the unaffected alveolar sacs) increase, ultimately progressing to a profoundly noncompliant, derecruited, and gas dysfunctional state.

The evaluation of respiratory failure includes the understanding of the following:

V̇/Q̇ Match
This general term refers to the relationship of gas distribution (V̇) to the amount of blood (V̇/Q̇), which passes the total alveolar surface in 1 minute of time. Normal alveolar ventilation occurs at a rate of 4 L/min, and normal pulmonary vascular blood flow occurs at a rate of 5 L/min. The normal V̇/Q̇ ratio is therefore 4 L/min divided by 5 L/min, or a ratio of 0.8, almost in a 1:1 ratio. Any disease process that interferes with either side of the equation upsets the physiologic balance, causing a V̇/Q̇ mismatch.

Components of an abnormal V̇/Q̇ ratio
Alveolar dead space ventilation: This is a primary problem with pulmonary perfusion. Alveoli may be compliant and elastic, but in a condition where the alveoli are normal or hyperventilated, and the perfusion is proportionately lower than the ventilation, there is a primary gas exchange problem. This is measured or evaluated as a high V̇/Q̇ mismatch, wherein ventilation is proportionately greater than perfusion. This is frequently seen with low cardiac output states, or pulmonary embolus, and in overventilation of the independent lung surface.

Diffusion distance: O_2 and CO_2 must cross the barrier created by the alveolar epithelium, the interstitial space, and the capillary endothelium. That space between is typically fluid free and product free, allowing gas to move rapidly across. Diffusion is affected when an increase in anatomic distance and/or product (fluid, proteins, and neutrophils) alters the ability of gas exchange between alveoli and the capillary bed. Pulmonary edema is a major problem that interferes with diffusion.

Carbon dioxide production
The volume of CO_2 produced by the body tissues varies with metabolic rate (fever, pain, agitation, sepsis, and so forth). The $Paco_2$ must be interpreted in conjunction with the volume exhaled, especially in patients who are mechanically ventilated. Many vagaries of CO_2 flux can be eliminated by controlling ventilation and muscular activity. Current evidence supports that the overdistension and shear force of opening-closing also profoundly affect the healthy lung.

Intrapulmonary right-to-left shunt: Large amounts of blood pass from the right side of the heart to the left side of the heart and out into the general circulation without adequate oxygenation. This process occurs when alveoli are not recruited on inspiration resulting from atelectasis or the alveoli are flooded. Primary causes of intrapulmonary shunt are atelectasis and ARDS.

ARDS is primarily defined once the injury creates a hypoxemia requiring intubation and mechanical ventilation. The presence of refractory hypoxemia in conjunction with diffuse pulmonary infiltrates in the absence of left atrial hypertension is considered to be the primary indicator of the continuum of acute respiratory failure. Despite advances in the treatment of the primary inflammatory process and progress in the method of ventilatory support, the continuum of ALI/ARDS continues to be associated with high morbidity and mortality, reaching greater than 60%. Since 1964, when the continuum was first described, the understanding of the etiology, pathophysiology, and epidemiology, as well as the relationship of genetic prodrome and ventilator-induced lung injury process, has significantly increased (Table 4-5).

ASSESSMENT
GOAL OF SYSTEM ASSESSMENT
Evaluate for decreasing Pao_2/Fio_2 and increasing requirements for pressure control and PEEP. (See Acid-Base Imbalances, Chapter 1).

HISTORY AND RISK FACTORS
Shock: Trauma, hemorrhagic shock, sepsis, massive blood transfusion, and aggressive fluid replacement creating an extra vascular lung water excess.

Table 4-5	RISK FACTORS FOR ACUTE RESPIRATORY DISTRESS SYNDROME	
Direct Injury	**Indirect Injury**	
Pneumonia	Severe sepsis	
Aspiration	Trauma	
Lung contusions	Pancreatitis	
Inhalation/burn injury	Transfusion-related lung injury	
Severe acute respiratory syndrome	Ventilation-associated lung injury	

Respiratory: Inhalation of toxic substances, pneumonia, severe pneumonitis, aspiration of gastric contents, drowning, air or fat embolus, O_2 toxicity, ventilator-induced lung injury.

Other: Acute pancreatitis, postperfusion cardiopulmonary bypass, drug overdose, neurologic injury, immunosuppression, and malaria.

VITAL SIGNS

- If breathing spontaneously (with or without ventilation support), RR may be rapid and compensatory for metabolic acidosis.
- Rapid HR if not receiving beta-antagonist therapy.
- Spo_2 is lower than expected when reviewing the ventilation settings or O_2 support.

OBSERVATION: OXYGENATION FAILURE

- Nasal flaring and expiratory grunt may be present.
- Use of accessory muscles indicates respiratory distress.
- May appear fatigued, with or without diaphoresis.
- May present with ashen, pale, or gray/blue facial color, lip color, or nail beds.
- Chest expansion may be decreased, restricted, or asymmetrical with severe changes in one lung manifesting severe atelectasis or pleuritic pain.
- Altered level of consciousness (confusion, disorientation, and agitation) is more common with older adults but is a very significant sign in any age group.
- Agitation is more commonly associated with hypoxemia, whereas somnolence is associated with hypercarbia (elevated CO_2 level).

HYPOXEMIC HYPOXIA IN MILD ARDS

- Initially: Dyspnea, restlessness, hyperventilation, cough, increased work of breathing; chest may appear to be clear on auscultation or there may be late inspiratory crackles. The patient may be significantly agitated and if intubated may appear combative.
- Ventilator pressures: As most of these patients will already be ventilated, increasing peak airway pressure (pulmonary arterial wedge pressure [PawP] or peak inspiratory pressure [PIP]) and a validation of increased pressure measured during inspiratory hold ($P_{plateau}$) when administering a volume-controlled breath should be evaluated and documented. The rising pressure ($P_{plateau}$) indicates a loss of functional alveolar surface; and while the compliance of the lung decreases, the pressure measured when a volume breath is delivered will rise.
- The patient with a loss of lung function will have a decreased P/F ratio (defined later). Initially, there may be a shift from volume control ventilation to pressure control as well as an increase in PEEP (see Table 4-1).

HYPOXEMIC HYPOXIA IN MODERATE TO SEVERE ARDS

- Initially: Respiratory failure including cyanosis, pallor, grunting respirations, mid to late inspiratory rales, rapid and shallow breathing, intercostal-suprasternal retractions, tachypnea, tachycardia, diaphoresis, and mental obtundation.
- Ventilator pressures: The increasing peak and plateau pressures will be measured when the patient is given a volume control breath (cannot be measured during a pressure-controlled breath).
- The O_2 (P/F) ratio will decline further and generally requires a change in ventilation support to a mean airway pressure strategy.

AUSCULTATION
- Decreased or bronchial breath sounds.
- High-pitched inspiratory crackles heard best after the patient coughs.
- Low-pitched inspiratory crackles caused by airway secretions.

PALPATION
- Palpate chest wall for tenderness indicative of inflammation.
- Palpate to assess for symmetry of chest expansion.

PERCUSSION
- May reveal presence of consolidation or fluid (dullness) or hyperresonance (pneumothorax).

SCREENING LABWORK
- CBC: Evaluates for elevated WBCs indicative of infection. Bandemia (immature neutrophils) of greater than 10% is especially concerning.
- Sputum Gram stain, culture, and sensitivity: Identifies infecting organism.
- Blood culture and sensitivity: If result is positive, it may indicate that the organism has migrated into the bloodstream to cause a systemic infection.
- ABG analysis: Evaluates for hypoxemia and eventually hypercapnia.

A-a GRADIENT/A-aDo$_2$/P(A-a)o$_2$
- The A-a gradient for hypoxemia and eventually tension difference is a clinically useful calculation. The calculation is based on a model as though the lung were one large alveolus and the entire blood flow of the right side of the heart passed around it. Using the rules of partial pressure as well as the laws of CO_2 production at the cell and the content of CO_2 exerting alveolar pressure, the theoretical alveolar Po$_2$ (Pao$_2$) is calculated. Once the theoretical Pao$_2$ has been calculated, the gradient is achieved by subtracting the measured arterial Pao$_2$. The gradient is the difference between the calculated alveolar oxygen (Pao$_2$) and the measured arterial oxygen (Pao$_2$).
- When the Fio$_2$ is above 0.21, the arterial oxygen (Pao$_2$) is a measurement of proportional gas exchange, although the difference between alveolar and arterial values should always be less than 150 mm Hg.
- Extrapulmonary failure: The A-a gradient generally remains normal or narrow. With shunt or $\dot{V}/\dot{Q}$ mismatch, the gradient is usually wider than normal.
- P/F ratio: The Pao$_2$ divided by the Fio$_2$ (Pao$_2$/Fio$_2$ ratio known as the P/F ratio) can be used to more simply assess the severity of the gas exchange defect. The normal value for the ratio of the partial pressure of arterial blood O$_2$ to Fio$_2$ {Pao$_2$/Fio$_2$} (Fio$_2$ is expressed as a decimal ranging from 0.21 to 1.00) is 300 to 500. A value of less than 300 indicates gas exchange derangement, and a value below 200 or greater than 40% Fio$_2$ is indicative of severe impairment and is a major component of the diagnostic criteria for ARDS. The inverse relationship of the P/F and the A to a difference is important to consider when discussing the level of gas exchange failure.
- QS/QT: The shunt fraction compares the nonoxygenated (shunted: QS) blood exiting the pulmonary bed to the total blood flow (cardiac output: QT). This mathematical calculation, which requires mixed venous blood gas and pulmonary blood gas, evaluates total intrapulmonary shunting. Normal physiologic shunt is 3% to 4% and may increase to 15% to 20% or more in ARDS. Shunt may be present when the ECTo$_2$-Paco$_2$ ratio is greater than 10 mm Hg. The routine measurements of ABGs, chest radiograph, A greater than 10 mm Hg ratio, as well as the presence of refractory hypoxemia are much more routinely used to diagnose intrapulmonary shunting, a core feature of ARDS.

DIAGNOSTIC TESTS

Diagnostic Tests for Acute Respiratory Distress Syndrome

Test	Purpose	Abnormal Findings
Noninvasive Pulmonary Volumes and Pressures		
Pulmonary function studies	Evaluates inspiratory volumes and exhalation volumes as well as capacities of the lung.	Persons with acute respiratory distress syndrome (ARDS) have decreased inspiratory volume (tidal volume and inspiratory reserve) as well as exhalation volumes (tidal volume and expiratory reserve), because the functional lung surface is significantly reduced. The amount of volume that stays in the lung at the end of a normal exhalation is significantly reduced and promotes continuous alveolar collapse.
Pulmonary pressures measured during volume control breath	Measures the relationship of volume delivered and the compliance of the surface, which contains it. Normal pulmonary arterial wedge pressure (PawP) or PIP when receiving an 8 mL/kg/ideal body weight breath is <35 cm H_2O. Normal $P_{plateau}$ when inspiratory hold is applied after an 8 mL/kg/ideal body weight breath at the end of inspiration is <25 cm H_2O.	Patients presenting with lung injury and distress will have significant increases in $P_{plateau}$ pressures to more than 25 cm H_2O. This increase may or may not manifest as a proportional increase in peak inspiratory pressure (PIP). For example, with a 350 mL breath, the patient with ARDS may have a PIP of 48 and a $P_{plateau}$ of 43.
Blood Studies		
Arterial blood gas analysis	Evaluates the oxygenation of the arterial blood as well as the presence or absence of acid and the effect on the pH (environment of the cells). See Acid-Base Imbalances, Chapter 1.	Although not always predictable when in the disease process, changes will occur, generally patients will develop hypoxemia, which may initially be resolved by increasing the FIO_2, but eventually will require great increases in FIO_2 and ultimately will no longer respond to oxygen therapy.
Complete blood count (CBC) Hemoglobin (Hgb) Hematocrit (Hct) Red blood cell (RBC) count White blood cell (WBC) count	Assesses for anemia, inflammation, and infection.	Decreased RBCs, Hgb, or Hct reflects anemia; WBCs and shift to the left may indicate ongoing inflammation.
Coagulation profile Prothrombin time (PT) with international normalized ratio (INR) Partial thromboplastin time (PTT) Fibrinogen D dimer	Assesses for causes of bleeding, clotting, and disseminated intravascular coagulation indicative of the abnormal clotting present in shock or ensuing shock.	Decreased PT with low INR promotes clotting; elevation promotes bleeding. In severe sepsis, PT and INR may increase, but in the presence of ALI/ARDS, these measures along with elevated fibrinogen and D dimer reflect a microcoagulopathy.

Continued

Diagnostic Tests for Acute Respiratory Distress Syndrome—cont'd

Test	Purpose	Abnormal Findings
Radiology		
Chest radiograph	Assesses size of lungs, presence of fluids, abnormal gas or fluids in the pleural sac, diaphragmatic margins, the pulmonary hilum, as well as integrity of the rib cage.	Presence of fluids in the lung parenchyma initially presents as pulmonary edema. The continuous accumulation differentiates this edema formation to one that is not cardiac.
Computed Tomography (CT)		
Cardiac CT scan	Assesses the three-dimensional lung capacities, fluid load, and primary displacement of the fluid.	Normally a large gas-filled surface, the ALI/ARDS lung when seen on CT is frequently whited out, filled a quarter to three quarters with fluid that has extravagated through the endothelial deficits (capillary leak).
Invasive Measures		
Tracheal-protein/plasma-protein ratio	A relatively new diagnostic tool used to differentiate between cardiogenic and noncardiogenic pulmonary edema (ARDS). It compares total protein in tracheal aspirate with total protein in plasma.	Ratio in cardiogenic pulmonary edema is <0.5, whereas the ratio in ARDS generally is >0.7.

COLLABORATIVE MANAGEMENT

Maintaining adequate arterial oxygenation while protecting the functional lung is the highest priority in both traditional and more recent approaches to ventilator management for ARDS. Careful consideration should be given to evaluate neurologic conditions and OSA because these are commonly overlooked causes of respiratory failure. In addition, the primary goal is to determine and treat the underlying pathophysiologic condition.

CARE PRIORITIES

1. Augment oxygen content with oxygen therapy

The goal is to provide acceptable Pao_2 levels (greater than 60 mm Hg) with Fio_2 less than 0.50, but Fio_2 up to 1.00 may be necessary for a short time while other adjustments are made. If an increase in Fio_2 exceeds 50%, clinicians should consider increasing PEEP (by increments of 2 to 5 cm H_2O every 1 to 2 hours, until 15 or 20 cm H_2O of PEEP is reached) to reduce the right-to-left shunt and promote oxygenation. For those on mechanical ventilation PEEP improves arterial oxygenation, primarily by recruiting collapsed and partially fluid-filled alveoli, therefore increasing the functional residual capacity at end-expiration, which decreases the effort and sheer stress (which may damage the alveoli) of opening the alveoli again during the next inspiration. This strategy is referred to as a mean airway pressure or open lung strategy, that is, by increasing the mean airway pressure, the lung will be constantly maintained in an open state.

2. Facilitate ventilation and gas exchange

Mechanical ventilation: Provide mechanical ventilation with moderate to high levels of PEEP (to prevent tidal collapse) and low tidal volumes of approximately 6 mL/kg IBW, to protect the functional lung from overdistension. This lung-protective ventilatory strategy has been shown to ensure adequate gas exchange, decrease the levels of intra-alveolar and systemic mediators, and improve outcomes in patients with ALI and ARDS. Many clinicians have successfully used strategies to treat ARDS by reducing the delivered tidal volume (from 8 to 10 mL/kg IBW to 4 to 6 mL/kg IBW) balanced with an RR (12 to 40 breaths/min) necessary to maintain adequate minute ventilation. This decrease of volume in the noncompliant lung reduces both peak inspiratory and plateau pressures. At the same time, the use of a lower tidal volume protects the functional lung surface from volutrauma and pressure trauma, both of which cause overdistension and stimulation of inflammation. Lung-protective ventilator strategies are considered standard practice in the care of patients with ARDS. To minimize ventilator-induced lung injury, attention is directed at avoidance of alveolar overdistension and cyclical opening and closing. The lowest possible plateau pressure and tidal volume should be selected. A reasonable target tidal volume in patients who are mechanically ventilated is 6 mL/kg. A topic of much controversy is the optimal setting of PEEP.

RESEARCH BRIEF 4-2

Evidence suggests that higher positive end-expiratory pressure (PEEP) should be used for moderate and severe acute respiratory distress syndrome (ARDS), whereas lower PEEP may be more appropriate in patients with mild ARDS. PEEP should be set to maximize alveolar recruitment while avoiding overdistension. Volume and pressure limitation during mechanical ventilation can be described in terms of stress and strain. Fraction of inspired oxygen and PEEP are typically titrated to maintain arterial oxygen saturation (Spo_2) of 88% to 95% (Pao_2 55 to 80, mm Hg).

From Biehl M, Kashiouris MG, Gajic O: Ventilator-induced lung injury: minimizing its impact in patients with or at risk for ARDS. *Respir Care* 58:927-937, 2013.

If PEEP trials fail, other strategies designed to open and maintain opening of the alveoli may be considered. These methods such as airway pressure release ventilation, inverse ratio (I greater than E), and high-frequency oscillation are also mean airway pressure strategies, but the discussion of this type of advanced ventilation is beyond the scope of this book.

Patient positioning: Primary lung edema occurs most aggressively in the dependent areas of the lung. Repositioning the patient at least every 2 hours is indicated in patients with hypoxemia; however, if staffing allows and the patient can tolerate it, more frequent (every 30 minutes) turning could be beneficial. Continuous lateral motion therapy beds may also be used to continuously turn the patient. Motion therapy assists in the redistribution of interstitial edema and may improve oxygenation.

RESEARCH BRIEF 4-3

Successful early mobilization of patients who are critically ill can reduce several complications including atelectasis and ventilator-associated pneumonia and shorten ventilator time. In addition, evidence shows that cognitive and functional limitations may last 1 to 5 years after discharge from the intensive care unit (ICU).

A schedule of repositioning every 2 hours was not superior to every 4 hours to prevent pressure ulcers in ICU patients under mechanical ventilation and on modern support surfaces. These position changes require a higher nursing workload and increases the likelihood of an adverse effect.

From Manzano F, Colmenero M, Perez-Perez AM, et al: Comparison of two repositioning schedules for the prevention of pressure ulcers in patients on mechanical ventilation with alternating pressure air mattresses. *Intensive Care Med* 40:1679-1687, 2014.

Prone patient positioning: Prone positioning of the patient may improve the oxygenation of many patients with ARDS. There are various methods to turn the patient prone: staff generated with pillows, foam wedges, the Vollman prone positioner, or mechanically with the Roto-Prone bed.

3. Maintain adequate cardiac output with fluid therapy

Usually, the patient's cardiac output is supported with fluid therapy. The balance between dehydration and euvolemia is a difficult one to achieve. New measures of total blood volume and arterial stroke volume may assist the provider in achieving adequate fluid without causing volume overload. The use of crystalloid versus colloid fluids has been and remains controversial, but the SAFE Study Investigators (2004) validated that the use of colloids in the general population of patients did not improve outcomes but significantly increased cost. More recently, concerns have been studied regarding the presence of extravascular lung water.

RESEARCH BRIEF 4-4

Managing thirst in the patient who is mechanically ventilated can be challenging. Thirst is a prevalent, intense, and distressing symptom in patients in the intensive care unit. Simple bundled therapies including ice water spray, mouth hygiene, and lip wetting reduced the perception and memory of severe thirst. Integrating this practice with routine thirst assessment can relieve one of the most distressing symptoms experienced by patients who are critically ill.

From Rose L, Nokoyama N, Rezai S, et al: Psychological wellbeing, health related quality of life and memories of intensive care and a specialised weaning centre reported by survivors of prolonged mechanical ventilation. *Intensive Crit Care Nurs* 30:145-151, 2013; Puntillo K, Arai SR, Cooper BA, et al: A randomized clinical trial of an intervention to relieve thirst and dry mouth in intensive care unit patients. *Intensive Care Med* 40:1295-1302, 2014.

---

4. Reduce anxiety

Before any medication is administered, the provider must ascertain that the ventilation is tailored to the patient. This can best be evaluated by analyzing the volume-pressure loop and the flow/time graph. The respiratory therapist is an invaluable resource for this method of evaluation. After ensuring adequate ventilation, many patients will require anxiety reduction with medication such as fentanyl and anxiolytics. Those patients who cannot be adequately oxygenated and ventilated with mechanical ventilation may be given anxiety-reducing agents such as propofol and dexmedetomidine. A sedation scale and protocol should be used to standardize this practice. The use of sedating agents has been linked to ICU delirium and post-ICU syndrome. In addition, the bedside nurse must ascertain if the patient is in pain and administer analgesics appropriately. A wide variety of pain scales can be used effectively.

Patients who are unable to achieve appropriate ventilation as a result of agitation and dyssynchrony or are hemodynamically unstable may require heavy sedation with agents such as propofol (Diprivan) or, in extreme cases, the diaphragm may need to be paralyzed with a neuromuscular blocking agent such as vecuronium bromide (Norcuron) or cisatracurium (Nimbex). Although very user-dependent, train of four should be performed when evaluating level of pharmacologic paralysis. The caregiver must recognize that, although the patient who is pharmacologically paralyzed may appear to be resting quietly or may even be comatose, he or she may be alert and extremely anxious because of the total lack of muscle control. These patients must receive appropriate sedation (e.g., lorazepam [Ativan]) and analgesia (e.g., morphine), and they will require expert psychosocial nursing interventions. (See Sedating and Neuromuscular Blockade, Chapter 1.) When patients appear agitated, ventilation should be evaluated first (as long as the patient is not in danger of extubation or self-harm) followed by pain evaluation and analgesia, followed by anxiety-relieving medications. Neuromuscular paralysis should be performed as a last resort and only when necessary to control ventilation.

5. Provide nutrition support

Energy outlay with respiratory failure is high, in part because of the increased work of breathing. If the patient is unable to consume adequate calories with enteral feedings, total parenteral nutrition is added. It is important to perform an occasional evaluation of the patient's caloric and metabolic needs to make certain that the patient is being adequately nourished but not overfed. All efforts should be made to feed enterally so that the gut is used. Newer elemental feedings require no digestion and can be used in the stomach, duodenum, or jejunum. (See Nutrition Support, Chapter 1.)

RESEARCH BRIEF 4-5

Risk Factors for Physical Impairment After Acute Lung Injury in a National Multi-center Study

The investigators of this study set out to determine what risk factors could be found that predicted physical impairment after acute lung injury/acute respiratory distress syndrome (ALI/ARDS). They evaluated patients enrolled from the ARDS Network studies around the United States using the physical measures from the Short Form-36 (SF-36). At 6 and 12 months, strength was 92% and 93% of maximal strength, 6-minute walk distance was 64% and 67% of predicted values, and SF-36 Physical Function Score was 61% and 67% of predicted values.

When adjusted for risk and acuity, corticosteroid dosage and intensive care unit length of stay were highly associated with poor or reduced physical outcomes.

From Needham DM, Wozniak AW, Hough CL, et al: National Institutes of Health NHLBI ARDS Network. *Am J Respir Crit Care Med* 189:1214-1224, 2014.

CARE PLANS FOR ARDS

IMPAIRED GAS EXCHANGE *related to alveolar-capillary membrane changes secondary to increased permeability with alveolar injury and collapse.*

Goals/Outcomes: On initiation of therapy, and the titration of ventilatory support, the patient has adequate gas exchange, as evidenced by the following ABG values: PaO_2 greater than 60 mm Hg, $PaCO_2$ less than 45 mm Hg, pH 7.35 to 7.45. Success is achieved when the patient can maintain his or her PaO_2 even with FIO_2 decreases.

NOC Respiratory Status: Ventilation, Vital Signs Status; Respiratory Status: Gas Exchange, Symptom Control Behavior, Comfort Level, Endurance.

Respiratory Monitoring

1. Assess and document characteristics of respiratory effort: rate, depth, rhythm, and use of accessory muscles of respiration.
2. Assess the patient for signs and symptoms of respiratory distress: restlessness, anxiety, confusion, tachypnea (RR greater than 20 breaths/min), and use of accessory muscles.
3. Assess breath sounds with each vital signs check. Adventitious sounds, which are usually present in the later stages of ARDS, are not as likely to occur during the early stage.
4. Monitor serial ABG values and consult the advanced practice provider for significant changes. Explain the need for frequent analysis to the patient and significant others.
5. Compare ABG saturation with pulse oximetry saturation for accuracy. Consult the Change to advanced practice provider for pulse oximetry values less than 90%.
6. Administer O_2 and monitor FIO_2 as prescribed.
7. Measure and compare $ECTO_2$ and arterial CO_2.
8. Monitor and record pulmonary function tests as prescribed, especially tidal volume and minute ventilation. Expect decreased tidal volume and increased minute ventilation with respiratory distress.
9. Position the patient for comfort and to promote adequate gas exchange: usually semi-Fowler position.
10. Keep oral airway and self-inflating manual ventilating bag at the bedside for emergency use. Keep emergency intubation equipment at the bedside.

RISK FOR INJURY *related to dislodging of life-sustaining equipment during positioning or repositioning.*

Goals/Outcomes: The patient can be turned, placed prone, or repositioned without dislodging life-sustaining equipment or devices.

NOC Personal Safety Behavior; Risk Control.

Environmental Management: Safety
1. Secure the endotracheal (ET) tube/other devices to prevent accidental movement or dislodging.
2. Provide the appropriate length ventilator tubing to facilitate positioning of the patient without risk of pulling on the ET tube.
3. Facilitate tolerance of rotational therapy by managing anxiety and promoting sleep with medications.
4. When proning, assess oxygenation. Typical responders will demonstrate at least 10 mm Hg increase in Pao$_2$ within 10 minutes of being placed prone.
5. Collaborate with the respiratory care practitioner to decrease the delivered O$_2$ while the patient improves.

NIC Acid-Base Management; Airway Management; Bedside Laboratory Testing; Laboratory Data Interpretation; Mechanical Ventilation; Oxygen Therapy; Positioning; Respiratory Monitoring; Ventilation Assistance; Vital Signs Monitoring.

ADDITIONAL NURSING DIAGNOSES

Also see nursing diagnoses and interventions in Nutrition Support, Mechanical Ventilation, Prolonged Immobility, Acid-Base Imbalances, and Emotional and Spiritual Support of the Patient and Significant Others (Chapters 1 and 2).

ACUTE PNEUMONIA

PATHOPHYSIOLOGY

Pneumonia is the ninth leading cause of death in the United States and the leading cause of death as a result of infectious disease (www.cdc.gov/Features/Pneumonia/). The hallmark pathophysiology of pneumonia is inflammation of the lung parenchyma, which include the alveolar spaces, respiratory bronchioles, and interstitial tissue. Pneumonia can be classified as community-acquired pneumonia (CAP) or hospital-acquired pneumonia (HAP).

Predisposing factors in the development of pneumonia are immunosuppression and neutropenia. The microorganisms involved include bacteria, protozoa, fungi (*Candida*, *Aspergillus*), and viruses (cytomegalovirus). Patients who have a severely compromised immune system, that is, acquired immune deficiency syndrome, are most often infected by *Pneumocystis jirovecii*, a fungus.

Sepsis, septic shock, respiratory failure, ARDS, emphysema, or lung abscesses are complications of pneumonia that may require intensive critical care. Those with the highest risk are older adults, the very young, and those with chronic medical conditions. Common disorders include COPD, cardiac disease, diabetes mellitus, liver disease, renal disease, or cerebrovascular disease, malignancy, or an immunocompromised state.

COMMUNITY-ACQUIRED PNEUMONIA

Pneumonia that occurs outside of the inpatient or "in facility" healthcare environment is associated with high mortality and morbidity rates. The most common pathogen is *Streptococcus pneumoniae*. Approximately 4 million patients develop CAP annually, resulting in 600,000 hospitalizations at a cost of approximately $23 billion. Mortality rates range from 5.1% for patients who are hospitalized and ambulatory to 36.5% for patients requiring critical care. The disease occurs in all age groups but is most common in those from the mid-50s to the late 60s.

NOSOCOMIAL PNEUMONIA

Nosocomial pneumonia is the second most common cause of hospital infections and has proven to be a fatal complication for many patients, especially the critically ill. The three types of nosocomial pneumonia are *hospital acquired pneumonia* (HAP), which transpires 48 hours or more after hospital admission noting that the infection was not incubating at the time of admission. *Healthcare-associated pneumonia* includes patients with recent hospitalization within 90 days of infection, exposure to healthcare environments such as nursing homes, long-term care facilities, and chronic hemodialysis; and receiving IV antimicrobial therapy, chemotherapy, or wound care with 30 days of pneumonia. The final type is *ventilator-associated pneumonia* (VAP), which develops 48 or more hours after ET intubation. VAP has been very difficult to define, resulting in inconsistent tracking and reporting of the hospital-acquired condition. VAP is now part of a broader classification of conditions associated with mechanical ventilation termed ventilator-associated events (VAEs). For practical purposes, HAP is the term used in this chapter to cover all the aforementioned types.

A diagnosis of HAP requires new or advanced infectious infiltrate on chest imaging and the presence of two of the following: fever, leukopenia and leukocytosis (which is WBC count less than 5000 cells/mm^3 or 10,000 cells/mm^3), or purulent-appearing sputum or ET aspirate. Other clinical manifestations used by the Centers for Disease Control and Prevention (CDC) include change in mental status, increase in respiratory secretions, new onset of dyspnea or cough, rales, and adventitious bronchial lungs sounds. Another criterion by the CDC is at least one positive result from a blood culture or pleural fluid, or bronchoalveolar culture. The risk factors for HAP are multifactorial from severe illness related to comorbidities, hemodynamic compromise, and depressed immune system. The use of conventional treatment modalities such as antibiotics, corticosteroids, sedatives, and acid-relieving medications (proton pump inhibitors and histamine blockers), which increase gram-negative colonization of the aerodigestive tract, artificial airway in the trachea, and respiratory therapy equipment (e.g., mechanical ventilation where bacteria can be inhaled from aerosols) also increase the risk of HAP.

ASPIRATION PNEUMONIA

Aspiration pneumonia occurs when oropharyngeal flora or gastric material are aspirated into the lower respiratory tract resulting from dysphagia or impaired coughing mechanisms. Aspiration pneumonia can lead to ALI, ARDS, empyema, or lung abscess. The patient population at highest risk is the older adult population. Other predictors of aspiration pneumonia in older adults include COPD, congestive heart failure, tube feeding, delirium, immobility, cerebrovascular accident, GERD, and obesity. Pathogens associated with aspiration pneumonia are gram-negative bacilli, given gastric pH-altering medications, anaerobes, and *Staphylococcus aureus*.

VENTILATOR-ASSOCIATED PNEUMONIA

A patient who acquires pneumonia more than 48 hours following ET intubation and initiation of mechanical ventilation may be classified as having VAP. VAP is associated with increased duration of ET intubation, mechanical ventilation, intensive care stay, and hospital cost (approximately $99,600 per case). Hospital mortality of mechanically ventilated patients who develop VAP is 46% compared with 32% for those without VAP, with 4.4% of deaths occurring at day 30 and 5.9% on day 60 in 2011. In 2010, the National Healthcare Safety Network (NHSN) facilities reported more than 3525 VAP cases. VAP incidence for hospital units ranged from 0.0 to 5.8 per 1000 ventilator days; a very broad range, indicative of a problem with consistency of reporting. Currently, there is no valid, reliable definition for VAP. The most widely used VAP definitions and criteria were evaluated and were found to be neither sensitive nor specific.

VENTILATOR-ASSOCIATED EVENTS

Surveillance for VAEs by the NHSN was limited to VAP until 2013. In 2011, the Centers for Disease Control and Prevention composed a Working Group of key stakeholder organizations to evaluate the limitations of the NHSN pneumonia definitions and to develop a more reliable approach to VAE surveillance by the NHSN. A VAE surveillance algorithm was developed by the Working Group and implemented by the NHSN in January 2013. The approach is based on measurable, simplified, and "automation-friendly" criteria designed to identify a comprehensive list of conditions and complications associated with adult patients who are mechanically ventilated. The three tiers of the VAE algorithm include: ventilator-associated condition, infection-related ventilator-associated complication, and possible and probable VAP. The Centers for Medicare and Medicaid Services has recognized VAP as a preventable illness when appropriate patient care is provided. The key components for improvement in outcomes of patients who are mechanically ventilated are defined within the "ventilator bundle" developed by the Institute for Healthcare Improvement. The evidence-based practices include elevation of the head of the bed, daily sedation vacation and assessment of readiness to extubate, peptic ulcer disease prophylaxis, daily oral care with chlorhexidine, and deep venous thrombosis (DVT) prophylaxis.

ASSESSMENT

GOAL OF SYSTEM ASSESSMENT

Identify ineffective breathing patterns, impaired gas exchange, and airway obstruction. Findings are influenced by the patient's age, extent of the disease process, underlying medical condition, and pathogen involved. Severity of pneumonia should be determined following initial assessment and diagnostic testing.

HISTORY AND RISK FACTORS

In addition to the risk factors listed in Table 4-5, any factor that alters the integrity of the lower airways, thereby inhibiting ciliary activity, increases the likelihood of pneumonia. Impairment of the "mucociliary elevator" system impairs the ability of the patient to move secretions from the airways to the oral cavity for expectoration. These factors include hypoventilation, hyperoxia (increased FIO_2), hypoxia, airway irritants such as smoke, and the presence of an artificial airway.

COUGH

· Can be unrelenting and severe; may induce vomiting in some patients.
· May be productive, weak, strong, or dry (nonproductive).
· Sputum varies in color depending on pathogen and degree of inflammation (yellow, green, rust, brown; blood-tinged with severe inflammation).
· May be associated with pleuritic chest pain.

CHEST RADIOGRAPH

· Determines presence of pneumonia, but initial radiograph finding is often negative if the patient is dehydrated.
· Reflects infiltrates (abnormal "white" areas) in various patterns, reflective of abnormal fluid distribution in the lungs; can be mistaken for heart failure.

VITAL SIGNS

· Fever occurs in response to infection; some patients are not febrile, especially if being cooled or on continuous renal replacement therapy.
· Pulse oximetry: Oxygen saturation is decreased from the patient's normal baseline value.
· P/F ratio (ratio of arterial O_2 tension to fractional inspired O_2) is decreased when O_2 therapy is applied.
· Tachycardia and tachypnea are present if pneumonia is moderate to severe.
· Hypotension may be present if sepsis is ensuing; hypotension is exacerbated by underlying dehydration often present in patients with pneumonia.
· Hypovolemia alone may prompt tachycardia.

OBSERVATION

· Nasal flaring and expiratory grunt may be present.
· Use of accessory chest and abdominal muscles indicates respiratory distress.
· May appear fatigued, with or without diaphoresis if coughing has been relentless.
· Ashen, pale, or gray/blue facial color, lip color, or nail beds.
· Chest expansion may be decreased, restricted, or asymmetrical with severe pneumonia in one lung manifesting severe atelectasis or pleuritic pain.
· Altered level of consciousness (confusion, disorientation, and agitation) is more common with older adults.
· Agitation is more commonly associated with hypoxemia, whereas somnolence is associated with hypercarbia (elevated CO_2 level).

AUSCULTATION

· Decreased or bronchial breath sounds.
· High-pitched inspiratory crackles heard best after the patient coughs.
· Low-pitched inspiratory crackles caused by airway secretions.

PALPATION
- Palpate chest wall for tenderness indicative of inflammation.
- Palpate to assess for symmetry of chest expansion.

PERCUSSION
- May reveal presence of consolidation or fluid (dullness) or hyperresonance (pneumothorax).

SCREENING LABWORK
- CBC: Evaluates for elevated WBCs indicative of infection.
- Sputum Gram stain, culture, and sensitivity: Identifies infecting organism.
- Blood culture and sensitivity: If result is positive, it indicates that the pneumonia organism has migrated into the bloodstream to cause a systemic infection.
- ABG analysis: Evaluates for hypoxemia and hypercapnia.

Diagnostic Tests for Acute Pneumonia		
Test	**Purpose**	**Abnormal Findings**
Arterial blood gas (ABG) analysis	Oxygenation status and acid-base balance are evaluated with ABGs.	*pH changes:* Acidosis may reflect respiratory failure; alkalosis may reflect tachypnea. *Carbon dioxide:* Elevated CO_2 reflects respiratory failure; decreased CO_2 reflects tachypnea. *Hypoxemia:* Pao_2 less than 80 mm Hg. *Oxygen saturation:* Sao_2 less than 92%. *Bicarbonate:* HCO_3 less than 22 mEq/L. *Base deficit:* less than -2.
Complete blood count (CBC)	Evaluates for presence of infection.	*Increased white blood cell (WBC) count:* less than $11,000/mm^3$ is seen with bacterial pneumonias. *Normal or low WBC count:* Seen with viral or mycoplasma pneumonias.
Sputum Gram stain, culture, and sensitivity	Identifies infecting organism. A sputum culture should be obtained from the lower respiratory tract before initiation of antimicrobial therapy. The most reliable specimens are obtained via bronchoalveolar lavage (BAL) during bronchoscopy, suctioning with a protected telescoping catheter (mini-BAL), or open-lung biopsy (used occasionally to reduce contamination of specimen with oral flora).	*Gram stain positive:* Indicates organism is present. *Culture:* Identifies organism. *Sensitivity:* Reflects effectiveness of drugs on identified organism.
Blood culture and sensitivity	Identifies whether pneumonia organism has become systemic; blood cultures help to identify the causative organism.	*Secondary bacteremia:* A frequent finding; patients with bacteremia are at higher risk for developing respiratory failure.
Serologic studies	Acute and convalescent titers are drawn to diagnose viral pneumonia. Both serologic and urine tests are available for Legionnaires' pneumonia.	*Increased antibody titers:* A positive sign for viral infection.
Acid-fast stain	To rule out mycobacterial infection (e.g., tuberculosis).	*Positive:* Mycobacterial infection is present.

Continued

Diagnostic Tests for Acute Pneumonia—cont'd

Test	Purpose	Abnormal Findings
Chest radiograph	Identifies anatomic involvement, extent of disease, presence of consolidation, pleural effusions, or cavitation.	*Lobar:* Entire lobe involved. *Segmental (lobular):* Only parts of a lobe involved. *Bronchopneumonia:* Affects alveoli contiguous to the involved bronchi.
Diagnostic fiber optic bronchoscopy using a PSB (protected specimen brush) and BAL	Obtains specimens during simple bronchoscopy without contaminating the aspirate; modified technique (mini-BAL) is also effective without the need of full bronchoscopy.	*Gram stain positive:* Indicates organism is present. *Culture:* Identifies organism. *Sensitivity:* Reflects effectiveness of drugs on identified organism.
Thoracentesis	Removal of pleural effusion fluid from the pleural space using a needle to drain the chest cavity. Pleural effusion fluid may be cultured following thoracentesis to identify the causative organism.	*Gram stain positive:* Indicates organism is present. *Culture:* Identifies organism. *Sensitivity:* Reflects effectiveness of drugs on identified organism.

Pneumonia management strategies are based on the recommendations of the Infectious Disease Society of America (IDSA), the American Thoracic Society (ATS), the American Society of Emergency Room Physicians, The Joint Commission as part of the Core Measures (revised July 25, 2014), and are endorsed by the Centers for Medicare and Medicaid Services.

PNEUMONIA MEASURES*

Indicators	Measure
Appropriate antibiotic selection	PN-6: Initial antibiotic is appropriate for community-acquired pneumonia in immunocompetent patients
Appropriate antibiotic selection	PN-6A: Initial antibiotic selection for community-acquired pneumonia in an immunocompetent patient-intensive care unit patient
Appropriate antibiotic selection	PN-6B: Initial antibiotic selection for community-acquired pneumonia in an immunocompetent patient-non—intensive care unit patient
Blood cultures drawn	PN-3A: Blood cultures performed within 24 hours before or 24 hours after hospital arrival for patients who were transferred or admitted to the intensive care unit within 24 hours of hospital arrival

*Criteria to include vaccinations PN-2 (pneumococcal vaccination) and PN-7 (influenza vaccination) were retired effective 1 January 2012. These measures have been replaced with the two immunization measures from The Joint Commission that are applicable to all patients regardless of diagnosis, rather than restricting the need for the vaccinations to patients with community-acquired pneumonia.

Retrieved from www.jointcommission.org/pneumonia/

COLLABORATIVE MANAGEMENT
CARE PRIORITIES
1. Relieve hypoxemia
- Oxygen therapy: Administered when the patient has an SpO_2 less than 92% or exhibits symptoms of air hunger or respiratory distress. Hypoxic drive, which contributes to the

compensatory mechanisms needed for effective breathing in patients with COPD who retain CO_2, can be lost with aggressive oxygen therapy. For patients with chronic CO_2 retention, O_2 is delivered in low concentrations while O_2 saturation (SpO_2) is closely monitored. Once the patient's SpO_2 exceeds the 88% to 92% range, the contributions of both hypoxic drive and hypoxic pulmonary vasoconstriction to maintaining stability are lost. Carbon dioxide dilates the pulmonary vasculature, while pulmonary arteries constrict in the presence of hypoxia. Identifying and maintaining the individual patient's balance between ventilation and perfusion optimizes gas exchange. The healthcare provider should be consulted for measurements of "acceptable" O_2 saturation values in any patient with CO_2 retention. Patients in need of higher-level O_2 may be considered for noninvasive, positive-pressure ventilation to help reduce work of breathing. Increased work of breathing indicates that the patient is having difficulty supporting ventilation.

- Intubation and mechanical ventilation: Intubation may be necessary if a patient experiences progressive respiratory distress despite treatments or if the patient becomes severely hypercapnic (CO_2 level greater than 50 mm Hg in normal patients; CO_2 level possibly greater than 70 mm Hg in patients who retain CO_2). Mechanical ventilation is indicated if the patient in respiratory distress is unable to maintain an adequate PaO_2 (PaO_2 greater than 60 mm Hg) with supplemental O_2. High concentrations of O_2 and PEEP may be necessary in severe cases of pneumonia that lead to acute respiratory failure. (See the section on Acute Respiratory Failure.)

2. Determine severity of pneumonia

Mortality rates for severe pneumonia range from 20% to 53%. The IDSA/ATS criteria for severe CAP are the presence of any single measurement as follows:

- RR greater than 30 breaths/min.
- Systolic BP less than 90 mm Hg.
- Diastolic BP less than 60 mm Hg.
- Bilateral or multilobar involvement on chest radiograph.
- P/F ratio (ratio of PaO_2 to FIO_2) less than 250.
- Confusion/disorientation.
- Urine output less than 20 mL/h or a total output of less than 80 mL/h over 4 hours.
- Acute renal failure.
- A 50% increase in size of the pulmonary infiltrate during the first 48 hours following diagnosis.
- Thrombocytopenia.
- The patient requires ET intubation and mechanical ventilation.
- Septic shock.
- Leukopenia.
- Hypothermia (core temperature less than 36° C).

3. Control infection

- Antibiotics or antiinfectives: Prescribed empirically on the basis of presenting signs and symptoms, clinical findings, and chest radiograph results until sputum or blood culture results are available. *Pneumococcus* is the most common pathogen associated with CAP, whereas enteric gram-negative bacteria are the most common pathogens identified with HAP. *Pseudomonas aeruginosa* and methicillin-resistant *Staphylococcus aureus* are the most common organisms seen in patients on long-term mechanical ventilation. Antimicrobial therapy in patients who are critically ill is usually parenteral and guided by sensitivity of the causative organism. Many of the organisms responsible for nosocomial pneumonias are resistant to multiple antibiotics or antimicrobials. Proper identification of the organism, determination of sensitivity to the medication, and attainment of therapeutic drug levels are crucial for effective therapy.
- Isolation: Some patients with pneumonia may require isolation and transmission-based precautions.

4. Control cough

Antitussives are used to relieve coughing. Occasionally, narcotics such as codeine are required if coughing is unrelieved by other agents. Patients receiving narcotics for pleuritic or other pain control may experience a reduction in coughing as a beneficial side effect of the narcotics. If cough is productive, adding an expectorant to help manage thicker secretions may assist the patient. Additional IV or enteral fluids may also help thin secretions by augmenting overall hydration. Coughing should be controlled to a reasonable level, but not at the expense of expectorating sputum.

5. Provide hydration

IV fluids may be necessary to replace insensible fluid loss and help thin secretions (e.g., tachypnea, diaphoresis with fever), in addition to providing enteral fluids. Volume resuscitation for dehydration must be done carefully to avoid volume overload in patients with multiple comorbidities. Dehydration causes secretions to become thick, tenacious, and difficult to expectorate.

6. Reduce fever

Analgesic antipyretics such as acetaminophen are used to reduce body temperature. Aspirin is generally not used for temperature control.

7. Provide pain relief

Analgesics are used to relieve pleuritic pain. Patients with pneumonia may have substantial pleuritic pain that requires administration of narcotic analgesics for relief. When opiates (e.g., codeine, morphine sulfate, and meperidine) are given, varying degrees of respiratory depression occur, but these agents are also generally effective in controlling severe coughing, which contributes to pain and discomfort. Careful and frequent monitoring of the patient's RR and depth, as well as O_2 saturation via pulse oximetry, is necessary.

8. Support nutritional status

Malnutrition is a causative factor in the development of infections. In patients who are severely ill, enteral nutrition may provide the best protection against the development of sepsis, owing to probable prevention of bacterial translocation from the gut. A nutritional therapy consultation is warranted for all patients who have developed an infection and those at high risk of infection.

9. Relieve congestion

Percussion and postural drainage are indicated if deep breathing, coughing, hydration (either enteral or parenteral fluids), and moving about in bed or ambulation are found to be ineffective in raising and expectorating sputum. Consult with the respiratory care provider as indicated.

INSTITUTE FOR HEALTHCARE IMPROVEMENT (IHI) VENTILATOR-ASSOCIATED PNEUMONIA (VAP) BUNDLE

The IHI has composed a group of interventions for all patients on mechanical ventilation that when implemented together result in better outcomes than when implemented individually. Reducing mortality resulting from VAP requires an organized approach to early recognition and consistent use of evidence-based practices

Indicator	Measure
Hand hygiene	Handwashing and hygiene are considered first-line defense for preventing infection. Lateral transmission of pathogens from the healthcare provider to the patient resulting in nosocomial infections including VAP can be prevented by ensuring the use of handwashing and hygiene.
Avoid circuit changes	No more than every 7 days unless soiled (not on the IHI bundle but recommended guidelines).
Elevation of head of the bed	Head of the bed is elevated at 30 degrees for the majority of the day (unless medically contraindicated).

INSTITUTE FOR HEALTHCARE IMPROVEMENT (IHI) VENTILATOR-ASSOCIATED PNEUMONIA (VAP) BUNDLE — cont'd

Indicator	Measure
Daily "sedation vacation" with assessment for readiness to extubate Adequate pain/sedation control but avoid oversedation	Sedation is interrupted until the patient is able to follow commands and can be assessed for discontinuation of mechanical ventilation.
Daily evaluation for weaning/extubation	Endotracheal intubation and mechanical intubation is a risk factor for VAP. Use a protocol for weaning from the ventilator and assess daily the possibility of weaning with the use of a spontaneous breathing trial.
Peptic ulcer disease prophylaxis	Gastric acid–controlling medications are administered to increase gastric pH. H_2-blockers are preferred over sucralfate. Proton pump inhibitors have not been fully studied.
Deep venous thrombosis prophylaxis	Thrombin-inhibiting medications or mechanical devices are used to reduce the risk of clot development in lower extremities.
Daily oral care with chlorhexidine	The oral cavity is a reservoir for pathogens with the potential to colonize into the upper respiratory tract. Daily oral hygiene can help to reduce the potential of VAP development of patients on the ventilator. The recommended chlorhexidine solution strength is 0.12%.

Retrieved from www.jsicm.org/pdf/VAPbundle2010kaitei_ENGLISH.pdf .

CARE PLANS FOR ACUTE PNEUMONIA

RISK FOR INJURY *related to respiratory compromise present with pneumonia*

Goals/Outcomes: The patient is free of infection reflected by normothermia and negative culture results; WBC count is within normal limits for the patient; and sputum is clear to white in color.
NOC Infection Severity, Infection Protection.

Infection Control
1. Implement standard precautions for infection prevention.
2. Provide additional infection control measures if infecting organism requires isolation.
3. Maintain a closed or in-line suction system or an aseptic environment when suctioning the secretions from the patient.
4. Inform visitors of effective precautions or pertinent isolation procedures.
5. Encourage and help provide turning, coughing, deep breathing, and use of incentive spirometer. Educate significant others to assist with these activities.
6. Encourage and assist with ambulation as soon as possible.

Infection Risk
1. Identify presurgical patients at increased risk for nosocomial pneumonia.
2. Provide presurgical patients and significant others with verbal and written instructions and demonstrations of turning, coughing, and deep-breathing exercises performed after surgery to prevent atelectasis, which may lead to pneumonia.
3. Postoperatively encourage lung expansion: turning and repositioning in bed, deep breathing, and coughing at frequent intervals. Mobilization of secretions is facilitated by movement.
4. Encourage and assist with ambulation as soon as possible.
5. Recognize the following ways in which nebulizer reservoirs can contaminate the patient: introduction of nonsterile fluids or air; manipulation of nebulizer cup; or backflow of condensation into reservoir or into the patient when delivery tubing is manipulated.

6. Use only sterile fluids and dispense them aseptically.
7. Recognize and manage risk factors for patients with tracheostomy or ET tubes and patients who are mechanically ventilated:
   - Presence of underlying lung disease or other serious illness.
   - Colonization of oropharynx or trachea by aerobic gram-negative bacteria.
   - Greater access of bacteria to lower respiratory tract.
   - Cross-contamination is more likely with manipulation of these tubes.
   - Change breathing circuits when visibly dirty or damaged; frequent changes to circuits is not advisable.
   - Use "no-touch" technique, or use sterile gloves on both hands until a new tracheostomy wound has healed or formed granulation tissue around the tube.
   - Suction on an "as needed" rather than a routine basis. Frequent suctioning increases the risk of trauma and cross-contamination.
8. For patients who cannot remove secretions effectively by coughing, perform procedures that stimulate coughing such as chest physiotherapy, which includes breathing exercises, postural drainage, and percussion.
9. If pain interferes with lung expansion, control it by administering as-needed analgesics approximately 30 minutes before deep-breathing exercises, and provide splint support of wound areas with hands or pillows placed firmly across site of incision.
10. Identify patients at risk for aspiration, such as those with a decreased level of consciousness or dysphagia or who have a nasogastric or gastric tube in place.
11. For patients with decreased level of consciousness who are unable to eat normally, consult with the physician regarding the need for a method of enteral feeding in which risk of aspiration is minimal such as postpyloric feeding (e.g., weighted small-bore feeding tube that imports enteral feeding to the duodenum) or percutaneous endoscopic gastrostomy (PEG tube).
12. Elevate the head of the bed to at least 30 degrees during feedings and for 1 hour after any feeding or medication to reduce the risk of aspiration.

DEFICIENT FLUID VOLUME *related to insensible fluid losses associated with pneumonia*

Goals/Outcomes: The patient is normovolemic reflected by no clinical evidence of hypovolemia (e.g., furrowed tongue), stable weight, BP within the patient's normal range, if available central venous pressure (CVP) 2 to 6 mm Hg, pulmonary artery pressure (PAP) 15 to 30/8 to 15 mm Hg, cardiac output 4 to 8 L/min, mean arterial pressure 70 to 105 mm Hg, HR 60 to 100 bpm, and systemic vascular resistance (SVR) 800 to 1200 dynes/s/cm^{-5}.
NOC Fluid Balance; Electrolyte; Acid-Base Balance.

Fluid Management
1. Identify patients at risk for dehydration, including those with poor nutritional status, reduced fluid intake, history of severe coughing (may be associated with inability to eat and/or vomiting), increased insensible loss secondary to hyperventilation, fever, and use of supplemental O_2.
2. Monitor input and output hourly. Initially, intake should exceed output during volume replacement therapy. Consult appropriate provider for urine output less than 0.5 mL/kg/h for 2 consecutive hours.
3. Monitor vital signs and hemodynamic pressures for signs of continued hypovolemia. Be alert to decreased values in BP, CVP, PAP, cardiac output, and mean arterial pressure, as well as increased HR and SVR.
4. Weigh the patient daily, at the same time of day (preferably before breakfast), on a balanced scale, with the patient wearing the same type of clothing. Use the same number of linens and equipment in place for bed weights.
5. Administer fluids by mouth (PO) and IV as prescribed. Document the patient's response to fluid replacement therapy.
6. Monitor for signs and symptoms of fluid overload or too-rapid fluid administration: crackles (rales), shortness of breath, tachypnea, tachycardia, increased CVP, increased PAPs, jugular vein distention, and edema.

NIC Aspiration Precautions; Chest Physiotherapy; Cough Enhancement; Environmental Management; Fluid/Electrolyte Management; Fluid Monitoring; Hypovolemia Management; Infection Control; Intravenous Therapy; Mechanical Ventilation; Nutrition Management; Positioning; Surveillance; Respiratory Monitoring; Vital Signs Monitoring.

ADDITIONAL NURSING DIAGNOSES
Also see Drowning (Chapter 3), and Acute Asthma Exacerbation (Chapter 4). As appropriate, see nursing diagnoses and interventions in Nutrition Support (Chapter 1), Acute Respiratory

Failure (Chapter 4), Mechanical Ventilation (Chapter 1), Prolonged Immobility (Chapter 1), and Emotional and Spiritual Support of the Patient and Significant Others (Chapter 2).

ACUTE RESPIRATORY FAILURE

PATHOPHYSIOLOGY

The primary goal of the pulmonary system is to promote appropriate and reasonable gas exchange at the alveolar-capillary surface, which is most often measured by pulse oximetry and ABGs. Acute respiratory failure is a general term that identifies a primary lung dysfunction, resulting in failure to remove CO_2 (known as hypoventilation) and/or failure to promote appropriate, proportionate O_2 uptake at the alveolar-capillary interface. Ventilation and perfusion must "match" to ensure the oxygen is able to appropriately diffuse across an intact alveolar-capillary membrane and attach to the hemoglobin carried on red blood cells. Saturation of hemoglobin with oxygen (oxyhemoglobin) in the lungs is the first step to oxygen delivery to the tissues. Carbon dioxide must also diffuse from the bloodstream into the alveoli to be exhaled. Type I respiratory failure (hypoxemic) is oxygenation failure, whereas type II (hypercapnic) is ventilation failure. Many patients manifest respiratory failure of types I and II simultaneously. Clinically, type I failure exists when Pao_2 is less than 50 mm Hg with the patient at rest and breathing room air (Fio_2 0.21 or 21% of the atmospheric pressure, which is 760 mm Hg at sea level). $Paco_2$ greater than 50 mm Hg is significant for acute ventilation failure or hypercapnia. The Pao_2 provides the "driving pressure" for the saturation of hemoglobin. Without adequate pressure (Pao_2), the hemoglobin is inadequately saturated. Approximately 98% of the oxygen delivered to tissues is provided by oxyhemoglobin. The amount of oxygen combined with hemoglobin depends on the Pao_2. The relationship is articulated within the oxyhemoglobin dissociation curve.

Carbon dioxide is transported in three main forms: (1) in simple solution, (2) as bicarbonate, and (3) combined with protein of hemoglobin as a carbamino compound. Under healthy conditions, the amount of carbon dioxide produced by the tissues is constant and equals the amount of carbon dioxide eliminated by the lung. A wide variety of disease states creates a single or mixed respiratory failure; some affecting ventilation, others, perfusion. One of the simplest methods of evaluating patients relates to the understanding of basic gas exchange. Oxygenation occurs primarily during inspiration and the removal of CO_2 occurs during exhalation. The basic concepts applied here include compliance and recoil. Lung compliance is the measure of expansion of the alveoli (the gas-exchanging surface), which occurs on inspiration, whereas elasticity refers to the ability of the alveoli to recoil, as they do on exhalation. Restrictive airway diseases [generally] present with significant hypoxemia, whereas obstructive disorders are more likely to develop a persistent and chronic hypercapnia. See Box 4-1 for a description of some of the disease processes that can lead to acute respiratory failure.

The evaluation of respiratory failure includes the understanding of the following:

VENTILATION AND PERFUSION MATCHING ($\dot{V}/\dot{Q}$ MATCH)

This general term refers to the relationship of gas distribution ($\dot{V}$) to the amount of blood ($\dot{Q}$), which passes the total alveolar surface in 1 minute of time. Normal alveolar ventilation occurs at a rate of 4 L/min, and normal pulmonary vascular blood flow occurs at a rate of 5 L/min. The normal $\dot{V}/\dot{Q}$ ratio is therefore 4 L/min divided by 5 L/min, or a ratio of 0.8, almost in a 1:1 ratio. Any disease process that interferes with either side of the equation upsets the physiologic balance, causing a $\dot{V}/\dot{Q}$ mismatch.

Components of an abnormal $\dot{V}/\dot{Q}$ ratio

Alveolar dead space ventilation: This is a primary problem with pulmonary perfusion. Areas where alveoli expand, but have less than normal blood surrounding the alveoli are called "dead spaces" because gas exchange is impaired rendering the area functionally "dead." Alveoli may be compliant and elastic, normal or hyperventilated, with perfusion proportionately lower than the ventilation. The imbalance is measured or evaluated as a high $\dot{V}/\dot{Q}$ mismatch, wherein ventilation is proportionately greater than perfusion. Because perfusion is the problem, underlying causes are often low cardiac output states resulting from pump impairment, or vascular occlusion impairing blood flow, such as seen with pulmonary embolus. Ventilatory causes involve overventilation of the independent lung surface.

Diffusion distance: Governed by the "thickness" of the alveolar-capillary membrane. O_2 and CO_2 must cross the barrier created by the alveolar epithelium, the interstitial space, and the capillary endothelium. That space between is typically fluid-free and product-free, allowing gas to move rapidly across. Diffusion is affected when an increase in anatomic distance and/or product (fluid, proteins, and neutrophils) alters the ability of gas exchange between alveoli and the capillary bed. Pulmonary edema is a major problem that interferes with diffusion, because it increases the "diameter" or thickness of the alveolar-capillary membrane.

Volume of CO_2: The volume of CO_2 produced by the body tissues varies with metabolic rate (fever, pain, agitation, sepsis, and so forth). The $Paco_2$ must be interpreted in conjunction with the volume exhaled, especially in patients who are mechanically ventilated. Many of the variables impacting CO_2 flux can be eliminated by controlling ventilation and muscular activity. Current evidence supports that the overdistension and shear force of opening-closing also profoundly affect the healthy lung.

Intrapulmonary right-to-left shunt: Large amounts of blood pass from the right side of the heart (receives the deoxygenated venous blood) to the left side of the heart without adequate saturation of hemoglobin with oxygen in the lungs. Poorly oxygenated blood passes in and out of the general circulation, impacting the amount of oxygen available to the cells. This process occurs when alveoli are not recruited on inspiration resulting from atelectasis or the alveoli are flooded with fluid. Primary causes of intrapulmonary shunt are atelectasis and ARDS.

ASSESSMENT

GOAL OF SYSTEM ASSESSMENT

To evaluate for poor gas exchange and increased ventilatory support requirements (see sections on Acid-Base Balance and Mechanical Ventilation, Chapter 1).

HISTORY AND RISK FACTORS

Indicators of acute respiratory failure vary according to the underlying disease process and severity of the failure. Acute respiratory failure is one of the most common causes of altered mental status and agitation. Respiratory failure is often associated with heart failure, pneumonia, or stroke. Sometimes, the onset of acute respiratory failure is so insidious it is missed or misinterpreted, similar to the insidious onset of shock in some patients. A patient may be somnolent attributable to hypercapnia (CO_2 retention causing elevated CO_2) from ventilatory failure, or agitated and combative as a result of hypoxia. Patients with COPD have reduced airway diameter as well as chronic inflammation and airway remodeling, and when the underlying chronic condition is exacerbated, mucus hypersecretion and airway edema compound the initial condition. Increased effort is needed to mobilize gas in and out of the lungs, particularly during exhalation. The failure to exhale leads to air trapping and hyperinflation, which further compromise inspiratory effort and contribute to increasing hypoxia and hypercapnia. Patients with impending shock are at high risk for respiratory failure. Inhalation of toxic substances, pneumonia, severe pneumonitis, aspiration of gastric contents, drowning, and air or fat embolus may prompt respiratory failure. Other causes include acute pancreatitis, drug overdose, neurologic injury, hemorrhage, sepsis, extreme obesity, or any condition that has enlarged the abdomen to the point of exerting upward pressure on the diaphragm.

VITAL SIGNS

- Early indicators: Dyspnea, restlessness, anxiety, headache, fatigue, cool and dry skin, increased BP, tachycardia, and persistent rapid RR, which indicate hypoxia. Hypercapnia results in slurred speech and headache.
- Intermediate indicators: Confusion, profound lethargy, tachypnea, hypotension and somnolence (if pH is less than 7.25), and cardiac dysrhythmias.
- Late indicators: Cyanosis, diaphoresis, coma, and respiratory arrest.

| Safety Alert | *A patient with a history of chronic obstructive pulmonary disease may increasingly or excessively use inhaled beta$_2$-agonists. If this is the case, evaluation of tachycardia may be indicative of recent medication use.* |

VITAL SIGNS
* RR is rapid. If the patient is experiencing impending shock, RR is compensatory for metabolic acidosis.
* Rapid HR if not receiving beta-antagonist therapy (beta-blockers).
* Spo_2 is lower than expected when reviewing O_2 support. Analysis of the Pao_2/Fio_2 ratio may reveal a value of less than 300.

A-a GRADIENT/A-aDo$_2$/P(A-a)o$_2$
* The A-a gradient or alveolar-arterial O_2 tension difference is a clinically useful calculation. The calculation is based on a model as though the lung were one large alveolus and the entire blood flow of the right side of the heart passed around it. Using the rules of partial pressure as well as the laws of CO_2 production at the cell and the content of CO_2 exerting alveolar pressure, the theoretical alveolar Po_2 (Pao_2) is calculated. Once the theoretical Pao_2 has been calculated, the gradient is achieved by subtracting the measured arterial Pao_2. The calculated "gradient" represents the difference between the calculated alveolar oxygen (Pao_2) and the measured arterial oxygen (Pao_2).
* When the Fio_2 is greater than 0.21, the A-a gradient becomes less accurate as in the measurement of proportional gas exchange, although the difference should always be less than 150 mm Hg.
* Extrapulmonary failure: The A-a gradient generally remains normal or narrow.
* With shunt or $\dot{V}/\dot{Q}$ mismatch, the gradient is usually wider than normal. The A-a gradient also measures the severity of gas exchange impairment. At any age, an A-a gradient greater than 20 mm Hg on room air or greater than 100 mm Hg on increased Fio_2 should be considered abnormal and indicative of pulmonary dysfunction.

OBSERVATION
* Nasal flaring and expiratory grunt may be present.
* Use of accessory muscles indicates respiratory distress.
* May appear fatigued, with or without diaphoresis.
* May present with ashen, pale, or gray/blue facial color, lip color, or nail beds.
* Chest expansion may be decreased, restricted, or asymmetrical with severe changes in one lung manifesting severe atelectasis or pleuritic pain.
* Altered level of consciousness (confusion, disorientation, and agitation) is more common with older adults but is a very significant sign in any age group.
* Agitation is more commonly associated with hypoxemia, whereas somnolence is associated with hypercarbia (elevated CO_2 level).

AUSCULTATION
Evaluate the presence of normal breath sounds and synchronous lung expansion. Auscultate for the presence of:
1. Late inspiratory rales (crackles): Anterior, lateral, and posterior: alveolar fluid or late opening.
2. Midinspiratory rales (crackles): Anterior, lateral, and posterior alveolar consolidation.
3. Early loud, coarse rales (bubbles or rhonchi): Anterior, lateral, and posterior: conducting airway inflammation and mucus secretion.
4. Inspiratory wheezes: Anterior, lateral, and posterior: early airway narrowing.
5. Expiratory wheezes: Anterior, lateral, and posterior: late airway narrowing.

PALPATION
* Palpate chest wall for tenderness indicative of inflammation.
* Palpate to assess for symmetry of chest expansion.

PERCUSSION
* May reveal presence of consolidation or fluid (dullness) or hyperresonance (pneumothorax).

SCREENING LABWORK
* Blood gas evaluation can determine primary and secondary problems, or primary problems with compensation (see Acid-Base Balance, Chapter 1).

- Pulse oximetry is used for continuous monitoring of O_2 saturation.
- Sputum Gram stain, culture, and sensitivity: Identifies infecting organism.
- Blood culture and sensitivity: If result is positive, it may indicate that the organism has migrated into the bloodstream to cause a systemic infection.
- ABG analysis: Evaluates for hypoxemia and eventually hypercapnia.

Diagnostic Tests for Acute Respiratory Failure

Test	Purpose	Abnormal Findings
Blood Studies		
Arterial blood gas analysis	Assesses adequacy of oxygenation and effectiveness of ventilation. Evaluates the oxygenation of the arterial blood as well as the presence or absence of acid and the effect on the pH (environment of the cells).	Typical results predicting respiratory failure are Pao_2 less than 60 mm Hg, $Paco_2$ greater than 45 mm Hg, with a pH that may be within normal range consistent with compensation via an increase in HCO_3 (bicarbonate), or the pH may be less than 7.35 consistent with acute (uncompensated) respiratory acidosis. Although changes are not always predictable in the disease process, generally patients will develop hypoxemia, which may initially be resolved by increasing the Fio_2 but eventually will require great increases in Fio_2 and ultimately will no longer respond to oxygen therapy.
Pao_2/Fio_2 ratio	The Pao_2 divided by the Fio_2 (Pao_2/Fio_2 ratio, or more simply P/F) can be used to more simply assess the severity of the gas exchange defect. The normal value for the ratio of the partial pressure of oxygen in arterial blood to Fio_2 (Pao_2/Fio_2) (Fio_2 is expressed as a decimal ranging from 0.21 to 1.00) is 300 to 500.	A value of less than 300 indicates gas exchange derangement, and a value less than 250 is indicative of severe impairment, and compliance calculations should be performed to encourage alveolar recruitment strategies. A value less than 200 or greater than 40% Fio_2 is indicative of severe impairment.
Radiology		
Chest radiograph	Assesses the size of lungs, presence of fluids, abnormal gas or fluids in the pleural sac, diaphragmatic margins, the pulmonary hilum, and the integrity of the rib cage.	The presence of fluids in the lung parenchyma initially presents as pulmonary edema. The continuous accumulation differentiates this edema formation to one that is not cardiac.
Computed tomography (CT) lung scan	Assesses the three-dimensional lung capacities, fluid load, and primary displacement of the fluid.	Normally a large gas-filled surface, the ALI/ARDS lung when seen on CT is frequently fluffy and white resulting from fluid that has extravasated through the endothelial deficits (capillary leak).

COLLABORATIVE MANAGEMENT

Careful consideration should be given to evaluate neurologic conditions and OSA because these are commonly overlooked causes of respiratory failure. In addition, the primary goal is to determine and treat the underlying pathophysiologic condition.

CARE PRIORITIES

1. Correction of hypoxemia: First treatment priority

Pao_2 levels less than 30 mm Hg for longer than 5 minutes may cause permanent brain damage or death. High-concentration O_2 therapy, in conjunction with pharmacotherapy (e.g., bronchodilators, steroids, antibiotics), often improves ABG levels sufficiently to remove the patient from danger, but increasing FIO_2 is a temporary solution and does not actually treat the problem. Adding additional molecules of oxygen improves the diffusion gradient from the alveolus into the capillary, and provides "driving pressure" for the saturation of hemoglobin with oxygen. Patients with COPD who chronically retain CO_2 (chronic hypercapnia) are unable to receive high concentrations of O_2 unless ventilation is highly supported with an underlying rate control strategy such as NPPV or NiPPV, CPAP or BiPAP, or invasive mechanical ventilation.

2. Correction of respiratory acidosis (hypercapnia)
May be corrected using NPPV such as BiPAP, or invasive mechanical ventilation following ET intubation. Exhalation time should be increased and particular attention to that time must be applied when altering tidal volume or RR. Because CO_2 is removed during exhalation time in the respiratory cycle, any patient with CO_2 retention must be provided with a longer E time.

- Noninvasive (NPPV): Ventilator support that is given without ET intubation or tracheotomy. Administered via a face or nasal mask. Requires skilled management but not necessarily intensive care admission. NPPV or invasive mechanical support is used as a continuous replacement for normal lung function until the underlying cause of the failure can be corrected and the patient can resume ventilatory efforts independently.
- Invasive: Mechanical ventilation delivered using an ET tube or tracheotomy; requires intensive or high-acuity care. The purposes of intubation and mechanical ventilation are to restore alveolar ventilation and systemic oxygenation, provide compensation in metabolic acidosis/alkalosis, and decrease work of breathing. Early intubation can prevent further airway collapse and tissue injury. In most cases of respiratory failure, the patient will require intubation and mechanical ventilation to support adequate respiratory function and stabilize ABG levels. (See Mechanical Ventilation, Chapter 1.)

3. Correction of acidotic pH as a result of hypercapnia (hypoventilation)
Adequate cellular and metabolic functioning are hindered when pH level remains outside the normal range of 7.35 to 7.45. When the pH is less than 7.20, evaluate for signs of systemic compromise such as failure to maintain vascular tone and therefore BP. After efforts to correct ventilation have failed or if the patient presents with clinical symptoms such as hypotension refractory to volume and vasopressors, IV sodium bicarbonate may be used conservatively to return the pH to a level higher than 7.25. The use of sodium bicarbonate is a short-term solution for most acid-base disturbances and its use may actually make the overall situation worse.

4. Correction of alkalotic pH as a result of hypocapnia (hyperventilation)
A pH greater than 7.45 may indicate primary hyperventilation with a high minute ventilation (F or V_T). If possible, assess the patient for anxiety and rapid RR. If the patient is intubated, assess the settings on the ventilator to assure that an appropriate method is being used.

If the minute ventilation is not the causative problem or cannot be adjusted, evaluate for a primary metabolic alkalosis. Causative factors of primary metabolic alkalosis may be overdiuresis, diarrhea, or aggressive nasogastric drainage. The pH may be managed by compensation with CO_2 retention via a rebreathing mask, decreasing minute ventilation, or by increasing dead space on mechanical ventilator circuitry.

5. Provide nutrition support
Energy outlay with respiratory failure is high, in part because of the increased work of breathing. If the patient is unable to consume adequate calories with enteral feedings, total parenteral nutrition is added. It is important to perform an occasional evaluation of the patient's caloric and metabolic needs to make certain that the patient is being adequately nourished but not overfed. All efforts should be made to feed enterally so the gut is used. Newer elemental feedings require no digestion and can be used in the stomach, duodenum, or jejunum. (See Nutrition Support, Chapter 1.)

RESEARCH BRIEF 4-6

Clinical research to evaluate the effectiveness of life support systems in acute fatal illness has unique problems of logistics, ethics, and consent. There have been 10 prospective comparative trials of extracorporeal membrane oxygenation in acute fatal respiratory failure, using different study designs. The trial designs were prospective controlled randomized, prospective adaptive randomized, sequential, and matched pairs. The trials were reviewed with regard to logistics, ethics, consent, statistical methods, economics, and impact. The matched pairs method is the best study design for evaluation of life support systems in acute fatal illness.

From Bartlett RH: Clinical research in acute fatal illness: lessons from extracorporeal membrane oxygenation. *J Intensive Care Med* Sep 15;pii: 0885066614550278 [Epub ahead of print], 2014.

CARE PLANS FOR ACUTE RESPIRATORY FAILURE

IMPAIRED GAS EXCHANGE *related to disease process underlying impending respiratory failure.*

Goals/Outcomes: Within 2 to 4 hours of initiation of treatment, the patient has adequate gas exchange reflected by PaO_2 greater than 80 mm Hg, $PaCO_2$ 35 to 45 mm Hg, and pH 7.35 to 7.45 (or ABG values within 10% of the patient's baseline), with mechanical ventilation, if necessary. Within 24 to 48 hours of initiation of treatment, the patient is weaning or weaned from mechanical ventilation, and RR is 12 to 20 breaths/min with normal baseline depth and pattern.

NOC Respiratory Status: Ventilation, Vital Signs Status; Respiratory Status: Gas Exchange, Symptom Control Behavior, Comfort Level, Endurance.

Respiratory Monitoring
1. Monitor for signs of increasing hypoxia at frequent intervals: restlessness, agitation, and personality changes are indicative of severe exacerbation. Cyanosis of the nail beds (peripheral) and/or lips (central) is an early and late indicator of hypoxia, respectively.
2. Monitor for signs of hypercapnia at frequent intervals: confusion, listlessness, and somnolence may indicate respiratory failure or near-fatal asthma exacerbation.
3. Monitor ABGs when continuous pulse oximetry values or patient assessment reflects progressive hypoxemia or development of hypercapnia. Be alert to decreasing PaO_2 and increasing $PaCO_2$ or decreasing O_2 saturation levels, indicative of impending respiratory collapse.
4. Monitor for synchronous, bilateral lung expansion, decreased breath sounds, or changes in wheezing at frequent intervals. Absent breath sounds in a distressed patient with asthma may indicate impending respiratory arrest.

Anxiety Reduction
1. Ascertain and alleviate the cause of restlessness to decrease metabolic demands (e.g., if restlessness is related to anxiety, help reduce anxiety by providing reassurance, enabling family members to stay with the patient, and offering distractions such as soft music or television).
2. Be aware that restlessness may be an early sign of hypoxemia.
3. Explain all procedures and offer support to minimize fear and anxiety, which can increase O_2 demands.

Oxygen Therapy
1. Provide humidity in O_2 if used for more than 12 hours to help thin secretions.
2. Administer supplemental O_2 using liter flow device as ordered.
3. Document pulse oximetry with O_2 liter flow in place at time of reading as ordered. Oxygen is a drug; the dose of the drug must be associated with the O_2 saturation or the reading is meaningless.
4. Monitor for skin breakdown where O_2 devices are in contact with the skin, such as nares, and around edges of mask devices.
5. Monitor FIO_2 to ensure that O_2 is within prescribed concentrations. If the patient does not retain CO_2, a 100% nonrebreather mask may be used to provide maximal O_2 support. If the patient retains CO_2 and is unrelieved by positioning, lower-dose O_2, bronchodilators, steroids, intubation, and mechanical ventilation may be necessary sooner than in patients who are able to receive higher doses of O_2 by mask.

Ventilation Assistance
1. Obtain ABGs if the patient experiences behavioral changes or respiratory distress to check for hypoxia or hypercapnia.
2. Monitor for induced hypoventilation, especially in patients with COPD.
3. Monitor for changes in chest radiograph and breath sounds indicative of O_2 toxicity and absorption atelectasis in patients receiving higher concentrations of O_2 (greater than 45% FIO_2) for longer than 24 hours. The higher the O_2 concentration, the greater is the chance of toxicity.
4. Position the patient for comfort and to promote optimal gas exchange. High-Fowler's position, with the patient leaning forward and elbows propped on the over-the-bed table to promote maximal chest excursion, may reduce use of accessory muscles and diaphoresis resulting from work of breathing.
5. Consider use of NPPV before ET intubation and mechanical ventilation.

NIC Acid-Base Management; Acid-Base Monitoring; Airway Management; Bedside Laboratory Testing; Cough Enhancement; Emotional Support; Energy Management; Fluid Management; Fluid Monitoring; Laboratory Data Interpretation; Mechanical Ventilation; Oxygen Therapy; Positioning; Respiratory Monitoring; Vital Signs Monitoring.

ADDITIONAL NURSING DIAGNOSIS

See sections relating to underlying pathologic condition of patients. Refer to Mechanical Ventilation, Chapter 1, for further information.

PNEUMOTHORAX

PATHOPHYSIOLOGY

Pneumothorax is an accumulation of air between the parietal and visceral pleura with secondary lung collapse. There are three types of pneumothorax: spontaneous, traumatic, and tension.

SPONTANEOUS

A portion of the lung may spontaneously collapse, while the chest wall remains intact with no leak to the atmosphere. Both primary and secondary spontaneous pneumothoraces may result from the rupture of a bleb or bullae on the visceral pleural surface, usually near the apex, resulting in air entering the thorax. A primary spontaneous pneumothorax is rarely life threatening and generally occurs in healthy, 20- to 40-year-old lean, thin men who smoke. The cause of the bleb/bullae rupture is unknown, although it may result from a weakness related to a respiratory infection. Symptoms most often occur at rest rather than with vigorous exercise or coughing. There is a high probability for recurrence within 2 to 3 years.

A secondary spontaneous pneumothorax may occur in all age groups resulting from an underlying lung disease (COPD, cystic fibrosis, tuberculosis, malignant neoplasm). Symptoms are more likely to be life threatening than with a primary spontaneous pneumothorax, and recurrence rates are high in this population. The rate of reabsorption of spontaneous pneumothoraces is 1.25% to 1.8% of the volume of the hemithorax every 24 hours. A 15% pneumothorax requires 8 to 12 days to fully resolve without treatment.

TRAUMATIC

The integrity of the chest wall may or may not be disrupted before lung collapse in a pneumothorax resulting from trauma. An open pneumothorax occurs when air enters the pleural space from the atmosphere through an opening in the chest wall, such as with a penetrating injury (includes stabbing, gunshot wound to the chest) or an invasive medical procedure (e.g., lung biopsy, thoracentesis, placement of a central line into a subclavian vein). A closed pneumothorax occurs when the visceral pleura is penetrated but the chest wall remains intact, with no atmospheric leak. Closed chest wall lung collapse occurs with blunt trauma, including cardiopulmonary resuscitation, when an external impact on the chest fractures and dislocates the ribs (i.e., motor vehicle crash with the chest hitting the steering wheel). It may also occur from the use of high-level PEEP therapy. For more information about blunt chest injuries, see Chest Trauma, Chapter 3.

TENSION

Tension pneumothorax is a life-threatening medical emergency most often associated with trauma or infection. Tension can ensue with a spontaneous pneumothorax or during positive-pressure mechanical ventilation. The integrity of the chest wall may or may not be disrupted before lung collapse. Air enters the pleural space during inspiration through a pleural tear and continues to accumulate inside the pleural cavity. The air cannot escape during expiration because the intrapleural pressure is greater than alveolar pressure, which creates a one-way or flap-valve effect. The increasing intrathoracic pressure is transmitted to the mediastinum, resulting in a mediastinal shift toward the unaffected side. The encroachment of the enlarging affected side makes it impossible for the unaffected side to fully expand. The increased pressure also compresses the vena cava, which impedes venous return, and reduces preload/end-diastolic volume. Cardiac output is progressively reduced while intrathoracic pressure and compression of the vena cava increases, leading to circulatory collapse if not promptly diagnosed and managed. Bilateral tension pneumothoraces may occur and generally result in cardiac arrest shortly after the lungs collapse.

ASSESSMENT

GOAL OF SYSTEM ASSESSMENT

Identify ineffective breathing patterns and impaired gas exchange. The clinical presentation will vary in degree, depending on the type and size of the pneumothorax. With tension pneumothorax, evaluate for decreased cardiac output and decreased tissue perfusion. See the section on Respiratory Assessment General: (earlier in Chapter 4), and Cardiac Assessment: General (Chapter 5).

HISTORY AND RISK FACTORS

Trauma, pulmonary infection, high-level positive-pressure mechanical ventilation: Nearly 46% of patients with primary pneumothoraces do not seek medical advice for more than 2 days. Assessing for delay is important because the occurrence of reexpansion pulmonary edema after reinflation may be related to the length of time the lung has been collapsed.

CHEST RADIOGRAPH

- Determines presence of pneumothorax, usually estimated in percentages depending on the size of the lung collapsed.
- Reflects absence of lung markers; includes absence of "white" blood vessels.
- No circulation is present in collapsed area filled with air (black).

VITAL SIGNS

- Tachycardia, tachypnea.
- Possible fever.
- BP may increase or decrease, depending on response to any changes in cardiac output, which are profound with tension pneumothorax.
- Small pneumothoraces may not affect vital signs at all.

OBSERVATION/INSPECTION

Spontaneous or traumatic pneumothorax

- Sudden onset of sharp, stabbing chest pain on the affected side, radiating to the shoulder if pneumothorax is large enough (greater than 20% collapse).
- The British Thoracic Society 2010 guidelines define "small" as a pneumothorax of less than 2 cm and "large" as a pneumothorax of greater than 2 cm between the lung margin and the chest wall (at the level of the hilum). Percentages of lung that have collapsed are also used to quantify the extent of lung collapse in clinical practice.
- Moderate to severe dyspnea and anxiety may be present if pneumothorax is large enough (greater than 30% collapse).
- Decreased chest wall movement on the affected side if the pneumothorax is large enough (greater than 40% collapse).
- Pale appearance is likely with a larger pneumothorax (greater than 50% collapse).
- With a small pneumothorax (10% to 20% collapse), the patient may have no pain and no abnormality in chest wall movement and be unaware that lung collapse has occurred.

Tension pneumothorax

- Severe dyspnea.
- Chest pain on affected side.

- Pale progressing to gray/blue, cool, clammy, mottled skin.
- Anxiety and restlessness resulting from progressive hypoxemia.
- Decreased chest wall movement on affected side.
- Expansion of affected side throughout respiratory cycle, rather than expansion and relaxation.
- Progressively increasing jugular vein distention as vena cava is compressed.
- Cardiac arrest is possible with bilateral tension pneumothoraces.

PALPATION
Spontaneous or traumatic pneumothorax
- Subcutaneous emphysema (crepitus).
- Tactile and vocal fremitus decreased or absent on affected side.

Tension pneumothorax
- Tracheal shift toward unaffected side.
- Subcutaneous emphysema in neck and chest.

PERCUSSION
Spontaneous or traumatic pneumothorax
- Hyperresonance on affected side.

Tension pneumothorax
- Hyperresonance on affected side.

AUSCULTATION
Spontaneous or traumatic pneumothorax
- Absent or decreased breath sounds on affected side.
- Increased RR.
- Moderate tachycardia (HR greater than 140 bpm) may be present.

Tension pneumothorax
- Absent or decreased breath sounds on affected side.
- Distant heart sounds.
- Tachypnea/increased RR (greater than 30 breaths/min).
- Hypotension/decreased BP (more than a 20% drop from previous BP).
- Tachycardia/increased HR (greater than 140 bpm).

Safety Alert   *Tension pneumothorax is life threatening. Immediate medical intervention is crucial.*

Diagnostic Tests for Pneumothorax		
Test	**Purpose**	**Abnormal Findings**
Chest radiograph A lateral chest or lateral decubitus radiograph should be done if the clinical suspicion of pneumothorax is high, but a posterior-anterior radiograph is normal. Expiratory chest radiographs are not recommended for the routine diagnosis of pneumothorax.	Reveals the size of the pneumothorax and presence of tracheal shift.	Affected side: Air is present in the pleural space (black); lung markings are absent in area of collapse (black); abnormal expansion of the chest wall with tension pneumothorax with lowering/flattening of the diaphragm.

Continued

Diagnostic Tests for Pneumothorax — cont'd

Test	Purpose	Abnormal Findings
Chest computed tomography (CT) scan	CT scanning is recommended when differentiating a pneumothorax from bullous lung disease, when incorrect tube placement may be present, and when the chest radiograph is obscured by surgical emphysema.	The presence of blackened areas is indicative of air, with the absence of white areas indicative of blood circulating in tissues, which may have been obliterated or unclear on the chest radiograph.
Arterial blood gas (ABG) analysis	Assesses for hypoxemia and acidosis.	Hypoxemia (Pao_2 <80 mm Hg on room air) is generally present with a 20% or greater lung collapse. Mild hypoxemia is present with smaller pneumothoraces. Tension pneumothoraces may cause both respiratory and lactic acidosis (pH <7.35) from impending respiratory failure and circulatory collapse. Elevated carbon dioxide and lactate lower the blood pH.
12-Lead ECG (electrocardiogram)	Rules out acute coronary syndrome as a cause for chest pain with vital sign changes indicative of deterioration.	Vena cava compression from tension pneumothorax affects perfusion of the coronary arteries if pneumothorax is not diagnosed and managed promptly. ST segment depression, indicative of myocardial ischemia, may be present, along with decreased QRS amplitude/decreased R waves, rightward axis deviation.
Pulmonary function tests	Pulmonary function tests provide minimally sensitive data to validate presence or size of pneumothorax.	Not recommended.

COLLABORATIVE MANAGEMENT

CARE PRIORITIES

Patients with shortness of breath should not be left without intervention regardless of the size of the pneumothorax seen on the chest radiograph.

1. Relieve hypoxemia

- Oxygen therapy/adjustment in mechanical ventilation: Oxygen is administered when ABG values demonstrate the presence of hypoxemia. If the patient is already receiving mechanical ventilation, Fio_2 is increased while evaluation is done regarding amount of positive pressure used during inspiratory and expiratory phases of ventilation. If positive pressure is a suspected cause of the pneumothorax, positive pressure is reduced if possible.
- High-flow O_2: If a patient with a pneumothorax is admitted for observation, high-flow (10 L/min) O_2 should be administered, with appropriate caution in patients with COPD with sensitivity to high concentrations of O_2. Use of high-flow O_2 has resulted in a fourfold increase in the rate of pneumothorax reabsorption while the therapy is in progress.

2. Reexpand the collapsed lung

- **Observation:** No treatment may be required for small, closed pneumothoraces without significant dyspnea or breathlessness.

- **Simple aspiration:** Recommended as first line of treatment for all primary pneumothoraces in need of intervention. Performed immediately in tension pneumothorax to remove air from the chest cavity. A large-bore needle is inserted into the second intercostal space, midclavicular line, which correlates with the superior portion of the anterior axillary lobe. A sudden rushing out of air confirms the diagnosis of tension pneumothorax. To decrease the risk of further pleural laceration while the chest reexpands, a stylet introducer needle with a plastic sheath may be used. The needle is removed after penetration, and the plastic catheter sheath is left in place to allow decompression of the chest cavity. Simple aspiration is less likely to succeed in secondary pneumothoraces and is recommended as an initial treatment in small (less than 2 cm) pneumothoraces in patients younger than 50 years with mild shortness of breath. Large secondary pneumothoraces (larger than 2 cm), especially in patients older than 50 years, are generally not successfully managed using simple aspiration and are at high risk for recurrence. Intercostal/chest tube drainage is recommended as appropriate initial treatment. Once air is removed from the pleural space, the lung is able to reexpand.
- **Catheter aspiration:** Catheter aspiration of the trapped air in a simple pneumothorax is done by passing a small (approximately 8 Fr) catheter over a guide wire into the pleural space. A three-way stopcock is attached and air may be aspirated via a 50-mL syringe. Addition of a Heimlich valve and suction may improve success rates to over 60%. If simple aspiration or catheter aspiration drainage is unsuccessful, a chest/intercostal tube should be inserted.
- **Chest tube placement/tube thoracostomy:** Recommended in secondary pneumothorax except in patients who are symptomatic with a very small (less than 1 cm or apical) pneumothorax. Chest tubes cause inflammation, ultimately scarring the pleura to help prevent recurrent spontaneous pneumothoraces. Patients with recurrent lung collapse or extensive lung disease generally require chest tubes rather than needle decompression because their visceral pleura does not seal promptly. Chest tubes are inserted in the second or third lateral intercostal space, midclavicular line, or near the fifth intercostal space at the midaxillary line to promote fluid evacuation. Abdominal viscera may be punctured with placement below the fifth intercostal space. During insertion, the patient should be in an upright position so that the lung falls away from the chest wall. A small (1 to 2 cm) incision is made, and the chest tube is placed, sutured in place, and connected to an underwater-seal drainage system. Usually simple underwater-seal drainage is all that is necessary for 6 to 24 hours. A one-way flutter valve may be placed on the chest tube instead of the underwater-seal drainage system, to allow air to escape while preventing reentry. After chest tube insertion and removal of air from the pleural space, the lung begins to reexpand. There is no evidence that large tubes (20 to 24 Fr) are more effective than small tubes (10 to 14 Fr). The initial use of large (20 to 24 Fr) intercostal tubes is not recommended. If a persistent air leak is present, it may be necessary to replace a small chest tube with a larger one. Suction may be used, depending on the size of the pneumothorax, the patient's condition, and the amount of drainage. Suction can be applied with a flutter valve in place.
- **Chest tube suction:** Suction should not be applied directly after tube insertion, but rather added after 48 hours if persistent air leak is present or the pneumothorax fails to reexpand. High-volume, low-pressure (greater than 10 to less than 20 cm H_2O) suction systems are recommended. Patients requiring suction should be managed by physicians and nurses who have experience managing complex pneumothoraces. There is no evidence to support routine use of immediate suction with chest drain systems in the treatment of spontaneous pneumothorax.
- **Chemical pleurodesis:** The instillation of caustic substances into the pleural space, resulting in aseptic inflammation with formation of dense adhesions, which can seal persistent air leaks. Pleurodesis is associated with a high recurrence rate of primary and secondary pneumothoraces, despite use of various sclerosants to reduce these rates. The chemicals are instilled either through chest tubes or during surgery. Doxycycline and talc slurry are the preferred sclerosing agents. Few usage guidelines are available for physicians. Prevention of additional recurrent pneumothoraces should be managed surgically in most cases.

3. Relieve pain

- Analgesic: Provides relief of pain of pneumothorax or its treatment. A chest tube may cause pleuritic pain, slight temperature elevation, and pleuritic friction rub. The nurse should administer analgesics and monitor the patient's response to the analgesics administered during the procedure.

4. Remove chest drainage device

- Stepped/staged approach: Remove chest tube using a stepped/stage approach to ensure that the air leak has resolved. A chest radiograph demonstrating complete resolution of the pneumothorax with no clinical evidence of air leak should be done first. Secondly, chest tube suction is discontinued. Clamping before discontinuation of the chest tube is controversial and performed by only half of trained practitioners.
- Chest radiograph before tube removal: Chest radiographs are obtained following the last evidence of air leak but before chest tube removal at intervals ranging from less than 4 to 24 hours after the last air leak assessment. Nearly two thirds of practitioners wait 5 to 12 hours after last evidence of air leak before obtaining the preremoval radiograph. Practices range from less than 4 to 24 hours.

5. Manage persistent air leak

- Continued observation: Patients should be observed for 4 days to assess for spontaneous closure of a pneumothorax caused by bronchopleural fistula. If the air leak persists longer than 4 days, patients should be evaluated for surgery to close the air leak with additional pleurodesis procedure to prevent recurrence. Thoracoscopy is the preferred management procedure.
- Additional closure techniques: Use of an additional chest tube or bronchoscopy in an attempt to seal endobronchial sites of air leakage is not indicated. Except in special circumstances where surgery is contraindicated or a patient refuses surgery, chemical pleurodesis should not be used.

6. Provide surgical intervention for recurrent pneumothoraces

- Thoracoscopy: Can be performed with or without video assistance. Intraoperative bullectomy should be performed by staple bullectomy in patients with apical bullae visualized at surgery.
- Thoracotomy: May be indicated when a patient is at high risk for repeated recurrence and is not successfully managed by thoracoscopy. High-risk status is present when at least two spontaneous pneumothoraces occurred in the same lung or if resolution of the pneumothorax has not occurred within 7 days. Thoracotomy may involve mechanical abrasion or decortication of the pleural surfaces with a dry, sterile sponge or chemical abrasion via an agent such as tetracycline (e.g., doxycycline) solution or talc, both of which result in pleural adhesions to prevent recurrence. A partial pleurectomy may be performed instead of mechanical or chemical abrasion.

CARE PLANS FOR PNEUMOTHORAX

IMPAIRED SPONTANEOUS VENTILATION AND IMPAIRED GAS EXCHANGE

related to collapsed lung

Goals/Outcomes: Within 2 to 6 hours of initiation of treatment, the patient exhibits adequate gas exchange, as evidenced by $Pao_2 \geq 60$ mm Hg and $Paco_2 \leq 45$ mm Hg (or values within 10% of the patient's baseline values, which depend on the underlying pathophysiology), RR less than 20 breaths/min with normal depth and pattern, and orientation to time, place, and person.

NOC Respiratory Status: Ventilation, Vital Signs Status; Respiratory Status: Gas Exchange, Symptom Control Behavior, Comfort Level, Endurance.

Ventilation Assistance

1. Position the patient to allow for full expansion of unaffected lung. Semi-Fowler position usually provides comfort and allows adequate expansion of chest wall. The patient can also be turned unaffected side-down with the head of the bed elevated to ensure a better $\dot{V}/\dot{Q}$ match.
2. Change the patient's position every 2 hours to promote drainage and lung reexpansion and to facilitate alveolar perfusion.
3. Encourage the patient to take deep breaths, providing necessary analgesia to decrease discomfort during deep-breathing exercises. Deep breathing will promote full lung expansion and may decrease the risk of atelectasis.
4. Ensure delivery of prescribed concentrations of O_2.

Environmental Management: Safety
1. Assist the advanced practice provider with chest tube insertion according to institutional guidelines.
2. Assess and maintain closed chest drainage system:
   - Closed chest drainage systems are typically a single disposable "dry" suction, plastic unit. They have one, two, or three collection chambers to accommodate large amounts of drainage. The amount of fluid evacuated is easily measured by graduated measurements on the collection chambers.
   - While fluid accumulates in the chambers, hydrostatic resistance increases while air also leaves the pleural space. Air passing through the water seal provides a flutter valve, thus minimizing resistance to pressure changes in the pleural space and reducing the resistance to the flow of drainage.
   - Avoid all kinks in the tubing, and ensure that the bed and equipment are not compressing any component of the system.
   - Closed systems must remain intact/airtight to maintain negative pressure and avoid air entrapment in the pleural space.
   - Stabilize the chest drainage system with appropriate device/holder on the floor to prevent tipping or other disruption, which may open the system to air.
   - Ensure that the system is appropriately vented at all times to help prevent the possibility of tension pneumothorax should the system be disrupted. Air should be released if the system is vented.
   - The drainage system should be kept below the level of the chest to maintain appropriate pressure dynamics.
   - Maintain fluid in underwater-seal chamber, and suction chamber at appropriate levels. Check the water level in "wet" suction controlled units at least every shift, because the water evaporates.
   - Be aware that the suction apparatus does not regulate the amount of suction applied to the closed drainage system. The amount of suction is determined by the water level in the suction control chamber. Minimal bubbling is optimal. Excessive bubbling causes rapid evaporative loss.
   - Suction aids in the reexpansion of the lung. Removing suction for short periods of time will not be detrimental to the patient as long as the system is appropriately vented to allow for the escape of air.
   - Fluctuations in the underwater-seal chamber indicate the tube is patent. Fluctuations stop when either the lung has reexpanded or there is a kink or obstruction in the chest tube.
   - Bubbling in the underwater-seal chamber occurs only during expiration and reflects air is leaving the pleural space through the drainage system.
   - Continuous bubbling on both inspiration and expiration in the underwater-seal chamber is a signal that air is leaking into the drainage system. Locate and seal the system's air leak, if possible.

> **Safety Alert** *A bubbling chest tube should never be clamped. Chest tubes should generally remain unclamped. Clamping a chest tube inserted for pneumothorax should be done under the supervision of a respiratory physician or thoracic surgeon if required. If a patient with a clamped drain experiences shortness of breath or develops subcutaneous emphysema, the tube must be unclamped immediately.*

3. Keep necessary emergency supplies at the bedside: (1) petroleum gauze pad to apply over insertion site if the chest tube becomes dislodged and (2) sterile water in which to submerge the chest tube if it becomes disconnected from the underwater-seal system. Never clamp a chest tube without a specific directive from the physician: clamping may lead to tension pneumothorax because the air can no longer escape.
4. Assist with chest tube removal in accordance with institutional guidelines.

Oxygen Therapy
1. Provide humidity in O_2 if used for more than 12 hours to help thin secretions.
2. Administer supplemental O_2 using liter flow device as ordered.
3. Document pulse oximetry with O_2 liter flow in place at time of reading as ordered. Oxygen is a drug; the dose of the drug must be associated with the O_2 saturation or the reading is meaningless.
4. Monitor for skin breakdown where O_2 devices are in contact with the skin, such as nares, and around edges of mask devices.

NIC Cough Enhancement; Oral Health Maintenance.

Respiratory Monitoring
1. Obtain ABGs if the patient experiences behavioral changes or respiratory distress to check for hypoxia or hypercapnia.

2. Monitor for induced hypoventilation, especially in patients with COPD.
3. Monitor for changes in chest radiograph and breath sounds indicative of O_2 toxicity and absorption atelectasis in patients receiving higher concentrations of O_2 (greater than 45% FiO_2) for longer than 24 hours. The higher the O_2 concentration, the greater the chance of toxicity.

NIC Acid-Base Management.

ACUTE PAIN *related to chest tube placement and pleural irritation*

Goals/Outcomes: Within 1 to 2 hours of initiating analgesic therapy, the patient's subjective evaluation of discomfort improves as documented by a pain scale. Nonverbal indicators of discomfort, such as grimacing and splinting on inspiration, are absent.
NOC Comfort Level; Pain Control Behavior; Pain Level.

Pain Management
1. At frequent intervals, assess the patient's degree of discomfort, using the patient's verbal and nonverbal cues. Devise a pain scale with the patient, rating discomfort on a scale of 0 (no pain) to 10 (worst pain). Medicate with analgesics as prescribed, evaluating and documenting the effectiveness of the medication on the basis of the pain scale.
2. Position the patient on unaffected side to minimize discomfort from chest tube insertion site. Administer medication 30 minutes before initiating movement.
3. Teach the patient to splint affected side during coughing, moving, or repositioning. Move the patient as a unit to enhance stability and comfort.
4. Schedule activities to provide for periods of rest, because fatigue may lower the patient's pain threshold.
5. Stabilize the chest tube to reduce pull or drag on latex connector tubing. Tape the chest tube securely to thorax, and loop latex tubing on the bed beside the patient.

Self-Responsibility Facilitation
1. Teach the patient to maintain active range of motion on the involved side to prevent development of a stiff shoulder from the immobility.
2. Give the patient and significant others appropriate information regarding chest tube placement and maintenance.

NIC Acid-Base Management; Acid-Base Monitoring; Analgesic Administration; Environmental Management: Comfort; Exercise Promotion; Laboratory Data Interpretation; Medication Administration; Medication Management; Oxygen Therapy; Pain Management; Positioning; Respiratory Monitoring; Vital Signs Monitoring.

ADDITIONAL NURSING DIAGNOSES

Also see the section on Activity Intolerance in Acute Asthma Exacerbation. See appropriate nursing diagnoses and interventions in Chapter 2 on Emotional and Spiritual Support of the Patient and Significant Others.

RESEARCH BRIEF 4-7

A faster and more efficient method for assessing pneumothorax progression in patients receiving positive-pressure mechanical ventilation would certainly lead to earlier intervention and improved patient safety. Ultrasonography is a common bedside tool that can offer clinicians a less expensive and more accessible alternative to computed tomography scanning in the assessment of pneumothorax. Research using animal models has provided reliable evidence that could possibly contribute to the development of best practice. Pneumothorax progression is known as the best indicator for the need for chest tube placement.

From Oveland NP, Lossius HM, Wemmelund K, et al: Using thoracic ultrasonography to accurately assess pneumothorax progression during positive pressure ventilation: a comparison with CT scanning. *Chest* 143:415-422, 2013.

PULMONARY EMBOLISM

PATHOPHYSIOLOGY

Pulmonary embolism (PE) is a blockage in the pulmonary circulation created by a lodged blood clot, vasculitis from fatty acids, or presence of air or other endogenous substances. Pulmonary emboli resulting from DVT affect from 300,000 to 600,000 patients (1 to 2 per 1000 patients; and in those older than 80 years, 1 per 100 patients) annually in the United States. It is estimated that from 60,000 to 10,000 people die of DVT/PE, with 10% to 30% dying in the first 30 days. Sudden death is the first symptom of a problem in approximately 25% of patients. PE occurs in nearly 70% of patients with venous thrombosis in veins proximal to the knee and is less common with more distal thrombosis. PE is associated with recurrent embolic events (within 10 years) in over 33% of affected patients. Venous thromboembolism (VTE) prevention augments both public health and patient safety. Despite efforts to prevent hospital-acquired VTE, the number of secondary diagnoses has increased. During 2007 to 2009, the data from each year revealed that approximately 550,000 adult hospital stays had a discharge diagnosis of VTE. Prevention of VTE has recently been the focus of attention from both researchers and quality improvement organizations as a leading strategy to help reduce morbidity and mortality in patients who are hospitalized. Acute right ventricular failure with resultant low cardiac output is the leading cause of death related to PE. Despite strong evidence, recommended evidence-based practices are inconsistently implemented. VTE rates are increasing as the U.S. population ages, is progressively obese, and is living longer with chronic diseases, which may promote thrombus formation. Venous thrombosis is the most common cause of PE, followed by fat emboli. Emboli related to venous air, foreign bodies, and other sources (amniotic fluid, sepsis/infection, and tumors) occur more rarely.

VENOUS THROMBOEMBOLISM

A formed blood clot from a large vein dislodges and travels to the pulmonary circulation, where it may obstruct one (massive PE) or both branches (saddle emboli) of the pulmonary artery or a smaller, distal vessel. Blood clots typically originate in the deep veins of the legs, the iliofemoral system, or pelvis. Many patients with VTEs have no symptoms of DVT. Thrombus formation can result from blood stasis, alterations in clotting factors, and injury to vessel walls. Emboli are classified by size and location and include submassive, massive, and saddle emboli. Total obstruction of blood flow leading to pulmonary infarction is rare. Prevention, early diagnosis, and appropriate treatment may reduce development of DVT and PE by 68% and mortality to less than 10%. Although most thrombotic emboli resolve completely, leaving no residual deficits, some patients may be left with chronic pulmonary hypertension (Table 4-6).

Table 4-6	INCIDENCE OF VENOUS THROMBOEMBOLISM IN HOSPITALIZED PATIENTS
Incidence	**Patient Type**
10% to 26%	Medical/nonsurgical
11% to 75%	Stroke
15% to 40%	Major surgery: general, gynecologic, urologic
15% to 40%	Neurosurgery
15% to 80%	Critically ill patients admitted to intensive care units
40% to 60%	Hip or knee surgery/orthopedic surgical patients
40% to 60%	Major trauma
60% to 80%	Spinal cord injury

Composite of statistics from the British Thoracic Society (2003), American College of Chest Physicians (2008), European Society of Cardiology (2008), and IMPROVE (2007) registry data on prevention of venous thromboembolism.

FAT EMBOLISM/FAT EMBOLISM SYNDROME

The most common nonthrombotic cause of PEs is fat emboli, which occur in less than 1% of patients. Fat emboli can result from trauma (fracture of long bones, accidents, or soft tissue injury) or nontrauma (burns or fatty liver). The event and subsequent syndrome most often occurs within 12 to 36 hours after skeletal trauma or major orthopedic surgery, but may be fulminant, with rapid embolization of fat into the pulmonary and systemic circulation, followed by right ventricular failure and cardiovascular collapse. Fat emboli most often result from the release of free fatty acids during a surgical procedure, prompting toxic vasculitis followed by thrombosis and obstruction of small pulmonary arteries by fat. More recently, fat embolism has been reported following liposuction, with lipid and propofol infusions, fatty liver, and hepatic necrosis.

VENOUS AIR EMBOLISM

Venous air embolism is almost always an iatrogenic complication caused by a large volume of air that enters the venous circulation and travels to the pulmonary circulation. The incidence of venous air embolism can range between 10% (penetrating chest trauma, during invasive monitoring catheter placement) and 80% (during laparoscopic surgical procedures). Smaller amounts of air may be completely unproductive of symptoms, because air can be rapidly resorbed. Surgical procedures, insertion of pulmonary artery catheters, central venous catheters, hemodialysis, endoscopy, and use of automatic injectors such as those used for contrast media can prompt symptomatic air emboli. A larger bolus of air into the right ventricle may completely obstruct pulmonary blood flow, leading to cardiac arrest. In severe cases, venous air embolus has a mortality rate greater than 50%. Rapid diagnosis and treatment are essential. Case reports describe the adult lethal volume of air as approximately 200 to 300 mL delivered rapidly. Air occludes the right ventricular pulmonary outflow tract, or the smaller pulmonary arteriole with a mixture of air and fibrin clots, which results in right ventricular failure and cardiogenic shock.

INTRAVASCULAR FOREIGN BODIES

Most foreign bodies in the central circulation are parts of intravascular catheters, a guide wire, or an inferior vena cava (IVC) filter that has accumulated a clot and migrated. More recently, coils for embolization and endovascular stenting have also migrated from their desired position. Most foreign bodies travel to the pulmonary arteries, with the right side of the heart and vena cava being the secondary locations.

OTHER TYPES OF PULMONARY EMBOLISM

Amniotic fluid embolism occurs in less than 1:8000 to 80,000 women as a result of amniotic fluid being forced into the central circulation through tears in the uterine veins that may occur during normal labor. Death of both the mother and fetus may result during the delivery. Septic pulmonary emboli are infected clots dislodged from either the peripheral or abdominal vein, or septic thrombophlebitis, or right-sided endocarditis. Prognosis is dependent on the overall patient condition and severity of the sepsis. Tumor embolism occurs with many types or carcinoma and sarcoma but causes significant respiratory symptoms in less than 3% of affected patients. Talc embolism results from drug users grinding up and injecting oral medications that are made with talc particles, which lodge in the small vessels of the pulmonary system.

ASSESSMENT

GOAL OF SYSTEM ASSESSMENT

Evaluate for ineffective breathing patterns and impaired gas exchange. The clinical presentation will vary in degree, depending on the type and size of the embolus. With a submassive or massive embolism, evaluate for decreased cardiac output and decreased tissue perfusion. Massive embolism may prompt cardiogenic shock. For saddle emboli, identifying pulmonary embolus as the cause for acute cardiopulmonary decompensation is of paramount importance so that life-saving treatments can be provided. (See the section on Respiratory Assessment: General, and Cardiac Assessment: General in Chapter 5.)

HISTORY AND RISK FACTORS FOR VENOUS THROMBOEMBOLISM

The American College of Chest Physicians, American Thoracic Society, American College of Physicians, American Academy of Family Physicians, European Society of Cardiology,

British Thoracic Society, and an array of medical and surgical specialty organizations have created guidelines for VTE prophylaxis and management. VTE prophylaxis protocols should be initiated when patients are admitted to the hospital, to help prevent development of DVT (Tables 4-7 and 4-8).

DETERMINE PROBABILITY BASED ON RISK FACTORS

- Helps determine presence of pulmonary embolus: More than six factors is considered high, two to six is moderate, and less than two is considered low probability.
- Diagnostic tests chosen are dependent on the probability that a DVT or VTE is present; a scoring system may be developed based on number of risks present. Reveals the presence of the infiltrates.

VITAL SIGNS

- Severity of all findings varies with size of the embolus; patients with small emboli may be asymptomatic.

Table 4-7	RISK FACTORS FOR VENOUS THROMBOEMBOLISM IN HOSPITALIZED PATIENTS*	
Age >50 years	Previous history of venous thrombo-embolism (VTE)	Myocardial infarction
Myeloproliferative disease	Impaired mobility, paresis, or paralysis	Acute or chronic lung disease
Dehydration	Recently bedridden >3 days	Obesity
Congestive heart failure	Inflammatory bowel disease	Known thrombophilic stroke
Active malignancy/cancer	Active rheumatic disease	Varicose veins or chronic venous stasis
Moderate to major surgery	Nephrotic syndrome	Pregnancy
Hormone replacement therapy	Sickle cell disease	Recently postpartum with immobility
Central venous catheter in place		Estrogen therapy or estrogen contraceptives

*Patients who have more than a single condition are at increased risk of developing venous thromboembolism. The more conditions present, the higher the risk.

Table 4-8	RISK FACTORS FOR VENOUS THROMBOEMBOLISM	
Strong Risk Factors	**Moderate Risk Factors**	**Weak Risk Factors**
Fracture (hip or leg)	Arthroscopic knee surgery	Prolonged bed rest
Hip or knee replacement	Central venous lines	Immobility
Major general surgery	Chemotherapy/cancer	Age >40 years
Major trauma	Congestive heart or respiratory failure	Laparoscopic surgery
Spinal cord injury	Estrogen	Obesity
	Age >65 years	Pregnancy
	Paralytic stroke	Varicose veins
	Postpartum period	
	Previous venous thromboembolism	
	Thrombophilia	

From Anderson FA Jr, Spencer FA: Risk factors for venous thromboembolism. *Circulation* 107(23 Suppl 1): 9-16, 2003.

- Tachycardia (HR greater than 100 bpm), tachypnea (RR greater than 20 breaths/min), fever (greater than 99.5° F or 37.5° C).
- Massive embolus: Hypotension (BP decreases by greater than 20%).
- Saddle embolus: May result in immediate cardiopulmonary arrest.

OBSERVATION/INSPECTION
- Dyspnea, nonproductive cough, and nausea.
- Syncope, pallor, and palpitations.
- Restlessness and anxiety.
- Diaphoresis, cool and clammy skin.
- Pleuritic chest pain and hemoptysis.
- Signs of lower limb DVT: Leg/calf tenderness, swelling, and/or edema.
- Submassive embolus: Any combination of the symptoms listed above.
- Massive embolus: Severe chest pain, cyanosis, and acute respiratory distress.
- Saddle embolus: Sudden-onset acute respiratory distress with cyanosis, which may progress to cardiopulmonary arrest.

PALPATION
- Possible reduced chest excursion on affected side attributable to splinting for pain.

PERCUSSION
- Unchanged.

AUSCULTATION
- Crackles.
- S3 and S4 gallop rhythms.
- Transient pleural friction rub may be present.

HIGH ALERT! Saddle pulmonary embolus is life threatening. Immediate medical or surgical intervention is crucial. Thrombolysis directed at the pulmonary embolus will also prompt lysis of other clots and may lead to other bleeding complications. If thrombolysis is contraindicated, surgical or percutaneous catheter-mediated embolectomy is performed immediately.

FAT EMBOLISM
HISTORY AND RISK FACTORS
- Multiple long bone fractures, particularly the femur and pelvis.
- Lower limb amputation.
- Trauma to adipose tissue or liver.
- Burns, see Chapter 3.
- Hemolytic crisis, see Chapter 10.
- Osteomyelitis.

OBSERVATION/INSPECTION
Patients are often asymptomatic for 12 to 24 hours after the embolization occurs. This period ends with a sudden deterioration in cardiopulmonary and neurologic status.
- Dyspnea and acute respiratory distress.
- Restlessness, confusion, delirium, and coma.
- Petechial rash may appear especially over the upper torso and axillae, secondary to thrombocytopenia. The platelets aggregate in the presence of circulating fats.

VITAL SIGNS
- RR greater than 20 breaths/min and HR greater than 100 bpm.
- Increased BP and elevated temperature.

AUSCULTATION
- Inspiratory crowing and expiratory wheezes.

VENOUS AIR EMBOLISM
HISTORY AND RISK FACTORS
* Recent surgical procedure.
* Pulmonary artery/central venous catheter insertion.
* Misuse of closed-wound suction unit.
* Cardiopulmonary bypass.
* Hemodialysis.
* Endoscopy.

CLINICAL PRESENTATION
Depends on severity of the bolus.

OBSERVATION/INSPECTION
Agitation, confusion, cough, dyspnea, and chest pain.

VITAL SIGNS
RR greater than 20 breaths/min, HR greater than 100 bpm, and hypotension.

AUSCULTATION
Wheezing, "mill wheel heart murmur," which can be defined as a temporary loud, machinery-like sound resulting from right ventricular blood mixing with air.

FOREIGN BODIES
HISTORY AND RISK FACTORS
* Advanced practice provider accidentally lets go of the guide wire during central line insertion.
* Vena cava filter has not been retrieved within recommended time frame.
* Intravascular catheter breaks during insertion.
* Coils or stent components are accidentally released or not properly secured during insertion.

Diagnostic Tests for Venous Thrombotic Pulmonary Embolism

Test	Purpose	Abnormal Findings
D-dimer Several assays are available with variable levels of sensitivity and specificity. This test may not be needed in high-risk or high-probability patients. Hospitals should provide information on specificity and sensitivity of test used.	Predicts likelihood that a thrombus is present in low-risk or intermediate-risk patients. When the value exceeds the cutoff, the test is positive. A negative D-dimer test reliably excludes pulmonary embolism (PE) in patients with low or intermediate clinical probability.	Positive: A thrombus is present. Scales range from 250 to 1000 ng/mL; the most common cutoff value is 500 ng/mL. Low-risk and intermediate-risk patients do not require imaging for venous thromboembolism (VTE) if the [D-dimer] is negative.
Lower extremity duplex ultrasound imaging A single normal test cannot be used to rule to subclinical deep venous thrombosis (DVT).	Reveals slow or obstructed flow in the venous system. Test is done on patients at high or moderate risk of DVT.	Positive: Reduced or obstructed blood flow is detected.
Chest radiograph: posterior-anterior and lateral chest radiograph Cannot be used alone to diagnose pulmonary embolus	Reveals abnormal lung markings and fluid shifts that occur during flow obstruction and pulmonary infarction. A baseline chest radiograph is helpful for comparison with subsequent films to identify changes.	Affected side: Initially the chest radiograph shows normal findings or an elevated hemidiaphragm. After 24 hours, small infiltrates secondary to atelectasis from decrease in surfactant may develop. If pulmonary infarction is present, infiltrates and pleural effusions may be seen within 12 to 36 hours.

Continued

Diagnostic Tests for Venous Thrombotic Pulmonary Embolism—cont'd

Test	Purpose	Abnormal Findings
Spiral CT angiography with contrast Current technology is nearly 100% accurate. Older technology may be insufficient to rule out PE.	Reveals flow obstruction in pulmonary circulation. Recommended for patients with intermediate-to-high probability of lower extremity DVT.	Generally reveals right ventricular dilatation. Patients with intermediate or high pretest probability of PE require diagnostic imaging studies.
Ventilation-perfusion lung scan The patient inhales radioactive-tagged gases, and radioactive particles are injected peripherally.	Assesses for $\dot{V}/\dot{Q}$ or ventilation/perfusion mismatching; a good alternative for patients who cannot receive contrast needed for spiral CT angiography.	If there is a mismatch of ventilation and perfusion (e.g., normal ventilation with decreased perfusion), vascular obstruction is likely. Results may not be definitive. False-positive results are more common than false-negative results.
Arterial blood gas (ABG) analysis Pulse oximetry may be used to monitor O_2 saturation changes. CO_2 increases and pH changes require ABG analysis.	Assesses for hypoxemia and acidosis. Saddle embolus may cause both respiratory and lactic acidosis (pH <7.35) from impending respiratory failure and circulatory collapse.	Initially, hypoxemia (Pao_2 <80 mm Hg), hypocapnia ($Paco_2$ <35 mm Hg), and respiratory alkalosis (pH >7.45). A normal Pao_2 does not rule out the presence of VTE. Mild hypoxemia may be present with smaller emboli.
12-Lead ECG (electrocardiogram) Vitally important because chest pain can mimic severe angina or acute myocardial infarction	Rules out acute coronary syndrome as a cause for chest pain with vital sign changes indicative of deterioration.	If VTE is extensive, signs of acute pulmonary hypertension may be present: right-shift QRS axes, tall and peaked P waves, ST segment changes, and T wave inversion in leads V_1 to V_4.
Echocardiogram	Diagnoses the presence of right ventricular impairment or failure as part of risk stratification.	May reveal right ventricular hypokinesis, dilatation, or elevated pressures. Right ventricular dilatation is found in >25% of patients with PE.
Pulmonary angiography The Miller (European) and Walsh (United States) scores were used to define the amount of luminal obstruction. Improved accuracy with current CT angiography has markedly reduced the need for this invasive procedure.	A definitive study for VTE. The right ventricle is catheterized and dye is injected into the pulmonary artery to visualize pulmonary vessels. Formerly, the gold standard for definitive diagnosis.	An abrupt vessel "cutoff" may be seen at the site of embolization. Usually, filling defects are seen. Used when other tests are inconclusive, because the procedure has a 0.2% mortality rate.
Hemodynamic studies	To determine if obstruction of blood flow is significant enough to cause pulmonary hypertension or right ventricular failure.	PA pressures increase (>20 mm Hg) if 30% to 50% of the pulmonary arterial tree is affected. Massive VTEs cause pressure increases to >40 mm Hg, resulting in right ventricular failure, decreased cardiac output, and hypotension.

FAT EMBOLISM
- ABG values: Hypoxemia (Pao_2 less than 80 mm Hg) and hypercapnia ($Paco_2$ greater than 45 mm Hg) will be present with respiratory acidosis (pH less than 7.35).
- Chest radiograph: A pattern similar to ARDS is seen: diffuse, extensive, bilateral interstitial, and alveolar infiltrates.
- CBC with WBC differential: May reveal decreased hemoglobin and hematocrit secondary to hemorrhage into the lung, thrombocytopenia, and possibly mild leukocytosis.

VENOUS AIR EMBOLI
- ABG values: Hypoxemia (Pao_2 less than 80 mm Hg), hypercapnia ($Paco_2$ greater than 45 mm Hg), and respiratory acidosis (pH less than 7.35) are generally present in severe cases.
- Chest radiograph: Reveals changes consistent with pulmonary edema or air-fluid levels in the main pulmonary artery system.
- Pulmonary artery pressure: Systolic, diastolic, and mean pressures are acutely elevated, but slight elevation of pulmonary artery wedge pressure remains within normal limits.

FOREIGN BODIES
- Chest radiograph: All devices are radiopaque for easy identification using radiographs. The "lost" device should be easily visible using a chest radiograph.

COLLABORATIVE MANAGEMENT

CARE PRIORITIES: VENOUS THROMBOEMBOLISM
Patients with shortness of breath should not be left without intervention regardless of the probability that VTE is present.

1. Relieve hypoxemia
Patent foramen ovale (or atrial septal defect) may augment hypoxemia if right atrial pressure exceeds left atrial pressure, causing deoxygenated blood to shunt from the right to the left atrium.
- Oxygen therapy/adjustment in mechanical ventilation: Oxygen is administered when ABG values demonstrate the presence of hypoxemia. If the patient is already receiving mechanical ventilation, Fio_2 is increased while evaluation is done regarding amount of positive pressure needed during inspiratory and expiratory phases of ventilation.

2. Manage right ventricular failure in patients with hypotension or shock
Hemodynamic stabilization is achieved using a combination of fluid therapy to increase the end-diastolic volume in the right ventricle and positive inotropic agents to increase the force of right ventricular contraction. Management of right ventricular failure is complex. Efforts should be directed at restoring patency of pulmonary circulation in patients with VTE. When the obstruction is relieved, the patient generally improves rapidly. See the sections on Heart Failure and Cardiogenic Shock in Chapter 5.
- Initiate cardiopulmonary resuscitation if the patient arrests with saddle embolus. Generally, these patients require pulmonary embolectomy because VTE has resulted in lethal cardiogenic shock. Sophisticated centers can use extracorporeal devices as a bridge to clot removal.

3. In patients who are less severely ill, or those in need of VTE prophylaxis, prevent clot development or clot extension
Pharmacologic therapy: All patients at risk of developing VTE should be screened for bleeding risk before implementing prophylaxis using medications, because all agents have the potential to cause bleeding. Thromboprophylaxis medications include low–molecular-weight heparin (enoxaparin [Lovenox], dalteparin [Fragmin]), low-dose unfractionated heparin, fondaparinux (Arixtra), direct thrombin inhibitors (argatroban, lepirudin, bivalirudin), and warfarin (Coumadin). Warfarin requires 3 and 5 days of oral therapy to attain therapeutic effect, during which time the patient requires an injectable medication as a "bridge" to warfarin. Ongoing therapy may include low-dose or regular-dose aspirin.

VENOUS THROMBOEMBOLISM PROPHYLAXIS: CONSIDERATIONS FOR CONTRAINDICATIONS/COMPLICATIONS

Absolute Contraindications	Relative Contraindications	Other Conditions That May Complicate Therapy
Active hemorrhage Allergy	Intracranial hemorrhage within the past year	Immune-mediated heparin-induced thrombocytopenia
Severe head or spinal cord trauma within 4 weeks	Craniotomy within 2 weeks	Epidural analgesia; catheter present, or will be present in the spine
Note: Absolute contraindication means that therapy should not be administered to the affected patients under any circumstances, because the risk of bleeding outweighs the benefits of clot prevention.	Intraocular surgery within 2 weeks Active intracranial lesions or neoplasms Thrombocytopenia (platelets <50,000) Coagulopathy (prothrombin time >18 seconds) End-stage liver disease Gastrointestinal, genitourinary hemorrhage within 1 month Current hypertensive urgency or emergency Current postoperative bleeding	Note: Unfractionated heparin and low–molecular-weight heparins can stimulate heparin-induced thrombocytopenia, an immune response that destroys platelets. Non–heparin anticoagulants: Argatroban (Argatroban) Bivalirudin (Angiomax) Fondaparinux (Arixtra) Lepirudin (Refludan) Danaparoid (Orgaran) (unavailable in the United States)

- Risk stratification: Provide appropriate therapy based on evaluation for level of risk of development of VTE and risk of bleeding.

VENOUS THROMBOEMBOLISM PROPHYLAXIS BASED ON LEVEL OF RISK (SELECT ONE DRUG/ONE DOSAGE REGIMEN)

Low Risk	Intermediate Risk	High Risk
Early aggressive ambulation Short-term mechanical thromboprophylaxis may be recommended for "borderline"-risk patients	Heparin 5000 units subcutaneously (SC) every 8 hours Heparin 7500 units SC every 12 hours Heparin 5000 units SC every 12 hours (if <50 kg or >75 years old) Enoxaparin 40 mg SC daily Dalteparin 2500 units daily for low or intermediate risk Consider adding sequential compression devices	Enoxaparin 30 mg SC every 12 hours Enoxaparin 40 mg SC daily Dalteparin 5000 units SC daily Fondaparinux 2.5 mg SC daily Warfarin until international normalized ratio is 2 to 3 Add sequential compression devices

- **Mechanical prophylaxis:** Sequential compression devices may be used as the sole preventive strategy in patients at low risk and in patients at moderate to high risk who are not able to receive thromboprophylaxis drugs because of risk for bleeding. Plexipulse and elastic compression stockings are not considered sufficient as a sole VTE prophylaxis strategy for patients who are hospitalized. Compression stockings with a pressure of 30 to 40 mm Hg at the ankle may be implemented before discharge and used posthospitalization.

4. Prevent clot extension or migration in patients with DVT or VTE

- **Pharmacologic therapy:** To inhibit thrombus growth, promote resolution of the formed thrombus, and prevent further embolus formation. The goals are achieved by keeping the activated partial thromboplastin time (aPTT) at 1.5 to 2.5 times the normal. Platelet counts should be obtained every 3 days, to monitor for thrombocytopenia and paradoxical arterial thrombosis associated with heparin therapy in predisposed patients. (See Bleeding and Thrombotic Disorders, p. 837.)

- **Weight-based IV heparin (unfractionated) therapy:** Treatment of choice; started immediately in patients without bleeding or clotting disorders and in whom signs and symptoms of VTE are present. Initial dose: 80 units/kg IV bolus. Dosage should be given based on the patient's weight.
  - **Maintenance dose:** Following initial dose, a continuous IV infusion is usually begun at 18 units/kg/h and titrated by serial aPTT values to determine level of anticoagulation. Titration is done according to institutional protocol (see Table 4-9).
  - **Heparin requirements** are the largest in the initial 72 hours of therapy. Maintenance continues for 7 to 14 days, during which time the patient is placed on bed rest to ensure that the thrombus is firmly attached to the vessel wall before ambulation. Platelets should be monitored, because patients sometimes experience heparin-induced thrombocytopenia (HIT) or low platelets. Protamine sulfate is a heparin antidote, which should be readily available during heparin therapy. Fatal hemorrhage occurs in 1% to 2% of patients undergoing heparin therapy. Risk of bleeding is greatest in women older than 60 years.
- **Subcutaneous low–molecular-weight heparin (dalteparin, enoxaparin):** An alternative to unfractionated heparin with longer half-life, greater bioavailability, and more predictable anticoagulant activity. Enoxaparin is given 1 mg/kg subcutaneously (SC) every 12 hours or 1.5 mg/kg SC daily. Dalteparin is given 200 units (international units)/kg SC daily to a maximum daily dose of 18,000 international units, while the patient is being bridged to warfarin.
  - SC Tinzaparin: A heparin alternative given 175 units SC daily.
  - SC Fondaparinux: Dose is given based on three body sizes.
  - 5 mg SC daily: Weight less than 50 kg.
  - 7.5 mg SC daily: Weight 50 to 100 kg.
  - 10 mg SC daily: Weight greater than 100 kg.

Inferior vena cava (IVC) filter: Also known as a "Greenfield filter," the devices are designed to trap emboli before they enter the heart and pulmonary arteries. Various types of IVC filters are available, with different recommendations governing the removal/retrieval of each device. The filter is inserted through an introducer sheath into the femoral vein, threaded through the venous system, and deployed below the level of the renal veins in the IVC. The American College of Chest Physicians recommends that most retrievable devices are removed approximately 2 weeks following insertion. Many devices are left in place for longer periods, with associated complications of device thrombosis and migration in 10% of patients. Permanent IVC filters are associated with recurrent DVT (in 20% of patients) and postthrombotic syndrome (in 40% of patients). Routine use is not recommended for management of VTE.

Table 4-9	UNFRACTIONATED HEPARIN INTRAVENOUS INFUSION DOSAGE TITRATION
Activated Partial Thromboplastin Time (aPTT; in Seconds)	**Dosage Titration**
Less than 35 (<1.2 times the control)	80 units/kg bolus; begin infusion at 18 units/kg/h; increase infusion rate by 4 unit/kg/h
35 to 45 (1.2 to 1.5 times the control)	40 units/kg bolus; increase infusion rate by 2 units/kg/h
46 to 70 (1.6 to 2.3 times the control)	No change; this is the desirable range
71 to 90 (2.4 to 3 times the control)	Decrease infusion rate by 2 units/kg/h
>90 (>3 times the control)	Hold/stop infusion for 1 hour; then restart at 3 units/kg/h less than when stopped
Active hemorrhage	Vitamin K, fresh-frozen plasma, and protamine sulfate may be used to help reverse heparin effects.

5. Dissolve clot using thrombolytic drugs in patients with massive or saddle embolus

These "clot buster" drugs lyse clots via conversion of plasminogen to plasma and may be given within 72 hours of VTE to speed the process of clot lysis. These medications are not often used but can be used immediately when severe cardiopulmonary compromise or arrest has occurred. Heparin therapy is used following thrombolytic infusion. As many as 33% of patients who receive thrombolytic therapy have hemorrhagic complications. The drug should be discontinued and fresh-frozen plasma infusion may be initiated for severe bleeding complications.

- Streptokinase: Loading dose of 250,000 international units in normal saline or D_5W given IV over a 30-minute period. Maintenance dose is 100,000 international units per hour given IV for 12 to 24 hours.
- Tissue plasminogen activator (Alteplase, rTPA): 100 mg IV infusion over 2 hours, or 0.6 mg/kg over 15 minutes (maximum dose 50 mg).
- Urokinase: 4400 international units/kg as a loading dose over 10 minutes, followed by an infusion of 4400 international units/kg/h for 12 to 14 hours.

6. Remove thrombus with an invasive procedure

- **Surgical pulmonary embolectomy:** Often reserved for patients in cardiopulmonary arrest; can also be used for patients with contraindications to thrombolytic therapy, those with patent foramen ovale, and those with intracardiac thrombi. Anesthesia is rapidly induced, a median sternotomy performed, and the pulmonary artery incised to remove the clot. Cardiopulmonary bypass should be avoided in patients with patent foramen ovale or intracardiac thrombi.
- **Percutaneous catheter embolectomy with fragmentation:** A possibly life-saving measure wherein a Greenfield suction embolectomy catheter (or other Roto-Blade cardiac catheter) is inserted through an introducer sheath, threaded through the pulmonary valve into the pulmonary artery, wherein the clot is macerated and fragmented, with the fragments immediately suctioned from the vessel to avoid distal embolization.
- **Endovascular ultrasound delivered thrombolysis:** Intended for controlled and selective infusion of thrombolytics in the peripheral vasculature for treatment of DVTs and PE including "saddle emboli." This therapy may be used in veins, arteries, behind valves, and through IVC filters. Ultrasonic energy prepares the clot by thinning fibrin, which increases permeability of the clot and creates a pressure gradient to transport clot-dissolving drugs inside the thrombus. This form is used in difficult-to-reach areas such as behind valves, reduces the risk of thrombus breakages and emboli, and uses less drug as the thrombus is directly exposed to the lytic, preventing hemolysis.

7. Long-term anticoagulation to prevent recurrence of VTE

Active cancer places a patient at high risk of recurrence of PE, with 20% of patients having another VTE within the first year. Other patient populations have lower, variable rates of recurrence based on whether the precipitating event was attributable to a modifiable risk factor or isolated event such as trauma or surgery. Patients with idiopathic PE are more difficult to stratify for risk of recurrence. Risk of bleeding must be considered when prescribing the duration of therapy.

- **Low–molecular-weight heparin:** SC injections may be indicated for a period of 6 months following hospitalization when a patient is at high risk for repeated recurrence.
- **Vitamin K antagonists (VKAs):** Oral warfarin (Coumadin) is prescribed at doses to keep the international normalized ratio (INR) at 2 to 3. It is started within 24 hours of initiation of heparin therapy. An average initial dose is 5 to 10 mg. Both agents are given simultaneously for 4 to 6 days to allow time for warfarin to inhibit vitamin K–dependent clotting factors before heparin is discontinued. Daily warfarin dose is adjusted according to INR, and correct dosage is individualized per patient based on frequent INR determinations.
  - **Prothrombin time (PT):** Monitored daily, with a goal of 1 to 1.5 times normal. Once the patient's condition has stabilized and the heparin is discontinued, weekly monitoring of INR is acceptable. After hospital discharge the PT should be monitored every 2 weeks for as long as the patient continues to take warfarin.
  - **Maintenance:** May be approximately 10 mg/day, but dosage varies greatly depending on the patient's age, weight, other medications taken, diet, and other factors. Warfarin is continued for 3 to 6 months and based on the continued presence of risk factors.
  - **Vitamin K administration:** For bleeding emergencies, reverses the effects of warfarin in 24 to 36 hours. Fresh-frozen plasma may be required in cases of serious bleeding.

- **Caution:** Warfarin crosses the placental barrier and can cause spontaneous abortion and birth defects.

8. Special considerations during pregnancy

Getting an accurate diagnosis is of paramount importance, because a prolonged course of heparin or low–molecular-weight heparin therapy is needed to resolve the emboli. Neither drug crosses the placental barrier or is found in breast milk in significant amounts. All diagnostic modalities, including computed tomography scanning, may be used without putting the fetus at significant risk for harm. Use of SC low–molecular-weight heparin has been increasingly recommended while evidence evolves. Warfarin or another VKA is not recommended during the first and third trimesters and is used with caution during the second trimester. Anticoagulant therapy should be continued for 3 months postpartum.

CARE PRIORITIES: FAT EMBOLI
1. Manage hypoxemia
Concentration of O_2 is based on clinical presentation, ABG results, and the patient's previous respiratory status. Intubation and mechanical ventilation may be required.

2. Control toxic vasculitis
Corticosteroids including cortisone and methylprednisolone have been used to decrease local injury to pulmonary tissue and pulmonary edema.

3. Manage pulmonary edema
Pulmonary edema develops in approximately 30% of patients with fat emboli, necessitating use of diuretics to remove fluid from the vascular system.

4. Manage right ventricular failure and cardiogenic shock
Although rare, fulminant, sudden onset cases of cardiovascular collapse have been reported. See the sections on Heart Failure and Cardiogenic Shock in Chapter 5.

CARE PRIORITIES: VENOUS AIR EMBOLI

> **Safety Alert** *Emphasis is on prevention. Ensure that the central venous catheter is inserted with the patient in the Trendelenburg position. Use Luer-Lok connectors on all intravenous tubing to prevent a disconnection. Should venous air embolus occur despite precautions, the following measures are anticipated.*

1. Prevent further air entry
If central line is being inserted, catheter hub should be occluded using a clamp, or the inserter's gloved finger.

2. Manage hypoxemia
Oxygen using 100% FIO_2 is initiated immediately.

3. Minimize dispersion of air bolus into central circulation
Place the patient in the Trendelenburg position with a left decubitus tilt (turned to left side, bed in "head-down" position) to minimize further movement of air bolus through the heart and into the pulmonary vasculature and beyond.

4. Remove air, if possible
If a central venous catheter is in place near the right atrium, an attempt is made to aspirate the air using a syringe.

5. Hyperbaric oxygen therapy
Case reports reveal the therapy to be beneficial with all types of air embolization. Impressive results have been gleaned with cerebral air embolization.

CARE PRIORITIES: INTRAVASCULAR FOREIGN BODIES
1. Remove the foreign body
The advanced practice provider retrieves the migrated device or part of a device using a snare.

CARE PLANS FOR PULMONARY EMBOLISM
RISK FOR INEFFECTIVE CARDIOPULMONARY TISSUE PERFUSION *related to partial to complete obstruction of the lumen of one/both pulmonary arteries or smaller pulmonary vessels: the nurse will identify and provide preventive measures and appropriate treatments for patients at risk of DVT and/or VTE and other pulmonary emboli.*

Goals/Outcomes: The patient is free of hemodynamic instability and shortness of breath reflected by normal (return to the patient's stable baseline) vital signs and normal work of breathing. Within 12 hours of initiation of therapy, the patient has adequate gas exchange reflected by the following ABG values: PaO_2 greater than 60 mm Hg, $PaCO_2$ 35 to 45 mm Hg, and pH 7.35 to 7.45. Within 2 to 4 days of initiating anticoagulant therapy, the patient's RR is 12 to 20 breaths/min with normal depth and pattern. Unobstructed, unidirectional blood flow at an appropriate pressure is restored through large vessels of the pulmonary and systemic circuits.

NOC Circulation Status; Cardiac Pump Effectiveness; Respiratory Status: Gas Exchange.

Embolus Precautions
1. Assess the patient for risk factors associated with VTE (see Table 4-7).
2. Implement VTE precautions appropriate for the patient's risk level.
3. Instruct the patient not to cross legs, either when in bed or sitting in a chair.
4. Apply sequential compression hose for patients who are bedridden. If the patient is aggressively ambulating, use of sequential compression hose is not necessary.
5. Aggressively ambulate all appropriate patients following surgical procedures.
6. Administer SC anticoagulants as ordered or according to VTE prophylaxis protocol/guidelines.

Embolus Care: Pulmonary
1. Evaluate chest pain for intensity, location, and precipitating and relieving factors.
2. Auscultate breath sounds to assess for presence of crackles or other changes that may account for shortness of breath.
3. Monitor respiratory pattern for increased work of breathing.
4. Monitor the determinants of tissue O_2 delivery as possible (cardiac output, hemoglobin level, O_2 saturation/pulse oximetry/ABGs).
5. Evaluate ABGs for decreased PaO_2 (hypoxemia), increased level of CO_2 (hypercapnia), and decreased pH (acidosis).
6. Assess for symptoms of respiratory failure and inadequate tissue oxygenation including altered mental status, anxiety, restlessness, increased work of breathing, pallor, cyanosis, and inability to maintain O_2 saturation without repeated increases in amount of supplemental O_2.
7. Instruct the patient/family/support system regarding diagnostic tests needed as part of differential diagnosis.
8. Screen the patient for risk of bleeding (see the VTE prophylaxis chart) in preparation for anticoagulant and possibly thrombolytic drug administration.
9. Administer anticoagulants as ordered and monitor for bleeding complications. If unfractionated or low–molecular-weight heparin is used, monitor for decreased platelet count, which may signal development of heparin-induced thrombocytopenia.
10. Administer thrombolytic agents as ordered and monitor for bleeding complications.
11. Consult with the dietician to ensure that the patient maintains a diet with consistent intake of vitamin K if VKAs, such as warfarin (Coumadin) are initiated. Varying vitamin K intake may have a marked effect on the ability to regulate the appropriate dose of medication to avoid bleeding and clotting complications.
12. Consult with the pharmacist about use of IV protamine sulfate, if the patient has the need for heparin reversal as a result of severe bleeding.
13. To avoid negative interactions with anticoagulants or thrombolytic therapy, establish compatibility of all drugs before administering them:
    - Heparin: Digitalis, tetracyclines, nicotine, and antihistamines decrease the effect of heparin therapy. Establish compatibility before infusing other IV drugs through heparin IV line.

- Warfarin sodium: Numerous drugs result in a decrease or an increase in response to treatment with warfarin. Consult with the pharmacist to obtain specific information about the patient's medication profile.
- Thrombolytic therapy: Do not infuse other medications through the same IV line.
14. Monitor PT with INR when using warfarin and aPTT when using heparin. Adhere carefully to drug titration and/or dosage guidelines.
15. Monitor neurologic status for deterioration because recurrent embolism, shock attributable to bleeding, cardiogenic shock, and intracranial bleeding are possible. Neurologic changes are the first subtle sign that shock may be ensuing.
16. Medicate for pain as needed.

Hemodynamic Regulation

1. Recognize presence of BP alterations.
2. Auscultate heart and breath sounds.
3. Monitor SVR and pulmonary vasculature resistance (PVR). PVR will be elevated with massive or saddle embolus, and can prompt right ventricular failure. SVR changes with the stages of shock. Initially, SVR is high while the body attempts to raise BP in the presence of cardiogenic shock if right ventricular failure has ensued.
4. Implement recommendations for managing right ventricular failure as ordered.
   - Systemic hypotension should be managed to avoid progression of right ventricular failure.
   - Regulate vasoactive drugs. Vasopressor drugs such as dopamine or Levophed will increase afterload and may worsen heart failure. Inodilator drugs such as milrinone, amrinone, and, to a lesser extent, dobutamine may not work well, because all decrease venous return, which may also worsen right ventricular failure.
   - Aggressive fluid challenge is not recommended, despite some evidence of efficacy in right ventricular failure. Hemodynamics of right ventricular failure differs in the scenario of acute PE, because heart disease is not the root cause of the problem.
5. Monitor for hypovolemic shock resulting from excessive bleeding when using thrombolytics or anticoagulants. Patients may develop either hypovolemic or cardiogenic shock in the setting of PE. Differential diagnosis of shock states may be assisted by examining PAPs and cardiac output.
   - Cardiogenic shock/right ventricular failure related to PE: Elevated CVP, elevated PVR, and decreased cardiac output.
   - Hypovolemic shock related to hemorrhage: Decreased CVP, decreased PVR, and decreased cardiac output.
   - Combined right ventricular failure and bleeding: Because CVP and PVR effects are opposite, hemodynamic readings may be difficult to interpret.

Bleeding Precautions

1. Maintain bed rest during active bleeding.
2. Administer blood products (fresh-frozen plasma, platelets, cryoprecipitate) as ordered.
3. Protect the patient from trauma, which may cause bleeding.
4. Avoid taking rectal temperatures.
5. Avoid puncturing the skin for injections, blood samples, and starting IV lines as much as possible.
6. The patient should wear shoes when ambulating, to avoid injuring the feet.
7. The patient should use a soft toothbrush for oral care.
8. The patient should use an electric razor for shaving.
9. Coordinate timing of invasive procedures with administration of fresh-frozen plasma and platelets as much possible to lessen the chance of bleeding.
10. Refrain from inserting devices into bleeding orifices.

Bleeding Reduction

1. Identify the cause of bleeding.
2. Note hemoglobin/hematocrit levels before and after blood loss.
3. Maintain patent IV access so that transfusions can occur quickly if needed.
4. Arrange for the availability of blood products, possibly using blood typing, screening, and holding the sample until products are needed.
5. Administer blood products if needed and monitor for transfusion reaction.
6. Instruct the patient and family regarding signs of bleeding (bruising, nosebleeds, bleeding gums) and to notify the nurse if bleeding ensues.
7. Instruct the patient on activity restrictions and how to apply direct pressure if bleeding ensues before the nurse arrives.
8. Discuss severity of bleeding and measures being provided to manage the situation.

9. Avoid use of drugs containing aspirin and NSAIDs (e.g., ibuprofen), which are platelet-aggregation inhibitors that prolong episodes of bleeding.

10. Monitor serial coagulation or thrombin times. Report values outside the desired therapeutic ranges. Optimal range for aPTT is 1.5 to 2.5 times control value. A therapeutic INR is 2 to 3. Optimal range for thrombin time is 2 to 5 times normal.

11. Ensure easy access to antidotes for prescribed treatment:
   - Protamine sulfate: 1 mg counteracts 100 units of heparin. Usually, the initial dose is 50 mg.
   - Vitamin K: 20 mg given SC.
   - Epsilon-aminocaproic acid (e.g., Amicar): Reverses the fibrinolytic condition related to thrombolytic therapy.

Teaching: Oral Anticoagulant Therapy
1. Determine the patient's knowledge of oral anticoagulant therapy.
2. Discuss the drug name, purpose, dosage, schedule, potential side effects, and complications of therapy.
3. Inform the patient of the potential side effects and complications of anticoagulant therapy: easy bruising, prolonged bleeding from cuts, spontaneous nosebleeds, black and tarry stools, and blood in urine and sputum.
4. Teach the rationale and application procedure for antiembolism stockings. Explain that the patient should put them on in the morning before getting out of bed.
5. Stress the importance of preventing impairment of venous return from the lower extremities by avoiding prolonged sitting, crossing the legs, and wearing constrictive clothing.
6. Teach the patient about foods high in vitamin K (e.g., fish, bananas, dark-green vegetables, tomatoes, cauliflower), which can interfere with anticoagulation. The patient must understand the importance of a consistent intake of foods high in vitamin K to avoid bleeding or clotting complications.
7. Caution the patient that a soft-bristle toothbrush, rather than a hard-bristle one, and an electric razor, rather than a safety razor, should be used during anticoagulant therapy while at home.
8. Instruct the patient to consult with the advanced practice provider before taking any new over-the-counter or prescribed drugs. The following are among many drugs that enhance the response to warfarin: aspirin, ibuprofen, cimetidine, and trimethoprim. Drugs that decrease the response include antacids, diuretics, oral contraceptives, and barbiturates, among others.

NIC Acid-Base Management; Acid-Base Monitoring; Bedside Laboratory Testing; Health Education; Oxygen Therapy; Respiratory Monitoring; Surveillance; Teaching: Individual; Teaching: Prescribed Medication; Respiratory Monitoring; Vital Signs Monitoring.

PULMONARY HYPERTENSION

PATHOPHYSIOLOGY

Pulmonary hypertension and pulmonary arterial hypertension (PAH) are complex, progressive, often fatal diseases caused by elevated pulmonary pressures. PAH is defined as a mean pulmonary artery pressure (MPAP) greater than 25 mm Hg, pulmonary capillary wedge pressure (PCWP) or left atrial pressure or left ventricular end-diastolic pressure less than 15 mm Hg, and PVR greater than 3 Wood units. Wood units are a calculated PVR that is obtained by subtracting the PCWP from the PAP systolic and dividing by the cardiac output. The pulmonary vasculature is normally a highly distensible, low-resistance system. All types of pulmonary hypertension or PAH may result in right ventricular failure, because the right ventricle is under constant strain to pump into the highly resistant pulmonary vasculature. (See Table 4-10 for World Health Organization classifications.) Each classification of pulmonary hypertension has a different cause and different approach to therapy.

Idiopathic pulmonary arterial hypertension (IPAH) is rare, has a poor prognosis, and affects primarily middle-aged and young women. Causes of IPAH are unclear. Heritable PAH is thought to be familial with a link to germline mutations, such as bone morphogenetic receptor 2 (BMPR2) or other causes. Associated pulmonary arterial hypertension (APAH) is attributable to secondary causes such as scleroderma or portopulmonary hypertension. Other causes of pulmonary hypertension are more common, with management directed at treating the underlying cause and lowering PAPs using vasodilator drugs. IPAH and APAH are often unresponsive to conventional treatments and may require specialty therapies.

In PAH, there is dysfunction and imbalance between vasodilation and vasoconstriction of the pulmonary vasculature from the right side of the heart to the lungs resulting in chronic

Table 4-10	WORLD HEALTH ORGANIZATION CLINICAL CLASSIFICATION OF PULMONARY HYPERTENSION
World Health Organization Class/Group	**Subsets/Examples of Causes**
1. Pulmonary arterial hypertension (PAH)	1.1 Idiopathic PAH (IPAH): Occurs at random. Also known as primary pulmonary hypertension. 1.2 Heritable: Formerly familial PAH; includes two types of PAH. 1.3 Drug- and toxin-induced: Includes antiobesity drugs such as [fen-phen] (fenfluramine + phentermine), methamphetamine, and cocaine. 1.4 Associated with other disorders: Diseases include connective tissue diseases, human immunodeficiency virus (HIV), portal hypertension, congenital heart disease, schistosomiasis, chronic hemolytic anemia, and persistent pulmonary hypertension of the newborn.
2. Pulmonary hypertension (PH) with left-sided heart disease	2.1 Systolic dysfunction 2.2 Diastolic dysfunction 2.3 Valvular disease
3. PH associated with lung diseases and/or hypoxemia	3.1 Chronic obstructive pulmonary disease 3.2 Interstitial lung disease 3.3 Other pulmonary diseases with mixed restrictive and obstructive pattern 3.4 Sleep-disordered breathing 3.5 Alveolar hypoventilation disorders 3.6 Chronic exposure to high altitude 3.7 Developmental abnormalities
4. Chronic thromboembolic pulmonary hypertension	Pulmonary thromboembolism or embolism attributable to fat, tumor, parasites, and foreign material.
5. Unclear multifactorial mechanisms	5.1 Hematologic disorders 5.2 Systemic disorders: sarcoidosis, pulmonary Langerhans' cell histiocytosis, lymphangioleiomyomatosis, neurofibromatosis, and vasculitis. 5.3 Metabolic disorders: glycogen storage disease, Gaucher disease, and thyroid disorders. 5.4 Others: tumoral obstruction, fibrosing mediastinitis, and chronic renal failure on dialysis.

From Simonneau G, Robbins IM, Beghetti M, et al: Updated clinical classification of pulmonary hypertension. *J Am Coll Cardiol* 54 S43-S54, 2009.

vasoconstriction. The vessel walls thicken and hypertrophy causing vascular remodeling from a non–muscular low-pressure system to a high-pressure, low-flow system. The endogenous vasodilators, nitric oxide and prostacyclin production, are impaired. In addition, endothelin-1, a potent endogenous vasoconstrictor, is increased. This increase in PVR and impedance to flow causes right ventricular strain, impaired filling, and increased right ventricular dilatation. This then leads to right ventricular ischemia. Eventually, the right side of the heart weakens and is unable to accommodate venous blood returning to the heart. PAH is generally a primary disease of the right side of the heart.

The pathophysiology of pulmonary hypertension differs from PAH in that it is generally attributable to primary disease of the left side of the heart such as left ventricular diastolic dysfunction or valvular heart disease. See the section on Heart Failure (Chapter 5) for further discussion of left-sided to right-sided heart failure.

Pulmonary hypertension may also be caused by chronic pulmonary diseases such as COPD or PE leading to cor pulmonale. The pulmonary vasculature responds to alveolar hypoxia by vasoconstriction, a beneficial mechanism that shunts blood away from underventilated areas to better ventilated areas in the lungs, thereby improving oxygenation. The resulting rise in PAP and increase in PVR from acute hypoxia are completely reversible once the hypoxia has been resolved. However, in the presence of chronic hypoxia, the pulmonary vasculature undergoes permanent changes similar to the changes in PAH, causing vascular remodeling. The right ventricle dilates and hypertrophies under the constant strain and workload. Eventually, the right side of the heart weakens and is unable to accommodate venous blood returning to the heart. As a result, pressure in the systemic venous circulation increases, causing cor pulmonale, or right-sided heart failure.

ASSESSMENT
GOAL OF ASSESSMENT
Because the low-resistance pulmonary vascular bed is clinically silent until late in the disease process, onset is insidious. Assessment before late stages of the disease should focus on discerning the cause of early indicators and classifying functional status (Box 4-2) so that an appropriate plan of care is created.

HISTORY AND RISK FACTORS
Factors associated with PAH and pulmonary hypertension include familial, exposure to amphetamines, connective tissue diseases, congenital anomalies (patent foramen ovale or ventricular septal defect) by which additional blood is shunted from the left side of the heart to the right side of the heart, left ventricular failure, acidemia, COPD, sleep apnea, interstitial lung disease or pulmonary fibrosis, massive PE, ARDS resulting in noncardiogenic pulmonary edema, and an array of other causes. See Table 4-10 for etiologic factors.

CLINICAL PRESENTATION
Early indicators
Exertional dyspnea, fatigue, and weakness.

Late indicators
Chest pain, dizziness, syncope, palpitations, and lower extremity edema.

VITAL SIGNS
- Tachycardia and tachypnea.
- BP may increase or decrease, depending on response to any changes in cardiac output, which may be significant with markedly elevated PAPs.

Box 4-2	WORLD HEALTH ORGANIZATION CLASSIFICATION: FUNCTIONAL STATUS OF PATIENTS WITH PULMONARY HYPERTENSION

Class I: Patients with pulmonary hypertension (PH) but without resulting limitation of physical activity. Ordinary physical activity does not cause undue dyspnea or fatigue, chest pain, or near syncope.

Class II: Patients with PH resulting in slight limitation of physical activity. They are comfortable at rest. Ordinary physical activity causes undue dyspnea or fatigue, chest pain, or near syncope.

Class III: Patients with PH resulting in marked limitation of physical activity. They are comfortable at rest. Less than ordinary activity causes undue dyspnea or fatigue, chest pain, or near syncope.

Class IV: Patients with PH with inability to carry out any physical activity without symptoms. These patients manifest signs of right-sided heart failure. Dyspnea and/or fatigue may even be present at rest. Discomfort is increased by any physical activity.

OBSERVATION/INSPECTION
- Cyanosis of the lips and nail beds.
- Peripheral edema.
- Hepatic enlargement and ascites.
- Anasarca (generalized, massive edema).
- Distended jugular veins.

PALPATION
- Right ventricular heave (visible left parasternal systolic lift).

AUSCULTATION
- Accentuated pulmonary component of the second heart sound.
- Right ventricular heave at the left parasternal area.
- Systolic murmur of tricuspid regurgitation.
- S3 or S4.
- Distant breath sounds.
- Clear or basilar crackles in lung fields.

SCREENING DIAGNOSTIC TESTS
- Chest radiograph: Validates presence of underlying pathology, which may have prompted development of pulmonary hypertension.
- 12-Lead electrocardiogram (ECG): Assesses if the patient has an acute myocardial infarction associated with heart failure. May show right ventricular hypertrophy or strain, right-axis deviation, right bundle branch block, and enlarged P waves.

Diagnostic Tests for Pulmonary Hypertension

Test	Purpose	Abnormal Findings
Arterial blood gas (ABG) values	Important to the differential diagnosis of the cause of pulmonary hypertension.	*Values vary:* Generally Pao_2 will be less than 60 mm Hg. $Paco_2$ will be within normal limits (35 to 45 mm Hg) unless chronic obstructive pulmonary disease is the cause of the pulmonary hypertension, in which case $Paco_2$ is usually elevated.
Chest radiograph	Will confirm anatomic abnormalities associated with chronic right ventricular failure.	Right ventricular dilation or hypertrophy, enlarged pulmonary artery secondary to increased pressure, and diminished diaphragmatic excursion.
Computed tomography scan	Helps to identify specific pathology.	Will confirm the presence of interstitial lung disease.
Hemodynamic measurements	Helps to confirm the presence of elevated pulmonary artery pressures and monitor treatment effectiveness. Pressures in the pulmonary vasculature are measured by a pulmonary artery (e.g., Swan-Ganz) catheter.	Cardiac output can be a better measure of disease severity than the pulmonary artery pressures. Used for definitive diagnosis of pulmonary hypertension.
Right heart catheterization	Gold standard for definitive diagnosis.	Data will differentiate or quantify the contribution of the left or right ventricular failure and measure the response to pharmacotherapy.
Echocardiography	Assesses for elevated pulmonary artery systolic pressure, but not the mean pulmonary artery pressure. Hemodynamic monitoring is used for definitive diagnosis.	May reveal enlarged right atrium and right ventricle, diminished wall motion, and pulmonic valve malfunction (midsystolic closure or delayed opening). Unfortunately, false-positive results are common with echocardiography.

Continued

Diagnostic Tests for Pulmonary Hypertension — cont'd

Test	Purpose	Abnormal Findings
Pulmonary function tests	Important for differential diagnosis of the underlying pathologic condition.	Will vary according to cause.
Pulmonary angiography and perfusion scans	To rule out an embolic event as the underlying cause.	Will not be positive if the cause is pulmonary hypertension.
Red blood cell/ hematocrit values	Screens for polycythemia associated with chronic hypoxia.	May be increased above normal.
Type B natriuretic peptide level	Monitors the progress of any associated heart failure.	Will be progressively elevated as heart failure worsens.
Other blood tests	Used to rule out other possible diagnoses, such as liver disease, human immunodeficiency virus (HIV), and autoimmune disease.	Various values will be positive for specific pathologies.

COLLABORATIVE MANAGEMENT

The goal of interdisciplinary management is to diagnose and treat the underlying disorder or process causing the pulmonary hypertension and improve the patient's symptoms, functional status, quality of life, and survival. Treatment is directed primarily toward preventing progression of the disease, preventing thrombi in situ, and reducing pulmonary artery vasoconstriction.

CARE PRIORITIES

1. Relieve hypoxemia and improve gas exchange
- Oxygen therapy: To eliminate hypoxia, a cause of pulmonary vascular vasoconstriction, and the resulting right ventricular afterload.

2. Promote dilation of the pulmonary vasculature to promote blood flow and better gas exchange
- **Nitric oxide therapy:** Nitric oxide gas is administered through either a face mask or artificial airway to promote pulmonary vasodilation. The vasodilation reduces BP in the pulmonary circulation. Owing to the short half-life of nitric oxide, chronic therapy is not available. It is currently under research as a portable device.
- **Vasodilators:**
  - Calcium channel blockers: Are used to reverse pulmonary vasoconstriction, reduce right ventricular afterload, and enhance pulmonary blood flow in a small subset of patients who show a positive vasoreactive response during cardiac catheterization.
  - Endothelin blockers: Medications such as bosentan (Tracleer), ambrisentan (Letairis), and macitentan (Opsumit) block endothelin, which contributes to vasoconstriction and vascular remodeling. Liver function tests must be performed monthly. Note: Endothelin blockers are contraindicated for use in pregnancy as a result of teratogenic effects.
  - Prostacyclin (PGI$_2$) analogues: Produced in endothelial cells from prostaglandin H2, PGI$_2$ vasodilates the pulmonary vessels. Prostacyclin also prevents formation of platelet plugs. Synthetic prostacyclin analogues (epoprostenol [Flolan], epoprostenol room temperature stable [Veletri], iloprost [Ventavis], treprostinil [Remodulin, Tyvaso]) are given IV, SC, or by inhalation. These medications require specialized infusion or inhalation devices. The first PO prostacyclin medication has recently been approved, treprostinil (Orenitram). Note: Prostacyclin is inhibited by NSAIDs, so the patient must be educated to avoid them.
- **Phosphodiesterase-5 (PDE-5) inhibitors:** Vasodilates the pulmonary vessels. Sildenafil (Revatio) and tadalafil (Adcirca) while used for pulmonary hypertension are also marketed under the trade names of Viagra and Cialis at much lower doses for erectile dysfunction.

- **Guanylate cyclase stimulator:** New classification of medication that is specifically for use in chronic thromboembolic pulmonary hypertension. Riociguat (Adempas) is an oral medication and works by stimulation of the enzyme, which is responsible for the production of nitric oxide.

3. Reduce circulating blood volume to reduce strain on the right side of the heart
- Diuretics: Reduce circulating volume via loss of sodium and water, which may decrease PAP and right ventricular workload. In turn, this reduces leftward septal bulging seen with right ventricular overload. Carefully evaluate response; if the patient's condition declines, a volume infusion may be needed if the patient is in right ventricular failure. Higher right ventricular pressure may be needed to overcome the elevated PAP to promote right ventricular ejection.

4. Enhance myocardial contractility to improve blood flow through the pulmonary and systemic circulation:
- Digitalis: Generally used only with biventricular failure when other therapies have not been sufficient. The inotropic effects of digitalis can increase cardiac output and pulmonary resistance, which are deleterious in the presence of right ventricular failure.

5. Prevent pulmonary thromboembolism:
- Anticoagulants: Warfarin is used for ongoing prevention of pulmonary emboli (blood clots in the lungs).

HIGH ALERT! Complex Parenteral Therapy

Epoprostenol and treprostinil are the only intravenous medications delivered in nanogram per kilogram per minute (1,000,000 [1 million] nanograms = 1 milligram). Because of the high risk of dose errors, verification of correct dose and dose weight should occur with the patient and family, specialty pharmacy, inpatient pharmacy, pulmonary arterial hypertension team if the institution has one, and provider team. Parenteral therapy should not be stopped, flushed, or diluted for any reason, and must be infused in a dedicated line without any flush bag. Owing to the short half-life of the medication epoprostenol, there must be an immediate backup bag available at all times. Any interruption or error in calculation can lead to rebound pulmonary hypertension and risk of death.

CARE PLANS FOR PULMONARY HYPERTENSION

RISK FOR INEFFECTIVE CARDIOPULMONARY TISSUE PERFUSION *related to blood flow anomalies stemming from pulmonary hypertension and right ventricular strain.*

Goals/Outcomes: Within 24 hours of initiating vasodilator medications, diuretics, and inotropic agents, PAPs are reduced by at least 10%, CVP or right atrial pressure is maintained at a level that facilitates forward flow of blood if the patient has right ventricular failure, PVR is reduced below 3 Wood units or below 300 dynes/s/cm^{-5}, and cardiac index is at least 2 L/min/m^2. Systemic BP is maintained at no less than 90 mm Hg systolic, with diastolic pressure at least 50 mm Hg.

NOC Tissue Perfusion: Pulmonary; Tissue Perfusion: Cardiac; Cardiac Pump Effectiveness; Respiratory Status: Gas Exchange; Circulation Status.

Hemodynamic Regulation
1. If present, monitor PAPs and cardiac output in response to vasodilator medications, diuretics, and inotropic medications.
2. Monitor invasive or noninvasive BP for improvement. Owing to the vasodilatory effects of acute and chronic PAH therapies, the patient may be normally hypotensive and the normal BP for the patient must be established. Medications and intravascular volume regulation may help improve cardiac output and systemic circulation. Those with right ventricular failure require a delicate balance between medication administration and volume regulation.
3. Auscultate breath sounds to assess for crackles at least every 2 hours.
4. Monitor for decreased urine output every 2 hours. Improvement in urine output is reflective of improved systemic circulation, resulting in improved renal blood flow.

5. If available, judiciously monitor CVP or right atrial pressure if the patient has right ventricular failure. Preload must be maintained at a sufficient level to be able to overcome the increased resistance to ejection (right ventricular afterload) created by pulmonary hypertension. The patient may require a CVP that is considerably higher than normal to facilitate forward flow of blood. If diuretics worsen hemodynamics, a volume infusion may be attempted to see if the cardiac output improves.

IMPAIRED GAS EXCHANGE *related to altered blood flow secondary to pulmonary capillary constriction and fluid, which may be present in the alveoli secondary to heart failure.*

Goals/Outcomes: Gas exchange improves within 12 hours of initiating therapies, toward a goal of at least 90%. Those who are O_2-dependent must be assessed using their baseline value coupled with their activity tolerance, because both are lower than expected for the general population.

NOC Respiratory Status: Gas Exchange.

Oxygen Therapy
1. Administer O_2 as prescribed. Advance O_2 delivery devices as needed. If the patient requires consistent increases in FIO_2 to maintain the same O_2 saturation, notify the advanced practice provider, because this is a sign of deteriorating gas exchange.
2. Assess respiratory pattern, rate, and depth; chest excursion and use of accessory muscles.
3. Monitor ABG results for hypoventilation, a sign of impending respiratory failure. (See Acute Respiratory Failure).

Ventilation Assistance
1. Monitor for changes in O_2 saturation and work of breathing in response to pulmonary vasodilator medications. If the patient fails to improve and respiratory distress increases, the patient must be intubated and placed on mechanical ventilation. (See Mechanical Ventilation for detailed information.)
2. Provide emotional and spiritual support for the patient and his or her support system. (See Emotional and Spiritual Support of the Patient and Significant Others, Chapter 2.)
3. Once the patient is on mechanical ventilation, strategies such as nitric oxide therapy can be initiated for patients who are severely ill and unresponsive to other vasodilator medications. Patients receiving nitric oxide should improve their O_2 saturation within 24 hours of initiating treatment. In addition, optimal ventilation management in the patient with right ventricular failure may include low tidal ventilation and low PEEP. Hyperinflation and increased PEEP can lead to excessive PVR and fatal drop in cardiac output.
4. If the patient is unable to sustain an improved O_2 saturation on nitric oxide, the advanced practice provider may need to approach the patient (if aware and oriented) and support system about extracorporeal membrane oxygenation if they are a candidate for heart-lung transplantation. If there are no further options available, discontinuation of life support may need to be addressed (see Ethical Considerations in Critical Care, Chapter 2).

DEFICIENT KNOWLEDGE *related to disease process and treatment of pulmonary hypertension and associated underlying diseases if present.*

Goals/Outcomes: Throughout the hospitalization, the patient and support system voice understanding of the plan of care; within 24 hours of hospital discharge, the patient and support system verbalize sufficient knowledge of management of the disease process(es) and treatments to sustain the patient outside the hospital.

NOC Knowledge: Disease Process; Knowledge: Treatment and Procedure(s).

Teaching: Treatments and Procedures
1. Explain all steps in the process of providing various O_2 delivery and ventilatory support strategies.
2. Discuss the selection of various modalities of vasodilator therapies. Inhaled medications and SC and IV infusions that will be continued outside the hospital require more extensive education and patient demonstration of independence before discharge. Owing to the high cost of medications and long-term care restrictions, patients may not be discharged to rehabilitation or skilled nursing facilities.
3. Involve case manager who is specialized in PAH if available and discharge planner in discussions of medications, so that all resource options are clarified. Many of the medications used are obtained from specialty pharmacies only and must be preapproved financially and clinically before administration and/or discharge.
4. If the patient requires mechanical ventilation, ensure that the patient understands how to communicate with care providers (see Mechanical Ventilation care plans for further details).

5. When preparing for discharge home, discuss the purpose of medications designed to reduce the workload on the heart (vasodilators), relax the heart (calcium channel blocking agents), and prevent fluid accumulation (diuretics). Include teaching and discussion of two forms of birth control for all women of child-bearing years because of the high maternal mortality between (30% and 50%), along with teratogenic effects of warfarin and endothelin blockers.

6. Ensure that the patient is familiar with the home health providers who will provide O_2 therapy and other ventilation strategies, such as a nebulizer or aerosol, if needed.

Teaching: Disease Process

1. Assess the patient's level and key support system members' level of understanding of the disease process.
2. If the cause of pulmonary hypertension has been identified, discuss appropriate management strategies of the associated disease process.
3. Discuss lifestyle changes that could prevent further complications.
4. Explain the value of learning relaxation therapy, including various breathing and visualization exercises, listening to music, meditation, and biofeedback.
5. Explain how smoking and second-hand smoke increase the workload of the heart by causing vasoconstriction. The patient should be encouraged to live in a smoke-free environment. Support system members who smoke should be given the opportunity to understand this vital information. Smoking cessation information should be provided.
6. If activity has been progressively impaired, consult with a physical therapist and respiratory therapist regarding an appropriate exercise program.
7. Have a dietician visit the patient to offer assistance with meal planning.

NIC Activity Therapy; Airway Management; Acid-Base Monitoring; Anxiety Reduction; Cardiac Care: Acute; Coping Enhancement; Invasive Hemodynamic Monitoring; Medication Administration: Intravenous; Medication Administration: Inhalation; Medication Administration: Oral; Self-Care Assistance; Sleep Enhancement; Support Group.

SELECTED REFERENCES

Abdo WF, Heunks LMA: Oxygen induced hypercapnia in COPD: myths and facts, *Crit Care* 16:323, 2012.

Abroug F, Ouanes-Besbes L, Dachraoui F, Brochard L: An updated study-level meta-analysis of randomized controlled trials on proning in ARDS and acute lung injury, *Crit Care* 15:R6, 2011.

Akinbami LJ, Moorman JE, Bailey CM, et al: National surveillance of asthma: United States, 2001-2010. In *Vital health statistics*, series 3, number 35, Maryland, 2012, National Center for Health Statistics, pp. 1-67.

American Thoracic Society: Patient information series: pulmonary arterial hypertension, *Am J Respir Crit Care Med* 187:P1-P2, 2013.

Apter A: Advances in adult asthma diagnosis and treatment in 2013, *J Allergy Clin Immunol* 133:49-56, 2014.

ARDS Definition Task Force, Ranieri VM, Rubenfeld GD, Thompson BT, et al: Acute respiratory distress syndrome: the Berlin definition, *JAMA* 307:2526-2533, 2012.

Attridge RT, Frei CR: Health care-associated pneumonia: an evidence-based review, *Am J Med* 124:689-697, 2011.

Badesch DB, Abman SH, Simonneau G, et al: Medical therapy for pulmonary arterial hypertension: updated ACCP evidence-based clinical practice guidelines, *Chest* 131:1917-1928, 2007.

Badesch DB, Champion HC, Sanchez MAG, et al: Diagnosis and assessment of pulmonary arterial hypertension, *J Am Coll Cardiol* 54:S55-S66, 2009.

Beckman MG, Hooper WC, Critchley SE, Ortel TL: Venous thromboembolism: a public health concern, *Am J Prev Med* 38(Suppl 4):S495-S501, 2010.

Bickley L: *Bates guide to physical examination and history taking*, ed 11, Philadelphia, 2013, Wolters Kluwer Health/Lippincott Williams & Wilkins.

Biehl M, Kashiouris MG, Gajic O: Ventilator-induced lung injury: minimizing its impact in patients with or at risk for ARDS, *Respir Care* 58:927-937, 2013.

Bonatti HJR, Sawyer RG, Pruett TL: Infection control in immunosuppressed patients. In *Critical Connections Newsletter*, February 2009, Society of Critical Care Medicine. Retrieved April 10, 2015, from http://www.sccm.org/Communications/Critical-Connections/Archives/Pages/Infection-Control-in-Immunosuppressed-Patients.aspx.

Booker S, Murff S, Kitko L, Jablonski R: Mouth care to reduce ventilator-associated pneumonia, *Am J Nurs* 113:24-30, 2013.

Braaten J, Goss R, Francis C: Ultrasound reversibly disaggregates fibrin fibers, *Thromb Haemost* 78:1063–1068, 1997.

Briel M, Meade M, Mercat A, et al: Higher vs lower positive end expiratory pressure in patients with acute lung injury and acute respiratory distress syndrome: systematic review and meta-analysis, *JAMA* 303:865–873, 2010.

British Thoracic Society, Scottish Intercollegiate Guidelines Network: *British guideline on the management of asthma, Quick reference guide*, May 2008. Retrieved May 17, 2014, from http://www.brit-thoracic.org.uk/ClinicalInformation/Asthma/AsthmaGuidelines.

Caironi P, Cressoni M, Chiumello D, et al: Lung opening and closing during ventilation of acute respiratory distress syndrome, *Am J Respir Crit Care Med* 181:578–586, 2010.

Centers for Disease Control and Prevention: CDC grand rounds: preventing hospital associated venous thromboembolism, *MMWR Morb Mortal Wkly Rep* 63:190–193, 2014.

Cepkova M, Matthay MA: Pharmacotherapy of acute lung injury and the acute respiratory distress syndrome, *J Intensive Care Med* 21:119–143, 2006.

Chalmers JD, Rother C, Salih W, Ewig S: Healthcare-associated pneumonia does not accurately identify potentially resistant pathogens: a systematic review and meta-analysis, *Clin Infect Dis* 58:330–339, 2014.

Chalmers JD, Taylor JK, Mandal P, et al: Validation of the Infectious Diseases Society of America/American Thoracic Society minor criteria for intensive care unit admission in community-acquired pneumonia patients without major criteria or contraindications to intensive care unit care, *Clin Infect Dis* 53:503–511, 2011.

Chan MC, Tseng JS, Chiu JT, et al: Prognostic value of plateau pressure below 30 cm H2O in septic patients with acute respiratory failure, *Respir Care* 60:12–20, 2015.

Chiumello D, Cressoni M, Carlesso E, et al: Bedside selection of positive end-expiratory pressure in mild, moderate, and severe acute respiratory distress syndrome, *Crit Care Med* 42:252–264, 2014.

Colleton LG: Beyond the stethoscope: respiratory assessment of the older adult, *Nursing Made Incredibly Easy* 6:11–14, 2008.

Dasenbrook E, Needham DM, Brower RG, Fan E: Higher positive end expiratory pressure in patients with acute lung injury: a systematic review and meta-analysis, *Respir Care* 56:568–575, 2011.

Dellinger RP, Levy MM, Rhodes A, et al: Surviving Sepsis Campaign Guidelines Committee including The Pediatric Subgroup: Surviving Sepsis Campaign: International Guidelines for Management of Severe Sepsis and Septic Shock, 2012, *Intensive Care Med* 39:165–228, 2013.

Dhar R: Pneumonia: review of guidelines, *J Assoc Physicians India* 60:25–28, 2012.

Dickinson S, Zalewski CA: Oral care during mechanical ventilation: critical for VAP prevention. In *Critical Connections Newsletter*, February 2008, Society of Critical Care Medicine. http://www.sccm.org/Communications/Critical-Connections/Archives/Pages/Oral-Care-During-Mechanical-Ventilation—-Critical-for-VAP-Prevention.aspx.

DPDx – Laboratory Identification of Parasitic Diseases of Public Health Concern: *Pneumocystis*, 2013. http://www.cdc.gov/dpdx/pneumocystis/index.html.

Eisenstadt E: Dysphagia and aspiration pneumonia in older adults, *J Am Acad Nurse Pract* 22:17–22, 2010.

Eriksson EA, Pellegrini DC, Vanderkolk WE, et al: Incidence of pulmonary fat embolism at autopsy: an undiagnosed epidemic, *J Trauma* 71:312, 2011.

Francis CW, Blinc A, Lee S, Cox C: Ultrasound accelerates transport of recombinant tissue plasminogen activator into clots, *Ultrasound Med Biol* 21:419–424, 1995.

Frederick D: Pulmonary issues in older adult, *Crit Care Nurs Clin North Am* 26:91–97, 2014.

Geerts WH, Bergqvist D, Pineo GF, et al: Prevention of venous thromboembolism: American College of Chest Physicians evidence-based clinical practice guidelines, ed 8. *Chest* 133(Suppl 6):S381–S453, 2008.

Goldhill DR, Imhoff M, McLean B, et al: Rotational bed therapy to prevent and treat respiratory complications: a review and meta-analysis, *Am J Clin Cardiol* 16:50–62, 2007.

Goligher EC, Kavanagh BP, Rubenfeld GD, et al: Oxygenation response to positive end-expiratory pressure predicts mortality in acute respiratory distress syndrome. A secondary analysis of the LOVS and ExPress trials, *Am J Respir Crit Care Med* 190:70–76, 2014.

Goodrich C: Needle thoracostomy (perform). In Weigand DJLM, editor: *AACN procedure manual for critical care*, ed 6, Philadelphia, 2011, Elsevier Saunders, pp. 204–207.

Goss L: A close up view of pneumococcal disease, *Nurse Pract* 36:41–45, 2011.

Gould MK, Garcia DA, Wren SM, et al: Prevention of VTE in nonorthopedic surgical patients: antithrombotic therapy and prevention of thrombosis, *Chest* 141:e227S-e277S, 2012.

Guerin C, Reignier J, Richard JC, et al: Prone positioning in severe acute respiratory distress syndrome, *N Engl J Med* 368:2159–2168, 2013.

Heppner H, Cornel S, Peter W, et al: Infections in the elderly, *Crit Care Clin* 29:757–774, 2013.

Herridge MS, Tansey CM, Matté A, et al; Canadian Critical Care Trials Group: Functional disability 5 years after acute respiratory distress syndrome, *N Engl J Med* 364:1293–1304, 2011.

Hess DR: Approaches to conventional mechanical ventilation of the patient with acute respiratory distress syndrome, *Respir Care* 56:1555–1572, 2011.

Hess DR: Noninvasive ventilation for acute respiratory failure, *Respir Care* 58:950–972, 2013.

Hill N: Noninvasive ventilation in critical care. In *Critical Connections Newsletter.* February 2008, Society of Critical Care Medicine. http://www.sccm.org/Publications/Critical_Connections/Archives/February_2008/Pages/NoninvasiveVentilation.aspx.

Institute for Healthcare Improvement: How-*to guide: prevent ventilator-associated pneumonia*, Cambridge, 2012, Institute for Healthcare Improvement. http://www.ihi.org/resources/Pages/Tools/HowtoGuidePreventVAP.aspx.

Institute for Healthcare Improvement: *Ventilator-associated pneumonia (VAP) bundle: Daily Oral Care with Chlorhexidine.* http://www.ihi.org/resources/Pages/Changes/ImplementtheVentilatorBundle.aspx. Accessed April 20, 2014.

Johnstone J, Mandell L: Guidelines and quality measures: do they improve outcomes of patients with community-acquired pneumonia, *Infect Dis Clin North Am* 27:71–86, 2013.

Kahn SR, Morrison DR, Cohen JM, et al: Interventions for implementation of thromboprophylaxis in hospitalized medical and surgical patients at risk for venous thromboembolism, *Cochrane Database Syst Rev* 7:CD008201, 2013.

Kahn SR, Lim W, Dunn AS, et al: Prevention of VTE in nonsurgical patients: antithrombotic therapy and prevention of thrombosis, *Chest* 141:e195S–226S, 2012.

Kalanuria AA, Zai W, Mirski M: Ventilator-associated pneumonia in the ICU, *Crit Care* 18:1–8, 2014.

Kaynar AM, Pinsky MR: Respiratory failure. In *Medscape*, New York, 2014, WebMD. http://www.emedicine.medscape.com/article/167981-overview.

Kesslert R, Ståhi E, Vogelmeier C, et al: Patient understanding, detection, and experience of COPD exacerbations, *Chest* 130:133–142, 2006.

Kieninger A, Lipsett P: Hospital acquired pneumonia: pathophysiology, diagnosis and treatment, *Surg Clin North Am* 89:439–461, 2009.

Killeen K, Skora E: Pathophysiology, diagnosis and clinical assessment of asthma in the adult, *Nurs Clin North Am* 48:11–23, 2013.

Kirkwood P: Chest tube removal (perform). In Weigand DJLM, editor: *AACN procedure manual for critical care*, ed 6, Philadelphia, 2011, Elsevier Saunders, pp. 171–177.

Klingman MS, Chin K: Safety recommendations for administering intravenous prostacyclins in the hospital, *Crit Care Nurse* 33:32–41, 2013.

Kollef MH: Ventilator-associated complications, including infection-related complications the way forward, *Crit Care Clin* 29:33–50, 2013.

Lemiale V, Resche-Rigon M, Azoulay E: Early non-invasive ventilation for acute respiratory failure in immunocompromised patients (IVNIctus): study protocol for a multicenter randomized controlled trial, *Trials* 15:372, 2014.

Lusardi PA, Scott SS, Scott F: Chest tube placement (perform). In Weigand DJLM, editor: *AACN procedure manual for critical care*, ed 6, Philadelphia, 2011, Elsevier Saunders, pp. 154–163.

MacDuff A, Arnold A, Harvey J: Management of spontaneous pneumothorax: British Thoracic Society pleural disease guideline 2010, *Thorax* 65(Suppl 2):ii18–ii31, 2010.

Mandel J, Poch D: Pulmonary hypertension, *Ann Intern Med* 158:ITC-1-ITC-16, 2013.

Manzano F, Colmenero M, Perez-Perez AM, et al: Comparison of two repositioning schedules for the prevention of pressure ulcers in patients on mechanical ventilation with alternating pressure air mattresses, *Intensive Care Med* 40:1679–1687, 2014.

Marik PE, Pastores S, Annane D, et al: Clinical practice guidelines for the diagnosis and management of corticosteroid insufficiency in critical illness: recommendations of an international task force, *Crit Care Med* 36:1937–1949, 2008.

Maynard G, Jenkins IH, Merli GJ: Venous thromboembolism prevention guidelines for medical inpatients: mind the (implementation) gap, *J Hosp Med* 8:582–588, 2013.

Muscedere J, Sinuff T, Heyland D, et al: The clinical impact and preventability of ventilator-associated conditions in critically ill patients who are mechanically ventilated, *Chest* 144:1453–1460, 2013.

Nair GB, Niederman MS: Nosocomial pneumonia, *Crit Care Clin* 29:521–546, 2013.

Nava S, Hill N: Non-invasive ventilation for acute respiratory failure, *Lancet* 374:250–259, 2009.

Needham DM, Wozniak AW, Hough CL, et al: National Institutes of Health NHLBI ARDS Network. Risk factors for physical impairment after acute lung injury in a national multicenter study, *Am J Respir Crit Care Med* 189:1214–1224, 2014.

Niederman M: Community acquired pneumonia, *Ann Intern Med* 151:ITC4-2-ITC4-14–quiz ITC4-16, 2009.

Niederman MS: Hospital-acquired pneumonia, health care associated pneumonia, ventilator-associated pneumonia, and ventilator-associated tracheobronchitis: definitions and challenges in trial design, *Clin Infect Dis* 51:S12–S17, 2010.

Nurses Learning: *Physical assessment: assessment of the lungs and thorax.* http://www.nurseslearning.com/courses/nrp/NRP-1616/Section2/index.htm.

Oba Y, Thameem DM, Zaza T: High levels of PEEP may improve survival in acute respiratory distress syndrome: a meta-analysis, *Respir Med* 103:1174–1181, 2009.

Ozsancak A, D'Ambrosio C, Hill NS: Nocturnal noninvasive ventilation, *Chest* 133:1275–1286, 2008.

Parikh S, Motarjeme A, McNamara T, et al: Ultrasound-accelerated thrombolysis for the treatment of deep vein thrombosis: initial clinical experience, *J Vasc Interv Radiol* 19:521–528, 2008.

Patadia MO, Murrill LL, Corey J: Asthma: symptoms and presentation, *Otolaryngol Clin North Am* 47:23–32, 2014.

Pelosi P, Gama de Abreu M, Rocco PR: New and conventional strategies for lung recruitment in acute respiratory distress syndrome, *Crit Care* 14:210, 2010.

Phoenix SI, Paravastu S, Columb M, et al: Does a higher positive end expiratory pressure decrease mortality in acute respiratory distress syndrome? A systematic review and meta-analysis, *Anesthesiology* 110:1098–1105, 2009.

Pickett JD: Closed chest drainage system. In Weigand DJLM, editor: *AACN procedure manual for critical care*, ed 6, Philadelphia, 2011, Elsevier Saunders, pp. 184–203.

Pieracci FM, Barle PS, Pomp A: Critical care of the bariatric patient, *Crit Care Med* 34:1796–1804, 2006.

Puntillo K, Arai SR, Cooper BA, et al: A randomized clinical trial of an intervention to relieve thirst and dry mouth in intensive care unit patients, *Intensive Care Med* 40:1295–1302, 2014.

Putensen C, Theuerkauf N, Zinserling J, et al: Meta-analysis: ventilation strategies and outcomes of the acute respiratory distress syndrome and acute lung injury, *Ann Intern Med* 151:566–576, 2009.

Reddel HK, Taylor DR, Bateman ED, et al: An official American Thoracic Society/European Respiratory Society statement: asthma control and exacerbations, *Am J Respir Crit Care Med* 180:59–99, 2009.

Rose L, Nokoyama N, Rezai S, et al: Psychological wellbeing, health related quality of life and memories of intensive care and a specialised weaning centre reported by survivors of prolonged mechanical ventilation, *Intensive Crit Care Nurs* 30:145–151, 2013.

Rubenfeld GD, Caldwell E, Peabody E, et al: Incidence and outcomes of acute lung injury, *N Engl J Med* 353:1685–1693, 2005.

Santos CL, Moraes L, Santos RS, et al: Effects of different tidal volume in pulmonary and extrapulmonary lung injury with or without intraabdominal hypertension, *Intensive Care Med* 38:499–508, 2012.

Scott SS, Kardos CB: Community-acquired, health care associated and ventilator-associated pneumonia: three variations of a serious disease, *Crit Care Nurs Clin North Am* 24:431–441, 2012.

Scott SS, Lusardi PA, Scott F: Chest tube placement (assist). In Weigand DJLM, editor: *AACN procedure manual for critical care*, ed 6, Philadelphia, 2011, Elsevier Saunders, pp. 164–170.

Shaikh N, Ummunisa F: Acute management of vascular air embolism, *J Emerg Trauma Shock* 2: 180–185, 2009.

Sligl W, Marrie T: Severe community acquired pneumonia, *Crit Care Clin* 29:563–601, 2013.

Soltani A, Volz KR, Hansmann DR: Effect of modulated ultrasound parameters on ultrasound-induced thrombolysis, *Phys Med Biol* 53:6837–6847, 2008.

Soltani A, Singhal R, Garcia JL, Raju NR: Absence of biological damage from prolonged exposure to intravascular ultrasound, *Ultrasonics* 46:60–67, 2007.

Sona C, Schallom L: Nursing practice excellence: a key to infection prevention. In *Critical Connections Newsletter*, February 2009, Society of Critical Care Medicine. Retrieved from Song WJ, Chang YS: Magnesium sulfate for acute asthma in adults: a systematic literature review, *Asia Pac Allergy* 2:76–85, 2012.

Sweet DD, Naismith A, Keenan SP, et al: Missed opportunities for noninvasive positive pressure ventilation: a utilization review, *J Crit Care* 23:111, 2008.

Tang B, Craig J, Eslick G, et al: Use of corticosteroids in acute lung injury and acute respiratory distress syndrome: a systematic review and meta-analysis, *Crit Care Med* 37:1594–1603, 2009.

Tapson VF, Decousus H, Pini M, et al: Venous thromboembolism prophylaxis in acutely ill, hospitalized medical patients: findings from the International Medical Prevention Registry on Venous Thromboembolism, *Chest* 132:936–945, 2007.

Taylor DR, Bateman ED, Boulet L-P, et al: A new perspective on concepts of asthma severity and control, *Eur Respir J* 32:545–554, 2008.

The ARDS Clinical Trials Network, National Heart, Lung, and Blood Institute; National Institutes of Health: Effects of recruitment maneuvers in patients with acute lung injury and acute respiratory distress syndrome ventilated with high positive end-expiratory pressure, *Crit Care Med* 31:2592–2597, 2003.

The Joint Commission: *Pneumonia measures.* http://www.jointcommission.org/pneumonia/.

The NHLBI ARDS Clinical Trials Network: Comparison of two fluid-management strategies in acute lung injury, *N Engl J Med* 354:2564–2575, 2006.

Torbicki A, Perrier A, Konstantinides S, et al: The Task Force for the Diagnosis and Management of Acute Pulmonary Embolism of the European Society of Cardiology: Guidelines on the diagnosis and management of pulmonary embolism, *Eur Heart J* 29:2276–2315, 2008.

United States Department of Health and Human Services, National Institutes of Health; National Asthma Education and Prevention Program Expert Panel Report 3: *Guidelines for the diagnosis and management of asthma (summary report 2007).* http://www.nhlbi.nih.gov/guidelines/asthma/index.htm.

United States Department of Health and Human Services: *The Surgeon General's call to action to prevent deep vein thrombosis and pulmonary embolism,* Washington, 2008, United States Department of Health and Human Services. http://www.surgeongeneral.gov/topics/deepvein.

Vollman, KM: Understanding critically ill patients hemodynamic response to mobilization: using the evidence to make it safe and feasible, *Crit Care Nurs Q* 36:17–27, 2013.

Watkins R, Lemonovich T: Diagnosis and management of community acquired pneumonia in adults, *Am Fam Phys* 83:1300–1306, 2011.

Wei C, Cheng Z, Zhang L, Yang J: Microbiology and prognostic factors of hospital- and community-acquired aspiration pneumonia in respiratory intensive care unit, *Am J Infect Control* 41:880–884, 2013.

Yarmus L, Feller-Kopman D: Pneumothorax in the critically ill patient, *Chest* 141:1098–1105, 2012.

Yeager S: Thoracentesis (assist). In Weigand DJLM, editor: *AACN procedure manual for critical care,* ed 6, Philadelphia, 2011, Elsevier Saunders, pp. 219–224.

Yeager S: Thoracentesis (perform). In Weigand DJLM, editor: *AACN procedure manual for critical care,* ed 6, Philadelphia, 2011, Elsevier Saunders, pp. 208-218.

Zamanian RT, Haddad F, Doyle RL, Weinacker AB: Management strategies for patients with pulmonary hypertension in the intensive care unit, *Crit Care Med* 35:2037–2050, 2007.

Zehtabshi S, Rios CL: Management of emergency department patients with spontaneous pneumothorax: needle aspiration or tube thoracostomy, *Ann Emerg Med* 51:91–100, 2008.

5

Cardiac and Vascular Disorders

CARDIOVASCULAR ASSESSMENT: GENERAL

GOAL OF SYSTEM ASSESSMENT
Evaluate for decreased cardiac output (CO) and decreased tissue perfusion.

VITAL SIGN ASSESSMENT
Measure heart rate (HR), heart rhythm, and blood pressure (BP) to evaluate CO and perfusion.
* Measure BP on both arms using an appropriate sized cuff. Use the higher reading to monitor BP.
* Compare cuff BP to arterial line BP if arterial line is in place; decide which pressure is the most accurate; treat BP using that value.
* Note pulse pressure.
* Considerations for the bariatric patient: Use appropriate BP cuff. Avoid using thigh cuff on the bicep or forearm.

12-LEAD ELECTROCARDIOGRAM
Evaluate for changes from last electrocardiogram (ECG) to assess for worsened heart disease (myocardial damage) or for electrolyte imbalances, which may decrease CO; this should be done on every patient to use for comparison.
* Heart rate: diagnose type of tachycardia, bradycardia, or irregular rhythm
* PR, QRS, and QT intervals
* ST segment and T wave changes such as depression or elevation
* Pacing and conduction: Regular, normal rate and velocity
* Considerations for the bariatric patient: Low voltage may be noted on the ECG tracing.

OBSERVATION
* Evaluate for facial and lip color, appearance of skin and nails, and patterns of edema (especially dependent areas) to evaluate for decreased tissue perfusion.
* Considerations for the bariatric patient: The bariatric patient may have excess tissue and "stretch marks" because of increased body surface area.
* Inquire about the presence of chest, arm, and jaw discomfort.
* Inquire about compliance with taking cardiac medications as prescribed.
* Considerations for the bariatric surgery patient: For those patients who have bariatric bypass surgery, note that pills must be crushed. Find alternatives to sustained-release tabs/capsules as they will not be absorbed.

PALPATION
Pulse assessment to evaluate for decreased tissue perfusion:
* Pulse quality and regularity bilaterally (scale 0 to 4+)
* Edema (scale 0 to 4+: Extremities, back, and sacrum)
* Capillary refill
* Evaluate all peripheral pulses to assess for vascular disease.

AUSCULTATION

- Heart sounds to evaluate for contributors to decreased CO (note changes with body positioning and respirations):
    Considerations for the bariatric patient: Heart sounds may be distant because of large body habitus
- Aortic, pulmonic, Erb point, tricuspid, mitral
- S_1 (lub) and S_2 (dub): Quality, intensity, pitch
- Extra sounds: S_3 (after S_2), S_4 (before S_1) indicative of heart failure (HF)
- Extra sounds: Murmurs, clicks (may indicate valve disease)
- Extra sounds: Friction rub indicative of pericarditis

LABWORK

Blood studies can reveal causes of dysrhythmias or changes in pacing/conduction or HR changes:

- Electrolyte levels: ↑ or ↓ potassium, magnesium, sodium, chloride, and calcium
- Complete blood counts: Anemia, ↑ white blood cells (WBCs)
- Coagulation studies
- Lipid profile
- Cardiac enzymes/isoenzymes/troponin
- B-type natriuretic peptide (BNP)
- Levels of cardiac medications

CARE PLANS FOR GENERALIZED CARDIOVASCULAR DYSFUNCTIONS

ACTIVITY INTOLERANCE *related to decreased cardiac output (CO)*

Goals/Outcomes: Within the 12- to 24-hour period before discharge from the critical care unit (CCU), the patient exhibits cardiac tolerance to increasing levels of activity as evidenced by respiratory rate (RR) less than 24 breaths per minute (breaths/min), normal sinus rhythm (NSR) on ECG, BP within 20 mm Hg of the patient's normal range, HR less than 120 beats per minute (bpm) (or within 20 bpm of resting HR for patients on beta-blocker therapy), and absence of chest pain.

NOC Endurance

Energy Management
1. Determine patient's physical limitations.
    Considerations for the bariatric patient: Assess the previous level of functioning before hospitalization. Fatigue can be common in a bariatric patient.
2. Determine causes of fatigue and perceived causes of fatigue.
3. Monitor cardiorespiratory response to activity (tachycardia, other dysrhythmias, tachypnea, dyspnea, diaphoresis, pallor) and hemodynamic response (elevated pulmonary artery pressures [PAPs], central venous pressure [CVP], or no change/little increase in CO) if a pulmonary artery catheter or bioimpedance device is in place.
4. Monitor for chest discomfort during activity.
5. Reduce all causes of discomfort, including those induced by the patient's environment, such as uncomfortable room temperature or position, thirst/dry mouth, and wrinkled or damp bedding.
6. Provide alternating periods of rest and activity.

Self-Care Assistance: Instrumental Activities of Daily Living
1. Determine need for assistance with Instrumental Activities of Daily Living (IADLs) including walking, cooking, shopping, housekeeping, transportation, and money management.
2. Provide for methods of contacting support/assistance (such as lifeline services and emergency response services including readily accessible telephone numbers if the patient's area is not 911 accessible).
3. Determine financial resources and personal preferences for modifying the home to accommodate any disabilities.

DECREASED CARDIAC OUTPUT *related to altered cardiac pump function.*

Goals/Outcome: Within 24 hours of this diagnosis, the patient exhibits adequate CO, as evidenced by BP within normal limits for the patient, HR 60 to 100 bpm, NSR on ECG, peripheral pulses greater than 2+ on a 0 to 4+ scale, warm and dry skin, hourly urine output greater than 0.5 mL/kg, measured CO 4 to 7 L/min, CVP 4 to 6 mm Hg, PAP

20 to 30/8 to 15 mm Hg, pulmonary artery wedge pressure (PAWP) 6 to 12 mm Hg, and patient awake, alert, oriented, and free from anginal pain.

Considerations for the bariatric patient: Preload and after load may be increased because of increased blood volume.

NOC Circulation Status

Cardiac Care: Acute

1. Palpate and evaluate quality of peripheral pulses, for presence of edema, capillary refill, and skin color and temperature of extremities.
2. Monitor ECG continuously, noting HR and rhythm. Select the most diagnostic lead(s) for monitoring patient. Consider use of ST-segment monitoring if available.
3. Compare current ECG readings with past readings and report abnormal findings that create instability or have the potential to create instability.
4. Use a 12- or 15-lead ECG to diagnose heart rhythm changes, because one or two leads are often insufficient to fully diagnose ECG changes.
5. Provide antidysrhythmic medications as appropriate to abate heart rhythms that prompt hypotension, chest discomfort, or fatigue. Consult with advanced practice provider for symptomatic ECG rhythm changes.
6. Provide positive inotropic drugs as appropriate to help increase CO to maintain stable BP.
7. Monitor effects of negative inotropic medications (e.g., beta blockers) carefully, as the decreased myocardial workload may prompt hypotension.
8. Evaluate chest pain for location, radiation, intensity, duration, and precipitating factors. Emphasize to the patient the importance of reporting all instances of chest pain and pressure and arm, neck, and jaw pain.
9. Apply oxygen when chest pain is present, according to Advanced Cardiac Life Support (ACLS) guidelines.
10. Monitor pacemaker function as appropriate to insure device is sensing, pacing, and capturing appropriately.
11. Auscultate heart tones; be alert for development of new S3 and S4, new "split" sounds, or pericardial friction rubs.
12. Auscultate lungs for rales, crackles, wheezes, rhonchi, pleural friction rubs, or other adventitious sounds indicative of fluid retention.
13. Monitor for diminished level of consciousness or altered mental status, which may signal cerebral perfusion is compromised secondary to decreased CO.
14. Auscultate abdomen and monitor for decreased bowel sounds and/or abdominal distention, which may indicate abdominal perfusion is compromised.
15. Record intake and output (I&O), urine output, and daily weight and evaluate for fluid retention, which may indicate compromised renal perfusion.
16. Note electrolyte values at least daily, monitoring closely for changes in potassium, magnesium, sodium, chloride, and calcium, which may prompt dysrhythmias; increased blood urea nitrogen (BUN) or increased creatinine, which may indicate low CO is causing renal insufficiency; and hyperglycemia, which may indicate patient has underlying diabetes.
17. Monitor for increasing activity intolerance, dyspnea, excessive fatigue, and orthopnea, which may all indicate CO is lessening.
18. Keep head of the bed (HOB) elevated if the patient is unable to breathe comfortably when flat in bed.
19. Insert urinary catheter if the patient is unable to void without markedly increasing activity level, or anuria is noted, as appropriate.

Hemodynamic Regulation

1. Monitor values generated by pulmonary artery catheter to directly assess CO. Considerations for the bariatric patient: CO is increased because of oxygen demands of an increased body mass index. Monitor the bariatric patient responses to cardiac-altering medications carefully.
2. Assess for further decreases in CO reflected by elevated pulmonary artery occlusive/wedge pressure, elevated CVP, and elevated pulmonary vascular resistance (PVR), which may signal right- and/or left-sided HF.
3. Monitor for fluid overload by assessing for elevated systemic vascular resistance (SVR).
4. Monitor the effects of all medications on hemodynamic readings, including effects of positive or negative inotropic agents, antidysrhythmics, and vasodilating or vasoconstricting medications.

IMPAIRED GAS EXCHANGE *related to decreased lung perfusion*

Goals/Outcome: Within 12 to 24 hours of treatment, the patient has adequate gas exchange as evidenced by PaO_2 greater than 80 mm Hg, $PaCO_2$ 35 to 45 mm Hg, pH 7.35 to 7.45, presence of normal breath sounds, and absence of adventitious breath sounds. RR is 12 to 20 breaths/min with normal pattern and depth.

NOC Respiratory Status: Ventilation

Airway Management

1. Assess for patent airway; if snoring, crowing, or strained respirations are present, indicative of partial or full airway obstruction, open airway using chin-lift or jaw-thrust. Considerations for the bariatric patient: Sleep apnea is very common. Patients who are not intubated may require noninvasive positive pressure ventilation (NIPPV: CPAP or BiPAP) when sleeping.
2. Insert oral or nasopharyngeal airway if the patient cannot maintain patent airway; if severely distressed, the patient may require endotracheal intubation.
3. Position the patient to alleviate dyspnea and ensure maximal ventilation—generally in a sitting upright position unless severe hypotension is present.
4. Clear secretions from airway by having patient cough vigorously, or provide nasotracheal, oropharyngeal, or endotracheal tube suctioning as needed.
5. Have patient breathe slowly or manually ventilate with Ambu bag slowly and deeply between coughing or suctioning attempts.
6. Assist with use of incentive spirometer as appropriate.
7. Turn patient every 2 hours if immobile. Encourage patient to turn self or get out of bed as much as tolerated if able.
8. Provide mucolytic and bronchodilating medications orally, intravenously (IV), or by inhaler, aerosol, or nebulizer as ordered to assist with thinning secretions and relaxing muscles in lower airways.
9. Provide chest physical therapy as appropriate, if other methods of secretion removal are ineffective.

Oxygen Therapy

1. Provide humidity in oxygen or bilevel positive airway pressure (BiPAP) device if used for longer than 12 hours to help thin secretions.
2. Administer supplemental oxygen using liter flow and device as ordered.
3. Prohibit patient and visitors from smoking while oxygen is in use.
4. Document pulse oximetry with oxygen liter flow in place at time of reading as ordered. Oxygen is a drug; the dose must be associated with the oxygen saturation reading or the reading is meaningless.
5. Obtain arterial blood gases (ABGs) if the patient experiences behavioral changes or respiratory distress to check for hypoxemia or hypercapnia.
   Considerations for the bariatric patient: There may be increased CO_2 levels, which may be the normal state because of abnormal diaphragm position and upper airway obstruction caused by the structure of the neck.
6. Monitor for oxygen-induced hypoventilation, especially in patients with chronic obstructive pulmonary disease (COPD).
   Considerations for the bariatric patient: ABGs may be similar to those of a COPD patient, without ever using tobacco.
7. Monitor for changes in chest radiograph and breath sounds indicative of oxygen toxicity and absorption atelectasis in patients receiving higher concentrations of oxygen (greater than Fio_2 45%) for longer than 24 hours. The higher the oxygen concentration, the greater the chance of toxicity.
8. Monitor for skin breakdown where oxygen devices are in contact with skin, such as nares and around edges of mask devices.
9. Provide oxygen therapy during transportation and when patient gets out of bed.
10. If the patient is unable to maintain an Spo_2 of greater than 88% off oxygen, consult with respiratory care practitioner and physician about the need for home oxygen therapy.

Respiratory Monitoring

1. Monitor rate, rhythm, and depth of respirations.
2. Note chest movement for symmetry of chest expansion and signs of increased work of breathing such as use of accessory muscles or retraction of intercostal or supraclavicular muscles. Consider use of BiPAP for impending respiratory failure.
3. Note that trachea remains midline, as deviation may indicate the patient has a tension pneumothorax.
4. Auscultate breath sounds following administration of respiratory medications to assess for improvement.
5. Note changes in oxygen saturation (Sao2), pulse oximetry (Spo2), end-tidal CO_2, and ABGs as appropriate. Obtain arterial blood gas if validity of noninvasive monitoring of O_2 and CO_2 is questionable.
6. Monitor for dyspnea and note causative activities or events.
7. If increased restlessness or unusual somnolence occur, evaluate patient for hypoxemia and hypercapnia. Consult with advanced practice provider about escalating current therapies from simple oxygen therapy (if present) to either NiPPV or endotracheal intubation with mechanical ventilation to help support the work of breathing.
8. Monitor chest radiograph reports as new films become available.

HEART FAILURE

PATHOPHYSIOLOGY

Heart failure (HF) is the inability of the heart to adequately fill with blood or pump blood through the body. Effective pumping of the heart is determined by the components of CO: preload (end-diastolic volume in the ventricles, which stretches the myocardial fibers); afterload (resistance to ejection); and contractility of the myocardium. Myocardial contractility depends heavily on the delivery of oxygen and nutrients to the heart.

Functional and structural factors that affect any component of CO can lead to impaired cardiac function and eventual HF. Preload may be impacted by valvular disorders, cardiac tamponade, pericarditis, or cardiac arrhythmias such as atrial fibrillation. Conditions that may increase afterload include aortic stenosis and hypertension. Contractility may be reduced by direct damage to the cardiac muscle during myocardial infarction, myocarditis, cardiomyopathy, or during times of increased metabolic demand such as thyroid storm. Damaged areas of myocardium can become hypokinetic (weakly contractile), akinetic (noncontractile), or dyskinetic (moving opposite from the normal cardiac muscle).

SYSTOLIC AND DIASTOLIC DYSFUNCTION

HF may be described as systolic or diastolic dysfunction. Systolic failure results from reduced cardiac contractility, commonly described as ejection fraction (EF), or the percent of blood ejected by the left ventricle with each beat. Normal EF is 55% to 70%, with a value of 40% or less considered to be diagnostic of HF. Common causes of systolic dysfunction include coronary artery disease (CAD), ischemic cardiomyopathy, hypertension, idiopathic cardiomyopathy, and valvular heart disease. Less common causes include alcohol- and substance-induced cardiomyopathy, viral cardiomyopathy, and peripartum cardiomyopathy.

In diastolic failure, cardiac relaxation and ventricular filling are impaired but EF is preserved. Common causes of diastolic dysfunction include CAD, ischemic cardiomyopathy, hypertension, arrhythmias, and aging. Some patients manifest the symptoms of HF without evidence of systolic or diastolic dysfunction. Obesity, chronic lung disease, pulmonary embolism, or acute coronary ischemia can be alternate causes of these symptoms.

LEFT- VERSUS RIGHT-SIDED HEART FAILURE

Heart failure is described as left-sided or right-sided depending on which ventricle is impacted. Left ventricular (LV) failure may be caused by ischemic heart disease, systemic hypertension, mitral or aortic valve disease, arrhythmias, myocarditis, or substance abuse. Causes of right ventricular (RV) failure include pulmonary hypertension, obstructive sleep apnea, tricuspid or pulmonic valve disease, atrial or ventricular septal defect, and RV infarction. Right-sided HF can also develop in patients with left-sided HF, as increased pressure in the left ventricle backs up into the lungs and increases RV afterload.

HEART FAILURE PROGRESSION

HF is a progressive condition that results from prolonged neurohormonal activation. Stress induced by underlying causes leads to activation of the renin-angiotensin-aldosterone system (RAAS). Catecholamines cause peripheral vasoconstriction, increased resistance to ventricular ejection, increased HR, and increased myocardial oxygen consumption, and may precipitate myocardial ischemia and ventricular arrhythmias. Prolonged activation of the RAAS leads to sodium retention, vasoconstriction, hypertension, and eventual ventricular remodeling. In remodeling, the affected ventricle dilates, hypertrophies, and becomes more spherical. The remodeling process itself increases wall stress, causing further remodeling. Early identification of HF and evidence-based medications to reduce remodeling are key components of effective HF management. The progression of HF symptoms varies with each patient.

Death results from HF-related complications (such as lethal dysrhythmias) before some patients develop symptoms, while others are managed for years with an effective medical regimen. Patients with EF less than 35% are at significantly increased risk of sudden cardiac death. Advanced HF is classified by severity of symptoms, cardiac dysfunction, frequency of hospitalization, and reduction in functional status. Patients with advanced or end-stage HF may require advanced intervention such as implanted defibrillator, cardiac resynchronization therapy, inotropic therapy, ventricular assist device, or cardiac transplantation.

CARDIOVASCULAR ASSESSMENT: HEART FAILURE

GOAL OF SYSTEM ASSESSMENT

- Patients should be assessed for signs and symptoms of left- and right-sided HF as outlined in Table 5-1. Table 5-2 outlines the American Heart Association/American College of Cardiology HF classes. These classes group patients by disease state and symptoms.

Table 5-1	HEART FAILURE ASSESSMENT
Left-Sided Heart Failure Pulmonary Edema and Congestion	**Right-Sided Heart Failure Cor Pulmonale and Systemic Congestion**
Symptoms	

• Decreased exercise tolerance
• Fatigue
• Weakness
• Anxiety
• Dyspnea
   At rest
   On exertion
   Orthopnea (inability to lie flat)
   Paroxysmal
   nocturnal dyspnea (awakening from sleep with significant dyspnea)
• Cough (possibly moist with frothy sputum)
• Diaphoresis
• Palpitations
	• Decreased exercise tolerance
	• Fatigue
	• Peripheral edema (legs, hands, abdomen, sacrum)
	• Weight gain
	• Decreased urination
	• Abdominal tenderness
	• Nausea, vomiting, constipation, and anorexia

Physical Assessment	

• Tachypnea
• Rales (most often dependent, in lung bases)
• Unilateral or bilateral diminished lung sounds at the base (pleural effusion)
• Hypertension or hypotension
• Orthostasis (drop in BP ≥20 mm Hg with sitting or standing)
• Tachycardia
• Atrial or ventricular arrhythmia
• S_3
• Cyanosis or pallor
• Cardiogenic shock in acutely ill patients (significant hypotension, tachycardia, altered mental status, significant dyspnea)
• The combination of skin and pulmonary assessment can provide information about perfusion and volume status:
  • Warm and dry
  • Well-perfused and euvolemic
  • Warm and wet
  • Well-perfused with volume overload
  • Cold and dry
  • Hypoperfused without volume overload
  • Cold and wet
  • Hypoperfused with volume overload
	• Dependent pitting edema
	• Jugular venous distention
	• Hepatomegaly
	• Splenomegaly
	• Ascites
	• Positive hepatojugular reflex
	• Cardiogenic shock in acutely ill patients (significant hypotension, tachycardia, altered mental status)

Heart Failure

Continued

Table 5-1	**HEART FAILURE ASSESSMENT — cont'd**
Left-Sided Heart Failure Pulmonary Edema and Congestion	**Right-Sided Heart Failure Cor Pulmonale and Systemic Congestion**
Monitoring	

Daily weight
Arrhythmias
SpO$_2$ less than 90%
Signs of decreased cardiac output:
    Hypotension
    Tachycardia
    Decreased urine output
Weak peripheral pulses
In patients with advanced hemodynamic monitoring:
   • Decreased CO/CI
   • Decreased Svo$_2$
   • Elevated pulmonary artery pressures and pulmonary artery wedge pressure
   • Elevated systemic vascular resistance
	Daily weight
	Arrhythmias
	
	In patients with advanced hemodynamic monitoring:
	    Elevated right atrial pressure and central venous pressure
	Decrease in Svo$_2$ with minimal activity
	Possible decrease in CO/CI caused by right ventricular failure causing reduced left ventricular preload

CI, Cardiac index; *CO*, cardiac output; *Svo$_2$*, venous O$_2$ saturation.

Table 5-2	**AMERICAN COLLEGE OF CARDIOLOGY/AMERICAN HEART ASSOCIATION HEART FAILURE CLASSES**
Heart Failure Class	**Defining Characteristics**
A	Patients at high risk for heart failure without heart disease or symptoms
B	Structural heart disease without prior or current symptoms of heart failure
C	Structural heart disease with prior or current symptoms of heart failure
D	Refractory heart failure requiring specialized interventions

- Evaluate for decreased CO and decreased tissue perfusion initially with General Assessment, (Chapter 4).
- If a patient has developed HF secondary to ACS, see Assessment in Acute Coronary Syndromes (Chapter 4).

HISTORY AND RISK FACTORS
- History of HF, CAD, myocardial infarction (MI), hypertension, hypercholesterolemia, obstructive sleep apnea, diabetes, arrhythmias, and recent viral illness.
- Familial history of CAD and MI
- Age older than 65 years
- Obesity
- History of HF symptoms including fatigue, weight gain, decreased exercise tolerance, dyspnea, or peripheral edema
- In patients with previously diagnosed HF, compliance with low-sodium diet, weight monitoring, fluid restriction, medications, and exercise recommendations

Diagnostic Tests for Acute Heart Failure

See diagnostic tests in *Acute Coronary Syndromes*.

Test	Purpose	Abnormal Findings
Noninvasive Cardiology		
12-, 15-, or 18-lead electrocardiogram (ECG). Consider a right sided 12-Lead ECG.	Assess for signs of acute and chronic cardiac conditions.	Myocardial Ischemia/Infarct: • T wave inversions • ST depression • ST elevation • Q waves (completed infarction) Arrhythmia: • Atrial or ventricular arrhythmia • Heart block Left Ventricular Hypertrophy: • Large R/S waves in the v leads
Blood Studies		
Digoxin levels	Digoxin levels are often difficult to manage in heart failure patients. Levels should be obtained for patients with decompensated CHF, patients with acute renal failure, and any time digitalis toxicity is a concern. (Digoxin levels are not accurate after the administration of digoxin immune fab (Digibind) for elevated digitalis levels.)	Elevated levels in renal failure, overdose, decompensated heart failure. Signs of digoxin toxicity: • Ventricular arrhythmias • Progressive bradycardia • Heart block • Neurologic symptoms (confusion, visual disturbances)
Complete blood count (CBC) Hemoglobin (Hgb) Hematocrit (Hct) RBC count (RBCs) WBC count (WBCs)	Assess for anemia, infection, or volume overload in heart failure patients.	Decreased Hgb/Hct: • Anemia • Volume overload WBC: • Normal or elevated with infection
Electrolytes Potassium (K^+) Magnesium (Mg^{2+}) Calcium (Ca^{2+}) Sodium (Na^+)	Assess for possible causes of arrhythmias and evaluate volume status.	Hypokalemia: • Often related to diuretic use • Diarrhea Hyperkalemia: • Renal failure • Medication side effect (ACEIs, angiotensin receptor blockers, aldosterone antagonists) • Rhabdomyolysis • Acidosis Hyponatremia • Volume overload • Medication side effect Hypernatremia • Dehydration
Coagulation profile Prothrombin time (PT) with international normalized ratio (INR), partial thromboplastin time (PTT), fibrinogen, D-dimer	PT/INR: Assess for coagulation with warfarin therapy, coagulopathy with hepatic congestion in heart failure. D-dimer: Assess for signs of increased fibrinolysis and determine level of suspicion for blood clots	Elevated PT/INR: • Anticoagulation • Hepatic vascular congestion • Liver failure Elevated D-dimer: • Presence of disease process or blood clot (an elevated D-dimer is a finding that must be further evaluated for life-threatening diagnoses such as pulmonary embolism).

Heart Failure

Continued

Diagnostic Tests for Acute Heart Failure—cont'd

Test	Purpose	Abnormal Findings
B-type natriuretic peptide (BNP) and pro-BNP	BNP is a hormone secreted by the ventricles in response to increased blood volume and subsequent stretch. The patient's baseline BNP level is helpful in determining current heart failure status. Serial BNP measurements in the hospitalized patient are not helpful in reducing mortality or improving outcomes.	Normal BNP: • Helpful in ruling out heart failure in a patient with heart failure symptoms Elevated BNP: • CHF • Acute renal failure • Sleep apnea • Hyperthyroid
Arterial blood gas (ABG) analysis	Assesses oxygenation, ventilation, and acid-base balance.	Hypoxemia: • Pulmonary edema • Pulmonary embolism Respiratory acidosis: (elevated CO_2, low pH) • Pulmonary edema • Pulmonary embolism • COPD exacerbation Respiratory alkalosis: • Hyperventilation Metabolic acidosis: • Hypo perfusion/shock (lactate level is helpful in assessing hypo perfusion) Metabolic alkalosis: • Excessive diuretic use
Hepatic enzymes and serum bilirubin levels	Serum glutamate oxaloacetate transaminase/aspartate aminotransferase (SGOT/AST) Serum glutamate pyruvate transaminase/alanine aminotransferase (SGPT/ALT) Serum bilirubin	Elevation: • Acute GI illness • Hepatic congestion resulting in increased hepatic enzymes and bilirubin.
Blood urea nitrogen (BUN) and creatinine levels	Assessment of renal function	Elevation: • Medication side effect (diuretics, ACEIs, angiotensin receptor blockers, aldosterone antagonists) • Chronic renal failure • Acute renal failure • Dehydration
Radiology		
Chest radiograph (CXR)	• Cardiac size and position • Thoracic cage • Lungs	Cardiac enlargement • Hypertension • Heart failure Thoracic cage • Fractures • Widened mediastinum (suggestive of aortic dissection) Lungs
Cardiac magnetic resonance imaging (MRI)	Assesses ventricular size, morphology, function, status of cardiac valves, and circulation.	• Enlarged or remodeled heart • Incompetent or stenotic heart valves • Narrowed or occluded coronary arteries • Myocarditis or pericarditis • Cardiac tumors

Diagnostic Tests for Acute Heart Failure—cont'd

Test	Purpose	Abnormal Findings
Cardiac computed tomography (CT scan)	Assesses ventricular size, morphology, function, status of cardiac valves, and circulation.	• Enlarged or remodeled heart • Incompetent or stenotic heart valves • Narrowed or occluded coronary arteries Chest CT can be used to diagnose pulmonary embolism and aortic dissection, but specific protocols must be used or these findings may be missed.
Transthoracic echocardiogram (cardiac ultrasound)	Mechanical and structural assessment of the heart. • Left and right ventricular function • Ventricular wall motion • Ventricular size • Valve function • Estimation of pulmonary artery pressures • Intracardiac thrombus or tumors • Pericardial effusion	Reduced ejection fraction: Heart failure Wall motion abnormality: • Myocardial infarction (acute or remote) • Conduction abnormality Valvular dysfunction • Stenosis or insufficiency of any of the cardiac valves Pulmonary hypertension: • COPD • Primary pulmonary hypertension • Pulmonary embolism • Left heart failure Intracardiac thrombus or tumor
Transesophageal echocardiogram	Similar to the transthoracic echocardiogram, but invasive as it uses an endoscope. Enhanced views of the heart valves and the posterior wall.	Same as transthoracic echocardiogram
Single photon emission computed tomography (SPECT)	A radioactive tracer is injected into the blood. Living heart muscle takes up the tracer. A camera picks up the signals from the tracer and pictures are created that show blood flow to the heart muscle. Cardiac wall motion and ejection fraction are also assessed. At rest, the viability of cardiac muscle can be assessed. A stress test involves the comparison of rest and stress (exercise- or chemical-induced) scans to determine cardiac ischemia with stress.	Reversible ischemia: • Viable areas of myocardium are not getting adequate blood flow with stress, suggestive of significant coronary artery disease Fixed ischemia: • Completed infarction, with blood flow absent in one or more areas of the heart at rest and with stress
Invasive Cardiology		
Coronary angiography/ cardiac catheterization	• Presence and extent of coronary artery disease • Left ventricular function • Valvular disease Uses a radiopaque catheter inserted through a peripheral vessel and advanced into the heart and coronary arteries	Reduced ejection fraction • Heart failure Impaired coronary blood flow: • Coronary artery disease • Coronary artery dissection Pulmonary hypertension Valvular disorders

Heart Failure

COLLABORATIVE MANAGEMENT

CARE PRIORITIES

1. Treat the underlying cause and precipitating factors

Initial therapy focuses on stabilizing the hemodynamic and respiratory status and searching for reversible causes of HF. Ischemic heart disease should always be considered in a patient with newly diagnosed heart failure. Use diagnostic tools including laboratory values and echocardiography to determine cardiac function and possible etiology (Table 5-3). The goals of long-term therapy focus on improvement of the quality of the patient's life and management of the compensatory mechanisms causing the patient's symptoms. Angiotensin converting enzyme inhibitors (ACEIs)/angiotensin receptor blockers (ARBs), and beta blockers have been shown to improve mortality and morbidity and are now the standard of care in patients with systolic HF.

2. Provide oxygen therapy and support ventilation

Supplemental oxygen is required to optimize the patient's oxygen saturation.

 Safety Alert *Pulse oximetry is done in combination with respiratory assessment, as use of pulse oximetry alone is an inaccurate reflection of efficacy of oxygenation at the cellular level. If patient is tachypneic with increased work of breathing, noninvasive positive pressure ventilation (NiPPV or NPPV; bilevel positive airway pressure [BiPAP]) may be used to reduce the work of breathing, and thus relieve additional stress associated with heart failure (see Acute Respiratory Failure, p. 383, for additional information regarding NiPPV, mechanical ventilation, and oxygen therapy).*

- Pulse oximetry (Spo_2): External monitoring of patient's hemoglobin saturation. Spo_2 does not provide information about ventilation and CO_2 retention

3. Provide evidence-based pharmacotherapy to help improve long-term prognosis, relieve symptoms, and promote stabilization during acute episodes

Medications help reduce intravascular volume, promote vasodilation to reduce resistance to ventricular ejection, and promote enhanced myocardial contractility. HF patients should have their medication regimen reviewed during hospitalization to ensure optimal medical therapy.

- **Evidence-Based Therapy to Improve Morbidity and Mortality in Systolic Dysfunction**
  - Beta-adrenergic blocking agents: The HF clinical guidelines specify the use of three beta blockers that have been shown to improve survival (carvedilol, metoprolol succinate, and bisoprolol). All stable patients with current or prior symptoms of HF and reduced EF should receive a beta blocker unless contraindicated. These drugs block the pathologic

Table 5-3	DIURETIC DOSING IN HEART FAILURE	
Type of Diuretic	**Generic (Trade Name) and Initial Dose**	**Usage Information**
Loop	Furosemide (Lasix) 20 mg	Given per os (PO) or intravenously (IV); PO dosage is doubled for the equivalent effect of IV dosing.
	Bumetanide (Bumex) 0.5 mg	PO and IV administrations result in the same effects from the same dosage.
	Torsemide (Demadex) 10 to 20 mg	Given PO or IV. Has the strongest PO effects of all loop diuretics.
	Ethacrynic acid (Edecrin) 50 mg	Given IV to patients who are allergic to furosemide or other loop diuretics.
Thiazide	Hydrochlorothiazide 12.5 mg	Given PO mainly to manage hypertension; can easily lead to hypokalemia, hyponatremia, and dehydration.
	Metolazone (Zaroxolyn) 2.5 mg	Given PO; should be given 30 minutes before furosemide if used together; has high incidence of hypokalemia.

effects of circulating catecholamines (epinephrine and norepinephrine) in patients with HF. Beta blockers reduce contractility and HR, resulting in decreased myocardial oxygen consumption and demand. While a reduction in HR and CO seems counterintuitive for a patient with HF, allowing the heart more time to fill and pump with each beat leads to more effective function. COPD is not a contraindication to beta-blocker therapy in patients without significant active wheezing. A cardioselective beta blocker such as metoprolol succinate or bisoprolol would be preferable in patients with a history of COPD. The combination of ACEI, diuretics, and beta blockers administered together may cause hypotension. Spacing medication administration and indicating clear "hold" parameters for BP in hospitalized patients can help to reduce this effect.

- ACEIs (benazepril, captopril, enalapril, fosinopril, lisinopril, perindopril, quinapril, ramipril, trandolapril): ACEIs affect the renin-angiotensin system by inhibiting the conversion of circulating angiotensin I into angiotensin II. They reduce remodeling, preload, and afterload to decrease the work of the ventricles. This results in increased CO and systemic tissue perfusion. Treatment with an ACEI has been shown to reduce mortality and HF symptoms while improving exercise tolerance and LVEF. All patients with an EF ≤ 40% should be treated with an ACEI unless they have a contraindication or intolerance. ACEIs are considered reasonable therapy and likely beneficial in all other patients with HF, regardless of EF. They help prevent HF in patients at high risk with atherosclerosis, diabetes mellitus, or hypertension with other cardiovascular risk factors. ACEI dose should be titrated to the maximum tolerated; however, 10% to 20% of patients are ACEI intolerant. The most troubling side effect from ACEIs is cough, which may prompt a change to an ARB or a combination of hydralazine and a nitrate. Most patients who cough on ACEIs are doing so because of HF rather than intolerance to the ACEI. Cough may disappear with increased diuresis. Development of either angioedema or acute renal failure requires that the drug be stopped immediately.

- ARBs (candesartan, eprosartan, irbesartan, olmesartan, losartan, telmisartan): ARBs have been shown in clinical trials to be noninferior to ACE inhibitors for patients with HF. The clinical guidelines indicate that patients who are ACEI intolerant can be placed on ARB therapy. ARBs do not cause the side effects of cough or angioedema, but they do have similar contraindications in renal failure and hyperkalemia.

- Aldosterone antagonists (spironolactone, eplerenone): Aldosterone inhibition reduces sodium and water retention, endothelial dysfunction, and myocardial fibrosis. Hyperkalemia is a significant potential side effect of aldosterone blockade. Serum potassium levels must be closely monitored, and the medications should not be used in patients with impaired renal function. When added to baseline therapy of a beta blocker and ACEI/ARB, aldosterone antagonists have been shown to improve HF morbidity and mortality in patients with moderately severe to severe symptoms of HF. The newest clinical guidelines outline the role of aldosterone antagonists in HF. These agents should not be used in patients who will not undergo close monitoring of renal function and potassium levels as part of outpatient management, or those with creatinine greater than 2.5 mg/dL.

- Hydralazine and isosorbide dinitrate: The combination of hydralazine and isosorbide dinitrate is shown to reduce morbidity and mortality in specific patient populations. Patients who self-identify as African American benefit from the addition of hydralazine and isosorbide dinitrate to beta blocker and ACEI/ARB therapy. In patients who are unable to take ACEI/ARB medications caused by renal insufficiency or hyperkalemia, hydralazine with isosorbide dinitrate is an alternative therapy.

- **Symptom Management in Heart Failure:**
  - Diuretics: Reduce blood volume and decrease preload. Diuretics effectively manage respiratory distress caused by pulmonary edema, but have not been shown to improve survival in HF patients. Diuretics are the only medications used in HF therapy that can control the retention of fluid. Diuretic therapy should be used in conjunction with evidence-based HF therapy (including beta blocker and ACEI/ARB.) A loop diuretic is first-line for patients with volume overload, while thiazide diuretics may be beneficial in patients with significant hypertension (Table 5-1). Diuretics may cause azotemia, hypokalemia, metabolic alkalosis, hypotension, and elevation of neurohormone (e.g., BNP) levels. See Table 5-3 for diuretic dosing.

- Digoxin: Slows HR, giving the ventricles more time to fill, strengthens contractions, and improves CO. Digoxin may be prescribed for patients with LV end-systolic dimension who remain symptomatic on standard therapy, especially if they develop atrial fibrillation. Digoxin controls ventricular response in atrial fibrillation without decreasing BP. Digoxin is excreted by the kidneys, and so is used cautiously in patients with impaired renal function. Bradycardia and heart block are contraindications to digoxin therapy.
- Inodilators (milrinone and inamrinone): Phosphodiesterase-inhibiting drugs increase myocardial contractility and lower SVR through vasodilation. This allows the failing heart to pump against less pressure (reduced afterload), resulting in increased CO. Milrinone is used for hypotensive patients with low-CO HF and pulmonary hypertension. It is a more potent pulmonary vasodilator than dobutamine. Milrinone is superior to dobutamine for patients on chronic oral beta-blocker therapy who develop acute hypotensive HF.
- Morphine: Used to reduce anxiety and relieve distress in patients with pulmonary edema. Morphine has been associated with poorer outcomes in patients with acute decompensated HF. Morphine is used in end-stage HF to relieve the symptoms of severe pulmonary edema.
- Vasodilators: Used for the management of dyspnea and volume overload in patients with stable BP. Vasodilators do not improve morbidity or mortality in HF.
  - Intravenous nitroglycerin (NTG) is beneficial in patients with hypertension, coronary ischemia, or severe mitral regurgitation. Nitroprusside reduces preload and afterload, and is beneficial in patients with severe hypertension or mitral regurgitation.
  - Nitroprusside can induce significant hypotension and must be titrated carefully. Nitroprusside is ideally used only for a short time in patients with advanced renal disease to avoid thiocyanate toxicity, resulting from an accumulation of this byproduct of the hepatic metabolism of nitroprusside. Nitroprusside should also be avoided in patients with ACS because it may cause coronary steal syndrome, which shunts blood away from the ischemic myocardium to better-perfused muscle.
  - Nesiritide is a vasodilator that has demonstrated no impact on hospitalizations, mortality, or renal failure. The longer half-life of nesiritide increases the chance for prolonged hypotension.

4. Manage acute pulmonary edema; include the following immediate interventions
- Monitor for signs and symptoms of acute respiratory failure
- Titrate supplemental oxygen to maintain adequate oxygenation
- Provide NiPPV for patients with increased work of breathing
- Elevate head of bed (HOB) as needed to promote oxygenation
- If NiPPV is unsuccessful, consider endotracheal (ET) intubation with mechanical ventilation (see Acute Respiratory Failure, Chapter 4).
- Diuretic therapy: In severely ill patients, furosemide or bumetanide may be used as continuous IV infusion to assist with constant fluid removal. Patients with renal impairment/failure may require infusions of appropriate diuretics.
- In patients refractory to diuretic therapy, ultrafiltration may be utilized for isotonic fluid removal.
- Pharmacologic therapy, including continuous IV infusions of inotropic agents, vasodilators, beta blockers, and IV morphine. If CS ensues, vasopressors and intra-aortic balloon pumping (IABP) may also be necessary. Adjustment or discontinuation of medications that affect renal function (such as ACEI/ARB) should be considered in patients with worsening BUN/creatinine.

5. Initiate a low-cholesterol and low-sodium diet
- Extra salt and water are held in the circulatory system, causing increased strain on the heart. Limiting sodium (Table 5-4) will reduce the amount of fluid retained by the body. In addition, fluids may be limited to 1500 to 2000 mL/day in patients who are hyponatremic.

6. Consider an implanted cardiac device
- Implanted cardioverter defibrillator (ICD): Systolic dysfunction places patients at increased risk of sudden cardiac death. Implantation of an ICD is indicated for patients

Table 5-4	REDUCING DIETARY SODIUM
Foods High in Sodium*	**Foods Low in Sodium**
Beans and frankfurters	Bread
Bouillon cubes	Cereal (dry or hot); read labels
Canned or packaged soups	Fresh fish, chicken, turkey, veal, beef, and lamb
Canned, smoked, or salted meats; salted fish	
Dill pickles	Fresh fruits and vegetables
Fried chicken dinners and other fast foods	Fresh or dried herbs
Monosodium glutamate (e.g., Accent)	Gelatin desserts
Olives	Oil, salt-free margarine
Packaged snack foods	Peanut butter
Pancake or waffle mix	Tabasco sauce
Processed cheese	Low-salt tuna packed in water
Seasoned salts (e.g., celery, onion, garlic)	
Sauerkraut	
Soy sauce	
Vegetables in brine or cans	
Additional suggestions	
Do not add table salt to foods.	Do not buy convenience foods; remember that fresh is best.
Season with fresh or dried herbs.	Read all labels for salt, sodium, and sodium chloride content.
Avoid salts or powders that contain salt.	

*Many of these foods now are available in low-salt or salt-free versions

with LVEF ≤35% and HF symptoms. Patients must be on optimal medical therapy and at least 40 days post-MI before implantation. (In some instances, LVEF will improve with medical therapy and/or treatment of CAD.) ICD therapy has been shown to significantly reduce mortality in patients with reduced LVEF. Patients should have a life expectancy of at least 1 year before implantation. In patients with end-stage HF symptoms who have an ICD in place, the decision can be made to deactivate the defibrillator to avoid unnecessary discomfort at end of life.

- Cardiac resynchronization therapy (CRT): Approximately one third of HF patients develop a widened QRS complex, indicating asynchronous ventricular function. Implantation of biventricular pacing allows coordination of the right and left ventricles. CRT is indicated for patients with LVEF ≤35%, and a QRS duration of 150 ms or greater with HF symptoms. CRT can improve contractility and EF, and decrease cardiac remodeling. CRT can be combined with an ICD as a single device if the patient meets the requirements for both therapies.

7. Initiate advanced heart failure therapy

- Patients with advanced HF are defined as those with refractory symptoms despite optimal goal-directed medical therapy. Indicators of advanced HF include two or more hospitalizations for HF in the past year, progressive renal dysfunction, and intolerance of evidence-based medical therapy caused by hypotension or renal failure.
- Inotropic agents: Dopamine, dobutamine, and milrinone are inotropic agents used to treat advanced HF. Inotropes may be used acutely in the patient with CS or as a bridge to transplant or other advanced therapy. Inotropic therapy may also be used as a palliative measure in patients with end-stage HF for symptom relief. Although hemodynamic status may be improved with inotropes, there is no demonstrated improvement in patient

outcomes with their use. Inotropic therapy should only be used in patients with severe hemodynamic compromise and evidence of systemic hypoperfusion. Medications should be titrated to the lowest dose needed to obtain clinical improvement.

- LV assist devices (LVADs): Some patients with CS unresponsive to intraaortic balloon counterpulsation and IV inotrope therapy may be referred for mechanical circulatory support. LVADs may be used as a bridge to cardiac transplantation or as a destination therapy for those ineligible for transplant. The inflow cannula of an LVAD is connected to the apex of the left ventricle. Blood is pumped by the device via the outflow cannula to the aorta. Complications include stroke, infection, coagulopathy with bleeding, multiple organ dysfunction syndrome (MODS), and prosthetic valve insufficiency. Most modern LVADs have continuous flow, leaving the patient without a palpable pulse despite adequate perfusion.
- Cardiac transplantation: Indicated for end-stage HF patients with symptoms refractory to guideline-based medical therapy. Cardiac transplantation has been shown to improve symptoms and quality of life. Patients are not transplant candidates if they have significant comorbidities including pulmonary hypertension, active infection, significant psychosocial issues, or history of medical noncompliance. Following cardiac transplantation, patients must maintain lifelong immunosuppression to prevent rejection, which places them at high risk for opportunistic infections and malignancies.

8. Patient education and psychosocial support

- Self-care: HF patients should be educated on self-care of their HF. This education includes daily weight monitoring, symptom management, follow-up care, and dietary and medication compliance.
- Advance directives: Patients with advanced HF should have a discussion about plan of care, including resuscitation status.
- Palliative care: Care to manage physical and psychosocial symptoms of HF should be incorporated in conjunction with goal-directed medical therapy. In patients with advanced HF who enter palliative or hospice care, evidence-based therapy such as beta blockers, ACEIs, and symptom management should be continued to prevent abrupt worsening of clinical condition.

CARE PLANS FOR HEART FAILURE

EXCESS FLUID VOLUME *related to compromised regulatory mechanism secondary to decreased cardiac output.*

Goals/Outcomes: Within 24 hours of treatment, the patient becomes normovolemic as evidenced by absence of adventitious lung sounds, decreased peripheral edema, increased urine output, and weight loss. In patients with advanced hemodynamic monitoring, goals include PAWP less than 18 mm Hg, SVR less than 1200 dynes/sec/cm^{-5}, and CO greater than 4 L/min.

NOC Fluid Overload Severity; Fluid Balance; Electrolyte and Acid-Base Balance

Fluid/Electrolyte Management
1. Pulmonary edema: Auscultate lung fields for presence of crackles and rhonchi or other adventitious sounds.
2. Decreased renal perfusion: Monitor I&O closely. Report positive fluid state or decrease in urine output to less than 0.5 mL/kg/h.
3. Third spaced fluid: Weigh patient daily; report increases in weight. An acute gain in weight of 1 kg can signal a 1 L gain in fluid.
4. Note changes from baseline assessment to detect worsening of HF, such as increased pedal edema, increased jugular venous distention, development of S_3 heart sound or new murmur, and dysrhythmias.
5. Monitor hemodynamic status every 1 to 2 hours and on an as-needed basis. Note response to drug therapy as well as indicators of the need for more aggressive therapy, including increasing PAWP and SVR and decreasing CO.
6. Administer medications as prescribed.
7. Fluid restriction as prescribed, particularly for patients with hyponatremia

NIC Invasive Hemodynamic Monitoring; Medication Management; Nutrition Counseling; Surveillance; Teaching: Disease Process; Hemodialysis Therapy

DECREASED CO *related to disease process that has resulted in decreased ability of the heart to provide adequate pumping to maintain effective oxygenation and nutrition of body systems.*

Goals/Outcomes: Within 24 hours of initiating treatment, the patient has attained a cardiac index (CI) of at least 2.0, PAP is reduced to within 10% of patient's normal baseline, BP has stabilized to within 10% of baseline, and HR is controlled to within 10% of normal baseline.

NOC Cardiac Pump Effectiveness; Circulation Status

Cardiac Care: Acute Hemodynamic Regulation
1. Manage CO: Monitor cardiac rhythm and rate continuously. Control tachycardia as soon as possible with beta blockers or other appropriate measures as determined by the physician and ACLS guidelines.
2. Obtain 12/15/18-lead ECG to assess new dysrhythmias or profound instability.
3. Monitor CO, CI, pulmonary and systemic vascular pressures, and other hemodynamic values at least hourly, as appropriate. Implement continuous CO and Svo_2 monitoring if available.
4. Decreased cerebral perfusion: Monitor neurologic status to assess for adequate cerebral perfusion.
5. Decreased renal perfusion: During periods of instability, monitor renal function (BUN and creatinine) daily.
6. Hepatic congestion: Monitor liver function (SGOT/AST, SGPT/ALT, and/or bilirubin), as appropriate.
7. Oxygen delivery: Monitor the other determinants of oxygen delivery, including level of hemoglobin (Hgb) and oxygen saturation.
8. IABP may be necessary; prepare needed equipment for insertion of the balloon catheter and implementation of pumping.
9. If the patient has atrial fibrillation, ensure that appropriate anticoagulants or antiplatelet agents to prevent thrombus formation are given.

NIC Cardiac Care: Acute; Circulatory Care: Mechanical Assist Device; Hemodynamic Regulation; Shock Management: Cardiac; Neurologic Monitoring; Medication Management; Dysrhythmia Management

IMPAIRED GAS EXCHANGE *related to alveolar-capillary membrane changes secondary to fluid collection in the alveoli and interstitial spaces.*

Goals/Outcomes: Within 24 hours of initiation of treatment, the patient has improved gas exchange as evidenced by Pao_2 at least 80 mm Hg, RR 12 to 20 breaths/min with normal pattern and depth, and absence of adventitious breath sounds.

NOC Respiratory Status: Gas Exchange; Mechanical Ventilation Response: Adult

Respiratory Monitoring
1. Monitor respiratory rate, rhythm, and character every 1 to 2 hours. Be alert to RR greater than 20 breaths/min, irregular rhythm, use of accessory muscles of respiration, or cough.
2. Auscultate breath sounds, noting presence of crackles, wheezes, and other adventitious sounds.
3. Provide supplemental oxygen as prescribed and titrate to Spo_2 of 90% or greater.
4. Monitor Spo_2 for decreases to less than 90%.
5. Assess ABG findings; note changes in response to oxygen supplementation or treatment of altered hemodynamics.
6. Suction patient's secretions as needed.
7. Establish a protocol for deep breathing, coughing, and turning every 2 hours.
8. Place patient in semi-Fowler or high-Fowler position to maximize chest excursion.
9. If mechanical ventilation is necessary, monitor ventilator settings, endotracheal tube function and position, and respiratory status.

NIC Airway Management; Anxiety Reduction; Cardiac Care: Acute; Medication Management; Oxygen Therapy; Respiratory Monitoring

ACTIVITY INTOLERANCE *related to imbalance between oxygen supply and demand secondary to decreased functioning of the myocardium.*

Goals/Outcomes: Within the 12- to 24-hour period before discharge from the critical care unit, the patient exhibits cardiac tolerance to increasing levels of activity as evidenced by RR less than 24 breaths/min, NSR on ECG, and HR 120 bpm or less (or within 20 bpm of resting HR).

NOC Activity Tolerance; Energy Conservation

Heart Failure

Energy Management
1. Balance rest and activity: Maintain prescribed activity level, and teach the patient the rationale for activity limitation. Organize nursing care so that periods of activity are interspersed with extended periods of uninterrupted rest.
2. To help prevent complications of immobility, assist patient with active/passive range-of-motion exercises, as appropriate. Encourage the patient to do as much as possible within prescribed activity allowances.
3. Activity intolerance: Note patient's physiologic response to activity, including BP, HR, RR, and heart rhythm. Signs of activity intolerance include chest pain, increasing shortness of breath (SOB), excessive fatigue, increased dysrhythmias, palpitations, HR response greater than 120 bpm, systolic BP greater than 20 mm Hg from baseline or greater than 160 mm Hg, and ST-segment changes. If activity intolerance is noted, instruct patient to stop the activity and rest.
4. Blood pressure: Administer medications as prescribed, and note their effect on patient's activity tolerance.
5. Physical therapy: As needed to help prevent muscle loss and wasting, refer patient to physical therapy department.

NIC Activity Therapy; Energy Management; Teaching: Prescribed Activity/Exercise; Dysrhythmia Management; Pain Management; Medication Management

DEFICIENT KNOWLEDGE *related to disease process with HF; need to stop smoking, if applicable; activity requirements and limitations; need for daily weight log; symptoms to report; prescribed diet and fluid restriction and medications.*

Goals/Outcomes: Within the 24-hour period before discharge from the critical care unit, the patient and significant others verbalize understanding of the disease, as well as the prescribed diet and medication regimens.
NOC Knowledge: Cardiac Disease Management

Teaching: Disease Process
1. Pathophysiology: Using appropriate language, teach the patient the physiologic process of HF and how fluid volume increases because of poor heart function.
2. Smoking cessation: Teach the patient about the adverse effects of smoking and how smoking cessation may benefit him or her. Provide information about smoking cessation classes and nicotine patches and medications prescribed to help people stop smoking, such as varenicline and bupropion.
3. Restrict sodium: Teach the patient about the importance of a low-sodium diet to help reduce volume overload. Provide him with a list of foods that are high and low in sodium. Teach patient how to read and evaluate food labels.
4. Fluid volume excess: Teach the patient the signs and symptoms of fluid volume excess that necessitate medical attention: irregular or slow pulse, increased SOB, orthopnea, decreased exercise tolerance, and steady weight gain ($\geq$1 kg/day for 2 successive days). The importance of daily weights should be stressed.
5. Daily weight: Advise the patient about the need to keep a journal of daily weight. Explain that an increase of $\geq$1 kg/day on 2 successive days of normal eating necessitates notification of advanced practice provider.
6. Device management: Teach the patient how to manage any advanced therapy that may be used, e.g., biventricular pacemaker or internal cardiac defibrillator, ventricular assist device (VAD), or heart transplant.
7. Activity tolerance: Instruct the patient regarding the prescribed activity progression after hospital discharge, signs of activity intolerance that signal the need for rest, and the need to report worsening symptoms with activity to their physician. General activity guidelines are as follows:
   - Get up and get dressed every morning.
   - Weigh yourself before breakfast.
   - Space your meals and activities to allow time for rest and relaxation.
   - Perform activities at a comfortable, moderate pace. If you get tired during any activity, stop to rest for 15 minutes before resuming.
   - Avoid activities that require straining or lifting.
   - Plan at least 30 minutes of exercise on most days of the week
   - Warning signals to stop your activity and rest: chest pain, SOB, dizziness or faintness, unusual weakness.

NIC Cardiac Care: Rehabilitation; Exercise Promotion; Smoking Cessation Assistance; Teaching: Prescribed Activity/Exercise; Emotional Support; Progressive Muscle Relaxation; Weight Management; Mutual Goal Setting; Teaching: Prescribed Diet; Teaching: Prescribed Medication

ADDITIONAL NURSING DIAGNOSES

Also see nursing diagnoses and interventions in Hemodynamic Monitoring (Chapter 1), Prolonged Immobility (Chapter 1), and Emotional and Spiritual Support of the Patient and Significant Others (Chapter 2).

ACUTE CORONARY SYNDROME

PATHOPHYSIOLOGY

Acute coronary syndrome (ACS) consists of diagnoses related to myocardial ischemia, a decrease in blood flow through the coronary arteries that results in insufficient perfusion of the myocardium. ACS includes unstable angina (UA), non-ST-elevation myocardial infarction (NSTEMI), and ST-segment elevation myocardial infarction (STEMI). Angina pectoris, or angina as it is commonly called, is chest discomfort or pain associated with myocardial ischemia. Angina may be caused by reduced coronary blood flow as a result of vessel lumen narrowing by plaque or vasospasm. It can also occur when perfusion pressure is low, as in sudden hypotension, or when there is increased myocardial workload, as in aortic stenosis caused by the tremendous resistance to ejection created by the narrowed aortic valve. Dysrhythmias may also cause chest discomfort caused by either increased workload (e.g., with tachycardias) or coronary perfusion deficit (e.g., with bradycardias). If the chest pain has a predictable pattern, such as being triggered by increased demand as in exertion (e.g., exercise), it is considered stable. Those with chest pain or chest discomfort that occurs at rest or with normal activity, as well as with exertion, have UA. There is also a variant form of angina, called Prinzmetal angina, which is caused by vasospasm of the coronary arteries.

Acute myocardial infarction (AMI), either ST elevation or non-ST elevation, results from necrosis of myocardial tissue caused by relative or absolute lack of blood supply to the myocardium. Most AMIs are caused by atherosclerosis, which results in plaque formation within the coronary arteries. Plaque deposition results in endothelial changes, which over time cause narrowing of the lumen of the coronary artery. If an unstable plaque ruptures, the immune system responds with localized inflammation: platelets aggregate at the site of the injured plaque, and a thrombus forms. If the lesion is large enough to fill the vessel lumen, this process results in total occlusion of blood flow. Occlusion can also be caused by coronary artery vasospasm. The site of the MI is determined by the location of the arterial occlusion. In addition to known biomarkers that are used to diagnose MI, novel biomarkers to help predict plaque instability that can lead to ACS are being researched.

American Heart Association (AHA)/American College of Cardiology (ACC) standards recommend treatment protocols for three types of ACSs: UA, MI with ST-segment elevation (STEMI), and MI without ST-segment elevation (NSTEMI or non-STEMI). Patients with STEMI evolve to an ECG with Q waves. Infarcts with Q waves are larger, although Q waves resolve in 15% of STEMIs. ECGs in patients with NSTEMIs do not show Q waves. The type of clot present in the coronary artery may determine the type of event that evolves. Platelet-rich clots often result in UA or NSTEMI, but as the rupture of the plaque leads to thrombus formation, it may result in a STEMI.

The cause of acute chest pain may not be related to myocardial ischemia. Differential diagnosis of cardiac pain versus other origins is critical and can challenge the most experienced clinician. Extracardiac causes of chest pain include pulmonary embolus, pneumonia, bronchitis, pneumothorax, pleurisy, aortic arch or high thoracic aortic aneurysm, esophagitis, esophageal motility disorders, hiatal hernia, cholecystitis, cholelithiasis, gastroesophageal reflux disease, costochondritis, musculoskeletal strain, anemia, hypoglycemia, fractured ribs or sternum, thyroid disease, anxiety disorder, obstipation, and bowel obstruction. Cardiac causes of chest pain not directly related to ischemia include valvular disease, aortic dissection, cardiac trauma, cardiac tamponade, pericarditis, and endocarditis.

The diagnostic process should initially focus on ruling out MI. It is the most common cause of severe, unrelieved chest pain and requires immediate intervention to minimize loss of myocardium. Left unchecked, patients with large areas of necrosis can progress to cardiogenic shock (CS) quickly. The patient's history and physical examination provide the initial framework for treatment decisions, coupled with the initial diagnostic ECG and assessment of serum biomarkers. If MI does not appear likely from these findings, differential diagnosis of chest pain should then focus on identification of other life-threatening events such as dissecting thoracic or aortic arch aneurysms, large pulmonary embolism, or cardiac tamponade.

Acute Coronary Syndrome

CARDIOVASCULAR ASSESSMENT: ACUTE CORONARY SYNDROME
GOAL OF SYSTEM ASSESSMENT
- Evaluate for decreased CO and decreased tissue perfusion initially with General Assessment, (Chapter 4).

HISTORY AND RISK FACTORS
- Family history of CAD, age older than 70 years, male sex, postmenopausal females, cigarette smoking, dyslipidemia, hypertension, hyperglycemia, increased waist circumference, diabetes, obesity, increased stress, sedentary lifestyle.

CHEST PAIN: ANGINA
- May result from exertion or emotional stress
- Onset can be abrupt or gradual
- Stable angina: Gradually increases in severity during episodes over several months; does not occur with rest; subsides gradually with rest
  - Lasts for 1 to 4 minutes; can last up to 30 minutes
  - Should be relieved by NTG in 45 to 90 seconds
- Unstable angina: Pain that has changed significantly from past patterns and can occur at rest; includes Wellens syndrome (left anterior descending coronary artery lesion), rest angina, preinfarction (crescendo) angina (may cause slight ST elevation and increased troponin level), Prinzmetal angina (from coronary artery vasospasms at rest), and new-onset angina
- Most common feelings: Substernal pressure, chest tightness, heaviness or squeezing in the chest
- Extreme pain: Crushing substernal chest pain radiating down the left arm, or up to the jaw with shortness of breath
- Variations: Jaw or arm pain only, shoulder pain, right- or left-sided chest discomfort, pain in the teeth, nausea, epigastric pain, syncope, extreme sudden fatigue, or SOB
- No pain: Does not rule out ischemia; common in elders, women, and diabetics

CHEST PAIN: ACUTE MYOCARDIAL INFARCTION
- Onset can be abrupt or gradual
- Does not subside with rest
- Lasts for longer than 30 minutes
- NOT relieved by sublingual NTG
- Most common feelings: Continuous substernal pressure, chest tightness, heaviness, or squeezing in the chest
- Extreme pain: Continuous crushing substernal chest pain radiating down the left arm or up to the jaw, nausea, vomiting, SOB, orthopnea, anxiety, apprehension, diaphoresis, cyanosis, syncope, stroke-like symptoms
- Variations: Jaw or arm pain only, shoulder pain, right- or left-sided chest discomfort, pain in the teeth, epigastric pain
- No pain: Does not rule out infarction; 25% of MIs are "silent" or without pain; common in older adults, women, and diabetic persons who may feel extreme, sudden-onset fatigue rather than pain

12-LEAD ELECTROCARDIOGRAM: ANGINA AND ACUTE MYOCARDIAL INFARCTION
- Compare current ECG with past ECG
- Angina: Review for ST-segment depression in at least two contiguous leads, which indicates myocardial ischemia
- AMI: Review for ST-segment elevation in at least two contiguous leads, which indicates active myocardial damage (acute infarction); Q waves may or may not form
- Evaluate pacing and conduction: Rhythm regularity, rate, and conduction velocity (PR, QRS, QT intervals)
- Dysrhythmias: New bundle branch block (especially left) is diagnostic for MI; sinus bradycardia, atrioventricular (AV) heart blocks, and ventricular ectopy may also be present

VITAL SIGNS
- Possible fever in patients with AMI

- BP may increase or decrease, depending on sympathetic nervous system (SNS) response to change in CO
- HR may increase or decrease depending on SNS response and ensuing damage to the conduction pathway, hypoxia; SNS response is blunted by beta-adrenergic blocking agents

OBSERVATION
Evaluate for facial and lip pallor, ashen or diaphoretic appearance of skin, ashen or cyanotic nail beds, and edema (especially in dependent areas) to determine decreased tissue perfusion
- Instruct patient to report any discomfort immediately
- Evaluate telemetry for dysrhythmias

PALPATION
Pulse amplitude may be increased or decreased, depending on SNS response; evaluate for:
- Pulse quality and regularity bilaterally (scale 0 to 4+)
- Edema (scale 0 to 4+): extremities and sacrum
- Slow capillary refill (longer than 2 seconds)

AUSCULTATION
Heart sounds to evaluate for contributors to decreased CO (note changes with body positioning and respirations):
- S_1 and/or S_2 split indicative of altered conduction
- S_3 indicative of HF (systolic)
- S_4 indicative of HF (diastolic)
- Murmurs, clicks indicative of valve disease
- Friction rub indicative of pericarditis

LABWORK
Blood studies can indicate MI and reveal causes of dysrhythmias or changes in pacing/conduction or HR changes:
- Cardiac enzymes/isoenzymes: Elevated troponin, CPK-MB if MI has occurred
- Complete blood counts: Possible anemia, ↑WBCs
- Electrolyte levels: ↑ or ↓ potassium or magnesium
- BNP: Elevated if HF is present
- Levels of cardiac medications (digoxin): Low levels may reveal noncompliance with ordered medications

Diagnostic Tests for Acute Coronary Syndrome		
Test	**Purpose**	**Abnormal Findings**
Noninvasive Cardiology		
12-, 15-, and 18-lead electrocardiogram (ECG): must be obtained during an episode of chest pain for full benefit of help with diagnosis; should be done in a series to view evolving changes; may not reveal changes if not during an episode of chest pain.	Assess for ischemic heart disease and acute or older myocardial infarction (MI); helps identify ST-segment elevation MI (STEMI) versus non-ST-segment elevation MI (NSTEMI); frames needed for antiplatelet drugs versus thrombin inhibitors versus thrombolytic drugs or percutaneous coronary intervention (PCI) for STEMI.	Presence of ST segment depression or T wave inversion (myocardial ischemia), ST elevation (acute MI), new bundle branch block (especially left BBB) or pathologic Q waves (resolving/resolved MI) in 2 contiguous or related leads. Contiguous leads indicative of location of ischemia or infarction: *V1 and V2:* Intraventricular septum *V3 and V4:* Anterior wall of left ventricle *V5 and V6:* Lateral wall of left ventricle *V7 to V9:* Posterior wall of left ventricle *II, III, AVF:* Inferior wall of left ventricle *V1, V2, V1R to V6R:* Right ventricle

Continued

Acute Coronary Syndrome

Diagnostic Tests for Acute Coronary Syndrome — cont'd

Test	Purpose	Abnormal Findings
Stress tests Stress test on a treadmill with or without nuclear imaging Pharmacologic stress test with nuclear imaging	Assess for cardiac ischemia by monitoring ECG changes and chest pain during exercise on a treadmill. Done once MI has been ruled out. Adenosine or dobutamine is injected intravenously, used for patients who cannot walk on a treadmill. Thallium or technetium is injected intravenously and scan is done following the exercise/injection of medication to further assess for ischemic areas.	ST depression on ECG, chest pain during exercise. Abnormal thallium/technetium scan does not accumulate normally in ischemic or infarcted areas (cold spots) of the heart. A single photon emission computed tomography (SPECT) camera is used.
Stress echocardiography	Assess for cardiac ischemia by monitoring ECG changes and chest pain during exercise on a treadmill. Can be done using dobutamine for patients who cannot walk on a treadmill. Done once MI has been ruled out. Echocardiography is done immediately before and after treadmill test. Assess myocardial perfusion to determine areas of infarction and ischemia.	Wall motion abnormalities that correspond to areas of ischemia or infarction are noted on echocardiography.
Blood Studies		
Serial cardiac enzymes CK-MB Troponin I Troponin T	Assess for enzyme changes indicative of myocardial tissue damage; diagnostic for MI; should be done at least every 8 hours during the first 24 hours following severe chest pain.	Elevated enzymes reflect muscle damage; if CK-MB and troponins are elevated, MI has occurred. *CK-MB:* Elevation begins in 3 to 12 hours, peaks at 24 hours, subsides in 48 to 72 hours. *Troponin I:* Elevation begins in 3 to 12 hours, peaks at 24 hours, subsides 5 to 10 days. Tropon*in T:* Elevation begins in 3 to 12 hours, peaks at 12 to 48 hours, subsides 5 to 10 days.
Complete blood count (CBC) Hemoglobin (Hgb) Hematocrit (Hct) RBC count (RBCs) WBC count (WBCs)	Assess for anemia, inflammation and infection; assists with differential diagnosis of chest pain.	Decreased RBCs, Hgb, or Hct reflects anemia, which exacerbates chest pain; MI may increase WBCs.
Electrolytes Potassium (K^+) Magnesium (Mg^2) Calcium (Ca^{2+}) Sodium (Na^+)	Assess for possible causes of dysrhythmias and/or heart failure.	Decrease in K^+, Mg^{2+}, or Ca^{2+} may cause dysrhythmias; elevation of Na^+ may indicate dehydration (blood is more coagulable); low Na^+ may indicate fluid retention and/or heart failure.
Coagulation profile Prothrombin time (PT) with international normalized ratio (INR) Partial thromboplastin time (PTT) Fibrinogen D-dimer	Assess for causes of bleeding, clotting, and disseminated intravascular coagulation (DIC) indicative of abnormal clotting present in shock or ensuing shock.	Decreased PT with low INR promotes clotting; elevation promotes bleeding; elevated fibrinogen and D-dimer reflect abnormal clotting.

Diagnostic Tests for Acute Coronary Syndrome—cont'd

Test	Purpose	Abnormal Findings
B-type natriuretic peptide (BNP)	Assess for heart failure.	Elevation indicates heart failure is present.
Lipid profile and lipoprotein-cholesterol fractionation Total cholesterol High-density lipoprotein (HDL) cholesterol Low-density lipoprotein (LDL) cholesterol Very-low-density lipoprotein (VLDL) cholesterol Triglycerides	Assess for causes of arterial plaque formation contributing to coronary artery disease (CAD). Total cholesterol measures circulating levels of free cholesterol and cholesterol esters. Triglycerides assess storage form of lipids.	Elevation of total cholesterol, LDL, VLDL, and triglycerides indicates a greater potential for developing CAD; elevated HDL lowers probability of CAD. New guidelines recommend moderate- versus high-dose statins based on risk factors rather than targeting a specific LDL goal.
C-reactive protein (CRP)	Assess for inflammation of coronary plaque.	Elevation places patients at higher risk for acute MI.
Homocysteine	Assess for potential of accelerated plaque formation.	Elevation places patients at higher risk for acute MI.
Radiology		
Chest radiograph (CXR)	Assess size of heart, thoracic cage (for fractures), thoracic aorta (for aneurysm) and lungs (pneumonia, pneumothorax); assists with differential diagnosis of chest pain.	Cardiac enlargement, increased vascular markings, and bilateral infiltrates reflect heart failure (pulmonary edema).
Magnetic resonance imaging (MRI) Cardiac MRI Cardiac MR angiography (MRA)	Assesses ventricular size, morphology, function, status of cardiac valves and blood vessels Contrast is injected intravenously	Enlarged heart, remodeled heart, incompetent stenotic heart valves, narrowed or occluded coronary arteries
Computed tomography (CT) Cardiac CT scan Cardiac CT angiography (CTA)	Assesses ventricular size, morphology, function, status of cardiac valves and blood vessels Contrast is injected intravenously	Enlarged heart, remodeled heart, incompetent stenotic heart valves, narrowed or occluded coronary arteries; technology is improving in accuracy
Echocardiogram (echo)	Assess for mechanical and structural abnormalities related to all four heart chambers and valves.	Abnormal ventricular wall movement or motion, low ejection fraction, incompetent or stenosed heart valves, abnormal intracardiac chamber pressures
Transesophageal echocardiogram (TEE)	Assess for mechanical and structural abnormalities related to all four heart chambers and valves using a transducer attached to an endoscope.	As above but can provide enhanced views, particularly of the posterior wall of the heart. Especially useful in obese patients or patients with COPD where it is difficult to get adequate views because of body habitus.
Positron emission tomography (PET) scan, cardiac	Isotopes are used to assess for infarct and/or ischemia.	Decreased viability. Can be used in conjunction with pharmacologic stress testing or with cardiac CT

Acute Coronary Syndrome

Continued

Diagnostic Tests for Acute Coronary Syndrome — cont'd

Test	Purpose	Abnormal Findings
Invasive Cardiology		
Coronary angiography cardiac catheterization	Assesses for presence and extent of CAD, left ventricular function, and valvular disease using a radiopaque catheter inserted through a peripheral vessel and advanced into the heart and coronary arteries.	Low ejection fraction indicates heart failure, stenotic or incompetent heart valves can decrease CO, narrowed or occluded coronary arteries cause chest pain and impaired circulation, elevated pressures inside the chambers of the heart indicate heart failure, abnormal ventricular wall motion decreases CO, and elevated pulmonary artery pressures indicate heart failure. Test is used to prescribe the most appropriate treatment: medical management, stents, or cardiac surgery.

ELECTROCARDIOGRAPHIC MONITORING AND INTERPRETATION
First ECG
The first ECG is done immediately upon complaint of chest pain and is used as part of the process to differentiate STEMI from NSTEMI/UA or other causes of chest pain and to help determine diagnosis. It is also helpful in determining the possible need for thrombolytic therapy or percutaneous coronary intervention (PCI) for STEMI or antiplatelet medications for patients with NSTEMI/UA. Reperfusion strategies should be implemented immediately for STEMI patients.

Standard 12-lead ECG
The standard 12-lead ECG is designed for evaluation of the anterior, inferior, and lateral walls of the left ventricle. Infarcts that extend to the right ventricle and/or the posterior wall of the left ventricle cannot be clearly detected by the 12-lead ECG.

15- to 18-lead ECG
Indications for performing additional ECG evaluation with 15 or 18 leads include ST-segment elevation suggestive of an inferior wall MI (II, III, AVF); isolated ST-segment elevation in V_1 or ST-segment elevation in V_1 greater than in V_2; borderline ST-segment elevation in V_5 and V_6 or in V_1 through V_3; and ST-segment depression or suspicious isoelectric ST segments in V_1 through V_3.

Serial ECGs
ECGs are then done in a series (initially and then every 30 minutes for the first 2 hours). Characteristic changes in certain lead groups identify the area and evolution of infarct. After the initial evaluation phase, ECGs may be done every 8 to 24 hours and as needed for complaints of chest pain.

SIGNIFICANT ELECTROCARDIOGRAM CHANGES
ST-segment changes and new bundle branch block
The presence or absence of ST-segment elevation is used to stratify risk and determine the best treatment plan. ST segments are elevated in the leads "over" or facing the infarcted area. Reciprocal changes (ST-segment depressions) will be found in leads 180 degrees from the area of infarction. New left bundle branch block, coupled with other findings, may also indicate that MI is present. Patients with STEMI are candidates for emergency reperfusion strategy. PCI within 90 minutes of arrival to a PCI-capable hospital is the ideal therapy. Patients who are admitted to a non-PCI-capable hospital should receive fibrinolytic therapy (unless contraindicated) as the primary reperfusion therapy within 30 minutes of arrival.

Not all patients experience STEMI. The 2012 ACCF/AHA practice guidelines outline treatment options for UA/NSTEMI patients. They include treatment with P2Y12 receptor inhibitors such as clopidogrel, prasugrel, or ticagrelor.

 Safety Alert *Geriatric alert: Prasugrel is not recommended in patients older than 75 years. Also contraindicated in patients who weigh less than 60 kg or have a history of stroke/ transient ischemic attack (TIA).*

Q waves

Q waves are a later ECG change and may or may not be present in patients presenting with an MI. Q waves are indicative of MI and are "pathologic" if they meet the following criteria: wider than 0.03 seconds, $\geq$ 1 mm in depth, and present in 2 contiguous leads. Q waves may develop later, or the tissue necrosis may extend itself if a reperfusion strategy is withheld.

Safety Alert *ST segment elevation myocardial infarction accounts for 25% to 40% of hospital presentations for acute myocardial infarction (AMI). Left bundle branch block (and, to a lesser extent, right bundle branch block) can distort the 12-lead ECG, making recognition of ST segment elevation difficult to impossible. Rarely, hyperacute T wave changes can occur before ST elevation.* Twelve-lead ECG diagnosis of posterior wall myocardial infarction (MI) can only be made by noting that the reciprocal change is the anterior leads (V1 to V3). Lead V1 is the only lead that may indicate an isolated right ventricle (RV) MI. Use of 15- or 18-lead ECGs that provide a more direct view of the posterior and RV walls of the heart is recommended for more accurate diagnosis of both posterior wall and RV MI.

T-wave changes

Within the initial hour of infarction, tall, peaked, "hyperacute" upright T waves may be seen in leads over the infarct. Within several hours to days, the T wave becomes inverted. Gradually over time, the ST segment becomes isoelectric and the T wave may remain inverted. T-wave changes may last for weeks and return to normal or remain inverted for the rest of the patient's life. T-wave changes reflective of posterior and RV MI are not clearly seen on the 12-lead ECG. Use of 15- or 18-lead ECGs should provide better information about these areas (Table 5-5).

Table 5-5	12- TO 18-LEAD ECG LOCATION OF MYOCARDIAL INFARCTION (MI)		
MI Location	**Leads Reflecting MI**	**Reciprocal Leads**	**Affected Artery(ies)**
Intraventricular septum	V_1, V_2	Not seen	Left coronary, LAD septal branch
Anterior LV	V_3, V_4	II, III, AVF	Left coronary, LAD diagonal branch
Lateral LV	V_5, V_6	V_1 to V_3	Left coronary circumflex branch
Posterior LV	V_7 to V_9*	V_1 to V_4	Right coronary or circumflex branch
Right ventricle	V_{1R} to V_{6R}*	Not seen	Right coronary with proximal branches
Inferior LV	II, III, AVF	I, AVL	Right coronary posterior descending branch

*Leads must be added to normal 12-lead ECG.
LAD, Left anterior descending artery; *LV*, left ventricle.

Acute Coronary Syndrome

COLLABORATIVE MANAGEMENT

ACUTE MYOCARDIAL INFARCTION HOSPITAL QUALITY ALLIANCE INDICATORS

The American Hospital Association (AHA), Federation of American Hospitals (FAH), and Association of American Medical Colleges (AAMC) launched the Hospital Quality Alliance (HQA), an initiative to provide the public with specific reported information about hospital performance. This national public-private collaboration encourages hospitals to voluntarily collect and report quality performance information. The Centers for Medicare and Medicaid Services (CMS) along with The Joint Commission participate in the HQA. Hospitals are expected to track and analyze their performance ratings and use the information to improve quality. The table reflects HQA measures considered essential when caring for patients following an acute myocardial infarction (AMI). All indicators are evidence-based actions that should be included in the plan of care. The measurement describes the details of each indicator. Evidence of performance is derived from review of each patient's medical record following hospital discharge.

Indicators	Measure
Aspirin at arrival	AMI patients without aspirin contraindications who received aspirin within 24 hours before or after hospital arrival
Aspirin at discharge	AMI patients without aspirin contraindications who were prescribed aspirin at hospital discharge
Angiotensin-converting enzyme inhibitor (ACEI) or for left ventricular systolic dysfunction	AMI patients with left ventricular systolic dysfunction (LVSD) and without both ACEI and ARB contraindications who were prescribed an ACEI or an ARB at hospital discharge
Beta blocker on admission	AMI patients without beta-blocker contraindications who were prescribed a beta blocker on admission
Beta blocker at discharge	AMI patients without beta-blocker contraindications who were prescribed a beta blocker at hospital discharge
Fibrinolytic agent received within 30 minutes of hospital arrival	AMI patients receiving thrombolytic therapy during hospital stay with a time from hospital arrival to thrombolysis of 30 minutes or less
Percutaneous coronary intervention (PCI) received within 90 minutes of hospital arrival	AMI patients receiving a PCI during the hospital stay with a time from hospital arrival to PCI of 90 minutes or less
Smoking cessation advice/counseling	AMI patients with a history of smoking cigarettes who are given smoking cessation counseling during a hospital stay
30-day risk-adjusted myocardial infarction mortality	The measures comply with standards for publicly reported outcomes models that have been endorsed by the American Heart Association and the American College of Cardiology. These measures have been published in peer review literature and approved by the rigorous process of the National Quality Forum.

CARE PRIORITIES FOR ALL ACUTE CORONARY SYNDROMES

Prevention of initial or further coronary thrombus formation may include administration of anticoagulant/antithrombin medications (i.e., unfractionated or low-molecular-weight heparin [LMWH]) and antiplatelet drugs (e.g., aspirin, clopidogrel, or glycoprotein [GP] IIb/IIIa inhibitors such as abciximab, eptifibatide, or tirofiban). In patients evolving toward AMI, these agents are thought to abate complete closure of the coronary arteries or to prevent more extensive clot formation. Cardiac catheterization is often performed to assess the size and location of coronary lesions. If significant lesions are found, PCI can immediately follow catheterization in facilities that offer PCI.

1. Relief of acute ischemic pain

Drugs are administered and titrated to reduce or eliminate chest pain. Morphine, oxygen, nitrates, and aspirin (MONA) are considered primary treatment modalities. The preferred order of these basic interventions is oxygen, aspirin (if not already given), nitrates, and morphine.

- Oxygen: Usually 2 to 4 L/min by nasal cannula, or mode and rate as directed by ABG values, to promote both myocardial and generalized increases in oxygenation. As oxygen delivery to the heart is enhanced, pain can be relieved. If the patient deteriorates, other methods of oxygen delivery may be implemented (e.g., nonrebreather mask with reservoir and mechanical ventilation for those who deteriorate markedly).
- Aspirin: 162 to 325 mg ideally chewed should be given immediately if the patient has not been given aspirin before arrival at the hospital.
- Oral, sublingual, and other forms of nitrates/NTG: Can be used for short-term therapy or longer-lasting prophylactic effects. These non-IV medications are used for management of myocardial ischemia or angina pectoris rather than for MI.
- IV nitrates/NTG: For UA or evolving MI, titrated until relief is obtained, generally up to 200 µg/min as long as the patient maintains a systolic BP of at least 80 mm Hg.
- IV or oral immediate-release morphine sulfate: Given in small increments (e.g., 2 mg) until relief is obtained. This medication is usually not necessary unless an MI is occurring. Low BP may contraindicate administration.

2. Prevention of coronary artery clot formation

- Antiplatelet therapy: Aspirin is the initial treatment as indicated above. P2Y12 inhibitors such as clopidogrel, prasugrel, or ticagrelor are recommended as soon as possible. Infusion of GP IIb/IIIa inhibitors (e.g., abciximab, eptifibatide, tirofiban) is used in patients undergoing angiography.
- Antithrombin therapy: Unfractionated heparin (UFH) or LMWH is sometimes implemented to prevent clot extension and/or formation, particularly during PCI. UFH should be weight-based and follow a titration protocol based on ongoing studies of partial thromboplastin time/activated partial thromboplastin time (PTT/aPTT). LMWH, such as enoxaparin, can be administered subcutaneously or IV and does not require monitoring of PTT/aPTT. Fondaparinux, an LMWH, cannot be administered as the only anticoagulant during PCI because of the increased risk of catheter thrombosis.
- Direct thrombin inhibitors (DTIs): An anticoagulant that binds directly to thrombin and blocks its interaction with its substrates. DTIs act independently of antithrombin, so they can inhibit thrombin bound to fibrin or fibrin degradation products. Bivalirudin is commonly used during PCI because its duration of action is short. Coagulation times return to baseline approximately 1 hour following cessation of administration.

3. Reduction of myocardial workload and myocardial oxygen consumption

- Limit activities: Restrictions are based on patient's activity tolerance. Bed rest with bedside commode privileges generally is recommended for patients with AMI for up to 12 hours after symptom onset although there is no good data to support this. Longer periods of bed rest can promote development of orthostatic intolerance, which is prevented by elevation of the HOB, dangling the lower extremities, and other low-exertion activities. Patients should be instructed to avoid the Valsalva maneuver when toileting, because it may predispose them to ventricular dysrhythmias.
- Administer medications:
    - Beta-adrenergic blocking agents (e.g., metoprolol, carvedilol, propranolol): To decrease HR, BP, and myocardial contractility. Recommended as part of primary pharmacologic therapy for AMI patients.
    - ACEIs (e.g., enalapril, ramipril, quinapril): To decrease BP and thus reduce the resistance to ventricular ejection. Used to reduce LV remodeling and if long-term BP control is needed. Effective in prevention and treatment of HF. Should be used for patients with diabetes, chronic kidney disease, and/or reduced EF unless contraindicated.
    - ARBs (candesartan, eprosartan, irbesartan, olmesartan, losartan, telmisartan): Have similar effects to ACEIs but have not been proved to reduce mortality. ARBs are used in patients who are ACEI intolerant.
    - CCBs (e.g., nifedipine, diltiazem): No longer recommended for management of patients with ACS unless coronary artery spasms are strongly suspected.

4. Prevention, recognition, and treatment of dysrhythmias

Beta blockers should be prescribed within the first 24 hours unless contraindicated.
ACLS algorithms should be used.

Acute Coronary Syndrome

HIGH ALERT! Caution should be exercised in the use of antiarrhythmic agents in patients with acute myocardial infarction (AMI), especially to manage reperfusion dysrhythmias, because instability of the conduction system with AMI is sometimes aggravated by use of antiarrhythmic agents. Electrical therapies such as synchronized cardioversion, defibrillation, external/transthoracic pacing, or transvenous pacing may provide a safer management strategy for these patients.

---

5. Prevention of contrast-induced nephropathy related to use of contrast during coronary angiography/PCI
- Hydration using IV and oral fluids is paramount.

ADDITIONAL TREATMENTS
1. Management of unstable AMI with ST-segment elevation (STEMI)
- Hemodynamic monitoring: Used in a patient with a complicated MI resulting in ventricular failure with threat of CS. Pulmonary artery (PA) and capillary pressures are measured, along with CO and SVR. Unstable patients may manifest increased PAP, increased PAWP, decreased CO, and increased SVR.

2. Acute STEMI: PCI procedures
- Primary PCI: A balloon-tipped catheter is inserted into the coronary arterial lesion, and the balloon is inflated to compress the plaque material against the vessel wall, thereby opening the narrowed lumen. Primary PCI is performed on individuals with STEMI. Elective PCI may be performed on patients with postinfarction angina, postcoronary angina, and UA. The ideal candidate for primary PCI has single-vessel disease with a discrete, proximal, noncalcified lesion. While PCI may be done on noninfarct arteries electively, primary PCI should target only the infarct artery. During the procedure, the patient is sedated lightly and is given a local anesthetic at the insertion site, either the radial or femoral artery. ECG electrodes are placed on the chest. An introducer sheath is inserted into the femoral or radial artery, a guidewire is passed into the aorta and coronary artery, and the balloon catheter is passed over the guidewire to the stenotic site. The patient may be asked to take deep breaths and cough to facilitate passage of the catheter. Heparin, GP IIb/IIIa inhibitor, and/or a direct thrombin inhibitor, such as bivalirudin, is administered to prevent clot formation. The balloon is inflated repeatedly for 60 to 90 seconds at a pressure of 4 to 15 atmospheres. Subsequently, radiopaque dye is injected to determine whether the stenosis has been reduced to less than 50% of the vessel diameter, which is the goal of the procedure. The femoral artery site may be closed using a device, or the introducer sheath is left in the femoral artery until the effect of anticoagulant medications has diminished. In the case of radial access, a radial artery band is applied.
  - Complications after PCI: These include acute coronary artery occlusion, coronary artery dissection, reocclusion in AMI patients, AMI, coronary artery spasm, bleeding, circulatory insufficiency, pseudoaneurysm, allergic or renal hypersensitivity to contrast material, hypokalemia, vasovagal reaction, dysrhythmias, and hypotension. Restenosis can occur 6 weeks to 6 months after PCI, although the patient may not experience angina.
  - Intracoronary stent procedure: A PCI wherein endovascular stents (metal-mesh tubes) are used to keep arteries open. Can be done during primary PCI or electively. A variety of designs, materials, and deployment procedures are available. Bare metal stents were the first stents developed, have an increased risk of restenosis, and are used in patients who cannot tolerate dual antiplatelet therapy. Drug-eluting stents are coated with antiproliferative drugs that elute into the coronary artery wall to reduce scar tissue formation and restenosis.
  - Aspiration thrombectomy: This may be done during primary PCI. Catheter is advanced with guidewire that has a distal lumen attached to a suction device to vacuum thrombus out.
  - Coronary artery atherectomy: A PCI that removes atherosclerotic plaque from coronary arteries using a special catheter equipped with a cutting device that shaves the lesion. Three types are directional, rotational, and laser.

3. Surgical revascularization

* Surgical revascularization procedures are rarely used as the primary management strategy for AMI unless primary PCI has failed, there is persistent ischemia causing hemodynamic instability, and the anatomy is amenable to CABG. CABG is usually done electively. Several approaches are available for myocardial revascularization, including CABG via median sternotomy or minimally invasive technique. Patients with multivessel or diffuse CAD are the most appropriate candidates for these procedures. Surgical indications include (1) stable angina with 50% stenosis of the left main coronary artery, (2) stable angina with three-vessel CAD, (3) UA with three-vessel disease or severe two-vessel disease, (4) recent MI, (5) ischemic HF with CS, and (6) signs of ischemia or impending MI after angiography. Robotics can be used to assist the surgeon with the procedure. Cardiac surgery should be readily available for patients who experience complications undergoing any diagnostic or treatment procedures in the cardiac catheterization laboratory.

4. Acute STEMI: Thrombolytic therapy

* Thrombolytic therapy (lysis of coronary arterial clot): Used for reperfusion of the occluded coronary vessel(s) causing the AMI. Streptokinase and anisoylated plasminogen streptokinase activator complex (APSAC) are first-generation, nonfibrin-specific agents. They are no longer available in the United States. Second-generation drugs that are fibrin specific include tenecteplase, alteplase, and reteplase (Box 5-1 and Table 5-6). Thrombolytic therapy is an AHA/ACC class I intervention for patients with ST-segment elevation in two or more contiguous leads, new left bundle branch

---

Box 5-1   THROMBOLYTICS

First-generation (nonselective) thrombolytics

Streptokinase: An enzyme derived from group C beta-hemolytic streptococci. Because it is an antigen, patients who have had previous exposure to streptococcal organisms may have antibodies against streptokinase. Therefore steroids or antihistamines are administered before streptokinase therapy to prevent a hypersensitivity reaction.

Anistreplase: A plasminogen activator that induces clot lysis with fewer systemic lytic effects than streptokinase. Allergic and anaphylactic reactions are possible.

Second-generation (fibrin-selective) thrombolytics

These fibrin-specific agents decrease the systemic activation of plasminogen and the resulting degradation of circulating fibrinogen compared with first-generation thrombolytics. They are also nonantigenic.

Alteplase: A recombinant tissue plasminogen activator (rtPA) with the same amino acid sequence as endogenous tissue plasminogen activator (tPA). Has a shorter half-life, 4 to 6 minutes, than other agents. Several dosage regimens are approved for coronary thrombolysis.

Reteplase: A recombinant deletion mutein of tPA, reteplase catalyzes cleavage of endogenous plasminogen to generate plasmin. It is not clot-specific, so fibrinogen levels fall to lower levels than those seen with rtPA (alteplase), with a return to baseline value within 48 hours after infusion. The half-life is 13 to 16 minutes, and the drug is cleared by the liver and kidneys. It is given as two boluses 30 minutes apart, each over 2 minutes.

Tenecteplase: A modified form of human tPA that binds to fibrin and converts plasminogen to plasmin. In the presence of fibrin, conversion of plasminogen to plasmin is increased relative to its conversion in the absence of fibrin. Following administration of tenecteplase, there are decreases in circulating fibrinogen and plasminogen. It has a half-life of up to 130 minutes for final clearance and is mostly metabolized through the liver. There are less bleeding complications than with alteplase. Tenecteplase is given as a single 5-second bolus and is dosed by weight.

Table 5-6 THROMBOLYTIC DOSAGE REGIMENS

Name of Agent: Generic and Trade Names	Streptokinase (Streptase)	Anistreplase (APSAC, Eminase)	Reteplase (Retavase)	Alteplase (Activase)	Alteplase (Activase)	Tenecteplase (TNKase)
Regimen	Original	Original	Double bolus	Accelerated	Original	Single bolus
Total time of regimen	30 to 60 minutes	2 to 5 minutes	30 minutes	90 minutes	180 minutes	5 seconds
Initial IV bolus		30 units over 2 to 5 minutes	10 units over 2 minutes	15 mg	6 to 10 mg	Weight / Dose
						>60 kg → 30 mg
						60 to 69 kg → 35 mg
						70 to 79 kg → 40 mg
						80 to 89 kg → 45 mg
						90 kg → 50 mg
Second IV bolus at time: 30 minutes			10 units over 2 minutes			
Infusion from time 0 to <30 minutes	1.5 million units IV over 30 to 50 minutes			0.75 mg/kg, max dose 50 mg		
Infusion from time 0 to 60 minutes					50 to 54 mg: 1 hour total 60 mg	
Infusion from 30 to 90 minutes				0.50 mg/kg, max dose 35 mg		
Infusion from 60 to 120 minutes					20 mg	
Infusion from 120 to 180 minutes					20 mg	
Total dose	1.5 million units	30 units	20 units	Varies by weight, max dose 100 mg	100 mg	50 mg

Box 5-2	CONTRAINDICATIONS AND WARNINGS FOR THROMBOLYTIC THERAPY

Absolute contraindications
- Known hypersensitivity to thrombolytic agents
- Suspected aortic dissection
- Active internal bleeding
- History of stroke (except ischemic stroke within 4.5 hours)
- Recent intracranial or intraspinal surgery or trauma
- Known bleeding diathesis
- Severe, uncontrolled hypertension

Warnings (risks may be increased and should be weighed against anticipated benefits)
- Recent major surgery (e.g., coronary artery bypass graft, obstetric delivery, organ biopsy)
- Previous puncture of noncompressible vessels
- Cerebrovascular disease
- Recent internal bleeding (within 2 to 4 weeks)
- Recent trauma
- Hypertension (systolic blood pressure >180 mm Hg and/or diastolic blood pressure >110 mm Hg)
- History of chronic, severe, poorly controlled hypertension
- Dementia
- Hemostatic defects including those secondary to severe hepatic or renal disease
- Severe hepatic or renal dysfunction
- Pregnancy
- Diabetic hemorrhagic retinopathy or other hemorrhagic ophthalmic conditions
- Active peptic ulcer
- Advanced age
- Currently receiving anticoagulants (e.g., warfarin)
- Any other condition in which bleeding constitutes a significant hazard or would be particularly difficult to manage because of its location

block (obscuring ST-segment analysis), and history suggestive of AMI who present within 12 hours of symptom onset and are younger than 75 years of age. Patients must be carefully screened for risk of bleeding before administration of these IV medications (Box 5-2). Time from the patient's entry into the emergency department to treatment with thrombolytics should be within 30 minutes.

CARE PLANS FOR ACUTE CORONARY SYNDROMES

ACTIVITY INTOLERANCE *related to imbalance between oxygen supply and demand secondary to decreased cardiac output associated with coronary artery disease.*

Goals/Outcomes: Within the 12- to 24-hour period before discharge from the CCU, the patient exhibits cardiac tolerance to increasing levels of activity as evidenced by RR less than 24 breaths/min, NSR on ECG, BP within 20 mm Hg of patient's normal range, HR less than 120 bpm (or within 20 bpm of resting HR for patients on beta-blocker therapy), and absence of chest pain.

NOC Energy Conservation, Instrumental Activities of Daily Living (IADL)

Energy Management
1. Assist patient with identifying activities that precipitate chest pain, and teach patient to use NTG prophylactically before the activity.
2. Assist patient as needed in a progressive activity program, beginning with level I and progressing to level IV, as tolerated (Table 5-7).

Table 5-7	ACTIVITY LEVEL PROGRESSION FOR HOSPITALIZED PATIENTS*	
Level	**Activity**	
I	Bed rest	Flexion and extension of extremities 4 times daily, 15 times each extremity; deep breathing 4 times daily, 15 breaths; position change from side to side every 2 hours
II	Out of bed to chair	As tolerated, 3 times daily for 20 to 30 minutes
III	Ambulate in room	As tolerated, 3 times daily for 20 to 30 minutes
IV	Ambulate in hall	Initially, 50 to 200 ft twice daily; progressing to 50 to 200 ft 4 times daily

*Signs of activity intolerance: Decrease in blood pressure less than 20 mm Hg; increase in heart rate to greater than 120 bpm (or more than 20 bpm above resting heart rate in patients receiving beta-blocker therapy).

3. Assess patient's response to activity progression. Be alert to presence of chest pain, SOB, excessive fatigue, and dysrhythmias. Monitor for a decrease in BP greater than 20 mm Hg and an increase in HR to greater than 120 bpm (greater than 20 bpm above resting HR in patients receiving beta-blocker therapy).
4. Teach the patient about measures that prevent complications of decreased mobility, such as active ROM exercises. (For additional details, see Prolonged Immobility, Chapter 1).

NIC Energy Management, Self-Care Assistance: IADL

RISK FOR DEFICIENT FLUID VOLUME *related to increased risk of bleeding*

Goals/Outcomes: The patient will not experience bleeding or a decrease in Hgb or hematocrit (Hct).
NOC Fluid Balance

Bleeding Precautions
1. Monitor dosing of all drugs known to increase bleeding, including aspirin and other antiplatelet drugs, GP IIb/IIIa inhibitors, direct thrombin inhibitors, and thrombolytics.
2. Monitor Hgb and Hct closely. Report Hgb drop greater than 2 g to physician immediately.
3. Monitor vital signs closely. Drop in BP and increase in HR may indicate developing shock, which may be cardiogenic or indicate hidden bleeding.
4. After PCI via femoral sheath, keep HOB less than 30 degrees and affected leg straight as ordered.
5. After PCI, monitor vital signs, sheath site, and distal pulses every 15 minutes until sheath is removed, then every 15 minutes x2, then every 30 minutes x2, then every 4 hours.
6. Carefully follow provider's orders for sheath removal after PCI.
7. If bleeding occurs at the insertion site, position the patient flat and apply pressure until hemostasis is achieved and obtain stat CBC. Notify provider of drop in Hgb.
8. Instruct the patient to report any discomfort. Groin pain may indicate pseudoaneurysm; back pain may indicate retroperitoneal bleed.

NIC Bleeding Reduction; Surveillance; Hemorrhage Control; Neurologic Monitoring

DECREASED CO (OR RISK FOR SAME) *related to alterations in rate, rhythm, and conduction secondary to increased irritability of ischemic tissue during reperfusion (usually occurs within 1 to 2 hours after initiation of therapy); reocclusion of thrombolysed vessels; negative inotropic changes secondary to cardiac disease; hypotension secondary to blood loss.*

Goals/Outcomes: Within 12 hours of initiation of thrombolytic therapy or PCI, the patient has adequate CO as evidenced by normal HR (60 to 100 bpm), peripheral pulses greater than 2+ on a 0 to 4+ scale, warm and dry skin, and hourly urine output >0.5 mL/kg/h. Patient is awake, alert, and oriented without palpitations, chest pain, or dizziness. Within 48 hours, the patient maintains stability as just described.

Safety Alert *Reocclusion occurs in as many as 16% of patients within 24 to 48 hours after thrombolysis.*

NOC Circulation Status

 Cardiac Care
1. Monitor ECG continuously for evidence of dysrhythmias. Consult provider for significant dysrhythmias or new or worsening ST-segment elevation.
2. With any dysrhythmia, check vital signs and note accompanying signs and symptoms such as dizziness, light-headedness, syncope, and palpitations.
3. Ensure availability of emergency drugs and equipment: atropine, isoproterenol, epinephrine, amiodarone, adenosine, vasopressin, procainamide, sotalol, lidocaine (use cautiously with AMI), defibrillator-cardioverter, and external and transvenous pacemaker.
4. Evaluate patient's response to medications and emergency treatment.
5. Monitor patient for signs of reocclusion: chest pain, nausea, diaphoresis, and dysrhythmias.
6. Consult provider for any signs of reocclusion.
7. Obtain 12/15/18-lead ECG if reocclusion is suspected.
8. Anticipate and prepare patient for cardiac catheterization, PCI with stent, or repeated thrombolytic therapy.
9. Monitor for signs of bleeding and bleeding complications: bleeding at sheath site or at IV sites, back pain (may indicate retroperitoneal bleed), signs and symptoms of cerebrovascular accident (CVA)/stroke (see Stroke: Acute Ischemic and Hemorrhagic, Chapter 7).

NIC Hemodynamic Regulation; Circulatory Care; Dysrhythmia Management; Cardiac Care: Acute

RISK FOR INJURY *related to potential for allergic or anaphylactic reaction to streptokinase or anistreplase secondary to antigen/antibody response.*

Goals/Outcomes: Patient has no symptoms of allergic response as evidenced by normothermia, RR 12 to 20 breaths/min with normal pattern and depth, HR less than 100 bpm, BP at baseline or within normal limits, natural skin color, and absence of itching, urticaria, headache, muscular and abdominal pain, and nausea.
NOC Risk Control

 Risk Identification
1. Before treatment, question the patient about history of previous streptokinase therapy or streptococcal infection. Consult provider for positive findings.
2. Administer prophylactic hydrocortisone as prescribed.
3. Monitor patient during and for 48 to 72 hours after infusion for indicators of allergy: hypotension (brief or sustained), urticaria, fever, itching, flushing, nausea, headache, muscular pain, bronchospasm, abdominal pain, dyspnea, or tachycardia. These indicators can appear immediately after or as long as several days after streptokinase therapy.
4. If hypotension develops, increase rate of IV infusion/administer volume replacement as prescribed. Prepare for vasopressor administration if there is no response to volume replacement.
5. Treat allergic response with diphenhydramine or other antihistamine as prescribed.

NIC Shock Management: Vasogenic; Shock Management

DECREASED CARDIAC OUTPUT *related to cardiac dysfunction following acute coronary event.*

Goals/Outcomes: Within 24 hours of this diagnosis, the patient exhibits adequate CO, as evidenced by BP within normal limits for patient, HR 60 to 100 bpm, peripheral pulses greater than 2+ on a 0 to 4+ scale, warm and dry skin, hourly urine output greater than 0.5 mL/kg, measured CO 4 to 7 L/min, right atrial pressure (RAP) 4 to 6 mm Hg, PAP 20 to 30/8 to 15 mm Hg, PAWP 6 to 12 mm Hg, and the patient awake, alert, oriented, and free from anginal pain.
NOC Tissue Perfusion: Cardiac

Cardiac Care, Acute

1. See Care Plans for Generalized Cardiovascular Dysfunctions, (Chapter 5).
2. Monitor for ST-segment elevation indicative of myocardial injury, ST depression indicative of myocardial ischemia, new left bundle branch block, and Q waves indicative of MI. All ECG changes must be present in at least two contiguous leads.
3. Collaborate with provider if decreased CO does not respond to acute cardiac care interventions.
4. Maintain fluid balance carefully, with close assessment for need for fluids versus diuretics. Patients with right-sided HF may require support with IV fluids, while those with left-sided HF may respond better to diuretics.
5. Provide patient with platelet-inhibiting (e.g., clopidogrel, aspirin, abciximab) and thrombin-inhibiting medications (e.g., heparin, enoxaparin, fondaparinux, bivalirudin) as appropriate, according to AHA guidelines for STEMI or NSTEMI.

Hemodynamic Regulation

1. Monitor for unstable BP and use hemodynamic readings to help assess need for titration of vasoactive, inotropic, and antiarrhythmic medications.
2. Collaborate with provider to assess if the patients with severe bundle branch block might benefit from biventricular cardiac pacing to improve synchrony of ventricular contraction.
3. Assess effects of fluid challenges on CVP and pulmonary artery occlusive pressure (PAOP), especially in patients with RV infarction.
4. Elevate legs rather than placing patients in Trendelenburg position to help augment venous return to increase BP.

Circulatory Care: Mechanical Assist Device

1. Assess peripheral circulation meticulously when intra-aortic balloon catheter is in place.
2. Evaluate impact of changes in balloon counterpulsation settings on CO, CI, all hemodynamic pressures, and BP.
3. Examine all cannulas for kinking or disconnection if the patient becomes suddenly unstable without other notable cause.
4. Use strict aseptic technique when changing device-related dressings.
5. Administer anticoagulants or thrombolytics as appropriate.
6. Collaborate with provider regarding need for further interventions if the patient remains unstable despite mechanical assist device and vasoactive, inotropic, and antiarrhythmic medications.

DEFICIENT KNOWLEDGE: CORONARY ARTERY DISEASE PROCESS AND ITS LIFESTYLE IMPLICATIONS *related to the need to help prevent further incidence of heart disease.*

Goals/Outcomes: Within the 24-hour period before discharge from the step-down unit, the patient verbalizes understanding of his or her disease, as well as the necessary lifestyle changes that may modify risk factors.
NOC Knowledge: Disease Process; Knowledge: Medication; Knowledge: Diet; Knowledge: Energy Conservation; Sexual Identity: Acceptance; Knowledge: Sexual Functioning

Teaching: Cardiac Disease Process

1. Teach the patient about ischemia and its resultant chest pain, referred to as angina pectoris.
2. Discuss the pathophysiologic process underlying patient's angina, using drawings or heart models as indicated.
3. Assist the patient in identifying his or her own risk factors (e.g., cigarette smoking, high-stress lifestyle, hyperglycemia, high-fat diet).
4. Teach the patient about risk factor modification:
   - Smoking cessation: Teach the patient that smoking causes the coronary arteries to constrict, thus decreasing blood flow to the heart.
   - Stress management: Discuss the role that stress plays in angina. Explain that stress increases sympathetic tone, which can cause the BP and HR to increase, resulting in increased oxygen demand. By using relaxation techniques such as imagery, meditation, or biofeedback, one can decrease the effects of stress on the heart. For a sample relaxation technique, see Appendix 7.

NIC Teaching: Individual; Teaching: Disease Process, Thrombolysis

ALTERED PROTECTION *related to risk of bleeding/hemorrhage secondary to nonspecific thrombolytic effects of therapy.*

Goals/Outcomes: Symptoms of bleeding complications are absent as evidenced by BP within patient's normal range, HR less than 100 bpm, blood-free secretions and excretions, natural skin color, baseline or normal level of consciousness (LOC), and absence of back and abdominal pain, hematoma, headache, dizziness, and vomiting.
NOC Risk Control

Risk Identification
1. When patient is admitted, obtain a thorough history, assessing for the following:
   * Risk factors for intracranial hemorrhage: uncontrolled hypertension, cerebrovascular pathology, central nervous system (CNS) surgery within previous 6 months
   * Bleeding risks: recent or active gastrointestinal (GI) bleeding, recent trauma, recent surgery, bleeding diathesis, advanced liver or kidney disease
   * Risk of systemic embolization: suspected left-sided heart thrombus
   * History of streptococcal infection or previous streptokinase therapy
2. Monitor clotting studies per hospital protocol. Regulate heparin drip to maintain PTT at 1.5 to 2 times control levels or according to protocol. Never discontinue heparin without consulting with the provider.
3. Apply pressure dressing over puncture sites. If cardiac catheterization was performed, inspect site at frequent intervals for evidence of hematoma formation. Immobilize extremity for 6 to 8 hours after catheterization procedure.
4. Avoid unnecessary venipunctures, IM injections, or arterial puncture. Obtain laboratory specimens from heparin-lock device.
5. Monitor patient for indicators of internal bleeding: back pain, abdominal pain, decreased BP, pallor, and bloody stool or urine. Report significant findings to provider.
6. Monitor patient for signs of intracranial bleeding every 2 hours: change in LOC, headache, dizziness, vomiting, and confusion.
7. Test all stools, urine, and emesis for occult blood.
8. Use care with oral hygiene and when shaving patient. For more information about safety precautions, see Pulmonary Embolus, (Chapter 4).

Teaching: Diet and Prescribed Medications
1. Diet low in cholesterol and saturated fat: Provide sample diet plan for meals that are low in cholesterol and saturated fat. Teach the patient about foods that are high or low in cholesterol and saturated fat. Stress the importance of reading food labels.
2. BP control: If the patient was found to have hypertension associated with MI, the patient should be taught the importance of taking appropriate medications to control BP and to follow recommended dietary guidelines to minimize sodium intake. Sodium promotes water retention, which can increase BP. Higher systemic BP increases the workload of the heart, demanding that more myocardial oxygen be consumed.
   * Teach the patient about the prescribed medications, including name, purpose, dosage, action, schedule, precautions, and potential side effects.
   * Teach the patient the actions that should be taken if chest pain is unrelieved or increases in intensity.

Teaching: Activity/Exercise
If chest pain occurs:
1. Stop and rest.
2. Take 1 tablet of NTG; wait 5 minutes. If pain is not relieved, take a second NTG; wait 5 minutes. If pain is not relieved, take a third NTG and call 911 or local emergency number.
3. Lie down if headache occurs. The vasodilation effect of NTG causes a decrease in BP, which may result in orthostatic hypotension and transient headache.
4. Explain to the patient that it is no more beneficial to be in the emergency department than it is to be at home during episodes of chest pain caused by angina and therefore traveling to a hospital at the first sign of chest pain usually is unnecessary.
5. Review activity limitations and prescribed progressions (see Tables 5-3 and 5-6). Provide the following information:
   * When you are discharged from the hospital, it is important that you continue your walking program. Do not overestimate your ability; rather, start off slowly and build up. Depending on how you feel, you may only be able to stay at one level or you may progress to 2 miles quickly. Remember to warm up and cool down with stretches for 5 to 7 minutes and to walk 3 to 5 times each week.

- Avoid sudden energetic activities.
- Plan for regular rest periods in the afternoon.
- Let your body guide you regarding whether to increase or decrease activity.
- Inform your provider of any changes in activity tolerance, such as the development of new symptoms with the same activity.

6. Avoid exercising outdoors in very cold, hot, or humid weather. Extreme weather places an additional stress on the heart. If you do exercise in extremes of weather, decrease the pace and monitor your response carefully.
7. Pulse monitoring: Teach the patient how to take pulse, including parameters for target HRs and limits.

Teaching: Sexuality

Sexual activity guidelines: Because sexual activity is a physical activity, certain guidelines can help the patient and his or her partner enjoy a satisfying sexual relationship while minimizing the workload of the heart:

1. Rest is beneficial before engaging in intercourse.
2. Find a position that is comfortable for you and your partner. Assuming a different position that is uncomfortable to both may increase the workload of the heart.
3. Medications such as NTG may be taken prophylactically by the patient before intercourse to prevent chest pain.
4. Postpone intercourse for 1 to 2 hours after eating a heavy meal.
5. Report the following symptoms to your physician if they are experienced after sexual relations: SOB, increased HR that persists for longer than 15 minutes, unrelieved chest pain.
6. Do not take phosphodiesterase type-5 (PDE-5) inhibitors (sildenafil, vardenafil) if taking nitrates.

NIC Teaching: Disease Process; Teaching: Prescribed Activity/Exercise; Teaching: Prescribed Medication; Teaching: Sexuality

ACUTE PAIN (CHEST) *related to biophysiologic injury related to decreased oxygen supply to the myocardium.*

Goals/Outcomes: Within 30 minutes of intervention, the patient's subjective evaluation of discomfort improves, as documented by a pain scale. Nonverbal indicators, such as grimacing, are absent. Vital signs return to baseline. ECG changes present during the event resolve.

NOC Pain Control

Pain Management

1. Assess and document the character of the patient's chest pain, including location, duration, quality, intensity, precipitating and alleviating factors, presence or absence of radiation, and associated symptoms. Devise a pain scale with the patient, rating discomfort from 0 (no pain) to 10 or using a system that assists in objectively reporting pain level.
2. Measure BP and HR with each episode of chest pain. BP and HR may increase because of sympathetic stimulation as a result of pain. If the chest pain is caused by ischemia, the heart muscle may not be functioning normally and CO may decrease, resulting in a low BP. In addition, dysrhythmias such as bradycardia and ventricular ectopy may be noted with ischemia. If BP is low, it may not be advisable to administer nitrates and morphine, which can further reduce BP, adding to myocardial ischemia.
3. After each titration of IV NTG, evaluate patient's BP and the effects of therapy in relieving patient's chest pain. If slight hypotension occurs (80 to 90 mm Hg systolic), reduce the flow rate to one-half or less of the infusing dose. If severe hypotension (less than 80 mm Hg systolic BP) occurs, stop the infusion and contact the provider for further directions.

Safety Alert *Cardiogenic shock occurs in 5% to 10% of acute myocardial infarctions.*

---

4. Monitor for side effects of NTG, including headache, hypotension, syncope, facial flushing, and nausea. If side effects occur, place the patient in a supine position and consult physician for further interventions.
5. Administer heparin, GP IIb/IIIa inhibitors (abciximab, tirofiban, eptifibatide), and aspirin as prescribed. Heparin infusion usually should be administered using a weight-based protocol, which is titrated according to PTT results. These patients are predisposed to bleeding and may need to be given bleeding precautions.
6. Maintain a quiet environment and group patient care activities to allow for periods of uninterrupted rest. Consider healing touch therapy, relaxation exercises, or music therapy.

7. Position patient according to his or her comfort level.
8. Provide care calmly and efficiently; reassure patient during chest pain episodes.
9. Ensure that activity restrictions and bed rest are maintained; teach patient about activity limitation and its rationale; to minimize oxygen requirements and thus decrease chest pain. Reassure patient that activities are allowed based on individual response. Often, patients may be afraid to engage in activities for fear of further deterioration.
10. Instruct the patient to report any further episodes of chest pain.

Dysrhythmia Management

1. Obtain a 12/15/18-lead ECG during patient's episode of chest pain. During angina, ischemia usually is demonstrated on the ECG by ST-segment depression and T-wave inversion.
2. Administer nitrates as prescribed, titrating IV NTG so that chest pain is relieved yet systolic BP remains greater than 90 mm Hg. NTG drip is usually 50 mg NTG in 250-mL D5W. Begin with 6 mL/h, which is 5 µg/min. Titrate by increments of 10 to 20 mL every 5 minutes (or 10 to 20 µg/min every 5 minutes) up to a maximum dosage determined by agency protocol, physician, or midlevel practitioner.
3. As prescribed, administer beta blockers and possibly calcium channel blockers (CCBs), which relieve chest pain by (1) diminishing coronary artery spasm, causing coronary and peripheral vasodilation, and (2) decreasing myocardial contractility and oxygen demand. Monitor for side effects, including bradycardia and hypotension. Be alert to indicators of HF, including fatigue, SOB, weight gain, and edema, and to indicators of heart block, such as syncope and dizziness.
4. Administer oxygen per nasal cannula at 2 to 4 L/min, as prescribed.

NIC Analgesic Administration; Cardiac Care: Acute; Hemodynamic Regulation

CARE PLANS FOR PATIENTS UNDERGOING PERCUTANEOUS CORONARY INTERVENTION

DEFICIENT KNOWLEDGE *related to angioplasty procedure and postprocedure care*

Goals/Outcomes: Within the 24-hour period before the procedure, the patient describes the rationale for the procedure, how it is performed, and postprocedure care. Patient relates discharge instructions within the 24-hour period before discharge from the CCU.

NOC Knowledge: Treatment Procedure(s); Knowledge: Medications; Knowledge: Disease Process

Teaching: Cardiac Disease Process

1. Assess patient's understanding of CAD and the purpose of angioplasty. Evaluate patient's style of coping and degree of information desired.
2. As appropriate for coping style and using a heart drawing, discuss the location of the patient's CAD with the patient and significant others.

Teaching: Procedure/Treatment

1. Use of local anesthesia and sedation during procedure
2. Insertion site of catheter: groin or arm
3. Sensations that may occur: mild chest discomfort, a feeling of heat as the dye is injected
4. Use of fluoroscopy during procedure. Determine patient's history of sensitivity to contrast material or allergy to iodine/shellfish
5. Ongoing observations made by nurse after procedure: BP, HR, ECG, leg or arm pulses, and lab work
6. Importance of lying flat in bed for 6 to 12 hours after procedure if a femoral approach is used, unless a vascular closure device is used. Patients are able to get out of bed sooner when a closure strategy is used
7. Necessity for nursing assistance with eating, drinking, and toileting needs after procedure
8. Need for increased fluid intake after procedure to flush contrast from system
9. If the patient and significant others express or exhibit evidence of anxiety regarding the procedure, try to arrange for them to meet with another patient who has had a successful intervention.

Teaching: Prescribed Medication

Discharge instructions:

1. Importance of taking antiplatelet drugs to prevent restenosis
2. Importance of taking statins and other antilipid drugs to prevent progression of CAD

3. Avoidance of strenuous activity during first few weeks at home
4. Follow-up visit with cardiology 1 week after hospital discharge
5. Signs and symptoms to report to healthcare professional (e.g., GI upset, repeat of angina, fainting)

NIC Teaching: Procedure/Treatment; Anxiety Reduction; Support Group

ADDITIONAL NURSING DIAGNOSES
Also see nursing diagnoses and interventions as appropriate in Nutritional Support (Chapter 1), Mechanical Ventilation (Chapter 1), Hemodynamic Monitoring (Chapter 1), Prolonged Immobility (Chapter 1), Emotional and Spiritual Support of the Patient and Significant Others (Chapter 2), Acute Cardiac Tamponade (Chapter 5), Heart Failure (Chapter 5), and Dysrhythmias and Conduction Disturbances (Chapter 5).

ACUTE INFECTIVE ENDOCARDITIS
PATHOPHYSIOLOGY
Infective endocarditis (IE) is infection of the endocardium (the innermost layer of the heart), often involving the natural or prosthetic valve; *Staphylococcus aureus* is considered the primary pathogen; others are *Staphylococcus epidermis*, *Streptococcus* species: Group A, B, C, G and D, *Viridans*, *Bovis*. Enterococci: alpha-hemolytic, *Intermedius*, *Lugdunensis*, Enterococcal gram-negative bacilli, *Legionella*, *Haemophilus*, *Aphrophilus*, *Actinobacillus*, *Actinomycetemcomitans*, *Cardiobacterium hominis*, *Eikenella corrodens*, *Kingella kingae*, *Bartonella*, *Candida*, *Aspergillus*, and *Pseudomonas aeruginosa*. Forty percent of patients with IE have no underlying heart disease. Despite diagnosis and treatment strategies, the fatality rate has not decreased since the 1970s. The age of a patient, proliferation of implanted biomechanical devices, rise in resistant organisms, and the incidence of hospital-associated infection may have influenced that. Antibiotic prophylaxis has had little effect on decreasing the incidence.

Portals of entry for the infecting organism include the mouth and GI tract, upper airway, skin, and external genitourinary (GU) tract. All heart valves are at risk for infection, but the aortic and mitral valves are more commonly affected than the right-sided pulmonic and tricuspid valves. IV drug abuse, along with right-side insertion of invasive lines increases the possibility of tricuspid IE. Once the infection process begins, valvular dysfunction, manifested by insufficiency with regurgitant blood flow, can occur, ultimately resulting in a decrease in CO. The vegetation may enlarge and obstruct the valve orifice, further reducing CO. The vegetation may break apart and embolize to vital organs. In severe cases, the affected valve may necrose, develop an aneurysm, and rupture; or the infection may extend through the myocardium and epicardium to cause a pericarditis (see Acute Pericarditis, Chapter 5). If the conduction system is affected by the spreading infection, bundle branch block may occur. The chordae tendineae can become infected and rupture, resulting in severe acute mitral or tricuspid regurgitation. Complications of IE occur suddenly, with a dramatic change in the clinical picture. Mortality rates between 20% and 50% have been reported. The infection recurrence rate is 10% to 20%. The incidence of IE is higher in patients older than 50 years of age, is more common in men than in women, and is uncommon in children.

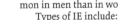

Types of IE include:
- Native valve endocarditis, acute and subacute
- Prosthetic valve endocarditis, early and late: 10% to 20%
- IV drug abuse
- Pacemaker
- Nosocomial

ASSESSMENT
GOAL OF ASSESSMENT
The goal is to identify the severity of symptoms. The severity of symptoms varies depending on the infective organism. (For example, *Staphylococcus aureus* infection is more severe than that with *Streptococcus viridans*.) Acute presentation is defined as onset within 1 week of infection, while subacute infections may take up to 4 weeks to present.

HISTORY AND RISK FACTORS

Patients at higher risk for bacteremia leading to IE include those with valvular disease undergoing invasive procedures and insertion of devices including temporary pacemakers, PA catheters, and central IV catheters or ports; those undergoing endoscopy, surgery, or dental work; and immunosuppressed patients (e.g., with organ transplants, carcinoma, burns, or diabetes mellitus). Users of illicit IV drugs are at risk of tricuspid valve disease.

VITAL SIGNS

- Fever, tachycardia, possible dysrhythmias, possible hypotension, fatigue, and valvular dysfunction

HEMODYNAMIC MEASUREMENTS

Invasive monitoring devices are used cautiously with these patients, as they may cause further valvular dysfunction, embolization, and infection.

- PA catheters are used to assess hemodynamic function if necessary.
- Elevations of PAP and CVP, with reduced CO, are expected in most patients with IE.

OBSERVATION

- The skin is often pale.
- If right-sided HF is present, skin and sclera may be jaundiced and edematous, with neck vein distention, a positive hepatojugular reflex, and ascites.
- Late assessment findings include anemia, petechiae, and clubbing of the fingers.
- Splenomegaly occurs by 10 days because of the activation of the reticuloendothelial system. If marked, a splenic infarct may have occurred.
- Acute infective stage: Diaphoresis, fatigue, anorexia, joint pain, weight loss, abdominal pain, flulike symptoms, pleuritic pain, headache.
- Splinter hemorrhages: Small red streaks on the distal third of the fingernails or toenails
- Janeway lesions: Painless, small, hemorrhagic lesions found on the fingers, toes, nose, or earlobes, probably occurring as the result of immune complex deposition with inflammation
- Osler nodes: Painful, red, subcutaneous nodules found on the pads of the fingers or on the feet, probably occurring as a result of emboli producing small areas of gangrene or vasculitis
- Roth spots: Retinal hemorrhages with pale centers seen on funduscopic examination

Safety Alert   *If emboli of the vegetations occur in other areas, signs and symptoms of stroke or peripheral, myocardial, renal, or mesenteric arterial insufficiency, occlusion, or infarct will be seen.*

AUSCULTATION

- A new or changed murmur may be heard as a result of the valvular dysfunction.
- If HF is present, fine crackles may be auscultated at the lung bases, and an S_3 or S_4 heart sound may be audible.

SCREENING LABWORK

Blood studies can reveal presence of infection or further and progressive worsening heart status, such as HF, conduction problems, or ischemia.

- Cardiac enzymes/isoenzymes: To rule out MI as a cause of chest discomfort or SOB
- BNP: Elevated if HF is present
- Levels of cardiac medications: Low levels may reveal noncompliance with ordered medications.

12-LEAD ELECTROCARDIOGRAM

Evaluates for changes from last ECG to assess for worsening of heart disease (myocardial damage). ECG changes resulting from electrolyte imbalances may also decrease CO. An initial 12-lead ECG should be done on every patient and used for comparison over the course of hospitalization.

- Heart rate: Diagnose type of tachycardia, bradycardia, or irregular rhythm. During acute episodes, atrial dysrhythmias such as paroxysmal atrial tachycardia, premature atrial contractions, atrial flutter, or atrial fibrillation may occur.

Acute Infective Endocarditis

- PR, QRS, QT intervals: May increase, but may be regular with a normal rate and conduction velocity.
- ST-segment and T-wave changes: Depression or elevation

Diagnostic Tests for Infective Endocarditis

Test	Purpose	Abnormal Findings
Noninvasive Cardiology		
12-lead electrocardiogram (ECG) Consider 15- or 18-lead ECG for tricuspid valve (right heart) involvement.	Frequently performed to determine if ischemia or conduction system defects are present.	Heart block may manifest if the AV node or His bundle is affected by the infection. Atrial and/or ventricular enlargement may be seen from the prolonged effects of valvular disease. Chambers may be enlarged or muscle walls thickened (see Table 5-8). Atrial dysrhythmias including premature atrial contractions (PACs), paroxysmal atrial tachycardia (PAT), and atrial fibrillation (AF) are frequently seen as chambers enlarge from volume overload (see Table 5-9).
Blood Studies		
Serial cardiac enzymes CK-MB isoform CK-MB Troponin I	Assess for enzyme changes indicative of myocardial tissue damage; diagnostic for MI; rule out MI.	Elevated if MI occurs from embolization of vegetations into the coronary arteries
Complete blood count (CBC) RBC count WBC count	Assess for signs of infection.	Increased WBCs and eosinophils, with reduced RBCs/possible anemia
Electrolytes Potassium (K^+) Magnesium (Mg^{2+}) Calcium (Ca^{2+}) Sodium (Na^+)	Assess for electrolyte imbalance, which helps with differential diagnosis.	May be normal. Potassium or magnesium is sometimes increased or decreased.
ABGs	Determine effectiveness of oxygenation.	Indicative of cardiac and pulmonary status (see *Acid-Base Imbalances*, Chapter 1)
Coagulation profile Prothrombin time (PT) with international normalized ratio (INR) Partial thromboplastin time (PTT) Fibrinogen D-dimer	Assess for causes of bleeding, clotting, and disseminated intravascular coagulation (DIC) indicative of abnormal clotting present in shock or ensuing shock.	Decreased PT with low INR promotes clotting; elevation promotes bleeding; elevated fibrinogen and D-dimer reflects abnormal clotting. In the presence of effusions, anticoagulants are contraindicated because of the high risk of cardiac tamponade, which can result from bleeding into the pericardium.

Diagnostic Tests for Infective Endocarditis — cont'd

Test	Purpose	Abnormal Findings
Blood cultures For low suspicion of IE: 3 to 6 sets of aerobic and anaerobic blood cultures should be drawn from different venipuncture sites. Drawn 1 hour apart over 3 hours and then, more than 12 hours apart following the hourly samples. If suspicion is high, cultures should be drawn within 1 to 2 hours of presentation and empiric antibiotic treatment begun. If considered prevalent in the area, also consider antibody detection of *Coxiella burnetii*, *Bartonella* spp., *Brucella* spp., *Chlamydia* spp., *Mycoplasma pneumoniae*, *Legionella pneumophila*, and *Aspergillus* spp. May also culture the valve tissue by polymerase chain reaction (PCR)	Can provide definitive diagnosis of the infecting organism. Antibiotics are prescribed based on organism sensitivity. Cultures can be negative when IE is present as a result of slow-growing organisms, prior antibiotic use, failure to obtain adequate number of specimens, or the organism's failure to grow in standard culture media.	The most common bacteria found in native (the patient's) valve IE are *Staphylococcus aureus*, *Streptococcus viridians*, and the HACEK group (*Haemophilus*, *Actinobacillus*, *Cardiobacterium*, *Eikenella*, and *Kingella* spp.). Manipulations of the gastrointestinal (GI) or genitourinary (GU) tract may result in IE from *Enterococcus faecalis*. Early prosthetic valve infections are caused by *Staphylococcus epidermidis*. Gram-negative bacteria. Candida is the most common fungal source of IE.
Additional studies Rheumatoid factor Erythrocyte sedimentation rate (ESR) IE gamma globulins B-type natriuretic peptide (BNP)	To identify the causes of IE and associated diseases	Rheumatoid factor and ESR are elevated. IE gamma globulins may be present. BNP will be elevated if heart failure is present.
Radiology		
Chest radiograph (CXR)	Assess size of heart, mediastinum, thoracic cage (for fractures), thoracic aorta (for aneurysm) and lungs (pneumonia, pneumothorax); assists with differential diagnosis of chest pain.	Cardiac enlargement may reflect widening mediastinum and pericardial effusion. Can be false negative
Computed tomography (CT) Cardiac CT scan	Assesses ventricular size, morphology, function, status of cardiac valves, and circulation. May be done to assess for embolization to other organs.	
Ultrasound Echocardiography (echo) Transesophageal echo (TEE)	Reveals valvular involvement and vegetation size and defines severity of valvular dysfunction. M-mode, 2-dimensional, Doppler, and TEEs are used. TEE is the preferred test.	Detects vegetation, especially with prosthetic valves. Obtained within 2 hours of acute presentation, the test is 90% specific and sensitive. Preexisting IE may be indistinguishable from new vegetations. Consider repeating once a week to assess progress.
Arteriograms: renal, mesenteric, and peripheral	Assess for embolization.	If embolization is present, affected organs are compromised and may fail.

Table 5-8	ASSESSMENT FINDINGS WITH VALVULAR HEART DISEASE		
Valve Dysfunction	Murmur	Pathology	Hemodynamic Changes
Aortic stenosis	Systolic, blowing murmur at second ICS, RSB; may radiate to the neck.	Reduced flow across aortic valve with ↑ LV volume and pressure, with ↓ CO; LV hypertrophy eventually occurs	↑ LV pressure; ↑ PAEDP; ↓ CO and aortic pressure with a narrow pulse pressure reflecting decreased stroke volume
Aortic insufficiency	Diastolic blowing murmur at second ICS, RSB, beginning immediately with S₂	Regurgitant blood flow from aorta to LV during diastole	↑ LV pressure and PAEDP; ↓ CO; ↓ systolic BP and widened pulse pressure
Mitral stenosis	Loud, long, diastolic rumbling murmur at fifth ICS, MCL; may radiate to axilla; S₁ is loud and there is an opening snap with S₂	Reduced flow across mitral valve with left atrial and pulmonary congestion	↑ Mean PAP; ↓ CO
Mitral insufficiency	Systolic murmur at fifth ICS, MCL	Regurgitant blood flow from LV to left atrium, resulting in pulmonary congestion	Giant V waves in the PA occlusive tracing; ↑ systolic PAP; ↓ CO; mean PAP may be normal.
Pulmonic stenosis	Systolic blowing murmur at second ICS, LSB; may radiate to neck	Reduced flow across pulmonic valve with ↑ RV volume and pressure; diminished LV return, resulting in ↓ CO	↑ RV systolic pressure, mean RAP, PAEDP, and mean PAP
Pulmonic insufficiency	Diastolic murmur at second ICS, LSB that starts later and is lower pitched than aortic murmur	Regurgitant blood flow from pulmonary artery to RV during diastolic, resulting in RV overload	↑ systolic RV pressure with wide pulse pressure; LVEDP and CO often normal but may ↓ if disorder is severe.
Tricuspid stenosis	Diastolic murmur at fourth ICS	Reduced flow across tricuspid valve with ↑ right atrial and venous congestion	↑ CVP with accentuated A wave on the RA waveform
Tricuspid insufficiency	Pansystolic murmur at fourth ICS, LSB that increases in intensity with inspiration	Regurgitant blood flow from RV to RA; right atrial and venous congestion occurs.	↑ CVP with prominent V wave on the RA tracing; normal or low PAP, LVEDP, and CO

BP, Blood pressure; *CO,* cardiac output; *CVP,* central venous pressure; *ICS,* intercostal space; *LSB,* left sternal border; *LV,* left ventricle/ventricular; *LVEDP,* left ventricular end-diastolic pressure; *MCL,* midclavicular line; *PA,* pulmonary artery; *PAEDP,* pulmonary artery end-diastolic pressure; *PAP,* pulmonary artery pressure; *RA,* right atrium; *RAP,* right atrial pressure; *RSB,* right sternal border; *RV,* right ventricle/ventricular.

COLLABORATIVE MANAGEMENT

CARE PRIORITIES

1. Prevent infective endocarditis in patients undergoing invasive procedures

- The AHA recommends prophylactic antibiotics for high-risk patients only: Those with a prosthetic heart valve or who have had a heart valve repaired with prosthetic material.
- A history of endocarditis
- A heart transplant with abnormal heart valve function
- Certain congenital heart defects including:
- Cyanotic congenital heart disease (birth defects with oxygen levels lower than normal), that has not been fully repaired, including children who have had a surgical shunts and conduits.

Table 5-9	ECG CHANGES FREQUENTLY FOUND WITH VENTRICULAR AND ATRIAL HYPERTROPHY
Chamber	**ECG Change**
Left ventricular enlargement	"R" voltage increases in V_4 to $_6$; "S" voltage increases (deeper inflection) in V_1 to $_2$; the sum of "S" in V_1 or V_2 and "R" in V_5 or V_6 will be more than 35 mm, or "R" in any V lead will be more than 25 mm.
Left atrial enlargement	"P mitral" in leads II, III, aV_F, and V_1; P wave is m-shaped with a duration more than 0.1 second.
Right ventricular enlargement	"R" voltage increases in V_1 or V_2; "S" voltage increases in V_5, V_6; sum of "R" in V_1 or V_2 and "S" in V_5 or V_6 will be more than 35 mm.
Right atrial enlargement	"P pulmonale" in leads II, III, aV_F, and V_1; P wave is 2.5 mm voltage and 0.1 second duration.

- A congenital heart defect that has been completely repaired with prosthetic material or a device for the first 6 months after the repair procedure.
- Repaired congenital heart disease with residual defects, such as persisting leaks or abnormal flow at or adjacent to a prosthetic patch or prosthetic device.
- Prophylaxis treatment: Amoxicillin 2 g in a single dose before the procedure. If penicillin-allergic, use clindamycin 600 mg orally in a single dose or azithromycin 500 mg orally in a single dose.
- Treatment with confirmation: Patients may be treated IV for at least 2 weeks in the hospital and observed for cardiac and noncardiac complications. The patient may be a candidate for outpatient and home parenteral antibiotic therapy.

2. Treat infection and prevent further complications, such as septic emboli, HF, or cardiogenic shock

- Antibiotics: Treatment of the infection: prompt and accurate treatment has an important effect on outcomes. It is initially empiric in nature and then modified based on blood cultures; penicillin G and gentamicin are given for streptococci coverage. With recent history of antibiotics and possible resistance to antibiotics (methicillin-resistant *Staphylococcus aureus* and penicillin-resistant streptococci), empiric treatment strongly leans toward vancomycin over penicillin for initial therapy. Patients usually require 4 to 8 weeks of IV antibiotics. The first 2 weeks may be initiated during hospitalization and the remaining therapy given on an outpatient basis. The vegetation must be sterilized, abscesses treated, and spread of infection prevented. Initial antibiotic selection is empiric followed by therapy based on the results of the blood/tissue culture and sensitivity studies.
- Fluid and sodium restriction: Used for optimal fluid balance with reduced heart function or HF. Specific restrictions must be individualized and based on severity of symptoms.
- Bed rest: May be used initially, with activity as tolerated for the remainder of treatment
- Diet: High in protein and calories to prevent cardiac cachexia and support the immune system
- Watch for signs of embolization during the first 3 months of treatment: Monitor renal status, vital signs, and oxygenation.

3. Pharmacotherapy

- Oxygen therapy with pulse oximetry (SpO_2): Oxygen (FIO_2) to maintain PaO_2 at 80 mm Hg or higher and pulse oximetry to monitor oxygen saturation continuously or intermittently to keep SpO_2 at 95% or higher
- Diuretics: May be used to decrease symptoms of HF by reducing intravascular volume
- Positive inotropic agents (e.g., digoxin, dobutamine, milrinone): Used to increase contractility and CO
- Vasodilators (nitroprusside, NTG): Reduce cardiac work and improve coronary arterial perfusion. Both preload and afterload (end-diastolic ventricular volume and pressure)

may be reduced to help relieve symptoms of HF. Aggressive vasodilation is not well tolerated by all patients.
- Sedation: May be necessary to allay anxiety and to reduce myocardial oxygen consumption

4. Manage HF and/or cardiogenic shock
See Heart Failure (Chapter 5) and Cardiogenic Shock (Chapter 5).

5. Consider surgical valve replacement
Required when HF worsens or if the infection fails to respond to antibiotics (see Valvular Heart Disease, Chapter 5). An abscess or infected tissue may be surgically removed if there is no response to long-term antibiotics. If the patient is hemodynamically stable, surgery may not be needed. A surgeon is usually consulted in case of an HF emergency. Early surgical intervention with severe valvular damage may decrease hospital mortality.
- **Indications for urgent native valve replacement include**:
  - Heart failure: Caused by acute aortic or mitral regurgitation
  - Persistent fever and bacteremia: For longer than 8 days despite adequate antimicrobial therapy
  - Local spread of infection: Includes abscesses, pseudoaneurysms, abnormal communications (i.e., fistulas) or rupture of one or more valves, conduction disturbances, and myocarditis
  - Virulent organisms: Antibiotic-resistant microorganisms (e.g., fungi, *Brucella* and *Coxiella* spp.) or microorganisms with a high potential for rapid destruction of cardiac structures (e.g., *Staphylococcus lugdunensis*)
- Indications for replacement of prosthetic valves: Complications that may prompt the need to replace a prosthetic valve include primary valve failure, prosthetic valve endocarditis, prosthetic valve thrombosis, thromboembolism, and mechanical hemolytic anemia.
  - Prosthetic valve endocarditis (PVE): The hallmark sign of PVE in mechanical valves is ring abscesses. Ring abscess may lead to valve dehiscence, perivalvular leakage, and formation of myocardial abscesses. Extension to the conduction system may prompt a new atrioventricular block. Valve stenosis and purulent pericarditis are seen less often. Valve stenosis is more common with bioprosthetic valves than mechanical valves. Bioprosthetic valve PVE results in leaflet tears or perforations. Ring abscesses, purulent pericarditis, and myocardial abscesses are seen less often in bioprosthetic valve PVE.
- Early PVE: Occurs within 60 days of valve insertion and is usually the result of perioperative contamination
- Late PVE: Occurs 60 days or later after insertion and is usually the result of transient bacteremia from dental or GU sources, GI manipulation, or IV drug abuse

CARE PLANS FOR ACUTE INFECTIVE ENDOCARDITIS
DECREASED CARDIAC OUTPUT *related to altered preload, afterload, or contractility secondary to valvular dysfunction.*

Goals/Outcomes: Within 72 hours after initiation of therapy, the patient has adequate hemodynamic function with NSR or controlled atrial fibrillation as evidenced by the following: HR less than 100 bpm, BP greater than 90/60 mm Hg, stable weight, intake equal to output plus insensible losses, RR less than 20 breaths/min with normal depth and pattern, and absence of S_3 or S_4 heart sounds, crackles, distended neck veins, and other clinical signs of HF. Optimally, the following normal parameters will be achieved: CO 4 to 7 L/min, CVP 4 to 12 mm Hg, and MAP 60 to 105 mm Hg.
NOC Cardiac Pump Effectiveness; Circulation Status

Cardiac Care
1. Monitor for valvular dysfunction: Assess heart sounds every 2 to 4 hours. A change in the characteristics of a heart murmur may signal progression of valvular dysfunction, which can occur with insufficiency, stenosis, dislodgment of vegetation, or unseating of a prosthetic valve. A new S_3 or S_4 sound may signal HF.
2. Monitor for new dysrhythmias that may contribute to HF: Report new dysrhythmias, which may indicate the spread of infection to the conduction system or atrial volume overload. Correlate dysrhythmias with changes in BP and CO.

3. Monitor for signs of left-sided HF: Crackles, S_3 or S_4 sounds, dyspnea, tachypnea, digital clubbing, decreased BP, increased pulse pressure, increased serum BNP levels, increased LVEDP, and decreased CO.

4. Monitor for signs of right-sided HF: Increased CVP, distended neck veins, positive hepatojugular reflex, edema, jaundice, increased serum BNP levels, and ascites.

5. Monitor for renal dysfunction, fluid volume overload, and third spaced fluids: Measure I&O hourly, and weigh at a consistent time each day, with the same scale and amount of clothing for accuracy. Consult physician or advanced practice provider if patient's weight increases by more than 1 kg per day.
   - Optimize ventricular filling pressures: If the patient's CVP or PAWP is elevated and CO decreases, decrease preload (filling pressures) by limiting fluid and sodium intake and administer diuretics and venous dilators (e.g., NTG) as prescribed. Filling pressures may need to be higher to optimize CO.
   - Reduce resistance to ventricular ejection: If the patient's MAP is high, decrease afterload with prescribed arterial dilators (e.g., nitroprusside).
   - Optimize volume status: For low CVP or BP, consult with advanced practice provider. Vasopressors may be prescribed. Patient may be developing sepsis, so monitor carefully.
   - Optimize coronary artery perfusion: If diastolic BP is low, coronary artery perfusion may be reduced. Prevent further reductions by avoiding administration of morphine sulfate or rapid warming of hypothermic patients. Increase contractility with inotropic drugs, as prescribed.

6. Balance rest and activities: Intolerance indicates ineffective oxygenation.

7. Manage stress: Help the patient reduce stress and myocardial oxygen consumption by teaching stress-reduction techniques such as imagery, meditation, or progressive muscle relaxation. For description of a relaxation technique, see Appendix 7.
   - Provide sedation as needed for anxiety and/or agitation after ruling out the patient is NOT hypoxic.

8. Prevent orthostatic hypotension: Change patient's position from lying to sitting to standing slowly.

See Cardiogenic Shock, Chapter 5, for a discussion of preload and afterload medications.

NIC Energy Management

IMPAIRED GAS EXCHANGE *related to alveolar-capillary membrane changes with decreased diffusion of oxygen secondary to pulmonary congestion.*

- -

Goals/Outcomes: Within 24 hours of initiation of oxygen therapy and during the weaning process, the patient has adequate gas exchange as evidenced by RR less than 20 breaths/min with normal pattern and depth, SvO_2 60% to 80%, PaO_2 greater than 80 mm Hg, SaO_2 greater than 95%, and natural skin color.

NOC Respiratory Status: Gas Exchange; Tissue Perfusion: Pulmonary

Ventilation Assistance

1. Monitor for and manage pulmonary congestion: Assess rate, effort, and depth of respirations. RR increases in response to inadequate oxygenation. Assess color of skin and mucous membranes. Pallor signals impaired oxygenation. Auscultate lungs every 2 hours. Report crackles, rhonchi, and wheezing.

2. Monitor for signs of impending instability: If hemodynamic monitoring with oximetry is used, monitor for decreased SvO_2 prompted by increased metabolic demands or from increased extraction as a result of reduced perfusion/oxygen delivery. SvO_2 values may fall before the patient is symptomatic; the values correlate with CO.

3. Monitor for and manage hypoxemia: Monitor ABG values for PaO_2 less than 80 mm Hg, respiratory acidosis ($PaCO_2$ greater than 45 mm Hg, pH less than 7.35) indicative of respiratory insufficiency or respiratory alkalosis ($PaCO_2$ less than 35 mm Hg, pH greater than 7.45) from tachypnea.
   - Deliver oxygen as prescribed. COPD patients may require NiPPV or intubation and mechanical ventilation to tolerate aggressive oxygen therapy. Oxygen alone may prompt hypoventilation and/or respiratory arrest.
   - Assess arterial oxygen saturation with pulse oximetry. Normal oxygen saturation is 95% to 99%. Levels of 90% to 95% necessitate frequent assessment. Oxygen levels that trend down to less than 90% require aggressive interventions to increase oxygen saturation. Consider increasing FiO_2, decreasing preload, and taking measures to improve ventilation.
   - Place patient in high Fowler position to facilitate gas exchange as tolerated.
   - Have patient cough, deep breathe, and use incentive spirometry to prevent atelectasis.

NIC Invasive Hemodynamic Monitoring; Oxygen Therapy; Respiratory Monitoring

RISK FOR INFECTION (SYSTEMIC) *related to presence of invasive catheters and lines; inadequate secondary defenses secondary to prolonged antibiotic use.*

Goals/Outcomes: The patient is free of secondary infection as evidenced by clear urine with normal odor, wound healing within acceptable time frame, and absence of erythema, warmth, and purulent drainage at insertion sites for IV lines. On resolution of acute stage of IE, the patient remains normothermic with WBC count less than 11,000/mm^3, negative culture results, and HR less than 100 bpm. CO is less than 7 L/min, and Svo$_2$ is 60% to 80%. No yeast overgrowth infections are present. Patient and significant others verbalize rationale for antibiotic therapy and identify where and how to obtain guidelines.

NOC Infection Severity

Infection Protection

1. Prevent central line-associated bloodstream infection: Use strict aseptic technique to care for all invasive monitoring device insertion sites and IV lines. Rotate central lines per hospital protocol. Discuss feasibility of a tunneled catheter or peripherally inserted central catheter (PICC) line with advanced practice provider.
   - Change tubing, containers, and peripheral insertion sites per agency protocol. Inspect all catheter insertion sites daily for redness, drainage, or other evidence of infection. Rotate site immediately if infection is suspected.
2. Control secondary fungal infections: Provide oral care at least every 4 hours to minimize fungal and other infections. Women may require antifungal medications to manage vaginal yeast infections.
3. Prevent catheter-associated urinary tract infections (CAUTI): Implement the CAUTI prevention bundle. Assess ongoing need for a urinary catheter. Remove if possible. Provide perineal care with soap and water for patients with indwelling urinary catheters. Inspect urine for evidence of infection, such as casts, cloudiness, or foul odor. Be alert to patient complaints of burning with urination after catheter is removed.
4. Monitor temperature, WBC count, and HR. Increases may indicate signs of infection.
5. Monitor for signs of sepsis: Calculate SVR with CO measurements. Symptoms of sepsis include increased CO, decreased SVR, and increased Svo$_2$ during the early stages.
6. Teach patient and significant others the importance of reporting signs and symptoms of recurring infections (e.g., fever, malaise, flushing, anorexia) or HF (e.g., dyspnea, tachypnea, tachycardia, weight gain, peripheral edema).
7. Stress the importance of prophylactic antibiotics before invasive procedures such as dental examinations or surgery. The AHA publishes general guidelines for prophylactic antibiotic treatment to prevent IE.

NIC Fever Treatment; Surveillance; Infection Control

> **Safety Alert** *Unlike peripheral venous emboli, these emboli are caused by the vegetations; therefore, prevention is difficult. Interventions are aimed at early detection of embolization and supportive therapies.*

INEFFECTIVE TISSUE PERFUSION (OR RISK FOR SAME) RENAL, GASTROINTESTINAL, PERIPHERAL, CARDIOPULMONARY, AND CEREBRAL *related to interrupted arterial blood flow secondary to septic emboli caused by valvular vegetations.*

Goals/Outcomes: The patient has adequate perfusion as evidenced by urine output at least 0.5 mL/kg/h, at least 5 bowel sounds/min, peripheral pulses at least 2+ on a 0 to 4+ scale, warm and dry skin, BP at least 90/60 mm Hg, RR 12 to 20 breaths/min with normal pattern and depth, NSR on ECG, and orientation to time, place, and person.

NOC Circulation Status

 Hemodynamic Regulation

1. Monitor I&O at frequent intervals. Be alert to urinary output less than 0.5 mL/kg/h for 2 consecutive hours. Report oliguria, as it may signal impending acute renal failure.
2. Monitor bowel sounds every 2 hours. Report hypoactive or absent bowel sounds. Patients are at risk for decreased mesenteric perfusion and mesenteric or bowel infarction.
3. Assess peripheral pulses, color, and temperature of extremities. Weak pulses (2+ or less on a 0 to 4+ scale) with pale, cool limbs/hands/feet may denote peripheral embolization.
4. Monitor patient for confusion and changes in sensorimotor capabilities or cognition, which may signal cerebral emboli.

5. Assess for chest pain, decreased BP, SOB, ischemic or injury pattern on 12-lead ECG, or elevated cardiac enzyme levels indicative of MI caused by vegetation emboli that have migrated to the coronary arteries (see Acute Coronary Syndromes, Chapter 5).
6. Assess for and report appearance of splinter hemorrhages, Osler nodes, Janeway lesions, and Roth spots (see Endocarditis Observation, Chapter 5).

NIC Circulatory Care; Cardiac Care: Acute

ADDITIONAL NURSING DIAGNOSES

As appropriate, also see nursing diagnoses and interventions in Nutritional Support (Chapter 1), Hemodynamic Monitoring (Chapter 5), Prolonged Immobility (Chapter 1), Emotional and Spiritual Support of the Patient and Significant Others (Chapter 2), Acute Cardiac Tamponade (Chapter 5), Heart Failure (Chapter 5), and Cardiogenic Shock (Chapter 5).

ACUTE PERICARDITIS
PATHOPHYSIOLOGY

Pericarditis is the general term for an inflammatory process involving the pericardium and the epicardial surface of the heart. Inflammation can occur as the result of an AMI, an infection, chronic renal failure, or an immunologic, chemical, or mechanical event (Box 5-3). Often, early pericarditis manifests as a dry irritation, whereas late pericarditis (after 6 weeks) involves pericardial effusions that can lead to cardiac tamponade if severe. Pericarditis is often seen in the CCU as a secondary finding following coronary revascularization surgery or valve replacement or associated with chronic renal failure. A thorough assessment and recognition are essential for appropriate treatment, as symptoms can be masked by the primary condition. For example, patients are sometimes transferred into a CCU with acute cardiac decompensation resembling ACS, when in reality, the condition is caused by pericardial effusions.

The initial pathophysiologic findings of pericarditis include infiltration of polymorphonuclear leukocytes, increased vascularity, and fibrin deposition. Inflammation may spread from the pericardium to the epicardium or pleura. The visceral pericardium may develop exudates or adhesions. Large effusions can lead to cardiac tamponade. The excess fluid compresses the heart within the pericardial sac, which impairs filling of the chambers and ventricular ejection.

ASSESSMENT
GOAL OF ASSESSMENT

The goal is to assess severity of the symptoms and to rule out ACS as the cause of ECG changes (ST-segment elevation and/or depression) and chest pain. Acute pericarditis is characterized by chest pain, pericardial friction rub, and serial electrocardiographic changes. Severe pericardial effusions can cause cardiac tamponade.

Box 5-3	CAUSES OF PERICARDITIS
• Autoimmune cardiac injury	• Neoplasms
• Dressler syndrome (post acute myocardial infarction)	• Postpericardiotomy syndrome
	• Radiation injury
• Drug induced (e.g., hydralazine, phenytoin)	• Rheumatologic disease
	• Rheumatic fever
• Hypothyroidism	• Rheumatoid arthritis
• Idiopathic	• Systemic lupus erythematosus
• Infection (bacterial or viral)	• Sarcoidosis
• Myocardial infarction	• Trauma
• Metabolic disorders	• Uremia

HISTORY AND RISK FACTORS

Assess for AMI, recent bacterial or viral infection, chronic renal failure, autoimmune disease including rheumatoid arthritis and systemic lupus erythematosus, radiation therapy, cardiac surgery, or chest trauma. Viral infection is the more common cause (1% to 10%) of acute pericarditis, followed by bacterial infection, which can lead to purulent pericarditis (1% to 8%). Tuberculosis causes 1% to 4% of cases.

OBSERVATION

The patient presents with chest pain, but the location and quality can vary. Pain can be knife-like and stabbing and may radiate to the neck or shoulder. Usually the pain is aggravated by a supine position, coughing, deep inspiration, and swallowing. Pain may be lessened when leaning forward. Dyspnea develops because of shallow breathing to prevent pain.

Early indicators of pericarditis

Fatigue, pallor, fever, and anorexia

Late indicators and evidence of effusions

Increased dyspnea, crackles, and neck vein distention. Joint pain may be present when inflammation is generalized. Evaluate for signs of pain, distress, and tamponade.
- Dyspnea level and oxygen need
- Neck vein distention assessment
- Use of pain scale to determine progress of treatment

VITAL SIGN ASSESSMENT

HR, heart rhythm, and BP are used to evaluate CO and perfusion.
- BP elevated on right arm: When BP is taken on both arms, if cardiac tamponade is ensuing, blood cannot flow into and through the constricted heart.
- Narrowing pulse pressure: May indicate effusion is exerting pressure around the heart
- Pulsus paradoxus: BP should be checked for a paradoxic pressure greater than 10 mm Hg. Normally the systolic pressure is slightly higher during the expiration and lower during inspiration. When effusions are present, this difference in systolic pressure across the respiratory cycle will be greater than 10 mm Hg.
- Tachycardia: Heart rate is usually rapid and regular.
- Beck triad: Hypotension, elevated venous pressure with jugular venous distention, and muffled heart sounds may occur in patients with cardiac tamponade, especially if sudden intrapericardial hemorrhage occurs.

HEMODYNAMIC MEASUREMENTS

If used, the PA catheter reveals elevated CVP, PAP, and PAWP.
- As effusions increase: CO will decrease. If adhesions are present, the filling of the chambers may be restricted, resulting in reduced end-diastolic volumes and pressures.
- If cardiac tamponade is developing: Pressures in all heart chambers eventually equalize and the patient has a cardiac arrest.

AUSCULTATION

Heart sounds may reveal an intermittent pericardial friction rub. The pericardial friction rub has three components; one systolic and two diastolic: one early in diastole when the heart begins to stretch during ventricular filling and the other during late diastole when the ventricles are fully stretched. The first and second heart sounds are obscured by the rubbing sounds, which are sometimes described as the sound of squeaky leather shoes. S_1 and S_2 are no longer crisp and clear. If all three components of the rub are audible, S_2 may sound split.

Pericardial friction rub: The rub is heard best with the diaphragm of the stethoscope positioned at the left lower sternal border. The rub is often positional, so auscultation should be done with the patient in several positions (i.e., supine, sitting and leaning forward, lying on the left lateral side). A friction rub may not be heard, even in the presence of pericarditis.

SCREENING LABWORK
- CBC: May reveal elevated WBCs and anemia
- Cardiac enzymes: Isoenzymes may be elevated if the epicardium is inflamed.

Table 5-10	ECG CHANGES WITH PERICARDITIS	
Stage	Time of Change	Pattern
1	Onset of pain	ST segments have a concave elevation in all leads except AVL and V_1; T waves are upright
2	1 to 7 days	Return of ST segments to baseline with T wave flattening and invert
3	1 to 2 weeks	Inversion of T waves without R or Q changes
4	Weeks to months	ECG returns to prepericarditis state

12-LEAD ELECTROCARDIOGRAM

Evaluates for changes from last ECG; assesses for worsened heart disease (myocardial damage) or electrolyte imbalances that may decrease CO; should be done on every patient to use for comparison.

- HR: Diagnose type of tachycardia, bradycardia, or irregular rhythm. During acute episodes, atrial dysrhythmias such as PAT, PACs, atrial flutter, or atrial fibrillation may occur.
- PR, QRS, QT intervals: May lengthen or shorten
- ST-segment and T-wave changes: Depression or elevation
- Pacing and conduction: Regular, normal rate and velocity
- Late dysrhythmias: Include ventricular ectopy or bundle branch blocks if the inflammatory process involves the ventricles. Pericardial effusion may decrease the voltage of the QRS complex on the ECG. Diffuse ST-segment elevation can be documented as described in Table 5-10.

Diagnostic Tests for Acute Pericarditis		
Test	Purpose	Abnormal Findings
Noninvasive Cardiology		
12-, 15-, and 18-lead electrocardiogram (ECG)	Differentiate between ischemia and inflammation	Will show ST-segment or T-wave changes, which often are confused with ischemic changes. In pericarditis, they are more diffuse and follow a 4-stage pattern (see Table 5-9).
Blood Studies		
Serial cardiac enzymes CK-MB isoform CK-MB Troponin I	Assess for enzyme changes indicative of myocardial tissue damage; diagnostic for MI; rule out MI.	May reveal elevation of the CK and MB bands if the epicardium is inflamed
Complete blood count (CBC) Hemoglobin (Hgb) Hematocrit (Hct) RBC count (RBCs) WBC count (WBCs) Antistreptolysin O (ASO) titer C-reactive protein Sedimentation rate	Assess for anemia, inflammation, and infection; assists with differential diagnosis of chest pain.	Decreased RBCs, Hgb, or Hct reflects anemia from blood loss. ASO titer is elevated when the cause of the pericarditis is an immunologic disorder related to exposure to *Streptococcus*. If the pericarditis is the result of an infection, blood cultures will identify the infecting organism. Other markers of inflammation can be seen (elevated WBCs, C-reactive protein [CRP], lactate dehydrogenase [LDH], or erythrocyte sedimentation rate [ESR]) unless the pericarditis is secondary to uremia.

Continued

Acute Pericarditis

Diagnostic Tests for Acute Pericarditis — cont'd

Test	Purpose	Abnormal Findings
Electrolytes Potassium (K^+) Magnesium (Mg^{2+}) Calcium (Ca^{2+}) Sodium (Na^+)	Assess for electrolyte status.	Use to rule out other causes.
Coagulation profile Prothrombin time (PT) with international normalized ratio (INR) Partial thromboplastin time (PTT) Fibrinogen D-dimer	Assess for causes of bleeding, clotting, and disseminated intravascular coagulation indicative of abnormal clotting present in shock or ensuing shock.	Decreased PT with low INR promotes clotting; elevation promotes bleeding; elevated fibrinogen and D-dimer reflect abnormal clotting. In the presence of effusions, anticoagulants are contraindicated because of the high risk of cardiac tamponade, which can result from bleeding into the pericardium.
Radiology		
Chest radiography (CXR)	Assess size of heart, mediastinum, thoracic cage (for fractures), thoracic aorta (for aneurysm), and lungs (pneumonia, pneumothorax); assists with differential diagnosis of chest pain.	Cardiac enlargement may reflect widening mediastinum and pericardial effusion. False negatives are common. Cardiac enlargement is not always indicative of tamponade nor is it always present with tamponade.
Computed tomography (CT) Cardiac scan	Check for effusions, in both pericardium and epicardium. Assess ventricular size, morphology, function, status of cardiac valves, and circulation.	Will differentiate restrictive pericarditis from constrictive cardiomyopathy by means of the appearance of thickened pericardium on the cross-sectional views of the thorax, which occurs with pericarditis.
Ultrasound Echocardiography (echo) Transesophageal echo (TEE)	Assess for mechanical abnormalities related to effective pumping of blood from both sides of the heart. Assess for fluid in both the pericardial sac and pleural space.	Will show absence of echoes in the areas of effusion. This test, which is essential for quantifying and evaluating the trend of effusions, will appear normal if the pericarditis is present without effusions. TEE may be helpful in identifying some areas of effusion and provide an enhanced view of the posterior wall of the heart.
Magnetic resonance imaging (MRI)	Check for effusions, in both pericardium and epicardium.	

COLLABORATIVE MANAGEMENT

CARE PRIORITIES

1. Relieve acute pain

May experience retrosternal or left precordial chest pain, nonproductive cough, and SOB. Pleural effusion may be present.

- Oxygen: Usually 2 to 4 L/min by nasal cannula, or mode and rate as directed by ABG values or pulse oximetry. Used to promote both myocardial and generalized increases in oxygenation. As oxygen (O_2) delivery to the heart is enhanced, pain can be relieved. If the patient deteriorates, other methods of O_2 delivery may be implemented (e.g., non-rebreather mask with reservoir and mechanical ventilation for those who deteriorate markedly).

- Aspirin: 160 to 320 mg ideally chewed. Should be given immediately if the patient has not been given aspirin before admission to the hospital.
- Nonsteroidal anti-inflammatory drugs (NSAIDs): Preferred for reducing inflammation, particularly if the patient has had an MI or cardiac surgery, since these drugs do not delay healing as do corticosteroids. NSAIDs have fewer side effects than steroids. Examples include aspirin, indomethacin, and ibuprofen. NSAIDs can increase fluid retention and may cause renal insufficiency and worsen HF, as well as pose a risk for GI bleeding.
- Colchicine: Reduces inflammation in the body; may be prescribed as a first-line treatment for pericarditis or for recurrent symptoms. Colchicine can reduce the length of pericarditis symptoms and decrease the risk that the condition will recur. However, the drug is not safe for people with certain preexisting health problems, such as liver or kidney disease. Carefully check the patient's health history before prescribing colchicine.
- Prednisone: Given at 20 to 80 mg daily for 5 to 7 days if there is no response to NSAIDs. Corticosteroids are contraindicated if pericarditis occurs secondary to an AMI because they can cause thinning of the scar formation and increase risk of rupture.
- Medications to manage the cause: Antibiotics, immunoglobulin, antifungals, chemotherapy

2. Prevent cardiac damage and manage pericardial effusions to prevent cardiac tamponade

- Subxiphoid pericardiocentesis: Performed if effusions persist and cardiac status decompensates. A needle (used in a tamponade emergency) or catheter is used to remove the fluid compressing the heart. Echocardiography is used to guide the catheter tip and assess the amount of effusion remaining. The pericardial catheter may be removed after the fluid has been withdrawn or may be left in place for several days to allow for gradual removal of fluid. Usually 100 mL or more is withdrawn every 4 to 6 hours. The catheter is flushed with saline every 4 to 6 hours after withdrawal of the effusion to prevent clotting. Strict aseptic technique is essential for preventing infection.
- Pericardiectomy: A surgical procedure to prevent cardiac compression or relieve the restriction. It may be necessary in chronic pericarditis for patients with recurrent effusions or adhesions. This procedure is often required in severe and recurrent pericarditis associated with uremia.

CARE PLANS FOR ACUTE PERICARDITIS

INEFFECTIVE BREATHING PATTERN *related to guarding as a result of chest pain*

Goals/Outcomes: Within 48 hours of this diagnosis, the patient demonstrates RR 12 to 20 breaths/min with normal depth and pattern and reports that chest pain is controlled.
NOC Respiratory Status: Ventilation

Respiratory Monitoring
1. Assess rate and depth of respirations along with the character and intensity of the chest pain. Provide prescribed pain medication as needed.
2. Teach the patient to avoid aggravating factors such as a supine position. Encourage patient to alter his or her position to minimize the chest pain. The following positions may be helpful: side-lying, high Fowler, or sitting and leaning forward.
3. Assess lung sounds every 4 hours. If breath sounds are decreased, encourage patient to perform incentive spirometry exercises every 2 to 4 hours along with coughing and deep-breathing exercises.
4. To facilitate coughing and deep breathing, teach the patient to support the chest by splinting with pillows or by holding the arms around the chest.

NIC Positioning; Pain Management

ACTIVITY INTOLERANCE *related to bed rest, weakness, and fatigue secondary to impaired cardiac function, ineffective breathing pattern, or deconditioning.*

Goals/Outcomes: Within 72 hours of this diagnosis, the patient exhibits cardiac tolerance to increasing levels of exercise as evidenced by peak HR less than 20 bpm over patient's resting HR, peak systolic BP less than 20 mm Hg over patient's resting systolic BP, Svo₂ at least 60%, RR less than 24 breaths/min, NSR on ECG, warm and dry skin, and absence of crackles, murmurs, and chest pain during or immediately after activity.

NOC Energy Conservation; Endurance; Activity Tolerance

Energy Management

> **Safety Alert** *Steroid myopathy may develop in patients who receive high-dose or long-term steroid treatment. Muscle weakness occurs in the large proximal muscles. Patients experience difficulty lifting objects and moving from a sitting position to a standing position. Steroids also increase the risk of developing osteoporosis and bone fracture; therefore, when on long-term therapy, the patient should take recommended daily intake of calcium and vitamin D.*

---

1. Assess the patient for evidence of muscle weakness; assist with activities as needed.
2. Modify the activity plan for the patient with post-MI pericarditis who is receiving steroids. A lower activity level may help prevent thinning of the ventricular wall and reduce the risk of an aneurysm or rupture of the ventricle.
3. Teach the patient to resume activities as tolerated, resting between activities.
4. For other interventions, see this nursing diagnosis in Prolonged Immobility, Chapter 1.

NIC Cardiac Care: Rehabilitative; Teaching: Prescribed Activity/Exercise

ADDITIONAL NURSING DIAGNOSES

Also see Decreased Cardiac Output in Acute Cardiac Tamponade (Chapter 3). For other nursing diagnoses and interventions, see Prolonged Immobility (Chapter 1).

AORTIC ANEURYSM/DISSECTION
PATHOPHYSIOLOGY

The aorta is exposed to high pulsatile pressure, making it susceptible to injury and disease from mechanical trauma. Conditions that weaken the medial layer or increase stress on the vessel wall can lead to dilation, aneurysmal formation, and eventually rupture or dissection of the aorta. Pathologies related to the aorta can be life-threatening because of the potential for disruption of blood flow to a large portion of the body, including vital organs such as the brain, heart, kidneys, and GI tract. Symptoms may mimic other conditions, and survival depends largely on timely diagnosis and rapid intervention to preserve end-organ function.

An aortic aneurysm is an abnormal dilation of the vessel, with an increase of at least 50% its normal diameter. Aneurysms are usually described based on their location along the aorta (thoracic, abdominal) and their morphology. A true aneurysm involves all three layers of the arterial wall (intima, media, adventitia). The two forms of a true aneurysm are fusiform (symmetrical dilation of the entire circumference of the aorta) and saccular (eccentric ballooning of only a portion of the aortic wall). A false aneurysm or "pseudoaneurysm" is a hematoma caused by injury to the aortic wall, resulting in blood contained by the adventitia or surrounding tissue.

Most often aneurysms develop at the site of an atherosclerotic lesion, which precipitates degeneration of the tissue and allows the arterial wall to dilate. With advancing age, the elastin in the aorta is decreased, which further weakens the vessel wall. Hypertension increases mechanical stress on the vessel, promoting further expansion of the aneurysm. Smoking has been linked to accelerated expansion of both thoracic and abdominal aneurysms. The rate at which the aneurysm increases is not predictable; however, the likelihood of rupture or dissection increases dramatically when the size exceeds 6 cm. Aortic aneurysms result in approximately 17,000 deaths per year, the majority because of rupture.

An aortic dissection is a longitudinal tear in the intimal layer of the aortic wall. Dissection can occur without the presence of an aneurysm. As blood enters the tear, pulsatile pressure creates a false channel between the intimal and medial layers. The force of pressure generated by ventricular contraction and systemic BP can cause the dissection to extend either distally or proximally—compromising flow to structures perfused by that segment of the aorta. Precipitating factors for aortic dissection include medial degeneration from inherited (e.g., connective tissue diseases, congenital defects) or acquired (e.g., hypertension, inflammation) disorders, trauma, pregnancy, and cocaine abuse (see Hypertensive Emergencies, Chapter 5).

Aortic dissection is classified by location, using two different systems. The DeBakey classification defines a dissection as type I if it involves the entire aorta, type II if it is confined to the ascending aorta only, and type III if the dissection originates in the descending aorta, distal to the left subclavian artery. The Stanford system classifies dissections into two groups: type A, which involves both the ascending and descending aorta (DeBakey types I and II), and type B, which affects only the descending aorta (DeBakey type III). Ascending dissections occur much more frequently (65%) than descending dissections and are considered more lethal.

The morbidity and mortality associated with aortic dissection are greatest near the time of the initial injury. Patients who present for medical evaluation within 2 weeks or less of symptom onset are characterized as "acute," while a dissection diagnosed after this time is considered "chronic." Approximately 2000 episodes of acute aortic dissection occur annually, with mortality approaching 75% if left untreated.

ASSESSMENT
GOAL OF THE ASSESSMENT
Gather information that can assist in making the differential diagnosis so appropriate management can be initiated immediately.

HISTORY AND RISK FACTORS
Assess for hypertension, atherosclerosis, and related risk factors (e.g., smoking, CAD, hyperlipidemia), connective tissue disorders (e.g., Marfan syndrome, Ehlers-Danlos syndrome), congenital defects (e.g., coarctation of the aorta, bicuspid aortic valve), family history of aneurysm or dissection, blunt chest trauma, pregnancy, cocaine use, advanced age (older than 60 years), and male sex.

VITAL SIGNS
- Hypertension may be preexisting or an SNS response to pain; more common in descending dissections.
- Hypotension secondary to hemorrhage or complications is associated with ascending dissection (aortic regurgitation, MI, tamponade).
- BP differences between extremities reflect involvement of brachial arteries; variation of 20 mm Hg is considered significant.

OBSERVATION
Pain
- Intense pain of abrupt onset, often described as tearing, ripping, or sharp
- Midline, anterior pain is typical of type A dissection, while posterior (intrascapular), back, or abdominal pain is more common in type B dissection.
- With rupture of an abdominal aneurysm, pain will occur along the flank or lumbar back.
- Pain may radiate, following the path of the dissection.
- Vasovagal responses to intense pain: Diaphoresis, apprehension, nausea, vomiting, faintness may occur.
- Up to 10% of patients may have no pain

Impaired organ perfusion
- Symptoms vary based on location of the dissection and resultant compromise in tissue perfusion.
- Acute LV failure (SOB, chest pain): Results from involvement of coronary arteries or the aortic valve.
- Neurologic deficits: Syncope, confusion, sensorimotor changes, and lethargy result from involvement of branches of the ascending aorta.
- Paraplegia, paresthesia, or focal deficits: Result from involvement of spinal arteries.
- Decreased urine output: If dissection extends to renal arteries, it can cause impaired perfusion and decreased kidney function.

PALPATION
- Pulse deficits (difference in pulse volume or absent pulses) are considered a classic finding; they occur in only 30% of patients.

- Sudden loss of pulses indicates extension of dissection.
- Slow capillary refill and cool skin reflect diminished perfusion.

AUSCULTATION
- Diastolic murmur: With aortic regurgitation
- Muffled heart tones: With cardiac tamponade
- Development or progression of bruits: With turbulent flow through carotid, brachial, or femoral vessels
- Hyperactive bowel sounds: With mesenteric artery ischemia

DIAGNOSTIC TESTS

HIGH ALERT! Rapid diagnostic imaging is essential, because mortality from aortic dissection increases by the hour. Transesophageal echocardiography, CT angiography, and magnetic resonance imaging are all highly accurate in identifying the presence and extent of dissection. The choice of study is usually determined by the patient's clinical stability and the facility's resources. Although the definitive diagnosis is made by imaging studies, additional diagnostic tests may be helpful in ruling out other potential causes of chest pain (pulmonary embolism, MI, pericarditis) or evaluating the extent of end-organ involvement (see Diagnostic Tests Table).

Diagnostic Tests for Acute Aortic Dissection

Test	Purpose	Abnormal Findings
Blood Studies		
Cardiac enzymes	Assess for myocardial infarction.	Elevations indicate myocardial damage but cannot rule out dissection of the ascending aorta, which may involve the coronary vessels.
Complete blood count	Evaluate for infectious processes (pericarditis) and possible blood loss.	WBCs may be elevated secondary to the stress response. Decreased hemoglobin and hematocrit indicate blood loss with aortic dissection or rupture.
Blood urea nitrogen/ creatinine	Evaluate renal function.	Elevations may be seen with dissection involving the renal arteries or with prerenal failure secondary to blood loss.
D-dimer	Evaluate risk for aortic dissection and pulmonary embolism (PE).	A negative result can be used to rule out aortic dissection. Levels >500 mg/mL in the first 24 hours of symptoms support diagnosis of acute dissection (AD), but further studies are needed to distinguish between AD and PE.
Noninvasive Cardiology		
Electrocardiogram (ECG)	Evaluate for presence of myocardial ischemia and infarction.	Presence of ST-segment depression or T-wave inversion (myocardial ischemia), ST-elevation (acute MI), in two contiguous or related leads. Changes could indicate primary MI or dissection with coronary artery involvement.
Transesophageal echocardiogram (TEE)	Assess for presence of aneurysm or dissection, location along the aorta, involvement of other structures (aortic valve, coronary arteries), and presence of complications.	Hallmark of dissection is the presence of an intimal "flap" dividing a true and false lumen. May reveal aortic regurgitation or coronary artery damage if dissection involves ascending aorta. Cardiac tamponade and pericardial effusion may also be present.

Diagnostic Tests for Acute Aortic Dissection—cont'd

Test	Purpose	Abnormal Findings
Radiology		
Chest radiograph (CXR)	Assess for abnormalities of the ascending aorta and rule out other possible causes of chest pain.	Widened mediastinum or abnormal aortic contour may increase suspicion for aortic dissection. A normal CXR may be present in up to 16% of aortic dissections.
Computed tomography angiography (CTA)	Identify dissection and define sites of origin and termination. Also useful in determining branch vessel involvement and size of the aorta.	Visualization of intimal flap and dual lumens confirms dissection. Spiral CT provides rapid imaging of entire aorta, coronary arteries, and pulmonary vessels to differentiate among MI, AD, and PE.
Magnetic resonance imaging (MRI)	Delineate presence and extent of dissection, including site of entry and presence of thrombus.	Presence of an intimal flap, along with true and false lumens, confirms diagnosis of dissection.

COLLABORATIVE MANAGEMENT

Because of the emergent nature of this disorder, limited randomized controlled trials are available to guide the treatment of patients with aortic dissection or rupture. The establishment of the International Registry of Acute Aortic Dissection has provided valuable information regarding presentation, management, and outcomes for this patient population. This information was combined with an appraisal of available cohort studies and retrospective reviews to develop the practice guidelines described in the following table.

ACUTE AORTIC DISSECTION GUIDELINES

In 2010 the American College of Cardiology, American Heart Association, and a number of other professional groups issued guidelines for diagnosis and management of patients with thoracic aortic disease. Some of the class I recommendations for managing acute and chronic dissection are listed below:

Initial Management of Acute Dissection

1. Initial management of thoracic aortic dissection should be directed at decreasing aortic wall stress by controlling heart rate and blood pressure as follows:
   - In the absence of contraindications, intravenous beta blockade should be initiated and titrated to a target heart rate of 60 beats per minute (bpm) or less.
   - In patients with clear contraindications to beta blockade, nondihydropyridine calcium channel-blocking agents should be used as an alternative for rate control.
   - If systolic blood pressure remains greater than 120 mm Hg after adequate heart rate control has been obtained, then ACEIs and/or other vasodilators should be administered intravenously to further reduce blood pressure to a level that maintains adequate end-organ perfusion.
   - Beta blockers should be used cautiously in the setting of acute aortic regurgitation because they will block compensatory tachycardia.

Definitive Management of Acute Dissection

1. Urgent surgical consultation should be obtained for all patients diagnosed with thoracic aortic dissection regardless of the anatomic location (ascending versus descending) as soon as the diagnosis is made or highly suspected.
2. Acute thoracic aortic dissection involving the ascending aorta should be urgently evaluated for emergent surgical repair because of the high risk of associated life-threatening complications such as rupture.
3. Acute thoracic aortic dissection involving the descending aorta should be managed medically unless life-threatening complications develop (e.g., malperfusion syndrome, progression of dissection, enlarging aneurysm, inability to control blood pressure or symptoms).

Continued

ACUTE AORTIC DISSECTION GUIDELINES — cont'd

Management of Asymptomatic Descending and Thoracoabdominal Aneurysms

1. In patients with chronic dissection, especially those with connective tissue disorders, open repair is recommended for aneurysms measuring more than 5.5 cm.
2. In patients with degenerative or traumatic aneurysms of the ascending aorta measuring more than 5.5 cm, endovascular stent grafting should be considered when feasible.
3. In patients with thoracoabdominal aneurysms at high risk for surgery and limited stent options, open repair is recommended when the aneurysm is more than 6.0 cm.

Medical Treatment of Patients with Thoracic Aortic Diseases

- Stringent control of hypertension, with a goal of ≤140/90 mm Hg in patients without diabetes, or <130/80 mm Hg in patients with diabetes or chronic renal disease.
- Optimization of lipid profiles, smoking cessation, and other measures to reduce the risk of atherosclerosis.

From: Hiratzka LF, Bakris GL, Beckman JA, et al: 2010 ACCF/AHA/AATS/ACR/ASA/ SCA/SCAI/SIR/ STS/SVM guidelines for the diagnosis and management of patients with thoracic aortic disease: executive summary. *J Am Coll Cardiol* 55:1509-1544, 2010.

CARE PRIORITIES

The immediate goal of therapy for aortic dissection or rupture is to limit propagation of the dissection by reducing the shearing forces created by myocardial contractility and BP.

1. Preserve the tissue integrity of the aorta with beta-blocker therapy (e.g., metoprolol, esmolol)

To reduce the velocity of LV ejection, slow HR, and reduce BP. Usually administered intravenously, titrating to achieve an HR of 60 bpm or less. In patients unable to tolerate beta-blockers (because of asthma, bradycardia, or signs of HF), CCBs (diltiazem, verapamil) may be used as an alternative.

- Antihypertensive therapy: Initiated if the patient remains hypertensive after beta blockers. Usually nitroprusside or nicardipine is started, as described in Hypertensive Emergencies, Chapter 5. Labetalol is another option, with the added advantage of providing beta blockade. A systolic BP of less than 120 mm Hg is desired.

 Safety Alert *Initiation of a vasodilator before beta blockade can cause a reflexive increase in heart rate and contractility. This sympathetic nervous system-mediated response can lead to further dissection.*

2. Control pain

Usually achieved with IV morphine sulfate, 2 to 10 mg, since morphine helps diminish sympathetic outflow. If additional sedation is required, midazolam may be used.

3. Evaluate for and facilitate surgical or endovascular treatment

Urgent intervention is recommended for type A (ascending) dissection and type B (descending) dissection when impending rupture, significant organ ischemia, or refractory hypertension occurs. Surgery involves removal of the affected section of the aorta and replacement with a prosthetic graft. Repair or replacement of the aortic valve may also be needed. For patients who meet clinical and anatomic criteria, endovascular repair is increasingly an option. This involves placement of a stent graft to occlude the false lumen, thus restoring flow in the true lumen. Fenestration, a technique in which holes are created either in the dissection flap or in the graft to reestablish flow from the aorta into branching arteries, may also be used.

4. Continue medical management

Patients with stable type B dissections are generally managed medically. After control of BP is achieved with IV agents, oral antihypertensive therapy is initiated, along with gradual weaning from the IV infusion. The goal of chronic therapy is to maintain a systolic BP less than 130 mm Hg to prevent further dissection. Long-term management includes beta blockade, lipid control, smoking cessation, and serial imaging to evaluate for further changes in the aorta. This strategy may be evolving, however, since a recent study showed improved 5-year survival when thoracic endovascular repair was added to standard medical therapy.

CARE PLANS FOR AORTIC ANEURYSM/DISSECTION

INEFFECTIVE TISSUE PERFUSION: PERIPHERAL, CARDIOPULMONARY, RENAL, AND CEREBRAL *related to interruption of arterial blood flow secondary to narrowed aortic lumen.*

Goals/Outcomes: Within 48 hours of this diagnosis, the patient has adequate tissue perfusion as evidenced by distal pulses bilaterally equal and greater than 2+ on a 0 to 4+ scale, brisk capillary refill (less than 2 seconds), warm skin, bilaterally equal sensations in the extremities, bilaterally equal systolic BP less than 120 mm Hg, HR less than or equal to 60 bpm, NSR on ECG, urine output greater than 0.5 mL/kg/h, equal and normoreactive pupils, and orientation to time, place, and person.
NOC Circulation Status

Shock Prevention
1. Myocardial infarction: Assess cardiovascular status by monitoring HR and rhythm, ECG, and cardiac enzyme levels. A dissection along the coronary arteries will result in an MI.
2. Perfusion changes: Perform bilateral assessment of BP and distal pulses (particularly radial, femoral, and dorsalis pedis) hourly during initial phase of dissection and then every 4 hours as the patient's condition stabilizes. Report changes in strength or symmetry of distal pulses. Be alert to any change in color, capillary refill, and temperature of each extremity.
3. Emerging dissection: If the difference in systolic BP between the extremities exceeds 10 mm Hg, consult advanced practice provider immediately. Titrate vasodilators based on the highest arm BP.
4. Manage intravascular volume: Monitor hemodynamic parameters (BP, CVP, PAP) for signs of decreased intravascular volume. Establish separate IV lines for volume and medications.
5. Spinal perfusion pressure: Monitor for paresthesias of the extremities — a sign of diminished perfusion to the spinal arteries. Implement drainage of cerebral spinal fluid if available to improve spinal perfusion pressure.
6. Pericardial tamponade: Assess for signs of pericardial tamponade, e.g., distended neck veins, muffled heart sounds, decreased systolic BP (less than 90 mm Hg or greater than 20 mm Hg drop in systolic trend), and pulsus paradoxus.
7. Aortic regurgitation: Assess for signs of acute aortic regurgitation: diastolic murmur, dyspnea, decreased CO.
8. Decreased renal perfusion: Monitor urine output hourly. Consult advanced practice provider if urine output is less than 0.5 mL/kg/h for 2 consecutive hours.
9. Decreased cerebral perfusion: Assess neurologic status hourly. Report restlessness and changes in level of consciousness (LOC), pupil size, or reaction to light.

NIC Hemodynamic Regulation; Cardiac Care: Acute; Circulatory Care; Surveillance

ACUTE PAIN *related to biophysical injury secondary to necrosis at the aortic media and distal tissue hypoperfusion.*

Goals/Outcomes: Within 24 to 48 hours of this diagnosis, patient's subjective evaluation of pain improves, as documented by a pain scale. Nonverbal indicators, such as grimacing, are decreased or absent.
NOC Pain Control

Pain Management
1. Monitor patient at frequent intervals for the presence of discomfort. Devise a pain scale with the patient, rating discomfort from 0 (no pain) to 10 (severe pain). Medicate with analgesics as prescribed, and rate relief obtained using the pain scale.
2. During episodes of pain, assess for a change in peripheral pulses or altered hemodynamics (i.e., BP, PAP, PAWP, CO, SVR), because such changes often are associated with extension of the aortic dissection.

3. Control BP during episodes of pain by titrating vasodilator or use a beta blocker to maintain specified parameters.
4. Immediately consult advanced practice provider for any increase in the severity of pain, because it may indicate the need for emergency surgery.

ADDITIONAL NURSING DIAGNOSES

For other nursing diagnoses and interventions, also see the following as appropriate: Hemodynamic Monitoring (Chapter 1), Prolonged Immobility (Chapter 1), Emotional and Spiritual Support of the Patient and Significant Others (Chapter 2), and Chest Trauma (Chapter 3).

CARDIOGENIC SHOCK
PATHOPHYSIOLOGY

Cardiogenic shock (CS) represents the final pathway of a large number of pathologic conditions, which lead to severe impairment of CO (cardiac function) and result in significant impaired end-organ perfusion. Initial perfusion changes resulting from CS are associated with a cycle of inflammation, ischemia, and progressive myocardial dysfunction. Morbidity and mortality are the end result of severe LV failure. CS may be caused by several conditions: primary LV failure, RV failure, severe valvular regurgitation, or ventricular septal rupture, which may occur alone or in combination. Because of the wide spectrum of causes of CS, the true incidence is unknown; however, the most common cause of CS is AMI. CS occurs in 5% to 8% of patients experiencing an AMI, most commonly in patients with STEMI. Although uncommon, NSTEMI can result in CS. There are few studies characterizing the differences in shock in patients presenting with STEMI versus NSTEMI. Despite high mortality rates in all patients with shock, no definitive guideline recommendations exist for the management of shock in patients with NSTEMI.

CS is initiated by a severe impairment in CO leading to decreased perfusion of the coronary arteries. The result is ischemia, which further reduces myocardial performance, commonly known as "pump failure." Myocardial necrosis or stunning of the myocardium can occur from reperfusion injury during invasive intervention such as primary PCI or reocclusion of the infarcted artery. Next in the cascade of events is the compensatory neurohumoral response to reduced blood flow. Activation of the SNS and renin-angiotensin-aldosterone system result in vasoconstriction and salt and water retention. As resistance to ventricular ejection increases, the result is worsening myocardial ischemia and end-organ hypoperfusion, with an increased incidence of ventricular dysrhythmias. Catecholamine release from the SNS also induces tachycardia, which further increases myocardial oxygen demand and worsens pump failure. As perfusion continues to decrease, compensation fails and vascular beds begin dilating, resulting in anaerobic metabolism and lactic acidosis, which further decreases myocardial contractility. Inflammatory mediators including interleukin-6 and tumor necrosis factor-alpha are elevated, which adds to the negative inotropic effects. Nitric oxide level increases are the result of high levels of cytokines. Vasodilatation progressively increases, which results in hypotension and worsening of lactic acidosis.

Despite decades of studies, the mortality rate from CS remains high. In the future, improved outcomes for patients with CS will result from an improved understanding of the pathophysiology and advances in pharmacologic and mechanical therapies.

ASSESSMENT
GOALS OF ASSESSMENT

The goals are to identify the severity of symptoms and the stage of shock and provide the patient's clinical and laboratory data to assist with the differential diagnosis of the cause.

The diagnosis of CS is dependent on several findings.
- Hypotension: Noninvasive assessment or invasive assessment of BP
- Decreased CO: Tachycardia, low pulse pressure, weak pulses, distant heart sounds, displaced apical impulse, and S_3 or S_4. Systolic murmur may indicate mitral regurgitation or ventricular septal defect. LV or RV dysfunction can be detected through the use of angiography or electrocardiography

- Hypoperfusion: Cool clammy or cyanotic extremities, oliguria from renal hypoperfusion, disorientation, lethargy, elevated lactic acid indicating visceral hypoperfusion
- Pulmonary congestion: Elevated jugular venous pressure, rales, and/ or chest X-ray indicating pulmonary edema

OBSERVATION
As shock progresses from the low CO state, there is evidence of vital organ hypoperfusion: disorientation (altered mental status), oliguria, and acidosis. Skin is cool to cold (mottling may be present) and diaphoretic caused by decreased peripheral perfusion.

VITAL SIGNS AND DIAGNOSTIC CRITERIA FOR CS
1) Systolic BP less than 90 mm Hg for at least 30 minutes or the need for supportive measures to maintain systolic BP above 90 mm Hg
2) Cool extremities or a urine output $\leq$ 30 mL/hour
3) HR $\geq$ 60 bpm
4) Cardiac index $\leq$ 2.2 L/min/m^2 of body surface area
5) Capillary refill greater than 3 seconds (jugular venous distention)
6) Pulmonary capillary occlusion pressure $\geq$15 mm Hg

AUSCULTATION
- S_3 or S_4 heart sounds may be present resulting from an overdistended, noncompliant ventricle.
- Pulmonary congestion and tachypnea result in rales throughout lung fields.
- Mitral regurgitation if present will result in a murmur that is high pitched, holosystolic, and radiates to the axilla. The intensity of the murmur may not correlate with the severity of the regurgitation. Electrocardiographic changes in mitral regurgitation are nonspecific and are primary changes of LV hypertrophy and strain.

HEMODYNAMIC MEASUREMENTS
Hemodynamic monitoring
An arterial line is used to guide initial therapy. The role of invasive hemodynamic monitoring with a pulmonary artery catheter in patients with CS is uncertain. Although no clinical trial has established a clinical benefit from its use, it is still being recommended for use in this patient population. Currently less invasive methods are also being used including:
- Transpulmonary thermodilution
- Pulse contour analysis
- Thoracic electrical bioimpedance
- Bedside Doppler echocardiography

The pulmonary artery catheter may serve to assist with the following in CS patients:
- Diagnostic accuracy
- Help distinguish between LV failure and RV failure:
  - LV failure: high PAOP, low CO, high SVR
  - RV failure: high RA pressure and ratio of right atrial/PAOP greater than 0.8
- Large V wave in PAOP tracing indicates mitral regurgitation.
- Assisting in guiding fluid therapy and inotropic therapy
- Measuring mixed venous oxygen, Svo$_2$, which is an indicator of how well oxygen supply meets tissue demand for energy production

Measuring tissue perfusion
The major focus for the treatment of CS is the improvement and preservation of tissue perfusion. Adequate tissue perfusion depends on an adequate supply of oxygen being transported to the tissues and the cell's ability to use it. Oxygen transport is influenced by pulmonary gas exchange, CO, and Hgb levels. Oxygen use is influenced by the internal metabolic environment.

Improving cellular oxygen transport
Part of the management of CS focuses on improving oxygen transport to the tissues. Svo$_2$ falls below the normal range of 60% to 80% when oxygen supply is decreased or tissue demand in increased. Svo$_2$ has a positive correlation with CO. Continuous monitoring of Svo$_2$ provides an indirect but continuous assessment of CO and perfusion.

Cardiogenic Shock

DIAGNOSTIC TESTS

See Diagnostic Tests for Heart Failure page and Acute Coronary Syndromes (Chapter 5).

COLLABORATIVE MANAGEMENT

CARE PRIORITIES

Patients in CS have high mortality rates. Early and rapid relief of ischemia when the cause of CS is AMI is essential to avoid refractory multiorgan dysfunction and death. Treatment of CS is aimed at improving symptoms and stabilizing the hemodynamics. The goals are to:

- Maximize oxygen delivery at the cellular level
- Reduce causes of increased stress or workload, which increases oxygen demand.

Normalization of ventricular filling pressures and optimization of CO are critical for patient stabilization. The challenge is to augment ventricular filling pressures (preload) without increasing afterload (systemic BP/SVR and PAP) in the process. All measures aim to increase the CO, which is the primary cause of the hypotension associated with severe HF/CS.

INITIAL THERAPY

Limited fluid resuscitation is reasonable unless there is pulmonary edema upon presentation. The maintenance of adequate oxygenation and airway protection is required, along with mechanical intubation if needed. Excessive levels of positive end-expiratory pressure should be avoided to prevent oxygen toxicity. Hypokalemia and hypomagnesemia contribute to ventricular arrhythmias and should be treated immediately. Amiodarone can be used to prevent arrhythmia recurrence. Bradycardia caused by heart block or drug effects should be corrected. Anxiety and pain can be treated with narcotic analgesics as they will also reduce preload, afterload, and sympathetic activity.

PHARMACOLOGIC SUPPORT OF THE FAILING HEART

The major goals of pharmacologic therapy in CS are to maintain adequate arterial pressure and CO. Both inotropes and vasopressors are frequently required. These therapies in high doses are associated with worse outcomes; therefore the lowest possible doses should be used.

The following vasoactive drugs are used in CS:

Dobutamine: Dobutamine is a beta$_1$-agonist agent and is used to increase CO in an unstable patient when systolic BP is above 100 mm Hg.

Milrinone: Milrinone is a phosphodiesterase-3 inhibitor agent and is used to increase CO in a patient who is not critically unstable, and when the systolic BP is above 90 mm Hg.

Dopamine: Dopamine is used to increase CO and BP when the HR is below 110 bpm

Dopamine is used in both low and high doses:

- Low dose: Dopamine receptor agonist–beta$_1$ agonist
- High dose: Alpha agonist

Norepinephrine: Norepinephrine is an alpha agonist and limited beta$_1$ agonist. It is used to increase BP and CO when the systolic BP is less than 90 mm Hg and/or the HR is more than 110 bpm.

Epinephrine: Epinephrine is an alpha agonist and a beta$_1$ agonist. It is used to increase HR, contractility, and systolic BP when the patient is critical.

Isoproterenol: Isoproterenol is a beta$_1$ and beta$_2$ agonist and is used to increase HR when the systolic BP is not $\geq$ 120 mm Hg. Other agents are ideally used before isoproterenol, as the drug can significantly increase myocardial oxygen demand. Isoproterenol may be used more often in patients with a denervated heart following cardiac transplantation to increase HR.

Levosimendan: Levosimendan is an inodilator indicated for the short-term treatment of acutely decompensated severe chronic HF and in situations where conventional therapy is not adequate. Data describing the use of levosimendan in CS are scarce; however, the drug appears to be safe and improve some hemodynamic and ventricular indices.

The principle pharmacologic effects of levosimendan are:

- Increased cardiac contractility by calcium sensitization of troponin C
- Vasodilation
- Cardioprotection

The vasodilation and cardioprotection are related to the opening of sarcolemma and mito-chondrial potassium–ATP channels. Levosimendan improves hemodynamics in the HF patient with no significant increase in cardiac oxygen consumption and relieves symptoms of acute HF. It also has favorable effects on neurohormone levels in HF patients. Patients who are under beta blockade can also be treated with levosimendan as it does not lose effect in these patients. Hemodynamic effects are maintained up to 7 to 9 days after stopping levosimendan because of the formation of an active metabolite. Compared to dobutamine, it produces a slightly greater increase in CO and a greater decrease in PAOP. Severe renal failure is a contra-indication for levosimendan because of the absence of studies based on this risk element.

Vasopressin: In high doses vasopressin activates vascular smooth muscle and oxytocin receptors causing vasoconstriction. It is considered to be a reasonable drug in CS from RV failure. It also reverses hypotension when vasoplegia complicates LVAD surgery.

The American College of Cardiology Foundation/American Heart Association (ACCF/AHA) guidelines no longer recommend the use of any particular agent, although they do report that dopamine may be associated with more harm than other agents. Treatment decisions are therefore based on clinical experiences and the patient's presenting hemodynamic profile.

Table 5-11 provides a summary of the hemodynamic effects of drugs used in CS.

INTRAVASCULAR VOLUME OPTIMIZATION

Optimization of the filling pressures enhances hemodynamic improvement in CS. Hypovole-mia should be treated with crystalloids, colloids, and blood products. As CS is more often associated with hypervolemia in the HF population, diuretics are sometimes used to decrease resistance to ventricular ejection or extremely high filling pressures. The concept of managing hypotension because of hypervolemia is difficult for those inexperienced with CS and HF. Balancing use of diuretics to support reduction of resistance to ejection while maintaining functional filling pressures can be challenging.

LOOP DIURETICS

Furosemide is a loop diuretic that blocks the sodium potassium chloride transporter and increases urinary excretion of sodium and chloride. LV filling pressures are reduced because of the ability of furosemide to increase the systemic venous capacitance.

Other loop diuretics that can be used are bumetanide and torsemide.

MECHANICAL SUPPORT OF THE FAILING HEART

Reduce left ventricular afterload and increase coronary arterial perfusion using balloon counterpulsation therapy/IABP

IABP is the most widely used form of mechanical hemodynamic support in patients with CS. The IABP is a balloon inserted into the descending aorta between the arch vessels and renal

Table 5-11	HEMODYNAMIC EFFECTS OF DRUGS USED IN CARDIOGENIC SHOCK					
Medication	**Mechanism/Receptor**	**Therapeutic Dose**	**BP**	**HR**	**CO**	**SVR**
Dobutamine	$\beta_1 > \beta_2 > \alpha$	2 to 15 µg/kg/min	D	I	I	D
Milrinone	PDE-E inhibitor	0.375 to 0.75 µg/kg/min	D	I	I	D
Levosimendan	Calcium sensitizer	0.05 to 0.2 µg/kg/min	0	0	I	D
Epinephrine	$\beta_1 = \beta_2 > \alpha$	0.01 to 0.03 µg/kg/min	I	I	I	D
Nor-epinephrine	$\beta_1 > \alpha > \beta_2$	0.01 to 0.03 µg/kg/min	I	0 or D	0	I
Dopamine	Moderate dose β	2 to 5 µg/kg/min	I	I	I	0 or D
Dopamine	High dose α	5 to 15 µg/kg/min	I	I	I	I
Phenylephrine	α_1	40 to 60 µg/min	I	D	D	I
Vasopressin	Vascular smooth muscle	0.01 to 0.04 units/min	I	0	0	I

BP, Blood pressure; *CO*, cardiac output; *D*, decrease; *HR*, heart rate; *I*, increase; *O*, no effect; *SVR*, systemic vascular resistance.

arteries. The balloon inflates after cardiac ejection and deflates before the onset of the following systole. The balloon displaces blood proximally, increasing coronary perfusion pressure and raising diastolic aortic pressure. Deflation of the balloon during systole reduces end-diastolic pressure and LV afterload. The main aims of the use of IABP are to improve hemodynamics, increase perfusion of vital organs, and reduce myocardial oxygen consumption. Results of recent studies have resulted in the ACCF/AHA downgrading the use of the IABP to class IIa (can be useful) in the guidelines for the management of STEMI.

Advanced Mechanical Circulatory Support
Percutaneous Left Ventricular Assist Devices
There are currently two devices that can be used in CS patients who are refractory to standard therapy.
TandemHeart
The TandemHeart consists of an external centrifugal blood pump, a 21-French inflow cannula placed in the left atrium via transseptal puncture, and a 17-French outflow cannula inserted into the femoral artery. The system supports the failing LV by providing a 4 to 5 L/min flow. The improved hemodynamics from the Tandem Heart include increased CI, decreased PAOP, and increased MAP. Risks include leg ischemia and displacement of the inflow cannula into the right atrium.
Impella recover 2.5
The Impella device is minimally invasive and the least invasive of the LVADs. It consists of a catheter-based 12-French pump motor inserted via a femoral artery and positioned across the aortic valve. The pump pulls blood from the LV through an inlet area and expels blood into the proximal ascending aorta. The Impella can generate up to 2.5 L/min of forward flow into the systemic circulation. After the pump is inserted and positioned, an activated clotting time (ACT) between 160 and 180 seconds is required to prevent clot formation in the motor. The current ACCF/AHA guidelines provide a IIb recommendation (may be considered) for the use of alternative LVADs for patients with refractory CS.
Extracorporeal membrane oxygenation
Veno-arterial (V-A) extracorporeal membrane oxygenation (ECMO) can also be used to support the CS patient. The ECMO circuit consists of a centrifugal blood pump, a heater, and a membrane oxygenator. ECMO is deployed into the patient via a sternotomy or percutaneously inserted cannula placed in the right atrium (via the femoral vein) and the descending aorta (via the femoral artery). The maximum flow rate is 4 L/min. The use of V-A ECMO provides hemodynamic stabilization and resolution of organ dysfunction from hypoperfusion. The literature to date on the efficacy of ECMO in CS is limited.

Provide other treatments for cardiogenic shock after the cause of pump failure has been identified
1. Emergency CABG or surgical reperfusion
2. Emergency PCI with stent placement in the occluded artery
3. Heart transplantation

CARE PLANS FOR CARDIOGENIC SHOCK

DECREASED CO *related to increased afterload, increased preload, or decreased contractility secondary to loss of 40% or more of myocardial functional mass.*

Goals/Outcomes: The patient's hemodynamic function is optimized as evidenced by CO of at least 4 L/min, BP greater than 90/60 mm Hg, SVR less than 1200 dynes/sec/cm⁻⁵, and PAOP less than 18 mm Hg, before weaning from assist device or pharmacologic agents. PAOP may need to be higher in some patients to maintain the BP.
NOC Tissue Perfusion: Cardiac; Hemodynamic Regulation: Circulatory Care;

Shock Management: Cardiac
1. Monitor arterial vital signs and hemodynamics continuously.
2. Customize alarm parameters on patient monitoring systems to the parameters ordered by the advanced practice provider and the ICU's policy and procedures to decrease unnecessary and nonactionable alarms and noise for patient and family.

3. Titrate vasoactive drugs to achieve a CO between 4 and 7 L/min, arterial BP at least 90/60 mm Hg, and PAOP less than 18 mm Hg. If reduction of filling pressures results in worsening hypotension, filling pressures are generally maintained at the level that optimizes the BP.
4. Assess CO/CI and SVR every 1 to 4 hours and after titration of pharmacologic therapy. If SVR increases to greater than 1200 dynes/sec/cm⁻⁵, notify physician.
5. Auscultate lung sounds every 2 hours, and monitor urine output hourly. Report any change that is significantly different from previous assessment.
6. Keep HOB elevated at least 30 to 45 degrees if not contraindicated and if IABP not in place.
7. Ventricular dysrhythmias are treated only if compromising CO/CI.
8. Temporary cardiac pacing may be indicated for symptomatic bradycardia.
9. If medical management fails to improve hemodynamic profile, prepare patient and family for insertion of IABP or LVAD.

INEFFECTIVE TISSUE PERFUSION: ALTERED CARDIOPULMONARY, CEREBRAL, PERIPHERAL, AND OR RENAL TISSUE PERFUSION *related to interrupted arterial blood flow to vital organs secondary to inadequate arterial pressure.*

Goals/Outcomes: Within 96 hours of initial diagnosis of CS, the patient will have adequate tissue perfusion as evidenced by orientation time, place and person, equal and normoreactive pupils; normal deep tendon reflexes; urine output at least 0.5 mL/kg/h; warm and dry skin; peripheral pulses at least 2+ on a 0 to 4 scale; brisk refill; BP at least 90/60 mm Hg; and SVO₂ greater than 65% or within patient's normal range.
NOC Circulation status

Cardiac Care: Acute Hemodynamic Regulation
1. Check neurologic status every 2 hours to assess cerebral perfusion. Changes in LOC, orientation, perception, motor activity, reflexes, and pupillary response to light should be reported to the physician.
2. Monitor I&O hourly to assess renal perfusion; report urine output less than 0.5 mL/kg/h for 2 consecutive hours. Assess extremities every 2 hours for any changes in skin color, temperature, capillary refill, and distal pulses.
3. Titrate vasoactive drugs to maintain systolic BP at 90 mm Hg or above.

IMPAIRED GAS EXCHANGE *related to alveolar-capillary membrane changes secondary to pulmonary congestion; altered oxygen-carrying capacity of the blood secondary to acidosis occurring with anaerobic metabolism.*

Goals/Outcomes: Before weaning from supplemental oxygen or ventilator assistance is attempted, the patient will have adequate gas exchange as evidenced by Pao₂ of at least 80 mm Hg, RR 12 to 20 breaths/min with normal depth and pattern, oxygen saturation at least 95%, SVO₂ 60% to 80%, and Scvo₂ at least 80%.
NOC Tissue Perfusion: Pulmonary; Respiratory Status: Gas Exchange

Ventilation Assistance
1. Every hour assess rate, depth, and effort of patient's respirations. Note tachypnea or labored breaths. Inspect skin and mucous membranes for pallor or cyanosis, which indicates hypoxia. Consult advanced practice provider if any changes occur.
2. Auscultate lung fields every 1 to 2 hours.
3. Monitor ABG values for hypoxemia (Pao₂ less than 80 mm Hg) or metabolic acidosis (pH less than 7.35 and HCO₃⁻ less than 22 mEq/L may indicate lactic acidosis).
4. Administer oxygen as ordered.
5. Monitor oxygen saturation with a pulse oximeter. If less than 90%, notify physician.
6. Monitor and manage Svo₂ by supporting CO. When CO decreases, perfusion decreases and oxygen extraction increases, lowering Svo₂.
7. If the patient deteriorates, prepare for intubation and mechanical ventilation.

NIC For patients undergoing IABP procedure

DECREASED CARDIAC OUTPUT *related to negative inotropic changes and rates, rhythm and conduction alterations secondary to ischemia or injury.*

Goals/Outcomes: Within 24 hours of diagnosis of CS, patient's CO is effectively supported as evidenced by MAP at least 60 mm Hg to support peripheral perfusion, improved ECG rhythm, HR above 60 and less than 100 bpm or at a higher rate that optimizes the BP without prompting angina, peripheral pulses audible with Doppler or palpable, hourly urine output at least 0.5 mL/kg/h or renal support strategy in place, CI greater than 2.5 L/min/m^2, SVR less than 1200 dynes/sec/cm^{-5}, SVO$_2$ 60% to 80%, Scvo$_2$ at least 80%, and patient is able to awaken and maintain periods of alertness, is oriented or responds to reorientation, and has chest pain controlled.

NOC Hemodynamic Regulation: Circulatory Care; Cardiac Pump Effectiveness

Circulatory Care: Mechanical Assist Device
1. Monitor BP, CVP, PAP, RAP, SVO$_2$, and HR continuously. Monitor PAOP, SVR, and CO/CI hourly. Report increased PAOP, decreased CO, new ST-segment elevation or depression, deterioration in heart rhythm, decreased Svo$_2$, or elevated SVR to advanced practice provider.
2. Monitor hourly urine output. Report output less than 0.5 mL/kg/h for 2 consecutive hours. Monitor BUN and creatinine values daily. Report increased BUN (greater than 20 mg/dL) and serum creatinine (greater than 1.5 mg/dL) indicative of acute renal failure.
3. Monitor bilateral peripheral pulses along with color and temperature of extremities every 2 hours.
4. Maintain ventilator support or oxygen delivery as ordered.
5. Titrate inotropic agents to maintain CI at least 2.5 to 4 L/min/m^2. Monitor for drug side effects, including changes in heart rhythm.
6. Regulate afterload-reducing agents to maintain SVR less than 1200 dynes/sec/cm^{-5}. Monitor for side effects including hypotension, dizziness, headache, nausea and vomiting, and cutaneous flushing.
7. Administer diuretic agents as ordered for elevated PAOP (greater than 14 mm Hg). Monitor for signs and symptoms of hypokalemia caused by the diuretics.
8. Provide a quiet environment for the patient and family.
9. Administer pain medications as ordered and assess effectiveness using pain assessment tools/scales.
10. Monitor Hgb and Hct values daily as loss of blood reduces oxygen delivery to the cells, resulting in tachycardia and tachypnea.

INEFFECTIVE TISSUE PERFUSION: PERIPHERAL: INVOLVED LEG *related to interrupted arterial blood flow secondary to arterial wall dissection by sheath or thrombus formation.*

Goals/Outcomes: Throughout hospitalization, the patient has adequate perfusion in the involved leg as evidenced by Doppler or palpable peripheral pulses, normal color and sensation, warmth, full motor function, and absence of bleeding, abdominal pain, and tingling in the involved leg.

NOC Tissue Perfusion: Peripheral; Circulation Status

Circulatory Care: Arterial Insufficiency
1. Monitor circulation in affected leg every 30 minutes for 2 hours and every 2 hours thereafter if assessment is within normal limits. Assess pulses, temperature, color and sensation, and mobility of the toes in the involved leg. Consult physician or midlevel provider immediately if any changes occur.
2. Instruct patient to notify RN if pain, numbness, or tingling occurs in the involved leg.
3. Provide protection to heel of involved leg to prevent pressure ulcer and place protective material such as sheepskin between toes.
4. Have patient perform passive foot exercises at least 4 times daily without bending leg at the hip.
5. Administer IV medications as ordered to prevent clots from forming on the balloon. Monitor patient for signs of bleeding, including decreased Hct, abdominal pain, hematuria, oral bleeding, or blood-tinged mucus.
6. Keep HOB at least 30 degrees or less to prevent migration of the balloon catheter.
7. Assess the following for balloon migration: decreased left radial pulse, sudden decrease in urine output, flank pain, and dizziness. Notify advanced practice provider if changes are noted.

IMPAIRED TISSUE INTEGRITY *related to external factors (pressure and immobilization); internal factors (altered circulation, possible insulin resistance, and decreased nutritional intake).*

Goals/Outcomes: Throughout hospitalization, patient's tissues remain intact.

NOC Tissue Integrity: Skin and Mucous Membranes.

Pressure Ulcer Prevention:
1. Position patient on low-pressure protective bed to enhance blood flow to dependent areas and allow air circulation across the skin, promoting evaporation of moisture.

2. Reposition patient every 2 hours keeping involved leg extended and log-roll patient onto side.
3. Provide care to keep skin dry and clean, inspect pressure areas at the beginning of each shift.
4. Patient's diet should be high in protein and calories.
5. Keep glucose within recommended range (the American Association of Clinical Endocrinologists and American Diabetes Association consensus statement recommends a target glucose range of 140 to 180 mg/dL in critically ill patients).
6. Encourage ambulation after assessing patient utilizing an evidence-based mobility protocol if available or consulting with physician (if not on IABP or LVAD).

INEFFECTIVE BREATHING PATTERN *related to fatigue and decreased energy secondary to HF; decreased lung expansion secondary to medically imposed position (HOB at 30 degrees).*

Goals/Outcomes: Within 4 hours after diagnosis of HF, the patient has an effective breathing pattern as evidenced by Pao$_2$ at least 80 mm Hg, Spo$_2$ at least 90%, absence of adventitious breath sounds, and RR 12 to 20 breaths/min with normal pattern and depth.
NOC Respiratory Status: Ventilation; Respiratory Status: Gas Exchange

Respiratory Monitoring
1. Monitor breath sounds every 2 hours. Assess anterior and posterior lung fields for adventitious or absent sounds.
2. Monitor oxygen saturation continuously and maintain greater than 90%.
3. Monitor RR, rhythm, and breathing pattern hourly.
4. Assess for atelectasis and respiratory infection (increased temperature, SOB, increased sputum production or coughing, and altered color of sputum).
5. Monitor temperature every 4 hours and WBC daily for signs of infection.
6. Encourage patient to breathe deeply, cough, and use incentive spirometer every hour.
7. Reposition patient every 2 hours to minimize status of lung secretions.
8. Monitor I&O.
9. Elevate HOB 30 degrees or more as tolerated.
10. Prepare for intubation and mechanical ventilation if the patient's respiratory status deteriorates.

INEFFECTIVE PROTECTION *related to risk of bleeding secondary to coagulopathy or IV anticoagulants needed to maintain therapeutic equipment (left ventricular assist devices).*

Goals/Outcomes: Throughout hospitalization, patient's bleeding is controlled as evidenced by secretions and excretions negative for blood, chest tube drainage within acceptable amounts, and absence of abdominal pain or ecchymosis.
NOC Blood Coagulation

Bleeding Precautions
1. Monitor PTT, ACT (or other blood clotting labwork), and platelet levels daily.
2. Monitor Hct and Hgb daily.
3. Protect patient from injury and suction oral cavity carefully.
4. Administer gastric acid-neutralizing drugs as ordered.
NIC Bleeding Reduction

Patients with ventricular assist devices
RISK FOR COMPLICATIONS FROM IMMOBILITY *related to imposed restrictions against movement secondary to presence of assist device or debilitated state.*

Goals/Outcomes: Patient is able to retain baseline range of motion of joints affected by immobilization.
NOC Mobility.

Exercise Therapy: Joint Immobility
1. Turn patient every 2 hours with assist device in place if care is taken during turning.
2. Provide passive range of movement to extremities 4 times daily and encourage family to assist.

NIC Energy Management

DECREASED CARDIAC OUTPUT *related to altered preload and negative inotropic changes secondary to reduced right ventricular contraction occurring with left- sided heart assist device.*

This is a complication of left-sided heart assist devices, particularly when the outflow cannula is located in the left ventricle. When the left ventricle is decompressed, septal wall motion is diminished, reducing right ventricle contraction.

Goals/Outcomes: Within 24 of diagnosis of HF patient's CO will be adequate as evidenced by measured CO 4 to 7L/min, RAP 4 to 6 mm Hg, PVR 60 to 100 dynes/sec/cm⁻⁵, and LAP at least 10 mm Hg.
NOC Circulation Status; Cardiac Pump Effectiveness

Circulatory Care: Mechanical Assist Device
1. Monitor patient for decrease in CO with associated increases in RAP and PVR.
2. An adequate preload is necessary to prevent a vacuum effect from the device, thereby decreasing CO.

RISK FOR INFECTION *related to inadequate primary defenses secondary to presence of multiple invasive lines, movement restrictions, and stasis of body fluids.*

Goals/Outcomes: Patient is free of infection as evidenced by normothermia, WBC count 11,000/mm³ or less, negative culture results, and absence of swelling, warmth, tenderness, and purulent drainage at incision or cannulation sites.
NOC Immune Status

Infection Protection
1. Every day monitor vital signs temperature, WBC count, and observe incisions and cannulation sites for evidence of infection.
2. Culture any drainage that is purulent, and report positive findings.
3. Change IV tubing every 72 hours (or per protocol) using aseptic technique.
4. Change all dressings over catheter insertion sites as per protocol.
5. Administer antibiotics as ordered.
6. Attain nitrogen balance by providing adequate nutrition.
7. Monitor breath sounds every 2 hours; after extubation have patient perform coughing and deep breathing exercises and have him or her mobilize as soon as possible.
8. Provide gentle chest physiotherapy as ordered.

IMBALANCED NUTRITION LESS THAN BODY REQUIREMENTS *related to decreased intake secondary to oral intubation; increased nutrition needs secondary to debilitated state and impaired tissue perfusion with concomitant nitrogen malabsorption.*

Goals/Outcomes: Within the 24- to 48-hour period before discharge from the ICU, the patient will have adequate nutrition as evidenced by a balanced nitrogen state and stable weight.
(Optimal nutrition in the ICU patient is still being debated in the literature.)
NOC Nutritional Status: Nutrient Intake

Nutritional Management
1. Provide via tube feedings or total parental nutrition, to ensure minimum 1 to 5 g protein/kg/day. (In patients with body mass index [BMI] less than 30, protein requirements should be in the range of 1.2 to 2.0 g/kg actual body weight.) In the critically ill obese patient, permissive underfeeding or hypocaloric feeding is recommended. In obesity where BMI is greater than 30, the goal of the enteral feeding regimen should not exceed 60% to 70% of target energy requirements or 11 to 14 kcal/kg actual body weight/day (or 22 to 25 kcal/kg ideal body weight/day). Protein should be provided in a range of ≥ 2.0 g/kg ideal body weight/day for patients with BMI 30 to 40 and ≥ 2.5 g/kg ideal body weight/day for BMI ≥ 40.
2. A dietician should be monitoring the patient daily.
3. Weigh patient daily for trend.
4. Monitor I&O hourly.

CARDIOMYOPATHY
PATHOPHYSIOLOGY
Cardiomyopathy (CM) refers to a heterogeneous group of myocardial diseases that are often genetic and associated with mechanical and electrical dysfunction. Most types of CM result in

inappropriate ventricular hypertrophy or dilation. The AHA 2006 Expert Panel on Contemporary Definitions and Classification of Cardiomyopathy categorized CM into two major groups: primary and secondary CM. Primary CMs are caused by pathology confined to the heart muscle alone; whereas secondary CMs are caused by pathology from a variety of generalized systemic (multiorgan) disorders (Table 5-12). Some common disease entities involving the heart muscle have been excluded from the present contemporary CM classification. These include pathologic myocardial processes and cardiac dysfunction caused by another cardiovascular abnormality, such as valvular heart disease, systemic hypertension, congenital heart disease, and atherosclerotic CAD. Other conditions not included in this CM classification are cardiac tumors, diseases affecting the endocardium with little or no myocardial involvement,

Table 5-12	TYPES AND CAUSES OF CARDIOMYOPATHY
Primary Types of Cardiomyopathy	**Secondary Causes of Cardiomyopathy**
Genetic Hypertrophic cardiomyopathy Arrhythmogenic right ventricular cardiomyopathy/dysplasia Left ventricular noncompaction ***Mixed Type (Genetic and Nongenetic)*** Dilated cardiomyopathy Restrictive cardiomyopathy (nonhypertrophied and nondilated) ***Acquired Type*** Inflammatory (myocarditis) Stress-induced ("tako-tsubo" or "broken heart syndrome") Peripartum Tachycardia induced	*Autoimmune/Collagen* Systemic lupus erythematosus, dermatomyositis, rheumatoid arthritis, scleroderma, polyarteritis, nodosa
	Storage Hemochromatosis, Fabry disease, glycogen storage disease (type II, Pompe), Niemann-Pick disease
	Neuromuscular/Neurologic Friedreich ataxia, Duchenne-Becker muscular dystrophy, Emery-Dreifuss muscular dystrophy, myotonic dystrophy, neurofibromatosis, tuberous sclerosis
	Infiltrative Amyloidosis, Gaucher disease, Hurler disease, Hunter disease
	Inflammatory (Granulomatous) Sarcoidosis
	Endocrine Diabetes mellitus, hyperthyroidism, hypothyroidism, hyperparathyroidism, pheochromocytoma, acromegaly
	Cardiofacial Noonan syndrome, lentiginosis
	Endomyocardial Endomyocardial fibrosis, hypereosinophilic syndrome (Löeffler endocarditis)
	Nutritional Deficiencies Beriberi (thiamine), pellagra, scurvy, selenium, carnitine, kwashiorkor
	Toxicity Drugs, heavy metals, chemical agents
	Electrolyte Imbalance *Consequence of Cancer Therapy* Anthracyclines: doxorubicin (Adriamycin), daunorubicin, cyclophosphamide, radiation
	Infectious HIV, Lyme disease, Chagas, coxsackie, influenza

Note: This table lists common diseases associated with primary and secondary CM and is not intended to represent an exhaustive and complete list of conditions associated with CM. Some disagreement exists in the scientific community regarding the classification, definition, and nomenclature of CM; therefore, discrepancies and contradictions may occur among various scientific resources.

Cardiomyopathy

and hypertensive hypertrophic CM. Primary and secondary CMs included in the 2006 AHA definition of CM are further classified into the following: hypertrophic CM (HCM), dilated CM (DCM), arrhythmogenic RV CM/dysplasia (ARVC/D), and LV noncompaction (LVNC). Be aware that one disease, be it primary or secondary CM, may fall into more than one CM classification, causing confusion if there is an overlap between categories. For example, some genetic primary CMs are known to cause both DCM and HCM. Furthermore, a CM may evolve as a consequence of remodeling from one category to another as the disease progresses. CMs, whether confined to the heart (primary CM) or part of a generalized systemic disorder (secondary CM), often lead to cardiovascular death or progressive HF-related disability.

FUNCTIONAL CLASSIFICATIONS OF CARDIOMYOPATHY
Dilated cardiomyopathy
Dilated cardiomyopathy (DCM) is characterized by marked, progressive dilation of the ventricles, resulting in decreased myocardial contractility and a reduced systolic ejection fraction (less than 40%). DCM is the most common cause of cardiomyopathy. Infectious agents (particularly viruses producing myocarditis), cocaine, chronic excessive alcohol consumption, and chemotherapeutic agents are common causes of DCM, along with other autoimmune, neurologic, metabolic, endocrine, nutritional, and other systemic disorders. About 20% to 35% of DCM cases have been reported as familial, and they are frequently associated with skeletal muscle or neuromuscular disorders. In patients with severe dilation, the increase in total cardiac mass may lead to ventricular hypertrophy. Alternatively, DCM may occur as a late manifestation of hypertrophic heart disease. DCM may ultimately lead to a decline in LV contractile function, ventricular and supraventricular arrhythmias, conduction system abnormalities, thromboembolism, progressive HF, and sudden or HF-related death.

Hypertrophic cardiomyopathy
Hypertrophic cardiomyopathy (HCM) is characterized by inappropriate hypertrophy of the ventricular muscle, leading to LV stiffness and diastolic dysfunction. HCM is most often a genetically acquired illness and is the most common inherited heart defect. Approximately 60% to 70% of patients with HCM have familial HCM, an inherited autosomal dominant condition. Other cardiovascular diseases, including hypertension and aortic stenosis, are capable of producing the same magnitude of wall thickening seen with HCM. HCM is the most common cause of sudden cardiac death in the young, especially in athletes, but may lead to HF and disability at any age. Obstructive HCM (also called hypertrophic obstructive cardiomyopathy or HOCM) occurs when the enlarged heart muscle, usually the ventricular septum, obstructs the ventricular outflow channel. HOCM may result in angina, HF, and sudden death.

Restrictive cardiomyopathy
Restrictive cardiomyopathy (RCM) is less common than HCM or DCM and is characterized by nondilated ventricles with impaired ventricular filling from rigid or fibrotic ventricular walls. LV diastolic dysfunction occurs, often associated with very high end-diastolic pressures and moderate to marked biatrial enlargement secondary to elevated atrial pressures. Hypertrophy is typically absent, although the infiltrative and storage diseases (such as amyloid and hemochromatosis) may cause an increase in LV wall thickness. Systolic function usually remains normal, at least early in the disease. Treatment is difficult and prognosis is poor. Differentiating RCM from constrictive pericarditis is important since the two clinical pictures are similar, while management is markedly different.

Arrhythmogenic right ventricular cardiomyopathy/dysplasia
Arrhythmogenic right ventricular cardiomyopathy/dysplasia (ARVC/D) is an uncommon genetic disease characterized by progressive replacement of normal myocardial cells with fatty or fibrofatty tissue. Initially thought to be a disease isolated to the right ventricle, more recent evidence shows that the left ventricle is also involved in as many as 75% of cases. Clinical manifestations include ventricular arrhythmias and HF. In young adults, ARVC/D often presents with sudden death.

Left ventricular noncompaction
Left ventricular noncompaction (LVNC) is an anatomic abnormality of LV myocardial development characterized by a "spongy" and "noncompacted" morphologic appearance of the LV

myocardium. Noncompaction predominantly involves the apical portion of the LV chamber with deep intertrabecular recesses, or channels, in communication with the ventricular cavity and filled with blood from the ventricular cavity. LVNC has been associated with a high incidence of HF, thromboembolism, and ventricular arrhythmias in adults.

ASSESSMENT
GOAL OF ASSESSMENT
The physical assessment of patients with CM attempts to characterize the etiology and severity of cardiac dysfunction, the level of functional impairment, and the optimal therapeutic approach. Furthermore, the physical assessment should identify factors that precipitated clinical decompensation, for example, exercise or exacerbation of autoimmune disease. A good physical assessment will help differentiate heart and circulatory failure from entities that cause similar complaints and findings. During the course of treatment, the physical assessment will also provide feedback about the patient's response to therapies (Table 5-13).

OBSERVATION
A patient's clinical presentation will vary according to the type and extent of the CM and whether the patient has progressed to overt HF. The clinical presentation will reflect both the hemodynamic abnormalities caused by cardiac dysfunction and the degree of secondary compensatory mechanisms. Patients' presenting symptoms may range from asymptomatic to, unfortunately, symptoms continuous with cardiogenic shock (CS) or sudden death. Most commonly, patients will present with symptoms of HF or arrhythmias. Diagnostic tests used in patients with suspected cardiomyopathy are outlined in the following table.

Diagnostic Tests for Cardiomyopathy		
Test	**Purpose**	**Abnormal Findings**
Noninvasive Cardiology		
Transthoracic echocardiogram (noninvasive cardiac ultrasound)	Mechanical and structural assessment of the heart. • Left and right ventricular function • Ventricular wall motion • Ventricular size • Valve function • Estimation of pulmonary artery pressures • Intracardiac thrombus or tumors • Pericardial effusion	Reduced ejection fraction: • Heart failure • Cardiomyopathy Wall motion abnormality: • Myocardial infarction (acute or remote) • Conduction abnormality Valvular dysfunction: • Stenosis or insufficiency of any of the cardiac valves Pulmonary hypertension: • COPD • Primary pulmonary hypertension • Pulmonary embolism • Left heart failure Intracardiac thrombus or tumor
Holter monitoring (24 to 48 hours)	Can help detect the presence of intermittent arrhythmias, including dangerous ventricular arrhythmias	May reveal undiagnosed, significant, asymptomatic, or minimally symptomatic arrhythmias
12-, 15-, or 18-lead electrocardiogram (ECG)	An ECG provides valuable information about the heart rate, rhythm, electrical conduction system, electrical synchrony, and presence of hypertrophy, ischemia, or infarction.	The detection of LA enlargement, repolarization abnormalities, and pathologic Q waves is often the first clue to the presence of HCM. Low voltage is seen in patients with RCM.

Continued

Cardiomyopathy

Diagnostic Tests for Cardiomyopathy — cont'd

Test	Purpose	Abnormal Findings
Functional exercise testing (VO_2 Max testing)	Determines maximal myocardial oxygen consumption (VO_2 Max) defined as the greatest amount of oxygen a patient can take in, transport, and use while performing dynamic aerobic exercise.	This test quantifies a patient's functional limitations resulting from ventricular dysfunction and helps differentiate between cardiac and pulmonary causes. VO_2 Max is usually expressed as milliliters of oxygen consumed per kilogram of body weight per minute.

Blood/Laboratory Studies

Laboratory testing is individualized based on a patient's history, examination findings, and imaging tests. Specialized diagnostic laboratory testing, such as gene testing, hemochromatosis panel, autoimmune tests, and infection screening, might not always be necessary or may only be ordered on initial presentation.

Complete blood count (CBC) Hemoglobin (Hgb) Hematocrit (Hct) RBC count (RBCs) WBC count (WBCs)	Assesses for anemia, inflammation, and infection; assists with differential diagnosis of chest discomfort and fluid balance.	Decreased Hgb/Hct: • Anemia • Volume overload WBC: • Normal or elevated with infection
Electrolytes Potassium (K^+) Magnesium (Mg^{2+}) Calcium (Ca^{2+}) Sodium (Na^+)	Assesses for possible causes of arrhythmias and/or evaluate volume status.	Hypokalemia: • Often related to diuretic use • Diarrhea Hyperkalemia: • Renal failure • Medication side effect (ACEIs, angiotensin receptor blockers, aldosterone antagonists) • Rhabdomyolysis • Acidosis Hyponatremia: • Volume overload • Medication side effect Hypernatremia: • Dehydration
Digoxin levels	Digoxin levels are often difficult to manage in heart failure patients. Levels should be obtained for patients with decompensated CHF, patients with acute renal failure, and any time digitalis toxicity is a concern. (Digoxin levels are not accurate after the administration of digoxin immune fab (Digibind) for elevated digitalis levels.)	Elevated levels in renal failure, overdose, decompensated heart failure. Signs of digoxin toxicity: • Ventricular arrhythmias • Progressive bradycardia • Heart block • Neurologic symptoms (confusion, visual disturbances)
Coagulation profile Prothrombin time (PT) with international normalized ratio (INR) Partial thromboplastin time (PTT) Fibrinogen D-dimer	PT/INR: Assesses for coagulation with warfarin therapy, coagulopathy with hepatic congestion in heart failure. D-dimer: Assesses for signs of increased fibrinolysis and determine level of suspicion for blood clots.	Elevated PT/INR: • Anticoagulation • Hepatic vascular congestion • Liver failure Elevated D-dimer: • Presence of disease process or blood clot (an elevated D-dimer is a finding that must be further evaluated for life-threatening diagnoses such as pulmonary embolism)

Diagnostic Tests for Cardiomyopathy—cont'd

Test	Purpose	Abnormal Findings
B-type natriuretic peptide (BNP) and pro-BNP	BNP is a hormone secreted by the ventricles in response to increased blood volume and subsequent stretch. The patient's baseline BNP level is helpful in determining current heart failure status. Serial BNP measurements in the hospitalized patient is not helpful in reducing mortality or improving outcomes.	Normal BNP: • Helpful in ruling out heart failure in a patient with heart failure symptoms Elevated BNP: • CHF • Acute renal failure • Sleep apnea • Hyperthyroid
Blood urea nitrogen (BUN) and creatinine levels	Assessment of renal function	Elevation: • Medication side effect (diuretics, ACEIs, angiotensin receptor blockers, aldosterone antagonists) • Chronic renal failure • Acute renal failure • Dehydration
Hepatic enzymes and serum bilirubin levels	Serum glutamate oxaloacetate transaminase/aspartate aminotransferase (SGOT/AST) Serum glutamate pyruvate transaminase/alanine aminotransferase (SGPT/ALT) Serum bilirubin	Elevation: • Acute GI illness • Hepatic congestion resulting in increased hepatic enzymes and bilirubin
Troponin	Assesses for damage to myocardial cells.	Elevation: • Myocardial infarction • Demand ischemia in a hypoxic state (hypotension, sepsis, respiratory failure) • Renal failure • Pulmonary embolism
Thyroid function Thyroid-stimulating hormone (TSH) Free thyroxine index (FTI) or thyroxine (T_4)	Screens for thyroid disease, which may contribute to heart failure.	TSH may be elevated unless the disease is long-standing or severe. FTI and T_4 levels may be decreased (see Myxedema Coma, Chapter 8, for more information).
Urinalysis	Helps assess for renal and urologic disease, metabolic abnormalities, and infection that may be related to cardiomyopathy.	Findings will be patient-specific.
Radiology		
Chest radiograph (CXR)	• Cardiac size and position • Thoracic cage • Lungs	Cardiac enlargement • Hypertension • Heart failure Thoracic cage • Fractures • Widened mediastinum (suggestive of aortic dissection) Lungs

Continued

Diagnostic Tests for Cardiomyopathy—cont'd

Test	Purpose	Abnormal Findings
Cardiac magnetic resonance imaging (MRI)	Assesses ventricular size, morphology, function, status of cardiac valves, and circulation.	• Enlarged or remodeled heart • Incompetent or stenotic heart valves • Narrowed or occluded coronary arteries • Myocarditis or pericarditis • Cardiac tumors • Fatty infiltration • Inflammation • Scarring/fibrosis
Cardiac computed tomography (CT scan)	Assesses ventricular size, morphology, function, status of cardiac valves, and circulation	• Enlarged or remodeled heart • Incompetent or stenotic heart valves • Narrowed or occluded coronary arteries Chest CT can be used to diagnose pulmonary embolism and aortic dissection, but specific protocols must be used or these findings may be missed
Single photon emission computed tomography (SPECT)	A radioactive tracer is injected into the blood. Living heart muscle takes up the tracer. A camera picks up the signals from the tracer and pictures are created that show blood flow to the heart muscle. Cardiac wall motion and ejection fraction are also assessed. At rest, the viability of cardiac muscle can be assessed. A stress test involves the comparison of rest and stress (exercise- or chemical-induced) scans to determine cardiac ischemia with stress	Reversible ischemia: • Viable areas of myocardium are not getting adequate blood flow with stress, suggestive of significant coronary artery disease Fixed ischemia: • Completed infarction, with blood flow absent in one or more areas of the heart at rest and with stress

Invasive Cardiology

Test	Purpose	Abnormal Findings
Transesophageal echocardiogram	Similar to the transthoracic echocardiogram, but invasive as an endoscope is used. Enhanced views of the heart valves and the posterior wall. This procedure requires sedation.	Same as transthoracic echocardiogram
Coronary angiography/cardiac catheterization	• Presence and extent of CAD • Left ventricular function • Valvular disease • Pulmonary pressure Uses a radiopaque catheter inserted through a peripheral vessel and advanced into the heart and coronary arteries.	Normal pressures found with right heart catheterization and hemodynamic monitoring are in Chapter 1.
Endomyocardial biopsy (EMB)	EMB is used to determine the classification and/or cause of cardiomyopathy through histologic studies that may identify an infiltrative or genetic disorder.	EMB tissue can detect inflammation, metabolic abnormalities, the presence of fibrofatty infiltration, and many other abnormalities of the myocardium. EMB is performed during cardiac catheterization.

Table 5-13	**SIGNS AND SYMPTOMS OF CARDIOMYOPATHY**		
Source of Initial Cardiomyopathy		**Dilated**	**Hypertrophic**
Clinical presentation	• Signs and symptoms of CHF usually develop insidiously and are caused by LV failure, RV failure, or biventricular failure. • Common symptoms include exertional dyspnea, fatigue, weakness, dry cough, orthopnea, PND, ascites, peripheral edema. • Patients may also have changes in mentation; i.e., confusion, restlessness, lethargy.	• Wide spectrum of signs and symptoms, depending on extent and severity of dysfunction • Most patients have few symptoms or are asymptomatic. • Symptomatic patients present with signs and symptoms of heart failure: dyspnea, PND, angina (caused by hypertrophy and relative ischemia), palpitations, fatigue (caused by decreased CO), and syncope (caused by arrhythmias or obstructive HCM).	• The least common type of CM. Hallmark signs and symptoms are from ventricular stiffness caused by LVH and endocardial fibrosis, reducing ability of the ventricle to relax and fill during diastole. • Common presenting symptoms include exercise intolerance and exertional dyspnea. • In more advanced disease, orthopnea, PND, peripheral edema, ascites, fatigue, and weakness. • Angina if RCM caused by amyloidosis
Physical assessment	• Must estimate the severity of hemodynamic dysfunction. • Common exam findings associated with HF: tachycardia, JVD, PMI displaced down and to left; +S₃ and S₄ gallops, systolic murmurs of AV valves; basilar rales; ascites and hepatomegaly, especially if RV failure; extremities cool, mottled, cyanotic; peripheral pulses weak with pulsus alternans; BP normal or low • Sinus tachycardia, atrial fibrillation, and ventricular arrhythmias are common.	• May reveal the presence of an LV outflow tract obstruction by revealing a harsh left sternal border caused by turbulent flow through the outflow tract. • An S₄ gallop may be present. Supraventricular arrhythmias, especially atrial fibrillation, and ventricular arrhythmias are common. • Sudden death can be the first symptom.	• Usually a result of elevated venous pressure and include dependent peripheral edema, ascites, and an enlarged, tender, and pulsatile liver; JVD that does not fall normally or may rise with inspiration (Kussmaul sign) • Atrial fibrillation is common. • PMI is typically in normal position and of normal character. • Heart block may be evident in patients with amyloidosis or sarcoidosis. • There may also be a loud S₃ or murmur of tricuspid or mitral regurgitation.

AV, atrioventricular; CHF, congestive heart failure; CM, cardiomyopathy; CO, cardiac output; HCM, hypertrophic cardiomyopathy; HF, heart failure; JVD, jugular venous distention; LV, left ventricular; LVH, left ventricular hypertrophy; PMI, point of maximal impulse; PND, paroxysmal nocturnal dyspnea; RCM, restrictive cardiomyopathy; RV, right ventricular.

COLLABORATIVE MANAGEMENT
CARE PRIORITIES
1. Reduce activity level to decrease oxygen demand during periods of activity intolerance because of instability

When the patient stabilizes, increase activity gradually, as tolerated, to prevent complications of immobility. Document activity tolerance (including position in bed) to help reflect if treatments are effective.

2. Initiate pharmacotherapy to maintain or reestablish hemodynamic stability, control symptoms, and prevent cardiac remodeling, all of which aid in halting further disease progression

Medications commonly used in the treatment of CM and their nursing implications (also see Heart Failure, Chapter 5, and Cardiogenic Shock, Chapter 5):

- HCM: Beta blockers reduce myocardial oxygen demand and increase diastolic filling time by slowing the HR, relaxing cardiac muscle, and increasing CO. Also, beta blockers help decrease cardiac outflow obstruction during exercise and reduce sympathetic cardiac stimulation in patients with HCM.
- DCM: Beta blockers block the compensatory response of the adrenergic system to HF and increase CO/CI. Vital signs should be monitored to ensure patients do not develop symptomatic bradycardia or hypotension. Note: These effects are not immediate and may take days to weeks to occur. Initiating or increasing beta-blocker doses while a patient is experiencing signs and symptoms of HF may worsen dyspnea, edema, bradycardia, and vasodilation. Beta-blocker therapy should be started at a low dose and titrated up slowly to avoid exacerbation of acute HF symptoms. Not all patients with CM tolerate target doses of beta blockers and should be titrated individually while monitoring BP, HR, and signs and symptoms of worsening HF.

ACEIs/ARBs: Used in DCM to decrease preload and afterload and block the compensatory response of the renin-angiotensin system to HF. Goal systolic BP is greater than 90 mm Hg. Monitor patients for postural hypotension, hyperkalemia, and worsening renal function.

Diuretics: Diuretics reduce preload and pulmonary congestion. If a patient is hemodynamically monitored, diuretics will result in a decreased PAWP and help to achieve a negative fluid balance and ultimately a euvolemic state. Use diuretics cautiously for HCM since they are contraindicated in some patients with obstructive HCM. Monitor the patient for weakness, postural hypotension, hypokalemia (see Hypokalemia, Chapter 1), hypomagnesemia, dehydration, and worsening renal function.

Aldosterone antagonists: Aldosterone is a neurohormone shown to contribute to the development of LV hypertrophy and fibrosis involved in cardiac remodeling. Aldosterone antagonists are weak diuretic drugs that block the action of aldosterone. These drugs inhibit sodium reabsorption in the distal convoluted tubule of the kidney and cause retention of potassium and magnesium. Potassium levels must be closely monitored to avoid hyperkalemia or worsening renal function. Other side effects include postural hypotension and gynecomastia if taking spironolactone.

Potassium supplements: Potassium lost in the urine as a result of diuresis may necessitate replacement with potassium supplements. Maintain serum levels in the high normal range (4.2 to 5 mEq/L).

Vasodilators (hydralazine and nitrates): These drugs decrease preload and afterload in DCM, resulting in improved CO and enhanced nitric oxide availability. It is important to maintain a stable BP (keep MAP at 65 mm Hg or higher). Nitrates are not typically used in HCM. Side effects of vasodilators include postural hypotension, dizziness, headache, nausea, and vomiting.

Inotropic therapy (digoxin, dobutamine, milrinone): Inotropes enhance contractility. If a patient has hemodynamic monitoring, the goal of milrinone and dobutamine is to increase CO/CI and maintain a stable BP for adequate perfusion. Monitor for rhythm disturbances. Other potential side effects include headache and angina.

> **Safety Alert** *Digoxin is contraindicated in the treatment of obstructive hypertrophic cardiomyopathy, as it may be ineffective or worsen the condition. Digoxin is also contraindicated in patients with a diagnosis of amyloidosis.*

Antiarrhythmic agents: Medications used to control atrial and ventricular arrhythmias are common for patients diagnosed with DCM and HCM.

Anticoagulants: Anticoagulants are important to prevent thrombus formation related to atrial fibrillation or decreased ventricular contraction and emptying. INRs must be monitored with extra caution because of the potential for medication interactions that affect the INR (such as antibiotic use).

Calcium channel blockers (CCBs): Nonhydropyridine CCBs, such as verapamil or diltiazem, may be used to treat HCM by improving diastolic filling time, heart muscle relaxation, and exercise capacity. Most CCBs are contraindicated in DCM, except for hydropyridine CCBs (such as amlodipine), which are occasionally used to treat hypertension in patients with DCM.

4. Initiate electrical/device-based therapy to maintain or reestablish hemodynamic stability, control symptoms, and prevent cardiac remodeling

(For further information, also see Heart Failure, Chapter 5, and Cardiogenic Shock, Chapter 5.)

* Dual-chamber pacemaker: Implantation of a dual-chamber pacemaker may be performed to treat symptomatic bradycardia (including sick sinus syndrome or heart block).
* Implanted cardioverter defibrillator (ICD): Implantation of an ICD is indicated for patients with LVEF 35% or less and HF symptoms. Patients must be on optimal medical therapy and at least 40 days post-MI before implantation. (In some instances, LVEF will improve with medical therapy and/or treatment of CAD.) ICD therapy has been shown to significantly reduce mortality in patients with reduced LVEF. Patients should have a life expectancy of at least 1 year before implantation. In patients with end-stage HF symptoms who have an ICD in place, the decision can be made to deactivate the defibrillator to avoid unnecessary discomfort at end of life.
* Cardiac resynchronization therapy (CRT): Approximately one third of HF patients develop a widened QRS complex, indicating asynchronous ventricular function. Implantation of biventricular pacing allows coordination of the right and left ventricles. CRT is indicated for patients with LVEF 35% or less, and a QRS duration of 150 ms or greater with HF symptoms. CRT can improve contractility and EF and decrease cardiac remodeling. CRT can be combined with an ICD as a single device if the patient meets the requirements for both therapies.

5. Initiate hemodynamic monitoring to help evaluate intracardiac pressures during therapeutic interventions

Routine hemodynamic monitoring is not recommended for all patients with cardiomyopathy or decompensated HF. Hemodynamic monitoring should be considered in patients with persistent symptoms in whom renal function is worsening with therapy and inotropic or vasoactive agents are required, and those who are being considered for advanced therapies such as LVAD implantation or cardiac transplantation.

6. Initiate advanced therapies for symptom management and stabilization

Alcohol ablation: During a cardiac catheterization, ethanol is injected into the septal branches of the LAD. This purposeful reduction of myocardial tissue through a limited, therapeutic septal infarction will reduce outflow obstruction in HCM.

Ultrafiltration: Ultrafiltration, used to treat acute decompensated HF with volume overload, is the mechanical removal of excess body fluid by the generation of a convective gradient across the hemofilter membrane. The electrolyte concentration of the ultrafiltrate is equal to that of the plasma and avoids the stimulation of the renin-angiotensin-aldosterone axis.

Intraaortic balloon pump (IABP): In the presence of a failing myocardium, an IABP helps to decrease afterload and increase coronary artery perfusion

* Left ventricular assist devices (LVADs): Some patients with CS unresponsive to intra-aortic balloon counterpulsation and IV inotrope therapy may be referred for mechanical circulatory support. LVADs may be used as a bridge to cardiac transplantation or as a destination therapy for those ineligible for transplant. The inflow cannula of an LVAD is connected to the apex of the left ventricle. Blood is pumped by the device via the outflow cannula to the aorta. Complications include stroke, infection, coagulopathy with bleeding, multiple organ dysfunction syndrome (MODS), and prosthetic valve insufficiency. Most modern LVADs have continuous flow, leaving the patient without a palpable pulse despite adequate perfusion.

7. Provide surgical interventions to maintain or reestablish hemodynamic stability, control symptoms, and prevent cardiac remodeling

(For further information, also see Heart Failure, Chapter 5, and Cardiogenic Shock, Chapter 5.)

Ventricular septal myotomy-myectomy: During this procedure, the hypertrophied ventricular septum of obstructive HCM is removed.

Heart transplantation: Open heart transplantation is pursued for patients with advanced CM refractory to optimal medical therapy. Each institution has criteria that must be met before transplantation is considered a treatment option (see Organ Transplantation, Chapter 11).

CARE PLANS FOR CARDIOMYOPATHY

Nursing care must be based on the type of CM, its associated pathology, and the patient's clinical manifestations. Acute decompensated HF is a gradual or rapid change in HF signs and symptoms resulting in a need for urgent therapy because of elevated LV filling pressures and/or low CO. The primary aspects of care related to acute decompensated HF are outlined since this is the most common presenting problem, for this patient population, in the acute care setting.

DECREASED CARDIAC OUTPUT *related to disease process that has resulted in decreased ability of the heart to provide adequate pumping to maintain effective oxygenation and nutrition of body systems.*

Goals/Outcomes: Within the 24-hour period before discharge from the CCU, the patient has adequate CO as evidenced by:

NORMAL VALUES FOR HEMODYNAMIC MEASUREMENTS

Assessment Measure	Goal
SBP	At least 90 mm Hg
MAP	At least 65 mm Hg
CI	2.5 to 4 L/min/m^2
CO	4 to 7 L/min
PAWP	Less than 18 mm Hg
Right atrial pressure (RAP)/CVP	4 to 6 mm Hg
RR	12 to 20 breaths/min
HR	Less than 100 bpm
Urinary output	More than 0.5 mL/kg/hr
Skin assessment	Warm and dry
Peripheral pulses	At least 2+ on a 0 to 4+ scale
Mental status	Orientation to time, place, and person (assuming baseline orientation ×3)

SBP, Systolic blood pressure; *MAP*, Mean arterial pressure; *CI*, Cardiac Index; *CO*, Cardiac Output; *PAWP*, Pulmonary artery wedge pressure; *CVP*, Central venous pressure; *RR*, Respiratory Rate; *HR*, Heart rate.

NOC Cardiac Pump Effectiveness; Circulation Status

Cardiac Care: Acute Hemodynamic Regulation

1. Pulmonary artery pressures: Evaluate hemodynamic readings at least every 1 to 2 hours. Manage PAWP greater than 18 mm Hg and RAP/CVP greater than 6 mm Hg. Although normal PAWP is 6 to 12 mm Hg, these patients may need increased filling pressures for adequate preload, with wedge pressure at 15 to 18 mm Hg. Those with right-sided HF may need an RAP/CVP 8 to 12 mm Hg. Measure CO/CI every 2 to 4 hours and on an as-needed basis. Optimally, CO should be 4 to 7 L/min and CI should be 2.5 to 4 L/min/m^2; for some patients, the best CO/CI will be below expected normal values.

2. Electrolytes and renal function: Monitor I&O records and weigh the patient daily at the same time every day, noting trends and goal weight. Individuals with CM may be on a strict fluid-restricted (e.g., 1000 to 2000 mL/day) and sodium-restricted (e.g., less than 2000 mg/day) diet. Notify the advanced practice provider if urinary output is less than 0.5 mL/kg/h, or if urine output does not increase after diuretic therapy.

3. Dysrhythmias: Monitor ECG continuously for sinus or atrial tachycardias, atrial fibrillation, or ventricular ectopy, which may further decrease CO.
4. Mobility: Assist patients with activities of daily living (ADLs) and report worsening exercise tolerance. To prevent complications of immobility, perform or teach patients and significant others active, passive, and assistive ROM exercises. For a discussion of an in-bed exercise program, see Table 5-7 and interventions in Prolonged Immobility, Chapter 1.
5. Medication management: Administer prescribed medications in accordance with possible food and medication interactions. Administer the HF medications throughout the day rather than administering them all at once. Provide ongoing patient education regarding the purpose and common side effects for each medication.

NIC Cardiac Care: Acute; Circulatory Care: Mechanical Assist Device; Hemodynamic Regulation; Shock Management: Cardiac; Neurologic Monitoring; Medication Management; Dysrhythmia Management

ACTIVITY INTOLERANCE *related to imbalance between oxygen supply and demand secondary to decreased functioning of the myocardium.*

Goals/Outcomes: Within the 12- to 24-hour period before discharge from the CCU, patients should exhibit cardiac tolerance to increasing levels of activity as evidenced by respiratory rate less than 24 breaths/min, BP within 20 mm Hg of patient's normal range, HR within 20 bpm of patient's normal resting HR, return to a stable baseline ECG rhythm, and activity tolerance to a level without presence of angina/chest pain or worsening dyspnea.
NOC Activity Tolerance; Energy Conservation

Energy Management
1. Monitor the patient's physiologic response to activity, reporting any symptoms of chest pain, new or increasing SOB, increases in HR greater than 20 bpm above resting HR, and increase or decrease in systolic BP greater than 20 mm Hg.
2. Assess for and manage decreased CO, e.g., changes in mentation, cool-clammy skin, or tachycardia.
3. Plan nursing care so that the patient is assured of extended periods of rest (at least 90 minutes). Consult the advanced practice provider to ensure that exercises are within the patient's prescribed limitations.

NIC Activity Therapy; Energy Management; Teaching: Prescribed Activity/Exercise; Dysrhythmia Management; Pain Management; Medication Management

ADDITIONAL NURSING DIAGNOSES

Also see nursing diagnoses and interventions in Hemodynamic Monitoring (Chapter 1), Heart Failure (Chapter 5), Prolonged Immobility (Chapter 1), Emotional and Spiritual Support of the Patient and Significant Others (Chapter 2), and Cardiogenic Shock (Chapter 5).

DYSRHYTHMIAS AND CONDUCTION DISTURBANCES
PATHOPHYSIOLOGY

Cardiac dysrhythmias reflect abnormal function of the heart's electrical system. Cardiac electrical cells closely interface with the mechanical cells, which contain the contractile muscle filaments. Dysrhythmias may originate in any part of the electrical system, from the pacing cells (sinoatrial [SA] node, atrioventricular [AV] junction) to any portion of the conduction system (atria, His–Purkinje system, bundle branches, and ventricles). Sympathetic and parasympathetic nerve fibers influence the rate of discharge of the SA node, conduction through the AV node, and force of both atrial and ventricular contraction. The main parasympathetic influence is the vagus nerve, which slows the rate of pacing by the SA node and AV junction, and decreases force of contraction. Sympathetic nerve fibers originate from T1 to T5 and, when stimulated, produce the neurotransmitter norepinephrine, which increases HR during the stress response. Sympathetic stimulation also promotes production of catecholamines by the adrenal glands, and the hormones are received by catecholamine receptors (alpha receptors, beta receptors, dopaminergic receptors), which increase HR, force of contraction, BP, and CO. Electrical dysfunction can markedly change the CO and cause prompt deterioration in the patient's hemodynamic status (Figure 5-1).

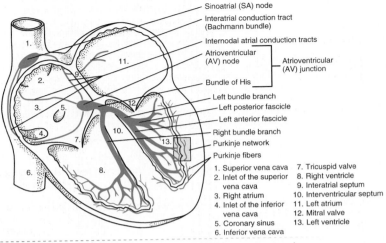

1. Superior vena cava
2. Inlet of the superior vena cava
3. Right atrium
4. Inlet of the inferior vena cava
5. Coronary sinus
6. Inferior vena cava
7. Tricuspid valve
8. Right ventricle
9. Interatrial septum
10. Interventricular septum
11. Left atrium
12. Mitral valve
13. Left ventricle

Figure 5-1 Electrical conduction system. (From Huszar RJ: *Basic dysrhythmias: interpretation and management,* ed 3, St. Louis, 2002, Mosby.)

Cardiac electrophysiology involves studying the electrical impulses and their conduction across the atria and throughout the ventricles to provide power and coordination for the cardiac cycle. Electrical impulses are created by ion exchange. Exchange of ions in the mechanical or muscle cells generates electrical activity. At rest, the muscle has slightly more positive ions (Na^+ and Ca^{2+}) on the outside of the cells and more negative ions inside the cells (resting membrane potential or polarization). K^+ is the most prevalent intracellular ion. The resting cells have a threshold for activation, based on the difference in the ion concentrations (action potential). Stimulation of a cardiac muscle cell, or depolarization, is created by a rapid influx of Na^+ followed by a slower influx of Ca^{2+} into the cell. Normally, the influx is followed by muscle contraction. The cell responds to the influx by K^+ diffusing out of the cell to help rebalance the positive ions (early repolarization and plateau phase) on both sides of the cell membrane. A slower efflux is followed by a rapid efflux of K^+ (rapid repolarization). Finally, the sodium-potassium pump must activate to fully rebalance the electrical potential of the cell, restore the ions to their original position, and achieve resting membrane potential or polarization.

Normal electrical activity of the heart produces waves or deflections on the ECG (Figure 5-2). The waves and intervals that comprise the components of the ECG make up one electrical cardiac cycle (Figure 5-3).

- **P wave:** Electrical impulse originating in the SA node, the heart's primary pacemaker, which prompts atrial depolarization or the spread of the impulse across the right and left atria. It is the first positive deflection from the isoelectric baseline in most ECG leads but may be positive, negative, or biphasic in leads III, aVL, and V1. The atria contract following the appearance of the P wave. The wave should be rounded, less than 0.11 second in duration (width), and no greater than 2.5 mm in height (voltage).
- **PR interval:** The P wave plus the isoelectric line extending to the beginning of the QRS complex, wherein the impulse spreads through the AV node, the bundle of His, the right and left bundle branches, and Purkinje fibers. The interval measures 0.12 to 0.2 second in normal adults.
- **QRS complex:** A set of three combined waves (Q, R, and S) that represents ventricular depolarization, which stimulates ventricular contraction. The wave of atrial repolarization is hidden within this larger, dominant complex. The QRS complex should be 0.06 to 0.1 second in normal adults and varies in direction depending on the ECG lead but is most recognized as positive deflection (which represents the R wave, a positive deflection from the baseline). Some normal positive complexes are "missing" a distinct Q or S wave. The complex is predominantly negative in leads aVR, V_1, and V_2 and biphasic in

leads V_3, V_4, and, occasionally, lead III (which represents stronger Q- and S-wave activity, which are the negative deflections that precede and follow the R wave).

- **ST segment:** The isoelectric line between the end of the QRS complex and the T wave, which represents early ventricular repolarization. The segment changes in response to myocardial ischemia, injury, hypokalemia, pericarditis, and other ventricular tissue abnormalities. The "J" point is where the ST segment begins and the QRS complex terminates.
- **T wave:** Represents ventricular repolarization, wherein during the first part of the wave, the tissue is refractory to further stimulation (absolute refractory period). At the peak of the T wave, the tissue becomes sensitive to stronger electrical stimuli (relative refractory period), and ventricular dysrhythmias may occur.
- **QT interval:** Represents the depolarization and repolarization of the ventricle, measured from the beginning of the QRS complex to the end of the T wave. If no Q wave is present, the interval is measured from the beginning of the R wave to the end of the T wave. As the HR increases, the QT interval should decrease proportionately. There are tables available to reflect the duration of a normal QT interval for various HRs. When the duration of the QT interval is adjusted or corrected for HR, the interval is termed the QTc interval. A QT interval that is greater than half the RR interval (distance between two R waves) is considered prolonged.
- **U wave:** A small positive waveform that sometimes follows the T wave. The significance is unknown, but it is theorized to be a wave of Purkinje fiber repolarization.
- **TP segment:** A segment rarely used clinically when discussing the ECG. It is the isoelectric segment on the ECG between the end of the T wave and beginning of the P wave. It reflects the time the cardiac cells are electrically silent or neutral.

ABNORMAL ELECTROCARDIOGRAPHIC TRACINGS

Myocardial ischemia, electrolyte or other chemical imbalance, and an abnormally configured electrical system are factors likely to stimulate dysrhythmias. The normal flow of impulses depends on properly nourished, well-oxygenated electrical tissues with an anatomically correct pacing and conduction system. The cardiac cycle depends on a balance of basic regulatory substances including sodium, potassium, calcium, and glucose and appropriate amounts of catecholamines. Imbalance of these regulators can cause a disturbance in automaticity, conduction/conductivity, or myocardial contractility.

- **Automaticity:** The ability of cardiac cells to initiate an electrical impulse spontaneously, without stimulation by a nerve or other source. Hypokalemia and hypocalcemia increase automaticity. The SA node, AV junction, and Purkinje fibers possess automaticity. All cardiac muscle is electrically "irritable" or excitable because of the concentration of ions on both sides of the cell membranes, but not all cells possess automaticity. All cardiac cells are able to respond to external stimuli, including electrical and mechanical sources.
- **Conduction/conductivity:** All cardiac cells can receive electrical stimuli and transmit or conduct impulses to an adjacent cell. Intercalated disks in the cell membranes facilitate the transmission of impulses throughout the heart muscle. When impulses reach muscle cells, they stimulate muscle contraction.
- **Myocardial contractility:** Cardiac muscle cells "shorten" in response to electrical impulses, which manifests as a muscle contraction.

CAUSES OF ABNORMAL RHYTHMS
Disturbances in Automaticity

May involve an acceleration or deceleration in pacing or automaticity of the SA node, such as sinus tachycardia (HR greater than 100 bpm) or sinus bradycardia (HR less than 60 bpm). Premature beats or possibly an escape or compensatory heart rhythm may arise from the atria, junction, or ventricles if the SA node is dysfunctional or arrests. Without additional catecholamines prompted by the stress response, escape rhythms generated from the AV junction or the ventricles are usually bradycardic (HR less than 60 bpm). Abnormal rhythms, such as atrial or ventricular tachycardia, may also result from excessive sympathetic stimulation or electrolyte imbalance.

Disturbances in Conduction

Conduction may be too rapid, as in conditions that induce the stress response (e.g., severe/critical illness, certain endocrine diseases, profound emotional stress) or in the presence of an

(Text continued on p. 544)

Atrial
Depolarization

P wave

Atrial
Repolarization

Ta wave

Ventricular
Depolarization

QRS complex

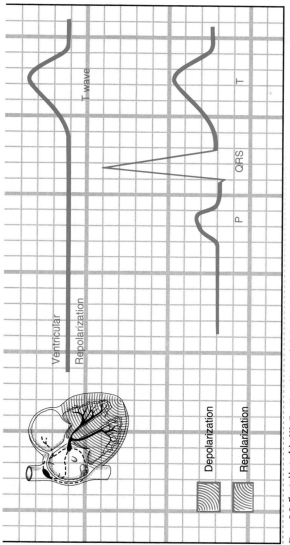

Figure 5-2 **Electrical basis of the ECG.** (From Huszar RJ: *Basic dysrhythmias: interpretation and management*, ed 3, St. Louis, 2002, Mosby.)

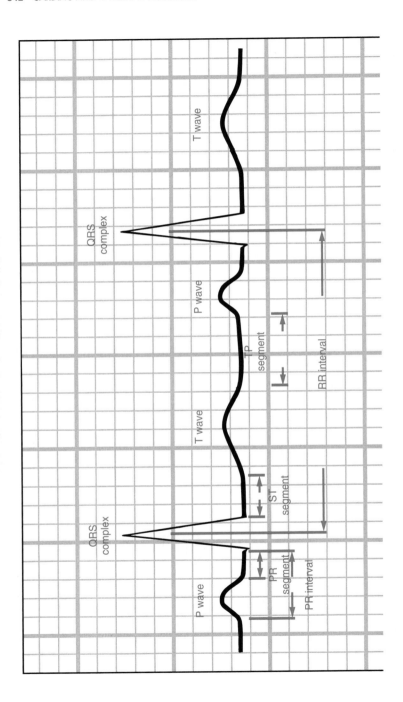

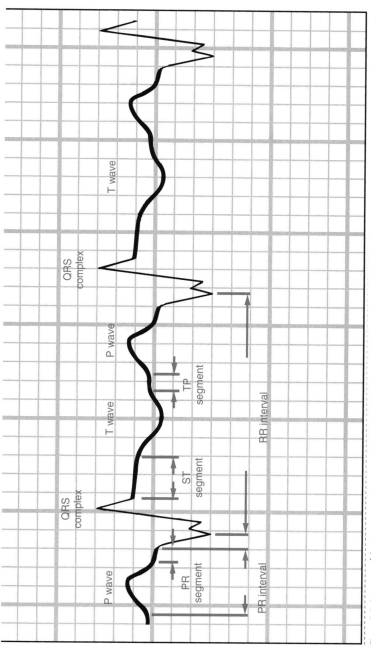

Dysrhythmias and Conduction Disturbances

Figure 5-3 Components of the ECG. (From Huszar RJ: *Basic dysrhythmias: interpretation and management,* ed 3, St. Louis, 2002, Mosby.)

accessory pathway (e.g., Wolff-Parkinson-White [WPW] syndrome). Accessory pathways are extraconduction fibers that provide a direct connection between the atria and the ventricles, circumventing the AV node. Rhythms generated from these anatomically incorrect conduction systems are called AV reciprocating tachycardias and may have rates greater than 250 bpm. Reentry is a situation in which a misdirected electrical impulse reexcites a conduction pathway through which it has already passed. Once started, this impulse may circulate through the same area repeatedly, prompting an AV reentrant tachycardia. The trapped impulse becomes the pacemaker in this circumstance. Impulse conduction may be delayed or too slow (e.g., first- and second-degree AV block), or become totally blocked from continuing down the pathway by abnormal electrical tissues (e.g., third-degree or complete heart block) (Figure 5-4).

Combinations of disturbed Automaticity and Conduction
Several dysrhythmias may occur simultaneously (e.g., first-degree AV block [disturbance in conductivity], premature atrial complexes [PACs] [disturbance in automaticity]).

ASSESSMENT
GOAL OF ASSESSMENT
To diagnose the type of dysrhythmia, the cause of the rhythm (electrolyte or acid-base imbalance, structural abnormality, heart and/or renal disease, nervous system or neuroendocrine dysfunction), the impact of the dysrhythmia on the CO (BP)/coronary artery perfusion (may prompt chest discomfort), and to determine the urgency and type of treatment. Lethal dysrhythmias result in cardiac arrest.

HISTORY AND RISK FACTORS
Assess for acidosis or alkalosis, ACS (CAD, angina, MI), or other heart disease or acute conditions (pericarditis, presence of accessory conduction pathways, cardiomyopathy, HF, valvular disease, cardiac tamponade), anemia, current use of antidysrhythmic or bronchodilating drugs, recreational drug abuse, drug overdose, use of catecholamines (epinephrine, dopamine, dobutamine, norepinephrine), use of tricyclic antidepressants, diuretics, exposure to other environmental toxins, electrolyte disturbances (especially hypokalemia, hypoglycemia, or hypomagnesemia), endocrine disease (posterior pituitary, thyroid, parathyroid, adrenal, or pancreas), hypothermia, hypoxia, hypotension, hypovolemia, hypervolemia, increased intracranial pressure, infection pneumothorax or tension pneumothorax, pulmonary disease including pulmonary embolism, peripheral vascular or peripheral arterial disease (PAD), respiratory failure, renal failure, and sepsis.

OBSERVATION
The patient's appearance varies from absence of symptoms to complete cardiopulmonary arrest. Common symptoms include activity intolerance, weakness, pallor, hypotension, dizziness, SOB, dyspnea, palpitations, chest discomfort or pressure, and sensation of "racing heart" or "skipped beats." More serious symptoms include altered mental status, anxiety, respiratory insufficiency, syncope, and seizures, which may lead to HF and cardiopulmonary arrest. Pulseless ventricular tachycardia, ventricular fibrillation, asystole, and pulseless electrical activity (PEA) result in immediate cardiac arrest.

VITAL SIGNS
Vary with type of dysrhythmia. Vital signs may be unaffected or affected slightly. Accelerated or decelerated HR may cause hypotension, result in HF, or deteriorate into pulselessness. Symptomatic dysrhythmias most often result in a very rapid, slow, or irregular pulse, changed pulse quality, hypotension, pallor, possibly a variable HR (fast, then slow), and tachypnea. If the CO is markedly decreased, shocklike symptoms ensue including cold, clammy skin, dusky or cyanotic appearance, decreased urine output, and feeling of impending doom or imminent death.

ELECTROCARDIOGRAPHIC AND HEMODYNAMIC MEASUREMENTS
Hemodynamic measurements will vary, depending on the effect of the dysrhythmia on the CO. If the patient has HF, CO is decreased and PAP may be elevated. Right- and left-sided HF

1. Prolonged PR interval (>0.20 sec)
(first-degree AV block)

Delay of
conduction of the
electrical impulse
through the:

AV node or
bundle of His

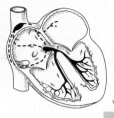

＼ Electrical impulse
Conduction delay

2. Absence of a QRS after a P wave
(second- and third-degree AV block)

Blockage of
conduction of the
electrical impulse
through the:

AV node or
bundle of His,
or bundle branches

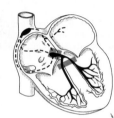

＼ Electrical impulse
Conduction delay

3. Short PR interval (<0.12 sec)

a. Ectopic
pacemaker in
the atria or
AV junction

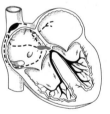

OR

b. Conduction of the
electrical impulse
through abnormal
AV conduction
pathways

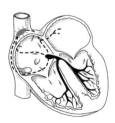

＼ Electrical impulse

Figure 5-4 Anomalous AV conduction. (From Huszar RJ: *Basic dysrhythmias: interpretation and management,* ed 3, St. Louis, 2002, Mosby.)

manifest differently (see Heart Failure, Chapter 5). Tachycardias usually increase CO initially, unless the rate is too fast to allow adequate ventricular filling, in which case CO decreases and may lead to HF. ECG findings seen with various dysrhythmias include abnormalities in rate such as sinus bradycardia or sinus tachycardia, irregular rhythm such as atrial fibrillation, extra beats such as PACs and premature junctional complexes, wide and bizarre-looking beats such as premature ventricular complexes (PVCs) and ventricular tachycardia (VT), a fibrillating baseline such as ventricular fibrillation (VF), and a straight line as with asystole. Figures 5-5 through 5-30 give an overview of common rhythms, dysrhythmias, conduction disturbances, and pacemaker rhythms and their treatment. Occasionally, patients have an electrical rhythm without corresponding mechanical pumping. This condition is known as PEA. Initially, the rhythm may appear nearly normal but rapidly deteriorates as the conduction pathway becomes hypoxic.

AUSCULTATION

If HF is present, heart sounds may include S_3 and S_4; basilar crackles or rales are audible with lung auscultation; and a wet cough with frothy sputum may be present. If atrial fibrillation or other dysrhythmias that prompt an irregular ventricular response are present, the irregularity is audible with auscultation.

PALPATION

With HF, jugular veins are distended and peripheral edema is present. ECG rhythms reflecting an irregular ventricular response will prompt an irregular pulse upon palpation. Electrical complexes that resulted in decreased stroke volume will be reflected as a lesser or absent pulse beat. (Text continued on p. 559)

Normal Sinus Rhythm

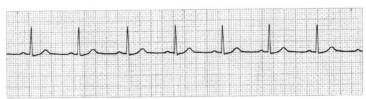

- Rhythm: regular
- Atrial rate: 60-100 beats/min
- Ventricular rate: 60-100 beats/min
- P waves: before each QRS
- QRS: normal and of normal width (less than .12 sec)
- PR interval: normal (.12-.20 sec)
- P: QRS: 1:1

Significance: Usual, normal rhythm and conduction.
Intervention: None.

Figure 5-5 **Normal sinus rhythm.** (From Huszar RJ: *Basic dysrhythmias: interpretation and management,* ed 3, St. Louis, 2002, Mosby.)

Sinus Tachycardia

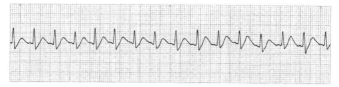

- Rhythm: regular
- Atrial rate: >100 beats/min; usually <160 beats/min
- Ventricular rate: >100 beats/min; usually <160 beats/min
- P waves: before each QRS
- QRS: normal duration
- PR interval: normal
- P: QRS: 1:1

Significance: Increased rate usually caused by sympathetic stimulation. Causes may include pain, fever, anxiety, hypovolemia, heart failure, caffeine intake, use of theophylline or sympathomimetic agents.

Intervention: Treat the cause. Increased rate is usually caused by sympathetic stimulation. Cause may include pain, fever, anxiety, hypovolemia, heart failure, caffeine intake, use of theophylline or sympathomimetic agents.

Figure 5-6 **Sinus tachycardia.** (From Huszar RJ: *Basic dysrhythmias: interpretation and management,* ed 3, St. Louis, 2002, Mosby.)

Sinus Bradycardia

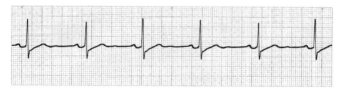

- Rhythm: regular
- Atrial rate: <60 beats/min
- Ventricular rate: <60 beats/min
- P waves: before each QRS
- QRS: normal duration
- PR interval: normal
- P: QRS: 1:1

Significance: Slow rate usually caused by increased parasympathetic stimulation. Causes may include vagal stimulation, β-adrenergic blocking agents and other drugs, AMI, increased intracranial pressure (IICP). This rhythm may be "normal" in some people.

Intervention: No treatment necessary unless patient's BP drops and/or LOC is altered or PVCs occur. Initial treatment is atropine and oxygen. Atropine 0.5 mg may be given and repeated up to a total dose of 3 mg if bradycardia is symptomatic (hypotension, chest discomfort). Transcutaneous pacing, epinephrine (2-10 mcg/min) or dopamine (2-10 mcg/kg/min) may also be considered.

Figure 5-7 **Sinus bradycardia.** (From Huszar RJ: *Basic dysrhythmias: interpretation and management,* ed 3, St. Louis, 2002, Mosby.)

Sinus Dysrhythmia

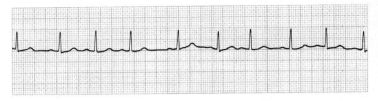

- Rhythm: irregular
- Atrial rate: 60-100 beats/min
- Ventricular rate: 60-100 beats/min
- P waves: before each QRS
- QRS: normal duration
- PR interval: normal
- P: QRS: 1:1

Significance: This rhythm usually increases in rate with respiration and decreases with expiration. It can be a normal finding in children. As an abnormal finding, it may be caused by drugs, IICP, or heart disease.

Intervention: Observation; usually no treatment necessary.

Figure 5-8 Sinus dysrhythmia. (From Huszar RJ: *Basic dysrhythmias: interpretation and management,* ed 3, St. Louis, 2002, Mosby.)

Sinus Arrest

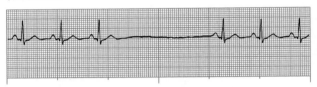

Significance: May indicate the sinus node is failing as a primary pacemaker.

Intervention: Observation; need for treatment is based on the frequency of sinus arrest occurrences. Increasing frequency should be reported to the advanced practice provider or physician.

Figure 5-9 Normal sinus rhythm with sinus arrest. (From Aehlert B: *ECGs made easy: pocket reference,* ed 2, St. Louis, 2002, Mosby.)

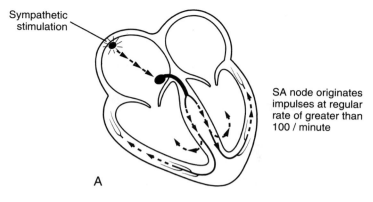

Sympathetic stimulation

SA node originates impulses at regular rate of greater than 100 / minute

A

Wandering Atrial Pacemaker

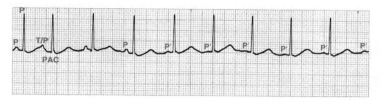

P   T/P   P   P'   P   P'   P   P'
PAC

- Rhythm: irregular
- Atrial rate: usually 60-100 beats/min
- Ventricular rate: usually 60-100 beats/min
- P waves: before each QRS
- QRS: normal duration
- PR interval: usually normal; some variation
- P: QRS: 1:1

Significance: An ectopic atrial focus. Causes may include drugs, COPD, inflammatory disorders.

Intervention: Observation. If cause can be determined, treat cause. If patient is receiving digoxin, check serum level.

Figure 5-10 Sinus tachycardia with premature atrial complexes (PACs). (Top, from *Emergency Nurses Association: Sheehy's manual of emergency care,* ed 6, St. Louis, 2005, Mosby. Bottom, from Aehlert B: *ECGs made easy: pocket reference,* ed 2, St. Louis, 2002, Mosby.)

Atrial Tachycardia

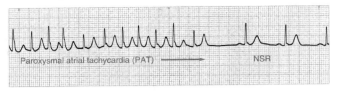

- Rhythm: mostly regular
- Atrial rate: 160-240 beats/min
- Ventricular rate: depends on AV conduction ratio
- P waves: may be difficult to identify because of fast rate
- QRS: normal; may be wide if aberrant conduction is present

Significance: Can precipitate chest pain and ischemia. Patients often experience dizziness, diaphoresis, and nausea. Many patients diagnosed with wide-complex atrial tachycardia (SVT) are found to have ventricular tachycardia when electrophysiology studies are done.

Intervention: Vagal maneuvers, diltiazem, adenosine. Other agents include digoxin, β-blockers, and procainamide. If the patient has an accessory pathway with AV reciprocating tachycardia, catheter ablation may be necessary to correct the problem.

Figure 5-11 **Atrial tachycardia.** (From Huszar RJ: *Basic dysrhythmias: interpretation and management,* ed 3, St. Louis, 2002, Mosby.)

Atrial Flutter (Type I)

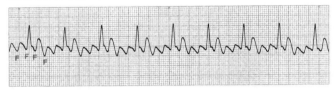

- Rhythm: regular if block is regular; may be irregular
- Atrial rate: 240-340 beats/min (type I); 340-430 beats/min (type II)
- Ventricular rate: depends on AV conduction
- P waves: saw-toothed; F waves
- QRS: normal
- PR interval: not measurable
- P: QRS: P > QRS

Significance: An atrial ectopic focus. AV conduction ratios can be variable, usually at least 2:1. The ineffective contraction can cause thrombus formation in the atria, which may subsequently embolize to the lungs, brain, and possibly other distal vessels.

Intervention: IV diltiazem, diltiazem, or β-blockers. For type I, rapid atrial pacing or cardioversion if unstable. Other agents may include IV ibutilide or amiodarone. PO flecainide, amiodarone, propafenone, or sotalol may also be used. Patients with an atrial rate of >240 may need to be anticoagulated to prevent atrial thrombus formation.

Figure 5-12 **Atrial flutter (type I).** (From Huszar RJ: *Basic dysrhythmias: interpretation and management,* ed 3, St. Louis, 2002, Mosby.)

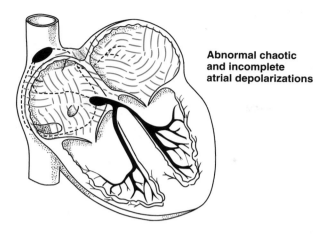

Abnormal chaotic and incomplete atrial depolarizations

Atrial Fibrillation

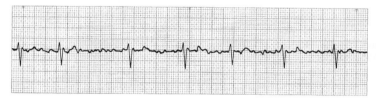

- Rhythm: irregularly irregular
- Atrial rate: >350 beats/min
- Ventricular rate: variable
- P waves: coarse or fine fibrillatory waves
- QRS: normal
- PR interval: not measurable
- P: QRS: P > QRS

Significance: Chaotic atrial firing and ineffective atrial contraction. Cardiac output usually drops because of loss of atrial "kick." Ineffective atrial contraction makes clot formation a danger.

Intervention: Management of atrial fibrillation is patient specific. New onset atrial fibrillation is managed the same as atrial flutter. The goal of therapy is to convert the rhythm to NSR as soon as possible, unless the rhythm is chronic. Patients should be anticoagulated to prevent embolization of blood trapped in the quivering atria, which will form thrombi if not managed. Treatment is targeted at managing the ventricular rate response. Cardioversion may be achieved using electrical or chemical therapy. Only patients with normal QTc intervals are eligible for use of ibutilide (Corvert) for chemical cardioversion. See page 522 for specific information.

Figure 5-13 **Atrial fibrillation (AF).** (From Huszar RJ: *Basic dysrhythmias: interpretation and management,* ed 3, St. Louis, 2002, Mosby.)

AV Junctional Rhythm or Junctional Escape Rhythm

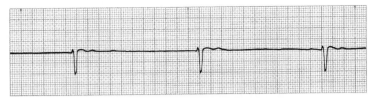

- Rhythm: regular
- Atrial rate: cannot determine
- Ventricular rate: 40-60 beats/min
- P waves: inverted before or after QRS or not present
- QRS: normal
- PR interval: <0.12 sec if P precedes QRS
- P: QRS: P ≤ QRS

Significance: AV node assumes primary pacing function from atria.

Intervention: Usually no specific therapy indicated. If patient becomes symptomatic because of a slow rate. Atropine 0.5 mg may be given, and repeated up to a total of 3 mg. Transcutaneous pacing, or continuous infusions of Epinephrine (2–10 mcg/min), or Dopamine (2–10 mcg/kg/min) may be considered.

Figure 5-14 **AV junctional rhythm or junctional escape rhythm.** (From Huszar RJ: *Basic dysrhythmias: interpretation and management,* ed 3, St. Louis, 2002, Mosby.)

Accelerated Junctional Rhythm

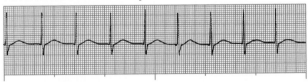

- Rhythm: regular
- Atrial rate: cannot determine
- Ventricular rate: 40-60 beats/min
- P waves: inverted before or after QRS or not present
- QRS: normal
- PR interval: <0.12 sec if P precedes QRS
- P: QRS: P ≤ QRS

Significance: AV node assumes primary pacing function from atria.
Intervention: Usually no specific therapy indicated.

Figure 5-15 **Accelerated junctional rhythm.** (From Aehlert B: *ECGs made easy: pocket reference,* ed 2, St. Louis, 2002, Mosby.)

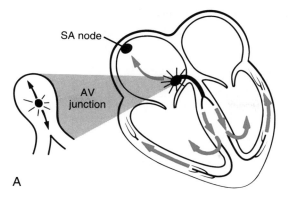

A

Premature Junctional Complexes

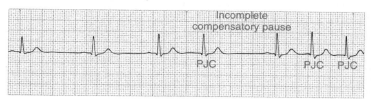

- Rhythm: irregular
- Atrial rate: cannot determine
- Ventricular rate: depends on underlying rhythm
- P waves: before, during, and after QRS
- QRS: normal
- PR interval: <0.12 sec if P precedes QRS
- P: QRS: P ≤ QRS

Significance: Less common than PACs; may precede blocks.
Intervention: Observation. Usually no treatment is necessary. If indicated, therapy is similar to that for PACs.

Figure 5-16 **Premature junctional complexes.** (Top, from *Emergency Nurses Association: Sheehy's manual of emergency care*, ed 6, St. Louis, 2005, Mosby. Bottom, from Huszar RJ: *Basic dysrhythmias: interpretation and management*, ed 3, St. Louis, 2002, Mosby.)

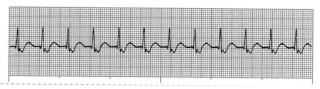

Figure 5-17 **Junctional tachycardia (JT).** (From Aehlert B: *ECGs made easy: pocket reference*, ed 2, St. Louis, 2002, Mosby.)

Dysrhythmias and Conduction Disturbances

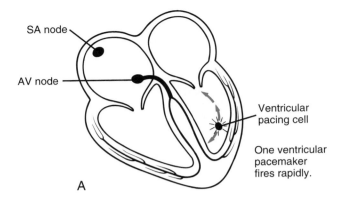

Ventricular Tachycardia

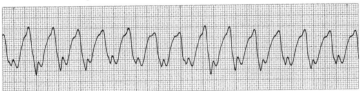

- Rhythm: slightly irregular
- Atrial rate: cannot determine
- Ventricular rate: 150-250 beats/min
- P waves: not visible
- QRS: wide (>0.12 sec)
- PR interval: cannot determine
- P: QRS: absent

Significance: Cardiac output falls significantly, cannot be tolerated for long, and will deteriorate into VF and asystole. May be monomorphic (same form repeated) or polymorphic (more than one type present).

Intervention: Current research indicates Amiodarone is useful in converting unstable VT to sinus rhythm. If pulseless, patient requires immediate defibrillation. Recent studies indicate patients who survive sudden cardiac death and those with sustained VT should be considered for an implantable cardioverter-defibrillator (ICD). For Torsades de Pointes, discontinue medications which cause prolonged QT Syndrome. Manage hypokalemia, hypomagnesemia and bradycardia. Rhythm is generally paroxysmal. Use defibrillation as a last resort.

Figure 5-18 Ventricular tachycardia. (Top, from *Emergency Nurses Association: Sheehy's manual of emergency care*, ed 6, St. Louis, 2005, Mosby. Bottom, from Huszar RJ: *Basic dysrhythmias: interpretation and management*, ed 3, St. Louis, 2002, Mosby.)

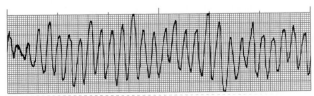

Figure 5-19 Torsade de pointes. (From Aehlert B: *ECGs made easy: pocket reference*, ed 2, St. Louis, 2002, Mosby.)

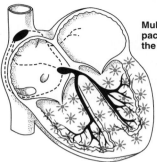

Multiple ectopic pacemaker in the ventricles

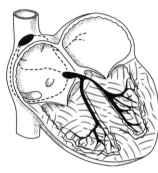

Abnormal, chaotic, and incomplete ventricular depolarizations

Ventricular Fibrillation

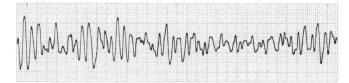

- Rhythm: irregular
- Atrial rate: cannot determine
- Ventricular rate: rapid
- P waves: not seen
- QRS: absent; fibrillatory waves
- PR interval: none
- P: QRS: none

Significance: Most common cause of sudden cardiac death. VF produces no cardiac output.

Intervention: Immediate defibrillation is required with 200 joules, or per other recommendation of the defibrillator manufacturer. Biphasic defibrillators may recommend an energy sequence beginning at 120 joules. Perform cardiopulmonary resuscitation until defibrillator is available. Repeat single shock defibrillation every 2 minutes while CPR continues between shocks, increasing energy to 300 joules after 2 minutes of CPR, then 360 joules for all subsequent shocks. Treatments should be revised if ACLS guidelines reflect a change in management is recommended. Patients who survive sudden cardiac death (VF) should be considered for an implantable cardioverter-defibrillator (ICD).

Figure 5-20 Ventricular fibrillation. (From Huszar RJ: *Basic dysrhythmias: interpretation and management,* ed 3, St. Louis, 2002, Mosby.)

Dysrhythmias and Conduction Disturbances

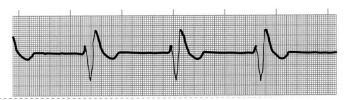

Figure 5-21   **Idioventricular rhythm.** (From Aehlert B: *ACLS Study Guide*, ed 3, St. Louis, 2007, Mosby.)

Asystole

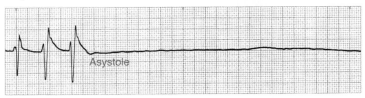

- No electrical activity
- May see a rare, wide, bizarre QRS

Significance: Mortality >95%. Always confirm asystole in 2 leads.
Intervention: Asystole means the heart is not beating or the pulse is absent. Perform cardiopulmonary resuscitation (CPR) according to current American Heart Association Basic Cardiac Life Support Guidelines, and initiate Advanced Cardiac Life Support as soon as possible.

Figure 5-22   **Asystole.** (From Huszar RJ: *Basic dysrhythmias: interpretation and management*, ed 3, St. Louis, 2002, Mosby.)

First-Degree AV Block

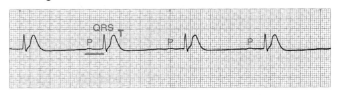

- Rhythm: regular
- Atrial rate: 60-100 beats/min
- Ventricular rate: 60-100 beats/min
- P waves: present; precede each QRS
- QRS: normal
- PR interval: prolonged (>0.2 sec)
- P: QRS: 1:1

Significance: Impulse conduction is delayed through the AV node. Causes are varied and may include heart disease, ischemia, digitalis toxicity, other drug effect, and myocarditis.
Intervention: Observation; usually no treatment needed. Atropine 0.5 mg may be given and repeated up to a total dose of 3 mg if bradycardia is symptomatic (hypotension, chest discomfort). Transcutaneous pacing, epinephrine (2-10 mcg/min), or dopamine (2-10 mcg/kg/min) may also be considered.

Figure 5-23   **First-degree AV block.** (From Huszar RJ: *Basic dysrhythmias: interpretation and management*, ed 3, St Louis, 2002, Mosby.)

Second-Degree AV Block Type I (Wenckebach)

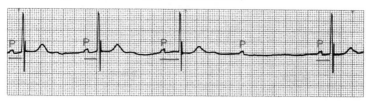

- Rhythm: irregular
- Atrial rate: exceeds ventricular rate
- Ventricular rate: less than sinus rate
- P waves: one P wave precedes each QRS except during nonconducted P waves, which occur regularly
- QRS: normal
- PR interval: lengthens progressively with each cycle until one is nonconducted

Significance: Usually a transient block that does not progress to complete heart block.

Intervention: Observation; treatment usually not necessary.
Atropine 0.5 mg may be given and repeated up to a total dose of 3 mg if bradycardia is symptomatic (hypotension, chest discomfort). Transcutaneous pacing, epinephrine (2-10 mcg/min), or dopamine (2-10 mcg/kg/min) may also be considered.

Figure 5-24 **Second-degree AV block (type I) (Wenckebach).** (From Huszar RJ: *Basic dysrhythmias: interpretation and management*, ed 3, St. Louis, 2002, Mosby.)

Second-Degree AV Block Type II

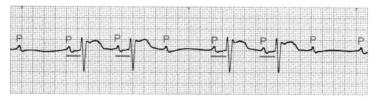

- Rhythm: irregular
- Atrial rate: exceeds ventricular rate
- Ventricular rate: depends on degree of block
- P waves: 2 or more for each QRS
- QRS: normal duration
- PR interval: normal or prolonged on the conducted complex
- P: QRS: P > QRS

Significance: This block may occur with anterior wall AMI and may progress rapidly to complete heart block.

Intervention: Observation if patient is asymptomatic. If symptoms occur, atropine 0.5 mg may be given and repeated up to a total dose of 3 mg if bradycardia is symptomatic (hypotension, chest discomfort). Transcutaneous pacing, epinephrine (2-10 mcg/min), or dopamine (2-10 mcg/kg/min) may also be considered.

Figure 5-25 **Second-degree AV block (type II).** (From Huszar RJ: *Basic dysrhythmias: interpretation and management*, ed 3, St. Louis, 2002, Mosby.)

Dysrhythmias and Conduction Disturbances

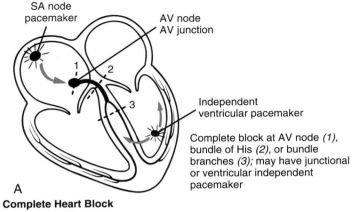

Complete Heart Block

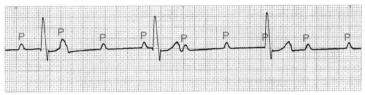

- Rhythm: usually regular
- Atrial rate: exceeds ventricular rate
- Ventricular rate: <60 beats/min
- P waves: occur at regular intervals
- QRS: <0.12 sec if pacemaker is in the AV node; >0.12 sec if ventricular pacemaker
- PR interval: no relationship between P and QRS
- P: QRS: no relationship

Significance: No conduction of SA node impulses. The atria and ventricles beat independently of each other. The slow rate can cause myocardial ischemia.

Intervention: Pacemaker insertion necessary.
Atropine 0.5 mg may be given and repeated up to a total dose of 3 mg if bradycardia is symptomatic (hypotension, chest discomfort). Transcutaneous pacing, epinephrine (2-10 mcg/min), or dopamine (2-10 mcg/kg/min) may also be considered.

Figure 5-26 **Complete (third-degree) AV block.** (Top, from *Emergency Nurses Association: Sheehy's manual of emergency care*, ed 6, St. Louis, 2005, Mosby. Bottom, from Huszar RJ: *Basic dysrhythmias: interpretation and management*, ed 3, St. Louis, 2002, Mosby.)

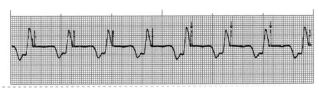

Figure 5-27 **Ventricular demand pacemaker (VVI).** (From Aehlert B: *ECGs made easy: pocket reference*, ed 2, St. Louis, 2002, Mosby.)

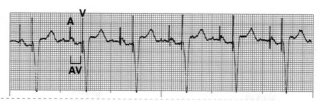

Figure 5-28 Dual-chambered pacemaker. (From Aehlert B: *ECGs made easy: pocket reference*, ed 2, St. Louis, 2002, Mosby.)

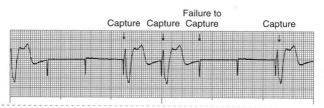

Figure 5-29 VVI pacemaker with failure to capture. (From Aehlert B: *ECGs made easy: pocket reference*, ed 2, St. Louis, 2002, Mosby.)

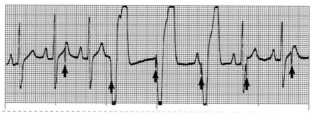

Figure 5-30 VVI pacemaker with failure to sense. (From Aehlert B: *ECGs made easy: pocket reference*, ed 2, St. Louis, 2002, Mosby.)

Dysrhythmias and Conduction Disturbances

Diagnostic Tests: Cause(s) of Dysrhythmias

Test	Purpose	Abnormal Findings
Noninvasive Cardiology		
12-lead electrocardiogram (ECG) or 15- or 18-lead ECG: Expanded method used to detect and analyze dysrhythmias, in which additional electrodes are placed on the skin of the right side of the chest and/or left posterior subscapular area to better detect problems with perfusion to the right ventricle and posterior wall of the left ventricle (see Figures 5-31 and 5-32)	12-lead ECGs are the accepted standard method for detecting and analyzing dysrhythmias, including those associated with myocardial ischemia, injury, and infarction. Twelve electrodes are placed on the skin of the patient's limbs and on the chest over the left ventricle.	Rapid tachycardias and profound bradycardias of all origins may prompt instability of hemodynamic status. Acute coronary syndrome manifests with presence of ST segment depression or T wave inversion (myocardial ischemia), ST elevation (acute MI), new bundle branch block (especially left BBB), or pathologic Q waves (resolving/resolved MI) in 2 contiguous or related leads. May be obtained during an episode of chest pain to help with establishing the relationship between the chest discomfort and the dysrhythmia.

Continued

Diagnostic Tests: Cause(s) of Dysrhythmias—cont'd

Test	Purpose	Abnormal Findings
Stress tests Stress test on a treadmill with or without thallium Thallium stress test using medications	Continuous ECG monitoring of the patient while a stressor (e.g., exercise on the treadmill; dipyridamole, dobutamine, or adenosine injection) is induced. The test continues until the patient reaches the target heart rate or becomes symptomatic (e.g., chest pain, severe fatigue, dysrhythmias).	Results determine the ability of the heart to compensate for various amounts of stress. Stress electrocardiography uses an echocardiogram immediately following the increase in heart rate to detect any regional wall motion abnormalities brought on by the tachycardia.
Ultrasound echocardiography (*ECHO*)	Assesses for mechanical and structural abnormalities related to effective pumping of blood from both sides of the heart.	Abnormal ventricular wall movement or motion, low ejection fraction, incompetent or stenosed heart valves, abnormal intracardiac chamber pressures
Transesophageal echocardiography (TEE)	Ultrasound technique to monitor atrial and ventricular wall motion through a high frequency two-dimensional transducer on the end of a gastroscope that allows the patient to swallow.	From this position in the esophagus, a high-resolution image of the posterior approach to the heart allows for better imaging of the aorta, valves, atria, and coronary arteries and can also detect clots that are present in the heart as a result of stasis of blood secondary to dysrhythmias (e.g., atrial fibrillation).
Ambulatory monitoring (e.g., 24-hour external Holter monitor or internal cardiac event [loop] recorder)	Continuous cardiac monitor worn externally (Holter) or for 24 hours so that ECG changes that occur during normal daily activities (including sleeping) can be determined	The loop recorder is implanted if the Holter monitor is ineffective in capturing dysrhythmias. The patient keeps a timed log of all activities/events/symptoms, which is later compared with the ECG recording to analyze the relationship of dysrhythmias to symptoms and activities. The loop recorder does not record continuously. Instead the patient activates the recorder when symptoms occur so that the cardiac "event" is recorded and then transmitted to monitoring agency via telephone.
Blood Studies		
Therapeutic drug levels	Assesses for effectiveness of antidysrhythmic drugs already prescribed, as well as other medications that may cause dysrhythmias.	Toxic levels of many cardiac, pulmonary, neurologic, and antidysrhythmic medications may prompt development of new, possibly more dangerous dysrhythmias. All antidysrhythmic agents are proarrhythmic, especially when certain electrolyte imbalances are present, particularly the class I agents (e.g., quinidine, mexiletine, disopyramide).
Complete blood count (CBC) Hemoglobin (Hgb) Hematocrit (Hct) RBC count (RBCs) WBC count (WBCs)	Assesses for anemia, inflammation, and infection; assists with differential diagnosis of chest pain.	Decreased RBCs, Hgb, or Hct reflects anemia, which often exacerbates dysrhythmias; MI, pericarditis, and endocarditis may increase WBCs.

Diagnostic Tests: Cause(s) of Dysrhythmias—cont'd

Test	Purpose	Abnormal Findings
Electrolytes Potassium (K^+) Magnesium (Mg^{2+}) Calcium (Ca^{2+}) Sodium (Na^+)	Both elevations and deficits of electrolytes can alter cardiac action potential, create an electrically unstable environment, and precipitate dysrhythmias.	Decrease in K^+, Mg^{2+}, or Ca^{2+} may cause dysrhythmias; elevation of Na^+ may indicate dehydration (blood is more coagulable); low Na^+ may indicate fluid retention and/or heart failure.
Toxicology screening Alterations in both automaticity and conduction can be prompted by recreational drugs.	Assesses for presence of drugs in the bloodstream and/or urine, which can alter various stages of cardiac action potential.	Toxic levels of "recreational" or "street" drugs (e.g., "crack," cocaine, amphetamines, barbiturates) or mood-altering drugs (e.g., tricyclic antidepressants, sedative/hypnotics) can induce lethal dysrhythmias.
ABG values	Screen for hypoxemia or acid-base imbalance, which may prompt dysrhythmias.	May reflect hypoxemia or pH abnormality that can interfere with electrolyte balance, both of which can cause dysrhythmias. Hypoxemia can also result from dysrhythmias that significantly decrease cardiac output.
B-type natriuretic peptide (BNP)	Assesses for heart failure.	Elevation indicates heart failure is present.
C-reactive protein (CRP)	Assesses for inflammation.	Elevation places patients at higher risk for acute MI, pericarditis, and endocarditis.
Radiology		
Chest radiograph (CXR)	Assesses size of heart, thoracic cage (for fractures), thoracic aorta (for aneurysm), and lungs (for pneumonia, pneumothorax).	Cardiac enlargement, increased vascular markings, and bilateral infiltrates reflect heart failure (pulmonary edema).
Magnetic resonance imaging (MRI) Cardiac MRI	Assesses ventricular size, morphology, function, status of cardiac valves, and circulation.	Enlarged heart, remodeled heart, incompetent stenotic heart valves, narrowed or occluded coronary arteries.
Computed tomography (CT) Cardiac CT scan	Assesses ventricular size, morphology, function, status of cardiac valves, and circulation.	Enlarged heart, remodeled heart, incompetent stenotic heart valves, narrowed or occluded coronary arteries; technology is improving in accuracy; may eventually reduce the need for cardiac catheterization.
Invasive Cardiology		
Electrophysiologic studies (EPSs) Invasive test in which 2 or 3 catheters are placed into the heart at the sinus node and along the conduction system	This test can help to assess the SA node, AV node, and the His-Purkinje system; determine the characteristics of reentrant dysrhythmias; and "map" the location of suspected proarrhythmic sites or accessory pathways.	Rapid pacing stimuli at those sites with various voltages of electricity can induce dysrhythmias. Results help to determine the type of device and medications the patient may need to maintain cardiac electrical stability. Various medications, electrical therapies, and ablation are then implemented to terminate the induced dysrhythmias.

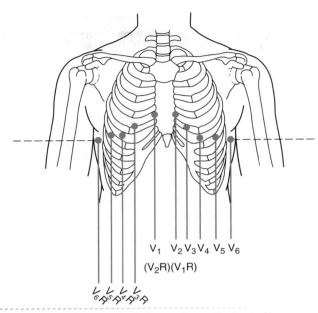

V_1 V_2 V_3 V_4 V_5 V_6

(V_2R) (V_1R)

V_6R V_5R V_4R V_3R

Figure 5-31 **Placement of the left and right chest leads.** (From Aehlert B: *ACLS study guide*, ed 3, St. Louis, 2007, Mosby.)

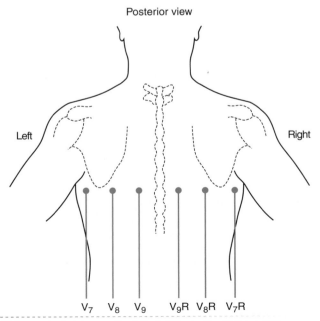

Posterior view

Left

Right

V_7 V_8 V_9 V_9R V_8R V_7R

Figure 5-32 **Posterior chest lead placement.** (From Aehlert B: *ACLS study guide*, ed 3, St. Louis, 2007, Mosby.)

COLLABORATIVE MANAGEMENT

CARE PRIORITIES

1. Identify the dysrhythmia and assess for symptoms

Diagnose the type of dysrhythmia and the effect of the rhythm on the patient's hemodynamic status. Rhythms resulting in hypotension, respiratory distress, chest discomfort, or pulselessness are considered unstable and require immediate management. When evaluating rhythms, the following basic assessments can be made before diagnosing the exact dysrhythmia:

Consciousness: Is the patient responsive or unconscious? If unconscious, is he or she breathing? If not breathing, open the airway and check the pulse. If still not breathing, and pulse is not present, the patient is in cardiac arrest (regardless of rhythm) and cardiopulmonary resuscitation (CPR) must be initiated while another person obtains the cardiac monitor, defibrillator, or automated external defibrillator (AED). An ECG rhythm is sometimes present without a pulse (PEA).

HR and rhythm: Too fast or too slow? Regular or irregular? When the HR exceeds 150 or is less than 50 bpm, patients are more likely to experience adverse effects. Fast rhythms include sinus tachycardia, atrial tachycardia, atrial flutter, atrial fibrillation, junctional tachycardia, and VT with a pulse. Slow rhythms include sinus bradycardia, junctional rhythms, ventricular or idioventricular rhythms, and second- and third-degree heart blocks.

Appearance of QRS complexes: Wide or narrow? Tachycardias with QRS that exceed 0.10 second in duration are more likely to originate from the ventricles, unless the patient has reason to have aberrant conduction or has a history of bundle branch block.

Presence of P waves/PR interval: Is there one P wave preceding each QRS complex? Is the P wave normal in appearance? Is the PR interval short, normal, or prolonged?

Stable or unstable vital signs and assessment: Unstable patients require immediate management. Symptomatic bradycardia resulting in hypotension may be best managed with transcutaneous cardiac pacing if atropine is ineffective. Symptomatic tachycardias may be best managed using synchronized cardioversion. Pulseless patients with tachycardia are managed with unsynchronized cardioversion/defibrillation.

Cardiopulmonary arrest: All patients receive CPR and IV or intraosseous (epinephrine 1 mg immediately, and every 3 to 5 minutes throughout resuscitation). Vasopressin 40 mg may be given instead of the first or second dose of epinephrine. Atropine 1 mg may be given to patients with slow-rate PEA or asystole every 3 to 5 minutes up to 3 mg total dose. Patients with pulseless VT or VF require immediate defibrillation.

2. Determine the urgency of correcting the dysrhythmia and whether drugs or electrical therapy is the most appropriate approach for the patient

The more unstable the patient, the more aggressive the treatment. There are situations wherein dysrhythmias do not readily respond to treatment, requiring further evaluation. Some lethal dysrhythmias may be resistant to correction, resulting in death. Generally, electrical therapies provide almost immediate correction of the instability associated with dysrhythmias, if the patient is able to respond to treatment. Boluses of medications such as atropine, adenosine, and ibutilide work quickly. Loading doses of medications that are followed by infusions such as amiodarone or diltiazem sometimes result in correction of rhythms but generally require the medication infusion to attain full correction and stability. Each patient's situation must be managed using a thorough evaluation of his or her history and under the guidance of the AHA guidelines for ACLS. A handbook of emergency cardiac care for health providers is updated regularly to reflect current research. The resource includes information reviewed by AHA Committee on Emergency Cardiovascular Care, and Subcommittees on Basic Life Support, Pediatric Resuscitation, and Advanced Cardiac Life Support.

3. Provide pharmacologic management to correct dysrhythmias if recommended as the first strategy by ACLS guidelines

Management of dysrhythmias is based on providing and/or balancing electrolytes, catecholamines, and other regulators of the cardiac cycle. Provision of antidysrhythmic drugs is done using an antidysrhythmic drug classification system, which has evolved from the original Vaughan Williams classification system. Toxic levels of any antidysrhythmic medication can prompt development of different and sometimes lethal dysrhythmias. All antidysrhythmic agents have the potential for proarrhythmic effects (Box 5-4).

Box 5-4 ANTIDYSRHYTHMIC DRUGS

Class I (sodium channel blockers)

Block the rapid, inward sodium current. Local anesthetics and other drugs that decrease automaticity of ventricular conduction, delay ventricular repolarization, decrease conduction velocity, increase conduction via AV node, and suppress ventricular automaticity. Class IA decreases depolarization moderately and prolongs repolarization. May prolong the QT interval. Class IB decreases depolarization and shortens repolarization. Class IC significantly decreases depolarization with minimal effect on repolarization.

Class IA	Class IB	Class IC
Disopyramide (PO)	Lidocaine (IV, IM)	Encainide (PO)
Procainamide (PO, IV, IM)	Mexiletine (PO)	Flecainide (PO)
Quinidine (PO, IV)	Phenytoin (PO)	Propafenone (PO)
	Tocainide (PO)	
	Moricizine (PO)	

Class II (beta-adrenergic blockers)

Block stimulation of beta$_1$ and beta$_2$ receptors by catecholamines. Slow sinus node automaticity and conduction via AV node, control ventricular response to supraventricular tachycardias, and shorten the action potential of Purkinje fibers.

Acebutolol (PO)	Carvedilol (PO)	Oxyprenolol (PO)*
Atenolol (PO)	Esmolol (IV)	Penbutolol (PO)
Betaxolol (PO)	Labetalol (PO, IV)	Pindolol (PO)
Bisoprolol (PO)	Metoprolol (PO,IV)	Propranolol (PO, IV)
Carteolol (PO)	Nadolol (PO, IV)	Timolol (PO, IV)

Class III (potassium channel/1K1 blockers)

Block the outward current of potassium. Increase the action potential and refractory period of Purkinje fibers, increase ventricular fibrillation threshold, restore injured myocardial cell electrophysiology toward normal, and suppress reentrant dysrhythmias. May prolong the QT interval.

Amiodarone (PO, IV)	Bretylium (IV, IM)	Ibutilide (IV)
Azimilide (PO)	Dofetilide (PO)	Sotalol (PO, IV)

Class IV (calcium channel blockers)

Depress automaticity in the SA and AV nodes, block the slow calcium current in the AV junctional tissue, reduce conduction via the AV node, and are useful in treating tachydysrhythmias caused by AV junctional reentry.
Diltiazem (PO, IV)
Verapamil (PO, IV)

Unclassified

Depress activity of the AV node.
Adenosine (IV)

AV, Atrioventricular; IV, intravenous; IM, intramuscular; PO, by mouth; SA, sinoatrial.
*Available in Great Britain.

4. Provide therapy for rapid HRs using current ACLS guidelines to manage ventricular tachycardias (monomorphic and polymorphic), ventricular fibrillation, and supraventricular tachycardias (atrial tachycardia, junctional tachycardia, atrial flutter, or atrial fibrillation)

Defibrillation and cardioversion: Delivery of electrical shocks to the heart through the chest wall via use of an external defibrillator used to convert symptomatic, rapid atrial, or ventricular rhythms to sinus rhythm. Shocks may be synchronized (cardioversion) with the patient's R waves (QRS complexes) or may be given as random/unsynchronized (defibrillation) countershocks. The operator must set the desired amount of electricity, apply the defibrillator paddles with conductive gel or hands-free gel patches to the patient's chest, and discharge the device. Defibrillators also provide the ability to provide electrical therapy "hands free." A special cable and multifunction/defibrillator pads are used instead of the conventional paddles.

- The placement of the pads or paddles is critical to deliver the electrical therapy to the heart muscle. The two pads are placed either on the anterior chest with one beneath the right clavicle and one on the left chest near the lower aspect of the heart, or with one pad over the heart anteriorly, and the other on the patient's back over the posterior side of the heart. Pads/paddles should not be placed over the larger bones (sternum and clavicle anteriorly, scapula and spinal column posteriorly), medication patches, or implanted electrical devices, including pacemakers and ICDs. Medication patches should be removed and residual medication wiped off. Defibrillators may use monophasic or biphasic technology. Biphasic defibrillation requires lower energy settings than recommended for monophasic defibrillation. Synchronized cardioversion also requires the additional step of synchronizing the patient's R waves with the cardioverter; lower energy is also required to convert the rhythm to NSR.
  - **Defibrillation:** Used for ventricular tachycardias without a pulse and ventricular fibrillation. Patients are in full cardiopulmonary arrest when defibrillation is used. Recommendations change for how electrical therapy should be performed. The energy sequence for biphasic defibrillators is initially 120 to 200 joules (manufacturer guidelines provide recommendations) followed by 2 minutes of CPR, then 300 joules followed by 2 minutes of CPR, then 360 joules (AHA, Advanced Cardiac Life Support guidelines, 2011). Torsades de Pointes is generally paroxysmal. Defibrillation should be used as a last resort, after managing the cause of prolonged QT syndrome.
  - **Cardioversion:** Used for all types of tachycardia with a pulse present, when patients have unstable vital signs or a high risk of developing unstable vital signs. Can be scheduled in advance for patients with a high risk of developing unstable vital signs. Short-acting sedation is used before discharging the energy, to render the patient unaware of the pain produced by the electrical shock received. The energy sequence may vary slightly for various tachycardias and recommendations change but, in general, it begins with 50 to 100 joules, followed by 200 joules, then 300 joules, then 360 joules. Energy is always increased with subsequent shocks (AHA Advanced Cardiac Life Support Guidelines, 2011.

Safety Alert *Defibrillation (Unsynchronized Cardioversion)*
Providers must clear the area by shouting "clear" before pressing the button to discharge the defibrillator. Ensure no one else is touching the patient/bed as shock is delivered. Anyone in contact with the bed is at risk of receiving the electrical shock. All fluids in contact with the patient should be considered electrical conductors. Every attempt must be made to wipe or dry fluids from the area surrounding the patient. It is unsafe to defibrillate or cardiovert a patient who is in a pool of liquid (water, therapeutic fluids, or body fluids) unless the care providers are NOT in contact with the fluids.

Safety Alert *Synchronized cardioversion*
The defibrillator will not discharge the energy until R wave synchronization is achieved, which sometimes takes several seconds. Providers need to exercise extreme caution to remain "clear" and not touch the patient, bed, or anything connected to the patient until the energy is delivered.

- AED: Defibrillation technique designed to provide ECG interpretation needed for the device to determine the need for electrical therapy. The device will give a series of voice prompts instructing the operator on how to connect the cable and apply defibrillator pads, assess the patient, and clear the area when the device analyzes the rhythm. When finished analyzing, the device will either automatically discharge if appropriate (fully automatic) or ask the provider to press a button to discharge if appropriate (semiautomatic). When providing basic life support, the sequence of actions includes defibrillation as the fourth step, after ensuring a patent airway, providing manual ventilation if breathing is absent, and providing cardiac compressions if the pulse is absent. The operator must be able to assess for pulselessness and apnea, along with applying hands-free defibrillator pads in the proper position at the right sternal border and anterior axillary line, fifth intercostal space. If healthcare providers are using the AED, the anterior-posterior pad position may also be used.

Safety Alert _AEDs_
Not all automated external defibrillators are programmed per current ACLS guidelines. Some still deliver three stacked shocks (per older ACLS guidelines) when it is time to defibrillate, rather than the currently recommended one shock. If a healthcare provider comes across this type of defibrillator, the provider is generally advised to follow the instructions and not interrupt the cycle. Interruption may cause the device to malfunction, resulting in the patient not receiving any further electrical therapy, or the device ceasing to give associated instructions regarding the proper steps of resuscitation.

- Life vest "wearable" cardioverter-defibrillator: The first defibrillator worn outside the body rather than implanted in the chest with continuous cardiac monitoring to detect life-threatening dysrhythmias, including VT and VF. The device uses nonadhesive sensing electrodes. If a life-threatening rhythm is detected, the device alerts the patient before delivering the shock, which allows time for a conscious patient to disarm the device before the shock. If the patient is conscious, the shock may not be necessary. If the patient is unconscious, the device releases a gel over the therapy electrodes and delivers the shock. The device is designed for home use, rather than as part of hospital management. The device may be used as a "bridge" to ICD implantation while patients are evaluated for appropriateness of the therapy.
- ICD: A battery-powered pulse generator (electrical device) implanted into the pectoral area, with a lead system and shocking coil positioned inside the heart and superior vena cava, which can recognize and terminate potentially lethal dysrhythmias. Risks and complications of thoracotomy versus nonthoracotomy implantation are outlined in Table 5-14.

Table 5-14	IMPLICATIONS FOR PATIENT CARE AND COSTS: IMPLANTABLE CARDIOVERTER-DEFIBRILLATORS (ICDs)		
Complication	**Thoracotomy (T)**	**Nonthoracotomy (NT)**	**Patient Care Implications**
Pneumothorax or hemothorax	Higher risk	Lower risk	ICU monitoring required for T. ICU unnecessary for NT. Length of hospital stay decreases with NT.
Pocket hematoma, seroma, wound adhesions	Higher risk	Lower risk	Wound care and home care less complex for NT.
Wound infection	Higher risk	Lower risk	If wound infection, T more likely to require IV antibiotics, which will increase costs and length of hospital stay.
Blood loss/bleeding	Higher risk	Lower risk	T may need type and screen for blood products. NT does not.
Pneumonia	Higher risk	Lower risk	T may have decreased activity tolerance and requires pulmonary toilet.
Pain	Higher risk	Lower risk	NT requires less analgesia to manage pain.

Newer, third-generation devices do not require thoracotomy for insertion. The devices are smaller and lighter, allowing prepectoral implantation. These devices may also provide antitachycardia pacing (ATP), low-energy cardioversion, high-energy cardioversion, antibradycardia pacing, and high-energy defibrillation along with the ability to score performance data. Algorithms for treatment of recognized dysrhythmias are programmed into the device. Maximal energy output is 30 to 40 joules, which can defibrillate malignant or lethal rhythms such as pulseless ventricular tachycardia and ventricular fibrillation. Magnets may be used for emergency deactivation/activation or suppression of all or part of programmed therapies in newer devices. If the patient has a combination ICD/pacemaker, the magnet will deactivate the ICD and change from demand (discharges electrical impulses or "fires" as needed to maintain the selected HR) pacing to fixed mode (discharges the selected number of impulses per minute, regardless of the patient's underlying heart rhythm). When the device discharges or fires, the patient's status should be documented in the medical record.

> **Safety Alert** *Immediate intervention is required for a device that is not delivering appropriate therapy. If the device does not deliver therapy, external cardioversion can be used. A patient with an implantable cardioverter defibrillator (ICD) who has a sustained hemodynamically unstable ventricular rhythm should be treated exactly as one who does not have an ICD. The placement of the external pads should not be over the ICD generator. When inappropriate firing occurs in the absence of a treatable dysrhythmia, there is a high probability that an ICD lead has become dislodged, a connection has become loose, or the device sensitivity setting is too "low," which causes the device to respond "too soon" to certain rhythm changes.*

- Catheter ablation: Before ablation, an electrophysiology study is done to evaluate the electrical activity of the heart. The "electrical map" guides the placement of the ablation catheters, which are placed in the heart during cardiac catheterization. The energy stimulus is then applied to the area in which the dysrhythmia originates or where an accessory pathway (bypassing AV node during conduction) is located. The energy causes controlled, localized necrosis of the area and may be applied via radiofrequency, thermal (heat), or cryo (cold) catheters. Bypass tracts (WPW) that produce AV reciprocating tachycardias and reentrant pathways that produce AV nodal reentrant tachycardias can be ablated to modify the heart tissue and stop abnormal rapid conduction in these areas, which produces supraventricular tachycardia. Ablation can be done as adjunctive therapy for management of monomorphic VT, following placement of an ICD to enhance rhythm control. Postablation assessment of the patient involves careful monitoring of the cardiac rhythm, vital signs, catheter insertion sites, LOC, and peripheral pulses. Complications include cardiac perforation, cardiac tamponade, coronary artery spasm, cerebral or pulmonary embolus, bleeding, thrombosis, and dysrhythmias including AV blocks.
- **Specific tachycardias:**
  - Sustained monomorphic VT: The VT ECG tracing has a regular rhythm, the QRS shape is wide and uniform, and the ventricular rate ranges from 130 to 250 bpm. The impulse is generated either from a single site of increased automaticity on one of the ventricles or is because of reentry. Scarring from prior MI often provides the setup for reentry, as the impulse attempts to travel around the infarcted tissue. Patients may be hemodynamically stable or may be pulseless, so proper assessment is crucial in deciding on therapy. Options for treatment include antidysrhythmic medication (amiodarone 150 mg IV over 10 minutes, repeated once if needed and followed by a continuous IV infusion at 0.5 mg/min; total dose should not exceed 2.2 g in 24 hours). Synchronized cardioversion is used for unstable tachycardia (hypotension or chest discomfort accompanies the rapid HR). Defibrillation is used if the patient is unconscious, apneic, and pulseless (cardiac arrest), with 120 to 200 joules using a biphasic defibrillator (or 360 joules using a monophasic device), along with CPR and advanced life support measures. See ACLS guidelines for tachycardia with pulses or pulseless arrest for specific management algorithms.
  - Sustained polymorphic VT includes Torsades de Pointes: Appears as a series of somewhat irregular, multishaped wide QRS "twisting" around the isoelectric line as seen on the ECG. It is important to try to determine if the patient's QT interval was

normal or prolonged just before the tachycardia ensued. If the QT interval was normal before onset of the tachycardia, the rhythm is simply called polymorphic VT. If polymorphic VT is sustained and the patient is symptomatic because of the tachycardia, treat any ischemia, correct electrolyte imbalances, and manage using guidelines for monomorphic VT. If the QT interval was prolonged, the patient has a particular type of polymorphic VT called torsade de pointes (TdP). Abnormal levels of potassium, magnesium, and calcium may contribute. Acquired TdP is usually related to drug toxicity or electrolyte abnormalities, or myocardial ischemia. Many patients with TdP experience cardiac arrest immediately. Regardless, when TdP is sustained and the patient is symptomatic, discontinue any medications (particularly continuous infusions) that may prolong the QT interval; correct electrolyte abnormalities; initially give magnesium sulfate IV if the patient is stable; if the patient is unstable, attempt defibrillation as for VF. These patients may be resistant to defibrillation. If the patient continues to experience TdP, an agent such as isoproterenol may be infused to increase the HR, thereby shortening the QT interval. This may be especially necessary if TdP is caused by medications with a long half-life. Antidysrhythmic drugs including class 3 amiodarone and sotalol prolong the QT interval and, like class 1 agents (e.g., quinidine, disopyramide), are proarrhythmic. Initiate a magnesium infusion if not done initially. Other drugs, including certain antibiotics and antihistamines, may promote polymorphic VT, particularly when used in combination. Congenital causes include long-QT syndrome, Brugada syndrome (possibly congenital), and catecholaminergic polymorphic VT.

- Atrial fibrillation: Atrial fibrillation with rapid ventricular response may result in progressive ventricular dysfunction and decreased CO. The "quivering" atria are not contracting, so the atrial contribution to ventricular filling is lost. Blood stagnates in the atria, often resulting in clot formation. Platelet activation occurs, making thromboembolic complications possible when the atria once again contract. The goal of therapy is to convert the rhythm to NSR as soon as possible unless the atrial fibrillation is chronic. Those with sustained, new-onset atrial fibrillation who become unstable (signs of decreased CO, congestive HF, or ACS) or become hemodynamically unstable are generally managed with synchronized cardioversion. Atrial fibrillation may occur post-CABG, producing CO compromise and danger of stroke. Rate control to slow the rapid ventricular response can be achieved by diltiazem. Loading dose is 0.75 mg/kg IV followed by a continuous infusion at 5 mg/h. If atrial fibrillation reoccurs or persists over a 24-hour period, warfarin anticoagulation for 4 weeks will be needed. For patients with normal QTc interval, immediate chemical conversion might be attained using ibutilide, 1 mg diluted in 10-mL IV solution given over 10 minutes, and repeated once if atrial fibrillation has been present for less than 48 hours. Ibutilide is reserved for patients with a normal QTc interval to avoid lethal ventricular dysrhythmias following administration. An alternative is amiodarone in a loading dose of 150 mg IV over 10 minutes followed by 1 mg/min drip for 6 hours and then 0.5 mg/min drip for 18 hours. For chronic atrial fibrillation patients, conversion to NSR without anticoagulation is not a goal because of the risk of atrial thrombus formation and possible embolization. If synchronized cardioversion is needed during the immediate postoperative period and anticoagulation is not an option, Doppler or transesophageal echocardiography may be used to check for atrial thrombus formation. In addition to cardioversion, other nonpharmaceutical treatments for atrial fibrillation include AV node and focal ablation, surgical correction such as the Maze procedure, and implanted permanent pacing with atrial fibrillation suppression algorithms.

5. Provide electrical therapy (cardiac pacing) to support unstable patients with slow HRs, and some rapid HRs if recommended as the most appropriate strategy by current ACLS guidelines

Management of symptomatic bradycardias includes heart blocks, slow junctional rhythms, and idioventricular rhythms or certain tachycardias (antitachycardia pacing) including atrial flutter, atrial tachycardia, reentrant tachycardias, and WPW. Cardiac pacing can be provided temporarily or permanently.

- Permanent cardiac pacing: A battery-powered device is implanted to provide an artificial pacing or electrical pacing stimulus for the heart. It is used for problems with either automaticity or conduction to either generate an appropriate number of pacing impulses or facilitate conduction of the impulses to all areas of the heart in a coordinated fashion to facilitate increased CO. Although most often used for management of symptomatic bradycardias including second- and third-degree heart block, it may also be used for patients with ventricular asynchrony (RV and LV contraction is uncoordinated). Specialized devices may also be used to correct rapid atrial and ventricular rhythms via ATP. Third-generation ICDs may also be programmed for cardiac pacing. Pacemakers are named or coded based on the functions they are able to perform (Table 5-15). If CO is disturbed by ventricular asynchrony, biventricular pacing or cardiac resynchronization therapy (CRT) may be used. CRT is recommended for patients with LVEF $\leq$ 35%, a QRS duration $\geq$ 0.12 second, and a sinus rhythm. CRT may also have an ICD added for treatment of patients with New York Heart Association (NYHA) functional class III or ambulatory class IV HF symptoms.

- Temporary cardiac pacing: Temporary pacing can be done using transthoracic, transcutaneous pacing pads applied to the skin on the chest (may be a dual pad used for either pacing or cardioversion [synchronized and unsynchronized]), via transvenous catheter insertion with positioning of leads into the endocardium, via a specialized pulmonary artery catheter with the capacity for transvenous cardiac pacing, or via surgically inserting epicardial wires with leads during open heart surgery.

Safety Alert *Patients in critical care often have electrolyte disturbances, are receiving antidysrhythmic medications, and are in acute coronary syndrome, acid-base imbalance, or hypotension/shock states. All of these conditions may alter the ability of the cardiac muscle to respond to a pacing stimulus and loss of capture may occur. Vigilance in watching for proper pacemaker function (pacing, capture, and sensing) is warranted in both temporary and permanent pacing.*

- Temporary epicardial pacing: Placement of temporary pacing wires on the epicardial surface of the heart while the chest is open during cardiac surgery so that cardiac pacing can be used in the postoperative period. Usually two atrial and two ventricular wires (pacing and ground wires) are attached to the outside surface of the heart and exit through the skin incision allowing attachment to a temporary pacing generator. The exposed pacing wires may be capped and later connected to a generator if pacing is needed. The end of the leads, connection points, and pacing generator terminals should be protected and insulated from electrical microshock. The temporary pacing wires are removed when

Table 5-15   NBG PACEMAKER CODES

The pacemaker code is written in a five-letter format as in the table, using no more letters than necessary. For example, the DDDR pacemaker is a dual-chamber paced, dual-chamber sensed, dual response, rate-modulated device. At least one pacemaker mode, the DVIC mode variation, does not conform to the NBG identification code and may sometimes be written DVI(C).

In the 1970s and 1980s, before the NBG codes came into being, the Inter-Society Commission for Heart Disease established standardized codes for pacemakers. Information on these older pacemaker codes can be found at NASPE.

Chambers Paced (1)	Chambers Sensed (2)	Modes of Response (3)	Programmable Functions (4)	Antitachycardia Functions (5)
V = ventricle	V = ventricle	T = triggered	R = rate modulated	0 = none
A = atrium	A = atrium	I = inhibited	C = communicating	P = paced
D = dual (A & V)	D = dual (A & V)	D = dual triggered/inhibited	M = multiprogrammable	S = shocks
0 = none	0 = none	0 = none	P = simple programmable	D = dual (P & S)
—	—	—	0 = none	—

NASPE, North American Society of Pacing and Electrophysiology.

no longer needed by slowly and gently pulling them out through the skin. The patient is monitored carefully after the pacing wires are removed for dysrhythmias, cardiac tamponade, hemorrhage, hematoma, and hemodynamic changes. If left in for a prolonged period of time, tissue may adhere to the wires and the provider may elect to cut the external wires at the level of the skin. The skin will then grow over the entry points and heal.

- Atrial overdrive pacing: ATP is used to control or terminate supraventricular dysrhythmias including atrial flutter, atrial tachycardia, reentrant tachycardias, and WPW. Atrial flutter and reentrant supraventricular tachycardias often result from electrical pathways or circuits set up around scarred or infarcted tissue. Using atrial pacing wires (transvenous or epicardial) connected to a pulse generator (pacemaker), the atria are rapidly paced by rapid bursts of electrical impulses during a 10- to 30-second period. The pacing rate selected is usually 20% to 30% faster than the rate of the tachydysrhythmia being treated. Successive bursts are performed at gradually increasing rates until termination of the tachycardia is achieved. The short bursts of rapid pacing create refractory cardiac tissue that interrupts the reentry circuit.

 Special care is given to proper connection of the atrial wires and to ensure against microshock. Rapid pacing of the atria can result in ventricular tachycardia or ventricular fibrillation.

- Transcutaneous, transthoracic cardiac pacing: Cardiac pacing performed with a device that delivers electrical stimulation to the heart via two conductive pads applied to the skin of the chest, positioned either anteriorly or over the anterior and posterior walls of the heart. Certain defibrillators include a capability for transcutaneous cardiac pacing. One pad is near the left sternal border and the other is near the left paraspinal line beneath the scapula for anterior-posterior position or in the same areas used for hands-free defibrillator pads in the proper position at the right sternal border and anterior axillary line, fifth intercostal space. Resistance of all muscles and bones of the chest wall must be overcome for impulses to reach the heart, requiring a higher milliampere to be used. Transcutaneous pacing will cause the muscles of the chest and back to contract, which can be quite uncomfortable for the patient, and sedation may be required.

 The pads cannot both sense and pace; therefore, the device includes an electrocardiogram (ECG) monitor so that efficacy (capture) of pacing can be assessed. Leads should be applied to the chest in addition to the pads to assess capture. Capture should reflect that the level of electrical stimulation (mA) provided was able to prompt ventricular contraction. The ECG tracing generally becomes larger and wider when capture is achieved. When pacing is effective, the patient's vital signs should improve. If the level of energy needed to achieve capture is high, sedation may be necessary for the patient to tolerate transcutaneous cardiac pacing.

6. Provide surgical procedures to help control dysrhythmias

- LV aneurysmectomy and infarctectomy: Excision of possible focal spots of ventricular dysrhythmias.
- Myocardial revascularization: Performed alone or in conjunction with electrophysiologic mapping, with excision or cryoablation of the dysrhythmia focus. Newer surgical techniques are less invasive than the standard median sternotomy approach.
- Maze procedure: Surgically placed incisions arranged in a pattern resembling a Maze in the atria to eliminate atrial fibrillation. Some Maze procedure variations use both surgical incisions and ablation of cardiac tissue in the electrophysiology laboratory (convergence procedure).
- Stellate ganglionectomy and block: Alters the electrical stability of the myocardium. Surgical option to treat inherited long-QT interval and predisposition to ventricular dysrhythmias.

7. Initiate anticoagulation for patients at higher risk for development of blood clots within the heart secondary to dysrhythmias that decrease either atrial or ventricular wall motion

Use of warfarin and/or platelet inhibitors (e.g., ticlopidine, clopidogrel) may be recommended.

8. Explain the content of dietary guidelines designed to help reduce stimulants normally consumed

Patients with recurrent dysrhythmias are usually placed on a diet that restricts or reduces caffeine and sodium and is low in fat and cholesterol (see Tables 5-5, 5-16, and 5-17). Dietary guidelines for patients at risk for or with heart disease require constant vigilance to stay informed of current recommendations. The DASH diet and the AHA diets (Mediterranean diet) outline other options that have proven successful in managing patients.

Table 5-16 LOW-CHOLESTEROL DIETARY GUIDELINES

Foods to Avoid	Foods Allowed
Egg yolks (no more than 3/week)	Egg whites; cholesterol-free egg substitutes
Foods made with many egg yolks (e.g., sponge cakes)	Lean, well-trimmed meats; minimize servings of beef, lamb, and pork
Fatty cuts of meat, fat on meats	Fish (except shellfish), chicken, and turkey (without the skin)
Skin on chicken and turkey	Dried peas and beans as meat substitutes
Luncheon meats and cold cuts	Nonfat (skim) or low-fat (2%) milk
Sausage, frankfurters	Low-fat cheese
Shellfish (e.g., lobster, shrimp, crab)	Ice milk, sherbet, low-fat yogurt
Whole milk, cream, whole milk cheese	Monosaturated oils for cooking and food preparation: canola, safflower, olive
Ice cream	Margarines that list one of the above oils as their first ingredients
Commercially prepared foods with hydrogenated shortening, which is saturated fat	Foods prepared "from scratch" with the above suggested oils
Coconut and palm oils and products made with them (e.g., cream substitutes)	Meats (in acceptable quantity) and vegetables prepared by broiling, steaming, or baking (never frying)
Butter, lard, hydrogenated shortening	Spices, herbs, lemon juice, wine, flavored wine vinegars
Meats and vegetables prepared by frying	
Seasonings containing large amounts of sugar and saturated fats	
Sauces and gravies	
Salad dressings containing cream, cheese, or mayonnaise	

Table 5-17 GUIDELINES FOR A DIET LOW IN SATURATED FAT

Foods to Avoid	Foods to Choose
Red meat especially when highly "marbled"; salami, sausages, bacon	Lean cuts of meat, fresh fish, poultry from which skin was removed before cooking; meats that have been grilled
Whole milk, whipping cream	Low-fat or skim milk
Tropical oils (coconut, palm oils; cocoa butter)	Monosaturated cooking oils, such as olive or canola oil
Candy	Fresh fruit, vegetables
Sweet rolls, donuts	Whole grain breads, cereals
Ice cream	Nonfat yogurt, sherbet
Salad dressings	Vinegar, lemon juice
Peanut butter, peanuts, hot dogs, potato chips	Unbuttered popcorn
Butter	Margarine (safflower oil listed as the first ingredient)

Dysrhythmias and Conduction Disturbances

CARE PLANS FOR DYSRHYTHMIAS AND CONDUCTION DISTURBANCES

DECREASED CARDIAC OUTPUT *related to altered rate, rhythm, or conduction or negative inotropic changes secondary to cardiac disease.*

Goals/Outcomes: Within 15 minutes of development of serious dysrhythmias, the patient has adequate CO as evidenced by BP at least 90/60 mm Hg or baseline, HR 60 to 100 bpm, and NSR on ECG. CVP is less than 7 mm Hg, and CO is 4 to 7 L/min.

NOC Circulation Status

Cardiac Care
1. Monitor the patient's heart rhythm continuously; note BP and symptoms if dysrhythmias occur or increase in occurrence.
2. If a PA catheter is present, note PAP, PAWP, and RAP; monitor for reduced CO in response to dysrhythmias.
3. Document dysrhythmias with a rhythm strip. Use a 12/15/18-lead ECG as necessary to identify the dysrhythmia.
4. Monitor patient's laboratory data, particularly K^+, Mg^{2+}, glucose, and digoxin levels.
5. Administer antidysrhythmic agents as prescribed; note patient's response to therapy.
6. Provide oxygen as prescribed. Oxygen may be beneficial if dysrhythmias are related to ischemia.
7. Maintain a quiet environment, and administer pain medications promptly. Both stress and pain can increase sympathetic tone and cause dysrhythmias.
8. If life-threatening dysrhythmias occur, initiate immediate unit protocols or standing orders for treatment, as well as CPR and ACLS algorithms as necessary.
9. When dysrhythmias occur, stay with patient; provide support and reassurance while performing assessments and administering treatment.
10. Administer inotropic agents (see Appendix 6) as prescribed to support patient's BP and CO.

NIC Hemodynamic Regulation; Medication Management; Oxygen Therapy; Respiratory Monitoring; Vital Signs Monitoring

RISK FOR ACTIVITY INTOLERANCE *related to imbalance between oxygen supply and demand secondary to dysrhythmias that reduce cardiac output.*

Goals/Outcomes: During activity, the patient rates exertion less than 3 on a scale of 0 to 10 and exhibits tolerance of the dysrhythmia by an RR less than 20 breaths/min, systolic BP within 20 mm Hg of baseline, HR within 20 bpm of resting HR, and absence of chest discomfort and/or new dysrhythmias.

NOC Activity Tolerance; Endurance; Energy Conservation

Energy Management
1. Monitor patient's response to activity. Instruct patient to report chest discomfort and SOB. Note new dysrhythmias associated with activity or other stressors.
2. Administer medications as prescribed.
3. Observe and report signs of acute decreased CO, including oliguria, decreasing BP, altered mentation, and dizziness.
4. Monitor BP and other vital signs frequently, and as soon as possible report to the advanced practice provider changes such as irregular HR, HR greater than 120 bpm, or decreasing BP.
5. Assess integrity of peripheral perfusion by monitoring peripheral pulses, distal extremity skin color, and urinary output. Report changes such as decreased pulse amplitude, pallor or cyanosis, and decreased urine output.

NIC Activity Therapy; Cardiac Care; Surveillance

DEFICIENT KNOWLEDGE OF DISEASE PROCESS OR OTHER MECHANISMS BY WHICH DYSRHYTHMIAS OCCUR *related to lifestyle implications.*

Goals/Outcomes: Within the 24-hour period before discharge from critical care, the patient and significant others verbalize knowledge about causes of dysrhythmias and the implications for modification of patient's lifestyle.

NOC Knowledge: Disease Process; Knowledge: Health Promotion; Knowledge: Medication

Teaching: Individual
1. Discuss causal mechanisms for dysrhythmias, including resulting symptoms. Use a heart model or diagrams as necessary.
2. Teach the signs and symptoms of dysrhythmias that necessitate medical attention: unrelieved and prolonged palpitations, chest pain, SOB, rapid pulse (greater than 150 bpm), dizziness, and syncope.
3. Teach the patient and significant others how to check pulse rate for 1 full minute.
4. Teach the patient and significant others about medications that will be taken after hospital discharge, including drug name, purpose, dosage, schedule, precautions, and potential side effects. Stress that the patient will be maintained on long-term antidysrhythmic therapy and that it could be life-threatening to stop or skip these medications without physician approval, because doing so may decrease blood levels required for dysrhythmia suppression.
5. Advise the patient and significant others about the availability of support groups and counseling; provide appropriate community referrals. Patients who survive sudden cardiac arrest may experience nightmares or other sleep disturbances at home. Explain that anxiety and fear, along with periodic feelings of denial, depression, anger, and confusion, are normal following this experience.
6. Stress the importance of leading a normal and productive life, even though the patient may fear breakthrough of life-threatening dysrhythmias. If the patient is going on vacation, advise him or her to take along sufficient medication and to be aware of healthcare facilities in the vacation area.
7. Advise the patient and significant others to take CPR classes; provide addresses of community programs.
8. Teach the importance of follow-up care; confirm date and time of next appointment, if known. Explain that outpatient Holter monitoring is performed periodically.
9. Explain that individuals with recurrent dysrhythmias should follow a general low-fat, low-sodium, and low-cholesterol diet (see Tables 5-5, 5-16, and 5-17) and reduce intake of products containing caffeine, including coffee, tea, chocolate, and colas. Dietary guidelines are dynamic. New recommendations frequently emerge. Patients may benefit from knowing changes in the recommendations, and more than one diet may be successful in preventing cardiovascular disease.
10. As indicated, teach patient relaxation techniques or guided imagery, which will reduce stress and enable patient to decrease sympathetic tone (see Appendix 7).

NIC Surveillance; Teaching: Prescribed Medication; Vital Signs Monitoring

INEFFECTIVE HEALTH MAINTENANCE *related to ineffective stress management and inability to relax.*

- -

Goals/Outcomes: Within the 24-hour period after instruction, the patient verbalizes and demonstrates the following relaxation technique.
NOC Health Promoting Behavior; Health-Seeking Behavior

Anxiety Reduction
1. Explain that to decrease sympathetic tone, some patients with dysrhythmias may benefit from practicing a relaxation response. Many different techniques can be used, including use of breathing alone or in conjunction with muscle group contraction and relaxation. Other techniques incorporate use of imagery.
2. Teach the patient a relaxation technique effective for stress reduction and facilitation of ability to take deep breaths slowly to relax. See Appendix 7 for a sample relaxation technique.

NIC Calming Technique; Meditation; Music Therapy; Simple Guided Imagery; Simple Relaxation Therapy; Teaching: Prescribed Activity/Exercise

FOR PATIENTS WITH AN ICD AND/OR PERMANENT PACEMAKER

DEFICIENT KNOWLEDGE: *ICD or related to pacemaker insertion procedure and follow-up care.*

- -

Goals/Outcomes: Within the 24-hour period before the procedure, the patient and significant others describe rationale for the procedure and method of insertion. Within the 24-hour period before discharge from ICU, the patient and significant others describe postinsertion care and need for continued advanced practice provider follow-up.
NOC Knowledge: Illness Care

Teaching: Procedure/Treatment

1. Assess patient's understanding of his or her medical condition (dysrhythmias) and the amount of detailed information desired.
2. Discuss the following with the patient and significant others:
   - Type of dysrhythmia the patient has, using rhythm strip and heart model or drawings/illustrations/charts to promote understanding.
   - Possible need for temporary transvenous pacemaker insertion before ICD or permanent pacemaker procedure.
   - Use of appropriate anesthesia throughout procedure.
   - Testing of the ability of the device to control lethal dysrhythmias, which will occur in the operating room/catheterization laboratory after implantation and before the incision is closed.
   - Reassurance that should the mechanism fail to control the dysrhythmia, the device can be adjusted or reprogrammed to do so.
   - Continuous observation of patient in a CCU for about 24 hours, with ongoing monitoring of BP, HR, and RR.
   - Importance of deep breathing, coughing (as necessary), and incentive spirometry exercises as appropriate. Explain that patient is at increased risk for respiratory tract and incisional infection if thoracic surgery was done, which tends to cause patient to avoid deep breathing and coughing to guard against pain. Have patient return demonstrations of breathing exercises. Reassure patient that analgesics can be administered before pulmonary toilet exercises, if needed.
   - No lifting of arm above level of shoulder for at least 4 weeks; may resume showering at 72 hours.
   - Discharge instructions: Follow-up visit within 10 to 14 days, need for obtaining an AED/home defibrillator, and importance of CPR/defibrillator classes for significant others.
3. Describe the procedure should ICD device deliver a shock. If the patient is aware of the shocks, the advanced practice provider should be notified as soon as possible that the device is firing. With newer devices, patients may be unaware of shocks but may become symptomatic (e.g., become intolerant of activity or dizzy, have chest discomfort) with prolonged or serious dysrhythmias. Teach the patient to record the number of shocks experienced.
4. Explain use of the AED/home defibrillator. These devices, which are available commercially from several companies, are designed to allow the nonmedical person or care providers untrained in dysrhythmia interpretation to effect defibrillation and to convert lethal dysrhythmias should the ICD fail. Provide information on Life Vest (as appropriate.).
5. Explain that shocks during sinus rhythm may indicate a lead fracture in the ICD system. Usually this is detected while the patient is being monitored (e.g., by ECG in physician's office, by hospital monitor, or by Holter monitor).

NIC Learning Facilitation; Learning Readiness Enhancement; Risk Identification; Teaching: Disease Process; Teaching: Prescribed Medication; Teaching: Psychomotor Skill

---

RISK FOR INFECTION *related to invasive procedure into thorax*

- -

Goals/Outcomes: Patient is free of infection as evidenced by normothermia, WBC count 11,000/mm³ or less, negative culture results, and absence of the clinical indicators of infection at the incision site and in the respiratory tract.
NOC Infection Severity

Infection Protection

1. Encourage and assist with deep breathing, coughing (if needed), and incentive spirometry exercises every 2 hours, and encourage early ambulation to the chair. As indicated, assist patient with splinting the incision site with hands or pillow to promote pain control. Administer prescribed analgesics 20 minutes before scheduled breathing exercises. For more information, see this nursing diagnosis in Acute Pneumonia, p. 373.
2. Assess incision site every 2 hours for warmth, erythema, swelling, and drainage. The presence of a seroma, which has the same symptoms as incision site infection, is confirmed by decubitus chest radiograph studies or CT.
3. Monitor patient's temperature every 2 to 4 hours, being alert to elevation greater than 38.6° C (101.5° F).
4. Monitor CBC for elevation of WBCs.
5. Consult advanced practice provider for significant findings.
6. Teach the patient and significant others the signs and symptoms of infection of both the incision site and the respiratory tract: cough, sputum production, fever, dyspnea, chills, headache, myalgia. Explain that the older adult with an infection may be confused and disoriented and may run low-grade fevers even though few other indicators are present.

NIC Infection Control; Cough Enhancement; Exercise Promotion; Surveillance; Medication Prescribing; Home Maintenance Assistance

FOR PATIENTS WITH A PACEMAKER (TEMPORARY OR PERMANENT) OR PATIENTS WITH THIRD-GENERATION ICDS WITH CARDIAC PACING

DECREASED CARDIAC OUTPUT *related to malfunction of cardiac pacemaker*

Goals/Outcomes: Within the 24-hour period preceding hospital discharge or throughout the duration of temporary cardiac pacing, the patient has adequate CO as evidenced by systolic BP at least 90 mm Hg, RR 12 to 20 breaths/min, HR less than 100 bpm, urinary output at least 0.5 mL/kg/h, warm and dry skin, and ECG indicative of effective capture, sensing, response to sensing, and function of antitachycardia pacing (if operational).

NOC Circulation Status

Cardiac Care: Acute

1. Recognize and document paced rhythms. Events to document include the following: (1) recognition of pacing spike preceding P wave and/or QRS complex as appropriate for settings; (2) sensing of patient's inherent pacing; (3) response of pacemaker when triggering and/or inhibiting pacing; (4) response of HR to activity if pacemaker is programmed "rate responsive"; and (5) initiation of antitachycardia pacing or electric shock (with ICD) for dysrhythmias.
2. Promptly detect problems with pacemaker functions. Include assessment of potential electromagnetic interference (EMI) (Table 5-18). Ensure that temporary pacemaker battery is still functional or changed as needed, and that cable connectors for temporary pacemakers are appropriately connected to the pulse generator (pacemaker box). For problems with functions of permanent pacemakers and ICDs, the advanced practice provider should be notified immediately.
3. Provide electrical safety measures for temporary cardiac pacing to include proper grounding and protection of exposed catheter tips and/or heart wires. Caregiver must wear nonconductive gloves when handling pacing lead wires/catheter so that microshocks are avoided. Microshocks can induce lethal dysrhythmias.
4. Observe for complications of temporary pacing, which include dysrhythmias, lead displacement or fracture, and lead perforation of the heart that could lead to cardiac tamponade, pericarditis, infection, and bleeding.
5. Perform threshold checks per hospital policy.

NIC Dysrhythmia Management; Vital Signs Management; Surveillance; Environmental Management: Safety

Table 5-18	ELECTROMAGNETIC INTERFERENCE AND THE THIRD-GENERATION ICDs AND SOME PROGRAMMABLE PACEMAKERS	
Unsafe Hospital Procedures/Equipment	**Unsafe Home Equipment: Use Caution**	**Safe Home Equipment**
MRI (magnetic resonance imaging)	Large magnets: junkyards, construction sites, other areas that may have large magnets	Microwave ovens
Nerve stimulator	Hand-held wands at airport security	Refrigerator magnets
Electrocautery	Bingo wands	Electric blankets
Diathermy	Certain slot machines	Tanning bed
Lithotripsy	Large stereo speakers (unsafe to carry) Cellular telephones High-tension wires Industrial transformers Robotic jacks Arc welders Power generators in dams Industrial motors Large boat motors	Riding lawnmower Jacuzzi CB radio HAM radio (except for antennas) Table saw Gas welder Electric drill Weed eater Small boat motors

ICD, Implantable cardioverter defibrillator.
Magnetic fields are measured in units (Gauss) or 1000th of a gauss, milliGauss (mG). Ten Gauss will affect an ICD or some programmable pacemakers. Common household electrical appliances (interferences) are less than 50 mG. Electrical fields are measured in volts per meter. 750 V is approximately 30 J.

Dysrhythmias and Conduction Disturbances

FOR PATIENTS WITH AN ICD

SEXUAL DYSFUNCTION (OR RISK FOR SAME) *related to fear of inducing dysrhythmias during sexual activity.*

Goals/Outcomes: Within the 24-hour period before discharge from the ICU, the patient and significant other verbalize understanding of interventions during and alternatives for sexual intercourse.

NOC Sexual Identity; Role Performance

Sexual Counseling

1. Ask patient to describe any symptoms of dysrhythmias during presurgical sexual experiences.
2. Explain the following interventions or alternatives that can be made if the patient continues to experience dysrhythmias during sexual intercourse:
   - Patient may need to take a less active role.
   - Patient may find that taking a prescribed vasodilator before engaging in sexual intercourse will prevent dysrhythmias. Should be advised not to take a vasodilator with NTG.
   - Suggest that during periods when dysrhythmias are a problem, less stressful forms of sexual activity, such as caressing and hugging, are positive alternatives.
3. As appropriate, advise patient that stressful situations, such as extramarital relations or unfamiliar environment/partner, may contribute to symptoms during sexual activity.
4. Explain that the device may shock at any time. If the patient's partner is in contact with the patient's body at that time, the shock may be experienced as a tingling sensation by the partner.

NIC Teaching: Sexuality; Anxiety Reduction; Coping Enhancement; Support Group

ADDITIONAL NURSING DIAGNOSES

The patient with ICD is at risk for pneumothorax. As indicated, also see Pneumothorax, Chapter 4, for information related to this disorder. Also see nursing diagnoses and interventions in Hemodynamic Monitoring (Chapter 1) and Emotional and Spiritual Support of the Patient and Significant Others (Chapter 2).

HYPERTENSIVE EMERGENCIES

PATHOPHYSIOLOGY

A hypertensive emergency is present when severely elevated BP results in end-organ damage. Severe hypertension adversely affects the CNS, cardiovascular, and renal systems. Both malignant hypertension and accelerated hypertension are considered emergencies, and they have similar outcomes and management strategies. Malignant hypertension is BP elevation with encephalopathy or nephropathy with papilledema. Progressive kidney failure and permanent blindness can occur if treatment is not provided. Accelerated hypertension is defined as a recent marked increase of BP over normal baseline pressure, associated with end-organ damage. Vascular damage is seen on funduscopic examination, including hemorrhages or exudates, but without papilledema.

Hypertensive urgency is managed differently from hypertensive emergency. Urgency is present when severely elevated BP is noted (e.g., systolic BP greater than 220 mm Hg or diastolic BP greater than 120 mm Hg) without end-organ damage. Signs and symptoms include severe headache, severe anxiety, and SOB. BP can be reduced within the subsequent 24 to 48 hours following diagnosis. IV treatment of BP is not necessary. Oral treatment is satisfactory.

Hypertensive emergencies require immediate management to reduce the BP. The patient may experience life-threatening signs and symptoms, such as severe pulmonary edema, cerebral edema, ischemia or hemorrhage of the brain, aortic dissection, AMI, and eclampsia (during pregnancy). Immediate vascular necrosis is possible if the diastolic pressure exceeds 120 mm Hg. Necrosis has also manifested with MAPs greater than 150 mm Hg. Conversely, no evidence suggests patients benefit from rapidly reducing BP in minutes to a few hours during hypertensive urgency. Aggressive therapy may result in cardiac, renal, or cerebral perfusion deficits resulting from low BP.

The morbidity and mortality of hypertensive emergencies depend on the extent of end-organ damage when the patient presents and subsequent BP control. Following a crisis, those with BP control and medication compliance have a 10-year survival rate of nearly 70%.

Hypertension causes more deaths and disease than any other cardiovascular risk factor worldwide. Hypertension prompts ventricular remodeling and increases the risk of heart attack, HF, stroke, and kidney failure. The Eighth Joint National Committee (8) did not define "hypertension," but rather prescribed thresholds for treatment applicable to all hypertensive populations except when the evidence supported variance in a particular subgroup. The guideline was submitted for external peer review in January 2013 by the National Heart, Lung, and Blood Institute (NHLBI) to 20 expert reviewers and 16 federal agencies. The guideline review focused on 3 key questions surrounding management of adults with hypertension: (1) Does initiating antihypertensive medications at specific BP thresholds improve outcomes? (2) Do medications targeted at a specific BP goal improve outcomes? (3) Do various classes of medications differ in benefits vs harms reflected in the outcomes? Lifestyle modifications were not revised, but rather, were supported by endorsing the evidence-based recommendations of the 2013 Lifestyle Work Group.

Following an exhaustive review of the literature, the following nine recommendations emerged from JNC-8:

- For those older than 60 years of age, initiate drug therapy for a systolic BP greater than 150 mm Hg and diastolic BP greater than 90 mm Hg. Goal: Systolic BP less than 90 mm Hg, diastolic BP less than 90 mm Hg.

    Corollary Recommendation: Those in this age group currently controlled at a lower BP do not need a medication adjustment to allow for a higher BP.

- For those younger than 60 years of age, initiate drug therapy for a diastolic BP above 90 mm Hg. Goal: Diastolic BP less than 90 mm Hg.

- For those younger than 60 years of age, initiate drug therapy for a systolic BP above 140 mm Hg. Goal: Systolic BP less than 140 mm Hg.

- For those older than 18 years of age with chronic kidney disease (CKD), initiate drug therapy to keep systolic BP below 140 mm Hg and diastolic BP below 90 mm Hg.

- For those older than 18 years of age with diabetes mellitus, initiate drug therapy to keep systolic BP below 140 mm Hg and diastolic BP below 90 mm Hg.

- In the general nonblack population, including those with diabetes mellitus, initial medications to control BP should include a thiazide-type diuretic, calcium channel-blocking agent, ACEI, or ARB.

- In the general black population, including those with diabetes mellitus, initial medications to control BP should include a thiazide-type diuretic or calcium channel-blocking agent.

- In those older than 18 years of age with CKD, initial (or added) medications should include an ACEI or ARB to improve kidney outcomes. This applies to people of all races, with or without diabetes mellitus.

- The main objective of hypertension treatment is to attain and maintain goal BP. If goal BP is not achieved within 30 days, the dose of the initial medication should be increased, or another medication from one of the four recommended classes (thiazide diuretic, CCB, ACEI, or ARB) should be added to the treatment plan. If the goal BP is not reached using two antihypertensive medications, a third drug may be added and titrated. If BP goal is not reached using careful monitoring of BP with three drugs, a drug from another class outside the four recommended classes may be used. Referral to a hypertension specialist may be needed when the patient's BP is not controlled with three medications.

The risk of death from ischemic heart disease and stroke increases in tandem with BP. The risk of heart attack or stroke increases several times when hypertension exists with obesity, smoking, high blood cholesterol levels, or diabetes. Patients with comorbidities such as diabetes or CKD are at higher risk of the cardiovascular complications of hypertension when systolic BP exceeds 140 mm Hg or DBP exceeds 90 mm Hg.

Elevation of systolic versus diastolic BP is related to age. Systolic BP and diastolic BP rise simultaneously until about 60 years of age, after which systolic BP continues to increase, while diastolic BP generally decreases. Age also affects the impact of systolic BP and diastolic BP as risk factors for heart attack and stroke. For persons younger than 60 years, diastolic BP is the main risk factor, while for those older than 60 years, systolic BP is more important.

PATHOPHYSIOLOGY

The pathophysiology of hypertensive emergencies is not well understood. Initially, there is a failure of the normal autoregulation and an abrupt rise in SVR. It is thought that the wall of a stressed vessel causes the release of humoral vasoconstrictors, which increases the SVR. The increased pressure within the vessel then starts a cycle of endothelial damage, local intravascular activation of the clotting cascade, fibrinoid necrosis of small blood vessels, and release of more vasoconstrictors. The cycle of vascular injury leads to tissue ischemia and autoregulatory dysfunction. Single-organ involvement is found in approximately 83% of patients presenting with hypertensive emergencies. Two-organ involvement is found in 14% of patients, and multiorgan involvement (more than three organ systems) is found in approximately 3% of patients presenting with a hypertensive emergency.

Hypertensive crisis can lead to hypertensive encephalopathy as cerebral blood vessels dilate resulting from inability to affect autoregulation. Cerebral autoregulation is the ability of the cerebral vasculature to maintain a constant pressure or cerebral blood flow (CBF). When autoregulation is disrupted, increased intercranial pressure and cerebral edema may result. Hallmark signs of hypertensive encephalopathy include cerebral edema and microhemorrhages, altered mental status, and papilledema. Blood flow is increased, and the excessive pressure drives fluid into the perivascular tissue, resulting in cerebral edema. The extreme pressure can cause arteriolar damage, as demonstrated by fibrinoid necrosis of the intima and media of the vessel wall. Although any organ is vulnerable, the eyes and the kidneys are most likely to suffer damage, leading to retinopathy, blindness, and renal failure. Patients with hypertension who are admitted to the ICU may have a rebound elevation of the BP if their usual antihypertensive regimen is interrupted. In addition, a loss of BP control can occur because of the nature of the primary disorder, trauma, or the stress of being in the ICU.

Patients also have increased cerebrovascular resistance and are more prone to ischemia when the BP decreases. Normotension achieved with BP control may result in decreased CBF. Rapid rises in BP can cause hyperperfusion with an increased CBF. The rapidity of the rise in pressure may be more destructive than the level of BP elevation. The 1-year mortality rate is 79% for patients with untreated hypertensive emergencies. The 5-year survival rate among all patients with treated hypertensive crisis is approximately 74%. Progressive stiffness occurs in the arteries, which increases systolic BP, resulting in a widened pulse pressure, which decreases coronary perfusion pressures, increases myocardial oxygen consumption, and causes the left ventricle to enlarge. The remodeled left ventricle is unable to compensate for an acute rise in SVR, leading to LV failure, pulmonary edema, and myocardial ischemia. Small renal arteries exhibit endothelial dysfunction and impaired vasodilation, which affects renal autoregulation. Once the renal autoregulatory system is disrupted, the intraglomerular pressure varies directly with the systemic arterial pressure. The kidney is no longer protected from fluctuations in perfusion caused by BP changes, resulting in acute renal ischemia during a hypertensive crisis.

ASSESSMENT

GOAL OF ASSESSMENT

The history and physical examination determine the nature, severity, and management of the hypertensive event. Patients should be questioned regarding compliance with antihypertensive drug therapy, intake of over-the-counter preparations and sympathomimetic agents, and illicit drug use. Identifying the presence of end-organ dysfunction, particularly renal and cerebrovascular disease, is of paramount importance. Duration and severity of preexisting hypertension and the degree of BP control should be clearly defined by the history.

HISTORY AND RISK FACTORS

The most common hypertensive emergency is a rapid unexplained rise in BP in a patient with chronic essential hypertension. Most patients who develop hypertensive emergencies have a history of inadequate hypertensive treatment or an abrupt discontinuation of their medications. Other causes include the following (see also Box 5-5):

- Coarctation of the aorta
- Drugs and drug interactions: Amphetamines, antidepressants, antihistamines, cocaine, clonidine withdrawal, cyclosporine, diet pills, monoamine oxidase inhibitors with tricyclic antidepressants, oral contraceptives, phencyclidine, recreational sympathomimetic drugs, serotonin syndrome, steroid use, tyramine-containing food

Box 5-5	CAUSES OF SECONDARY HYPERTENSION

Renal disease
- Acute glomerulonephritis
- Chronic pyelonephritis
- Hydronephrosis
- Renal tumors
- Renovascular hypertension

Endocrine disorders
- Cushing syndrome
- Pheochromocytoma
- Primary aldosteronism
- Thyroid/parathyroid disease

Congenital disorders
- Adrenal hyperplasia
- Coarctation of the aorta

Pregnancy-induced disorders
- Pregnancy-induced hypertension
- Preeclampsia
- Eclampsia

Drug-induced disorders
- Cyclosporine
- Oral contraceptives
- Steroids

Other
- Sleep apnea

- Endocrine: Cushing syndrome, pheochromocytoma, primary hyperaldosteronism
- Hypertension of pregnancy: Preeclampsia/eclampsia
- Neurologic disorders: CNS trauma or spinal cord disorders including Guillain-Barré syndrome
- Postoperative hypertension
- Renal parenchymal and renovascular disease: Chronic pyelonephritis, primary glomerulonephritis, tubulointerstitial nephritis (comprises 80% of all secondary causes), atherosclerosis, fibromuscular dysplasia, polyarteritis nodosa
- Systemic disorders with renal involvement: Systemic lupus erythematosus, systemic sclerosis, vasculitis
- Other factors: Hypertension is a familial disease; genetic and environmental factors contribute to its etiology. Psychologic stress, a diet high in sodium, and cigarette smoking increase the risk.

OBSERVATION
Early indicators
Although most patients are free of symptoms, vague discomfort, fatigue, dizziness, and headache can occur. The heart's initial response to systemic hypertension is to develop LV hypertrophy, which progresses to dilated cardiomyopathy.

Late indicators (nearly always present during a hypertensive crisis)
Throbbing suboccipital headache, irritability, confusion, somnolence, stupor, visual loss, focal deficits, and coma. Cardiac symptoms may include angina, MI, paroxysmal nocturnal dyspnea, congestive HF, pulmonary edema, and orthostatic hypotension. Chest pain may also indicate a dissecting aortic aneurysm. Renal symptoms include hematuria, nocturia, and azotemia. Nausea and vomiting also may occur.

Eye assessment
A funduscopic examination is performed to determine whether hemorrhage, fluffy cotton exudates, or arteriovenous nicking of the vessels has occurred. When these changes occur, visual perception is decreased. Nurses should assess the patient's gross visual acuity by the ability to read and recognize objects and people. Retinal hemorrhages and exudates as well as papilledema may occur.

Neurologic assessment
Assess level of consciousness, visual fields, and focal neurologic signs. May reveal evidence of a residual neurologic deficit from a cerebral infarct or ischemic event, as manifested by a positive Babinski reflex (upgoing toe), hemiparesis, hemiplegia, ataxia, confusion, or

cognitive alterations. Assessment should include any onset of headache, nausea, vomiting, lethargy, restlessness, or agitation. Neurologic presentations during crisis include occipital headache, stroke (infarction or hemorrhage), and visual disturbances. Hypertensive encephalopathy (severe hypertension, headache, vomiting, visual disturbances, altered mental status, seizures, and retinopathy with papilledema) may be present. A complete neurologic examination should be done to screen for localizing signs. Focal neurologic signs might not be attributable to encephalopathy; focal signs may reflect cerebral hemorrhage, infarct, or presence of a mass.

VITAL SIGNS
Blood pressure measurements
BP must be checked in both arms to screen for aortic dissection or coarctation of the aorta. Those with suspected coarctation should have BP measured in the legs. An accurate cuff pressure must be obtained after 5 minutes of rest, with 2 or more measurements taken at least 2 minutes apart. Average these readings unless there is a 5 mm Hg or greater difference. Greater differences warrant additional readings. A well-calibrated manometer with a properly fitting cuff or an automatic BP recorder should be selected for use. The bladder of the cuff must encircle 80% of the arm and cover two thirds of the length of the upper portion of the arm. BP measurement in both the supine and standing positions (if able) may help in assessment for volume depletion. A significant difference between the arms may be suggestive of an aortic dissection. Note when the patient last smoked or used any nicotine product, how much caffeine was consumed during the previous 4 hours, and whether adrenergic stimulants (e.g., over-the-counter decongestants or bronchodilators) have been used within the past 24 hours, as they elevate BP.

Pheochromocytoma assessment
Paroxysmal elevations of BP associated with palpitations, tachycardia, headache, diaphoresis, pallor, warmth or flushing, tremor, excitation, fright, nervousness, feelings of impending doom, tachypnea, abdominal pain, nausea, and vomiting. Episodes also are associated with hyperglycemia and hypermetabolism. Postural hypotension and paradoxic response to antihypertensive medications may occur.

Renal insufficiency assessment
Oliguria, hyperkalemia, anemia, or any of the typical features of kidney disease.

PALPATION
Evaluate for LV hypertrophy
Results from the need of the heart to pump against the high SVR or afterload. An LV heave or lift may be palpated with the palm of the hand at the mitral area (fifth intercostal space at the midclavicular line [MCL]). If cardiac failure is present or the left ventricle is enlarged, the apical impulse will be felt nearer to the anterior axillary line instead of the MCL.

Peripheral pulses
Pulsus alternans, an alteration in pulse pressure with a regular rhythm, may be palpated at any of the major pulse points. All peripheral pulses should be palpated bilaterally. With coarctation of the aorta, the femoral pulses will be bilaterally weak with a slow upstroke; whereas the radial and brachial pulses will be normal or bounding

AUSCULTATION
Heart sounds
When dilated cardiomyopathy is developing, an S_3 or S_4 heart sound may be auscultated in the mitral area with the bell of the stethoscope. Murmurs may be audible. In addition, crackles may be auscultated in the presence of cardiac failure along with jugular venous distention and peripheral edema.

Vascular sounds
Screen for carotid or renal bruits.

DIAGNOSTIC TESTS

The definitive test for hypertension is BP measurement. Once hypertension has been documented, many tests may be performed to determine the amount of end-organ damage or to diagnose the condition responsible for the development of secondary hypertension.

Diagnostic Tests for Hypertensive Urgencies and Emergencies

Test	Purpose	Abnormal Findings
Noninvasive Cardiology		
Cardiac echocardiography (ECHO)	Assesses for mechanical and structural abnormalities related to effective pumping of blood from both sides of the heart.	LVH with or without dilation will be demonstrated on echocardiogram by an increase in wall thickness with or without increased chamber size; a transesophageal echocardiography may be indicated if aortic dissection is suspected.
Blood and Urine Studies		
Complete blood count (CBC)	Assesses for anemia	CBC and smear to exclude microangiopathic anemia. The RBC count may fall because of hematuria caused by acute tubular necrosis.
Electrolytes Potassium (K^+) Magnesium (Mg^{2+}) Calcium (Ca^{2+}) Sodium (Na^+)	Assess for possible causes of dysrhythmias and/or heart failure.	Abnormal levels of K^+, Mg^{2+}, or Ca^{2+} may cause dysrhythmias. Elevation of Na^+ may indicate dehydration (blood is more coagulable); may reveal hyponatremia (dilutional); hypokalemia, which can result from use of diuretics; or hyperkalemia, if glomerular filtration is decreased. Hyperkalemia can also be a side effect of angiotensin-converting enzyme inhibitors (ACEIs) and potassium-sparing diuretics.
Blood urea nitrogen (BUN) and creatinine levels	Evaluate renal impairment.	If renal parenchymal disease is present, the patient may have serum creatinine above 1.3 mg/dL and BUN above 20 mg/dL.
Urinalysis (UA) and urine culture	Detects hematuria or proteinuria; microscopic UA to detect RBCs or RBC casts for renal impairment	Urinalysis results will be normal until hypertension causes renal impairment. Specific gravity may be low (<1.010). Glomerulonephritis is suspected if the urine contains granular or red cell casts or if the patient has hematuria. Pyelonephritis is suspected if there is bacterial growth in the urine.
24-hour urine collection Vanillylmandelic acid (VMA) and urinary catecholamines	Screens for abnormalities of the adrenal glands	Elevations of the 24-hour urine VMA and urinary catecholamines (10 to 50 times normal) are indicative of pheochromocytoma. The VMA level is elevated only during episodes of hypertension.
Urinary cortisol	Screens for defects in the adrenal cortex	If the patient has Cushing disease, the urine cortisol or adrenocorticotropic hormone level will be elevated.

Continued

Hypertensive Emergencies

Diagnostic Tests for Hypertensive Urgencies and Emergencies—cont'd

Test	Purpose	Abnormal Findings
Radiology		
Chest radiograph (CXR)	Assesses size of heart, thoracic cage (for fractures), thoracic aorta (for aneurysm).	CXR to detect dilation of the left ventricle; if present, the cardiac silhouette will be enlarged. If heart failure is present, there will be evidence of pulmonary congestion and pleural effusions. Notching of the aorta and a distended aortic root are indicative of coarctation of the aorta. If widening of the mediastinum is seen, a dissection of the aorta is suspected (see Aortic Aneurysm Dissection, Chapter 5). An intravenous pyelogram with nephrotomography or CT may identify the adrenal tumor and detect pheochromocytoma. Chest CT scan or aortic angiography is indicated in cases where the patient is being evaluated for aortic dissection.
Brain computed tomography (CT scan) or magnetic resonance imaging (MRI)	Indicated in patients with abnormal neurologic examinations or clinical concern for intracranial bleeding, edema, or infarction.	Presence of intracranial bleeding, cerebral edema, or infarction (acute ischemic stroke)
Abdominal aortic angiography or arteriogram	Identifies abnormal vascular anatomy of the aorta and abdominal vessels.	Angiography may identify an adrenal medullary tumor.

See diagnostic tests for patients with Acute Coronary Syndrome (Chapter 5), Aortic Aneurysm/Dissection (Chapter 5), Heart Failure (Chapter 5), Stroke: Acute Ischemic and Hemorrhagic (Chapter 7), and Acute Kidney Injury/Acute Renal Failure (Chapter 6). Additional studies such as a toxicology screen, pregnancy test, and endocrine testing may be necessary.

COLLABORATIVE MANAGEMENT
CARE PRIORITIES

In the treatment of hypertensive emergencies complicated by (or precipitated by) CNS injury, IV labetalol or nicardipine may be recommended, since they both are nonsedating and do not cause significant cerebral vasodilation, which can increase intracranial pressure (a potential problem with sodium nitroprusside). In hypertensive emergencies arising from catecholaminergic mechanisms, such as pheochromocytoma or cocaine use, beta blockers can worsen the hypertension because of unopposed peripheral vasoconstriction; phentolamine may be effective. Labetalol is useful in these patients if the HR must be controlled.

1. Control the BP within minutes to 2 hours during hypertensive crisis
The initial goal in hypertensive emergencies is to reduce the pressure by no greater than 25% (within minutes to 1 or 2 hours) and achieve a level of 160/100 mm Hg within 2 to 6 hours. Parenteral therapy is indicated in hypertensive emergencies associated with end-organ damage such as encephalopathy or aortic dissection. Constant BP monitoring is necessary. Rapid reductions in pressure may precipitate coronary, cerebral, or renal ischemia. The use of an antihypertensive that is titratable and predictable is preferred.

2. Manage patients with acute ischemic stroke according to the American Stroke Association (ASA)/AHA guidelines
With acute ischemic stroke, antihypertensives should only be used if the BP exceeds 220/120 mm Hg, and BP should be reduced cautiously by 10% to 15%. If thrombolytics are to be given, the BP should be maintained at less than 185/110 mm Hg during treatment and for 24 hours following treatment. In hemorrhagic stroke, the aim is to minimize bleeding with a target MAP of less than 130 mm Hg.

3. Manage patients with acute subarachnoid hemorrhage

For patients who will not undergo an intervention, the goal is to prevent further bleeding while maintaining cerebral perfusion in the face of cerebral vasospasm.

- **Parenteral antihypertensive therapy:**

    Nitroprusside: A short-acting, rapid arterial and venous dilator. BP will rise almost immediately if the drip is stopped. The usual initial dose is 0.3 to 0.5 µg/kg/min. AHA guidelines recommend beginning with 0.1 µg/kg/min and titrating upward every 3 to 5 minutes to desired effect. Usual dose is 3 µg/kg/min, rarely is more than 4 µg/kg/min needed, and maximum dose is 10 µg/kg/min. Direct arterial pressure monitoring is essential for titration of this drug, with constant vigilance to prevent hypotension. Nitroprusside is metabolized to thiocyanate, a toxin, which can cause fatigue, nausea, tinnitus, blurred vision, and delirium. Serum thiocyanate levels should be drawn after 48 hours of use and regularly thereafter, especially with patients with impaired renal function. Levels of less than 10 mg/dL are considered safe. Concomitant administration of parenteral and oral therapy should be initiated before weaning nitroprusside. When oral antihypertensives begin to reduce the BP, weaning is done carefully to prevent hypotensive episodes.

    Fenoldopam: A peripherally acting rapid-acting vasodilator and a selective dopamine$_1$ receptor agonist. Initial dose is 0.1 µg/kg/min and it can be increased by 0.05 µg/kg/min; the maximum recommended dose is 1.7 µg/kg/min. The half-life is 9.8 minutes. The patient must still be kept in the ICU and undergo arterial monitoring with this drug.

    Labetalol: A fast-acting alpha/beta-blocking agent, which also can be used to treat the patient in hypertensive crisis. Given slowly by IV push, beginning with a 20- to 80-mg dose, repeated every 10 minutes, or a continuous infusion of 2 to 8 mg/min can be administered. The usual cumulative dose is 50 to 200 mg. Do not exceed a total dose of 300 mg. Keep the patient supine during the injection and until stable. Check BP every 5 minutes and then every 30 minutes until blood pressure is stabilized. Monitor for bronchospasm, heart block, or orthostatic hypotension.

    Esmolol: A short/quick-acting beta-blocker with an onset of action of 1 to 2 minutes and a duration of 10 to 20 minutes. Initial dose is 250 to 500 µg/kg/min for 1 minute and then 50 to 100 µg/kg/min for 4 minutes. May repeat the sequence. Observe for hypotension, nausea, vomiting, and, with asthmatics, bronchospasm.

    Nicardipine: A potent CCB given at a rate of 5 to 15 mg/h. When desired BP reduction is achieved, consider reducing to the average maintenance dose of 3 mg/h. When discontinuing, can lose 50% of effect within 30 minutes, but gradually decreased effects persist for up to 50 hours. It may cause tachycardia, headache, flushing, and aggravation of angina. Do not exceed 150 mL/h (15 mg/h).

    Enalaprilat: An ACEI that reduces peripheral arterial resistance. The usual dose is 1.25 to 5 mg by IV bolus, administered over a 5-minute period. Dose may be repeated every 6 hours. Patients on diuretics should receive a lower standard dose. Initial response may take 15 minutes to 1 hour. Peak BP reduction occurs in 1 to 4 hours, and effects last up to 6 hours. Enalaprilat should be used with caution in patients with renal failure or those with bilateral renal artery stenosis (because of high renin states). Avoid in AMI.

    Hydralazine: A potent vasodilator administered as a 10 to 20 mg IV bolus or a 10 to 40 mg intramuscular injection. The onset is 10 to 30 minutes, with a duration of 2 to 6 hours. Adverse effects include tachycardia, headache, vomiting, and aggravation of angina.

    Nitroglycerin: A coronary and peripheral vasodilator supplied in a 50-mg vial, which is added to a 250-mL glass bottle of D5W. The IV infusion may be concentrated to prevent fluid overload if higher doses are needed to control BP. NTG is administered via an infusion pump starting at 5 µg/min. Onset is rapid, so BP must be monitored closely during titration. Increase by 5 to 10 µg every 3 to 5 minutes. Headache is common and controlled with analgesics.

    Phentolamine: An alpha adrenergic-blocking agent that reduces afterload and has minimal effect in reducing BP except for secondary hypertension caused by pheochromocytoma. A dose of 5 to 20 mg is administered via IV push. The onset is immediate, and the half-life is approximately 19 minutes. Use with caution in patients with CAD.

> **HIGH ALERT!** Nifedipine is no longer recommended for the management of hypertensive emergencies. Liquid nifedipine had been used for rapid treatment of hypertension; the capsule was pierced and the contents were squeezed out under the tongue, with rapid sublingual absorption the goal. However, the drug was not absorbed sublingually but rather was swallowed and absorbed in the stomach, producing a quick onset of action. Effects were varying and dangerous. Variations in dosage occurred, since the amount removed from the capsule by squeezing liquid from the small pierced hole was variable, as was the amount actually swallowed, versus that left pooled in the mouth. Serious side effects, including stroke, have been reported.

4. Facilitate adjustment to a routine antihypertensive regimen

As the patient is adjusted to a routine antihypertensive regimen, diuretics, ACEIs, CCBs, or ARBs may be used in various combinations. If ineffective in a combination of three of the four categories, medications in other categories, including beta blockers and alpha-adrenergic blockers, may be used. A hypertension specialist may be needed for optimal medication management for patients with resistant hypertension. For persons with severe hypertension, three to five medications are often needed to achieve normal BP. Resistant hypertension is defined as BP that remains above goal despite the concurrent use of three antihypertensive agents of different classes.

5. Provide patient education regarding lifestyle alterations

Behavioral changes are the cornerstone of medical treatment for early and established hypertension. Normal body weight should be achieved and maintained. Alcohol consumption should be less than 1 oz ethanol per day. Daily intake of sodium for the average adult should be modified to 2 to 3 g for the person with hypertension. Smoking cessation is imperative (1) to halt the injury to the intima of the coronary and peripheral vessels and (2) to reduce the workload of the heart. A regular aerobic program has been proven beneficial in maintaining better control of BP. This should consist of 30 minutes of exercise 3 to 5 times per week at a target HR of 60% to 80% of the anaerobic threshold (determined by an exercise physiologist). Maintenance of adequate potassium, calcium, and magnesium intake is important.

6. Educate patients regarding ongoing pharmacotherapy

Maintenance pharmacotherapy for hypertension is now approached by evaluating on an individual basis the best treatment option based on the patient's other disease states or demographic factors. For persons with severe hypertension, three to five medications are often needed to achieve normal BP. Patients must be informed that taking more than one drug is to be expected and not a sign of failure or worsening of disease. Healthcare providers must set patient expectations for compliance. This approach is promoted by the JNC-8 and the AHA. After an adequate trial of the first drug, a second drug from a different category may be tried.

7. Discuss surgical treatment of appropriate conditions that prompt hypertension

Although there is no surgical intervention for primary hypertension, several forms of secondary hypertension respond well to the surgical correction of the primary problem. A coarctation of the aorta can be repaired by removing the narrowed area of the vessel and inserting an aortic graft. Renal artery stenosis may be corrected by grafting or by renal artery angioplasty. For patients with pheochromocytoma, surgical removal of the tumor(s) will return the patient to a normotensive state.

CARE PLANS FOR HYPERTENSIVE EMERGENCIES

INEFFECTIVE TISSUE PERFUSION: CARDIOPULMONARY, CEREBRAL, AND RENAL *related to interruption of arterial flow secondary to vasoconstriction that occurs with interruption of the normal BP control mechanism; interruption of venous flow secondary to vasodilation or tissue edema that occurs with loss of autoregulation.*

Goals/Outcomes: Tissue perfusion is established within 24 hours as evidenced by systemic arterial BP 110 to 160/70 to 110 mm Hg (or within patient's normal range); MAP 70 to 105 mm Hg; equal and normoreactive pupils; strength and tone of the extremities bilaterally equal and normal for patient; orientation to time, place, and person;

urinary output 0.5 mL/kg/h or greater; and stable weight. Within 48 hours, systolic BP is less than 140 mm Hg and diastolic BP is less than 90 mm Hg, with MAP 70 to 105 mm Hg.
NOC Circulation Status

Hemodynamic Regulation
1. Monitor BP and MAP every 1 to 5 minutes during titration of the medications. As patient's condition stabilizes, perform these assessments every 15 minutes to 1 hour. Be alert to sudden drops or elevations in BP. As the oral medications begin to affect BP, gradually wean IV nitroprusside and other potent vasodilators to prevent hypotensive episodes. Continuous monitoring is recommended.
   • Correlate cuff pressure with pressure from arterial cannulation.
   • Determine ideal range for BP control and maximal nitroprusside dose with advanced practice provider. Usually the following guidelines are used: systolic BP less than 140 to 160 mm Hg; MAP less than 110 mm Hg; diastolic BP less than 90 mm Hg (see table 5-19.).
   • If hypotension develops, decrease or stop nitroprusside infusion until the pressure rises.
2. Assess patient for neurologic deficit by performing hourly neurostatus checks. Be alert to sensorimotor deficit if MAP is greater than 140 mm Hg. As patient's condition stabilizes and BP becomes controlled, perform neurostatus checks at least every 4 hours.
3. Monitor patient for changes in funduscopic examination. Consult advanced practice provider if hemorrhages or fluffy cotton exudates are present.
4. Assess patient for evidence of decreasing renal perfusion by monitoring I&O and weighing patient daily. Consult advanced practice provider if urinary output is less than 0.5 mL/kg/h for 2 consecutive hours or if weight gain is at least 1 kg (2.2 lb). Be alert to azotemia (increasing BUN), decreasing creatinine clearance, and increasing serum creatinine. Optimal laboratory values are BUN 20 mg/dL or less, creatinine clearance 9.5 mL/min or higher, and serum creatinine 1.5 mg/dL or less.

NIC Medication Administration; Cardiac Care; Circulatory Care

ACUTE PAIN *related to headache secondary to cerebral edema occurring with high perfusion pressures.*

Goals/Outcomes: Patient's subjective evaluation of pain improves within 12 to 24 hours, as documented by a pain scale. Nonverbal indicators, such as grimacing, are absent or diminished.
NOC Pain Control

Pain Management
1. Monitor patient for headache pain at frequent intervals. Devise a pain scale with patient, rating discomfort from 0 (no pain) to 10 (severe pain).
2. Provide pain medications as prescribed. A variety of analgesics may be used, ranging from acetaminophen with codeine to morphine, depending on the severity of the symptoms. Assess effectiveness of the pain medication, using the pain scale to determine degree of relief obtained.
3. Use of meperidine should be avoided.

Safety Alert *Concurrent use of meperidine and a monoamine oxidase inhibitor may result in hypertensive crisis, hyperpyrexia, cardiovascular collapse, and death.*

4. Teach the patient relaxation techniques to use in conjunction with the medications. Guided imagery, meditation, progressive muscle relaxation, and music therapy often are effective. Maintain a quiet, low-lit environment that is free of extensive distraction and stimulation. Limit visits as indicated.

NIC Analgesic Administration; Environmental Management: Comfort; Progressive Muscle Relaxation

DISTURBED SENSORY PERCEPTION *related to decreased visual acuity secondary to retinal damage occurring with high perfusion pressures; pain secondary to cerebral edema.*

Text is continued on page 589

Hypertensive Emergencies

Table 5-19	MEDICATIONS USED IN THE TREATMENT OF HYPERTENSION		
Drug Type	**Medication**	**Dosage/Schedule**	**Side Effects**
Diuretics			
Thiazides/related compounds (JNC-8 recommended)	Chlorothiazide (Diuril)	12.5 to 50 mg daily	Hypokalemia and hyperuricemia in thiazides and loop diuretics; hypercholesterolemia, hyperglycemia, increased type 2 diabetes, impotence, indigestion in all categories of diuretics
	Chlorthalidone (Hygroton)	12.5 to 25 mg daily	
	Cyclothiazide (Anhydron, Renazide)	1 to 2 mg daily	
	Hydrochlorothiazide (Hydrodiuril)	12.5 to 50 mg daily	
	Hydroflumethiazide (Aldactide)	12.5 to 50 mg daily	
	Indapamide (Lozol)	2.5 to 5 mg	
	Methylchlorthiazide (Enduron)	2.5 to 5 mg daily	
	Metolazone (Mykrox) *or*	0.5 to 1 mg daily	
	metolazone (zaroxolyn)	2.5 to 20 mg daily	
	Polythiazide (Renese)	2 to 4 mg daily	
Loop diuretics	Bumetanide (Bumex)	0.25 to 2.5 mg every 12 hours	
	Ethacrynic acid (Ethacrynate)	25 to 200 mg every 12 hours	
	Furosemide (Lasix)	20 to 200 mg every 6 to 24 hours	
	Torsemide (Demadex)	2.5 to 10 mg every 12 to 24 hour	
Potassium-sparing agents	Amiloride (Midamor)	5 to 10 mg every 12 to 24 hours	Hyperkalemia, gynecomastia, menstrual abnormalities
	Eplerenone (Inspra)	25 to 100 mg daily	
	Spironolactone (Aldactone)	25 to 200 mg every 8 to 24 hour	
	Triamterene (Dyrenium)	100 to 300 mg every 12 to 24 hour	
Adrenergic-Inhibiting Agents			
Beta blockers	Atenolol (Tenormin)*	25 to 100 mg daily	Fatigue, drowsiness, depression, fluid retention, heart failure, impotence, hypoglycemia, flushing, bronchospasm (diminished with cardioselective beta-blockers)
	Betaxolol (Kerlone)*	5 to 20 mg daily	
	Bisoprolol (Zebeta)*	2 to 20 mg daily	
	Metoprolol (Lopressor)*	50 to 100 mg every 12 to 24 hours	
	Metoprolol extended release (Toprol XL)	50 to 100 mg daily	
	Nadolol (Corgard)	40 to 120 mg daily	
	Nebivolol (Bystolic)	2.5 to 40 mg daily	
	Propranolol (Inderal)	40 to 160 mg every 12 hours	
	Propranolol long–acting (Inderal LA)	60 to 180 mg daily	

Table 5-19	MEDICATIONS USED IN THE TREATMENT OF HYPERTENSION—cont'd		
Drug Type	**Medication**	**Dosage/Schedule**	**Side Effects**
	Propranolol long-acting (InnoPran XL)	80 to 120 mg at bedtime	
	Timolol (Blocadren)	20 to 40 mg every 12 hours	
Beta blockers with ISA	Acebutolol* (Sectral)	200 to 800 mg every 12 to 24 hours	
	Carteolol (Cartrol)	2.5 to 10 mg daily	
	Penbutolol (Levatol)	10 to 40 mg daily	
	Pindolol (Visken)	10 to 40 mg twice daily	
Alpha and beta blocker	Labetalol (Normodyne, Trandate)	200 to 800 mg twice daily	May cause severe postural hypertension; dose adjustments should be made based on standing BP.
	Carvedilol (Coreg)	12.5 to 50 mg twice daily	
Alpha-receptor blocker	Alfuzosin (Uroxatral)	2.5 to 20 mg twice daily	Hypoglycemia, diarrhea, hypertension, flushing, first-dose syncope, blurred vision
	Doxazosin (Cardura)	1 to 16 mg daily	
	Phentolamine (Regitine)	50 mg twice daily	
	Prazosin HCl (Minipress)	1 to 7 mg 3 times daily	
	Terazosin (Hytrin)	1 to 20 mg daily	
Angiotensin-Converting Enzyme Inhibitors (ACEIs) (JNC-8 recommended)			
	Benazepril (Lotensin)	10 to 40 mg twice daily	To prevent severe hypotension, reduce dose of diuretic; may cause hyperkalemia in person with renal failure; may cause acute renal failure in bilateral renal artery stenosis; also may cause profound postural hypotension; dose adjustments should be made based on standing BP.
	Captopril (Capoten)	25 to 50 mg twice daily	
	Enalapril (Vasotec PO)	2.5 to 40 mg twice daily	
	Enalaprilat (Vasotec IV)	0.625 to 1.25 mg every 6 hours	
	Fosinopril (Monopril)	10 to 40 mg daily	
	Lisinopril (Prinivil, Zestril)	10 to 40 mg daily	
	Moexipril (Univasc)	7.5 mg daily	
	Perindopril (Aceon)	4 to 8 mg twice daily	
	Quinapril (Accupril)	10 to 40 mg daily	
	Ramipril (Altace)	25 mg daily	
	Trandolapril (Mavik)	1 to 4 mg daily	

Hypertensive Emergencies

Continued

Table 5-19	MEDICATIONS USED IN THE TREATMENT OF HYPERTENSION—cont'd		
Drug Type	**Medication**	**Dosage/Schedule**	**Side Effects**
Angiotensin Receptor Blockers (ARBs) (Angiotensin II Antagonists) (JNC-8 recommended)			
	Candesartan (Atacand)	8 to 32 mg daily	Hepatotoxicity, hyperkalemia, agranulocytosis, leukopenia, neutropenia. Less risk of angioedema and cough than with ACE inhibitors.
	Eprosartan (Teveten)	400 to 800 mg daily; may divide doses	
	Irbesartan (Avapro)	150 to 300 mg daily	
	Losartan (Cozaar)	25 to 100 mg daily; may divide doses	
	Olmesartan (Benicar)	20 to 40 mg daily	
	Telmisartan (Micardis)	20 to 80 mg daily	
	Valsartan (Diovan)	80 to 320 mg daily	
Calcium Channel Blockers (CCBs) (JNC-8 recommended)			
Nondihydropyridines	Diltiazem (Cardizem)	30 to 90 mg 4 times daily	Constipation, peripheral edema
	Verapamil (Calan, Isoptin)	80 to 120 mg 3 times daily	
Dihydropyridines	Amlodipine (Norvasc)	2.5 to 10 mg daily	Dihydropyridines are more potent peripheral vasodilators and may cause more flushing, peripheral edema, tachycardia, dizziness, and headache.
	Felodipine (Plendil)	5 to 50 mg daily	
	Isradipine (DynaCirc)	2.5 to 10 mg twice daily	
	Nicardipine (Cardene)	60 to 120 mg twice daily	
	Nifedipine LA (Procardia XL)	30 to 60 mg 3 times daily	
	Nisoldipine (Sular)	10 to 40 mg daily	
Direct Renin Inhibitors			
	Aliskiren (Tekturna)	Starting dose: 150 mg once daily. May titrate up to 300 mg daily. No dosage adjustment in the elderly. Concomitant use with cyclosporine is not recommended.	Addition of aliskiren to an ACEI (or ARB) and beta-blocker had favorable neurohumoral effects in heart failure and appeared to be well tolerated.
Miscellaneous Antihypertensives			
	Clonidine (Catapres)	0.2 to 2.4 mg daily in divided doses	Gradually withdraw over 1 week
	Guanabenz (Wytensin)	8 to 30 mg daily	Orthostatic hypotension, xerostomia
	Guanfacine (Tenex)	1 to 2 mg at bedtime daily	Orthostatic hypotension, xerostomia
	Methyldopa (Aldomet)	250 to 1000 mg daily in 2 divided doses	Peripheral edema; sedation with initial dosing

BP, Blood pressure; *ISA*, intrinsic sympathomimetic activity; *IV*, intravenous; *PO*, by mouth.
Some drug combinations available in multiple fixed doses. Each drug dose is reported in milligrams.
*Cardioselective.

Goals/Outcomes: Within 24 to 48 hours of this diagnosis, the patient reads print, recognizes objects or people, and demonstrates coordination of movement.

NOC Vision Compensation Behavior

Environmental Management: Safety

1. Assess patient for signs of decreased visual acuity by monitoring patient's ability to read and recognize objects or people. Evaluate patient's movement coordination to determine depth perception. Perform a funduscopic examination per institutional guidelines, if appropriate and allowable.

2. If the patient has decreased visual acuity, assist with feeding and other ADLs and keep patient's personal effects within his or her visual field.

3. Reassure patient and significant others that visual problems usually resolve when the BP is lowered sufficiently.

NIC Surveillance: Safety

ADDITIONAL NURSING DIAGNOSES

For other nursing diagnoses and interventions, see the following as appropriate: Hemodynamic Monitoring (Chapter 1) and Emotional and Spiritual Support of the Patient and Significant Others (Chapter 2).

PERIPHERAL VASCULAR DISEASE

PATHOPHYSIOLOGY

Peripheral vascular disease includes all vascular disorders of the blood vessel system outside of the heart. Both chronic disease states and acute disorders are included. This chapter discusses care of chronic diseases of the carotid arteries and lower extremity PAD and the acute development of critical limb ischemia.

Chronic, as well as many acute, vascular diseases develop from progressive atherosclerotic plaque formation in arterial walls throughout the body. The presence of PAD may indicate cardiovascular disease. Atherosclerosis, as defined by the World Health Organization, is a combination of changes in the intimal and medial layers of the vessel wall in which lipids, hemorrhage, fibrous tissue, and calcium deposits occur. The intima is the innermost layer composed of endothelial cells within a matrix of collagen and elastin fibers. The media is the thick middle layer of the vessel composed of varying amounts of smooth muscle, collagen, and elastic fibers. The adventitia is the outermost layer composed of collagen and elastin, making it a key element in providing the strength of the arterial wall.

Atherosclerotic plaque formation occurs in three stages. The early stage is development of fatty streaks during childhood or young adult life. The fatty streaks are formed from lipid-laden macrophages called foam cells. Low-density lipoprotein cholesterol is the main lipid component of the fatty streaks. The second stage is the appearance of fibrous plaque later in life from progression of the fatty streaks from foam cells to a more permanent fibrous plaque. These plaques are most often found at areas of bifurcation of the arterial vessels. The last stage occurs as the fibrous plaque develops into a complicated lesion with necrosis and ulceration of the plaque surface with exposure, leading to thrombogenesis through platelet aggregation and thrombus formation. Elasticity of the arterial wall is lost and there is progressive narrowing of the vessel lumen. The vessel wall may also degenerate and dilate, leading to aneurysmal development.

The primary risk factors known to accelerate this process are smoking, hypertension, hyperlipidemia, and diabetes mellitus. The presence of CAD and renal artery stenosis has been correlated with carotid artery disease of 50% stenosis or greater. Exercise and modification of risk factors can slow the progression and even promote regression of the fatty streaks.

Symptoms of atherosclerosis emerge over time with the progressive narrowing and occlusion of the arterial bed until the vessel that provides the main perfusion of a limb or tissue is critically narrowed to 50% or more of lumen diameter (noted as a hemodynamically significant stenosis). Symptoms of chronic progressive atherosclerosis include subtle changes in skin appearance, color, and temperature. Other factors, such as length of stenosis, blood viscosity, peripheral resistance, and acute versus chronic development, affect blood flow and tissue perfusion. As plaque progresses along the arterial walls in an uneven pattern, the laminar flow of blood becomes turbulent and can be heard with a stethoscope as a bruit. Generally, the progressive and chronic development of disease allows for the development of collateral blood flow and perfusion to be maintained at a minimal level for the person at rest without symptoms present at this time. Pain occurs when the tissue needs more oxygen, such as with walking or other exercises.

Autonomic neuropathy, which occurs when blood is shunted away from peripheral cutaneous capillary beds, may occur with PAD alone, or in conjunction with diabetes or other comorbidities. Motor neuropathy causes changes in gait and pressure distribution, which may lead to ulceration. Skin is less elastic with diminished capillary perfusion and reparative mechanisms. Loss of protective sensation and proprioception resulting in increased force with each step can lead to callus formation at pressure areas, which decreases elasticity and increases skin ischemia. Bone and joint changes occurring with comorbidities, such as diabetes, can add additional abnormal weight-bearing mechanisms to the feet, leading to callus and ulcer formation. This can become critical in the presence of PAD and diminished perfusion.

Sudden blockage of an artery presents with an acute onset of symptoms that are more pronounced. An acute blockage of a lower extremity artery (acute limb ischemia [ALI]) may present with pain, pallor, and neurosensory impairment in the lower limb, while an acute occlusion of a cerebrovascular artery may present as a stroke.

CAROTID ARTERY OCCLUSIVE DISEASE

The pathogenesis of atherosclerosis in the carotid arteries is very similar to the formation in all coronary and peripheral arterial vessels. Stenosis in the carotid arteries is not only associated with stroke or transient ischemic attacks (TIA), which are warnings of impending stroke, but it is also associated with an increased risk of MI and PAD. Ischemic stroke compose 87% of all strokes, and of those, carotid stenosis is associated with 15% to 20%. Additionally, the risk increases with the progressive increase in stenosis of the carotid artery, especially with ulcerative plaque. Other sources of ischemic stroke include thromboemboli from a variety of sources (see Box 5-6). Without intervention, significant carotid stenosis (greater than 70%) in a patient who has experienced a TIA or stroke is associated with an increased risk of a second stroke. Thus, the goal of treating significant carotid stenosis is to prevent stroke.

Stenosis of the carotid arteries is generally measured in the internal carotid arteries and described as a percentage of the artery measured at defined points. Flow velocities measured per Doppler ultrasonography at these points are used in defining the percentage of stenosis.

The internal carotid artery bifurcates at the distal common carotid (at the level of the thyroid cartilage), providing perfusion to the intercerebral circulation (the circle of Willis) and middle and anterior cerebral arteries. Bifurcations are common areas of plaque formation. Significant stenosis or occlusion of this artery may present with classic symptoms of TIA or stroke, consisting of transient monocular blindness (amaurosis fugax) on the side of the lesion relating to temporary reduction in blood flow to the ophthalmic artery off the internal carotid artery, contralateral neurosensory deficits (hemiparesis or hemiparesthesias), or difficulties with speech and/or swallowing. See Box 5-7 for a detailed listing of manifestations of TIA or stroke relating to stenosis of the right or left internal carotid artery. TIA or strokes may also occur from ischemia or infarction of the vertebrobasilar system secondary to stenosis of the vertebral arteries. Symptoms related to vertebral artery stenosis include cranial nerve deficits, visual field loss, ataxia, dizziness, imbalance, incoordination, and ataxic gait.

LOWER EXTREMITY PERIPHERAL ARTERY OCCLUSIVE DISEASE: ACUTE

Acute occlusion of a lower extremity artery may occur from chronic PAD with development of an acute thrombosis, referred to as "acute-on-chronic" disease. When the chronic development of peripheral artery occlusive disease in the lower extremity becomes severe, it is referred to as "critical limb ischemia" (CLI) and usually is manifested by rest pain and/or ischemic ulcers of the foot. Acute thrombosis of sites of stenosis in which the blood flow impairment was hemodynamically significant can occur and present with acute symptoms. However, most often ALI is caused by an embolic source. Cardiac disease is one of the most common embolic sources, with atrial fibrillation being one of the most frequent cardiac sources. Aneurysmal disease is another common embolic source. See Box 5-6 for a listing of

Box 5-6	CAUSES OF ACUTE ARTERIAL OCCLUSION

General pathologic processes

Arterial versus atheroembolization

Thrombosis of a diseased artery (acute-on-chronic disease)

Acute occlusion of a vascular bypass graft

Arterial traumas

Specific sources or processes

Cardiac Causes	Noncardiac Causes
Atherosclerotic heart disease (most common cardiac source) Arrhythmias — atrial fibrillation	Aneurysms (most common noncardiac source) • Abdominal aortic aneurysms • Peripheral aneurysms (such as femoral or popliteal)
Myocardial infarction (left ventricular mural thrombus formation) (second most common source)	Atherosclerotic plaque ulcers (in aorta or common iliac artery; also source of stroke in carotid artery disease)
Cardiomyopathy	Prosthetic grafts
Left ventricular aneurysms	Iatrogenic sources or arterial trauma (such as catheter-induced thrombus formation)
Endocarditis (valvular vegetation)	Paradoxical sources (secondary to an intracardiac defect and a patent foramen ovale)
Prosthetic cardiac valves	
Rheumatic heart disease	

Box 5-7	SYMPTOMS OF TIA AND ISCHEMIC STROKE RELATED TO STENOSIS OF THE CAROTID ARTERY

Right Internal Carotid Artery (RICA)	Left Internal Carotid Artery (LICA)
Right eye monocular blindness (amaurosis fugax)	Left eye monocular blindness (amaurosis fugax)
Right homonymous hemianopsia (visual loss involving right visual field)	Left homonymous hemianopsia (visual loss involving left visual field)
Aphasia in ambidextrous or left-handed persons	Aphasia
Left-sided weakness (hemiparesis)	Right-sided weakness (hemiparesis)
Left-sided sensory loss (paresthesia)	Right-sided sensory loss (paresthesia)

embolic sources. Diagnostic workup will include looking for the source of emboli, especially ruling out a cardiac or aneurysmal source.

The acute occlusion of a limb presents with a sudden onset of symptoms that are characteristic and essential in determining the diagnosis of ALI. These prominent symptoms, referred to as the six "P"s, include pain, pallor, paresthesias, paralysis, pulselessness, and poikilothermia. The severity of the symptoms depends on a number of factors, such as the acuteness of development of the vessel occlusion, presence of chronic disease with collateral circulation, and duration of the ischemic event. Symptoms of paresthesias and paralysis indicate advanced ischemia that is affecting nerve pathways of the extremity. Additionally, the presentation may include decreased sensation along the dorsum of the foot and loss of great toe or ankle dorsiflexion.

With acute disease, critical ischemia develops within hours and is associated with irreversible anoxic injury to skeletal muscle or peripheral nerves within 4 to 6 hours. Skin and subcutaneous tissue remain viable for longer periods because of increased tolerance to ischemia. In less than 8 hours' duration of acute ischemia, the limb may appear pale, waxy white with a cadaveric appearance. At 8 to 12 hours, areas of local stasis develop with bluish skin mottling followed by blebs, superficial skin necrosis, and dry gangrene mummification of toes.

Evaluation and diagnosis of the cause of ALI are crucial to prevent tissue injury and necrosis. In general, an onset of symptoms indicative of ALI presenting within the past 14 days is considered acute. Early diagnosis would include duplex ultrasound or vascular noninvasive Doppler studies, angiography, echocardiogram, and possible magnetic resonance angiography (MRA) or computer tomography angiography (CTA). Treatment will include a number of options including anticoagulation, thrombolytic therapy, surgical thromboembolectomy, endovascular procedures of stent, angioplasty, or atherectomy, and surgical bypass or amputation of the limb. Complications include those secondary to the treatment, as well as complications related to the acute ischemic event and reperfusion injury. These include catheter-induced vessel injury, bleeding, reocclusion, compartment syndrome, and reperfusion injury.

Compartment syndrome and reperfusion injury occur when ischemia to a limb is absent for an extended period of time. Compartment syndrome is defined by the swelling of tissues within closed fascial compartments leading to increased pressure, compression, and further necrosis and nerve injury. In anticipation of this, a fasciotomy of the involved limb may be performed at the time of surgical thromboembolectomy or at a later time. Reperfusion injury also involves the development of severe acidosis, hyperkalemia, renal failure secondary to myoglobinuria, and pulmonary insufficiency (see Compartment Syndrome Ischemic Myositis, Chapter 3).

PERIPHERAL VASCULAR ASSESSMENT: ARTERIAL OCCLUSIVE DISEASE

GOAL OF SYSTEM ASSESSMENT

- Evaluate for decreased blood flow and tissue perfusion so as to evaluate for focal diminished perfusion of the cerebrovascular or lower extremity peripheral arterial systems.

HISTORY AND RISK FACTORS

- Family or personal history of tobacco abuse, hyperlipidemia, hypertension, diabetes, obesity, stress, sedentary living, cardiovascular disease, renal insufficiency, clotting disorders, foot ulcers, or noncompliance with medical management (daily antiplatelet inhibitors, statins, or other medications to control above risk factors).
- Age younger than 50 years, with diabetes and one other atherosclerosis risk factor (smoking, dyslipidemia, hypertension, or hyperhomocysteinemia)
- Age 50 to 69 years with history of smoking or diabetes
- Age 70 years and older
- Leg symptoms with exertion (suggestive of claudication) or ischemic rest pain
- Abnormal lower extremity pulse examination
- Known atherosclerotic coronary, carotid, or renal artery disease

CAROTID ARTERY OCCLUSIVE DISEASE

- CAD and renal artery stenosis greater than 60% are associated with increased risk for carotid disease.
- Retinal ischemic events, especially in the absence of migraine or cardiac embolic events, warrant evaluation for carotid artery disease.
- Patients with a bruit and/or two or more risk factors for PAD should be evaluated for carotid stenosis.
- Significant stenosis may be present without symptoms.
- Symptomatic carotid stenosis or occlusion may present with TIA symptoms.
  - TIA is defined by symptoms that last less than 24 hours.
  - TIA symptoms indicative of stenosis or occlusion of the internal carotid artery (see Box 5-7).
- Atypical symptoms of dizziness, vertigo, syncope, unsteady gate, bilateral paresthesias/paresis may be attributed to other causes, such as cardiac disease, hypovolemia, medication side effects, vertebrobasilar insufficiency, and others.

PERIPHERAL ARTERY OCCLUSIVE DISEASE WITH OR WITHOUT DISTAL LIMB INVOLVEMENT, CHRONIC

* Associated with the presence of CAD.
* May be chronic or acute-on-chronic disease.
* Intermittent claudication is the most common manifestation of PAD.
    * The calf, thigh, hip, or buttock develops tightening or cramping pain with exertion, such as walking a predictable distance, and is relieved with rest.
    * The site of claudication is indication of the location of occlusion, which will be above the presentation of pain.
* Claudication that is considered to be lifestyle limiting is significant to the point that it substantially interferes with the person's ability to perform ADLs or to work.
* Symptoms may also be described as "fatigue" or "numbness" of the extremity that occurs with walking.
* Nocturnal rest pain indicates a worsening of the disease. It occurs at night and is usually relieved by sitting, standing, or dangling the affected limb, using gravity to increase perfusion.
* Rest pain, which is present all the time without relief, indicates a critically ischemic limb and is generally present in the distal foot, forefoot, and toes.
* Most common symptom of rest pain is a burning sensation across the dorsum of the foot.
* Chronic symptoms may be masked by the presence of other diseases limiting the ability to walk, such as cardiac or respiratory disease causing fatigue or dyspnea before lower extremity symptoms are present or the presence of neuropathy.

PERIPHERAL ARTERY OCCLUSIVE DISEASE WITH OR WITHOUT DISTAL LIMB INVOLVEMENT, ACUTE

* Acute occlusions are commonly associated with a thromboembolic source, which needs to be identified.
* Hallmark signs: The six "P"s (pain, pallor, pulselessness, paresthesia [numbness], poikilothermia [coldness], and paralysis).
    * Paralysis is a late and grave sign; the limb already has necrotic muscle and will not likely regain function, resulting in foot drop. It may require amputation.
* Presence of "blue toe syndrome" is indicated by bluish, mottled spots scattered over the toes and represents an embolic process.
* Outcome depends on duration of tissue ischemia, site of obstruction, extent of thrombus propagation, adequacy of collateral circulation, and hemodynamic state of the patient.

OBSERVATION

Symptoms of PAD may vary depending on the vessels involved and may include intermittent claudication if it involves the limbs or TIAs if it involves the carotid arteries, which provide perfusion to the brain. Most patients with intermittent claudication require no intervention, approximately 20% require surgical reconstruction, and approximately 5% to 10% progress to require an amputation. The presence of pain at rest or a nonhealing necrotic ulcer defines CLI and indicates disease in greater than one artery and impending loss of the limb without treatment. Evaluate blood flow quality and tissue perfusion of cerebrovascular and peripheral vascular vessels:

* Cerebrovascular perfusion
    * Level of consciousness, alertness, speech, responsiveness
    * Neurologic assessment of cranial nerve function
    * Extremity strength, movement
* Lower extremity perfusion
    * Look for decreased hair growth, shiny skin, nail changes, distal joint abnormalities, or skin ulcers.
    * Evaluate for change in skin color in neutral, elevated, and dependent positions (pallor with limb elevation versus rubor with dependency).
    * Neurosensory function of peripheral nerves: sensation, strength

Carotid artery occlusive disease

* Evaluate for cranial nerve (CN) deficit, presenting with unilateral paralysis of extremities or facial features, or gait ataxia (see chapter on stroke for details of CN assessment)

- Evaluate for CN damage status post carotid procedure.
  - CN VII: facial movement, symmetry of face (as in drooping at the corner of the mouth), unable to smile symmetrically.
  - CN IX: taste to posterior third of tongue, gag reflex; injury may cause mild dysphagia or loss of taste.
  - CN X: palatal, pharyngeal, and laryngeal, gag movement; injury may affect tongue movement, dysphagia, or dystonia.
  - CN XI: sternocleidomastoid, trapezius muscle movement; injury may cause an inability to shrug shoulders or move head side to side against resistance.
  - CN XII: tongue movement; injury may cause an inability to move the tongue from side to side or dysarthria.

Peripheral artery occlusive disease
- Presence of pallor in the foot when the extremity is elevated 30 to 45 degrees for several seconds to a minute.
- Presence of dependent rubor (intense deep red color) in the foot when it is dependent for several minutes.
- Presence of bluish or deep purple, mottled discolorations of the foot or toes.
- Ulceration, fissures, or gangrene lesions present at the digits, interdigits, or heel.
- Presence of extremity paralysis, or gait ataxia.

VITAL SIGNS
Check temperature, HR, BP, and peripheral pulses to evaluate blood flow quality and tissue perfusion.
- Temperature: Possible fever if cellulitis or infected wounds are present.
- HR: Symptomatic bradycardia may develop post carotid procedure caused by vagal stimulation.
- BP: Unequal BP in arms may indicate carotid or subclavian artery disease. Arm with the lower pressure indicates a possible subclavian stenosis. The higher of the two arm pressures should be considered the accurate pressure.
- BP may increase or decrease with stimulation of baroreceptors in the carotid bulb during or following carotid procedures.
- Severe hypertension or hypotension is worrisome for impending stroke or MI and will need immediate attention.
- Obtain an ankle-brachial index (ABI), see Box 5-8. Decreased ABI can indicate presence of PAD. The ABI is also used to assess perfusion in the lower extremity and checks for changes in perfusion to a limb after an endovascular or surgical intervention to a limb.
- Monitor for changes in BP, HR, and RR after the carotid procedure to assess for increased intracranial pressure secondary to hemorrhage, edema, or ischemia.
- May also represent reperfusion injury following carotid procedures; hemorrhage or headache may occur with increased blood flow, usually after repair of a high-grade stenosis.

PALPATION
- Check skin temperature and pulse assessment to evaluate for decreased tissue perfusion.
- Check bilateral pulse quality and regularity (scale of 0 to 4+; 0=absent pulse to 4+=bounding pulse).

Box 5-8 | ANKLE-BRACHIAL INDEX

To obtain an ankle-branchial index (ABI):
- With the patient lying flat, measure blood pressure (BP) of both arms. If the BP differs between arms, use the higher reading.
- Apply BP cuff over ankles. Take BP reading over dorsalis pedis (DP) and posterior tibial (PT) arteries of both legs using a Doppler ultrasound.
- Calculate the ABI by dividing the systolic reading at the DP/PT level by the systolic reading at the arm (brachial artery).
- Normal ABI ranges from 1.0 − 1.4; Pressure is normally higher in the ankle than the arm.

- Pulse amplitude may be increased or decreased depending on disease process. Change in pulse is palpable below the level of disease.
- Decrease in pulse quality or absent pulse may indicate occluded or stenotic arteries.
- Bounding pulses may be indicative of aneurysmal development of the artery.
  - Palpate the femoral and popliteal arteries for presence of an aneurysm affecting distal circulation.
  - Aneurysmal arteries have an increased diameter and may have an easily palpable or bounding pulse.
  - Pseudoaneurysm can occur because of injury of an artery such as the catheter insertion point for angiogram or thrombolysis.
- Presence of edema (scale 0 to 4+) of extremities is indicative of other secondary problems (such as HF, liver or renal disease, venous insufficiency, or venous thrombosis)
  - Edema with erythema may be indicative of infection.
  - Lymphedema may be present after bypass procedure because of disruption of the lymph system when making incision or creating vein graft (not caused by arterial disease).
- Slow capillary refill (greater than 2 seconds) is indicative of sluggish circulation and arterial occlusions.
- Temperature changes: increased warmth may indicate tissue inflammation or infection. Coolness may be present distal to the site of occlusion.
- After repair of an acutely ischemic limb, palpate affected limb for compartment syndrome. Most common site is the anterior compartment of the lower leg. Presents with tightness of the skin and muscle pain to a higher degree than expected.

AUSCULTATION

Listen for presence of bruits, which indicate disturbances in flow (plaque formation).
- Bilateral carotid arteries
- Abdominal aortic and bilateral femoral
- Bruits in the carotid arteries, the aorta, or the renal arteries may be indicative of stenosis or dilation of arteries.
  - Bruits are high-pitched pulsations (similar to a murmur) best heard with the bell of the stethoscope and correlate with the presence of turbulent flow.
  - Carotid bruits are assessed by auscultation of the carotid artery from the base of the neck to the angle of the jaw; they are usually loudest in the upper third of the neck in the area of the carotid bifurcation.
  - Renal and aortic bruits are assessed in the midabdominal or epigastric area of the abdomen.
- Doppler auscultation of the peripheral pulses for quality of pulse signal.
  - A healthy artery has 3 phases (sounds) heard when using a Doppler for assessment of pulses. A repaired or diseased artery may have 1 or 2 phases.
  - A change in the Doppler signal from 3 (triphasic) or 2 phases (biphasic) to only 1 (monophasic) may be indicative of complications.

SCREENING LABWORK

Blood studies can help to determine risk of vascular disease or its complications.
- Chemistries: checking for blood glucose and renal function (elevated creatinine, BUN, potassium).
- CBC: anemia, high or low platelet level evaluating for increased clotting/bleeding propensity.
- Coagulation studies: PT/INR or PTT evaluating for increased clotting/bleeding propensity.
- $HgbA_{1c}$: evaluating risk factor control (presence of, or uncontrolled diabetes).
- Lipid profile: evaluating for control of risk factor (presence of, or uncontrolled hyperlipidemia).

POSTPROCEDURAL SCREENING LABWORK

Blood studies can reveal postprocedural or surgical complications such as bleeding, fluid overload, early infection, renal insufficiency, or muscle damage associated with reperfusion injury.
- CBC: possible anemia related to surgical blood loss or postoperative bleeding; increased WBCs indicating possible infection.
- Electrolytes: fluid shift or volume changes with increased use of IV fluids;

- Blood glucose: HbAIC indicates long-term effectiveness of blood glucose control in patients with diabetes, and should be reviewed along with blood glucose level to anticipate the probability of complications.
- Creatinine, BUN: possible changes in perfusion of the kidneys.
- Liver enzymes, CPK: possible muscle injury related to reperfusion or compartment syndromes.
- Coagulation panel: protime, INR, partial thromboplastin time to evaluate anticoagulation management.

Diagnostic Tests for Arterial Disease

Test	Purpose	Abnormal Findings
Noninvasive Vascular Studies		
Ultrasound carotid duplex	Assess for presence and degree of carotid stenosis, location of bifurcation. Used for screening or diagnostic. PSV and EDV are measured in the common carotid, proximal to distal internal carotid arteries, and external carotid arteries. A ratio is also measured using the PSV in the internal and compared with PSV in the common carotid artery.	Evidence of plaque is determined by the velocities. The percentage of stenosis caused by plaque accumulation must be considered relative to presence or absence of symptoms. In general, plaque <50% is considered mild-moderate, >50% to 69% is considered moderate, and >70% is significant plaque. A ratio between 2 and 4 is abnormal, relating to significant stenosis.
Ankle-brachial index (ABI)	Quick, cost-effective method to establish or refute presence of LE PAD. Surveillance of disease progression before and after intervention. Pressures at the ankle are divided by brachial pressures, which result in the index (see Box 5-8). Toe pressures and toe-brachial index (TBI) may also be included.	Normal ABI 1.00 to 1.40 Abnormal ABI ≤0.90 Borderline disease 0.91 to 0.99 Mild disease 0.91 to 0.80 Moderate disease 0.75 to 0.40 Severe disease <0.40 (<0.40 is indicative of ischemic limb or threatened limb loss.) Normal TBI 0.70 or above Disease <0.70 Absolute toe pressures of at least 50 mm Hg are required for wound healing.
Doppler waveforms	Assess for LE stenosis, useful in conjunction with ABIs, especially patients whose ABI is >1.4, which indicates arterial calcification or noncompressible vessels.	Normal arteries have a sharp systolic component and one or more diastolic components (referred to as triphasic). As the vessel becomes narrowed, the diastolic components are absent and the systolic component widens (referred to as biphasic or monophasic). An abnormal waveform indicates disease proximal to the site where the signal was obtained.
LE continuous-wave Doppler ultrasound or duplex ultrasound	Provide quantitative data after a successful LE endovascular or surgical revascularization; provide graft surveillance of recurrence of disease. ABI and TBI are usually included with this study.	Stenosis of artery, stent, or bypass graft as an explanation for symptoms or poor wound healing of an ulcer. Stenosis is identified by elevated PSV in an area of the vessel, stent, or graft that is two times higher than the prior or following PSV. The effect on the ABI and presence of symptoms are taken into consideration.

Diagnostic Tests for Arterial Disease—cont'd

Test	Purpose	Abnormal Findings
Blood Studies		
Glycosylated hemo-globin (A_{1c})	Assess for presence or control of diabetes	Increase in fasting glucose may indicate diabetes. Increase of $HgbA_{1c} > 6.5$ indicates diabetes, > 7.0 indicates uncontrolled diabetes. Diabetes increases the risk of PAD and affects healing.
Liver enzymes AST, CPK LDH	Assess for presence of rhabdomyolysis associated with compartment syndrome or reperfusion injuries.	Increased levels may indicate damage to skeletal muscles.
Lipid profile and li-poprotein-choles-terol fractionation Total cholesterol, HDL-C, LDL-C , VLDL cholesterol, and tri-glycerides	Assess for causes of arterial plaque formation contributing to PAD or carotid stenosis. Assess for 10-year risk factors for ASCVD.	Elevation of total cholesterol, LDL-C, VLDL, and triglycerides indicates a greater potential for developing atherosclerosis. Elevated HDL-C lowers probability of arterial stenosis.
	Total cholesterol: Measures circulating levels of free cholesterol and cholesterol esters	2013 ACC/AHA Blood Cholesterol Guidelines recommend not focusing on cholesterol level numbers but on identifying persons in whom the potential for an ASCVD risk reduction benefit clearly exceeds the potential for adverse effects of statin use in adults with: • Clinical ASCVD • Primary elevations of LDL-C ≥190 mg/dL • Individuals 40 to 75 years of age with diabetes with LDL-C between 70 and 189 mg/dL • Individuals without clinical ASCVD or diabetes who are 40 to 75 years old with LDL-C between 70 and 189 mg/dL and an estimated 10-year ASCVD risk of 7.5% or higher.
	Triglycerides: Assesses storage form of lipids	
Radiology		
MRI Cerebral MRI	Assesses for presence of old or new signs of stroke.	Any signs of intracranial lesions indicating old or new infarcts
CT Cerebral CT scan	Assesses for presence of old or new signs of stroke.	Any signs of intracranial lesions indicating old or new infarcts
Magnetic resonance angiography (MRA)	Assesses vascular anatomy, presence and degree of stenosis or vessel occlusions with reconstruction images of vascular anatomy. Similar to MRI with vascular imaging obtained with gadolinium injected for contrast.	Arterial stenosis or occlusions; may suggest presence of aneurysms (will need to corroborate with CT scan). NOTE: MRA may be contraindicated in individuals in renal failure or with significant chronic kidney disease caused by increased risk of nephrogenic systemic fibrosis.
CT angiography (CTA)	Assess vascular anatomy, presence and degree of stenosis or vessel occlusions with reconstruction images of vascular anatomy. Provides associated soft tissue diagnostic information, acute emboli or aneurysms. Radiopaque contrast media is injected peripherally for vascular imaging.	Arterial stenosis or occlusions; presence of aneurysms; presence of acute emboli

Peripheral Vascular Disease

Continued

Diagnostic Tests for Arterial Disease—cont'd

Test	Purpose	Abnormal Findings
Invasive Vascular Studies		
Contrast angiography with digital subtraction	Assesses for presence and extent of arterial stenosis or occlusions using a radiopaque catheter inserted through a peripheral vessel advanced into the carotid, aortic, or distal arteries; allows more accurate imaging of peripheral vessels and determining significant stenosis by pressure differences. It also allows for direct injection of thrombolytic drugs and/or endovascular treatment of flow-limiting stenosis.	Arterial stenosis; presence of intracranial, aortic, iliac, femoral, or popliteal aneurysms; presence of arteriovenous malformations or fistulas. Test is used to prescribe the most appropriate treatment: endovascular (including thrombolytic, angioplasty, atherectomy, or stent placement) or surgical.

ALI, acute limb ischemia; *ASCVD,* atherosclerotic cardiovascular disease; *AST,* aspartate aminotransferase; *CLI,* critical limb ischemia; *CPK,* creatine phosphokinase; *CT,* computed tomography; *EDV,* end-diastolic velocity; *HDL-C,* high-density lipoprotein cholesterol; *LDH,* lactate dehydrogenase; *LDL-C,* low-density lipoprotein cholesterol; *LE,* lower extremity; *PAD,* peripheral artery disease; *PSV,* peak systolic velocity; *TBI,* toe brachial index; *VLDL,* very low-density lipoprotein.

CAROTID DUPLEX AND ARTERIOGRAM

Carotid duplex ultrasound (DUS) is used to detect the presence of carotid artery stenosis. At centers where the DUS has been internally validated in comparison with angiography and a comparable level of performance has been documented, surgeons may choose to proceed with surgery based on the DUS without the extra risks of a carotid angiogram. At centers where the DUS results are less reliable, it is used as a screening tool for carotid artery disease. Stenosis greater than 70% may indicate the need for CTA or angiogram, especially if symptoms are present. A CTA may also be used if unilateral symptoms are present and there are conflicting findings on the DUS.

ANKLE-BRACHIAL INDEX

BP is taken in both arms, with the highest pressure used for calculating indices (unequal arm pressures may indicate the presence of carotid or subclavian artery disease and the need for a carotid/subclavian DUS). Segmental pressures are also taken with a thigh cuff placed above the knee for a low thigh pressure and above the ankle to obtain ankle pressures of the dorsalis pedis and posterior tibial artery. A hand-held Doppler is used to acquire the dorsalis pedis and posterior tibial pulses. Normally, the pressure in the leg is equal to or slightly higher than brachial pressure. A difference of greater than 30 mm Hg between segments indicates disease of the artery proximal to where the pressure was taken. The ankle pressure is divided by the brachial pressure to obtain the ABI. Calcification of the arterial wall provides a falsely high measurement preventing compression of the vessel to obtain the pressure; this is referred to as a "noncompressible" vessel. In these patients, diagnosis must be based on Doppler waveform analysis.

COLLABORATIVE MANAGEMENT
CARE PRIORITIES: PERIPHERAL ARTERY OCCLUSIVE DISEASE

Priorities for the care of a patient with chronic peripheral artery occlusive disease should focus on early identification of disease and prevention of disease progression, disability secondary to ischemic injury, and thrombotic ischemic events. Prevention of disease progression would include the control of risk factors, prevention of thrombus formation (i.e., antiplatelet therapy or other anticoagulants), and management of medications to control risk factors.

To assist and guide the identification and management of patients with PAD, many national organizations have collaborated to produce evidence-based guidelines. Selective recommendations from the guidelines that are related to acute care settings are outlined in the following tables.

GUIDELINES FOR THE MANAGEMENT OF PATIENTS WITH PERIPHERAL ARTERY DISEASE

In 2011, the American College of Cardiology Foundation (ACCF) and the American Heart Association (AHA) Task Force on Guidelines approved the work of a collaborative effort of multiple vascular-associated organizations in the evaluation of multiple evidence-based studies and trials and development of nationally recognized evidence-based guidelines for the management of patients with PAD. This effort was also endorsed by many additional organizations not able to participate in the development activities.

NOTE: Abbreviations are detailed at the end of the table.

Lower Extremity Artery Occlusive Disease With or Without Symptoms

Intervention	Rationale
Assess for risk and presence of PAD in individuals with 1 or more of the following: • Exertional leg symptoms (claudication) • Nonhealing wounds • Age 70 years or older • Age 65 years or older with history of smoking or diabetes • Age 50 years with a history of smoking and one other risk factor.	History evaluation to include questions regarding presence of risk factors, walking impairment, claudication, ischemic rest pain, and/or nonhealing wounds. Patients with LE PAD have an increased risk for stroke or cardiovascular ischemic events caused by coronary artery disease and cerebrovascular disease, which are more frequent than ischemic limb events.

Treat and modify risk factors:
• Uncontrolled diabetes
• Control HTN*
  • <60 years old, diabetic, or renal disease, BP goal <140/90 mm Hg
  • >60 years old, BP goal <150/90 mm Hg
  • HLD† target 50% reduction in LDL (between 70 and 189 mg/dL), depending on risk factors for ASCVD*
Optimize cardiac disease management
Smoking cessation, if needed, use of pharmacotherapy (varenicline, bupropion, and nicotine replacement) and/or smoking cessation program.
	Uncontrolled diabetes, HTN, HLD, smoking and other risk factors increase the risk of cardiovascular events. HLD: Use of a hydroxymethyl glutaryl coenzyme-A reductase inhibitor (statin) is the recommended therapy, especially in patients with CV disease, 40 to 75 years of age, and/or diabetes. Statins have demonstrated a positive effect on CV disease. Smoking: Studies have demonstrated that in individuals who continue to smoke, the risk of death and/or MI is substantially greater. Additionally, the patency rate of angioplasty, stent, or surgical bypass is lower.

Ensure patient is on antiplatelet therapy to decrease risk of stroke, MI, or CV death. Aspirin 75 to 325 mg as a monotherapy is recommended in individuals with ASCVD, ABI <0.90, and/or symptomatic PAD (claudication, CLI, prior LE revascularization procedure, or amputation because of PAD). If high CV risks are present, a combination of aspirin and clopidogrel may be considered, if no increased risk of bleeding. Antiplatelet therapy may be considered in individuals with asymptomatic PAD with an ABI ≤0.90.	Use of daily antiplatelet therapy (low-dose aspirin, or the alternatives of clopidogrel 75 mg or Persantine) demonstrated a 35% risk reduction in nonfatal stroke, MI, and vascular death. One trial demonstrated only incremental benefit of clopidogrel over aspirin. Individuals at high risk of acute ischemic or thromboembolic event may be considered for aspirin and clopidogrel therapy based on trial findings. Antiplatelet therapy for individuals with an ABI between 0.91 and 0.99 to reduce CV events is not well established. Use of warfarin is of no benefit and may be harmful. Use of newer antithrombotic medications has not undergone adequate research to demonstrate benefit at this time.
Identify persons with risk factors for PAD, but who are *asymptomatic* by physical examination and ABI. If ABI is above 1.40, use TBI, PVR, or Doppler waveforms to assess for PAD.	Exercise ABI measurement can be useful to diagnose LE PAD in individuals at risk who have a normal ABI without classic claudication symptoms and no other clinical evidence of atherosclerosis. TBI, PVR, or Doppler waveform measurement can be useful to diagnose LE PAD in individuals at risk with calcified noncompressible vessels (ABI greater than 1.40) and no other clinical evidence of atherosclerosis.

Continued

Peripheral Vascular Disease

GUIDELINES FOR THE MANAGEMENT OF PATIENTS WITH PERIPHERAL ARTERY DISEASE—cont'd

Intervention	Rationale
Evaluate for evidence of other disorders that may cause significant functional impairment (e.g., angina, heart failure, chronic respiratory disease, or orthopedic limitations) before revascularization surgery or endovascular procedures.	Patients with symptoms of intermittent claudication should have significant functional impairment with a reasonable likelihood of symptomatic improvement and absence of other disease that would comparably limit exercise before undergoing revascularization.

Critical Limb Ischemia (CLI) and Acute Limb Ischemia (ALI)

Recommendation	Supporting Data
In patients with CLI, initiate an expedited evaluation and treatment of factors known to increase the risk of amputation: vascular history, ASCVD risk factor assessment for arterial disease in other areas, and specific precipitating factors, trauma, or infection.	The natural history of untreated, severe PAD would lead to major limb amputation within 6 months. Determine the time and course of development of the ischemia. If history and examination suggest rapid progression, early revascularization may be required to prevent further deterioration and irreversible tissue loss. Revascularization of an ischemic extremity may be complicated by reperfusion injury to the damaged tissues and precipitate systemic responses, including cardiac, renal, and pulmonary dysfunction.
Immediately assess patients at risk for CLI who develop acute limb symptoms. Ensure emergent assessment and treatment by a specialist competent in treating vascular disease.	Patients at risk for CLI (patients with diabetes, neuropathy, chronic renal failure, or infection) are at risk to develop vascular emergencies. In the individual whose life expectancy is less than 2 years with no autogenous vein conduit available for bypass, an endovascular procedure, such as balloon angioplasty, may be considered before any other intervention.
Ensure that patients with CLI in whom open surgical repair is anticipated undergo assessment of cardiovascular risk.	Patients with LE PAD and CLI have an increased risk for stroke or cardiovascular ischemic events caused by coronary artery disease and cerebrovascular disease. A detailed coronary assessment may be performed in selected patients in whom coronary ischemic symptoms would merit such an assessment if CLI were not present; such assessments should not impede care.
Evaluate all patients with CLI or ALI for aneurysmal disease of proximal arteries.	Patients with CLI or ALI who present with clinical features to suggest atheroembolization should be evaluated for more proximal aneurysmal disease (e.g., abdominal aortic, popliteal, or femoral aneurysms). Atheroembolism is suggested by the onset of signs and symptoms of CLI after recent endovascular catheter manipulation.
Establish regular intervals of direct examination of the feet after successful treatment of CLI or ALI.	Patients at risk of CLI (ABI less than 0.4 in a nondiabetic individual or any diabetic individual with known LE PAD) should undergo regular inspection of the feet to detect objective signs of recurrent or new CLI.
Promptly initiate systemic antibiotics in patients with CLI, skin ulcerations, and evidence of limb infection.	Patients with CLI, skin ulcerations, and infections are at risk for potential development of vascular emergencies. Infections increase the metabolic demand of the tissue and could worsen ischemia.

GUIDELINES FOR THE MANAGEMENT OF PATIENTS WITH PERIPHERAL ARTERY DISEASE—cont'd

Intervention	Rationale
In CLI and ALI, perform emergent arterial Doppler/ABI studies and imaging studies, such as angiography, CTA, or MRA with gadolinium enhancement. Document evidence of previous history of contrast reaction or renal insufficiency before imaging studies and after angiography.	Patients with ALI should undergo an emergent evaluation that defines the anatomic level of occlusion and lead to prompt endovascular or surgical revascularization. If baseline renal insufficiency is present, hydration before undergoing contrast angiography is recommended. Follow-up evaluation postangiography is recommended to evaluate renal function after contrast is used.
If not contraindicated, initiate catheter-based thrombolysis in patients with ALI of less than 14 days' duration. Mechanical thrombectomy can be used as an adjunctive therapy for acute peripheral arterial occlusion. Above therapies may be considered in patients with ALI of <14 days' duration.	Analysis of controlled trials indicate that catheter-based, intra-arterial thrombolytic therapy is effective and beneficial in ALI of <14 days' duration; is comparable to surgery (embolectomy) as a low-risk alternative to open surgery in complex patients with severe comorbidities; and may enhance long-term patency relative to the clearing of intra-arterial thrombus from the distal runoff vessels.
In patients with combined inflow and outflow disease with CLI, inflow lesions should be addressed first with endovascular or surgical approach.	Patients with profound limb ischemia may not tolerate the time required to perform thrombolysis. In infrainguinal or distal arterial occlusions, thrombolysis may have worse outcomes than more proximal or iliofemoral occlusions. Mechanical thrombectomy may avert the need for thrombolysis or allow the use of lower doses of thrombolytic drugs. A significant improvement in inflow may diminish the symptoms of rest pain; however, pulsatile flow to the foot may be needed for ischemic ulcers or ischemic gangrene.
Surgical revascularization, consisting of bypass with vein or prosthetic conduit, may be considered in patients with CLI and both inflow and outflow blockage to the LE. Reconstructive surgery requiring a synthetic graft significantly increases the risk of survival and amputation. An endovascular revascularization is recommended over use of a synthetic graft.	Comparative studies of vein to prosthetic conduit (graft) for LE arterial reconstruction demonstrate vein to be superior in patency. Prosthetic conduit (PTFE or Dacron) may be used with acceptable patency rate for above-the-knee bypasses; however, patency is significantly lower when used for below-the-knee reconstruction. Vein bypass is associated with a significant increase in overall survival and decreased amputations in certain specifically selected patients.
Primary limb amputation may be considered in patients with an unsalvageable limb.	Unsalvageable limb may be considered in a limb with significant necrosis of weight-bearing areas of the foot, uncorrectable flexion contracture, refractory ischemic rest pain, sepsis or presence of significantly limited life expectancy because of comorbid conditions.
Initiate ongoing graft or stent patency surveillance at least every 6 months in all patients treated for CLI or ALI.	Long-term patency of bypass grafts and endovascular treatments should be evaluated via a surveillance program at regular intervals (e.g., interval vascular history, resting ABIs, physical examination, and a duplex ultrasound).

Peripheral Vascular Disease

ABI, Ankle-brachial index; ACEI, angiotensin-converting enzyme inhibitor; ASCVD, atherosclerotic cardiovascular disease; CHF, congestive heart failure; CV, cardiovascular; DM, diabetes mellitus; HLD, hyperlipidemia; HTN, hypertension; LDL-C, low-density lipoprotein cholesterol; LE, lower extremity; MI, myocardial infarction; PAD, peripheral artery disease; PTFE, polytetrafluoroethylene; PVR, pulse volume recording; TBI, toe-brachial index.

*2014, JNC-8 Guidelines for Management of Hypertension in Adults
†2013, ACC/AHA Task Force Cholesterol Management Guidelines

LOWER EXTREMITY PERIPHERAL ARTERY OCCLUSIVE DISEASE: CRITICAL LIMB ISCHEMIA

In CLI, rest pain and/or ischemic ulcers are present. For a patient with ischemic ulcers, specific care priorities would include wound care, preventing or treating infection, and protecting the limb to prevent further tissue damage. Additional measures would include the following.

1. Relief of ischemic pain

In general, relieving ischemic pain requires improving perfusion to the limb. However, depending on the length of ischemic time and amount of ischemic nerve injury, administration of a narcotic analgesic is usually required.

2. Prevention of injury to the ischemic limb

Pressure to an already ischemic limb diminishes perfusion even further, leading to tissue breakdown. Maintain the heel and other pressure points of the extremity free from sustained pressure.

In the surgical or endovascular management, care priorities should focus on promoting perfusion to the extremity, preventing infection, and promoting wound healing. Promotion of perfusion in an extremity includes preventing limb edema that could impair graft perfusion and wound healing, maintaining perfusion of the stent or graft, and preventing thrombus or occlusion of the stent or graft. For more information and description of endovascular techniques and instruments, such as intra-arterial stent placement, balloon angioplasty, or atherectomy (see Acute Coronary Syndromes, Chapter 5).

3. Promoting perfusion of the extremity

Activities include keeping the extremity warm to prevent vasoconstriction, maintaining hydration, preventing hypotension, and preventing edema to the limb. If a surgical incision has been made to the limb, the limb will have a propensity for edema to develop, which not only promotes graft compression, but also impairs wound healing. Elevation of the extremity will help prevent or diminish edema.

 Safety Alert   *Maintaining hydration and preventing hypotension in a patient who has undergone lower extremity bypass or stent placement are important to prevent graft occlusion. Hypotension decreases perfusion to the graft and dehydration increases blood viscosity, leading to thrombosis and graft or stent occlusion.*

4. Prevention of peripheral artery clot formation

Antiplatelet therapy is the recommended medication used to prevent thrombus formation in individuals with PAD and no history of an event. However, antithrombotics may be required in those persons with a history of a thrombotic event or hypercoagulable condition. Antithrombotics include warfarin, direct factor X inhibitor (such as rivaroxaban or betrixaban), UH, and LMWH (such as enoxaparin, fondaparinux, or dalteparin). A direct thrombin inhibitor, such as argatroban, may be used if allergic to heparin or if there is a history of heparin-induced thrombocytopenia. Antiplatelet therapy includes the use of the following:

- Aspirin: Low doses of 75 to 325 mg orally are given on a daily basis.
- Clopidogrel: The standard dose is 75 mg daily. If a stent has been placed, clopidogrel is recommended. For patients who have not been on a regimen of daily clopidogrel and are about to undergo a carotid or peripheral stent, a loading dose of 300 mg of clopidogrel before stent placement is required.
- In patients who are unable to take aspirin or clopidogrel, other antiplatelet drugs will be considered, such as ticlopidine. Ticlopidine is not used as a first-line drug because of the adverse effects of life-threatening neutropenia, agranulocytosis, and thrombotic thrombocytopenia purpura.
- Dipyridamole and aspirin combination may be used for arterial graft patency but is most often used in stroke prevention. It is considered to be a third-line treatment option.
- Ticagrelor is a newer antiplatelet medication that is currently recommended only for coronary patients as there is no data on its use in PAD patients.

5. Prevent contrast-induced nephropathy (CIN) secondary to contrast during angiography

Prevention is required for endovascular intervention, especially in patients with evidence of renal insufficiency (serum creatinine levels greater than 1.4 mg/dL and/or glomerular filtration rate less than 60 mL/min/1.73 m^2). Additional measures may be taken if glomerular filtration rate is less than 40 mL/min/1.73 m^2.

- Hydration is paramount and is accomplished with IV fluids. Normal saline is recommended for 12 hours before and after the contrast study. In addition to IV hydration, administration of the following medication is generally used:
- N-acetylcysteine: Although previously used as a standard protocol for CIN in the recent past, it is now fallen out of favor and its efficacy is controversial in preventing CIN. Currently, it is suggested for use in patients with baseline serum creatinine above 2.0 mg/dL. If given, the dosing is 600 mg as an oral solution or a compounded tablet twice daily for 4 doses, starting the day before the procedure.
- $NaHCO_3$ infusion: Infusion rate of 3 mL/kg/h for 1 hour before the procedure, then 1 mL/kg/h for 6 hours after the contrast procedure.

6. Endovascular or surgical treatment of CLI/ALI

- A significant arterial stenosis or occlusion is performed using endovascular techniques of angioplasty, atherectomy, or stent placement. Surgical treatments include thromboendarterectomy or bypass around occluded vessels.
- Angioplasty, atherectomy, and/or stent placement (see Acute Coronary Syndromes, Chapter 5)
- Thromboendarterectomy or endarterectomy: This procedure is similar to that described above with a carotid endarterectomy (CEA). An incision is made along the length of the artery where the stenosis is located. The plaque is removed and the artery is sewn closed. A vein patch may be placed in the vessel during closure to provide an adequate size for blood flow. This is generally performed on the proximal vessels of the distal aorta, iliac, or femoral arteries. A shunt, as may be used in the CEA to ensure cerebral perfusion, is not required in the distal limbs.
- Surgical placement of a bypass graft or reconstruction: Through surgical incisions, a conduit is surgically attached forming an anastomosis that is end-to-end or end-to side to the artery above the site of an occlusion or hemodynamically significant lesion to provide "inflow" of blood to the extremity. The distal graft is surgically attached below the occlusions to provide "outflow" of blood to the extremity. Synthetic material, such as Dacron or polytetrafluoroethylene, is often used as a conduit for bypasses above the knee, since the patency rate is equal to that of vein. This preserves the vein for future need. A vein, usually the greater saphenous vein (GSV), is the conduit of choice for a bypass extending below the knee. The patient's vein may be harvested by excising the GSV and placing it in a reversed position to allow blood flow to pass valves. The GSV may also be used in situ, without completely excising, after a valvulotome is used to destroy the 1-way flow of the valve leaflets. The bypass is referred to by its anatomic placement. For example, an aortobifemoral bypass indicates that the proximal graft is attached at the aorta and bifurcated grafts are inserted bilaterally into each femoral artery. A femoropopliteal bypass indicates that the proximal graft is sewn to the femoral artery and the distal end of the graft is attached at the popliteal artery.

LOWER EXTREMITY PERIPHERAL ARTERY OCCLUSIVE DISEASE: ACUTE LIMB ISCHEMIA

In ALI resulting from acute arterial occlusion, the care priorities are similar to those of CLI, which would include early identification of an acutely ischemic limb and early intervention to diminish ischemic time and restore blood flow to the ischemic limb. In the limb with an acute arterial occlusion, thrombolysis is the recommended emergent procedure used to dissolve the arterial clot and restore limb perfusion. Time is of great concern in an acute arterial occlusion. Anticoagulation may be initiated with a heparin bolus and continuous infusion. If the patient is unable to undergo thrombolytic therapy, a thromboembolectomy may be performed to treat an acute arterial occlusion to quickly restore perfusion of the limb.

1. Thrombolysis

See Acute Coronary Syndromes Chapter 5, for a complete discussion of this procedure and care priorities related to its use. Care priorities for a patient undergoing thrombolysis for an acute peripheral artery occlusion are essentially the same as in the patient with an acute coronary thrombus.

2. Thromboembolectomy

A surgical arteriotomy is performed and an embolectomy balloon catheter is passed past the thrombus, the balloon is inflated, and the clot is extracted. Neighboring arteries are checked for clot. Distal embolization is of great concern with this procedure because of the manipulation of the catheter around the thrombus.

Care priorities for ALI also include monitoring and early recognition of compartment syndrome, thromboembolic injury, and neuromuscular injury. For a full discussion and care priorities of compartment syndrome, see Compartment Syndrome/Ischemic Myositis, Chapter 3.

In ALI, care priorities would also include facilitating the identification of the source of emboli. Given that the heart is a common source, an echocardiogram will be performed as soon as perfusion to the limb has been restored. Additional studies that would be considered include an abdominal/pelvic CTA scan or angiogram to look for any aneurysmal source. A lower extremity ultrasound may be performed to look for peripheral aneurysms of the femoral or popliteal arteries.

 High potential for distal emboli to the foot, referred to as "trashed foot" or "blue toe syndrome." The risk for distal embolism from dislodgment of thrombus or thrombotic plaque is significant in any procedure in which catheters are manipulated around or through the clot, causing clot fragmentation, such as with thrombolysis, thromboendarterectomy, angioplasty, or stenting. Incorporate monitoring for distal emboli into care priorities.

COLLABORATIVE MANAGEMENT
CARE PRIORITIES: CAROTID ARTERY OCCLUSIVE DISEASE

The focus of care is similar to PAD but includes the early recognition and intervention of carotid artery stenosis to reduce progression of disease and to prevent stroke. Multiple large randomized trials have demonstrated an association between carotid stenosis and other significant risk factors (ischemic heart disease, TIA/stroke, PAD, hypertension, dyslipidemia, and smoking). Many of these same trials have demonstrated a decreased risk of stroke and MI with medical management. Several trials have evaluated the risk of stroke in asymptomatic persons with carotid artery stenosis, finding that persons with 60% to 80% stenosis had higher stroke rates. Many trials have demonstrated decrease in stroke and cardiovascular events with management of the risk factors. Treatment of carotid disease includes medical management and possibly a surgical approach of CEA or endovascular placement of a carotid artery stent.

CLINICAL PRACTICE GUIDELINES FOR THE MANAGEMENT OF ATHEROSCLEROTIC CAROTID ARTERY DISEASE

The American College of Cardiology Foundation (ACCF), American Heart Association (AHA), and American Stroke Association, along with many other cardiovascular organizations, periodically review and revise evidence-based clinical practice guidelines for the management of carotid artery disease and prevention of stroke. These multiorganizational committees evaluate the outcomes of a large number of large clinical trials and systematic reviews to summarize the best available evidence to a grading scheme to grade the quality of evidence. Below are the recommendations from these collaborative efforts.

Carotid Artery Occlusive Disease With or Without Symptoms

Intervention	Rationale
Optimize medical management in all patients with asymptomatic or symptomatic carotid stenosis and the following risk factors: • Control HTN <140/90 mm Hg • JNC-8, 2014 recommendations* • <60 years old, diabetic or renal disease, BP goal is <140/90 mm Hg • >60 years old, BP goal 150/90 mm Hg • HLD† (LDL-C above 100 mg/dL) with a statin, if tolerated, with or without ASCVD. 2013 guidelines do not recommend use of a specific LDL or HDL treatment target. Moderate risk reduction is defined as a lowering of LDL by 30% to <50% and high-intensity reduction is 50%, depending on risk factors for ASCVD. Use of statins is the recommended therapy, especially in patients with CV disease, 40 to 75 years of age, and/or diabetes (ACC/AHA, 2013 Guidelines)† • Increase physical activity • Manage diabetes. Control glucose (target HbA1c is <7%) • Smoking cessation • Antiplatelet therapy with low-dose aspirin (75 to 325 mg) or clopidogrel daily. Dipyridamole may be used if unable to tolerate aspirin or clopidogrel.	In patients with low-grade carotid stenosis, the risk of disabling stroke or death was increased by 20%. Treatment of asymptomatic patients with >60% stenosis was of benefit. HTN: The risk of stroke is lowered by 33% for each 10 mm Hg decrease in systolic blood pressure (BP) to 115/75 mm Hg. Benefit of lowering BP below 140/90 mm Hg is not well known in the hyperacute period, relative to inducing more additional cerebral ischemia, especially in individuals with significant carotid stenosis. In patients with severe carotid stenosis, the effect of BP reduction is unknown and may confer harm because of reduction in cerebral perfusion. HLD: Stroke risk was reduced by 15% for each 10% reduction in LDL and evidence of decreased carotid plaque. SPARCL trial demonstrated a relative risk reduction of ischemic stroke of 22% with atorvastatin. Statins reduce the risk of MI by 23% and cardiovascular death by 19% in patients with CAD. Physical activity: Referral to a program that is comprehensive and behaviorally oriented may be beneficial. Diabetes: Ischemic stroke was found to increase by two- to five-fold in individuals with diabetes. Smoking: Stroke risk decreases substantially within 5 years of quitting smoking. Medications: Use of antiplatelet therapy has been shown to decrease stroke incidence by 25%.
DUS of the carotid is recommended in an asymptomatic individual with the following: • ASCVD • Carotid bruit • Carotid disease of <50% stenosis (evaluate for progression annually) • Individuals with TIA symptoms of transient monocular vision dysfunction and/or unilateral hemispheric symptom • Consider in asymptomatic individuals with CV risk factors or family history of early PAD before age 60 years or ischemic stroke DUS of the carotid is recommended in an individual with symptoms of amaurosis fugax and/or hemispheric TIA symptoms. An MRA or CTA should be done when the DUS is indeterminate.	The DUS should be done by a qualified technologist in a certified laboratory to detect hemodynamically significant disease. Carotid artery disease has been found in 15% to 20% of ischemic strokes. The benefit of screening asymptomatic individuals continues to be an area in which there has not been strong consensus. However, carotid stenosis is a marker of ASCVD and the DUS is widely available, having negligible risks or discomfort making the recommendations reasonable. The IMT of the carotid artery is a marker for CAD and stroke.

Continued

Peripheral Vascular Disease

CLINICAL PRACTICE GUIDELINES FOR THE MANAGEMENT OF ATHEROSCLEROTIC CAROTID ARTERY DISEASE—cont'd

Intervention	Rationale
Consideration for CEA or CAS in asymptomatic individuals should include assessment of comorbid conditions, life expectancy, and other individual factors. It should also include discussion of the risks and benefits of the procedure, and consideration of patient preferences.	The risk of stroke or death after a CEA is relative to the preoperative comorbid conditions and clinical status. Complications associated with CEA include hyper- and hypotension, hemorrhage, stroke, MI, cranial nerve palsies, and death. CAS risks include stroke, vessel injury/dissection/perforation, thrombotic events, MI, hypotension, transient bradycardia, and pseudoaneurysm at catheter access site.
Consideration for CEA versus CAS is based on each patient's surgical or procedural risks, age, and documentation of one of the following: • Carotid stenosis of >70% on DUS or 50% on angiogram and symptomatic with TIA or ischemic stroke within 6 months • Asymptomatic carotid stenosis >70% • May be considered in symptomatic carotid stenosis >50% and medically optimized (2014 Stroke Prevention Guidelines do not recommend intervention if stenosis is between 50% and 69%, even in presence of TIA/stroke, because of low stroke rate with medical management). • CEA may be considered in the older patient (i.e., 70 years or older) with an indication for intervention, an arterial anatomy not amenable for CAS, and the surgeon's anticipated rate of periprocedural stroke/death is <6%. • Consider CAS in the patient with a neck pathology/anatomy not amenable for CEA CEA versus CAS should consider high-risk factors in patients with renal failure on dialysis, extremely low LVEF, oxygen- or corticosteroid-dependent chronic lung disease, etc., and an endovascular approach may be considered in patients at high risk for a surgical approach.	Multiple multicenter trials have demonstrated no significant difference in outcome between CEA and CAS. CEA demonstrated a higher risk of MI and lower stroke, while CAS demonstrated a higher risk of stroke and lower risk of MI. Women faced a higher risk than men. Results of multiple multicenter randomized trials showed the risk of ischemic stroke after a CEA versus a CAS versus medical management. Some of the outcomes were: • For both CEA and CAS, the 1-year ipsilateral stroke rate after the first 30 days was 1% to 2% in symptomatic and <0.5% to 0.8% in asymptomatic patients. • For CEA performed in asymptomatic patients, risk of ischemic stroke reported at <0.5%. • 1.1% stroke risk per year after CEA, and 5-year stroke rate of 10%. • 5-year stroke rate after CEA was 5.1% to 10% versus 11% to 20% for those medically managed (date from multiple trials). • Asymptomatic, moderate to severe carotid stenosis demonstrated a 30-day perioperative stroke or death rate of 2.8% in the CEA group versus medical management. • Meta-analysis of 10 randomized trials of 3182 patients with >50% stenosis comparing CAS and CEA concluded a "nonsignificant" risk reduction of stroke with CAS.
Postop/procedure management: • Assessment and documentation of neurologic status • Immediately post-CAS: frequent assessment of BP and heart rate; assessment of catheter access site. • Risk factor control as before CEA/CAS, especially including HTN control • CEA: antiplatelet restarted 1 month after surgery • CAS: dual antiplatelet therapy with clopidogrel and aspirin for 30 days, then monotherapy with aspirin • 1-month DUS assessment • Routine, long-term imaging is not recommended.	CAS postop complications include neurologic deficits (TIA, stroke rate reported at 1% to 2%), carotid vessel injury, catheter access vessel injury, and pseudoaneurysm. CV complications postop CAS include an increased risk of hypotension and bradycardia caused by vasovagal and vasodepressor reactions in the periprocedure period. CEA complications include HTN or hypotension, hemorrhage, acute arterial occlusion, stroke, MI, venous thromboembolism, cranial nerve palsy, and infection.

ASCVD, Atherosclerotic cardiovascular disease; *BP*, blood pressure; *CAD*, coronary artery disease; *CAS*, carotid artery stent; *CEA*, carotid endarterectomy; *CTA*, computed tomography angiography; *CV*, cardiovascular; *DUS*, duplex ultrasonography; *HTN*, hypertension; *IMT*, intramural thickness; *LDL-C*, low-density lipoprotein cholesterol; *LVEF*, left ventricular ejection fraction; *MI*, myocardial infarction; *MRA*, magnetic resonance angiography; *TIA*, transient ischemic attack.
*2014, JNC-8 Guidelines for Management of Hypertension in Adults
†2013, ACC/AHA Task Force Cholesterol Management Guidelines

Provide management of patients to help prevent stroke and to manage patients following preventive procedures.

1. Facilitate recovery from CEA

- Prevent impaired cerebrovascular perfusion secondary to hypotension, hypertension, or bradycardia.

- Prevent respiratory impairment secondary to bleeding or hematoma formation at the incision leading to tracheal deviation and respiratory distress.
- Postoperative complications of a CEA related to the surgical approach include neurologic deficits, hypertension, bradycardia, neck hematoma with potential for airway obstruction, and local nerve injuries of the laryngeal or hypoglossal nerves that require prompt treatment.

2. Facilitate recovery from an endovascular stenting

- Monitor for potential embolic TIA or stroke, as is done with the surgical approach.
- Monitor for bradycardia or hypotension relative to vasovagal stimulation.
- Observe for and prevent limb ischemia related to the access site for the endovascular procedure.
- For patients with a carotid stent: Continue antiplatelet therapy (generally with clopidogrel) to prevent stent occlusion.

3. In a patients undergoing CEA or carotid artery stent with 100% occlusion of the contralateral carotid artery, prevent hypotension

- After revascularization in a patient with 100% occlusion of the contralateral carotid artery, a hyperemia can occur secondary to increased cerebral perfusion. The hyperemia can lead to increased intracranial pressure. This may occur immediately postoperatively, but may also occur days later. Manifestations to observe for include headache, cloudy thinking, or altered mental status.

4. Initiate medical management, including antiplatelet medications

> **Safety Alert**
> *There is a relationship between the presence of cerebrovascular disease and coronary artery disease (CAD). The most common cause of mortality following carotid endarterectomy is myocardial infarction; the highest risk after a carotid stent placement is for stroke. There is also a relationship between peripheral arterial disease (PAD) and CAD. The prognosis of patients with lower extremity PAD is characterized by an increased risk for cardiovascular ischemic events caused by concomitant CAD and cerebrovascular disease. Cardiovascular ischemic events are more frequent than ischemic limb events in any patient with lower extremity PAD and/or carotid stenosis.*

CARE PLANS FOR GENERALIZED PERIPHERAL VASCULAR DISEASE

ACTIVITY INTOLERANCE *related to compromised tissue perfusion and pain*

Goals/Outcomes: Within the 12- to 24-hour period before discharge from the ICU, the patient exhibits tolerance to increasing levels of activity as evidenced by RR less than 24 breaths/min, NSR on ECG, BP within 20 mm Hg of patient's normal range, HR less than 120 bpm (or within 20 bpm of resting HR for patients on beta-blocker therapy), and generalized pain less than 4 on a 1 to 10 scale.

NOC Endurance; Energy Conservation; Activity Tolerance

Energy Management
1. Determine patient's physical limitations.
2. Determine causes of fatigue and perceived causes of fatigue.
3. Monitor for muscle pain during activity.
4. Reduce all causes of discomfort, including those induced by the patient's environment, such as uncomfortable room temperature or position, thirst/dry mouth, and wrinkled or damp bedding.
5. Provide alternating periods of rest and activity.
6. Assist patient in prioritizing activities to accommodate energy levels.

Self-Care Assistance: Instrumental Activities of Daily Living (IADLs)
1. Determine need for assistance with IADLs including walking, bathing, dressing, cooking, shopping, housekeeping, transportation, and money management.
2. Provide for methods of contacting assistance support (such as home health nursing, lifeline services, emergency response services, including readily accessible telephone numbers if the patient is not within 911 access area).
3. Determine financial resources and personal preferences for modifying the patient's home to accommodate any disabilities or assisting with medication costs or other home healthcare costs.

DEFICIENT FLUID VOLUME *related to procedure-related blood loss or inadequate hydration.*

Goals/Outcomes: Within the 12-hour period before discharge from the ICU, the patient exhibits a normal fluid balance as evidenced by normal laboratory results of Hgb, Hct, potassium, sodium, creatinine, BUN; good skin turgor; warm, pink skin; normal level of consciousness (or maintenance of preprocedure LOC if baseline is impaired); normal vital signs and weight.
NOC Fluid Balance

Fluid/Electrolyte Management
1. Maintain adequate fluid volume.
2. Assess urine output, condition of skin, wound drainage, and I&O.
3. Monitor potassium, sodium, creatinine, and BUN; notify advanced practice provider if abnormal.
4. Monitor vital signs, weight, restlessness, skin temperature, and decreased LOC.

Hemorrhage Control
1. Monitor vital signs, Hgb, and Hct; notify advanced practice provider if abnormal.
2. Assess for excess drainage from dressing or drains (if present).
3. Assess for restlessness, pallor, skin temperature, decreased capillary refill, or decreased tissue perfusion.
4. Check operative site for bruising or excessive swelling.

INEFFECTIVE TISSUE PERFUSION: PERIPHERAL *related to reduced circulation resulting from vascular disease.*

Goals/Outcomes: Within 12 to 24 hours of treatment, the patient has adequate tissue perfusion as evidenced by warm, dry skin; brisk capillary refill; normal color, temperature, and sensory and motor function; RR less than 24 breaths/min; NSR on ECG; BP within 20 mm Hg of patient's normal range; HR less than 120 bpm (or within 20 bpm of resting HR for patients on beta-blocker therapy).
NOC Circulation Status; Tissue Perfusion: Peripheral

Circulatory Care: Arterial Insufficiency
1. Monitor vital signs.
2. Assess skin color, temperature; peripheral pulses as appropriate.
3. Provide warmth; avoid prolonged exposure to cold temperatures.
4. Promote smoking cessation and decreased caffeine intake.
5. Encourage activity as tolerated; passive and active ROM exercises if confined to bed.

Peripheral Sensation Management
1. Assess neurologic functions; decreased sensations.
2. Avoid constrictive clothing around operative site.
3. Minimize external pressure points.

DEFICIENT KNOWLEDGE: PERIPHERAL VASCULAR DISEASE PROCESS *related to lifestyle implications.*

Goals/Outcomes: Within the 24-hour period before discharge from the hospital, the patient verbalizes understanding of his or her disease, as well as the necessary lifestyle changes that may modify risk factors.
NOC Knowledge: Diabetes Management; Knowledge: Diet; Knowledge: Disease Process; Knowledge: Energy Conservation; Knowledge: Health Behaviors; Knowledge: Medication

Teaching: Peripheral Vascular Disease Process
1. Teach the patient about arterial stenosis or occlusion and its resultant symptoms such as TIAs, claudication, or rest pain.

2. Discuss the pathophysiologic process underlying the patient's arterial stenosis or occlusion, using drawings as indicated.
3. Assist patient in identifying his or her own risk factors (e.g., cigarette smoking, high-fat diet, hyperglycemia, high-stress lifestyle).
4. Teach the patient about risk factor modification:
   • Smoking cessation: Teach the patient that smoking causes arteries to constrict and increases platelet viscosity, thus decreasing blood flow to the brain, muscles, and tissues.
   • Hyperglycemia control: Discuss how high blood sugar levels accelerate the course of atherosclerosis; cause structural changes in the collagen of skin, joint capsules, and tendons leading to limitations of flexion and extension that result in increased foot pressures and risk of ulcerations; are associated with developing neuropathy; and accelerate wound sepsis.

Teaching: Diet and Prescribed Medications
1. Diet low in cholesterol and saturated fat: Provide sample diet plan for meals that are low in cholesterol and saturated fat. Teach the patient about foods that are high in cholesterol and low in cholesterol and saturated fat. Stress the importance of reading food labels. (See Tables 5-16 and Table 5-17 for more information.)
2. Blood pressure control: If the patient was found to have hypertension, he or she should be taught the importance of taking appropriate medications to control BP and to follow recommended dietary guidelines to minimize sodium intake. (See Table 5-4 for more information.) Sodium promotes water retention, which can increase BP. High BP may accelerate the process of atherosclerosis.
   • Teach the patient about the prescribed medications, including name, purpose, dosage, action, schedule, precautions, and potential side effects.

Teaching: Activity/Exercise
Discharge Instruction:
1. Increase activity slowly; do not push, pull, or lift anything over 10 lb for 2 to 6 weeks. Do not drive until you talk with your practitioner.
2. Try to develop a regular exercise and/or walking program. Start off slowly and build up.
3. Plan for regular rest periods; let your body guide you in decreasing or increasing activities.
4. Inform your practitioner of any changes in activity tolerance, such as the development of new symptoms with the same activity.

NIC Teaching: Disease Process; Teaching: Prescribed Diet and Medications; Teaching: Prescribed Activity/Exercise; Risk Identification

CARE PLANS FOR CAROTID ARTERY OCCLUSIVE DISEASE
INEFFECTIVE TISSUE PERFUSION: CEREBRAL *related to cerebral vascular disease.*

Goals/Outcomes: Within 12 to 24 hours of treatment, the patient has adequate cerebral perfusion as evidenced by RR less than 24 breaths/min, NSR on ECG, BP within 20 mm Hg of patient's normal range, HR less than 120 bpm (or within 20 bpm of resting HR for patients on beta-blocker therapy), and cranial nerves II to XII intact or equal to baseline.
NOC Circulation Status; Neurological Status; Tissue Perfusion: Cerebral

Cerebral Perfusion Promotion
1. Monitor vital signs per unit standards.
2. Assess for increased BP, decreased HR, and Cheyne–Stokes respiration (may indicate increased intracranial pressure secondary to hemorrhage).
3. Assess for decreased BP, increased HR, and increased respirations (may indicate cerebral ischemia).
4. Monitor for symptomatic bradycardia caused by vagal nerve stimulation.

Neurologic Monitoring
1. Monitor neurologic checks per unit standards.
2. Assess for presence of a gag reflex, difficulty swallowing, tongue deviation to one side, or biting of tongue when eating.
3. Assess for symmetry of lip movements by having the patient smile or show teeth.

4. Assess speech for hoarseness, and assess uvula for symmetry.
5. Assess shoulder alignment, strength of sternocleidomastoid muscle by having the patient shrug his or her shoulders and rotate his or her head to one side then the other while you provide resistance to the head and shoulder movements.

DEFICIENT FLUID VOLUME *related to surgical blood loss*

Goals/Outcomes: Within 12 to 24 hours of treatment, the patient has adequate fluid volume with no signs of hematoma or hemorrhage and normal Hgb and Hct.
NOC Fluid Balance; Electrolyte and Acid-Base Balance

Hemorrhage Control
1. Monitor vital signs, Hgb, and Hct.
2. Monitor dressing and drain (if present) for excessive drainage/output.
3. Assess operative site for bruising or excessive swelling.
4. Monitor airway for any respiratory compromise or tracheal deviation related to cervical hematoma.

CARE PLANS FOR PERIPHERAL ARTERY OCCLUSIVE DISEASE

INEFFECTIVE TISSUE PERFUSION: PERIPHERAL *related to decreased circulation resulting from atherosclerotic lower limb vascular disease.*

Goals/Outcomes: Within 12 to 24 hours of treatment, the patient has adequate peripheral perfusion as evidenced by warm, dry skin; normal or improved pedal pulses; normal color and temperature of skin; normal or improved sensory and motor function; and brisk capillary refill.
NOC Sensory Function: Cutaneous; Tissue Integrity: Skin and Mucous Membranes; Tissue Perfusion: Peripheral

Circulatory Care: Arterial Insufficiency
1. Palpate and/or auscultate per Doppler peripheral pulses distal to treatment site (also pulses distal to catheter insertion site for endovascular procedures). Report any decrease in pulse quality or strength immediately.
2. Monitor capillary refill and temperature and color of skin.
3. Position extremity to optimize circulation.
4. Encourage passive and active ROM exercises.
5. Provide warmth and avoid prolonged exposure to the cold.
6. Instruct patient to avoid crossing legs.

Neurologic Monitoring
1. Assess for decreased sensation of extremities and skin (skin immediately surrounding incisions may be numb if a skin nerve is cut during the incision).
2. Ask the patient to wiggle his or her toes and flex and extend foot and knee to assess motor function.

Skin Surveillance
1. Assess skin integrity of both extremities and pressure points; minimize external pressure points.
2. Change patient's position as appropriate.
3. Promote proper foot care for operative leg and opposite foot as opposite foot will be bearing more weight during convalescence.
4. Provide pressure-relieving mattress as appropriate.

IMPAIRED SKIN INTEGRITY *related to inadequate perfusion to maintain tissue integrity.*

Goals/Outcomes: Within 12 to 24 hours of treatment, the patient will maintain intact skin surfaces with healing wounds as evidenced by normal skin temperature, color, and sensation (or baseline); if open wound, minimal drainage present without odor; if open wound, granulation tissue will be present; normal vital signs and white blood count.
NOC Tissue Integrity: Skin and Mucous Membranes; Wound Healing: Primary Intention; Wound Healing: Secondary Intention

Pressure Management
1. Assess skin integrity of both extremities and pressure points; minimize external pressure points.
2. Change patient's position as appropriate.
3. Provide pressure-relieving mattress as appropriate.

Wound Care
1. Assess for decreased perfusion of the wound by assessing pain, swelling, erythema, and drainage.
2. Avoid further skin injury by not using tape directly on the skin.
3. Monitor for wound infection by assessing patient's temperature, WBC count, and exposure of bypass graft (if present).
4. Use aseptic technique for all dressing changes and incisional care.
5. Monitor incisions for drainage, erythema, tenderness, or separation of suture/staple sites.
6. Monitor nutritional status: assess weight, albumin, and prealbumin.

CARE PLANS FOR PATIENTS UNDERGOING ENDOVASCULAR REPAIR OF STENOSIS OR OCCLUSION

INEFFECTIVE TISSUE PERFUSION: PERIPHERAL *related to presence of a device within the vessel.*

Goals/Outcomes: See Goals/Outcomes and plan under Care Plans for Peripheral Vascular Disease, (Chapter 5).

DEFICIENT KNOWLEDGE *related to endovascular procedure and postprocedure care.*

Goals/Outcomes: Within the 24-hour period before the procedure, the patient describes the rationale for the procedure, how it is performed, and postprocedure care. Patient relates discharge instructions within the 24-hour period before discharge from the ICU.
NOC Knowledge: Treatment Procedures; Knowledge: Disease Process; Knowledge: Medication; Knowledge: Prescribed Activity

Teaching: Carotid/Peripheral Arterial Disease Process
1. Discuss location of the patient's disease using drawings as possible.
2. Assess patient's understanding of carotid/PAD and the purpose of the endovascular procedure. Evaluate patient's style of coping and degree of information desired.

Teaching: Procedure/Treatment
As appropriate for coping style, discuss the following with patient and significant others:
1. Use of local anesthesia and sedation during procedure
2. Insertion site of catheter: groin or arm
3. Sensations that may occur: mild pressure and/or a feeling of heat as the dye is injected
4. Use of fluoroscopy during procedure. Determine patient's history of sensitivity to contrast material and use of medications that may cause complications such as metformin.
5. Ongoing observations made by nurse after procedure: BP, HR, leg or arm pulses, blood tests, observation of insertion site, neuro checks as indicated, ABIs as indicated
6. Importance of lying flat in bed for 6 to 12 hours after procedure unless a vascular closure device is used. Patients are able to get out of bed sooner when a closure device is used.
7. Necessity for nursing assistance with eating, drinking, and toileting needs after procedure while lying flat
8. Need for increased fluid intake after procedure to flush dye from system
9. If the patient and significant others express or exhibit evidence of anxiety regarding the procedure, try to arrange for them to meet with another patient who has had a successful angioplasty.

Teaching: Prescribed Medications/Activity
Discharge Instructions:
1. Importance of taking antiplatelet medications to prevent restenosis
2. Avoidance of strenuous activity during the first few weeks at home
3. Follow-up visit with vascular surgeon/primary care provider 1 week after hospital discharge
4. Signs and symptoms to report to physician
   • Any pain or bruising at catheter insertion site
   • Fever or drainage from insertion site
   • Muscular pain or coolness in the extremity used for the catheter insertion, not experienced before the procedure
   • Any return of symptoms present before procedure

NIC Teaching: Disease Process; Teaching: Prescribed Activity/Exercise; Anxiety Reduction; Infection Protection; Decision-Making Support

Peripheral Vascular Disease

ADDITIONAL NURSING DIAGNOSES

Also see nursing diagnoses and interventions as appropriate in Nutritional Support (Chapter 1), Hemodynamic Monitoring (Chapter 1), Wound and Skin Care (Chapter 1), Pain (Chapter 1), Prolonged Immobility (Chapter 1), Emotional and Spiritual Support of the Patient and Significant Others (Chapter 2), Compartment Syndrome/Ischemic Myositis (Chapter 3), Stroke: Acute Ischemic and Hemorrhagic (Chapter 7), and Bleeding and Thrombotic Disorders (Chapter 10).

VALVULAR HEART DISEASE

PATHOPHYSIOLOGY

Valves facilitate the unidirectional flow of blood from atrium to ventricles (AV valves) or ventricles to pulmonary and systemic circulation (semilunar valves). Disease that alters the valve's structure can affect any or all of the cardiac valves, resulting in either stenosis or insufficiency. Stenosis results from the narrowing of the valve orifice because of the inability of the valve to open properly, causing partial obstruction. Insufficiency is the leaking of blood around the orifice when the valve does not close properly, resulting in regurgitation or backward flow of blood through the valve. Both conditions result in higher pressure behind the valve that reduces forward blood flow and CO. Stenosis and insufficiency can occur independently or together and affect a single or multiple valves.

ATRIOVENTRICULAR VALVES

AV valves are connected by chordae tendineae to papillary muscles, enabling the valve cusp to point in the direction of blood flow. Papillary muscle contraction holds the AV valves in place, preventing them from being forced into the atria by the increased ventricular pressure during contraction.

- Mitral: Has two leaflets/cusps and is located between the left atrium and the left ventricle.
- Tricuspid: Has three leaflets/cusps and is located between the right atrium and right ventricle.

SEMILUNAR VALVES

Semilunar describes the half-moon shape of the valves. When intraventricular pressures increase and exceed atrial and pulmonary pressures, valves open, allowing blood to flow forward into the pulmonary and systemic vasculature. Closure of the valves, after ventricular contraction and ejection, prevents blood from reversing or flowing backwards.

- Pulmonic: The pulmonic valve has three leaflets/cusps and is located between the right ventricle and the pulmonary artery.
- Aortic: The aortic valve has three leaflets/cusps and is located between the left ventricle and the aorta.

Valvular heart disease, whether from stenosis or insufficiency, results in decreased CO because of the increase in pressure behind the valve and reduced forward flow through the valve orifice. Narrowing of the valve opening because of stenosis requires the heart to pump harder through the smaller opening, thereby reducing CO and increasing myocardial oxygen demand. A stenotic aortic or pulmonic valve results in increased intramyocardial wall tension. Over time, the increased cardiac workload leads to thickening of the myocardial wall, reduced heart chamber size, and subsequent reduced volume capacity and CO. This persistent increase in wall tensions leads to ventricular hypertrophy and remodeling as the heart compensates for the excess workload. Atrial and ventricular dilatation caused by prolonged increased pressure increases the incidence of atrial fibrillation.

Insufficiency from inadequate closing of the valve leaflets causes reverse flow, which causes blood to accumulate in the pulmonary and systemic vasculature. Blood is unable to flow forward through the heart and systemic circulation, resulting in symptoms of fluid overload including orthopnea with pulmonary and peripheral edema. Impaired perfusion within the coronary vasculature results in decreased oxygen-rich blood within the myocardium, which causes chest pain, dysrhythmias, and dyspnea. When the demand for increased flow becomes greater than the supply during exertion or extreme stress, the result is fatigue and dyspnea.

MITRAL VALVE DISEASE

- Mitral stenosis: Mitral stenosis is most commonly caused by the inflammatory response to rheumatic heart disease resulting in thickening or stiffening of the valve leaflets, commissures, or chordae tendineae. The formation of small lesions known as Aschoff bodies and tiny pin-head size deposits called rheumatic vegetations embed in the endocardial, myocardial, and valvular structures and lead to stenosis of valve structures many years after the acute phase of rheumatic endocarditis. Diastolic doming of the anterior leaflet (hockey-stick deformity) and an immobile posterior leaflet give the valve a fish-mouth appearance and restrict the valve orifice. Pressure in the left atrium increases caused by the extra force needed to drive blood through the narrowed opening. Eventually, left atrial hypertrophy and stiffening of the left atrial wall change the surrounding structures and increase pulmonary artery pressure. Additionally, the structural abnormalities of the atria contribute to changes in atrial conduction patterns leading to atrial fibrillation in half of individuals with mitral stenosis.

- Mitral insufficiency/regurgitation (MR): Can be caused by injury or disruption to any part of the valve including the mitral annulus, the leaflets (a large anterior [aortic] leaflet and a small posterior [mural] leaflet), the chordae tendineae, and the papillary muscles. The most common etiologies of MR include mitral valve prolapse, rheumatic heart disease, infective endocarditis, annular calcification, cardiomyopathy, and ischemic heart disease. Pure MR is most commonly caused (71%) by a myxomatous (floppy, prolapse) process. Rheumatic heart disease (postinflammatory disease) accounts for 9% of cases. HF may occur acutely following rupture of an infarcted papillary muscle or chronically from papillary muscle fibrosis, hypertrophy, or LV dilatation.

TRICUSPID VALVE DISEASE

- Tricuspid stenosis: Usually associated with mitral stenosis resulting from rheumatic heart disease. In the absence of mitral stenosis, the possibility of right atrial myxoma (tumor) should be eliminated.
- Tricuspid regurgitation (TR)/insufficiency (TI): TR/TI is more common than tricuspid stenosis. Two types of patients are noted: those with normal leaflets and those with abnormal leaflets. Functional TR results from annular dilatation secondary to pulmonary hypertension associated with other valvular disorders. Acquired TR is less common, originating from an abnormality of the leaflets because of a variety of disease processes. Medications used to treat migraine (e.g., methysergide), Parkinson disease (e.g., pergolide), and obesity (e.g., fenfluramine) have been associated with TR.

AORTIC VALVE DISEASE

- Aortic stenosis (AS): A bicuspid (versus tricuspid) aortic valve is congenital and occurs predominantly in males and in 1% to 2% of the population. Most develop stenosis as a result of excess stresses on the valve from asymmetrical flow patterns and turbulence causing structural thickening, calcification, leaflet retraction, or aortic regurgitation. In adults, stenosis usually develops over a period of many years. Left ventricular diastolic dysfunction, reduced coronary reserve, and myocardial ischemia from longstanding systolic pressure overload eventually leads to depressed contractility and LV systolic dysfunction, HF, and finally sudden death. Often these patients remain symptom free until the late stage of the disease. The onset of symptoms (i.e., angina, syncope, and HF) depicts poor prognosis and mortality within 2 to 5 years. Mortality rates are worse for those with moderate to severe AS treated medically, at 25% and 50% at 1 and 2 years, respectively. Approximately 50% of deaths are from sudden cardiac death.
- Aortic insufficiency (AI)/regurgitation (AR): Acute AR results from a rapid increase in end-diastolic volume caused by regurgitant blood flow from endocarditis or aortic dissection. The left ventricle fills from both the left atrium and by retrograde or reverse flow from the aorta through the leaky aortic valve. In acute AR, the left ventricle does not have time to dilate in response to the volume load, resulting in chest pain and acute respiratory distress secondary to pulmonary edema. In severe cases, ventricular dilatation and hypertrophy cannot compensate for AI and HF develops, deteriorating to CS when CO no longer meets the systemic demand. Early surgical intervention should be considered. AR caused from aortic dissection requires immediate surgical intervention.
- Chronic AR occurs in response to gradual dilatation of the left ventricle and symptoms are masked by compensatory mechanisms. Once symptoms become severe, rapid decline follows.

PULMONIC VALVE DISEASE

- Pulmonic stenosis: Obstruction of the RV outflow tract may be acquired or congenital. Pulmonary stenosis accounts for 5% to 8% of all congenital heart defects. Mild pulmonary stenosis may not require intervention but is susceptible to infective endocarditis. Severe pulmonary stenosis (pulmonary atresia) is complete fusion of commissures with complete obstruction of the pulmonary artery outflow tract. An increased pressure gradient across the valve results in RV hypertrophy and right HF.
- Pulmonic insufficiency (PI)/regurgitation (PR): PI/PR causes include leaky valve after repair, RV conduit to pulmonary artery obstruction, pulmonary hypertension, congenital defects including large ducts (Ebstein anomaly), and tetralogy of Fallot with ventricular septal defect, pulmonary stenosis, RV hypertrophy, or overriding aorta. Abnormalities in sizes of heart structures cause variations in directional flow, vessel and heart chamber pressures, volume, and function, resulting in poor cardiac and systemic oxygenation and circulation.

ASSESSMENT: VALVULAR HEART DISEASE

GOAL OF SYSTEM ASSESSMENT

Evaluate for LV and RV failure, decreased CO, and decreased tissue perfusion. Many persons with longstanding valvular disease leading to atrial enlargement develop atrial fibrillation and should be monitored for the dysrhythmia, HF, and thrombosis. Cardiac cachexia may be seen in persons with longstanding valvular dysfunction as inflammatory processes release catecholamines, endotoxins, and tumor necrosis factors, causing cell breakdown, weight loss, and weakness. Early recognition of clinical changes and timely intervention are essential to improved outcomes.

HISTORY AND RISK FACTORS

Causes of valvular heart disease
- Rheumatic heart disease
- Congenital malformations
- Connective tissue disease (Marfan syndrome, systemic lupus erythematosus)
- Rheumatoid arthritis
- Chronic inflammatory disease (ankylosing spondylitis, giant cell arteritis)
- Acute myocardial infarction with papillary muscle rupture
- Drug use (intravenous drug abuse, combination weight loss drugs fenfluramine, dexfenfluramine, and phentermine)
- Advanced age
- Mitral valve prolapse
- Infective endocarditis
- Annular calcification
- Cancer
- Syphilis
- Pulmonary hypertension
- Cardiomyopathy
- Ischemic heart disease

PHYSICAL ASSESSMENT

Murmurs: Auscultation of heart sounds is the most effective screening tool for valvular disease. Evaluate changes in quality, pitch, and intensity to obtain insight into the patient's clinical condition, functional capacity, and quality of life. Changes in the quality and sound of murmurs can provide essential information regarding the clinical condition of patients with valvular heart disease.

Classifications of Murmurs: Murmurs are classified as systolic, diastolic, or continuous (throughout the cardiac cycle) with the characteristics described as holosystolic/pansystolic, midsystolic/systolic ejection, early, or late systolic. Diastolic murmurs are early, middiastolic, or presystolic.

MITRAL VALVE DISEASE

Assessment Findings	Mitral Stenosis	Mitral Insufficiency
Observation	Dyspnea, pulmonary congestion, edema, hemoptysis, slight cyanosis, fatigue, weakness	Dyspnea, pulmonary congestion, edema, fatigue, weakness, symptoms related to left-sided heart failure
Auscultation	Increased amplitude of S_1; opening snap and mid-diastolic murmur at the mitral area	Holosystolic murmur loudest in the mitral area and transmitted to the axilla or left sternal edge
Chest radiograph	Atrial enlargement	Left and right ventricular enlargement
12-lead ECG	Left atrial abnormality; humped or notched P wave (P "mitrale"); right ventricular hypertrophy; deep S in leads I and V_5, tall R in V_1; atrial fibrillation	Left ventricular hypertrophy; large S wave in V_1, large R wave in V_4, and minor atrial abnormality; atrial and ventricular arrhythmias
Hemodynamics	Elevated pulmonary artery occlusive pressure (PAOP), elevated pulmonary artery pressure (PAP), elevated venous pressure, decreased cardiac output (CO), elevated left atrial pressure (LAP). Patients will not experience valve-related symptoms until the valve area is >2 to 2.5 cm^2, when moderate exercise may cause exertional dyspnea. Severe mitral stenosis (valve area <1 cm^2) results in an increased resting diastolic mitral valve gradient and increased LAP. Pulmonary hypertension may develop. As PAP increases, the right ventricle (RV) dilates and tricuspid regurgitation may develop, resulting in increased jugular venous pressure, liver congestion, ascites, and pedal edema. LV end-diastolic pressure (LVEDP) and CO are often normal when only the mitral valve is stenosed. With progressive stenosis, the CO becomes subnormal at rest and fails to increase during exercise.	V waves in the pulmonary artery, increased systolic PAP, decreased CO. Acute mitral regurgitation (MR) causes increased preload and decreased afterload with an increase in end-diastolic volume (EDV) and decrease in end-systolic volume (ESV). The total stroke volume (TSV) is markedly increased, but forward stroke volume (FSV) is decreased because much of the TSV regurgitates, resulting in increased LAP. In chronic compensated MR, the left atrium and ventricle dilate to accommodate the regurgitant volume, so LAP may be normal or minimally elevated. In the chronic decompensated phase, muscle dysfunction decreases both TSV and FSV, but EF may be normal. ESV and EDV increase, then LAP and LVEDP increase, pulmonary edema may occur, and if unmanaged, cardiogenic shock ensues.

PULMONIC VALVE DISEASE

Assessment Findings	Pulmonic Stenosis	Pulmonic Insufficiency
Observation	Abnormal venous pulsations and elevated jugular pressure; hepatic tenderness and enlargement from venous congestion caused by right ventricular (RV) failure. Exertional dyspnea and fatigue. Commonly acquired in adults, congenital in children.	
Auscultation	Systolic blowing murmur at the second intercostal space, left sternal border that radiates to the neck.	Diastolic murmur at the second intercostal space at left sternal border, which starts later at lower pitch than aortic murmur. The Graham Steell murmur of pulmonary hypertension is a high-pitched, early diastolic decrescendo murmur heard over the left upper-to-left midsternal area.
Chest radiograph	Atrial enlargement, prominent pulmonary artery	Left and right ventricular enlargement

Valvular Heart Disease

Continued

PULMONIC VALVE DISEASE—cont'd

Assessment Findings	Pulmonic Stenosis	Pulmonic Insufficiency
12-lead ECG	R voltage increased in V_1; or increased S voltage in V_2; right axis deviation and RV hypertrophy	
Hemodynamics	Increased RV systolic pressure, mean RAP, PAWP, and mean PAP	Increased RV systolic pressure with wide pulse pressure; LVEDP and CO often normal but may decrease with wide pulse pressure

TRICUSPID VALVE DISEASE

Assessment Findings	Tricuspid Stenosis	Tricuspid Insufficiency
Observation	Abnormal venous pulsations and elevated jugular pressure; hepatic tenderness and enlargement from venous congestion caused by right heart failure, peripheral edema, dyspnea.	
Auscultation	Diastolic murmur at the 4th intercostal space, increases with inspiration	Pansystolic murmur at the 4th intercostal space; S_3 gallop is present.
Chest radiograph	Right atrial enlargement	
12-lead ECG	R voltage increased in V_1 or V_2; S voltage increased in V_5 or V_6; sum of R in V_1 or V_2 and S in V_5 or V_6 will be greater than 35 mm, atrial fibrillation	
Hemodynamics	Increased central venous pressure (CVP), accentuated A wave on the right atrial waveform	Increased CVP and prominent V wave on the right atrial waveform

AORTIC VALVE DISEASE

Assessment Findings	Aortic Stenosis	Aortic Insufficiency
Observation	Faint slow radial pulse, low blood pressure and pulse pressure, dizziness, fainting, syncope, pallor, dyspnea, fatigue; chest pain caused by coronary insufficiency, irregular heart sounds, and left-sided heart failure	Dyspnea, pulmonary congestion, edema, symptoms related to left-sided heart failure. Aortic regurgitation (AR) is indicated by three findings: Corrigan pulse is a palpated pulse with rapid and forceful distention of the artery followed by quick collapse. DeMusset sign is forward and backward bobbing of the head. Quincke sign is visible pulsation seen with slight compression of nail beds. Hill sign is popliteal cuff systolic blood pressure 40 mm Hg higher than brachial cuff systolic blood pressure.
Auscultation	Increased amplitude of S_1; opening snap and mid-diastolic murmur at the mitral area	Diastolic blowing murmur heard loudest at the second right intercostal space beginning with S_2. Duroziez sign is a systolic murmur over the femoral artery with proximal compression of the artery, and a diastolic murmur with distal compression of the artery.
Chest radiograph	Left ventricular (LV) enlargement and dilation of the ascending aorta	LV enlargement
12-lead ECG	LV hypertrophy; large S in V_2, large R in V_5; strain results in inverted T and depressed ST segments in I and II and V_I, V_5, and V_6, bradydysrhythmias	LV hypertrophy; large S in V_2, large R in V_5; strain results in inverted T and depressed ST segments in I and II and V_I, V_5, and V_6.

AORTIC VALVE DISEASE—cont'd

Assessment Findings	Aortic Stenosis	Aortic Insufficiency
Hemodynamics	Increased LV pressure, increased pulmonary artery end-diastolic pressure and wedge pressure; increased gradient across the aortic valve on pullback from LV end-diastolic pressure to aortic pressure; narrow pulse pressure, decreased cardiac output. LV systolic function is preserved and cardiac output is maintained for many years despite an elevated LV systolic pressure. Despite the cardiac output at rest being normal, it fails to increase appropriately during exercise, causing exercise-induced syncope or near syncope. With severe aortic stenosis, atrial contraction is vital to diastolic filling of the LV so atrial fibrillation can be catastrophic to maintaining stroke volume.	Increased LV pressure, increased peripheral artery disease (PAD) and pulmonary artery occlusive pressure (PAOP), decreased cardiac output; increased systolic blood pressure and widened pulse pressure. Peripheral pulses are prominent or bounding. Symptoms may result from the elevated stroke volume during systole and the incompetent aortic valve allowing significantly decreased aortic diastolic pressure (often <60 mm Hg), with pulse pressures often >100 mm Hg. During early chronic AR, the LV ejection fraction (EF) is normal or increased. As AR progresses, LV enlargement exceeds preload reserve and the EF decreases to normal and then subnormal levels. The LV end-systolic volume increases and reflects progressive myocardial dysfunction. The LV gradually transforms from an elliptical to a spherical configuration.

Diagnostic Tests for Evaluation of Valvular Disease

Diagnostic testing for the patient with a heart murmur varies considerably depending on when the murmur occurs in the cardiac cycle, location and possible radiation, and response to selected physiologic maneuvers used during evaluation. The presence/absence of cardiac and noncardiac symptoms, along with other findings on physical examination, will help determine if the murmur is clinically significant. Treatment is based on echocardiographic measurements of left ventricular (LV) size and systolic function. When determining recommendations, the accuracy and reproducibility of results are critical. Surgical recommendations for asymptomatic patients with mitral regurgitation (MR) or aortic regurgitation (AR) are often dependent on the reliability and validity of the measurements.

Test	Purpose	Abnormal Findings
• Echocardiography Doppler flow studies • Color flow mapping • Transesophageal echocardiography (TEE) • Dobutamine stress echocardiography	Recommended for evaluation of all patients with cardiac murmurs. Provides information on valve morphology and function, chamber size, wall thickness, ventricular function, and pulmonary and hepatic vein flow. Estimates of pulmonary artery pressures can be readily assessed.	Abnormal blood flow patterns, resulting in reduced forward flow of blood. Stenosis: Blood flow is somewhat occluded. Incompetency: Blood flows backward through the valve into the heart chamber preceding the valve. Echocardiography may not be necessary for the evaluation of asymptomatic younger patients with lower grade murmurs. Minimal or physiologic mitral, tricuspid, or pulmonic valve regurgitations may be detected by color flow imaging in many patients who have no heart murmur. Sensitive Doppler ultrasound devices may find trace or mild regurgitation through structurally normal tricuspid and pulmonic valves, as well as through normal left-sided heart valves (especially mitral) in young, healthy patients.
• Doppler flow studies	Continuous-wave or pulsed-wave frequencies used to determine blood flow.	
• Color flow mapping studies	Uses colors (red and blue) to enhance the image of blood flowing through the heart.	
• Transesophageal echocardiography (TEE)	Uses an endoscope to produce an image unimpeded by the chest wall. The esophagus is close to the heart, so images are clearer or less distorted.	

Valvular Heart Disease

Continued

Diagnostic Tests for Evaluation of Valvular Disease—cont'd

Dobutamine stress echocardiography	Uses a dobutamine infusion to increase heart rate and force of contraction during an echocardiogram to assess for changes in blood flow under more stressful conditions	Flow gradients across diseased valves may deteriorate under more stressful conditions. Assists in determining whether valve stenosis is moderate or severe in patients with aortic stenosis.
Chest radiograph	To evaluate the size of the heart to assist with assessment of degree of ventricular remodeling, indicative of possible heart failure	Cardiac enlargement, reflective of ventricular remodeling
Cardiac catheterization	Unnecessary in most patients with cardiac murmurs with normal or diagnostic echocardiograms. Provides information for patients with a discrepancy between echocardiographic and clinical findings. Gradients across valves can indicate severity of stenosis. Ventriculogram may assist in visualization of blood flow.	Describes presence and severity of valvular obstruction or regurgitation, and intracardiac shunting. Abnormal or giant V wave on the pulmonary artery occlusive pressure (PAOP) waveform (right-sided heart catheterization) is seen with mitral regurgitation. Visualizing the coronary arteries also provides information about concomitant CAD, which may require revascularization at the time of surgical valve repair or replacement.
Cardiac magnetic resonance imaging (MRI)	Provides an enhanced evaluation of patients for whom transthoracic Doppler flow studies are inadequate to describe valvular lesions.	Abnormal blood flow patterns, valvular stenosis or incompetency
Exercise testing	Provides information for patients whose symptoms are difficult to assess.	Ischemic ECG changes associated with exercise
B-type natriuretic peptide (BNP)	Helps to diagnose if valvular disease has reduced cardiac output resulting in heart failure.	Elevation may be an early marker of heart failure resulting from the valvular stenosis or regurgitation.

COLLABORATIVE MANAGEMENT
CARE PRIORITIES
1. Consider antibiotic prophylaxis for infective endocarditis and rheumatic fever

Prophylaxis, which was once mandatory for all patients, is now controversial. Providing prophylactic antibiotics has not been shown to prevent the development of endocarditis valve disease in all patient populations. Varying levels of evidence support the following recommendations from the 2014 ACC/AHA Task Force Writing Committee.

2014 ACC/AHA GUIDELINES FOR ANTIBIOTIC PROPHYLAXIS FOR INVASIVE DENTAL PROCEDURES

High-Risk Recommended	Not Recommended
• Patients with prosthetic valves • Prior infective endocarditis • Cardiac transplant patients with regurgitation caused by abnormal valve structure • Unrepaired and palliated cyanotic congenital heart defects (surgically constructed palliative shunts and conduits) • Repaired congenital heart defects (prosthetic material or devices) first 6 months postprocedure • Congenital heart defects with residual defects at or adjacent to the prosthetic patch or device that inhibits endothelialization	• Aggregated lifetime risk of endocarditis • GU and GI procedures (TEE, esophagogastroduodenoscopy, colonoscopy, cystoscopy) (See Acute Infective Endocarditis, Chapter 5).

Prevention of endocarditis continues to be important for all patients with valvular heart disease (VHD). Patient education including good daily oral hygiene and regular dental visits is essential. Additionally, aseptic measures during catheter manipulation or any invasive procedure, to reduce the rate of healthcare-associated infective endocarditis, have been included in the recommendations by the European Society of Cardiology (ESC).

2. Manage aortic stenosis

- Monitoring: Frequently for progression of the disease, including asymptomatic patients; stenosis requires initial and serial visits for grading severity and evaluation of symptoms. Echocardiography is indicated annually for severe AS, every 1 to 2 years for moderate AS, and every 3 to 5 years for mild AS.
- Medical management: The overall goal using medical therapy is to manage and treat related cardiovascular conditions and comorbidities that exacerbate AS. Patient education including lifestyle and behavioral modifications, infection prevention, and nutrition, as well as symptom recognition and self-management techniques, is essential in optimizing management and reducing hospital readmissions. Additionally, palliative care and end-of-life discussions should be included early in the plan of care.
- Hypertension: Use antihypertensive agents cautiously.
- Decision about surgery: Need is based largely on the patient's symptoms, rather than exclusively on the transvalvular pressure gradient. Angina, syncope, and HF can develop suddenly, sometimes following a lengthy asymptomatic period. Following onset of symptoms, survival averages 2 to 3 years.
- Aortic valve replacement (AVR): AVR was the first effective treatment shown to improve symptoms and long-term survival in patients with severe symptomatic AS, including the very elderly; it is the only class I recommendation by ACC/AHA and ESC (2013). Furthermore, patients undergoing coronary bypass surgery with known moderate AS should have the valve replaced simultaneously. Valve replacement during coronary bypass surgery for patients with mild AS is unsupported. According to the Society of Thoracic Surgeons (STS) registry, the mortality rate is less than 3% for all patients undergoing AVR. However, risk stratification is necessary especially in elderly patients with comorbid conditions. Valve types can be mechanical or bioprosthetic (tissue). Mechanical valves are preferred in younger patients because of the longevity of the valve. On the other hand, in the elderly, tissue valves have been favored over mechanical, because of improvements in valve durability and reduced need for anticoagulation.
- Transcatheter aortic valve replacement (TAVI/TAVR): First performed in 2002, TAVR using the transapical or transfemoral approach has become one of the most widely used methods to treat AS, especially in patients with high surgical risk. Procedural success rates are reported to be greater than 90%. Patients undergoing TAVR can have their valve repaired or replaced in the cardiac catheterization lab under moderate sedation. Currently, most data regarding TAVR are based on the use of two replacement valves, the

Sapien valve from Edwards Life Sciences, Inc., and the Core Valve from Medtronic, Inc. Data are limited as TAVR/TAVI is a relatively new procedure. However, there have been no reports of structural deterioration to date. Studies are ongoing and according to a multicenter randomized clinical trial comparing TAVR with standard therapy, benefits greatly outweigh risks in inoperable patients with severe symptomatic AS. Results show significantly improved quality of life during the first year following TAVR/TAVI.

- Aortic balloon valvotomy: In patients with a high risk for surgery, balloon aortic valvuloplasty may be a reasonable option of therapy. However, there is a high rate of recurrence of AS, and restenosis often recurs within 6 months.

3. Manage aortic insufficiency/regurgitation

- Crisis: Can occur acutely resulting in pulmonary edema and/or CS. Death from CS, ventricular dysrhythmias, and PEA is common with acute, severe AR.
- Urgent surgery: Inodilators such as milrinone and inamrinone are used to help increase CO. Dopamine and dobutamine may be used to increase contractility and, along with vasodilators such as nitroprusside, reduce LV afterload for preoperative stabilization. Immediate surgery is recommended for symptomatic patients with acute AR resulting from infective endocarditis.
- Balloon counterpulsation: NOT recommended for acute AR; may be harmful.
- Compensatory tachycardia: Vital for survival in acute AR; beta blockers must be used with caution, especially when treating aortic dissection.
- Medications: Vasodilators are used for those with chronic severe AR who are not surgical candidates. Diuretics, nitrates, and digoxin are sometimes used to help control symptoms, but there are insufficient data to justify recommending or discouraging these therapies.
- Chronic AR: Management is based on LV systolic function. If LV systolic dysfunction occurs (a reduced EF at rest) and cannot be controlled with antihypertensive therapy, patients may require AVR. Initially, the process of ventricular remodeling is reversible with management of afterload (BP/SVR) using vasodilators.

4. Manage mitral stenosis

- Monitoring: A progressive, lifelong disease generally resulting from rheumatic fever. Patients' symptoms can remain insignificant for up to 10 years then suddenly develop HF and decline rapidly. When severe pulmonary hypertension develops, average survival is 3 years.
- Atrial fibrillation: Up to 40% of patients develop atrial fibrillation. Anticoagulation, is recommended to avoid clot formation and thromboembolism. Heart rate can be controlled using amiodarone, CCBs, beta adrenergic-blocking agents, or digoxin. Cardioversion may be required if the patients are uncontrolled with oral medications and become symptomatic. Ablation may be an option for select patients.
- Percutaneous balloon mitral valvotomy (PBMV): Recommended for symptomatic patients without severe pulmonary hypertension. Moderate to severely symptomatic patients with PA systolic pressure of greater than 60 mm Hg may require a mitral commissurotomy or mitral valve replacement (MVR).

5. Manage mitral regurgitation

- Crisis: May occur acutely, as in AMI, resulting in CS. Sodium nitroprusside, NTG, or ACEIs are used in combination with inotropic agents (e.g., dobutamine or dopamine) to avoid severe hypotension.
- Balloon counterpulsation therapy: Provides stabilization by helping to increase forward blood flow, resulting in increased MAP and reducing the volume of regurgitation and LV preload (LV end-diastolic pressure).
- MVR: May be necessary for stabilization of severely symptomatic patients.
- Transcatheter interventions: Increasingly studied for carefully selected patients with severe MR. Data are limited and there is FDA approval for only one device to date. ACC, AATS, SCAIF, and STS recommendations and guidelines are in development.
- Mitral valve repair: Recommended for patients with a lesser degree of LV dysfunction.
- Chronic MR: Patients may remain in a stable, compensated state for many years. Incidence of sudden death in asymptomatic patients varies widely among documented studies. There is no universally recommended medical therapy.

- LV systolic dysfunction: Patients may benefit from ACEIs or beta adrenergic–blocking agents (e.g., carvedilol) and biventricular cardiac pacing to reduce regurgitant volume.
- Acute atrial fibrillation: Managed with CCBs, beta blockers, digoxin, and sometimes amiodarone to promote control of tachycardia.
- Chronic atrial fibrillation: May require a Maze procedure (ablation); may be done simultaneously with mitral valve repair to help prevent stroke. All patients with chronic atrial fibrillation require long-term anticoagulation with warfarin.

6. Manage tricuspid valve disease
- Surgery: Tricuspid valve repair, valve replacement, or annuloplasty for TR often occurs during mitral valve surgery.
- Severe TR: Patients have poor long-term outcomes because of RV dysfunction with or without systemic venous congestion.

7. Manage pulmonic valve disease
- Pulmonic valve stenosis: Pulmonic stenosis is usually congenital, not likely because of acquired heart disease, and managed with percutaneous balloon valvotomy. Most patients undergoing valvotomy for stenosis also have MR.
- Pulmonic regurgitation: Generally not seen unless other valve disease is present. It is also likely to be a congenital defect and typically managed with pulmonic valve replacement if HF is present.

8. Provide lifelong anticoagulation for patients with prosthetic heart valves
- Warfarin: Maintain the international normalized ratio (INR) as follows:
  - Aortic valve: INR 2.5 to 3.0
  - Mitral valve: INR 3.0
- Low-dose aspirin: 75 to 100 mg daily is recommended in addition to warfarin therapy for both aortic and mitral valves with or without risk factors for thromboembolism (e.g., atrial fibrillation, previous thromboembolism, or a hypercoagulable state, and older generation mechanical AVR).

9. Provide short-term anticoagulation for patients with biological heart valves
- Warfarin is recommended for the first 3 months following surgery, unless at higher risk of thromboembolism, wherein anticoagulation may be continued long-term.
- At least two-thirds of patients do not require lifelong anticoagulation.

10. Reverse excessive anticoagulation
- INR greater than 5: Increases the possibility of bleeding and/or hemorrhage
- Prosthetic heart valve: If the patient with an INR 5 to 10 is not bleeding, withholding warfarin and giving vitamin K (phytonadione) 1 to 2.5 mg orally daily until INR normalizes is appropriate. In the case of uncontrolled bleeding, fresh-frozen plasma or prothrombin complex concentrate is recommended over higher-dose parenteral (IV) vitamin K1, which often results in a hypercoagulable state. Low-dose IV vitamin K (1 mg) has been found to be safer, if needed. Aspirin should also be discontinued.

11. Manage thrombosis of prosthetic valves
- Emergency surgery: Recommended for patients with left-sided heart valves with NYHA class III to IV HF and a large clot burden.
- Fibrinolytic therapy: May be appropriate for patients with right-sided valves with class II to IV HF and large clot burden, or those with left-sided valves with NYHA class I to II HF and smaller clot burden.

SURGICAL INTERVENTIONS
- Valve replacement: Procedure with a mortality rate of about 6%, performed in patients with moderate to severe calcification, stenosis with insufficiency, and pure insufficiency. Three types of replacement valves are available: homografts and heterografts, which are tissue grafts, and mechanical valves. Homografts are specially treated human cadaver valves and are seldom used because of a lack of availability. The more commonly used heterograft is a specially prepared valve from an animal, usually a pig or a cow. These

valves are readily available and more advantageous because there is less of a tendency for clot formation and adherence to the valve structures. Thus, patients do not require anticoagulation therapy after valve replacement. The disadvantage is that they function for only 5 to 8 years. Mechanical valves are made from stainless steel, carbon, plastic, and other durable materials. Mechanical valves have a 10- to 15-year life span and require lifelong anticoagulation because of their susceptibility to clot formation. Postoperative care is similar to that of the patient who has undergone myocardial revascularization for CAD (see Acute Coronary Syndromes, Chapter 5). Patients undergoing valve surgery are at increased risk for thrombosis, embolism, and valvular endocarditis (particularly with mechanical mitral valves and patients with atrial fibrillation).

- Commissurotomy: A procedure in which the stenotic valve is opened using a dilating instrument. When performed early in the course of the disease, chances of success are good, although the procedure may result in valve regurgitation and recurrent stenosis.
- Reshaping: A portion of the diseased valve is removed and the valve is sewn back together to promote more effective closure.
- Decalcification: Calcium deposits are removed to allow the smooth surface of the valve to close more effectively.
- Patching: Covering damaged portions or "holes" in valves with tissue to improve valve closure.
- Surgical valvuloplasty: Valvular repair may be possible in select patients. In addition, insertion of a valvular ring can improve native valve function.
- Percutaneous balloon valvuloplasty: For dilation of stenotic heart valves. Candidates for this procedure may (1) be at high risk for surgery, (2) refuse surgery, (3) be older adults (often older than 80 years), or (4) be informed of treatment choices and choose this procedure over others. The procedure parallels the technique for percutaneous coronary intervention (see Acute Coronary Syndromes, Chapter 5). The patient undergoes this procedure in the cardiac cath lab, and a transfemoral approach is used. The femoral artery and vein are accessed and supravalvular and LV pressures are obtained. The valve gradient is measured pre- and postdilatation of the valve. Despite modifications in procedural techniques peri- and postprocedure complications and restenosis rates remain high. Complications include thromboembolic stroke, disruption of the valve ring, acute valve regurgitation, valvular restenosis, hemorrhage at the catheter insertion site, guidewire perforation of the left ventricle, and dysrhythmias.

CARE PLANS FOR VALVULAR HEART DISEASE

FOR PATIENTS UNDERGOING VALVE REPLACEMENT

INEFFECTIVE PROTECTION *related to risk of bleeding/hemorrhage secondary to anticoagulation.*

Safety Alert *Patients undergoing aortic valve replacement are at a higher risk for postoperative hemorrhage than are those undergoing coronary artery bypass grafting.*

Goals/Outcomes: Throughout hospitalization, the patient is free of symptoms of bleeding or hemorrhage as evidenced by RAP 4 to 6 mm Hg, PAWP 6 to 12 mm Hg, BP within patient's normal range, CO 4 to 7 L/min, CI 2.5 to 4 L/min/m², urine output 0.5 mL/kg/h or greater, urine specific gravity 1.010 to 1.030, and chest tube drainage 100 mL/h or less.
NOC Circulation Status

Circulatory Precautions
1. Monitor for hemorrhage and clotting: Monitor vital signs and measure chest tube drainage hourly. Report chest tube drainage greater than 100 mL/h. Maintain patency of chest tubes at all times.
2. Monitor clotting studies: Report and manage prolonged PT, PTT, and ACT and decreased platelet count. Optimal values are as follows: PT 11 to 15 seconds, PTT 30 to 40 seconds (activated), and ACT 120 seconds or less.

For a patient with prolonged PT, PTT, or ACT, administer IV protamine sulfate as prescribed if heparin was the anticoagulant used. After discharge from the hospital, the INR should be maintained at 2.5.

3. Monitor hemodynamics for hypovolemia: RAP less than 4 mm Hg, PAWP less than 6 mm Hg, decreased BP, decreased measured CO/CI, urine output less than 0.5 mL/kg/h, increased urine specific gravity, and excessive chest tube drainage (more than 100 mL/h). Be alert to a decreased Hct. Optimal values are Hct greater than 37% (female) and greater than 40% (male).

4. Assess postoperative chest radiograph for a widened mediastinum, which may indicate hemorrhage and possible cardiac tamponade.

5. Manage hemorrhage: Orders may include administration of platelets, fresh-frozen plasma, or cryoprecipitate to replace clotting factors and blood volume.

6. Administer packed RBCs as prescribed to replace blood volume or use chest tube drainage for autotransfusion.

7. Manage hyperfibrinolytic state (increased fibrin degradation products): Orders may include aminocaproic acid given slowly per IV bolus (Box 5-9).

NIC Bleeding Reduction; Autotransfusion; Hemorrhage Control

DECREASED CARDIAC OUTPUT (OR RISK FOR SAME) *related to negative inotropic changes secondary to intraoperative subendocardial ischemia and administration of myocardial depressant drugs.*

Safety Alert *After cardiac surgery, some myocardial depression is always present, usually lasting 48 to 72 hours. Patients with long-standing aortic stenosis or ventricular failure caused by mitral valve disease are at an even greater risk for postoperative low cardiac output.*

Goals/Outcomes: Within 48 to 72 hours, the patient has adequate CO as evidenced by NSR on ECG, measured CO of 4 to 7 L/min, CI greater than 2.5 L/min/m², BP within patient's normal range, PAP 20 to 30/8 to 15 mm Hg, PAWP 6 to 12 mm Hg (or range specified by physician), SvO_2 60% to 80%, SVR 900 to 1200 dynes/sec/cm⁻⁵, peripheral pulses greater than 2+ on a 0 to 4+ scale, warm and dry skin, and hourly urine output greater than 0.5 mL/kg/h. Patient is awake, alert, and oriented.

NOC Cardiac Pump Effectiveness

Shock Prevention
1. Monitor peripheral pulses and color and temperature of extremities every 2 hours.
2. Provide oxygen therapy as prescribed.

Box 5-9	NURSING IMPLICATIONS FOR ADMINISTRATION OF EPSILON-AMINOCAPROIC ACID

- Be aware that rapid administration may induce hypotension, bradycardia, or cardiac dysrhythmias.
- Monitor for and report the following side effects: nausea, cramps, diarrhea, dizziness, tinnitus, headache, skin rash, malaise, nasal stuffiness, postural hypotension.
- Be alert to clotting or thrombosis, which can be precipitated by this medication. Assess for indicators of thrombophlebitis: calf erythema, warmth, tenderness, or increase in size or positive reaction for Homan sign. Provide pneumatic compression stockings as prescribed.
- Assess for indicators of pulmonary emboli: chest pain, dyspnea, fever, tachycardia, cyanosis, falling blood pressure, restlessness, agitation.
- Monitor and report blood levels of epsilon-aminocaproic acid via use of chromatography, if available in the institution.
- Consult advanced practice provider promptly for significant findings.

3. Maintain an adequate preload (i.e., PAWP greater than 10 mm Hg, RAP 10 mm Hg) via administration of IV fluids.

> **Safety Alert** *With aortic stenosis and severe LV hypertrophy, a high filling pressure (i.e., pulmonary artery wedge pressure greater than 18 mm Hg) may be necessary to ensure an adequate cardiac output.*

4. Maintain a normal or reduced afterload (SVR less than 1200 dynes/sec/cm⁻⁵) by administering prescribed IV vasodilating drugs such as nitroprusside and NTG.
5. Maintain NSR by administering antidysrhythmic agents as prescribed. Atrial fibrillation is common in aortic and mitral valve disease and may result in a 20% to 50% decrease in CO. If a junctional rhythm or bradycardia occurs, a pacemaker may be necessary.
6. Administer inotropic agents as prescribed to maintain CI greater than 2.5 L/min/m² and systolic BP greater than 90 mm Hg. Commonly used agents include dobutamine, dopamine, milrinone, and amrinone. Monitor for side effects, including tachydysrhythmias, ventricular ectopy, headache, and angina.

NIC Cardiac Care; Hemodynamic Regulation

INEFFECTIVE TISSUE PERFUSION (OR RISK FOR SAME): CEREBRAL *related to impaired blood flow to the brain secondary to embolization resulting from cardiac surgery.*

> **Safety Alert** *An air embolus, particulate emboli from calcified valves, and thrombotic emboli from prosthetic valves may lodge in the brain, leading to varying degrees of stroke.*

Goals/Outcomes: Throughout hospitalization, the patient has adequate or baseline brain perfusion as evidenced by orientation to time, place, and person; equal and normoreactive pupils; and ability to move all extremities, communicate, and respond to requests (or comparable to patient's preoperative baseline).
NOC Neurologic Status

Neurologic Monitoring
1. Monitor patient immediately after surgery and hourly for signs of neurologic impairment: diminished LOC, pupillary response, ability to move all extremities, and response to verbal stimuli.
2. Assess patient's orientation and ability to communicate, answer yes/no questions, point to objects, write responses and requests, identify family members, and state his or her location. Inform other healthcare personnel about patient's LOC and communication deficits.
3. Assess patient's PT, PTT, and INR as heparin is tapered off and warfarin therapy is instituted. Heparin and warfarin may be initiated simultaneously to reduce the time needed to stabilize the lab values.
4. If CNS impairment is noted, report findings to the physician and administer medications for brain resuscitation as prescribed.
5. In the presence of CNS impairment, implement the following measures:
   • Assist patient with turning and moving as needed. Teach the patient to use unaffected extremities to assist with moving.
   • Perform ROM to all extremities 4 times daily. Have patient assist as much as possible.
   • Progress patient's activity level, as tolerated, with the assistance of a physical therapist.
6. Assess patient's ability to swallow food and fluids. If the patient's voice is hoarse or patient coughs when swallowing, consult advanced practice provider. Patient may require nothing-by-mouth status and an enteric tube until the swallowing reflex has improved.

NIC Surveillance; Cerebral Perfusion Promotion

DEFICIENT KNOWLEDGE *related to risk of infective endocarditis after valve surgery and preventive strategies.*

Safety Alert *All patients who have undergone valve surgery are at risk for infective endocarditis as a result of bacteria entering the bloodstream and traveling to the heart, leading to destruction of a new tissue valve or obstruction of a new artificial valve.*

Goals/Outcomes: Within the 24-hour period before discharge from the CCU, the patient verbalizes knowledge about the risk of IE after valve surgery and the precautions that must be taken to prevent it.
NOC Knowledge: Disease Process

Teaching: Disease Process
1. Teach the patient about IE (see Acute Infective Endocarditis, Chapter 5), describing what it is, how it develops, and how it may affect the repaired valve.
2. Teach the patient to caution dentists and other healthcare providers so antibiotics can be prescribed to prevent development of endocarditis after valve surgery. Antibiotics must be taken before any dental work or examination by instrument, including teeth cleaning, fillings, extractions, cystoscopy, endoscopy, or sigmoidoscopy.
3. Instruct patient to cleanse all wounds and apply antibiotic ointments to help prevent infection.

NIC Teaching: Prescribed Medication; Surveillance

DEFICIENT KNOWLEDGE *related to risk of bleeding or clotting caused by excessive or insufficient anticoagulation therapy.*

Safety Alert *It can be difficult to find and maintain the dosage of warfarin needed to maintain target international normalized ratio. Foods, medications, vitamins, and food supplements can enhance or inhibit efficacy.*

Goals/Outcomes: Within the 24-hour period before discharge from the hospital, the patient or significant others verbalize knowledge about the risk of warfarin therapy after valve surgery and the precautions that must be taken to prevent embolism or hemorrhage.
NOC Knowledge: Treatment Regimen

Teaching: Prescribed Medication
Teach the patient and significant others:
1. How to institute bleeding precautions after discharge. Shave with an electric razor. Take care when handling sharp objects. Prevent injury through an annual safety home check. Use a soft-bristle toothbrush.
2. To call advanced practice provider if bleeding or bruising is noted.
3. To report all changes in medication to healthcare provider who is managing warfarin or other anticoagulant therapy.
4. To avoid altering the intake of foods that may be high in vitamin K. Excessive intake of vitamin K can block warfarin and lower the INR.

NIC Teaching: Prescribed Diet; Surveillance

FOR PATIENTS UNDERGOING PERCUTANEOUS BALLOON VALVULOPLASTY
DEFICIENT KNOWLEDGE *related to procedure for percutaneous balloon valvuloplasty (PBV) and postprocedural assessment.*

Goals/Outcomes: Within the 24-hour period before PBV, the patient verbalizes rationale for the procedure, the technique, and postprocedural care.
NOC Knowledge: Treatment Regimen

Teaching: Preoperative
1. Assess patient's understanding of aortic stenosis and the purpose of valvuloplasty. Evaluate patient's style of coping and the degree of information desired.

2. Discuss with patient and significant others the valvuloplasty procedure, including the following:
    *   Location of diseased valve, using heart drawing
    *   Use of local anesthesia and sedation during procedure
    *   Insertion site of catheter: femoral artery and vein
    *   Use of fluoroscopy during procedure. Evaluate patient for a history of sensitivity to contrast material.
    *   Postprocedural observations made by nurse: BP, HR, ECG, pulses, and catheter insertion site
    *   Importance of lying flat for 6 to 12 hours after the procedure to minimize the risk of bleeding

NIC Teaching: Procedure/Treatment

DECREASED CARDIAC OUTPUT (OR RISK FOR SAME) *related to altered preload and negative inotropic changes associated with valve regurgitation or hemorrhage secondary to PBV; Altered rate, rhythm, or conduction associated with dysrhythmias secondary to PBV.*

Goals/Outcomes: Throughout the postoperative course, the patient has adequate CO as evidenced by NSR, CO 4 to 7 L/min, CI greater than 2.5 L/min/m², HR 60 to 100 bpm, RAP 4 to 6 mm Hg, PAWP 6 to 12 mm Hg, PAP 20 to 30/8 to 15 mm Hg, BP within patient's normal range, urinary output greater than 0.5 mL/kg/h, peripheral pulses greater than 2+ on a 0 to 4+ scale, orientation to time, place, and person; and absence of new murmurs, pulsus paradoxus, or jugular vein distention.
NOC Cardiac Pump Effectiveness

Shock Prevention
1. Monitor ECG continuously after procedure. Document any changes. Consult advanced practice provider for dysrhythmias, and treat according to hospital protocol.
2. Monitor CO/CI, HR, RAP, PAWP, and PAP hourly or as prescribed. Report a fall in CO/CI, a change in HR, and an increase or decrease in RAP, PAWP, or PAP.
3. Monitor Hct and electrolyte values. Observe for a decrease in Hct or any change in electrolyte levels (particularly potassium) that could precipitate dysrhythmias. Optimal values are Hct greater than 37% (female) or greater than 40% (male) and serum potassium 3.5 to 5 mEq/L.
4. Assess heart sounds immediately after procedure and every 4 hours. Report the development of a new murmur.
5. Monitor patient for evidence of cardiac tamponade: hypotension, tachycardia, pulsus paradoxus, jugular vein distention, elevation and plateau pressuring of PAWP and RAP, and possibly an enlarged heart silhouette on chest radiograph study. For more information, see Acute Cardiac Tamponade, Chapter 5.

NIC Cardiac Care; Hemodynamic Regulation

INEFFECTIVE PROTECTION *related to risk of hemorrhage or hematoma formation secondary to heparinization with PBV.*

Goals/Outcomes: Throughout the postoperative course, the patient has minimal or absent bleeding or hematoma formation at the catheter insertion site. PTT is within therapeutic anticoagulation range (as prescribed or according to institutional procedure).
NOC Circulation Status

Bleeding Precautions
1. Monitor catheter insertion site for evidence of bleeding. Report hematoma formation, and outline the bleeding on the dressing for subsequent comparison.
2. Keep patient's catheterized leg straight for the prescribed amount of time.
3. Monitor heparin drip as prescribed. Usually heparin drip is maintained until 1 to 2 hours before the sheaths are removed.
4. Monitor PTT for therapeutic range, which is usually 1.5 times that of normal.
5. When IV or invasive lines (arterial or venous sheaths) are removed, apply firm pressure either manually or with a mechanical clamp for 30 minutes.

NIC Surveillance; Bleeding Reduction: Wound

ADDITIONAL NURSING DIAGNOSES

Also see Deficient Knowledge in Pulmonary Embolus (Chapter 4). Also see Altered Tissue Perfusion in Acute Coronary Syndromes (Chapter 5). See all nursing diagnoses in the discussion of Coronary Artery Bypass Graft in Acute Coronary Syndromes (Chapter 5). Also see nursing diagnoses and interventions in Hemodynamic Monitoring (Chapter 1), Prolonged Immobility (Chapter 1), and Emotional and Spiritual Support of the Patient and Significant Others (Chapter 2).

SELECTED REFERENCES

2013 ACCF/AHA key data elements and definitions for measuring the clinical management and outcomes of patients with acute coronary syndromes and coronary artery disease. A Report of the American College of Cardiology Foundation/American Heart Association Task Force on Clinical Data Standards (Writing Committee to Develop Acute Coronary Syndromes and Coronary Artery Disease Clinical Data Standards), *Circulation* 127:1052–1089, 2013. http://my.americanheart.org/professional/StatementsGuidelines/ByTopic/TopicsA-C/ACCAHA-Joint-Guidelines_UCM_321694_Article.jsp.

ACCF/AHA guideline: 2013 ACCF/AHA guideline for the management of ST-elevation myocardial infarction: a report of the American College of Cardiology Foundation/American Heart Association Task Force on Practice Guidelines, *Circulation* 127:e362–e425, 2013.

Algorithms for advanced cardiac life support 2015. ACLS Training Center. http://www.acls.net/aclsalg.htm.

American Diabetes Association: Standards of medical care in diabetes—2013, *Diabetes Care* 36 (Suppl 1):S11–S66, 2013.

American Heart Association: *ACLS: principles and practice*, Dallas, 2011, American Heart Association.

American Heart Association: *Handbook of emergency cardiovascular care for healthcare providers*, Dallas, 2011, American Heart Association.

American Heart Association: *Pericardium and pericarditis*. http://www.americanheart.org/presenter.jhtml?identifier=4683.

American Heart Association: *Single photon computed tomography*. http://www.heart.org/HEARTORG/Conditions/HeartAttack/SymptomsDiagnosisofHeartAttack/Single-Photon-Emission-Computed-Tomography-SPECT_UCM_446358_Article.jsp.

Anderson JL, Halperin JL, Albert NM, et al: Management of patients with peripheral artery disease (compilation of 2005 and 2011 ACCF/AHA guideline recommendations): a report of the American College of Cardiology Foundation/American Heart Association Task Force on Practice Guidelines, *Circulation* 127:1–9, 2013. http://circ.ahajournals.org/content/early/2013/03/01/CIR.0b013e31828b82aa.citation.

Anderson JL, Halperin JL, Albert NM, et al: Management of patients with atrial fibrillation (compilation of 2006 ACCF/AHA/ESC and 2011 ACCF/AHA/HRS guideline recommendations): a report of the American College of Cardiology Foundation/American Heart Association Task Force on Practice Guidelines), *Circulation* 127:1916–1926, 2013.

Angeja BG, Grossman W: Clinician update: evaluation and management of diastolic heart failure, *Circulation* 107:659, 2003.

Baird MS, Bethel S: *Manual of critical care nursing: nursing interventions and collaborative management*, ed 6, St. Louis, 2011, Elsevier Mosby.

Balady GJ, Arena R, Sietsema K, et al: on behalf of the American Heart Association Exercise, Cardiac Rehabilitation, and Prevention Committee of the Council on Clinical Cardiology; Council on Epidemiology and Prevention; Council on Peripheral Vascular Disease; and Interdisciplinary Council on Quality of Care and Outcomes Research: Clinician's guide to cardiopulmonary exercise testing in adults: a scientific statement from the American Heart Association, *Circulation* 122:191–225, 2010.

Bart BA, Goldsmith SR, Lee KL: Ultrafiltration in decompensated heart failure with cardiorenal syndrome, *N Engl J Med* 367: 2286–2304, 2012.

Benham-Hermetz J, Lambert M, Stephens RCM: Cardiovascular failure, inotropes, and vasopressors, *Br J Hosp Med* 73:c74–c77, 2012.

Berg KB, Janelle GM: Descending thoracic aortic surgery: update on mortality, morbidity, risk assessment and management, *Curr Opin Crit Care* 18:393–398, 2012.

Bickley LS, Szilagyi PG: *Bates guide to physical examination and history taking*, ed 11, Philadelphia, 2013, Wolters Kluwer Health/Lippincott, Williams and Wilkins.

Bonatti J, Schachner T, Bonaros N, et al: Robotically assisted totally endoscopic coronary bypass surgery, *Circulation* 124:236–244, 2011.

Bonow RO, Mann DL, Zipes DP, editors: *Braunwald's heart disease: a textbook of cardiovascular medicine*, Philadelphia, 2012, Saunders Elsevier.

Brashers VL: Alterations of cardiovascular function. In McCance KL, Huether SE, editors: *Pathophysiology: the biologic basis for disease in adults and children*, ed 5, 2006, Elsevier Mosby.

Braverman AC: Acute aortic dissection: clinician update, *Circulation* 122:184–188, 2010.

Brodie BR: Aspiration thrombectomy with primary PCI for STEMI: review of the data and current guidelines, *J Invasive Cardiol* 22(10, Suppl B):2B–5B, 2010.

Brott TG, Halperin JL, Abbara S et al: 2011 ASA/ACCF/AHA/AANN/AANS/ACR/ASNR/CNS/SAIP/SCAI/SIR/SNIS/SVM/SVS Guideline on the management of patients with extracranial carotid and vertebral artery disease: a report of the American College of Cardiology Foundation/American Heart Association Task Force on Practice Guidelines, and the American Stroke Association, American Association of Neuroscience Nurses, American Association of Neuroradiology, Congress of Neurological Surgeons, Society of Atherosclerosis Imaging and Prevention, Society for Cardiovascular Angiography and Interventions, Society of Interventional Radiology, Society of NeuroInterventional Surgery, Society for Vascular Medicine, and Society for Vascular Surgery, *Circulation* 124:e54–e130, 2011.

Bruce CJ, Connolly HM: Right-sided valve disease deserves a little more respect, *Circulation* 119:2726–2734, 2009.

Brueck M, Cengiz H, Hoeltgen R, et al: Usefulness of N-acetylcysteine or ascorbic acid versus placebo to prevent contrast-induced acute kidney injury in patients undergoing elective cardiac catheterization: a single-center, prospective, randomized, double-blind, placebo-controlled trial, *J Invasive Cardiol* 25:276–283, 2013.

Brulotte V, Leblond FA, Elkouri S, et al: Bicarbonates for the prevention of postoperative renal failure in endovascular aortic aneurysm repair: a randomized pilot trial, *Anesthesiol Res Pract* 2013(467326), 2013. http://www.ncbi.nlm.nih.gov/pmc/articles/PMC3694372/.

Brusch J: *Infective endocarditis*. http://emedicine.medscape.com/article/216650–overview.

Bulechek GM, Butcher HK, Dochterman JM, et al, editors: *Nursing interventions classification*, St. Louis, 2013, Elsevier.

Buxton AE, Ellison KE, Lorvidhaya P, et al: Left ventricular ejection fraction for sudden death risk stratification ad guiding implantable cardioverter-defibrillators implantation, *J Cardiovasc Pharmacol* 55:450–455, 2010.

Cannon CP, Brindis RG, Chaitman BR, et al: 2013 ACCF/AHA Key data elements and definitions for measuring the clinical management and outcomes of patients with acute coronary syndromes and coronary artery disease: a report of the American College of Cardiology Foundation/American Heart Association Task Force on Clinical Data Standards (Writing Committee to Develop Acute Coronary Syndromes and Coronary Artery Disease Clinical Data Standards), *Circulation* 127:1052–1089, 2013.

Caputo R: *Currently approved vascular closure devices*, September/October 2012, Cardiac Interventions Today, pp 70–76.

Centers for Disease Control and Prevention: *Recommendations and Reports*, 62(RR03):26, March 29, 2013. Appendix B: Duke Criteria for Infective Endocarditis.

Cheng MJ, Den Uil CA, Hoeks ES, et al: Percutaneous left ventricular assist devices vs. intra-aortic balloon pump counterpulsation for treatment of cardiogenic shock: a meta-analysis of controlled trials, *Eur Heart J* 30(17):2102–2108, 2009.

Chernecky CC, Berger BJ: *Laboratory tests and diagnostic procedures*, ed 6, St. Louis, 2012, Elsevier.

Christensen CR, Lewis PA: *Core curriculum for vascular nursing*, Philadelphia, 2014, Lippincott, Williams & Wilkins.

Colucci WS: *Atlas of heart failure cardiac function and dysfunction*, ed 5, New York, 2009, Springer Publishing.

Connor JA: Alterations of cardiovascular function in children: In McCance KL, Huether SE, editors: *Pathophysiology: the biologic basis for disease in adults and children*, ed 5, 2006, Elsevier Mosby.

Constantinou J, Jayia P, Hamilton G: Best evidence for medical therapy for carotid artery stenosis, *J Vasc Surg* 58:1129–1139, 2013.

Cooper BE: Review and update on inotropes and vasopressors, *AACN Adv Crit Care* 19:5–15, 2008.

Cooper HA, Panza JA: Cardiogenic shock, *Cardiol Clin* 31:567–580, 2013.

Cooper LT: Definition and classification of the cardiomyopathies. In: Mckenna WJ, editor: *UpToDate*, Waltham, 2013, Wolters Kluwer.

Cunha B, D'Elia A, Pawar N, et al: Viridans streptococcal (*Streptococcus intermedius*) mitral valve subacute bacterial endocarditis in a patient with mitral valve prolapse after a dental procedure: the importance of antibiotic prophylaxis, *Heart Lung* 39:64–72, 2010.

Danyi P, Elefteriades JA, Jovin IS: Medical therapy of thoracic aortic aneurysms: are we there yet? *Circulation* 124:1469–1476, 2011.

Daughenbaugh LA: Cardiomyopathy: an overview, *J Nurse Practitioners* April 3:248–258, 2007.

Davis EL: Evaluation and management of the adult with bicuspid aortic valve disease, *J Nurse Practitioners* 6:349–357, 2010.

Den Uil AC, Lagrand KW, Valk SDA, et al: Management of cardiogenic shock: focus on tissue perfusion, *Curr Probl Cardiol* 34:330–349, 2009.

DeSimone D, Imad T, Correa de Sa D, et al: Incidence of infective endocarditis caused by Viridans, group streptococci before and after publication of the 2007 American Heart Association endocarditis prevention guidelines, *Circulation* 126:60–64, 2012.

Di Franco A, Vilano A, Di Monaco V, et al: Correlation between coronary microvascular function and angina status in patients with stable microvascular angina, *Eur Rev Medical Pharmacol Sci* 18:374–379, 2014.

Dixon M: Misdiagnosing aortic dissection: a fatal mistake, *J Vasc Nurs* 29:139–146, 2011.

Dolinger C, Strider DV: Endovascular interventions for descending thoracic aortic aneurysms: the pivotal role of the clinical nurse in postoperative care, *J Vasc Nurs* 28:147–153, 2010.

Dressler DK: Death by clot: acute coronary syndromes, ischemic stroke, pulmonary embolism, and disseminated intravascular coagulation, *AACN Adv Crit Care* 20:166–176, 2009.

Drozda J Jr, Messer JV, Spertus J, et al: ACCF/AHA/AMA-PCPI 2011 performance measures for adults with coronary artery disease and hypertension: a report of the American College of Cardiology Foundation/American Heart Association Task Force on Performance Measures and the American Medical Association–Physician Consortium for Performance Improvement, *Circulation* 124:248–270, 2011.

ECG Training Center: electrocardiogram center. http://www.practicalclinicalskills.com/ekg.aspx.

Eckel RH, Jakicic JM, Ard JD, et al: AHA/ACC guideline on lifestyle management to reduce cardiovascular risk: a report of the American College of Cardiology/American Heart Association Task Force on Practice Guidelines, *Circulation* 129:579–599, 2013.

Epstein AE, DiMarco JP, Ellenbogen KA, et al: American College of Cardiology Foundation, American Heart Association Task Force on Practice Guidelines, Heart Rhythm Society, 2012 ACCF/AHA/HRS focused update incorporated into the ACCF/AHA/HRS 2008 guidelines for device-based therapy of cardiac rhythm abnormalities: a report of the American College of Cardiology Foundation/American Heart Association Task Force, *J Am Coll Cardiol* 61:e6–75, 2013.

Fann JI, Ingels NB, Miller DC: Pathophysiology of mitral valve disease, chapter 41. In *Cardiac surgery in the adult*, ed 3, New York, 2008, McGraw-Hill.

Fihn SD, Gardin JM, Abrams J, et al: 2012 ACCF/AHA/ACP/AATS/PCNA/SCAI/STS guideline for the diagnosis and management of patients with stable ischemic heart disease: a report of the American College of Cardiology Foundation/American Heart Association Task Force on Practice Guidelines, and the American College of Physicians, American Association for Thoracic Surgery, Preventive Cardiovascular Nurses Association, Society for Cardiovascular Angiography and Interventions, and Society of Thoracic Surgeons, *Circulation* 126:e3, 2012.

Filippatos G, Farmakis D, Parissis J: Novel biomarkers in acute coronary syndromes: new molecules, new concepts, but what about new treatment strategies? *J Am Coll Cardiol* 63:1654–1656, 2014.

Fiore MC, Jaén CR, et al: *Clinical practice guideline, treating tobacco use and dependence: 2008 update*, May 2008, U.S. Department of Health and Human Services. http://www.surgeongeneral.gov/tobacco/treating_tobacco_use.pdf.

Flack JM, Sica DA, Bakris G, et al: International Society on Hypertension in Blacks. Management of high blood pressure in blacks: an update of the International Society on Hypertension in Blacks consensus statement, *Hypertension* 56:780–800, 2010.

Florian A, Slavich M, Masci PG, et al: Electrocardiographic Q-wave "remodeling" in reperfused ST segment elevation myocardial infarction: validation study with CMR, *JACC Cardiovasc Imaging* 5:1003–1013, 2012.

Francis GS, Greenberg BH, Hsu DT, et al: ACCF/AHA/ACP/HFSA/ISHLT 2010 clinical competence statement on management of patients with advanced heart failure and cardiac transplant: a report of the ACCF/AHA/ACP Task Force on Clinical Competence and Training, *Circulation* 122:644–672, 2010.

Gahart B, Nazaren A: *2014 intravenous medications: a handbook for nurses and health professionals*, St. Louis, 2013, Elsevier.

Garber AJ, Abrahamson MJ, Barzilay JI, et al: American Association of Clinical Endocrinologists' comprehensive diabetes management algorithm 2013 consensus statement—executive summary, *Endocr Pract* 19:536–557, 2013. doi: 10.4158/EP13176.CS.

Genereux P, Madhavan MV, Mintz GS, et al: Ischemic outcomes after coronary intervention of calcified vessels in acute coronary syndromes: pooled analysis from the horizons-AMI and acuity trials, *J Am Coll Cardiol* 63:1845–1854, 2014.

Gerber MA, Baltimore RS, Eaton CB, et al: Prevention of rheumatic fever and diagnosis and treatment of acute streptococcal pharyngitis: a scientific statement from the American Heart

Association Rheumatic Fever, Endocarditis, and Kawasaki Disease Committee of the Council on Cardiovascular Disease in the Young, the Interdisciplinary Council on Functional Genomics and Translational Biology, and the Interdisciplinary Council on Quality of Care and Outcomes Research: endorsed by the American Academy of Pediatrics, *Circulation* 119:1541-1551, 2009.

Gibbons GH, Harold JG, Jessup M, et al: The next steps in developing clinical practice guidelines for prevention, *J Am Coll Cardiol* 62:1399-1400, 2013.

Gibbons GH, Shurin SB, Mensah GA, et al: Refocusing the agenda on cardiovascular guidelines: an announcement from the National Heart, Lung, and Blood Institute, *Circulation* 128:1713-1715, 2013.

Go AS, Mozaffarian D, Roger VL, et al: on behalf of the American Heart Association Statistics Committee and Stroke Statistics Subcommittee: AHA statistical update: heart disease and stroke statistics—2014 update: a report from the American Heart Association, *Circulation* 129:e28-e292, 2014.

Goodlin SJ: Palliative care in congestive heart failure, *J Am Coll Cardiol* 54:386-396, 2009.

Haase J, Schafers HJ, Sievert H, et al, editors: *Cardiovascular interventions in clinical practice*, 2010, Wiley-Blackwell.

Habib G, Thuny F, Avierinos JF: Prosthetic valve endocarditis: current approach and therapeutic options, *Prog Cardiovasc Dis* 50:274-281, 2008.

Hagan PG, et al: International Registry of Acute Aortic Dissection (IRAD): new insights into an old disease, *JAMA* 283:897-903, 2000.

Halliday A, Bulbulia R, Gray W, et al: Status update and interim results from the asymptomatic carotid surgery trial-2 (ACST-2), *Eur J Vasc Endovasc Surg* 46:510-518, 2013.

Hanna EB, Glancy DL: ST-segment depression and T-wave inversion: classification, differential diagnosis, and caveats, *Cleve Clin J Med* 78:404-414, 2011.

Hancock EW, Deal BJ, Mirvis DM, et al: AHA/ACCF/HRS recommendations for the standardization and interpretation of the electrocardiogram: part V: electrocardiogram changes associated with cardiac chamber hypertrophy: a scientific statement from the American Heart Association Electrocardiography and Arrhythmias Committee, Council on Clinical Cardiology; the American College of Cardiology Foundation; and the Heart Rhythm Society: endorsed by the International Society for Computerized Electrocardiology, *Circulation* 119:e251, 2009.

Hazinski MF, Nolan JP, Billi JE, et al: Part 1: executive summary: 2010 international consensus on cardiopulmonary resuscitation and emergency cardiovascular care science with treatment recommendations, *Circulation* 122(Suppl 2):S250-S275, 2010.

Hazinski MF, Gilmore D: *American Heart Association handbook of emergency cardiovascular care for healthcare providers*, Dallas, 2011, American Heart Association.

Heart Failure Society of America, Lindfield J, Albert NM, et al: HFSA 2010 Comprehensive heart failure practice guideline, *J Card Fail* 16:e1, 2010.

Heart Sounds Easy Auscultation Web Sites.

Henderson R: Acute coronary syndrome: optimizing management through risk assessment, *Clin Med* 13:602-606, 2013.

Herkner H, Arrich J, Havel C, Mullner M: Bed rest for acute uncomplicated myocardial infarction, *Cochrane Database Syst Rev* (2):CD003836, 2007.

Hershberger R, Lindenfeld J, Mestroni L, et al: Genetic evaluation of cardiomyopathy—a Heart Failure Society of America practice guideline, *J Card Fail* 15:83-97, 2009.

Hillis LD, Smith PK, Anderson JL, et al: 2011 ACCF/AHA guideline for coronary artery bypass graft surgery: executive summary: a report of the American College of Cardiology Foundation/American Heart Association Task Force on Practice Guidelines, *Circulation* 124:2610-2642, 2011.

Hiratzka LF, Bakris GL, Beckman JA, et al: 2010 ACCF/AHA/AATS/ACR/ASA/ SCA/SCAI/SIR/STS/SVM guidelines for the diagnosis and management of patients with thoracic aortic disease: executive summary: a report of the American College of Cardiology Foundation/American Heart Association Task Force on Practice Guidelines, American association for Thoracic Surgery, American College of Radiology, American Stroke Association, Society of Cardiovascular Anesthesiologists, Society for Cardiovascular Angiography and Interventions, Society of Interventional Radiology, Society of Thoracic Surgeons, and Society for Vascular Medicine (developed in collaboration with the American College of Emergency Physicians), *J Am Coll Cardiol* 55:1509-1544, 2010.

Hirsch AT, Allison MA, Gomes AS, et al: A call to action: women and peripheral artery disease: a scientific statement from the American Heart Association, *Circulation* 125:1449-1472, 2012. http://circ.ahajournals.org/content/early/2012/02/15/CIR.0b013e31824c39ba.citation.

Holmes DR Jr, Mack MJ, Kaul S, et al: 2012 ACCF/AATS/SCAI/STS expert consensus document on transcatheter aortic valve replacement, *J Am Coll Cardiol* 59:1200-1254, 2012.

Htin A, Friedman N, Hughes A, et al: Outpatient parenteral antimicrobial therapy is safe and effective for the treatment of infective endocarditis: retrospective cohort study, *Int Med J* 43:700–705, 2013.

Hunt SA, Abraham WT, Chin MH, et al: 2009 focused update incorporated into the ACC/AHA 2005 guidelines for the diagnosis and management of heart failure in adults: a report of the American College of Cardiology Foundation/American Heart Association Task Force on Practice Guidelines, *Circulation* 119:e391–e479, 2009.

Hypertension Canada: *Hypertension without compelling indications: 2013 CHEP recommendations*, 2013. http://www.hypertension.ca /hypertension-without-compelling-indications.

Imazio M: *Evaluation and management of acute pericarditis.* http://www.uptodate.com/home/index. html.

Imazio M, Negro A, Belli R, et al: Frequency and prognostic significance of pericarditis following acute myocardial infarction treated by primary percutaneous coronary intervention, *Am J Cardiol* 103:1525–1529, 2009.

Isaac S: Contrast-induced nephropathy: nursing implications, *Crit Care Nurse* 32:41–48, 2012.

James PA, Oparil S, Carter BL, et al: 2014 evidence-based guideline for the management of high blood pressure in adults. Report from the panel members appointed to the Eighth Joint National Committee (JNC-8), *JAMA* 311:507–520, 2014.

Jellinger PS, Smith DA, Mehta AE, et al: American Association of Clinical Endocrinologists' guidelines for dyslipidemia and the prevention of atherosclerosis, *Endocr Pract* 18(Suppl 1):1–78. http://www.aace.com/files/lipid-guidelines.pdf.

Jennings GL, Esler MD: Circulatory regulation at rest and exercise and the functional assessment of patients with congestive heart failure, *Circulation* 81(Suppl 1):S115, 1990.

Jha AK, Li Z, Orav EJ, et al: Care in U.S. hospitals—the hospital quality alliance program, *N Engl J Med* 353:265–274, 2005.

Jneid H, Anderson JL, Wright RS, et al: 2012 ACCF/AHA focused update of the guideline for the management of patients with unstable angina/non-ST-elevation myocardial infarction (updating the 2007 guideline and replacing the 2011 focused update): a report of the American College of Cardiology Foundation/American Heart Association Task Force on Practice Guidelines, *Circulation* 126:875–910, 2012.

Kapelios CJ, Terrovitis JV, Nanas JN: Current and future applications of the intra-aortic balloon pump, *Curr Opin Cardiol* 29:258–265, 2014.

Kernan WN, Ovbiagele B, Black HR, et al: Guidelines for the prevention of stroke in patients with stroke and transient ischemic attack: a guideline for healthcare professionals from the American Heart Association/American Stroke Association, *Stroke* 45:2160–2236, 2014.

Kevin LJ, Barnard M: Right ventricular failure, *CEACCP* 7:89–94, 2007.

Kidney Disease; Improving Global Outcomes (KDIGO) Blood Pressure Work Group: KDIGO clinical practice guideline for the management of blood pressure in chronic kidney disease, *Kidney Int* 2(Suppl 5):337–414, 2012.

Kinlay S: Coronary artery spasm as a cause of angina, *Circulation* 129:1717–1719, 2014.

Krumholz HM, Normand SL: Public reporting of 30-day mortality for patients hospitalized with acute myocardial infarction and heart failure, *Circulation* 118:1394–1397, 2008.

Kuang XH, Zhang SY: Hyperthyroidism-associated coronary spasm: a case of non-ST segment elevation myocardial infarction with thyrotoxicosis, *J Geriatr Cardiol* 8:258–259, 2011.

Kumar A, Cannon CP: Acute coronary syndromes: diagnosis and management, part II, *Mayo Clin Proc* 84:1021–1036, 2009.

Kumar A, Cannon CP: Acute coronary syndromes: diagnosis and management, part I, *Mayo Clin Proc* 84:917–938, 2009.

Lalani T, Cabell C, Benjamin D, et al: Analysis of the impact of early surgery on the in-hospital mortality of native valve endocarditis: use of propensity score and instrumental variable methods to adjust for treatment-selection bias, *Circulation* 121:1005–1013, 2010.

Laslett LJ, Alagona P Jr, Clark BA III, et al: The worldwide environment of cardiovascular disease: prevalence, diagnosis, therapy, and policy issues: a report from the American College of Cardiology, *J Am Coll Cardiol* 60(Suppl 25):S1–S49, 2012.

Leeper B: Valvular disease and surgery. In Carlson KK, editor: *American Association of Critical Care Nurses: advanced critical care nursing*, 2009, Saunders Elsevier.

Leon MB, Smith CR, Mack M, et al: Transcatheter aortic-valve implantation for aortic stenosis in patients who cannot undergo surgery, *N Engl J Med* 363:1597–1607, 2010.

Libby P, Bonow RO, Mann DL, et al: *Braunwald's heart disease: a textbook of cardiovascular medicine*, ed 8, Philadelphia, 2008, Saunders Elsevier.

Libby P, Bonow RO, Zipes DP, et al: Valvular heart disease, chapter 62. In *Braunwald's heart disease*, ed 8, Philadelphia, 2008, Saunders Elsevier.

Valvular Heart Disease

Linde JJ, Kofoed KF, Sorgaard M, et al: Cardiac computed tomography guided treatment strategy in patients with recent acute-onset chest pain: results from the randomized, controlled trial: cardiac CT in the treatment of acute chest pain (CATCH), *Int J Cardiol* 168:5257–5262, 2013.

Luber S, Fischer D, Venkat A: Care of the bariatric surgery patient in the emergency department, *J Emerg Med* 34:13–20, 2008.

Mancia G, Fagard R, Narkiewicz K, et al: 2013 ESH/ESC guidelines for the management of arterial hypertension: the Task Force for the Management of Arterial Hypertension of the European Society of Hypertension (ESH) and of the European Society of Cardiology (ESC), *Eur Heart J* 34:2159–2219, 2013.

Maron BJ, Towbin JA, Thiene G, et al: Contemporary definitions and classification of the cardiomyopathies. An American Heart Association scientific statement from the Council on Clinical Cardiology, Heart Failure and Transplantation Committee; Quality of Care and Outcomes Research and Functional Genomics and Translational Biology Interdisciplinary Working Groups; and Council on Epidemiology and Prevention, *Circulation* 113:1807–1816, 2006.

Masoudi FA, et al: ACC/AHA statement on performance measurement and reperfusion therapy, *Circulation* 118:2649–2661, 2008.

Marshall K: Acute coronary syndrome: diagnosis, risk assessment and management, *Nursing Standard* 25:47–57, 2010.

Masse L, Antonacci M: Low cardiac output syndrome: identification and management, *Crit Care Nurs Clin North Am* 17:375–378, 2005.

McCance KL, Huether SE, editors: *Pathophysiology: the biologic basis for disease in adults and children*, ed 5, St. Louis, 2009, Elsevier Mosby.

McClave SA, Martindale RG, Vanek VW, et al: Guidelines for the provision and assessment of nutrition support therapy in the adult critically ill patient: Society of Critical Care Medicine (SCCM) and American Society for Parenteral and Enteral Nutrition (A.S.P.E.N.), *JPEN J Parenter Enteral Nutr* 33:277–316, 2009.

McHale Wiegand L: *AACN procedure manual for critical care*, ed 6, St. Louis, 2011, Elsevier.

Mead NE, O'Keefe KP: Wellen's syndrome: an ominous EKG pattern, *J Emerg Trauma Shock* 2:206–208, 2009.

Mehta SR, Granger CB, Boden WE, et al: Early versus delayed invasive intervention in acute coronary syndromes, *N Engl J Med* 360:2165–2175, 2009.

Moll FL, Powell JT, Fraedrich G, et al: Management of abdominal aortic aneurysms clinical practice guidelines of the European Society of Vascular Surgery, *Eur J Vasc Endovasc Surg* 41:S1–S58, 2011.

Morton PG, Fontaine DK: *Critical care nursing: a holistic approach*, ed 9, Philadelphia, 2009, Lippincott, Williams and Wilkins.

Mosca L, Banka CL, Benjamin EJ, et al: AHA guideline: evidence-based guideline for prevention of cardiovascular disease in women: 2007 update, *Circulation* 115:1481–1501, 2007.

Mosca L, Benjamin EJ, Berra K, et al: Effectiveness-based guidelines for the prevention of cardiovascular disease in women: 2011 update: guidelines from the American Heart Association, *Circulation* 123:1243–1262, 2011.

Moser D, Riegel B: *Cardiac nursing, a companion to Braunwald's heart disease*, St. Louis, 2008, Saunders Elsevier.

Mueller C: Biomarkers and acute coronary syndromes: an update, *Eur Heart J* 35:552–556, 2014.

Munro N: Cardiac surgery. In Morton PG, Fontaine DK, editors: *Critical care nursing: a holistic approach*, ed 9, Philadelphia, 2009, Lippincott Williams & Wilkins.

National Institute for Health and Clinical Excellence: *Hypertension (CG127)*, 2011. http://www.nice.org.uk/guidance/cg127.

National Heart Foundation of Australia (National Blood Pressure and Vascular Disease Advisory Committee): *Guide to management of hypertension 2008, quick reference guide for health professionals*, 2008. http://www.heartfoundation.org.au/Professional_Information/Clinical_Practice/Hypertension/Pages/default.aspx.

Nativi-Nicolau J, Selzman CH, Fang JC, et al: Pharmacologic therapies for acute cardiogenic shock, *Curr Opin Cardiol* 29:1–7, 2014.

Neergaard-Petersen S, Ajjan R, Hvas AM, et al: Fibrin clot structure and platelet aggregation in patients with aspirin treatment failure, *PLoS One* 8:e71150, 2013.

Nienaber CA, Kische S, Rousseau H, et al, for the INSTEAD-XL trial: Endovascular repair of type B aortic dissection: long-term results of the randomized investigation of stent grafts in aortic dissection trial, *Circ Cardiovasc Interv* 6:407–416, 2013.

Nishimura RA, Otto CM, Bonow RO, et al: 2014 AHA/ACC Guideline for the Management of Patients With Valvular Heart Disease: A Report of the American College of Cardiology/American Heart Association Task Force on Practice Guidelines, *J Am Coll Cardiol* 63(22):e57–e185, 2014. doi:10.1016/j.jacc.2014.02.536.

Nishimura RA, Otto CM, Bonow RO, et al: 2014 AHA/ACC guideline for the management of patients with valvular heart disease: executive summary: a report of the American College of Cardiology/American Heart Association Task Force on Practice Guidelines, *Circulation* 129:2440–2492, 2014.

O'Gara PT, Kushner FG, Ascheim DD, et al: 2013 ACCF/AHA guideline for the management of ST-elevation myocardial infarction: executive summary: a report of the American College of Cardiology Foundation/American Heart Association Task Force on Practice Guidelines, *Circulation* 127:529–555, 2013.

O'Malley RG, Bonaca MP, Scirica BM, et al: Prognostic performance of multiple biomarkers in patients with non-ST elevation acute coronary syndrome: analysis from Merlin-Timi 36, *J Am Coll Cardiol* 63:1644–1653, 2014.

Packer M, Colucci W, Fisher L, et al: Effect of levosimendan on short-term clinical course of patients with acutely decompensated heart failure, *JACC Heart Failure* 1:103, 2013.

Patarroyo M, Wehbe E, Hanna M, et al: Cardiorenal outcomes after slow continuous ultrafiltration therapy in refractory patients with advanced decompensated heart failure, *J Am Coll Cardiol* 60:1906–1912, 2012.

Perry JJ, Sharma M, Sivilotti ML, et al: A prospective cohort study of patients with transient ischemic attack to identify high-risk clinical characteristics, *Stroke* 45:92–100.

Petros S, Horbach M, Seidel F, et al: Hypocaloric vs normocaloric nutrition in critically ill patients: a prospective randomized pilot trial, *JPEN J Parenter Enteral Nutr,* published online 3 April 2014. doi: 10.1177/0148607114528980.

Pieracci F, Barie P, Pomp A: *Critical care of the bariatric patient,* 34:1796–1804, 2006.

Pinto DS, Kociol RD: Evaluation of acute decompensated heart failure. In Colucci WS, editor: *UpToDate,* Waltham, 2014, Wolters Kluwer.

Poole JE: Present guidelines for device implantation: clinical considerations and clinical challenges from pacing, implantable cardiac defibrillator, and cardiac resynchronization therapy, *Circulation* 129:383–394, 2014.

Pradhan D, Jian S, Shrestha R, et al: Clinical significance of ST segment elevation in posterior leads V7, V8 and V9 in patients with acute inferior wall myocardial infarction, *J Cardiovasc Dis Diagnosis* 1:2013. http://dx.doi.org/10.4172/2329-9517.1000106.

Pyeritz RE: Heritable thoracic aortic disorders, *Curr Opin Cardiol* 29:97–102, 2014.

Reiter MR, Twerenbold T, Reichlin P, et al: Early diagnosis of acute myocardial infarction in the elderly using more sensitive cardiac troponin assays, *Eur Heart J* 32:1379–1389, 2011.

Reiter R, Henry TD, Traverse JH: Pre-infarction angina reduces infarct size in ST-elevation myocardial infarction treated with percutaneous coronary intervention, *Circulation Cardiovasc Interv* 6:52–58, 2013.

Rennard S, Rigotti N, Daughton D: *Pharmacotherapy for smoking cessation in adults,* March 16, 2014, Up to Date. http://www.uptodate.com/contents/pharmacotherapy-for-smoking-cessation-in-adults.

Riegel B, Moser DK, Anker SD, et al: on behalf of the American Heart Association Council on Cardiovascular Nursing, Council on Clinical Cardiology, Council on Nutrition, Physical Activity, and Metabolism, and Interdisciplinary Council on Quality of Care and Outcomes Research: state of the science: promoting self-care in persons with heart failure: a scientific statement from the American Heart Association, *Circulation* 120:1141–1163, 2009.

Ristow B, Ali S, Ren X, et al: Elevated pulmonary artery pressure by Doppler echocardiography predicts hospitalization for heart failure and mortality in ambulatory stable coronary artery disease: the Heart and Soul Study, *J Am Coll Cardiol* 49:43–49, 2007.

Rivera-Bou WL: *Thrombolytic agents.* http://emedicine.medscape.com/article/811234-overview #aw2aab6b3.

Rivera-Bou WL: *Thrombolytic therapy for acute myocardial infarction.* http://emedicine.medscape.com/article/811234-overview#aw2aab6b4.

Rogers AM, Hermann LK, Booher AM, et al: Sensitivity of the aortic dissection risk score, a novel guideline-based tool for identification of acute aortic dissection at initial presentation: results from the international registry of acute aortic dissection, *Circulation* 123:2213–2218, 2011.

Rooke TW, et al: 2011 ACCF/AHA Focused update on the guideline for the management of patients with peripheral artery disease (updating the 2005 guideline): a report of the American College of Cardiology Foundation/American Heart Association Task Force on Practice Guidelines, *J Am Coll Cardiol* 58:2020–2045, 2011.

Sadanandan S: The obsession with finding ST segment elevation on a 12-lead EKG, *J Electrocardiol* 46:16–18, 2013.

Saw J: Carotid artery stenting for stroke prevention, *Can J Cardiol* 30:22–34, 2014.

Schey R, Villarreal A, Fass R: Non-cardiac chest pain: current treatment, *Gastroenterol Hepatol* 3:255–262, 2007.

Valvular Heart Disease

Schiffner A: Glucose management in critically ill medical and surgical patients, *Dimens Critical Care Nurs* 33:70–77, 2014.

Schindler TH, Schelbert HR, Quercioli A, et al: Cardiac PET imaging for the detection and monitoring of coronary artery disease and microvascular health, *JACC Cardiovasc Imaging* 3:623–640, 2010.

Schlett CL, Pursnani A, Marcus RP, et al: The use of coronary CT angiography for the evaluation of chest pain, *Cardiol Rev* 22:117–127, 2014.

Schocken D, et al: Prevention of heart failure, *Circulation* 119:e391–e479, 2009.

Shah PM, Raney AA: Tricuspid valve disease, *Curr Probl Cardiol* 33:47–84, 2008.

Shizuyuki S, Kajimoto K, Miyauchi K, et al: Comparing outcomes after off-pump coronary artery bypass versus drug eluting stent in diabetic patients, *J Cardiol* 59:195–201, 2012.

Silvain J, Beygui F, Barthelemy O, et al: Efficacy and safety of enoxaparin versus unfractionated heparin during percutaneous coronary intervention: systematic review and meta-analysis, *BMJ* 344:e553, 2012.

Simms AD, Batin PD, Kurian J, et al: Acute coronary syndromes: an old age problem, *J Geriatr Cardiol* 9:192–196, 2012.

Singer P, Pichard C: Reconciling divergent results of the latest parenteral nutrition studies in the ICU, *Curr Opin Clin Nutr Metab Care* 16:187–193, 2013.

Sismanoglu M, Sarikaya S, Onk OA, et al: Treatment of left anterior descending coronary artery stenosis: stent or surgery, *Asian Cardiovasc Thorac Ann* 21:528–532, 2012.

Skidmore-Roth L: *Mosby's 2014 nursing drug reference*, ed 27, St. Louis, 2014, Mosby.

Smith SC Jr, Benjamin EJ, Bonow RO, et al: AHA/ACCF secondary prevention and risk reduction therapy for patients with coronary and other atherosclerotic vascular disease: 2011 update: a guideline from the American Heart Association and American College of Cardiology Foundation, *Circulation* 124:2458–2473, 2011.

Spangler S, Fredi J: *Acute pericarditis treatment and management*, 2013. http://emedicine.medscape.com/article/156951-Treatment.

Stella LB: Understanding core measures for heart-failure treatment, *Am Nurse Today* 8:2013. http://www.americannursetoday.com/understanding-core-measures-for-heart-failure-treatment/.

Stevenson LW, Pagini FD, Young JB, et al: INTERMACS profiles of advanced heart failure: the current picture, *J Heart Lung Transplant* 28:535–541, 2009.

Stone NJ, Robinson J, Lichtenstein AH, et al: 2013 ACC/AHA Guideline on the treatment of blood cholesterol to reduce atherosclerotic cardiovascular risk in adults: A report of the American College of Cardiology/American Heart Association Task Force on Practice Guidelines, *Circulation* 129(Suppl 1):S1–S45, 2014.

Suryadevarra RS, Skelding K: Radial access for coronary angiography and percutaneous coronary artery intervention, *Cardiac Interv Today* 64–69, September/October 2012.

Tamis-Holland JE, O'Gara P: Highlights from the 2013 ACCF/AHA guidelines for the management of ST-elevation myocardial infarction and beyond, *Clin Cardiol* 37:252–259, 2013.

The Merck Manuals: *Pericarditis, the Merck manual for healthcare professionals*. http://www.merck.com/mmpe/sec07/ch078/ch078a.html.

The Task Force for the Diagnosis and Treatment of Acute and Chronic Heart Failure 2012 of the European Society of Cardiology: ESC guidelines for the diagnosis and treatment of acute and chronic heart failure 2012, *Eur Heart J* 33:1787–1847, 2012.

Thuny F, Grisoli D, Collart F, et al: Management of infective endocarditis: challenges and perspectives, *Lancet* 379:965–975, 2012.

Thomas RJ, King M, Lui K, et al: AACVPR/ACC/AHA 2007 performance measures on cardiac rehabilitation for referral to and delivery of cardiac rehabilitation/secondary prevention services, *Circulation* 116:1611–1642, 2007.

Tracy CM, Epstein AE, Darbar D, et al: 2012 ACCF/AHA/HRS focused update of the 2008 guidelines for device-based therapy of cardiac rhythm abnormalities: a report of the American College of Cardiology Foundation/American Heart Association Task Force on Practice Guidelines and the Heart Rhythm Society, *Circulation* 126:1784–1800, 2012.

Tsounis D, Deftereos S, Bouras G, et al: High sensitivity troponin in cardiovascular disease: is there more than a marker of myocardial death? *Curr Top Med Chem* 13:201–215, 2013.

Unger T: The role of the rennin-angiotensin-aldosterone system in heart failure, *J Renin-Angio-Aldo S* 5(Suppl 1):S7–S10, 2004.

Unverzagt SL, Wachsmuth K, Hirsch H, et al: Inotropic agents and vasodilator strategies for acute myocardial infarction complicated by cardiogenic shock or low cardiac output syndrome, *Cochrane Database Syst Rev* 1:CD009669, 2014.

Upadhye S, Schiff K: Acute aortic dissection in the emergency department: diagnostic challenges and evidence-based management, *Emerg Med Clin North Am* 30:307–327, 2012.

U.S. Department of Health and Human Services, Centers for Disease Control and Prevention, National Center for Chronic Disease Prevention and Health Promotion, Office on Smoking and Health: *How tobacco smoke causes disease: the biology and behavioral basis for smoking-attributable disease: a report of the surgeon general,* 2010. http://www.cdc.gov/tobacco/data_statistics/sgr/2010/index.htm?s_cid=cs_1843.

U.S. Preventive Services Task Force: *Screening for carotid artery stenosis: recommendation statement,* 2014. http://www.uspreventiveservicestaskforce.org/uspstf07/cas/casrs.htm.

Valenta I, Quericoli A, Schindler TH: Diagnostic value of PET measured longitudinal flow gradient for the identification of coronary artery disease, *JACC Cardiovascular Imaging* 7:387–396, 2014.

Velasco M, Rojas E: Non-Q-wave myocardial infarction: comprehensive analysis of electrocardiogram, pathophysiology, and therapeutics, *Am J Ther* 20:432–441, 2013.

Warkentin TE, Greinacher A, Koster A: Bivalirudin, *Thromb Haemost* 99:830–839, 2008.

Weintraub NL, Collins SP, Pang PS, et al, on behalf of the American Heart Association Council on Clinical Cardiology and Council on Cardiopulmonary, Critical Care, Perioperative and Resuscitation: acute heart failure syndromes: emergency department presentation, treatment, and disposition: current approaches and future aims: a scientific statement from the American Heart Association, *Circulation* 122:1975–1996, 2010.

White A, Broder J: Aortic emergencies—part 1, *Adv Emerg Nurs J* 34:216–229, 2012.

White A, Broder J: Aortic emergencies—part 2, *Adv Emerg Nurs J* 35:28–52, 2013.

Whitman I, Patel VV, Soliman EZ, et al: Validity of the surface electrocardiogram criteria for right ventricular hypertrophy: the MESA-right ventricle study, *Circulation* 63:672–681, 2013.

Wright P, Antoniou S: Acute coronary syndrome: potent oral antiplatelets, *Nurse Prescribing* 11:397–400, 2013.

Yancy CW, Jessup M, Bozkurt B, et al: 2013 ACCF/AHA guideline for the management of heart failure: a report of the American College of Cardiology Foundation/American Heart Association Task Force on Practice Guidelines, *J Am Coll Cardiol* 62(16):e147–239, 2013.

Yayan J: Emerging families of biomarkers for coronary artery disease: inflammatory mediators, *Vasc Health Risk Manag* 9:435–456, 2013.

Yilmaz A, Kindermann I, Kinderman M, et al: Comparative evaluation of left and right ventricular endomyocardial biopsy: differences in complication rate and diagnostic performance, *Circulation* 122:900, 2010.

Zwar N, Richmond R, Borland R, et al: *Supporting smoking cessation: a guide for health professionals,* Melbourne, 2011, The Royal Australian College of General Practitioners. http://www.treatobacco.net/en/uploads/documents/Treatment%20Guidelines/Australia%20treatment%20guidelines%20in%20English%202011.pdf.

Kidney Injury

GENITOURINARY ASSESSMENT: GENERAL

GOAL OF SYSTEM ASSESSMENT

Evaluate for decreased renal function and assess the severity of renal dysfunction.

DETAILED HEALTH HISTORY

- Chronic symptoms of fatigue, weight loss, anorexia, nocturia, and pruritus.
- Renal-related symptoms including dysuria, edema, frequency, hematuria, flank pain, pyuria, frothy urine, bloody urine, and renal colic.
- Presence of comorbidities: hypertension, congestive heart failure, diabetes, multiple myeloma, chronic infection, and myeloproliferative disorder.
- Current medications including over-the-counter medications.
- Exposure to chemicals.
- Recent trauma or unaccustomed exertion.
- Recent diagnostic studies requiring dye administration.
- **Considerations for the bariatric patient:** History of difficult urinary catheterization

OBSERVATION

Evidence of chronic versus acute process:
- Skin: petechiae, purpura, ecchymosis, livedo reticularis, dryness, pallor, yellowness, decreased turgor.
- Eyes: uveitis, ocular palsy, findings suggestive of hypertension, atheroembolic disease.
- Inspection of the flank area in a standing and supine position for raised masses or unusual pulsations.
- **Considerations for the bariatric patient**: Large folds of abdominal skin covering the genitourinary area causing retracted penis or vagina. Look for bulging areas that could be a hernia. Adequate urinary output is 0.5/kg/h.

VITAL SIGN ASSESSMENT

Evaluate for changes indicative of fluid volume excess or depletion and infection.
- Blood pressure (BP) and pulse both lying and standing.
- Respiratory rate (RR).
- Height and weight.
- Temperature.

PALPATION

Abdominal assessment to identify renal pathology:
- Costovertebral angle tenderness, which may occur with pyelonephritis.
- Enlarged liver, which may occur with congestive heart failure.
- Kidneys are difficult to palpate because of location. If they are enlarged and palpable, this could represent polycystic kidney disease or hydronephrosis.
- Ascites may occur with liver failure or acute renal failure.
- Lower extremity or sacral edema.
- Bladder tenderness and distension.

AUSCULTATION

- Cardiac auscultation for the presence of murmurs, pericardial friction rub, S_3 and/or S_4 and congestive heart failure.
- Lung auscultation for the presence of pleural rub, rales, decreased breath sounds, and volume excess states.

LABWORK

Renal dysfunction causes marked changes in fluid and electrolyte balance, acid-base balance, and red cell production, and increased concentrations of blood urea nitrogen (BUN) and creatinine.

- Complete blood count (CBC) to evaluate anemia.
- Electrolytes including calcium, phosphorus, and magnesium.
- BUN and creatinine.
- Estimated glomerular filtration rate (eGFR) to evaluate clearance.
- 24-hour urine collection for creatinine clearance, protein, and metanephrines.
- Urinalysis.
- Urine electrolytes.
- **Considerations for the bariatric patient**: Monitor creatinine levels.

ACUTE KIDNEY INJURY

PATHOPHYSIOLOGY

Acute kidney injury (AKI) is a complex syndrome characterized by a rapid decline in GFR that results in disturbances in fluid, electrolyte, and acid-base balances. The evolution of AKI can occur over a number of hours to days and is usually accompanied by a marked decline in urine output and retention of metabolic wastes including urea and creatinine. The Kidney Disease/Improving Global Outcomes (KDIGO) clinical practice guidelines define three stages of AKI that reflect changes in serum creatinine and urine output (Table 6-1). These stages provide the basis for early recognition and stage-based management of AKI.

Formation of urine is a three-step process consisting of (1) ultrafiltration of delivered blood by the glomeruli (renal cortex), (2) internal processing of the ultrafiltrate via tubular secretion and reabsorption (renal parenchyma), and (3) excretion of waste products from the kidneys through the ureters, bladder, and urethra. Corresponding to those steps, AKI is categorized as prerenal, intrarenal, and postrenal (Table 6-2).

Prerenal AKI, or azotemia, is the result of decreased blood flow to the kidneys below the limit of autoregulation. Autoregulation is the process by which the kidneys maintain a relatively constant level of renal blood flow and GFR. In response to low renal blood flow, preglomerular arterioles vasodilate whereas postglomerular arterioles vasoconstrict. The net

Table 6-1	KIDNEY DISEASE/IMPROVING GLOBAL OUTCOMES (KDIGO) CRITERIA FOR THE DIAGNOSIS OF ACUTE KIDNEY INJURY	
Stage	**Serum Creatinine**	**Urine Output Criteria**
1	1.5 to 1.9 baseline OR ≥ 0.3 mg/dL (≥ 26.5 μmol/L) increase	<0.5 mL/kg/h for 6 to 12 hours
2	2.0 to 2.9 times baseline	<0.5 mL/kg/h for ≥ 12 hours
3	3.0 times baseline OR Increase in serum creatinine to ≥ 4.0 mg/dL (≥ 353.6 μmol/L) OR Initiation of renal replacement therapy OR in patients <18 years, decrease in estimated glomerular filtration rate to <35 mL/min per 1.73 m²	<0.3 mL/kg/h for ≥ 24 hours OR Anuria for ≥ 12 hour

Table 6-2	CAUSES OF ACUTE KIDNEY INJURY	
Prerenal	**Intrarenal**	**Postrenal**
Decreased Effective Arterial Volume	*Tubular Injury*	*Bladder Neck*
• Hypovolemia	• Ischemia	• Prostatic disease
• Decreased cardiac contractility	• Toxins (drugs, pigments)	• Pelvic malignancies
• Systemic vasodilation (sepsis)	• Interstitial	• Bladder carcinoma
Renal Vasoconstriction	• Allergic: beta-lactams, sulfa drugs, NSAIDs	• Neurogenic bladder
• NSAIDs	• Infection: pyelonephritis	*Ureteral*
• ACEIs	• Infiltrative: sarcoid, lymphoma, leukemia	• Nephrolithiasis
• Angiotensin blockers	*Glomerular Diseases*	• Urethral strictures
• Calcineurin inhibitors	• Poststreptococcal glomerulone-phritis	• Blood clots
• Hypercalcemia	• IgA nephropathy (e.g., Berger's disease)	• Retroperitoneal disease
• Hepatorenal syndrome	• Lupus glomerulonephritis	*Tubular*
Large Vessel-Renal Artery Issues	*Renal Vessel Disease*	• Precipitation of crystals
• Renal artery stenosis	• Thrombosis	
• Thrombosis	• Vasculitis	
• Embolism	• Atheroembolic	
• Dissection	• Microangiopathy	
• Vasculitis		
Increased Intraabdominal Pressure		
• Intraabdominal compartment syndrome		

ACEIs, Angiotensin-converting enzyme inhibitors; *GI*, gastrointestinal; *IgA*, immunoglobulin A; *NSAIDs*, nonsteroidal antiinflammatory drugs.

effect is relatively constant glomerular capillary hydrostatic pressure. Autoregulation is effective until the mean arterial pressure (MAP) drops lower than 75 to 80 mm Hg. While autoregulation fails, there is a reduction in GFR. Drugs that interfere with autoregulation such as angiotensin-converting enzyme inhibitors (ACEIs) and nonsteroidal antiinflammatory drugs (NSAIDs) may provoke prerenal AKI through exacerbating renal hypoperfusion. In response to reduced perfusion, stretch receptors in the glomerular afferent arterioles cause vasodilation. Vasodilation is also enhanced by the production of prostaglandins, kallikrein, kinins, and nitric oxide. NSAIDs inhibit prostaglandin production, thereby diminishing afferent arteriole vasodilation prompting low filtration pressure. Efferent arterioles normally increase vasoconstriction in response to angiotensin II. Angiotensin II inhibitors and blockers interfere with the efferent arteriole response to hypoperfusion. Patients receiving ACEIs with a glomerular filtration critically dependent on the angiotensin II–regulated efferent arteriole vascular tone (patients with heart failure or severe volume depletion) can experience low efferent arteriolar pressure, which contributes to reduced filtration. Prerenal AKI is reversible if treated promptly. Treatment is directed at the underlying cause of decreased renal blood flow. Intravascular volume depletion, reduced cardiac output, systemic vasodilation, renal vasoconstriction, and increased intraabdominal pressure are causes of hypoperfusion. A consequence of prolonged hypoperfusion includes renal tissue ischemia and the subsequent development of intrarenal AKI.

Intrarenal AKI is caused by direct insults to the glomerular or tubular structures. The most common form of intrarenal AKI is acute tubular necrosis (ATN). In addition to renal ischemia, ATN may be the result of nephrotoxic injury produced by medications, radiocontrast media, infection, and exposure to toxic substances such as heavy metals, pesticides, and organic solvents. Conditions that produce myoglobinuria and hemoglobinuria can also lead to tubular injury. Contrast material–induced nephropathy (CIN) is a form of ATN that develops within 12 to 48 hours of contrast administration. Risk factors for CIN include diabetes mellitus, chronic kidney disease, hypotension, volume depletion, cirrhosis, heart failure, and administration of nephrotoxic agents. Although the development of low-osmolality contrast agents and prevention protocols have reduced the incidence of CIN, most patients in the intensive care unit would have one or more risk factors for the development of CIN. Clinicians weigh the diagnostic benefit of using contrast material during imaging procedures and the risk of CIN.

RESEARCH BRIEF 6-1

Purpose: The authors conducted a systematic review and metaanalysis of controlled studies comparing the incidence of acute kidney injury (AKI) in patients who received intravenous (IV) contrast media with patients who underwent an imaging procedure without contrast media.

Methods: MEDLINE, EMBASE, Scopus, and the Cochrane Library were searched for studies that compared the incidence of AKI in patients exposed to IV contrast medium with the incidence of AKI in unexposed patients. Changes in serum creatinine level or estimated glomerular filtration rate 48 to 72 hours following imaging procedures or admission were used for the detection of AKI. Relative risk was calculated and tested in subgroups of different patient comorbidities, contrast medium types, and AKI diagnostic criteria.

Results: Thirteen nonrandomized studies (25,950 patients) met inclusion criteria. The average rate of AKI was 6.4% in the contrast medium group and 6.5% in the noncontrast group. The risks of AKI, dialysis, and death were similar for both groups regardless of IV contrast medium type, diagnostic criteria for AKI, or whether patients had diabetes mellitus or renal insufficiency.

Conclusion: Controlled contrast medium–induced nephropathy studies demonstrate a similar incidence of AKI, dialysis, and death between the contrast medium group and control group.

From McDonald J, McDonald R, Comin J, et al: Frequency of acute kidney injury following intravenous contrast medium administration: a systematic review and meta-analysis. *Radiology* 267:119-128, 2013.

ATN is characterized by tubular cell necrosis, cast formation, and tubular obstruction caused by casts and cellular debris. Therapy is focused on maintenance of renal perfusion pressure, administering renal vasodilators to restore blood flow, and promoting diuresis to "wash out" the intratubular debris. ATN is sometimes nonoliguric. Oliguria may occur with both toxic ATN and ischemic ATN. Common nephrotoxic agents are found in Table 6-3.

Postrenal failure is the least common cause of AKI and may be either intrarenal (within the kidney) or extrarenal (outside the kidney in another area of the elimination tract) obstruction. Intrarenal obstruction is often attributable to crystal deposition caused by medications (e.g., acyclovir, indinavir, sulfonamides, methotrexate) or endogenous substances (oxalate, uric acid). Extrarenal obstruction may be related to bladder outlet problems (prostate and urethral obstruction) or stones, clots, pus, tumor, fibrosis, or ligation of or papilla within the ureters.

Fluid, electrolyte, and acid-base disorders that occur with AKI include hypervolemia, hyperkalemia, hyperphosphatemia, hypocalcemia, hypermagnesemia, and metabolic acidosis (Table 6-4). Phosphate levels rise because of impaired excretion of phosphorus by the renal tubules with continued gastrointestinal (GI) absorption. Hypocalcemia results from the lack of active vitamin D, which is activated by the kidney, which would otherwise stimulate absorption of calcium from the GI tract, or high phosphate levels, which inhibit absorption of calcium. Hypocalcemia triggers the parathyroid glands to secrete parathyroid hormone (PTH), which mobilizes calcium from the bone into the blood. Hypermagnesemia is generally moderate (2 to 4 mg/dL) and is rarely symptomatic unless the patient receives magnesium-containing antacids (e.g., Maalox, Milk of Magnesia).

Table 6-3	COMMON NEPHROTOXINS
Exogenous	**Endogenous**
Antineoplastics • Methotrexate • Cisplatin *Antimicrobials* • Amphotericin • Aminoglycosides • Acyclovir • Penicillins *Nonsteroidal Antiinflammatory Drugs* • Ibuprofen • Ketorolac *Chemicals* • Ethylene glycol • Pesticides • Organic solvents • Radiocontrast Medium	Rhabdomyolysis Hemolysis Tumor Lysis Syndrome

Table 6-4	ALTERED ELECTROLYTE BALANCE IN ACUTE KIDNEY INJURY
Condition/Cause	**Nursing Implications**
Hyperkalemia	
Decreased ability to excrete K^+; K^+ release with catabolism	• Monitor ECG for tall and peaked T waves, loss of P waves, prolonged PR interval, widened QRS when K^+ is greater than 6.5 mEq/L. Cardiac arrest is more likely seen with K^+ greater than 7.5 mEq/L. • Monitor serum K^+ levels for values greater than 5 mEq/L. • Monitor the patient for indicators such as paresthesias, muscle weakness or flaccidity, and HR less than 60 bpm. • Teach the patient and significant others the indicators of hyperkalemia and the importance of notifying the nurse promptly if they occur. • Provide a list of foods high in potassium and emphasize the importance of avoiding these foods. • Implement the following to help minimize the cellular release of potassium: • Ensure the patient consumes only the amount of protein prescribed by the advanced practice provider ; enforce sound infection control techniques to minimize risk of infection; and treat fevers promptly. Catabolism of protein, which occurs in these situations, causes potassium to be released from tissues. • Ensure the patient consumes the allotted amounts of carbohydrates, and limit strenuous patient activity as prescribed, both of which will spare protein. • Be aware that hyperkalemia can be a fatal complication, especially during the oliguric phase of AKI, because of its adverse effect on cardiac status. Keep emergency supplies (i.e., manual resuscitator, crash cart, emergency drug tray) readily available.

Table 6-4	ALTERED ELECTROLYTE BALANCE IN ACUTE KIDNEY INJURY — cont'd

Condition/Cause	Nursing Implications
Hypokalemia	
Prolonged, inadequate oral intake; use of potassium-losing diuretics without proper replacement; excessive loss from vomiting, diarrhea, or gastric or intestinal suctioning	• Monitor ECG for prolonged PR interval, flattened or inverted. • T wave, depressed ST segment, presence of U wave, and ventricular dysrhythmias; ECG changes are more likely to occur at serum K^+ levels less than 3 mEq/L. • Be alert to serum K^+ less than 3.5 mEq/L. • Monitor the patient for muscle weakness, soft and flabby muscles, paresthesias, decreased bowel sounds, ileus, weak and irregular pulse, and distant heart sounds. • Neuromuscular symptoms are seen at serum levels of approximately 2.5 mEq/L. • Teach the patient and significant others the indicators of hypokalemia and the importance of notifying the nurse promptly if they occur. • Provide a list of foods high in potassium and assist with planning menus that incorporate them. • Administer potassium-sparing diuretics (e.g., spironolactone, triamterene) as prescribed. • Administer oral or IV potassium supplements as prescribed; for oral route, administer with at least 4 oz water or juice to minimize gastric irritation.
Hypernatremia	
The inability of the kidneys to excrete excess sodium; decreased water intake; increased water losses via osmotic diuresis; excessive parenteral administration of sodium-containing solutions (e.g., sodium bicarbonate, 3% sodium chloride)	• Monitor serum sodium levels for serum Na^+ greater than 147 mEq/L. • Monitor VS and I&O hourly; weigh the patient daily. • Be alert to dry mucous membranes, flushed skin, firm and rubbery tissue turgor, hyperthermia, oliguria, or anuria. • Assess sensorium for restlessness and agitation; institute seizure precautions as indicated. • Administer prescribed IV replacement fluids. • Administer diuretics as prescribed.
Hyponatremia	
Loss through vomiting, diarrhea, profuse diaphoresis; use of potent diuretics; salt-losing nephropathies; administration of large amount of sodium-free IV fluids (may be associated with fluid volume excess or postobstructive diuresis)	• Monitor for serum Na^+ less than 137 mEq/L. • Monitor input and output hourly; record weight daily for trend. • Assess the patient for abdominal cramps, diarrhea, nausea, dizziness when changing position, postural hypotension, cold and clammy skin, and apprehension. • Provide parenteral replacement therapy as prescribed. • Institute a safe environment for individuals with altered LOC.

Continued

Table 6-4	ALTERED ELECTROLYTE BALANCE IN ACUTE KIDNEY INJURY — cont'd
Condition/Cause	**Nursing Implications**

Hypocalcemia

Poor absorption of dietary calcium; precipitation of calcium out of tissues in the presence of elevated phosphorus level; inadequate absorption and use of calcium occurring with lack of conversion of vitamin D to its usable form	• Monitor for serum Ca^{2+} less than 8.5 mg/dL. • Monitor for numbness and tingling around the mouth, muscle twitching, facial twitching, and tonic muscle spasms. • Assess for Trousseau sign (carpopedal spasm) and Chvostek sign (spasm of lip and cheek). • Administer calcium and vitamin D supplements as prescribed. • Reinforce the necessity of taking these medications as prescribed. • Teach the patient and significant others the indicators of hypocalcemia. • Teach the importance of continued medical follow-up to check serum Ca^{2+} levels.

Hyperphosphatemia

Abnormal retention of phosphates caused by the inability of the kidneys to excrete excess phosphorus	• Monitor for serum phosphate greater than 4.5 g/dL. • Although most foods contain generous amounts of phosphate, those especially high in phosphate include beef, pork, dried beans, dried mature peas, and dairy products. Monitor the patient's diet accordingly. • Administer phosphate binders as prescribed. Assess for constipation, which may result from use of phosphate binders. • Teach the patient and significant others the relationship between calcium and phosphate levels in the body. • Emphasize that maintaining good phosphate control and calcium balance may help control itching and prevent future problems with bone disease. • Reinforce the need for follow-up visits to check serum phosphate levels.

Hypermagnesemia

Administration of magnesium-containing medications to patients with impaired renal function	• Monitor serum Mg^{2+} levels greater than 2.5 mEq/L. • Assess for diaphoresis, flushing, hypotension, drowsiness, weak-to-absent DTRs, bradycardia, lethargy, and respiratory impairment. • Teach the indicators listed above to the patient and significant others. • Avoid giving medications that contain magnesium (see Box 1-7). Emphasize to the patient that such medications should not be taken without the physician's approval.

Metabolic Acidosis

The inability of the kidneys to excrete excess acid produced by normal metabolic processes; marked tissue trauma, infection, and diarrhea may contribute to a more rapid development of acidosis (often associated with K^+ greater than 5 mEq/L)	• Monitor for HCO_3^- less than 22 mEq/L and pH less than 7.35. • Monitor input and output, LOC, and VS. • Be alert to Kussmaul's respirations, SOB, anorexia, headache, nausea, vomiting, weakness, apathy, fatigue, and coma. • Institute seizure precautions in the presence of altered LOC. • Administer IV fluids and bicarbonate as prescribed. • Teach the patient the importance of dietary restrictions, particularly of protein, and of maintaining adequate carbohydrate intake to prevent worsening acidosis. • Emphasize that the patient should report to the advanced practice provider increased temperature and other signs of infection. • Teach the patient the importance of taking sodium bicarbonate as prescribed and of maintaining the dialysis schedule (both hemodialysis and peritoneal dialysis help correct acidosis)

Table 6-4	ALTERED ELECTROLYTE BALANCE IN ACUTE KIDNEY INJURY — cont'd
Condition/Cause	**Nursing Implications**
Uremia	
Failure of the kidneys to excrete urea, creatinine, uric acid, and other metabolic waste products	• Monitor the patient for chronic fatigue, insomnia, anorexia, vomiting, metallic taste in the mouth, pruritus, increased bleeding tendency, muscular twitching, involuntary leg movements, decreasing attention span, anemia, muscle wasting, and weakness. • Teach the patient and significant others that the indicators of uremia develop gradually and are very subtle. Explain the importance of notifying the nurse of sudden worsening of the symptoms that may be present. • Monitor and record dietary intake of protein, potassium, and sodium. • Use lotions and oils to lubricate the patient's skin and relieve drying and cracking. • Provide oral hygiene at frequent intervals, using a soft-bristle toothbrush and mouthwash, to help combat the patient's thirst and the metallic taste caused by uremia. Chewing gum and hard candy may also help alleviate thirst and the unpleasant taste. • Encourage isometric exercises and short walks, if the patient is able, to help maintain the patient's muscle strength and tone, especially in the legs. • Teach significant others that because of the patient's decreasing concentration level, they should communicate with the patient by using simple and direct statements. • Teach the patient to maintain good nutrition by ingesting the allotted amounts of carbohydrates and high–biological value protein to support cell rebuilding and decrease waste products from protein breakdown. • Explain that profuse bleeding can occur with uremia and that knives, scissors, and other sharp instruments should be used with caution. • Stress that OTC medications such as aspirin and ibuprofen may enhance bleeding tendency. • Emphasize the importance of follow-up visits to evaluate the progression of uremia. • Stress that the dialysis schedule should be maintained to decrease the symptoms of uremia and correct many of the metabolic abnormalities that occur.

AKI, Acute kidney injury; Ca^{2+}, calcium; *DTR*, deep tendon reflex; *ECG*, electrocardiogram; HCO_3^-, bicarbonate; *HR*, heart rate; *I&O*, intake and output; *IV*, intravenous; K^+, potassium; *LOC*, level of consciousness; Mg^{2+}, magnesium; Na^+, sodium; *OTC*, over-the-counter; *SOB*, shortness of breath; *VS*, vital signs.

There are three identifiable stages/phases of AKI:
1. Oliguric phase: A drop in the 24-hour urinary output to less than 400 mL lasting approximately 7 to 14 days. Approximately 30% of patients have nonoliguric kidney failure.
2. Diuretic phase: A doubling of the urinary output from the previous 24-hour total. During this phase the patient may produce as much as 3 to 5 L of urine in 24 hours.
3. Recovery phase: A return to a normal 24-hour volume (1500 to 1800 mL). Usually, kidney function continues to improve and may take 6 months to 1 year from the initial insult to return to baseline functional status.

ASSESSMENT
GOAL OF ASSESSMENT
AKI impacts most of the major organs and the focus of assessment is to determine how AKI is affecting these organs. Assessment findings contribute to the development of a treatment plan that manages fluid, electrolyte, and acid-base imbalances, as well as prevents or minimizes metabolic encephalopathy, anemia, and infection.

HISTORY AND RISK FACTORS

The assessment of AKI begins with a comprehensive history of the patient including the presence of chronic illness (e.g., diabetes mellitus, hypertension, heart failure, cancer, chronic kidney disease). Recent changes in urine patterns and weight as well as recent infections, trauma, procedures, or surgery may establish the risk as well as a time frame for the onset of AKI. A review of patient medications including prescriptions, over-the-counter medications, and herbal/complimentary practices is important in the development of the treatment plan. Some herbal products such as mu tong, fangchi, and *Aristolochia fangchi* contain aristolochic acid, which can cause acute interstitial nephritis. *A. fangchi* is listed as the ingredients "aristolochia," "bragantia," or "as arum" on the label. Aristolochia is sometimes substituted for other botanicals, including *Stephania tetrandra*, *Clematis armandii*, and *akebia* extract.

Juicing is a popular health practice that has been implicated in the development of AKI related to oxalate nephropathy. The practice of "juicing" or "juice cleansing" typically refers to a 3- to 10-day period where the diet consists of fruit and vegetable juice. Oxalate is a nephrotoxin found in fruits, vegetables, and nuts. Typically, oxalate absorption and secretion occurs in the GI tract. If the concentration of oxalates consumed during juicing exceeds the secretion capacity of the intestine, oxalate enters the circulatory system with subsequent renal tubular exposure. Recreational drug use (e.g., cocaine, methamphetamines, and bath salts) has also been implicated in the development of AKI.

SPECIAL POPULATIONS AT RISK

Morbid Obesity: According to the World Health Organization, morbid obesity is defined as a body mass index greater than 40 kg/m^2. This measure expresses weight in relation to height and provides an estimate of fat burden for the human body. The incidence of AKI among patients who are morbidly obese is unknown. Detection of AKI is complicated by an unclear association between weight and urine production. Weight-based formulas for collecting creatinine clearance have not been validated for this population. Several factors may contribute to the development of kidney dysfunction. Creatinine production is increased as a result of body mass. Structural and functional nephron changes include glomerular hyperfiltration, glomerulomegaly, and glomerulosclerosis. Comorbidities associated with obesity including chronic kidney disease, diabetes mellitus, sleep-disordered breathing, heart failure, and hypertension also increase the risk of AKI. The risk of increased intraabdominal pressure and abdominal compartment syndrome is greater in individuals who are obese. Orlistat is a GI lipase inhibitor prescribed for weight loss and has been associated with the development of acute oxalate nephropathy. Drug prescription based on actual weight may result in nephrotoxic doses of lipophilic drugs. The volume distribution of a drug is influenced by lipophilicity. The use of adjusted body weight (ABW) is recommended for lipophilic drugs including unfractionated heparin, aminoglycosides, corticosteroids, and propofol. The formula for ABW is:

$$ABW = (actual\ body\ weight - ideal\ body\ weight) \times 0.25 + ideal\ body\ weight.$$

Older Adult: Chronic illnesses, polypharmacy, impaired thirst sensation, and the structural /functional changes of aging increase the risk of AKI in older adult patients. There is a natural decline in kidney size, GFR, and renal blood flow with advancing age. An impaired ability to concentrate urine increases the risk of volume depletion and may predispose the older adult patient to prerenal azotemia. Diagnosis of AKI in older adults can be challenging. KDIGO guidelines use serum creatinine and urine production for staging AKI. Serum creatinine levels are influenced by age, muscle mass, hydration status, and race. AKI may be obscured by a low or normal serum creatinine level in the older adult population. Serial changes in creatinine values, urine output, and weight may be more helpful in the detection of AKI in the older adult.

PRERENAL PRESENTATION

- Oliguric or nonoliguric.
- Urinary sodium (Na$^+$) less than 20 mEq/L.
- Urine specific gravity greater than 1.020.
- Urine osmolality greater than 500 mOsm/L.
- Hyaline casts possible.
- Elevated plasma BUN/creatinine ratio (greater than 20:1).

- Fractional excretion of sodium (FE_{Na}) less than 1%. FE_{Na} is the ratio between urine sodium excretion and the filtered load of sodium. It reflects how well the kidney can concentrate urine and conserve sodium. It can be greater than 1% in prerenal AKI, with diuretic and bicarbonate use, and with chronic kidney disease.

Intrarenal Presentation
- Oliguric or nonoliguric.
- Urinary Na^+ greater than 20 mEq/L.
- Urine specific gravity 1.010.
- Urinary osmolality less than 350 mOsm/L.
- Abnormal sediment with red blood cell (RBC) casts and cellular debris in the urine.
- Decreased plasma BUN/creatinine ratio (10:1).
- Fractional excretion of sodium (FE_{Na}) greater than 1% FE_{Na} is the ratio between urine sodium excretion and the filtered load of sodium. It reflects how well the kidney can concentrate urine and conserve sodium. The ratio can be less than 1% in ATN associated with radiocontrast administration and rhabdomyolysis.

POSTRENAL PRESENTATION
- Likely oliguric but may be nonoliguric.
- Urinary chemical indices are typically normal.
- Normal or mildly abnormal sediment (hematuria, pyuria, and crystals).
- Often associated with urinary tract or pelvic cancer.
- Often associated with renal/ureteral calculi.

VITAL SIGNS
- BP may be elevated in states of fluid volume excess or decreased in states of fluid volume deficit.
- Heart rate (HR) may be increased or decreased with abnormal rhythms based on fluid and electrolyte abnormalities.
- Weight may be increased or decreased based on fluid volume status.
- Temperature: may be hyperthermic or hypothermic with sepsis.

OBSERVATION
- Peripheral edema and periorbital edema.
- Jugular venous distention.
- Shortness of breath.
- Kussmaul respirations associated with metabolic acidosis.
- Poor skin turgor, flushed skin, and dry mucous membranes.
- Pallor.
- Purpura.
- Weakness.
- Altered mental status and disorientation.
- Signs of central nervous system depression.
- Neuromuscular dysfunction.
- Dysrhythmias.

PALPATION
- Edema (scale 0 to 4+): extremities and sacrum.
- Muscle tenderness.
- Suprapubic tenderness or distention.
- Flank tenderness.

AUSCULTATION
- S3 and S4 gallops indicative of heart failure.
- Pericardial friction rub.
- Tachycardia or dysrhythmias.
- Pulsus paradoxus in the presence of pericardial effusion/cardiac tamponade.
- Crackles.
- Bruits over the renal arteries indicative of renovascular disease.

UREMIC MANIFESTATIONS

- Drowsiness, confusion, irritability, and coma.
- Anemia and bleeding tendencies.
- Pallor, yellow dry skin, pruritus.
- Hypertension.
- Heart failure.
- Pericarditis with cardiac tamponade.
- Pulmonary edema.
- Anorexia, nausea, vomiting.
- Tremors, twitching, seizures.
- Uremic halitosis and stomatitis.
- Increased susceptibility to infection.

SCREENING LABORATORY TESTS

- BUN and creatinine: Elevations indicative of renal impairment. Elevated BUN is an early indication of hydration and possible renal issues in the older adult.
- GFR: Most reliable estimation of GFR is the measurement of 24-hour creatinine clearance.
- Electrolyte levels: Elevated or decreased potassium, phosphorus, magnesium, and sodium.
- Urinalysis: Presence of sediment including tubular epithelial cells, debris, casts, protein, RBC casts, or myoglobin.
- Urinary sodium: Prerenal disease results in urinary sodium levels less than 10 mEq/L.
- Fractional excretion of sodium (FENa): Assesses how well the kidney can concentrate urine, it is affected by numerous conditions that affect the renal parenchyma and is not a sensitive indicator of AKI.
- CBC and coagulation studies (prothrombin time [PT], partial thromboplastin time [PTT]): Evaluate for hematologic complications.
- Arterial blood gas (ABG) values: Evaluate for metabolic acidosis associated with AKI.

Diagnostic Tests for Acute Kidney Injury		
Test	**Purpose**	**Abnormal Findings**
Ultrasonography	Provides general appearance of kidney; integrity of collecting system	Small scarred kidneys Renal mass Kidney stones Hydronephrosis
Computed tomography without contrast	Evaluates kidney and collection system	Renal mass Ureteral stones
Magnetic resonance imaging/Magnetic resonance angiography	More specific in detecting renal masses and vessel malformations	Tumors or cysts Vessel malformation
Cystoscopy	Diagnoses partial or complete obstruction	Bladder or ureteral stenosis or obstruction.
Renal angiography	Evaluates renal vessels	Thrombotic, stenotic lesions in the main renal vessels.
Renal biopsy	Determines intrarenal pathology	Acute glomerulonephritis, vasculitis, or interstitial nephritis.
Blood Studies		
Complete blood count (CBC) Hemoglobin (Hgb) Hematocrit (Hct) Red blood cell (RBC) count White blood cell (WBC) count	Assesses for anemia, inflammation, and infection; assists with differential diagnosis of septic cause of acute renal failure/acute kidney injury (ARF/AKI)	Decreased RBCs, Hgb, or Hct reflects anemia or recent blood loss.

Diagnostic Tests for Acute Kidney Injury—cont'd

Test	Purpose	Abnormal Findings
Coagulation profile: Prothrombin time (PT) with international normalized ratio (INR) Partial thromboplastin time (PTT)	Assesses for the presence of bleeding or clotting and disseminated intravascular coagulation (DIC)	Decreased PT with low INR promotes clotting; elevation promotes bleeding.
Blood urea nitrogen (BUN) Creatinine Estimated glomerular filtration rate (eGFR)	Assesses for the severity of renal dysfunction	Elevation indicates renal dysfunction. Creatinine may be markedly elevated in the presence of massive skeletal muscle injury (e.g., multiple trauma, crush injuries). BUN is influenced by hydration, catabolism, gastrointestinal bleeding, infection fever, and corticosteroid therapy. The eGFR in ARF/AKI is usually less than 50 mL/min. BUN may elevate before creatinine in the setting of dehydration or hypovolemia, particularly in older adults.
Electrolytes: Potassium (K^+) Sodium (Na^+) Calcium (Ca^{2+}) Magnesium (Mg^{2+})	Assesses for abnormalities associated with AKI	Increase or decrease in K^+ may cause arrhythmias. Elevated Na^+ may indicate dehydration. Decreased Na^+ may indicate fluid retention. Low Mg^{2+} or Ca^{2+} may cause dysrhythmias.
Arterial blood gases	Assesses for the presence of metabolic acidosis	Low $Paco_2$ and plasma pH values reflect metabolic acidosis.
Urinalysis	Assesses for the presence of sediment	Presence of sediment containing tubular epithelial cells, cellular debris, and tubular casts supports diagnosis of ARF/AKI. Increased protein and many RBC casts are common in intrarenal disease. Sediment is normal in prerenal causes. Large amounts of myoglobin may be present in severe skeletal muscle injury or rhabdomyolysis.
Urinary sodium	Differentiates prerenal from intrarenal cause; often overlooked as a significant finding	Urinary Na^+ is less than 20 mEq/L (prerenal). Urinary Na^+ is more than 20 mEq/L in intrarenal causes.

KIDNEY ATTACK: EARLY RECOGNITION OF AKI WITH URINARY AND SERUM BIOMARKERS

AKI is a global health problem associated with significant morbidity and mortality. Just as in the case of myocardial infarction and stroke, early recognition of AKI is crucial to reverse or limit the progression of injury. Changes in urine output and serum creatinine levels are evidence-based markers for the identification of AKI. However, these changes are measured over

Box 6-1	INVESTIGATIONAL BIOMARKERS FOR ACUTE KIDNEY INJURY

- Interleukin-18
- Neutrophil gelatinase-associated lipocalin
- Kidney injury molecule-1
- Cystatin C
- N-Acetyl-beta-d-glucosaminidase
- Urinary liver-type fatty acid–binding protein

time and can be affected by muscle mass, age, sex, medications, and hydration status. Several urinary and serum proteins are being investigated for early detection of AKI. Preliminary studies have been inconclusive. None have yet been approved for clinical use in the United States. See Box 6-1 for a listing of investigational markers.

COLLABORATIVE MANAGEMENT
CARE PRIORITIES FOR AKI
The management of AKI focuses on interventions to limit nephron damage and restore fluid, electrolyte, and acid-base balances. Supportive therapies are implemented to manage uremia and associated complications (Table 6-5).

Table 6-5	MANAGEMENT CONSIDERATIONS: ACUTE KIDNEY INJURY
Issue	**Treatment**
Intravascular volume overload	Restriction of salt (1 to 1.5 g/day) and water (1 L/day). Consider diuretic therapy to decrease filtrate reabsorption and enhance water excretion. Use only after adequate hydration to increase urine output or in an attempt to prevent onset of oliguria. If volume overload is present, they are used to prevent pulmonary edema. Osmotic diuretics such as mannitol may be used to increase intravascular volume, promote renal blood flow, increase glomerular filtration rate, and stimulate urinary output. Ultrafiltration may be considered for extracorporeal fluid removal. Hemodynamic monitoring of central venous pressure. Oxygen/high flow, continuous positive airway pressure
Rhabdomyolysis/Tumor lysis syndrome	Forced alkaline diuresis with isotonic sodium bicarbonate solution at 100 mL/h to manage pigmenturia (myoglobinuria, hemoglobinuria) resulting from rhabdomyolysis or severe crush or skeletal muscle injury. In addition, aggressive volume replacement to maintain renal perfusion pressure and reduce cast formation leading to renal tubular obstruction.
Hyponatremia	Restriction of oral and intravenous free water.
Hyperkalemia	Restriction of dietary potassium. Discontinuation of potassium supplements or potassium-sparing diuretics. Loop diuretics in diuretic-responsive patients. Potassium-binding resin. Glucose (50 mL of 50% with regular insulin 10 units intravenously). Calcium gluconate (10 mL of 10% solution over 5 minutes). Sodium bicarbonate (50 mEq intravenously): Sodium bicarbonate is given in acidosis to promote the shift of potassium back into the cells. Albuterol 20 mg nebulized. Renal replacement therapy.
Metabolic acidosis	Careful management of dietary protein. Renal replacement therapy. Sodium bicarbonate: Sodium bicarbonate is given to control metabolic acidosis and promote the shift of potassium back into the cells.

Table 6-5	MANAGEMENT CONSIDERATIONS: ACUTE KIDNEY INJURY — cont'd
Issue	**Treatment**
Management of hyper-phosphatemia	Restriction of dietary phosphate intake. Phosphate-binding agents: Phosphate binders (calcium carbonate antacids, calcium acetate) that bind phosphorus and control hyperphosphatemia and hypermagnese-mia are given with meals.
Hypermagnesemia	Discontinuation of magnesium-containing drugs such as antacids.
Prevention of contrast-induced nephropathy	Aggressive hydration with normal saline or bicarbonate solution 12 hours before con-trast administration. N-Acetylcysteine may be added with hydration for patients with glomerular filtration rate of less than 30 undergoing major procedures.
Uremic encephalopathy/ Uremic pericarditis	Renal replacement therapy. Monitor for high risk of bleeding and injury.
Nutrition therapy	Enteral feeding is preferred. Total energy intake of 20 to 30 kcal/kg/day. Protein intake of 0.8 to 1.0 g/kg/day for noncatabolic patients with acute kidney injury. Protein intake of 1.0 to 1.5 g/kg/day for patients with acute kidney injury receiv-ing renal replacement therapy. Higher amounts may be required for hypercatabolic patients.
Hematologic problems	Packed red blood cells are given to maintain hematocrit. Anemia caused by decreased erythropoietin, low-grade gastrointestinal bleeding from mucosal ulceration, blood drawing, and shortened life of the red blood cells. Erythropoietin is used for primary prevention and treatment of anemia. Prolonged bleeding time is caused by decreased platelet adhesiveness.
Drug dosage	Adjust all dosages for glomerular filtration rate and renal replacement therapy.
Relief of obstruction	Achieved via catheterization with indwelling urinary catheter or nephrostomy tube, or ureteral stent to relieve obstruction before surgical intervention or lithotripsy to disintegrate stones.

1. Maintain renal perfusion

a. Administer intravenous (IV) fluids to achieve/maintain central venous pressure (CVP) of 10 to 12 mm Hg and/or urine output greater than 0.5 mL/kg/h.

b. After volume repletion, consider vasopressor or inotropic support to achieve MAP greater than 60 mm Hg.

c. Low-dose dopamine is not recommended to prevent or treat AKI.

d. Treat underlying cause of volume depletion (e.g., hemorrhage, burns, GI losses, extrava-sation into extravascular compartments).

e. Correct underlying cause of renal hypoperfusion (e.g., sepsis, compartment syndrome, cardiogenic shock).

2. Minimize exposure to nephrotoxic agents

a. Review current medications for potential nephrotoxicity (e.g., NSAIDS, antibiotics, ACEIs/angiotensin blockers).

b. Aminoglycosides should be avoided unless a therapeutic alternative is not available.

c. Avoid diuretics unless in the management of fluid overload.

Safety Alert *See Table 6-6 Diuretic Use in Acute Kidney Injury.*

Table 6-6	DIURETIC USE IN ACUTE KIDNEY INJURY	
Types	**Mechanisms of Action**	**Potential Fluid and Electrolyte Abnormalities**
Osmotic Diuretics		
Mannitol Urea	Increase osmotic pressure of the filtrate, which attracts water and electrolytes and prevents their reabsorption	Hyponatremia Hypokalemia Rebound volume expansion
Loop Diuretics		
Furosemide Ethacrynic acid Bumetanide Torsemide	Inhibit reabsorption of Na^+ and Cl^- at the ascending loop of Henle in the medulla; they produce a vasodilatory effect on the renal vasculature	Hypokalemia Hyperuricemia Hypocalcemia Hyperglycemia and impairment of glucose tolerance Dilutional hyponatremia Hypochloremic alkalosis
Thiazides		
Bendroflumethiazide Benzthiazide Chlorothiazide sodium Hydrochlorothiazide Hydroflumethiazide Polythiazide Trichlormethiazide	Inhibit Na^+ in the ascending loop of Henle at the beginning of the distal loop	Hypokalemia Dilutional hyponatremia Hypercalcemia Metabolic alkalosis Hypochloremia Hyperuricemia Hyperglycemia and impaired glucose tolerance
Thiazide-like Diuretics		
Chlorthalidone Indapamide Metolazone Quinethazone	Action same as thiazides	Same as thiazides
Potassium-sparing Diuretics*		
Amiloride HCl Spironolactone Triamterene	Inhibit aldosterone effect on the distal tubule, causing Na^+ excretion and K^+ reabsorption	Hyperkalemia Hyponatremia Dehydration Acidosis Transient increase in BUN
Carbonic Anhydrase Inhibitors		
Acetazolamide sodium Dichlorphenamide Methazolamide	Block the action of the enzyme carbonic anhydrase, producing excretion of Na^+, K^+, HCO_3^-, and water	Hyperchloremic acidosis Hypokalemia Hyperuricemia

*Used with caution in patients with oliguria.
BUN, Blood urea nitrogen; Cl^-, chloride; $HCO3^-$, bicarbonate; K^+, potassium; Na^+, sodium.
Note: Loop or osmotic diuretics (or a combination of both) are used in patients with acute kidney injury to prevent hypervolemia and to stimulate urinary output.

d. Consider alkaline diuresis for patients with crush injuries or rhabdomyolysis.
e. Avoid radiocontrast material when possible. If necessary, administer isotonic saline at 1 mL/kg/h for 12 hours before and after contrast administration. An alternative regimen is 3 mL/kg/h for 1 hour before the procedure followed by 1 to 1.5 mL/kg/h for 6 hours after the procedure. Sodium bicarbonate is another strategy to prevent contrast induced nephropathy (CIN). A typical protocol is the addition of 150 mEq of sodium bicarbonate to 1 L of 5% dextrose administered at 3 mL/kg/h for 1 hour before contrast administration

and continued at 1 mL/kg for 6 hours after contrast administration. Risks associated with the addition of sodium bicarbonate are alkalemia, exacerbation of heart failure, and hypocalcemia. N-Acetylcysteine (NAC) has been used for the prevention of CIN. However, there is conflicting evidence regarding efficacy. The usual oral dose of NAC is 600 mg twice daily before and the day of contrast administration. It can also be administered IV as a one-time dose immediately before contrast administration. The most common side effects of NAC are nausea and vomiting. KDIGO guidelines do not recommend the use of NAC for postsurgical patients or patients with hypotension.

3. Provide nutrition support
a. Enteral feeding route is preferred.
b. Total energy intake of 20 to 30 kcal/kg/day.
c. Protein intake of 0.8 to 1.0 g/kg/day for noncatabolic patients with AKI; 1.0 to 1.5 g/kg/day for patients with AKI receiving renal replacement therapy; hypercatabolic patients may require up to 1.7 g/kg/day. Patients with diabetes mellitus with AKI require vigilant management to ensure a balance of both carbohydrates and proteins to meet the needs of both conditions.

4. Avoid hyperglycemia
Provide insulin therapy targeting plasma glucose 110 to 149 mg/day.

5. Continue assessment and monitoring of hemodynamic and oxygenation measurements
This is to prevent development or worsening of AKI in patients who are critically ill.

6. Initiate renal replacement therapy
Renal replacement therapies include hemodialysis and continuous renal replacement therapies.
a. Refractory fluid overload.
b. Hyperkalemia.
c. Metabolic acidosis.
d. Uncontrolled azotemia.
e. Drug overdose.

CARE PLANS FOR ACUTE KIDNEY INJURY
EXCESS FLUID VOLUME *related to inability of kidney to normally excrete urine*

Goals/Outcomes: Within 24 to 48 hours of onset, intravascular volume is stabilized, as evidenced by balanced intake and output (I&O), urinary output greater than 0.5 mL/kg/h, body weight within the patient's normal range, MAP greater than 60 mm Hg and within the patient's normal range, CVP 10 to 12 mm Hg, HR 60 to 100 beats/min (bpm), and improvement of edema, crackles, gallop, and other clinical indicators of fluid overload.
NOC Fluid Overload Severity; Fluid Balance.

> **Safety Alert** *Although the patient is retaining sodium, his or her serum sodium level may be within normal limits or decreased from baseline because of the dilution effect of the fluid overload.*

Fluid Management
1. Document input and output hourly. Consult the advanced practice provider if urinary output falls to less than 0.5 mL/kg/h.
2. Weigh the patient daily; consult the advanced practice provider regarding significant weight gain (e.g., 0.5 to 1.5 kg/24 h).
3. Assess for and report the presence of new or increased basilar crackles, jugular vein distention, tachycardia, pericardial friction rub, gallop, increased BP, increased CVP, or shortness of breath (SOB), any of which are indicative of fluid volume overload. Chronic heart failure may require additional support measures to help resolve AKI.
4. Assess for and report new or increasing peripheral, sacral, or periorbital edema.
5. Restrict total fluid intake to 1200 to 1500 mL/24 h or as prescribed. Measure all output accurately, and replace milliliter for milliliter at intervals of 4 to 8 hours or as prescribed.

Acute Kidney Injury

6. Provide ice chips, chewing gum, or hard candy to help quench thirst and moisten mouth.
7. Monitor serum osmolality and serum sodium values. Values are decreased in the setting of fluid overload resulting from dilution by excess volume.
8. Patients receiving total parenteral nutrition will receive the largest fluid intake volume. If total fluid intake is greater than 2000 mL/day, ultrafiltration with hemodialysis or continuous renal replacement therapy (CRRT) (continuous venovenous hemofiltration [CVVH], continuous venovenous hemodialysis [CVVHD], continuous venovenous hemodiafiltration [CVVHDF], slow continuous ultrafiltration [SCUF], or continuous arteriovenous hemofiltration) may be required to maintain fluid and electrolyte balance.
9. If the patient is retaining sodium, restrict sodium-containing foods, avoid diluting IV medications with saline diluents or intravenous solutionsand avoid sodium-containing medications such as sodium penicillin.

NIC Electrolyte Management: Hypokalemia; Electrolyte Management: Hyponatremia; Fluid/Electrolyte Management; Fluid Management; Fluid Monitoring. Additional, optional interventions include Dysrhythmia Management; Hemodialysis Therapy; Hemodynamic Regulation; Invasive Hemodynamic Monitoring; Medication Management; Positioning; Skin Surveillance; and Weight Management.

FLUID VOLUME DEFICIT *related to overdiuresis and/or dehydration resulting in AKI*

Goals/Outcomes: Within 24 hours of this diagnosis, volume status is stabilized, as evidenced by balanced I&O, urinary output greater than 0.5 mL/kg/h, CVP 10 to 12 mm Hg, HR 60 to 100 bpm, MAP greater than 60 mm Hg, absence of thirst, and other indicators of hypovolemia. Weight stabilizes within 2 to 3 days.
NOC Hydration; Fluid Balance.

Hypovolemia Management
1. Weigh the patient daily. Consult the advanced practice provider for weight loss of 1 to 1.5 kg/24 h. Weight is often the most reliable indicator of fluid status in patients with kidney impairment.
2. Assess for and manage dehydration and hypovolemia (e.g., poor skin turgor, dry and sticky mucous membranes, thirst, hypotension, tachycardia, decreasing CVP, increasing BUN and creatinine).
3. Promote hydration: Monitor and document I&O hourly. Report if the patient's output is less than 0.5 mL/kg/h. With a deficit, supplemental fluid intake should exceed output by 0.5 to 1 L/day (depending on severity of dehydration). Encourage oral fluids if allowed. Ensure that IV fluid rates are maintained as prescribed.
4. Monitor for additional fluid losses: Report increased losses from vomiting, diarrhea, wound drainage, or sudden onset of diuresis. Fluid intake may need to be increased.
5. Patients with AKI are at risk for GI bleeding related to uremia, which may cause platelet dysfunction, acidosis, and the stress of critical illness. Monitor hemoglobin (Hgb), hematocrit (Hct), and BUN levels. ABGs are drawn to assess pH, HCO_3^-, and CO_2 levels, reflective of acid-base balance.

 Safety Alert *A patient with acute kidney injury may have a hematocrit in the range of 20% to 30% if prerenal azotemia has occurred over time. Anemia occurs as a result of prolonged renal insufficiency leading to failure. Blood urea nitrogen will increase in the presence of gastrointestinal bleeding without a concomitant rise in serum creatinine level.*

6. Monitor for occult bleeding: Test all stools, emesis, and peritoneal dialysate drainage for occult blood. Check urine and dialysate drainage at least every 8 hours.
7. Minimize the risk of bleeding: Implement fall precautions, minimize invasive procedures, use small-gauge needles for injections, minimize blood drawing, and promote the use of electric razors and soft-bristle toothbrushes. If possible, avoid intramuscular (IM) or subcutaneous injections for 1 hour after hemodialysis. Apply gentle pressure to injection sites for at least 2 to 3 minutes.
8. Inspect hemodialysis insertion, peritoneal access sites, and other invasive sites for bleeding when interacting with the patient at least every 8 hours.

IMBALANCED NUTRITION, LESS THAN BODY REQUIREMENTS *related to the adverse effects of AKI on digestion and absorption of nutrients.*

Goals/Outcomes: Within 72 hours of this diagnosis, the patient has adequate nutritional intake, as evidenced by a caloric intake that ranges from 35 to 45 calories/kg normal body weight, a daily protein intake consisting of 50%

to 75% high–biological value proteins, and a nitrogen intake of 4 to 6 g greater than nitrogen loss (calculated from 24-hour urinary urea excretion and protein intake).
NOC Nutritional Status.

Nutrition Therapy
1. Augment nutritional intake: Administer nutritional supplements/enteral feedings as prescribed and record amount of intake every shift.
2. Reduce incidence of nausea: Present appetizing food in small, frequent meals. Provide a pleasant atmosphere; eliminate any noxious odors. Administer prescribed antiemetic 30 minutes before meals.
3. Control catabolism:
   - Manage fever: As prescribed, use cooling blanket or antipyretic agents to control fever. Fever increases tissue catabolism, which in turn increases metabolic needs. Patients who are critically ill are often catabolic and require careful nutrition management, especially when hemodialysis, peritoneal dialysis, or CRRT is implemented. Protein target is 0.8 to 1.0 g/kg/day to provide essential amino acids for a noncatabolic patient with AKI. The end products of protein metabolism that accumulate are reflected by an increase in BUN level. Ensure intake of protein with high biological value (e.g., eggs, meat, fowl, milk, fish), which contains essential amino acids necessary for cell building.
   - Provide adequate calories: Be sure that caloric intake ranges from 20 to 30 kcal/kg/day for a critically ill adult patient with AKI. The exact amount will vary with age, sex, activity, and the degree of preexisting malnutrition. Foods that may be used to increase caloric intake include fats and concentrated carbohydrates.
4. Manage electrolytes:
   - Restrict high-potassium foods such as bananas, citrus fruits, potatoes, fruit juices, nuts, tea, coffee, legumes, and salt substitute. In acute renal failure (ARF) or acute kidney injury (AKI), the kidneys are unable to excrete potassium effectively.
   - Assess sodium requirement, because it will vary greatly. If oliguria is present, sodium intake may be restricted in the diet. If diuresis is present, sodium intake may be increased because of excess sodium loss in the urine. Intervene accordingly.
   - Measure ionized calcium to avoid inappropriate treatment of malnourished patients whose values may appear falsely low as a result of serum calcium being bound to albumin, which is decreased in patients with renal failure.
   - Manage hypocalcemia: Reduced intestinal calcium absorption coupled with hyperphosphatemia is managed by replacing calcium orally (e.g., with dairy products, Tums) or IV. Administer phosphate binders as prescribed.
   - Recognize that catabolism of protein, which occurs with infection, causes potassium to be released from the tissues.

NIC Nutrition Management; Nutrition Monitoring; Fluid Management; Fluid Monitoring. Additional, optional Nursing Interventions Classification (NIC) interventions include: Bowel Management; Energy Management; Enteral Tube Feeding; Exercise Promotion; Gastrointestinal Intubation; Hyperglycemia Management; Hypoglycemia Management; Intravenous Insertion; Intravenous Therapy; Medication Management; Mutual Goal Setting; Phlebotomy: Venous Blood Sample; Positioning; Teaching: Individual; Teaching: Prescribed Diet; Total Parenteral Nutrition Administration; and Venous Access Devices Maintenance.

RISK FOR INFECTION *related to immunocompromised state associated with renal failure*

Goals/Outcomes: At the time of discharge from the intensive care unit, infection is controlled, as evidenced by normothermia, negative culture results of dialysate and body secretions, and white blood cell (WBC) count less than 11,000/mm^3.
NOC Immune Status.

Safety Alert *After the initial insult, infection is the primary cause of death in acute kidney injury.*

Infection Protection
1. Monitor and record the patient's temperature every 8 hours. If elevated (i.e., greater than 37° C [98.6° F]), monitor temperature every 4 hours. AKI may be accompanied by hypothermia. A slight rise in temperature of 1 to 2 degrees may be significant; especially if the patient is receiving CRRT (an extracorporeal therapy.)

2. Identify possible sources of infection: Inspect and record the color, odor, and appearance of all body secretions. Be alert to cloudy or blood-tinged peritoneal dialysate return, cloudy and foul-smelling urine, foul-smelling wound exudate, purulent drainage from any catheter site, foul-smelling and watery stools, foul-smelling vaginal discharge, or purulent sputum.

3. Vigilantly monitor open wounds: Recognize that uremia retards wound healing. All wounds (including scratches resulting from pruritus) should be assessed for infection. Send samples of any suspicious fluid or drainage for culture and sensitivity tests.

4. Monitor for infection: Monitor WBC count with differential analysis for elevation.

5. Prevent infection: Use aseptic technique when manipulating central lines, peripheral IV lines, and indwelling catheters. Avoid use of indwelling urinary catheter in patients with oliguria and anuria. The presence of a catheter further increases the risk of infection.

6. Provide oral hygiene every 2 to 4 hours to help maintain the integrity of the oral mucous membranes.

7. Reposition the patient every 2 to 4 hours to help maintain the barrier of an intact integumentary system. Provide skin care at least every 8 hours.

8. Encourage good pulmonary hygiene: Instruct the patient to practice deep-breathing exercises (and coughing, if indicated) every 2 to 4 hours. Implement ventilator-associated pneumonia (VAP) prevention (e.g., VAP Bundle) on patients who are mechanically ventilated.

NIC Infection Control. Additional, optional interventions include Airway Management; Exercise Promotion and Therapy; Medication Management; Respiratory Monitoring; Teaching: Disease Process; Tube Care: Urinary; and Vital Signs Monitoring.

KNOWLEDGE DEFICIT *related to disease process of AKI*

Goals/Outcomes: Within 72 hours of admission, the patient and significant others verbalize accurate information regarding AKI and the plan of care.
NOC Knowledge: Disease Process.

Teaching: Disease Process

1. Provide education regarding AKI including the signs and symptoms of the biochemical alterations (hyperkalemia, hypokalemia, hypernatremia, hyponatremia, hypocalcemia, hyperphosphatemia, hypermagnesemia, metabolic acidosis, and uremia) that can occur (see Table 6-4).

2. Provide lists of foods high in potassium, sodium, and magnesium that the patient should avoid when planning meals. Provide a list of medications that contain magnesium that should not be taken without approval of the advanced practice provider .

3. Explain the importance of consuming only the amount of protein prescribed by the advanced practice provider.

4. Discuss the need to avoid exposure to persons with infection or a febrile illness to prevent infection. Infection and strenuous activity promote protein catabolism, which causes potassium to be released from the tissues.

5. Teach the patient to report to the advanced practice provider an increase in temperature or other signs of infection.

6. Reinforce the importance of taking vitamin D and calcium supplements as prescribed.

7. Teach the relationship between calcium and phosphate levels. Emphasize that maintaining good phosphate control and calcium balance may help control itching and prevent future problems with bone disease.

8. Stress the importance of taking phosphate binders (e.g., Amphojel, Alternagel, PhosLo) as prescribed and to avoid antacids containing magnesium (e.g., Maalox, Milk of Magnesia).

9. Teach the patient not to take over-the-counter medications without first consulting the advanced practice provider. Aspirin, for example, exacerbates the bleeding tendency caused by uremia.

10. Instruct the patient about the importance of maintaining the prescribed dialysis schedule, because dialysis will help correct acidosis, uremia, and many of the metabolic abnormalities that occur.

11. Teach the patient to use lotions and oils to lubricate the skin and relieve drying and cracking.

12. Stress the importance of follow-up monitoring of serum electrolyte levels.

NIC Teaching: Individual; Teaching: Prescribed Medication. Additional, optional interventions include Discharge Planning; Medication Management; and Weight Management.

ACUTE CONFUSION *related to altered level of consciousness that results from fluid and electrolyte imbalance and/or uremia.*

Goals/Outcomes: Within 48 to 72 hours of onset, the patient verbalizes orientation to time, place, and person and maintains his or her normal mobility.
NOC Neurologic Status.

Neurologic Monitoring
1. Monitor the patient for the following mentation and motor dysfunctions associated with AKI:
   - Hyperkalemia (during oliguric phase): muscle weakness, irritability, paresthesias.
   - Hypokalemia (during diuretic phase): lethargy; muscle weakness, softness, flabbiness; paresthesias.
   - Hypernatremia: fatigue, restlessness, agitation.
   - Hyponatremia: dizziness when changing position, apprehension, personality changes, agitation, confusion.
   - Hypocalcemia: neuromuscular irritability, tonic muscle spasms, paresthesias.
   - Hyperphosphatemia: excessive itching, muscle weakness, hyperreflexia.
   - Hypermagnesemia: drowsiness, lethargy, sensation of heat.
   - Metabolic acidosis: confusion, weakness.
   - Uremia: confusion, lethargy, itching, metallic taste, muscle twitching.
2. Explain to significant others that the patient's decreasing attention level necessitates simple and direct communication efforts.
3. To alleviate the unpleasant metallic taste caused by uremia, provide frequent oral hygiene. Because the patient with uremia is at increased risk for bleeding, ensure the use of soft-bristle brushes.
4. Implement fall prevention interventions.
5. Promote early mobilization: Encourage isometric exercises and short walks, if the patient is able, to help maintain muscle strength and tone, especially in the legs.
6. Assess for delirium: Decrease environmental stimuli, and use calm, reassuring manner in caring for the patient.
7. Balance rest and activities: Encourage establishment of sleep/rest patterns by scheduling daytime activities appropriately and promoting relaxation methods.
8. Monitor for development of neuropathies: Assess for decreased tactile sensations in the feet and legs, which may occur with peripheral neuropathy. Be alert to the potential for pressure sores and friction burns, which may occur with peripheral neuropathy.
9. Use splints and braces to aid in mobility for patients with severe neuropathic effects.

NIC Nutrition Management; Nutrition Therapy; Nutrition Counseling; Pressure Management; Pressure Ulcer Prevention; and Teaching: Individual.

CONSTIPATION *related to fluid and electrolyte imbalance and reduced activity level.*

Goals/Outcomes: Within 48 hours of onset, the patient has bowel movements of soft consistency.
NOC Bowel Elimination.

Constipation/Impaction Management
1. Monitor and record the number and quality of the patient's bowel movements.
2. Administer prescribed stool softeners and bulking agents, such as psyllium husks.
3. Additional measures: Administer oil retention or tap water enemas as prescribed. Because excess fluid can be absorbed from the gut, avoid using large-volume water enemas.
4. Encourage moderate exercise on a routine basis.
5. Establish a regular schedule for fluid intake within the patient's prescribed limits.
6. Administer metoclopramide as prescribed to increase motility in the presence of autonomic neuropathy. Treatment with metoclopramide for more than 12 weeks is not recommended, given the risk of developing tardive dyskinesia.

NIC Exercise Promotion; Medication Administration: Oral; Medication Management; Pain Management; and Skin Surveillance.

IMPAIRED SKIN INTEGRITY *related to uremia*

Goals/Outcomes: The patient's skin remains intact.
NOC Tissue Integrity: Skin and Mucous Membranes.

Pruritus Management

1. Monitor the patient for presence of pruritus with resulting frequent and intense scratching. Pruritus decreases with reduced BUN level and control of hyperphosphatemia. Monitor laboratory values of BUN and phosphorus, and report levels outside the optimal range (BUN greater than 20 mg/dL and phosphorus greater than 4.5 mg/dL or less than 2.6 mEq/L). Pruritus increases in the presence of secondary hyperparathyroidism. Monitor serum calcium and PTH levels, and report elevations (Ca^{2+} greater than 10.5 mg/dL and PTH greater than 30% above the upper limit of the test used).
2. Administer phosphate binders (e.g., Alternagel) as prescribed, and, if possible, reduce the patient's dietary intake of phosphorus (see Box 1-6).
3. Ensure that the patient's fingernails are cut short and that the nail tips are smooth.
4. Because of reduced oil gland activity associated with uremia, the patient's skin may be very dry. Use skin emollients liberally, and avoid harsh soaps and excessive bathing.
5. Advise the patient of the potential for bruising because of clotting abnormality and capillary fragility.
6. Administer oral antihistamine, such as diphenhydramine, to relieve itching as prescribed.

NIC Skin Surveillance; Pressure Ulcer Prevention. Additional, optional interventions include Bathing; Bleeding Reduction; Cutaneous Stimulation; Exercise Promotion and Therapy (all listed); Electrolyte Monitoring; Exercise Promotion: Stretching; Fluid/Electrolyte Management; Infection Control; Infection Protection; Medication Management; Nail Care; Nutrition Management; Perineal Care; Surveillance; and Vital Signs Monitoring.

ADDITIONAL NURSING DIAGNOSES

For patients undergoing dialytic therapy (conventional hemodialysis), see nursing diagnoses and interventions in Continuous Renal Replacement Therapies, as follows.

CONTINUOUS RENAL REPLACEMENT THERAPIES

The patient with ARF or AKI may progress to a physiologic disequilibrium requiring support with renal replacement therapy to prevent metabolic complications. CRRT has gained acceptance throughout Europe and the United States for the treatment of hemodynamically unstable patients who may not tolerate or have not tolerated hemodialysis, or have not responded to conservative management and pharmacologic interventions. The initiation of this therapy is variable throughout institutions and physician practices. Patient characteristics that are considered include age, severity of illness, and existing comorbidities.

The goals of CRRT include:
1. Prevention of uremic complications.
2. Acid-base balance.
3. Electrolyte and fluid volume homeostasis.
4. Maintenance of cardiopulmonary function and hemodynamics.
5. Maintenance of adequate nutrition support.

The most common indications for CRRT include:
1. Hyperkalemia and other electrolyte disturbances refractory to medical management.
2. Metabolic acidosis unresponsive to medical therapy.
3. Intravascular volume excess refractory to diuretics.
4. Uremic intoxication.
   - Neurologic (encephalopathy).
   - Hematologic (bleeding caused by platelet dysfunction).
   - Gastrointestinal (anorexia, nausea, vomiting).
   - Cardiovascular (pericarditis).
5. Need for removal of dialyzable substances (metabolites, drugs, toxins).

Other indications for CRRT include:
1. Massive fluid overload: congestive heart failure, overaggressive fluid resuscitation in multiple trauma.
2. Fluid overload in the presence of hemodynamic instability.
3. Cardiogenic shock with pulmonary edema.
4. Oliguria unresponsive to diuretics.
5. Severe hypovolemia with anuria: helps stabilize fluid balance in patients with multiple organ dysfunction syndrome requiring aggressive volume resuscitation to stabilize hemodynamics.

Indications for early initiation of CRRT include:
1. Predicted impending electrolyte or acid-base disturbances.
2. Presence of oliguria and the need for infusion of large volumes of fluid.
3. Presence of ARF/AKI with a poor prognosis for immediate recovery.
4. ARF/AKI in the presence of sepsis or systemic inflammatory response syndrome.

PATHOPHYSIOLOGY

Historically, CRRT has evolved from an arteriovenous to a venovenous extracorporeal process to achieve solute and fluid removal in the patient who is critically ill. For this reason, arteriovenous therapy will not be included in this chapter. Venous access has proven to be safer, and the evolving technology has improved the efficacy of treatment. CRRT has been traditionally limited to the intensive care unit setting based on the requirement for close hourly monitoring and fluid adjustments. The multiple acronyms and description of therapies are available in Table 6-7.

The principles of solute and water removal during CRRT are similar to other methods of renal replacement therapy (e.g., hemodialysis) and include diffusion, ultrafiltration, and convection. These therapies provide solute clearance and fluid removal slowly and continuously. Conventional hemodialysis is more aggressive and may not be tolerated in unstable patients.

Diffusion: Movement of solutes, including high concentrations of waste products and excess electrolytes, from an area of greater concentration to an area of lesser concentration. Diffusion requires a concentration gradient. During CRRT, high concentrations of these excess particles diffuse into the dialysate/effluent, which contains much lower concentrations of these solutes.

Ultrafiltration: Removal of water from the blood compartment of the hemofilter by generating a lower pressure in the effluent compartment. In hemodialysis, lower or negative pressure in the dialysate facilitates more rapid removal of excess water from the blood compartment in which positive or higher pressure exists.

Convection: Removal of a solute along with fluid through a filter with a semipermeable membrane over time. This occurs in response to the pressure gradient across the filter. Small molecules freely pass into the ultrafiltrate. Large molecule removal is dependent on the pore size of the filter. Larger molecules tend to move through membranes in the filter more easily by using convection rather than diffusion. Various elements in plasma

Table 6-7	COMPARISON OF MODES OF CONTINUOUS RENAL REPLACEMENT THERAPY
SCUF	Slow continuous ultrafiltration: Indicated primarily to remove fluids. A filter with a large surface area, high sieving coefficient, and low resistance facilitates continuous fluid removal and minimal solute removal.
CVVH	Continuous venovenous hemofiltration: Ultrafiltration is used to remove fluid. Convective clearance is used to remove solutes. Replacement solution is infused via prefilter, postfilter, or both prefilter and postfilter to create a solute drag effect (a large volume of fluid is infused into the patient's bloodstream, which facilitates solutes to be returned or "dragged" to the filter. CVVH does not use dialysate solution.
CVVHD	Continuous venovenous hemodialysis: Ultrafiltration is used to remove fluid. Diffusive clearance is used to remove solutes. Dialysate solution is infused into the filter countercurrent to the blood flow. Solutes diffuse from the blood (high solute concentration) to the dialysate solution (low solute concentration). Replacement solution is not used.
CVVHDF	Continuous venovenous hemodiafiltration: Ultrafiltration is used to remove fluid. Both convective and diffusive clearance is used to remove solute so that both replacement and dialysis fluids are used.
SLED	Sustained low-efficiency dialysis: Hybrid form of continuous renal replacement therapy using a reduced blood flow and rate of dialysate infusion to remove both solute through diffusive clearance and fluid by ultrafiltration. Therapy is usually sustained 4 to 12 hours per day.

Continuous Renal Replacement Therapies

fluid (e.g., urea) are conveyed across the filter as a result of the differences in hydrostatic pressure. The removal of large amounts of plasma fluid results in the removal of large amounts of filterable solutes.

Improved and enhanced technology for CRRT has not resulted in standardization of when therapy should be initiated, dosage, choice of modality, or the intensity and duration of therapy. The use of a highly permeable filter, the infusion of various types of replacement solution, and the continuous nature of each of the techniques make them highly effective and versatile in managing the control of fluids. CRRT techniques can serve as a regulatory system for fluids without compromising the metabolic balance. More recent literature suggests that the use of daily hemodialysis may provide equally effective therapy in patients with AKI or for those with more complex disease processes who are unable to receive consistent therapy as a result of machine problems, such as clotting of the filter. Frequent machine alarms indicate that therapy has ceased or will cease shortly, which undermines the efficacy of CRRT. Continuous replacement requires a fully operational system that provides uninterrupted therapy. If the system is frequently alarming, diffusion, ultrafiltration, and convection are interrupted with the sounding of each alarm.

ASSESSMENT: PRE-CRRT
GOAL OF ASSESSMENT
Evaluate fluid, electrolyte, and acid-base balances to prevent the development of metabolic complications attributable to AKI.

HISTORY AND RISK FACTORS
Chronic illness (e.g., hypertension, diabetes, cardiomyopathy, peripheral vascular disease), recent infections or sepsis (e.g., streptococcal), recent episodes of hypotension (e.g., major bleeding, septic shock, major surgery), exposure to nephrotoxins (e.g., carbon tetrachloride, diuretics, aminoglycoside antibiotics, contrast media), recent blood transfusion, urinary tract disorders, toxemia of pregnancy or abortion, recent severe muscle damage (e.g., rhabdomyolysis with myoglobinuria), crush injury, and burn trauma.

VITAL SIGNS
- BP may be elevated in states of fluid volume excess or decreased in states of fluid volume deficit.
- HR may be increased or decreased with abnormal rhythms based on fluid and electrolyte abnormalities.
- Baseline electrocardiogram (ECG) and rhythm.
- Hemodynamic measurements of cardiac output, cardiac index, ejection fraction, CVP, and pulmonary artery occlusion pressure.
- Weight may be increased or decreased based on fluid volume status.
- Temperature may be hyperthermic or hypothermic if the patient is septic.
- Pulse oximetry.

OBSERVATION
- Peripheral edema and periorbital edema.
- Jugular venous distention.
- Dyspnea.
- Kussmaul respirations.
- Poor skin turgor, flushed skin, and dry mucous membranes.
- Pallor.
- Purpura.
- Weakness.
- Altered mental status and disorientation.
- Signs of central nervous system depression.
- Neuromuscular dysfunction.
- Asterixis.
- Mechanical ventilation measurements.
- Presence of any assist devices such as extracorporeal membrane oxygenator.

PALPATION
- Edema (scale 0 to 4$^+$): extremities and sacrum.
- Muscle tenderness.
- Suprapubic tenderness or distention.
- Flank tenderness.

AUSCULTATION
- S3 and S4 gallops indicative of heart failure.
- Pericardial friction rub.
- Tachycardia or dysrhythmias.
- Pulsus paradoxus in the presence of fluid volume excess.
- Crackles.
- Bruits over the renal arteries indicative of renovascular disease.

UREMIC MANIFESTATIONS
- Accumulation of urea, creatinine, and uric acid.
- Anemia and bleeding tendencies.
- Fatigue and pallor.
- Increased BP.
- Congestive heart failure.
- Pericarditis with tamponade.
- Pulmonary edema.
- Anorexia, nausea, vomiting, and diarrhea.
- Behavioral changes.
- Decreased wound-healing ability.
- Increased susceptibility to infection.

SCREENING LABWORK
Blood and urine tests will determine the level of renal dysfunction and can provide clues to the cause of ARF/AKI.
- BUN and creatinine: Elevations indicative of renal impairment.
- GFR: Most reliable estimation of renal function using 24-hour creatinine clearance or laboratory estimation, which is part of the renal panel in most laboratories.
- Electrolyte levels: Elevated or decreased potassium, phosphorus, magnesium, and sodium.
- Urinalysis: Presence of sediment including tubular epithelial cells, debris, casts, protein, RBC casts, or myoglobin.
- Urinary sodium: Prerenal disease results in urinary sodium less than 20 mEq/L.
- CBC and coagulation studies: Evaluate for hematologic complications.
- ABG values: Evaluate for metabolic acidosis associated with ARF/AKI.

Diagnostic Tests Used In Association With Continuous Renal Replacement Therapy Blood Studies

Test	Purpose	Abnormal Findings
Complete blood count (CBC) Hemoglobin (Hgb) Hematocrit (Hct) Red blood cell (RBC) count White blood cell (WBC) count	Assesses for anemia, inflammation, and infection. Assists with differential diagnosis of septic cause of acute renal failure/acute kidney injury (ARF/AKI).	Decreased RBCs, Hgb, or Hct reflects anemia or recent blood loss. Increased WBCs may be indicative of infection/sepsis.
Coagulation profile: Prothrombin time (PT) with international normalized ratio (INR) Activated partial thromboplastin time (aPTT)	Assesses for the presence of bleeding or clotting and disseminated intravascular coagulation (DIC).	Decreased PT, aPTT with low INR promotes clotting. Elevation promotes bleeding.

Continued

Diagnostic Tests Used In Association With Continuous Renal Replacement Therapy Blood Studies—cont'd

Test	Purpose	Abnormal Findings
Blood urea nitrogen (BUN) Creatinine Estimated glomerular filtration rate (eGFR)	Assesses for the severity of renal dysfunction.	Elevation indicates renal dysfunction. Creatinine may be markedly elevated in the presence of massive skeletal muscle injury (e.g., multiple trauma, crush injuries). BUN is influenced by hydration, catabolism, gastrointestinal bleeding, infection, fever, and corticosteroid therapy. The eGFR in ARF/AKI is usually less than 50 mL/min.
Electrolytes: Potassium (K^+) Sodium (Na^+) Calcium (Ca^{2+}) Magnesium (Mg^{2+})	Assesses for abnormalities associated with ARF/AKI.	Increase or decrease in K^+ may cause dysrhythmias. Elevated Na^+ may indicate dehydration. Decreased Na^+ may indicate fluid retention. Low Mg^{2+} or Ca^{2+} may cause dysrhythmias.
Arterial blood gases	Assesses for the presence of metabolic acidosis.	Low $Paco_2$ and plasma pH values reflect metabolic acidosis.
Urinalysis	Assesses for the presence of sediment.	Presence of sediment containing tubular epithelial cells, cellular debris, and tubular casts supports diagnosis of ARF/AKI. Increased protein and many RBC casts are common in intrarenal disease. Sediment is normal in prerenal causes. Large amounts of myoglobin may be present in severe skeletal muscle injury or rhabdomyolysis.
Urinary sodium	Differentiates prerenal from intrarenal etiology.	Urinary Na^+ <20 mEq/L indicates prerenal etiology. Urinary Na^+ >20 mEq/L indicates intrarenal etiology.

DETERMINING TYPE AND MODALITY OF CRRT USED

The availability of CRRT in the institution and the therapeutic options available on existing equipment are part of the considerations used to determine the modality of CRRT used. Treatment goals for removal of water and potentially toxic solutes are considered. Therapeutic options may target removal of water plus solutes, water only, or solutes only to be removed. All modalities use a highly permeable, hollow-fiber filter. The type of filter used is a crucial element contributing to efficacy of treatment when removing solutes, coupled with the functionality of the venous access device. Dysfunctional vascular access can undermine the best of technology and filters, given that the blood flow through the extracorporeal system must be adequate to achieve treatment goals. Solutes removed are generally unbound substances, including urea, calcium, sodium, potassium, chloride, vitamins, and unbound drugs with a molecular weight between 500 and 10,000 Da. Types/modalities of CRRT include:

- Slow continuous ultrafiltration (SCUF).
- Continuous venovenous hemofiltration (CVVH).
- Continuous venovenous hemodialysis (CVVHD).

- Continuous venovenous hemodiafiltration (CVVHDF).
- Sustained low-efficiency daily dialysis (SLEDD).

Indications, advantages, disadvantages, and complications of CRRT modes of therapies are found in Table 6-8. Approaches to troubleshooting major problems of CRRT are found in Table 6-9.

SCUF, CVVH, CVVHD, and CVVHDF are types of continuous renal replacement therapies used to manage fluid and solute overload in patients who are critically ill. Their advantage over conventional hemodialysis is that ultrafiltration occurs more gradually, thus avoiding large volume changes and rapid fluid shifts. A hybrid form of CRRT, SLEDD, is a modification to intermittent hemodialysis. The dialysis duration is 6 to 12 hours per day. CRRT duration will depend on the total amount of fluid and/or solute to be removed. The type best suited for

Table 6-8	INDICATIONS, ADVANTAGES, AND DISADVANTAGES/ COMPLICATIONS OF MODES OF CONTINUOUS RENAL REPLACEMENT THERAPY			
	SCUF	**CVVH**	**CVVHD**	**CVVHDF**
Indications	Patient is diuretic resistant, has volume overload, is hemodynamically unstable	Patient has volume overload, is hemodynamically unstable with azotemia or uremia	Same as CVVH	Same as CVVH plus catabolic acute renal failure, electrolyte imbalances/metabolic acidosis
Advantages	Continuous, gradual therapy, precise fluid control, ease of initiation	Same as SCUF	Same as SCUF	Same as SCUF, better solute clearance than CVVH or CVVHD
Complications and disadvantages	Anticoagulation, bleeding, hypotension, hypothermia, access complications (bleeding, clotting, infection), requires strict monitoring of fluid and electrolyte balance, minimal solute removal, poor control of azotemia	Anticoagulation, bleeding, hypotension, hypothermia, access complications (bleeding, clotting, infection), requires strict monitoring of fluid and electrolyte balance	Same as CVVH	Same as CVVH

CVVH, Continuous venovenous hemofiltration; CVVHD, continuous venovenous hemodialysis; CVVHDF, continuous venovenous hemodiafiltration; SCUF, slow continuous ultrafiltration.

Table 6-9	TROUBLESHOOTING MAJOR PROBLEMS IN CONTINUOUS RENAL REPLACEMENT THERAPY	
Problem	**Cause**	**Intervention**
Hypotension	Cardiac dysfunction Excessive intravascular volume removal	Cardiotonic and vasopressor support Fluid replacement Reduce ultrafiltration rate
Poor ultrafiltration	High hematocrit Clotted filter	Predilution fluid replacement Flush filter; replace if necessary
Clotted filter	Inadequate anticoagulation Poor blood flow rates Kinks in blood tubing	Consult the licensed independent practitioner to assess effectiveness of anticoagulation Check tubing hourly to guard against kinks Change filter and restart therapy

each situation is chosen based on clinical status, including the ability to safely provide anticoagulation therapy to the patient and the type of vascular access. Catabolism, for example, causes rapid rises in BUN, creatinine, and potassium values, thus requiring rapid removal of these metabolic wastes. For this reason, patients may require hemodialysis with supplemental CRRT (see Table 6-7).

PRINCIPLES APPLIED TO SPECIFIC THERAPIES

Ultrafiltration: For ultrafiltration to occur, there must be a pressure gradient across the filter compartments; the pressure in the blood compartment must exceed the pressure in the filtrate compartment. This pressure gradient is called transmembrane pressure (TMP). Its major determinants are hydrostatic pressure and oncotic pressure. The rate of ultrafiltration depends on the type of filter, the hydrostatic pressure of the blood, and blood flow. The hydrostatic pressure forces small and middle size molecules such as creatinine, urea, glucose, and cytokines from the blood across the filter. The longer it takes for blood to exit the filter, the longer the blood is in contact with the porous filter surface, the dialysate (if used), and the filtration pressure. Longer exposure increases the likelihood that the molecules of solute will be filtered from the patient's blood. Hydrostatic pressure from the dialysis system is opposed by oncotic pressure, which is maintained by plasma proteins that do not pass through the filter because of their larger size. When hydrostatic pressure exceeds oncotic pressure, filtration of water and solutes occurs.

Ultrafiltration Prescription: To achieve optimal fluid management, the right amount of ultrafiltration must be prescribed and delivered. The net ultrafiltrate (fluid loss) is the difference between the amount of urine output and plasma water removed and the amount of fluid administered to the patient. Fluid balance is normally calculated hourly and is adjusted in response to hemodynamic changes.

Calculation of the ultrafiltration prescription can be found in Box 6-2.

CRRT Dose Prescription: The CRRT dose prescription includes the flow rate of dialysate and replacement fluids, the rate of ultrafiltration, and the blood flow rate. Depending on the patient's condition, the licensed independent practitioner (LIP) may prescribe a higher intensity therapy (40 mL/kg/h) versus a lower intensity therapy (25 mL/kg/h) based on ideal body weight.

Sieving Coefficient (SC): Clearance of medication during CRRT is impacted by the SC of the drug while it passes through the membrane. The SC is equal to the ultrafiltrate concentration of the drug divided by the plasma concentration. Drugs that are more protein-bound have a lower clearance during CRRT. However, as a result of the long duration of CRRT, more of these drugs may be removed.

PROCEDURE

The filter and lines are primed with normal saline to remove all air bubbles before the treatment is initiated. A large, double-lumen catheter is placed in the internal jugular, subclavian, or femoral vein. The catheter must have radiographic confirmation of placement before

---

Box 6-2   ULTRAFILTRATION PRESCRIPTION

Example 1: Calculate ultrafiltrate based on anticipated fluid balance
- Anticipated fluid intake is 4 L/24 h
- Desired net fluid loss equals 2 L/24 h
- Ultrafiltration rate equals 6 L + 2 L/24 h
- 6 L/24 h = 250 mL/h
- Set ultrafiltration pump to remove 250 mL/h

Example 2: Calculate precise ultrafiltration balance
- Calculate hourly intake from previous hour = 200 mL
- Calculate hourly urine output from previous hour = 50 mL
- Subtract output from intake to obtain net volume = 150 mL
- Add desired hourly fluid loss = 100 mL to net volume = 250 mL
- Set ultrafiltration pump to remove 250 mL/h

beginning therapy. Although the system is driven by venous access, dialysis terminology states that blood flows from the patient into the "arterial" or proximal port of the vascular access through the filter and returns to the patient through the "venous" or distal port of the access. If the "arterial" or proximal lumen of the catheter becomes occluded by being pulled up against the vessel wall, the proximal and distal lumens may be interchanged so that the blood is being removed from the patient via the "venous" or distal lumen of the catheter and returned via the "arterial" or proximal lumen. This phenomenon is sometimes signaled by the presence of increased air in the system, or low-flow alarms, which indicate that lower blood volume is being filtered.

For most patients, a continuous method of anticoagulation is necessary to prevent clotting in the lines and filter, heparin or citrate is most commonly used. A pump is used to drive the blood flow. While the blood flows through the filter, water, electrolytes, and most drugs not bound to plasma protein diffuse across the filter and thus become part of the filtrate, referred to as effluent.

If the objective is the removal of large amounts of fluid and solute (e.g., urea, potassium, creatinine) through convective clearance, it is necessary to infuse large volumes of replacement fluid to maintain fluid and electrolyte balance. Nursing responsibilities include initiating treatment, monitoring the patient and the system, and discontinuing treatment. Tables 6-9 and 6-10 list the advantages, disadvantages, and complications of the various therapeutic CRRT modes. Table 6-9 evaluates troubleshooting major problems with CRRT.

The current preference of most practitioners is pump-assisted venovenous CRRT. The advancements in technology have provided several alternatives for automated devices that monitor system pressures, ultrafiltration rates, dialysate solution rates, and various alarm systems.

ANTICOAGULATION

Patients who are critically ill may have an increased tendency for coagulation and/or bleeding. All CRRT modalities require the patient's blood to be in contact with artificial tubing and membranes, which stimulates the coagulation cascade. The complement cascade may also be stimulated if a biocompatible filter is not used. The goal of anticoagulation is to prevent clotting in the CRRT circuit, preserve filter performance, and optimize survival of the circuit. Care providers strive to achieve a balance between preventing blood loss within the circuit as a result of clotting and preventing excessive anticoagulation leading to bleeding. Clotted blood remaining in the circuit is "lost" from the patient. The patient who is critically ill is at increased risk for bleeding as a result of coagulopathy and endothelial disruption. AKI/ARF may be associated with a procoagulant state because of downregulation of natural anticoagulants and inhibition of fibrinolysis. If AKI has evolved slowly resulting from an underlying disease, platelets may also be dysfunctional.

Table 6-10	APPROACHES TO CONTINUOUS RENAL REPLACEMENT THERAPY FILTRATION FLUID REPLACEMENT
Predilution: Replacement Fluid Infused Proximal to the Filter	**Postdilution: Replacement Fluid Infused Distal to the Filter**
Patient population: Those with elevated BUN and Hct levels	Patient population: All types
Replacement fluid infused into access line	Replacement fluid infused into return line
Used to enhance urea clearance to $\geq 18\%$; decreases oncotic pressure, increasing net TMP; moves urea from erythrocytes into plasma	Used to maintain fluid and electrolyte balance
Increases net fluid removal	Less replacement fluid required
Potentially increases filter life	Simplified clearance determination
*Urea clearance 12.5 mL/min	Urea clearance 10.6 mL/min

*If increased urea clearance is desired, predilution mode of fluid replacement is used.
BUN, Blood urea nitrogen; *Hct*, hematocrit; *TMP*, transmembrane pressure.

FACTORS RELATED TO COAGULATION
Patient Factors
- Decrease in natural anticoagulants.
- Platelet count and function.
- Transfusions.
- Fibrinolysis inhibition.

Vascular Access Factors
- Catheter characteristic (e.g., diameter and length).
- Kinking or malposition.
- Patient position change.

Treatment Variations
- Intermittent blood flow reductions.
- Predilution or postdilution fluid replacement.
- Reaction time to alarms.
- Blood–air contact in the system.

The choice of anticoagulation generally depends on patient condition, physician preference, and nursing staff experience with specific regimens. Collaboration between providers promotes patient safety and efficacy of treatment. Evidence supports three considerations in maintaining a clot-free system: type of renal replacement therapy, the anticoagulant, and the desired blood flow rate.

HEPARIN
Heparin is the most common and least expensive of the choices. It can be administered either systemically or regionally.

Systemic heparinization: Heparin can be infused in a separate IV line for systemic heparinization or into the "arterial" line of the CRRT device. In addition to the complication of bleeding, heparin-induced thrombocytopenia can occur. Potential for thrombocytopenia has limited the use of systemic heparin in recent years.

Regional heparinization: A relatively uncommon procedure that produces anticoagulation in the circuit but not systemically to the patient. There is little research available on regional heparinization. When done, it requires two infusion devices: one to infuse heparin prefilter (before the hollow-fiber filter) and another for protamine, a heparin antagonist that is run postfilter into the return line to neutralize the heparin. This process requires determining the activated PTT systemically from the patient and postfilter preprotamine infusion. The goal is to heparinize the circuit without systemically heparinizing the patient. This process is labor-intensive and requires meticulous monitoring and frequent dose adjustment of both the heparin and protamine. Use of protamine in this manner is rather uncommon, thus few centers engage in this method of anticoagulation.

DIRECT THROMBIN INHIBITORS
These agents are used for anticoagulation in patients with heparin-induced thrombocytopenia. The most common agents are Argatroban, Bivalirudin (e.g., Angiomax), and Lepirudin (e.g., Refludan). Argatroban is eliminated by the liver and is more suitable for most patients on CRRT. Lepirudin is excreted renally and therefore not the choice for patients with AKI/ARF. Bivalirudin is not widely used in this setting, but is under investigation. These agents are considerably more expensive than heparin, are generally administered systemically, and tend to exert prolonged anticoagulation in patients with renal impairment. Careful monitoring and dosage adjustments are required. Reversal of the effects of direct thrombin inhibitors cannot be achieved immediately, because there is no reversal agent available.

CITRATE
Citrate is a common alternative to heparin for regional anticoagulation. Citrate is infused into the arterial line to chelate or bind with calcium and magnesium, thus inhibiting the coagulation cascade in the extracorporeal circulation. The deficit in ionized calcium is present only outside the body in the extracorporeal circuit, because before reinfusion of the filtered blood, calcium is substituted into the venous line to target normal ionized calcium. The goal is

to maintain ionized calcium less than 0.35 mmol/L in the extracorporeal circuit to prevent clotting within the filter. It is important to infuse calcium systemically to maintain normal levels of ionized calcium in the patient's circulation. If dialysate and predilution replacement fluids are used, they should be calcium-free to prevent reversal of the citrate effect in the circuit. The amount of citrate infused into the preblood pump is determined by systemic ionized calcium levels, which are sampled every 6 hours. During regional citrate anticoagulation, a minimum amount of citrate enters the systemic circulation; however, a systemic calcium infusion is used to assure that normal levels of ionized calcium are maintained in the patient's circulation.

Monitoring all laboratory values, including ionized calcium, sodium, and acid-base balance, is essential.

ISOTONIC SODIUM CHLORIDE SOLUTION

If the patient's condition prohibits anticoagulation, this presents a challenge in maintaining circuit patency. The system may need to be flushed with small boluses of isotonic sodium chloride to reduce stagnation of blood in the system. Specific unit protocol may require flushing with 50 to 100 mL every hour to maintain patency and decrease the potential for clotting.

The use of predilution replacement fluid hemodilutes the blood, which decreases the chance for clotting. Predilution also helps separate all solute particles, making it easier for solutes to pass into the filter. The fluid provides continuous flushing of the circuit. Use of sodium chloride must be done judiciously, with monitoring of acid-base balance and electrolytes.

Chloride can accumulate, prompting acidosis.

REPLACEMENT FLUID

Electrolyte imbalances that may occur with CRRT include hypokalemia, hypocalcemia, hypophosphatemia, and hypoglycemia. Free water can be depleted. Use of large amounts of normal saline replacement fluid can prompt hyperchloremic acidosis. The replacement fluid may be infused prefilter or postfilter and is tailored to the specific needs of individual patients. Three types of solutions are available: citrate-based, lactate-based, and bicarbonate-based. Lactate solutions can prompt the development of acidosis, and are not used in patients with liver abnormalities or in patients with lactic acidosis. Citrate is generally not used in patients with liver dysfunction.

ASSESSMENT: DURING CONTINUOUS RENAL REPLACEMENT THERAPY

GOAL OF SYSTEM ASSESSMENT
Evaluate hemodynamic stability and maintain homeostasis.

HISTORY AND RISK FACTORS
- Events leading to the development of ARF/AKI.
- Underlying chronic kidney disease.
- Presence of cardiovascular disease.
- Presence of pulmonary compromise.
- Nutritional state.
- Neurologic status.

VITAL SIGNS
- BP may increase or decrease based on fluid volume status.
- HR may increase or decrease in response to fluid and electrolyte changes.
- A change in baseline temperature in the presence of sepsis.
- Hypothermia, a common complication of CRRT, increases energy demands.
- Cardiac dysrhythmias may occur with hypothermia.
- Pulmonary artery occlusion pressure and CVP will fluctuate in tandem with changing volume status.
- Oxygen saturation to assess respiratory status.
- Body weight to assess fluid balance.
- Urine output and other fluid losses (blood loss drainage fluid).

OBSERVATION
Hourly Monitoring of the CRRT Circuit
- Blood flow rate.
- Venous (return) pressure.
- Arterial (access) pressure.
- Filter pressures.
- Balance pressures.
- Effluent pressures.
- Color of the blood in the circuit.
- Presence of air in the system.
- Dialysate flow rate (if applicable).
- Replacement flow rate (if applicable).
- Transmembrane pressure.
- Ultrafiltration rate.
- Calculate fluid balance.
- Filter patency.
- Anticoagulation.

Hourly Monitoring of the Vascular Access
- Catheter patency.
- Access pressure.
- Return pressure.
- Access site for signs of bleeding or infection.

PALPATION
- Pulse quality and regularity bilaterally (scale 0 to 4+).
- Vascular access site for tenderness or expression of exudate.
- Edema extremities and sacrum (scale 0 to 4+).

AUSCULTATION
- Heart sounds to evaluate for contributors to decreased cardiac output.
- Friction rub indicative of pericarditis.
- S3 and S4 indicative of heart failure.
- Pleural rub indicative of pulmonary pathology.
- Bowel sounds to evaluate gastric motility.

SCREENING LABWORK
- Electrolytes, BUN, and creatinine to determine renal function and effectiveness of CRRT.
- CBC to assess for the presence of anemia.
- Ionized calcium if using citrate anticoagulation to assess for hypocalcemia.
- Coagulation profile to monitor effects of other anticoagulants.

COLLABORATIVE MANAGEMENT
Goals for patients undergoing CRRT: The goal is the removal of excess fluid and solutes, while maintaining electrolyte balance and adequate fluid intake for homeostasis. In the adult patient who is critically ill, catabolic rate is two to three times that of normal.

Key Considerations	Goals
Enteral nutrition	Maintain nutritional requirements
Predilution fluid replacement	Used if increased solute removal is required
Replacement fluid	Used for convective clearance and to maintain fluid and electrolyte balance
Anticoagulation	Used to prevent clotting in the circuit
Vasopressors	Used to maintain adequate blood pressure
Vascular access	Double-lumen catheter, preferably in the subclavian or internal jugular vein

CARE PRIORITIES

Prevention of hemodynamic instability and maintenance of homeostasis are the goals of CRRT. This includes fluid removal and electrolyte replacement. Continuous monitoring and frequent prescription changes based on patient condition and needs are required to meet the goal of therapy. Fluid removal, electrolyte balance, and maintaining nutrition in these catabolic patients who are critically ill present a major care challenge for the treatment team.

1. Maintain hemodynamic stability

Evaluate the volume status based on weight, pulmonary artery occlusion pressure, cardiac output, CVP, and the clinical signs of hypervolemia or hypovolemia. Determine electrolyte balance with particular attention to sodium, potassium, and calcium. Determine the state of catabolism based on BUN and creatinine levels, along with the presence of metabolic acidosis.

2. Provide adequate nutrition to promote healing

Assess the nutrition requirements based on the rate of catabolism, serum albumin, and loss of protein. Most patients will require enteral or parenteral nourishment to meet nutrition requirements. All forms of fluid intake (e.g., IV and enteral fluids) must be accounted for when calculating the desired fluid loss.

3. Replacement fluids

Use physiologic solutions (more chemically similar to normal body chemistry) to replace the majority of the filtrate removed hourly, maintain volume stability, and replace electrolyte losses. The use of plain normal saline may not be appropriate for patients with high-volume replacement fluid, because electrolyte imbalances or hyperchloremic acidosis may ensue. Determine hourly fluid balance to maintain hemodynamic stability. Frequent changes in the CRRT prescription (orders) may be necessary based on intake changes. If the patient is receiving citrate-based anticoagulation, systemic calcium must be measured by ionized calcium levels, and replaced by a calcium infusion to prevent hypocalcemia.

4. Vascular access adequacy

Maintain adequate flow rates. Inappropriate positioning may cause blood flow interruption from the patient into the device or from the CRRT circuit into the patient as a result of catheter movement against the vessel wall or kinking of the access device. Changing the patient's position may increase the ability of the device to maintain more adequate blood flow. Assess for alignment and signs of infection. Sterile technique is required when performing access care.

5. Maintain patency of the CRRT machine circuit

Monitor coagulation measurements every 6 hours or as prescribed in the presence of anticoagulant infusions. Check the circuit for any signs of blood stasis in lines or filter. Flush with normal saline if there is evidence of clotting. If using regional anticoagulation of the circuit, adjust the rate of the anticoagulant infusion as necessary to maintain blood flow within the circuit without causing systemic anticoagulation of the patient.

CARE PLANS FOR CONTINUOUS RENAL REPLACEMENT THERAPY

DECREASED CARDIAC OUTPUT *related to fluid overload creating heart failure*

Goals/Outcomes: The patient's cardiac output is adequate, as evidenced by stabilization of vital signs and heart rhythm to the patient's normal range. Classic measurements include systolic BP 100 mm Hg or greater, HR 60 to 100 bpm, RR 12 to 20 breaths/min, peripheral pulses greater than 2+ on a 0-to-4+ scale, brisk capillary refill (less than 2 seconds), and normal sinus rhythm.

NOC Circulation Status.

Hemodynamic Regulation

1. Promote hemodynamic stabilization: Before, during, and after CRRT, assess and document BP, HR, and RR every 15 minutes during periods of instability; and then hourly once stabilized. Indicators of fluid volume overload and deficit include decreased systolic BP to less than 100 mm Hg, tachycardia, and tachypnea.
2. Monitor perfusion: Assess for decreased amplitude of peripheral pulses, coolness, pallor, and delayed capillary refill in the extremities indicative of decreased perfusion every 4 hours.

3. Fluid removal: Measure and record I&O hourly. Consult the advanced practice provider for a loss of greater than 200 mL/h over desired fluid removal volume.
4. Dysrhythmia management: Monitor cardiac rhythm continuously; notify the advanced practice provider of a decrease in BP greater than 20 mm Hg from baseline resulting from a HR or rhythm change, including tachycardia, bradycardia, and depressed T waves and ST segments, associated with intravascular fluid volume or electrolyte changes.
5. Collaborate with all members of the healthcare team to ensure that the prescription of CRRT is achieving the desired results during the appropriate time frame.
6. Monitor for abnormalities and changes in serum electrolyte values (potassium, calcium, phosphorus, and bicarbonate). Normal ranges: potassium 3.5 to 5 mEq/L, calcium 8.5 to 10.5 mg/dL, phosphorus 2.5 to 4.5 mg/dL, and bicarbonate 22 to 26 mEq/L (see the sections on Fluid and Electrolyte Disturbances, and Acid-Base Imbalances, Chapter 1).

RISK FOR DEFICIENT FLUID VOLUME *related to ultrafiltration during CRRT*

Goals/Outcomes: The patient achieves normovolemia without further destabilization, as evidenced by a gradual weight loss (less than 2.5 kg/day) and recovery of a urinary output greater than 0.5 mL/kg/h in nonanuric patients. Ultrafiltration fluid removal rate remains within 50 mL of the desired hourly rate.
NOC Fluid Balance.

Fluid Monitoring
1. Measure and record I&O hourly. Ensure that it is within desired limits.
2. Weigh the patient daily. Be alert to a daily loss of greater than 2.5 kg.
3. Record ultrafiltrate hourly.
4. Check replacement fluid infusion hourly to ensure that it is within prescribed limits.
5. Check dialysate fluid infusion rate hourly to ensure that it is within prescribed limits.
6. Consult the LIP for unanticipated fluid loss from vomiting, diarrhea, fever, and wound drainage.

NIC Electrolyte Management: Hyperkalemia; Electrolyte Management: Hypermagnesemia; Electrolyte Management: Hypernatremia; Electrolyte Management: Hyperphosphatemia; Fluid Management; Fluid Monitoring; Hypovolemia Management; Intravenous Therapy. Additional, optional interventions include Dysrhythmia Management; Feeding; Fever Treatment; Gastrointestinal Intubation; Hemodynamic Regulation; Invasive Hemodynamic Monitoring; Medication Management; Nutrition Management; Weight Management; and Phlebotomy: Arterial Blood Sample and Venous Blood Sample.

EXCESS FLUID VOLUME *related to renal insufficiency*

Goals/Outcomes: The patient experiences a gradual fluid loss and stabilization of intravascular volume, as evidenced by vital signs achieving baseline range, CRRT system functioning effectively, CVP 4 to 8 mm Hg, improvement of edema, crackles, and other physical indicators of hypervolemia.
NOC Fluid Overload Severity.

Fluid/Electrolyte Management
1. Check tubes for kinks hourly.
2. Maintain anticoagulation therapy within prescribed goals. The system must be functional for the patient to get the full benefit of CRRT.
3. Inspect vascular access, filter, and lines for patency hourly. If clotting or clogging with protein is suspected, flush the system with 50 mL normal saline to check patency.
4. If clots are present, consult the advanced practice provider, change the filter as needed.
5. On an hourly basis, assess for and document the presence of physical indicators of hypervolemia: CVP greater than 10 mm Hg, BP elevated greater than 20 mm Hg over baseline, tachycardia, jugular venous distention, basilar crackles, increasing edema (peripheral, sacral, periorbital), and tachypnea.

NIC Electrolyte Management: Hypokalemia; Electrolyte Management: Hyponatremia; Fluid/Electrolyte Management; Fluid Management; Fluid Monitoring. Additional, optional interventions include Dysrhythmia Management; Feeding; Gastrointestinal Intubation; Hemodialysis Therapy; Hemodynamic Regulation; Invasive Hemodynamic Monitoring; Medication Management; Phlebotomy: Arterial and Venous Blood Samples; Positioning; Skin Surveillance; and Weight Management.

DEFICIENT KNOWLEDGE *related to CRRT procedure/treatment*

Goals/Outcomes: The patient or significant other verbalizes accurate information about the CRRT procedure within 24 to 48 hours of instruction.
NOC Knowledge: Treatment/Procedure.

Teaching: Procedure/Treatment
1. Assess the patient's knowledge of CRRT, explain necessity of vascular access and what can be expected during vascular access insertion. Typical access sites are the internal jugular or the subclavian vein. Occasionally femoral access is required.
2. Explain the importance of and rationale for limited movement of the area of catheter insertion following catheter placement.
3. Describe the equipment used for the procedure (e.g., CRRT machine, filter, lines). Explain that their blood will be visible in the filter and lines throughout therapy.
4. Discuss that vital signs will be assessed and blood tests will be performed at frequent intervals to monitor for stability throughout therapy. Reinforce that staff members are close at all times to provide support and additional information as needed.
5. Explain that the use of CRRT may require 24 hours or longer to attain fluid balance.

NIC Teaching: Disease Process; Teaching: Individual; Teaching: Prescribed Medication. Additional, optional interventions include Discharge Planning; Medication Management; and Weight Management.

IMPAIRED PHYSICAL MOBILITY *related to weakness ensuing with critical illness*

Goals/Outcomes: The patient exhibits ability to move about in bed with assistance without evidence of disruption of hemofiltration equipment. The patient's skin remains intact, no evidence of muscle atrophy or contracture formation caused by imposed immobility.
NOC Mobility.

Positioning
1. Secure the access device and tape to ensure safe movement without disruption of the catheter.
2. Explain to patient the need for care and assistance when moving.
3. Try to avoid use of physical restraint to restrict movement. If the access site is near or within a limb and movement prompts device occlusion, initiate a limb immobilizer.
4. Turn and reposition the patient at least every 2 hours, maintaining good body alignment.
5. Advance mobility as tolerated by the patient and position of catheter.
6. Massage bony prominences during every position change to promote comfort and circulation.
7. Support involved extremities with pillows.
8. Teach patient-assisted range-of-motion exercises on uninvolved extremities. Encourage isometric, isotonic, and quadriceps setting exercises on uninvolved extremities.

NIC Exercise Therapy: Ambulation; Exercise Therapy: Joint Mobility. Additional, optional interventions include Activity Therapy; Body Mechanics Promotion; Circulatory Care; Circulatory Precautions; Fall Prevention; Pain Management; Progressive Muscle Relaxation; Skin Surveillance; and Weight Management.

RISK FOR INJURY *related to CRRT equipment*

Goals/Outcomes: The patient's CRRT filter and line connections remain intact, and ultrafiltrate test results are negative for blood.
NOC Fluid Balance.

Fluid Monitoring
1. Secure all connections within the system and check hourly.
2. Avoid concealing lines, filter, or connections with linen.
3. Inspect ultrafiltrate hourly for blood. If unsure whether ultrafiltrate contains blood, check the solution for occult blood.
4. If the test result is positive for blood, clamp the ultrafiltrate port and consult the advanced practice provider for further interventions.

NIC Electrolyte Management: Hyperkalemia; Electrolyte Management: Hypermagnesemia; Electrolyte Management: Hypernatremia; Electrolyte Management: Hyperphosphatemia; Fluid Management; Fluid Monitoring; Hypovolemia Management; Intravenous Therapy. Additional, optional interventions include Dysrhythmia Management; Feeding; Fever Treatment; Gastrointestinal Intubation; Hemodynamic Regulation; Invasive Hemodynamic Monitoring; Medication Management; Nutrition Management; Weight Management; and Phlebotomy: Arterial Blood Sample and Venous Blood Sample.

ADDITIONAL NURSING DIAGNOSES

For more information about fluid and electrolytes, see sections on Fluid and Electrolyte Disturbances, and Prolonged Immobility, Chapter 1.

SELECTED REFERENCES

ACT Investigators: Acetylcysteine for prevention of renal outcomes in patients undergoing coronary and peripheral vascular angiography: main results from the randomized Acetylcysteine for Contrast-induced nephropathy Trial (ACT), *Circulation* 124:1250–1259, 2011.

Adedotun A, Perazella M: Recurrent acute kidney injury following bath salts intoxication, *Am J Kidney Dis* 59:273–275, 2012.

American Nephrology Nurses Association: *Core curriculum for nephrology nursing*, Pitman, 2008, Anthony J. Jannetti.

Bagshaw SM, Berthiaume LR, Delaney A, Bellomo R: Continuous versus intermittent renal replacement therapy for acute kidney injury: a meta-analysis, *Crit Care Med* 35:610–617, 2008.

Balemans C, Reichert L, vanSchelven B, et al: Epidemiology of contrast material-induced nephropathy in the era of hydration, *Radiology* 263:706–713, 2012.

Banks DS: Prescribing continuous renal replacement therapy using a JavaScript calculator improves delivered dose, *JICS* 12:289–292, 2011.

Bellomo R, Lipesey M, Calzavacca P, et al: Early acid-base and blood pressure effects of continuous renal replacement therapy intensity in patients with metabolic acidosis, *Intensive Care Med* 39:429–436, 2013.

Boling B: Renal issues in older adults in critical care, *Crit Care Nurs Clin North Am* 26:99–104, 2014.

Bouchard J, Mehta RL: Acid-base disturbances in the intensive care unit: current issues and the use of renal replacement therapy as a customized treatment tool, *Int J Artif Organs* 31:6–14, 2008.

Bouchard J, Mehta RL: Volume management in continuous renal replacement therapy, *Semin Dial* 22:146–150, 2009.

Bucaloiu I, Perkins R, DiFilippo W, et al: Acute kidney injury in the critically ill, morbidly obese patient: diagnostic and therapeutic challenges in a unique population, *Crit Care Clin* 26:607–624, 2010.

Cerda J, Lameire N, Eggers P, et al: Epidemiology of acute kidney injury, *Clin J Am Soc Nephrol* 3:881–886, 2008.

Chrysochoou G, Marcus RJ, Sureshkumar KK, et al: Renal replacement therapy in the critical care unit, *Crit Care Nurse Q* 31:282–290, 2008.

Cruz DN, Goh CY, Marenzi G, et al: Renal replacement therapies for prevention of radiocontrast-induced nephropathy: a systematic review, *Am J Med* 125:66–78, 2012.

Davenport M, Khlaltbari S, Dillman J, et al: Contrast material-induced nephrotoxicity and intravenous low-osmolality iodinated contrast material, *Radiology* 267:94–105, 2013.

Dennen P, Douglas I, Anderson R: Acute kidney injury in the intensive care unit: an update and primer for the intensivist, *Crit Care Med* 38:261–275, 2010.

Erdbruegger U, Okusa M: Investigational biomarkers and the evaluation of acute tubular necrosis. In Palevsky PM, editor: *UptoDate*, Waltham, 2014, Wolters Kluwer. http://www.uptodate.com/contents/investigational-biomarkers-and-the-evaluation-of-acute-tubular-necrosis/abstact/54. (Updated January 31, 2014).

Fiaccadori E, Regolisti G, Maggiore U: Specialized nutritional support interventions in critically ill patients on renal replacement therapy, *Curr Opin Clin Nutr Metab Care* 16:217–224, 2013.

Filiponi TC, de Souza Durao M: How to choose the ideal renal replacement therapy in sepsis? *Shock* 39:50–53, 2013.

Getting J, Gregoire J, Phul A, Kasten M: Oxalate nephropathy due to "juicing"; case report and review, *Am J Med* 126:768–772, 2013.

Ghossein C, Grouper S, Soong W: Renal replacement therapy in the intensive care unit, *Int Anesthesiol Clin* 47:15–34, 2009.

Himmelfarb J, Joannidis M, Molitoris B, et al: Evaluation and initial management of acute kidney injury, *Clin J Am Soc Nephrol* 3:962–967, 2008.

Honiden S: *Caring for the critically ill, obese patient*, Northbrook, 2011, American College of Chest Physicians. http://69.36.35.38/accp/pccsu/caring-critically-ill-obese-patient?page=0,3.

Honore PM, Jacobs R, Joannes-Boyau O, et al: Newly designed CRRT membranes for sepsis and SIRS – a pragmatic approach for bedside intensivists summarizing the more recent advances: a systematic structured review, *ASAIO J* 59:99–106, 2013.

Hoste E, Schurgers M: Epidemiology of acute kidney injury: how big is the problem? *Crit Care Med* 36(Suppl 4):S146–S151, 2008.

Kidney Disease/Improving Global Outcomes (KDIGO) Acute Kidney Injury Work Group: KDIGO clinical practice guidelines for acute kidney injury, *Kidney Int Suppl* 2:1–138, 2012.

Kinsey G, Okusa M: Pathogenesis of acute kidney injury: foundation for clinical practice, *Am J Kidney Dis* 58:291–301, 2011.

Lameire N, Bagga A, Cruz D, et al: Acute kidney injury: an increasing global concern, *Lancet* 382:170–179, 2013.

Legrand M, Darmon M, Joannidis M, Payen D: Management of renal replacement therapy in ICU patients: an international survey, *Intensive Care Med* 39:101–108, 2013.

Luber S, Fischer D, Venkat A: *Care of the bariatric surgery patient in the emergency department*, In Medscape, New York, 2008, WebMD. http://www.medscape.com/viewarticle/572923. Accessed on Feb. 20, 2014.

Lyndon WD, Wille KM, Tolwani AJ: Solute clearance in CRRT: prescribed dose versus actual delivered dose, *Nephrol Dial Transplant* 27:952–956, 2012.

Mayrtenson J, Martling C, Bell, M: Novel biomarkers of acute kidney injury and failure: clinical applicability, *Br J Anaesth* 109:843–850, 2012.

McDonald J, McDonald R, Comin J, et al: Frequency of acute kidney injury following contrast medium administration: a systematic review and meta-analysis, *Radiology* 267:119–128, 2013.

Oh JH, Shin DH, Lee MJ, et al: Urine output is associated with prognosis in patients with acute kidney injury requiring continuous renal replacement therapy, *J Crit Care* 28:379–388, 2013.

Palevsky P: Definition of acute kidney injury (acute renal failure). In Curhan GC, editor: *UptoDate*, Waltham, 2008, Wolters Kluwer. http://www.uptodate.com/contents/definition-of-acute-kidney-injury-acute-renal-failure.

Pannu N, Klarenbach S, Wiebe N, et al: Renal replacement therapy in patients with acute renal failure: a systematic review, *JAMA* 299:793–805, 2008.

Pieracci F, Barie P, Pomp A: Critical care of the bariatric patient. In *Medscape*, New York, 2006, WebMD. http://www.medscape.com/viewarticle/533570.

Ricci Z, Ronco C: Timing, dose and mode of dialysis in acute kidney injury, *Curr Opin Crit Care* 17:556–561, 2011.

Rosner M: Acute kidney injury in the elderly, *Clin Geriatr Med* 29:565–578, 2013.

Schefold JC, Haehling SV, Pschowski R, et al: The effect of continuous versus intermittent renal replacement therapy on outcome of critically ill patients with acute renal failure (CONVINT): a prospective randomized controlled trial, *Crit Care* 18:R11, 2014.

Scoville BA, Mueller BA: Medication dosing in critically ill patients with acute kidney injury treated with renal replacement therapy, *Am J Kidney Dis* 61:490–500, 2013.

Sharfuddin A, Weisbord S, Palevsky P, Molitoris B: Acute kidney injury. In Taal M, Chertow G, Marsden P, et al, editors: *Brenner & Rector's the kidney*, ed 9, Philadelphia, 2011, Saunders, pp 1044–1099.

Shashaty M, Meyer N, Localio A, et al: African race, obesity and blood product transfusion are risk factors for acute kidney injury in critically ill trauma patients, *J Crit Care* 27:496-504, 2012.

Shingarev R, Allon M: A physiologic-based approach to the treatment of acute hyperkalemia, *Am J Kidney Dis* 56:578–584, 2010.

Soto G: Body mass index and acute kidney injury in the acute respiratory distress syndrome, *Crit Care Med* 40:2601–2608, 2012.

Spahillari A, Parikh C, Sint K, et al: Serum cystatin C versus creatinine-based definitions of acute kidney injury following cardiac surgery: a prospective cohort study, *Am J Kidney Dis* 60:922–929, 2012.

The VA/NIH Acute Renal Failure Trial Network: Intensity of renal support in critically ill patients with acute kidney injury, *N Engl J Med* 359:7–20, 2008.

Tolwani A: Continuous renal replacement therapy for acute kidney injury, *N Engl J Med* 367:2505–2514, 2012.

Vanmassenhove J: Urinary and serum biomarkers for the diagnosis of acute kidney injury: an in-depth review of the literature, *Nephrol Dial Transplant* 28:254–273, 2013.

Venkataraman R: Can we prevent acute kidney injury? *Crit Care Med* 36(Suppl 4):S166–S171, 2008.

Waikar S, Liu K, Chertow G: Diagnosis, epidemiology and outcomes of acute kidney injury, *Clin J Am Soc Nephrol* 13:844–861, 2008.

Wang X, Yuan WJ: Timing of initiation of renal replacement therapy in acute kidney injury: a systematic review and meta-analysis, *Ren Fail* 34:396–402, 2012.

Zhang JD, Hongying M: Efficacy and safety of regional citrate anticoagulation in critically ill patients undergoing continuous renal replacement therapy, *Intensive Care Med* 38:20–28, 2012.

Neurologic Disorders

GENERAL NEUROLOGIC ASSESSMENT

LEVEL OF CONSCIOUSNESS

* Assess for orientation, drowsiness, inappropriate use of words, slurred speech, arousability, confusion, and amnesia.
* Close monitoring of level of consciousness (LOC) is essential to assess for determining deterioration, and even a slight change may indicate that emergent intervention is needed.
* For specifics of how to assess using levels of stimulation, refer to Appendix 2, Glasgow Coma Scale (GCS).
* Considerations for the bariatric patient: The increased ratio of adipose to lean body mass changes the volume of distribution of lipophilic drugs. Propofol and benzodiazepines used for sedation and control of anxiety are lipophilic. Increased adipose tissue prompts an accumulation of these and all lipophilic drugs. Increased dose is required to achieve the desired effects, and the elimination half-life is prolonged. The dose of many lipophilic medications in the bariatric population is considered more effective using the actual body weight rather than ideal body weight. If doses of propofol and benzodiazepines (e.g., lorazepam, diazepam, midazolam) are prescribed using actual body weight, the patient may remain agitated. Patients may also experience prolonged sedation, particularly with benzodiazepines, when the drugs are weaned. Underlying mood changes and memory loss may be present, because these conditions are associated with obesity.

VITAL SIGNS

Refer to specific sections for key vital sign changes specific for the type of neurologic disorder.

KEY CRANIAL NERVE ASSESSMENT

It is not always necessary to assess all 12 cranial nerves (see Appendix 3). Specific neurologic disorders will address cranial nerve impairments.

* Assess the nerves responsible for vision (optic), pupillary response (oculomotor), and eye movements (oculomotor, trochlear, abducens).
* Assess facial/corneal sensation and chewing (trigeminal) and facial muscle movement and taste (facial).
* All functions are evaluated bilaterally (e.g., both eyes, both sides of face, etc.).
* A full examination includes all 12 nerves.
* Considerations for the geriatric patient: Obesity accelerates aging, including changes seen in cranial nerve assessment in older adults. Diabetic neuropathy may manifest in patients who are insulin-resistant, with persistent hyperglycemia.

ASSESS MOTOR AND CEREBELLAR FUNCTION

Evaluate bilaterally (both sides of body, both arms and legs) for muscle size, strength, tone, and coordination. Note muscle atrophy or hypertrophy.

* If the patient can walk, assess gait.
* Ask the patient to walk heel to toe to check for balance and coordination.
* Perform Romberg test: Ask the patient to close eyes and stand with feet close together while you stand nearby in case the patient sways/falls (abnormal response indicative of cerebellar dysfunction).
* Ask the patient to squeeze your hands and push feet against your hands, to assess if strength is equal on both sides.

- Note any involuntary movements (tremors, jerking, fasciculations) and general posture.
- Move the patient's joints through passive range-of-motion (ROM) exercises, noting any tenderness of involved muscle groups.
- To further evaluate muscle strength, have the patient perform active ROM exercises while you apply resistance against the movements. Use the following rating scale for muscle strength:

MUSCLE STRENGTH RATING

Score	Description of Strength
5/5	Patient moves joint with full ROM against normal resistance and gravity
4/5	Patient moves joint with full ROM against mild resistance and gravity
3/5	Patient moves joint with full ROM against gravity only
2/5	Patient moves joint with full ROM but not against gravity
1/5	Patient's muscle contracts in an attempt to move joint; joint does not move
0/5	Patient does not visibly attempt to move; no muscle contraction; paralysis

ROM, Range of motion.

- Assess for abnormal motor movements unilaterally and bilaterally:
  - Decorticate posturing (abnormal flexion).
  - Decerebrate posturing (abnormal extension).
  - Flaccidity.

Motor deficits (weakness or paralysis) are caused by injury or edema to the primary motor cortex and corticospinal (pyramidal) tracts.

- Perform specific testing for abnormalities as appropriate:
  - Grasp: Place two fingers within the patient's palm and ask the patient to squeeze your fingers. Ask the patient to let go. Abnormal grasp: The patient cannot let go once grasp is in progress. May reflect frontal lobe disease; observed occasionally with occipital lobe disease, Alzheimer disease, or bilateral thalamic disease.
  - Babinski sign: Upward or dorsiflexion of the big toe when stroking the outer sole and ball of the foot can indicate a lesion of the pyramidal tract.
  - Kernig sign: Painful resistance to full extension of the leg at the knee when the hip is flexed; used in the diagnosis of meningitis resulting from meningeal irritation.
  - Brudzinski sign: Flexion of the hip and knee involuntarily with neck flexion and used in the diagnosis of meningitis resulting from meningeal irritation.
- Considerations for the bariatric patient: Assess exercise history, noting weakness in extremities. The spine and joints are burdened by the additional weight, and are at risk for deterioration and instability. Pain assessment may reveal the reasons for limited mobility, in addition to reduced level of endurance. Posture analysis is done to help classify the body type, which helps to anticipate risk factors. Functional ability, mobility, and disabilities should be noted, including simple findings such as the ability to transfer from bed to chair.

SENSORY ASSESSMENT

Sensory deficits occur when the primary sensory cortex, the sensory association areas of the parietal lobe, or the spinothalamic tracts are injured or edematous. Sensory deficits include inability to distinguish objects according to characteristics (e.g., size, shape, weight) and inability to distinguish overall changes in temperature, touch, pressure, and position.

- Assess perception of touch, proprioception, pain, temperature, and vibration (if possible). Ask the patient to close eyes while you apply stimuli. The patient should not be given the opportunity to anticipate your moves. Compare the same stimulus on the right side of the body to the identical location on the left side of the body. Note if the patient perceives stimuli symmetrically and appropriately (sharp versus dull using a needle versus a cotton swab, or hot versus cold). Compare proximal and distal parts of arms and legs when testing pain and touch.

- Superficial and deep reflexes are tested on symmetrical sides of the body and compared noting the strength of contraction.
- Test vibratory sense (with vibrating tuning fork) distally (on the tip of big toe or finger) and ask when the patient feels the vibration stop.
- For position sense, move distal joints about using very light touch and ask about the position the patient perceives of the joint.
- Two-point discrimination can be done using a bent paper clip. Note the smallest distance between the two points at which the patient senses two points are pressing on the skin. Document using a dermatome map.

Improvement in both motor and sensory perception may be seen while cerebral edema subsides.

FUNDOSCOPIC ASSESSMENT

Generally done by the advanced practice provider and may reveal retinal hemorrhage(s) at the side of the optic disc. Hemorrhage is caused by blood from the subarachnoid space (SAS) being forced along the optic nerve sheath under high pressure. The patient may complain of blurred vision or blind spots (scotomata). Terson hemorrhage associated with vitreous and/or subhyaloid hemorrhage has been seen as a subarachnoid complication and its presence has been noted with increased mortality and morbidity rates.

DYSPHAGIA SCREENING

Should be performed early, particularly when stroke has occurred, to prevent complications of aspiration and to initiate appropriate nutrition therapy. People with neurologic dysfunction are poor judges of their own ability to swallow, thus a thorough evaluation and intervention by a speech pathologist may be required, following routine screening procedures recommended by institutional protocol.

Diagnostic Tests for Neurologic Disorders		
Test	**Purpose**	**Abnormal Findings**
Cerebral angiography	Digital subtraction angiography visualizes blood flow. Involves use of intravascular catheter. The gold standard for evaluating cerebral vasculature. Invasive procedure with minimal risk used to visualize the cerebral blood vessels.	Areas of reduced cerebral blood flow, aneurysms, arteriovenous malformations (AVMs), vascular abnormalities. Used with interventional neuroradiologic procedures such as coiling, AVM embolization (gluing). Provides specific information on the cause of stroke by identifying the blood vessel involved
Computed tomography (CT) of brain	Performed emergently, is the gold standard of differentiating ischemic from hemorrhagic stroke; may be done at intervals to monitor progress. Assesses details of structures of bone, tissue, and fluid-filled space. Detects exudate, abscesses, and intracranial pathology (e.g., tumors, brain injury). Assesses for hydrocephalus.	Shift of structures caused by enlarged mass, edema, exudate, abscesses, fresh hemorrhage, hematomas, infarction, and hydrocephalus. Can visualize facial skeleton and soft tissue structures for abnormalities (e.g., tumors, brain injury). Within the first few hours after an acute ischemic stroke, the scan may appear normal. Intracranial hemorrhage is easily diagnosed on CT—blood appears as a bright white signal.
Continuous electrocardiographic monitoring	Evaluates cardiovascular status, especially during medication administration.	Phenytoin and other antiepileptic drugs can cause dysrhythmias and hypotension.
CT angiography	Less invasive than cerebral angiography; involves use of contrast media injection into peripheral vein and use of CT scanner.	Visualizes intraarterial clot, small intracranial aneurysm, and AVM.

Continued

Diagnostic Tests for Neurologic Disorders—cont'd

Test	Purpose	Abnormal Findings
CT perfusion or CT-xenon scan	Provides information related to cerebral blood flow (CBF) and volume. Used to guide clinical decision-making regarding the use of thrombolysis or interventional procedures.	Compromised blood flow; a limited test; cannot detect infarcted tissue.
Electroencephalography	Evaluates electrical activity of the brain for ongoing seizures, even if there are no clinical signs of seizures.	Diagnosis of seizures and localization of structural abnormalities. Also used as element of criteria for brain death.
Electromyography (EMG) or nerve conduction velocity (NCV)	Assesses NCV deficit as a result of the demyelination of peripheral nerves.	EMG and NCV demonstrate profound slowing of motor conduction velocities and conduction blocks several weeks into the illness.
Lumbar puncture (LP) with cerebrospinal fluid (CSF) specimen for analysis	Measures CSF pressures and obtains CSF specimen when infection, such as meningitis or neurosyphilis, is suspected. May be performed when subarachnoid hemorrhage is suspected and CT is normal.	Elevated protein, low glucose, elevated white blood cell count.
Magnetic resonance imaging (MRI) and arteriography (MRA) of brain	Minute oscillations of hydrogen atoms in the brain create graphic image of bone, fluid, and soft tissue. Provides a more detailed image. MRI is most useful for patients with ischemia in identifying the cause and area involved. Provides detailed information regarding the area of injury or its vascular supply (magnetic resonance arteriogram or MRA). Diffusion-weighted imaging is a measurement of edema, whereas perfusion-weighted imaging is a measurement of global CBF.	Infarcts, areas at risk or ischemic areas, vascular defects, stenosis, occlusion.
Positron emission tomography (PET) and single-photon emission computed tomography	To evaluate brain metabolism and blood flow using three-dimensional imaging produced using a radioactive tracer.	Demonstrates abnormal function of the brain by revealing abnormal structures, metabolism, and perfusion. Locates areas of brain causing seizures, head injury, and some disorders (e.g., Alzheimer disease).
Radioisotope brain scan	Examines areas of blood flow through concentration of isotope uptake in the brain.	Increased or decreased blood flow intraoperatively or assesses for postoperative cerebral infarction. Lack of uptake may indicate cerebral brain death.
Transcranial Doppler	Noninvasive and can be done serially at the bedside. Evaluates the intracranial vessels and assesses the velocity of blood flow in the anterior and posterior cerebral circulation. Also used to evaluate vasospasm, to determine brain death via detection of cerebral circulatory arrest, for intraoperative monitoring, and to locate emboli.	Arterial narrowing, vasospasm, cerebral circulatory arrest, emboli as a result of vasospasm. Can also be used to confirm absent blood flow in brain death.

BRAIN DEATH
PATHOPHYSIOLOGY

Brain death is defined as irreversible loss of function of the brain, including the brainstem and respiratory centers. Cardiac death is the cessation of mechanical action/pumping of the heart, resulting in absence of pulse, heart sounds, blood pressure (BP), and respirations. Brain death is most frequently the result of increased intracranial pressure (ICP) caused by severe traumatic head injury or hemorrhagic stroke caused by ruptured cerebral aneurysm with subarachnoid hemorrhage (SAH) or intracranial hemorrhage (ICH). A significant number of patients with large acute ischemic strokes (AIS) experience cerebral edema and herniation. Hypoxic-ischemic encephalopathy with massive brain swelling after prolonged cardiopulmonary resuscitation or asphyxia and encephalopathy with cerebral edema resulting from fulminant hepatic failure may also result in increased ICP, herniation, and brain death.

If brain death occurs quickly, cardiac death may occur immediately. If brain death occurs more slowly, with time to initiate mechanical ventilation before cardiac death, the heart can continue to beat/pump because the cardiac pacing cells operate independently from brain regulation. Mechanical ventilation provides the oxygen necessary to maintain viable cardiac pacing cells and conduction pathways if the patient is circulating adequate amounts of blood cells carrying oxyhemoglobin, acidosis is controlled, and electrolytes are managed. Over time, without a functional hypothalamus and pituitary gland, patients experience further instability of BP caused by loss of regulation of the thyroid and adrenal glands. Massive diuresis is common when the posterior pituitary gland ceases to function.

If the patient is an organ donor, the organs must be sustained before removal, requiring management of all sequelae of brain death. Guidelines for managing brain dead organ donors have common elements internationally, with most controversy stemming from the need to provide additional hormones to help control endocrine-related crises associated with loss of function of the pituitary and hypothalamus and use of prophylactic antibiotics to prevent infection.

The President's Commission report regarding "guidelines for the determination of death" drafted a proposal for a legal definition of death resulting in the Uniform Determination of Death Act (UDDA). The document states: "An individual who has sustained either (1) irreversible cessation of circulatory and respiratory functions, or (2) irreversible cessation of all functions of the entire brain, including the brainstem, is dead. A determination of death must be made with accepted medical standards." In the United States, the majority of state laws reflect the UDDA. Amendments including physician qualifications, confirmation by a second physician, or religious exemption have also been included by legislators in several states.

The UDDA does not define "accepted medical standards." The American Academy of Neurology (AAN) brain death practice guidelines were initially written in 1995 to define medical standards for determination of brain death. The guidelines highlighted that three key clinical findings must be present to confirm irreversible cessation of brain functions, including the brainstem: coma (with a known cause), absence of brainstem reflexes, and apnea. Despite the AAN guidelines, patients are inconsistently managed in U.S. hospitals and worldwide. Differences in prerequisites, the number of required physician assessments, the lowest "living person" core temperature, and other measurements varied. Medical record documentation of those diagnosed with brain death consistently reveals deficiencies in documentation.

In 2010, the AAN incorporated the majority of available evidence into updated guidelines. Five questions emerged, and were answered following a thorough review of the literature, to address variations in brain death determination and to facilitate more consistency in diagnosis:

- Question: Are there patients who fulfill the clinical criteria of brain death who recover brain function? Answer: In adults, recovery of neurologic function has not been reported after the clinical diagnosis of brain death has been established using the criteria given in the 1995 AAN practice parameter.
- Question: What is an adequate observation period to ensure that cessation of neurologic function is permanent? Answer: There is insufficient evidence to determine the minimally acceptable observation period to ensure that neurologic functions have ceased irreversibly.
- Question: Are complex motor movements that falsely suggest retained brain function sometimes observed in brain death? Answer: For some patients diagnosed as brain

dead, complex, non–brain-mediated spontaneous movements can falsely suggest retained brain function. Ventilator autocycling may falsely suggest patient-initiated breathing.

- Question: What is the comparative safety of techniques for determining apnea? Answer: Apneic oxygenation diffusion to determine apnea is safe, but there is insufficient evidence to determine the comparative safety of techniques used for apnea testing.
- Question: Are there new ancillary tests that accurately identify patients with brain death? Answer: Because of a high risk of bias and inadequate statistical precision, there is insufficient evidence to determine if any new ancillary tests accurately identify brain death.

Only one study has prospectively developed criteria for the determination of brain death. Despite the lack of evidence, the principles used for the development of "accepted medical standards" for declaration of brain death are easily understood, and derived from the definition of brain death within the UDDA. To determine "cessation of all functions of the entire brain, including the brainstem," physicians must diagnose unresponsive coma, absence of brainstem reflexes, and absence of respiratory drive after an apnea test/CO_2 challenge. To ensure cessation of brain function is "irreversible," physicians must diagnose the cause of coma, exclude other medical conditions, and evaluate the patient over time to exclude the possibility of recovery.

Despite having reasonably clear guidelines for evaluation, the lack of evidence prompts clinicians to exercise considerable judgment when using the criteria on each unique patient. Adherence to the AAN guidelines varies among the large medical centers in the United States. Diabetes insipidus, myxedema coma, and adrenal crisis may result from loss of the hypothalamic/pituitary regulatory axis as part of brain death. Large amounts of dextrose-containing intravenous (IV) fluids and insulin resistance may prompt hyperglycemia. Neurologists, neurosurgeons, and intensivists may diagnose brain death approximately two to three times monthly in large referral centers. Herniation, or displacement of a portion of the brain through openings in the intracranial cavity, results from increased ICP. Herniation occurs when there is a difference between the cranial compartment pressures above (supratentorial) and below (infratentorial) the tentorium, the rigid membrane that divides the skull. If additional blood or cerebrospinal fluid (CSF), edematous tissue, or tumor occupies space inside the skull, there is little ability to expand to "make room" for anything not normally present. These "mass lesions" or "space-occupying lesions" cause "crowding" within their cavity, which increases the pressure.

When pressure in one of the two compartments (supratentorial or infratentorial) is markedly elevated, the brain structures and blood vessels within the cavity are compressed, resulting in ischemia, hypoxia, and, if uncontrolled, cerebral anoxia. When blood flow is minimal to absent, the hypoxic/anoxic brain tissues become more edematous. Eventually, no space remains for further expansion. The skull cannot expand and the tentorium expands minimally, thus the brain is forced through the available openings. The movement or displacement through an opening causes further compression of blood vessels, with possible laceration and destruction, which leads to necrosis of brain tissues and brain death (see Traumatic Brain Injury, Neurologic Herniation Syndromes, Chapter 3).

NEUROLOGIC ASSESSMENT: BRAIN DEATH

GOAL OF SYSTEM ASSESSMENT

The assessment validates absence of function of the brain and brainstem. If mechanical ventilation is terminated, natural death results. Severity of brain injury should be determined following two expert clinical assessments and diagnostic testing.

HISTORY AND RISK FACTORS

- Severe traumatic head injury (motor vehicle accident, gunshot/other assault, recreational/industrial accidents).
- Ruptured cerebral aneurysm with SAH.
- ICH resulting in intracerebral hematoma.
- Large AIS resulting in massive cerebral edema and/or brain herniation.
- Prolonged cardiopulmonary resuscitation.

- Asphyxia (asthmatic cardiac arrest, drug overdose, hanging, carbon monoxide poisoning, drowning, meningitis).
- Fulminant hepatic failure.

APNEA TEST (CO$_2$ CHALLENGE)

- Determines absence of respirations when mechanically induced ventilations cease. Testing must be done carefully to avoid cardiac death during the test. If the patient begins to deteriorate while off the ventilator, the patient should be placed back on the ventilator.

VITAL SIGNS

- Mild hypothermia: Core temperature greater than 32° C (90° F), but less than 36.5° C (97° F).
- Hypotension: With mechanical ventilation in place, BP is greater than 90 mm Hg. Without mechanical ventilation, the heart rate (HR) will decrease, resulting in hypotension and eventually asystole.
- Apnea: No spontaneous respirations when mechanical ventilation is suspended. A formal apnea test is required to confirm the absence of respirations.

OBSERVATION/INSPECTION/PALPATION

- Coma: The patient does not respond to verbal stimuli, touch, or deep pain induced by pressure exerted on nail beds, the supraorbital area of the skull, or the temporomandibular joint or rubbing the sternum. The cause of coma is most often determined by history and physical examination, coupled with neuroradiologic imaging and laboratory testing. If the patient has received central nervous system (CNS) depressing medications, neuromuscular blocking agents, has consumed alcohol, has severe electrolyte, acid-base, or endocrine disease, diagnosis of brain death cannot be made until residual effects of the drugs or other conditions are fully resolved. Core temperature must be raised and maintained at $\geq$36° C. Two neurologic examinations should be done. Any physician is legally allowed to perform the examination in most U.S. states, but neurologists, neurosurgeons, and intensivists may have a great level of comfort and expertise in determining a brain death diagnosis.
- Brainstem reflexes/cranial nerve function: *Absent*
    - Pupils: Unresponsive to bright light.
    - Ocular movement: No oculocephalic reflex ("doll's eyes" negative). No oculovestibular reflex: No deviation of eyes toward irrigation of ear canal with 50 mL ice-cold water within 1 minute following irrigation. Irrigation of each ear canal should be done several minutes apart (cold caloric test).
    - Facial sensory and motor responses: No corneal reflex to touch with a cotton swab, no jaw reflex, no grimacing to deep pain, no facial muscle movement to noxious stimuli.
    - Pharyngeal and tracheal reflexes: No coughing or gagging when posterior pharynx is stimulated by a tongue blade; no cough response to bronchial suctioning. (See Appendix 5 Major Superficial Reflexes and Appendix 3 Cranial Nerves".)
- Apnea test/CO$_2$ challenge: No spontaneous respirations (absence of a respiratory drive). Paco$_2$ levels elevated above normal must be documented. Structured testing is required for diagnosis. Prerequisites for testing include normotension, normothermia, euvolemia, normal Paco$_2$ level, absence of hypoxia and no previous history of CO$_2$ retention (chronic obstructive pulmonary disease, severe obesity). All prerequisite conditions must be normalized before testing.

SCREENING LABWORK

- Toxicology screen: Evaluates for presence of toxic doses of recreational drugs, medications, or poisons (see Drug Overdose, Chapter 11).
- Basic metabolic panel/blood chemistry: Identifies electrolyte imbalance, including hypoglycemia, hyperglycemia, and acidosis (using bicarbonate/CO$_2$). May also reflect the patient's volume status, including dehydration and hypovolemia (see Fluid and Electrolyte Disturbances, Chapter 1).
- Arterial blood gas (ABG) analysis: Evaluates for hypoxia, acidosis, and hypercapnia (see Acid-Base Balance, Chapter 1).

Diagnostic Tests for Brain Death

Test	Purpose	Abnormal Findings
Arterial blood gas (ABG) analysis	Assesses for acidosis resulting from abnormal gas exchange or compensation for metabolic derangements.	Low pH: Acidosis may reflect respiratory failure or metabolic crisis. Carbon dioxide: Elevated CO_2 or hypercapnia reflects respiratory failure; decreased CO_2 may reflect compensation for metabolic acidosis. Hypoxemia: PaO_2 less than 80 mm Hg. Oxygen saturation: SaO_2 less than 92%. Bicarbonate: HCO_3^- less than 22 mEq/L. Base deficit: less than -2.
Apnea test Prerequisite conditions are met. The patient is preoxygenated for at least 10 minutes with 100% oxygen ($PaO_2 \uparrow$ to 200 mm Hg), ventilatory rate is reduced to 10 breaths/min, positive-end expiratory pressure $\downarrow$ to 5 cm H_2O. If the patient desaturates, apnea testing may be difficult. If SpO_2 remains 95%, obtain an ABG. The ventilator is disconnected. The patient is placed on 100% at 6 L/min oxygen via insufflation catheter in endotracheal tube at the level of the carina, or via T tube and observed for apnea. PaO_2, PcO_2, and pH are measured after approximately 8 to 10 minutes; the ventilator is reconnected after the ABG sample is drawn. Abort test for systolic blood pressure less than 90 mm Hg, SpO_2 less than 85% for 30 seconds. Retry with T piece, continuous positive airway pressure 10 cm H_2O, and 100% O_2 at 12 L/min.	Validates absence of spontaneous respirations while ventilator is disconnected; test is designed to be completed safely, to avoid inducing cardiopulmonary instability during the procedure: O_2 saturation is monitored continuously by pulse oximetry. Ventilator is reconnected if the patient becomes unstable (hypoxia, hypotension, or lethal dysrhythmias occur).	Confirmatory findings The apnea test result is positive if: No spontaneous chest or abdominal excursions that produce reasonably normal, effective tidal volumes occur. The arterial PcO_2 is either greater than 60 mm Hg or increased 20 mm Hg from the baseline PcO_2. The apnea test result is negative if: Effective respiratory movements are observed. PcO_2 does not increase by 20 mm Hg above baseline or is not greater than 60 mm Hg.

Note: If the patient has severe facial trauma, preexisting abnormal pupils, sleep apnea, severe lung disease resulting in chronic hypercapnia (CO_2 retention), or toxic levels of any sedative drugs, aminoglycosides, tricyclic antidepressants, anticholinergics, antiepileptic drugs, chemotherapeutic agents, or neuromuscular blocking agents, additional testing may be required to confirm brain death. Additional confirmatory tests are not mandatory if the clinical diagnosis is positive (patient is unresponsive/in a coma, brainstem reflexes are absent, apnea test result is positive).

Cerebral angiography using contrast medium under high pressure in both anterior and posterior circulation injections.	Assesses if cerebral perfusion is present. Carotid circulation must be patent.	Absent perfusion: No intracerebral blood filling is present at the level of the carotid or vertebral artery entry into the skull. Delayed filling may be noted in the superior longitudinal sinus.

Diagnostic Tests for Brain Death—cont'd

Test	Purpose	Abnormal Findings
Electroencephalography (EEG) using a minimum of eight scalp electrodes with distances of at least 10 cm. Sensitivity should be increased to at least 2 mV for 30 minutes with inclusion of appropriate calibrations.	Assesses level of electrical activity of the brain (brain wave analysis).	No signs of viability: No electrical activity during at least 30 minutes of recording, which meets the minimal technical criteria of EEG recording for brain viability; test adheres to the American Electroencephalographic Society criteria for those with suspected brain death.
Transcranial Doppler ultrasonography with bilateral insonation. The probe is placed at the temporal bone above the zygomatic arch or the vertebrobasilar arteries through the suboccipital transcranial window.	Assesses for presence of cerebral perfusion and degree of vascular resistance using Doppler signals. Positive findings indicate very high vascular resistance resulting from markedly increased intracranial pressure.	No functional blood flow: Small systolic peaks corresponding with early systole without diastolic flow or reverberating flow. Note: 10% of patients do not have temporal windows appropriate for transmitting ultrasound signals. Initial absence of Doppler signal does not confirm brain death.
Cerebral scintigraphy (perfusion scan) using technetium Tc-99m hexametazime.	Assesses for cerebral circulation and brain cell viability using uptake of isotope as the criteria.	No circulation/no uptake: No uptake of isotope by brain cells ("hollow skull phenomenon").

COLLABORATIVE MANAGEMENT

ORGAN DONOR MANAGEMENT FOLLOWING BRAIN DEATH

Once brain death has been diagnosed, the organ removal team may begin preparations for organ removal within 5 minutes under ideal conditions. If the death was unanticipated, or organ donation was not discussed or controversial, additional time is needed for approaching the donor's family/significant other(s) regarding donation. The measurements listed as follows must be managed to provide the best opportunity to recover viable organs from the donor.

Physiologic Measurement	Intervention
Maintain blood pressure.	Mean arterial pressure (MAP) ≥70 mm Hg: systolic pressure greater than 100 mm Hg. Maintain euvolemia administering intravenous (IV) or enteral fluids; central venous pressure 6 to 10 mm Hg. Administer vasopressor agents (e.g., norepinephrine) if needed. High doses of vasopressors should be avoided. Fluid overload should be avoided.
Monitor organ perfusion.	Monitor urine output and lactate level; urine output 0.5 to 3 mL/kg/h. Consider hemodynamic monitoring with a pulmonary artery (PA) catheter. PA pressures: pulmonary capillary wedge pressure: 6 to 10 mm Hg, cardiac index 2.4 L/min/m^2. Systemic vascular resistance 800 to 1200 dynes/s/cm^{-5}.
Balance electrolytes.	Monitor electrolytes (Na^{2+}, K$^+$) every 2 to 4 hours; correct to normal range. Avoid hypernatremia.
Control diabetes insipidus.	Suspected diabetes insipidus (urine output greater than 200 mL/h, rising serum sodium): administer DDAVP (e.g., 2 to 4 μg IV in adults) and replace volume loss with 5% dextrose.
Manage hyperglycemia.	Treat hyperglycemia: keep blood glucose 100 to 180 mg/dL or 4 to 8 mmol/L. Insulin infusion per institutional hyperglycemia protocol, or at least 1 unit/h.
Control hypothermia.	Keep temperature greater than 35° C. Early use of warming blankets to prevent declining temperature is helpful; hypothermia is difficult to reverse once developed.

Continued

ORGAN DONOR MANAGEMENT FOLLOWING BRAIN DEATH—cont'd

Physiologic Measurement	Intervention
Ventilate and oxygenate.	Provide ongoing respiratory care: frequent suctioning, positioning/turning, positive-end expiratory pressure 5 cm H_2O, alveolar recruitment strategies. Consider lower tidal volume (6 to 8 mL/kg) to improve lung preservation for transplant.
Manage anemia and coagulation.	Maintain hemoglobin at greater than 8 g/dL using red blood cell transfusions if necessary. Correct coagulation if actively bleeding. Maintain thromboprophylaxis, given there is a high incidence of pulmonary emboli found at organ retrieval.
Consider control of hormonal imbalances causing hemodynamic instability.	Consider hormonal replacement therapy if volume resuscitation and low-dose inotropes are ineffective for maintaining blood pressure and/or if cardiac ejection fraction is less than 45%. Typical regimens include: Triiodothyronine (T_3): 4 μg IV bolus, then 4 μg/h by IV infusion. Arginine vasopressin: 0.5 to 2.4 units/h to maintain MAP 60 to 70 mm Hg. Methylprednisolone: 15 mg/kg IV single bolus (may be given immediately following confirmation of brain death).

CARE PRIORITIES
1. Confirm a clinical diagnosis of brain death
Unresponsiveness or coma, absence of brainstem reflexes, and apnea. Complete additional diagnostics as needed.

2. Allay doubts about the diagnosis
When the patient manifests the three cardinal findings of brain death recognized by the AAN, the healthcare team should educate the patient's family members about signs and symptoms that may be present. The following findings commonly cause doubt about the diagnosis of brain death in both care providers and the patient's family:
- Spontaneous movement of limbs: spinal reflex movements may occur.
- Respiratory-like movements of the chest and abdomen: shoulder elevation and adduction, back arching, intercostal expansion, which do not produce effective tidal volume.
- Sweating, blushing, and tachycardia: residual autonomic responses.
- Normal BP without vasopressors or sudden increases in BP: residual autonomic responses.
- Absence of diabetes insipidus: does not occur in some patients.
- Reflexes are present: deep tendon, superficial abdominal, triple flexion, Babinski sign.

3. Discuss organ donation ONLY AFTER the clinical diagnosis of brain death has been made and the family understands the patient is dead
Contact with the organ procurement organization should be done in a timely manner when death is imminent. Collaborate with the organ procurement organization to enhance the experience of the donation process. Do not broach the subject of donation or hint about donation before the time the patient has been pronounced dead, unless the patient had resolved the issue of organ donation with the family before death. The subject of organ donation is generally better discussed after the patient has been pronounced dead and the family understands that despite the patient having a beating heart, without mechanical ventilation, cardiac death will ensue. Choose a quiet, private, comfortable place to discuss organ donation, ideally leaving the lead role to a professional from the organ procurement agency. The family requires privacy, so they can express their grief regarding the death and can be left alone to discuss donation, if needed. Ensure all members of the team participating in the discussion are introduced to family members. All family members/significant others should be introduced to the team by name, and their role in the family/life of the deceased should be explained. Only those whom the next of kin requests to be present should participate in the discussion. Adequate time should be given asking/answering questions. The words used during the discussion are very important:
- Words to avoid: harvest, cadaver, remains, breathing, respirator, corpse, or any complex medical terminology.
- Phrases to avoid: artificial life support, will live on in others, deeply comatose.

- Words to include: the deceased patient's name, ventilator, procurement, retrieval, donation, dead.
- Phrases to include: time of death, wishes regarding organ donation, reasons for declining the opportunity, religious beliefs on organ donation.

4. Maintain organs for donation if the family/significant others agree

If the family agrees to donation, the next of kin/others chosen by next of kin are interviewed by the organ procurement team regarding the patient's medical and social history. Reassure the family that the patient's body will be handled with utmost care/respect to maintain dignity and will not be visibly disfigured. Offer the opportunity to view the patient's body following donation. Major immediate threats to organ donation are development of pulmonary edema, hypotension, polyuria leading to dehydration from diabetes insipidus, and infection. Initiate measures discussed in the table on Diagnostic Tests for Brain Death in this chapter.

5. Discontinue life support after the family has had time to visit the patient, if the family declines the opportunity to donate the patient's organs

Weaning of mechanical ventilation and vasoactive drugs is unnecessary because the patient is dead. Reasons for declining donation generally relate to the wishes of the patient, religious convictions, fear of disfigurement/mutilation of the patient's body, and mistrust of the motives or anger with the procurement team members. Mistrust and anger often ensue if the family is improperly approached regarding organ donation. Involving the experienced healthcare professionals from the organ procurement team has been shown to yield a higher success rate with donation.

CARE PLANS FOR BRAIN DEATH

DECREASED INTRACRANIAL ADAPTIVE CAPACITY   related to increased ICP resulting from imminent brain death. When brain death is imminent, mechanisms that normally compensate for increases in ICP are failing. When failed, brain herniation occurs.

- -

Goals/Outcomes: The patient is maximally supported for reduction of ICP until efforts are proved futile, when brain herniation ensues, resulting in brain death. Following brain death, hemodynamic status is supported until decisions are made regarding organ donation and/or discontinuation of life support.

NOC Tissue Perfusion: Cerebral; Neurologic Status: Consciousness.

Cerebral Perfusion Promotion
1. Consult with the advanced practice provider to determine hemodynamic measurements.
2. Maintain hemodynamics within set measurements.
3. Administer osmotic diuretics/rheologic agents (e.g., mannitol, dextran) as ordered.
4. Administer vasopressin as ordered if diabetes insipidus ensues.
5. Keep blood glucose level within ordered range, avoiding hyperglycemia unless using medications that induce osmotic diuresis.
6. Avoid neck flexion or extreme hip/knee flexion.
7. Consult with the advanced practice practitioner regarding optimal elevation of the head of the bed (HOB).

Cerebral Edema Management
1. Monitor neurologic status closely and compare with baseline.
2. Monitor respiratory status: rate, rhythm, depth of respirations, Pao_2, Pco_2, pH, and bicarbonate.
3. Monitor ICP and cerebral perfusion pressure (CPP) at rest and in response to patient care activities. Minimize activities that result in further increases in ICP.

Neurologic Monitoring
1. Monitor pupillary size, shape, symmetry, and reactivity.
2. Assess LOC, orientation, and trend of GCS score.
3. Monitor vital signs: temperature, BP, pulse, and respirations.
4. Monitor for corneal reflex, and cough and gag reflexes.
5. Monitor extraocular movements and gaze characteristics.
6. Monitor Babinski response.
7. Monitor for the Cushing response; a late indicator of increased ICP.

DECISIONAL CONFLICT *related to the uncertainty regarding the proper course of action related to the discontinuation of life support and possible organ donation following brain death.*

Goals/Outcomes: Family/support system is maximally supported in making judgments, and choosing between immediate discontinuation of life support, organ donation, or possibly continuing life support until information about brain death can be processed and accepted.

NOC Decision-Making; Information Processing; Dignified Life Closure; Acceptance: Health Status.

Dying Care
1. If cerebral perfusion promotion measures fail and brain death ensues, provide care appropriate for the dying.
2. Encourage family to share feelings about death.
3. Monitor deterioration of the patient's physical (and mental) capabilities.
4. Facilitate obtaining spiritual support for the family/significant others.
5. Facilitate discussion of funeral arrangements.

Coping Enhancement
1. Assess the impact of the patient's life situation on roles and relationships within family/support system.
2. Use a calm, reassuring approach.
3. Provide factual information concerning diagnosis, treatment, and prognosis.
4. Seek to understand the family's perception of the stressful situation.
5. Acknowledge the patient and significant others' religious, spiritual, and cultural beliefs surrounding death, dying, and organ donation.
6. Encourage gradual mastery of the situation if resistance or denial is impacting the family's ability to accept the diagnosis of brain death.
7. Ensure that the family understands that brain dead patients are dead. Patients are no longer able to breathe without mechanical ventilation, will experience cardiac death when removed from mechanical ventilation, will never regain consciousness, will never interact with others, and have no ability to experience joy related to human life.
8. Explain the difference among brain death, persistent vegetative state, and cardiac death. The family and significant others may have difficulty understanding why brain dead patients are different than those in a coma who can recover from their insult/injury and those in a vegetative state who can recover brainstem function to begin breathing spontaneously. Families may not be able to comprehend why when the brain is dead, the heart still functions unless mechanical ventilation is removed. Guilt may be associated with removal of mechanical ventilation because the patient appears "alive" with mechanical ventilation in place.

NIC Emotional Support; Environmental Management; Fluid/Electrolyte Management; Fluid Monitoring; Hypovolemia Management; Infection Control; Intravenous Therapy; Mechanical Ventilation; Positioning; Surveillance; Respiratory Monitoring; Spiritual Support; Vital Signs Monitoring.

ADDITIONAL NURSING DIAGNOSES

As appropriate, see nursing diagnoses and interventions in Nutrition Support (Chapter 1), Acute Respiratory Failure (Chapter 4), Mechanical Ventilation (Chapter 1), Prolonged Immobility (Chapter 1), and Emotional and Spiritual Support of the Patient and Significant Others (Chapter 2).

CEREBRAL ANEURYSM AND SUBARACHNOID HEMORRHAGE

PATHOPHYSIOLOGY

A cerebral aneurysm is an abnormal, localized dilation of an artery within the cranial vault caused by weakness in the vessel wall. Ninety percent of cerebral aneurysms are saccular (berry) aneurysms, whereas the other 10% are fusiform, traumatic, septic, dissecting, and Charcot-Bouchard aneurysms. Recent research suggests that cerebral aneurysms result from degenerative vascular diseases complicated by hypertension and atherosclerosis. Cerebral aneurysms most often occur at the bifurcation and branches of the blood vessels of the circle of Willis, with 85% in the anterior cerebral circulation and 15% in the posterior cerebral circulation. Approximately 25% of patients have multiple aneurysms.

The critical care nurse may provide care patients with an unruptured aneurysm or those postrupture with a diagnosis of SAH. Unruptured aneurysms may be asymptomatic, but nearly half of the affected population experiences some warning sign or symptom before rupture as a result of expansion of the lesion and compression of cerebral tissue. When an aneurysm ruptures, a hemorrhage occurs in the SAS and basal cisterns. If the patient survives the initial compromise of cerebral circulation from the force of the arterial hemorrhage resulting in sharply increased ICP, the next challenges are surviving possible rebleeding and cerebral arterial vasospasms. The greatest incidence of rebleeding following SAH is between 3 and 11 days following the rupture, with the peak at day 7. Mortality is approximately 70% from SAH. Theories regarding the cause(s) of rebleeding propose a problem with the normal process of clot dissolution coupled with "spikes" in arterial pressure.

The major complication postrupture is the occurrence of delayed cerebral ischemia from cerebral arterial vasospasm. This occurs as a result of the constriction of the arterial smooth muscle layer of the major cerebral arteries and causes a dramatic decrease in cerebral blood flow that leads to cerebral ischemia and progressive neurologic deficit. Vasospasm occurs in as many as 60% of patients from 4 to 21 days following SAH, with incidence peaking between 7 and 10 days. The pathogenesis of the vasospasms is poorly understood, but ongoing research indicates a direct relationship to the amount of blood in the SAS and basal cisterns. The greater the volume of blood, the greater is the risk of vasospasm. While clots in the basal cisterns begin to hemolyze, substances may be released that prompt vasospasms. A current prophylactic treatment includes careful fluid balance and "triple H" (hypervolemia-hemodilution-hypertension) therapy. Recent evidence has suggested that intravascular volume management should target euvolemia and avoid prophylactic hypervolemic therapy. Aggressive administration of fluid aimed at achieving hypervolemia has been shown to be harmful by several studies. Other treatments include the use of calcium antagonists to relieve vasospasms, balloon or chemical angioplasty to normalize the vessel lumen, and possibly cisternal fibrinolytic drugs to alter the natural process of clot breakdown for those with a larger cisternal blood accumulation. The patient with a ruptured cerebral aneurysm and SAH is also at risk for communicating or obstructive hydrocephalus, hypothalamic dysfunction, and hyponatremia.

Some patients present with an obstructive hydrocephalus from intraventricular blood. However, communicating hydrocephalus develops in approximately 20% of patients with SAH as a result of the presence of blood in the SAS and ventricular system. Hydrocephalus may be acute (occurs within less than 24 hours), subacute (occurs within less than 4 hours to 1 week), or delayed (beginning 10 or more days after SAH). Blood in the SAS and ventricles obstructs the flow of CSF, interferes with circulation and resorption of CSF, and causes increased ICP, with concomitant worsening of neurologic status. Hydrocephalus sometimes produces minimal symptoms and resolves without medical intervention, whereas some patients may require temporary or permanent diversion of CSF circulation to achieve symptom relief.

Hypothalamic dysfunction, seen in approximately one third of patients with hydrocephalus after SAH, may result from mechanical pressure on the hypothalamus from a dilated third ventricle. The increased pressure causes an increase in the releasing hormones from the hypothalamus, which activates the hypothalamic-pituitary axis of the anterior pituitary, as well as stimulating the production of antidiuretic hormone (ADH) by the posterior pituitary gland. The response to the increased adrenocorticotropic hormone from the anterior pituitary gland mimics an exaggerated stress response, which includes a marked increase in serum catecholamines leading to overstimulation of the sympathetic nervous system. The vasoconstrictive response is severe enough in a subset of patients to cause "stunned myocardium," similar to what is seen with an acute myocardial infarction (MI).

The surge of ADH from the posterior pituitary results in syndrome of inappropriate antidiuretic hormone (SIADH), which may include hyponatremia caused by cerebral salt-wasting (CSW) syndrome, or a combination of factors influencing sodium and water metabolism (Table 7-1). Recent studies emphasize that the diagnosis of CSW requires the presence of hypovolemia versus SIADH, which usually results in euvolemia or moderate hypovolemia. Patients with an SAH may have CSW and SIADH occurring simultaneously, manifested by excessive urine output coupled with excessive free water retention. Fluid management strategies in this patient population may be difficult (see Syndrome of Inappropriate Antidiuretic Hormone, p. 734). Hyponatremia occurs in 30% to 50% of patients with SAH. Untreated hyponatremia may lead to intracranial hypertension, cerebral ischemia, seizures, coma, and death.

Table 7-1	CLINICAL PRESENTATION WITH CEREBRAL SALT-WASTING SYNDROME VERSUS SYNDROME OF INAPPROPRIATE ANTIDIURETIC HORMONE
Cerebral Salt-Wasting Syndrome	**Syndrome of Inappropriate Antidiuretic Hormone**
Hypotension	Normotension
Postural hypotension	Normotension
Tachycardia	Normal pulse rate or bradycardia
Elevated hematocrit	Normal or low hematocrit
Decreased glomerular filtration rate	Increased glomerular filtration rate
Normal or elevated blood urea nitrogen and creatinine	Normal or decreased blood urea nitrogen and creatinine
Normal or low urine output	Normal or low urine output
Hypovolemia	Normovolemia or hypervolemia
Dehydration	Normal hydration
True hyponatremia	Dilutional hyponatremia
Hypoosmolality	Hypoosmolality
Decreased body weight	Increased body weight

Note: Both hypothalamic dysfunction and hyponatremia are seen more frequently in patients with extensive SAH and are positively correlated with the subsequent development of cerebral vasospasm.

NEUROLOGIC ASSESSMENT: CEREBRAL ANEURYSM(S) AND SUBARACHNOID HEMORRHAGE

GOAL OF SYSTEM ASSESSMENT

Evaluate for key nursing diagnoses requiring emergent intervention: Alteration in cerebral tissue perfusion resulting from vasospasm of cerebral vessels, increased ICP as a result of decreased intracranial adaptive capacity, risk for seizure activity with potential impairment of cerebral tissue perfusion, impaired gas exchange or ineffective airway clearance attributable to altered LOC, potential need for management of hyperglycemia, and fluid volume imbalance and potential for aspiration.

HISTORY AND RISK FACTORS

Evidence reveals that outcomes for patients with ruptured aneurysms and SAH are affected by factors such as patient's age, having the worst clinical grade on the Fisher Scale, or other predictive scales including the World Federation of Neurosurgeons Scale (WFNS), the Claassen Scale, the Ogilvy and Carter Scale, or the commonly used Hunt and Hess Scale (see later). The Fisher Scale is predictive of the possibility of vasospasm, which is indicative of the amount of blood in the SAS. The Claassen Grading System quantifies the risk of delayed cerebral ischemia from vasospasm associated with SAH. Unlike the Fisher Scale, the Claassen Scale considers the additional risk of SAH and intraventricular hemorrhage. The Claassen Scale has not yet been prospectively validated. The WFNS Grading System is widely used and includes objective terminology to determine grades. Similar to the Hunt and Hess Scale, the predictive power of the WFNS Grades are inconsistent. The Ogilvy and Carter Scale includes several features that may affect the outcome, including age, Hunt and Hess Grade, initial presentation, Fisher Grade (SAH volume and vasospasm risk), and computed tomography (CT) scan findings. A noncontrast CT scan confirms the diagnosis of SAH by establishing the presence, amount, and location of blood in the SAS, the presence and degree of hydrocephalus, and the presence or absence of intraventricular hemorrhage or intraparenchymal hemorrhage.

The Ogilvy and Carter Scale is more complicated to administer than the Hunt and Hess Scale, and has been tested only on patients who have undergone aneurysm surgery. Patient outcomes are also affected by aneurysm size, occurrence of fever following the SAH, and new-onset hyperglycemia on admission with SAH.

Hunt and Hess classification system

Permits objective evaluation of progression of the patient's initial symptoms and is used to predict clinical outcomes and for choosing treatments. Critical care nurses can benefit from using this grading system. Grading is first determined by the initial symptoms and LOC upon presentation, and is used as a basis of comparison over time.

Grade I: Asymptomatic, alert, and oriented, minor headache, moderate nuchal rigidity.
Grade II: Alert, oriented, headache, and stiff neck.
Grade III: Lethargic or confused; minor focal deficit such as hemiparesis.
Grade IV: Stuporous, moderate to severe focal deficits, hemiplegia, possible early decerebrate rigidity, and vegetative disturbances.
Grade V: Deep coma, decerebrate rigidity, moribund appearance.

The critical care nurse must carefully review the patient's history and diagnostic findings to understand the potential risk for complications. Patients with unruptured aneurysms are at risk for rupture, depending on the location and size of the aneurysm. Unruptured aneurysms may be found during diagnostic testing for headaches or other neurologic symptoms and may produce symptoms of cerebral ischemia. A patient with new onset of oculomotor nerve palsy, visual field loss, or lower cranial nerve deficits should be evaluated for a potential aneurysm. Patients with unruptured aneurysms are typically encountered in the critical care setting after elective aneurysm securement (treatment). The two main options for aneurysm treatment are craniotomy with aneurysm neck clipping, wrapping or ligation; and the more recently developed option of a neurovascular interventionalist performing endovascular coiling or embolization ("chemical gluing"). Patients admitted for management of a ruptured cerebral aneurysm may have additional unruptured aneurysms, which will be secured at a later date.

The distinguishing characteristic of a ruptured aneurysm is often a patient who complains of the "worst headache of my life." This is usually accompanied by severe nausea and vomiting, nuchal rigidity, visual disturbances, and photophobia. There is a 2% to 4% risk for rebleeding within the first 24 hours. "Sentinel" or warning headaches are associated with an aneurysm that begins leaking days to weeks before rupturing. Very few patients report having a sentinel headache before aneurysm rupture.

Rupture results in hemorrhage producing seizures, neurologic deficits, deterioration in LOC, and a mortality rate of 20% to 50% if the aneurysm rebleeds. Vasospasms may ensue, which increases the probability for a negative outcome.

VITAL SIGNS

BP, HR, and respiratory rate (RR)/pattern may change secondary to altered cerebral tissue perfusion. BP control is an essential strategy to prevent rebleeding of an aneurysm. Continuous intraarterial monitoring is essential for prompt detection of subtle changes/trends. Many patients are hypertensive following hemorrhage. BP and headache may fluctuate in tandem; higher BP increases the severity of the headache. Treatment involving intravascular volume expansion can increase BP, and is generally withheld until after the aneurysm has been surgically clipped or managed with endovascular coils or chemical embolization. Conversely, hypotension can decrease cerebral blood flow and perfusion. Hypertension must be managed with great care to avoid creating hypotension. Temperature should be monitored closely to avoid worsening outcomes post-SAH. Fever increases cerebral metabolic rate, which can worsen cerebral ischemia, with resultant negative outcomes.

INTRACRANIAL PRESSURE

Blood in the SAS can produce acute hydrocephalus within the first 24 hours, which may result in increased ICP. Subacute, or chronic, hydrocephalus occurs in approximately 10% to 15% of patients, usually 10 or more days following the SAH. It is caused by a clot within the ventricular system that blocks the pathways for the resorption of CSF leading to ventricular enlargement and nonfocal neurologic deterioration. Intraventricular extension (distension of the ventricles) at the time of aneurysm rupture can result in acute hydrocephalus and requires temporary external ventricular drainage for management of ICP. Nuchal rigidity may be present. Indicators of increased ICP are listed in Box 7-1.

INDICATORS OF HYDROCEPHALUS

- Acute: Persistent or sudden onset of coma with loss of pupillary reflexes within 24 hours of SAH.
- Subacute: Gradual onset of confusion, drowsiness, lethargy, or stupor within 1 to 7 days of SAH.
- Delayed or chronic: Gradual onset of confusion, incontinence, or impaired balance, mobility, and gait; intellectual impairment (slowness, mutism); lack of affect; and presence of the grasp and sucking frontal lobe reflexes (abnormal in adults), at about 10 days following SAH.

OBSERVATION AND FUNCTIONAL ASSESSMENT

Diminished level of consciousness

Acute deterioration in a patient's neurologic function may signal rerupture in a patient with a ruptured, unsecured aneurysm or herald the onset of vasospasm. At the onset of significant hemorrhage, unconsciousness may occur with only reflexive or pathologic motor responses seen. Morbidity and mortality are high in those with massive hemorrhage. Approximately 10% to 30% of patients with an acute SAH will die before obtaining medical treatment. Of those who survive the initial hemorrhage, up to 30% to 60% will die from the initial hemorrhage or sequelae.

Pupillary changes

Depending on location of the aneurysm, visual changes may vary; assess for visual field loss, oculomotor palsy, diplopia, immobile eye, retroorbital pain, or hemianopsia.

Motor/sensory assessment

Fluctuating hemiparesis or aphasia with increasing confusion can be clinical symptoms of vasospasm. Hydrocephalus is generally not associated with focal neurologic deficits. Anxiety, confusion, agitation, disorientation, lethargy, stupor, and coma may indicate hydrocephalus, vasospasm, or early hyponatremia. Anorexia, nausea, vomiting, abdominal pain, cold and clammy skin, generalized weakness, and lower extremity muscle cramps are late signs of untreated hyponatremia. Flushing, diaphoresis, pupillary dilation, decreased gastric motility, increased serum glucose, fever, hypertension, tachycardia, cardiac dysrhythmias, ischemia, and infarction can be attributable to increased circulating catecholamines.

Box 7-1	**INDICATORS OF INCREASED INTRACRANIAL PRESSURE***

- Alterations in consciousness: increasing restlessness, confusion, irritability, disorientation, increasing drowsiness, and lethargy.
- Bradycardia.
- Increasing systolic blood pressure with a widening pulse pressure.
- Irregular respiratory patterns (e.g., Cheyne-Stokes respiration, ataxic, apneustic, central neurogenic, hyperventilation).
- Hemisensory changes and hemiparesis or hemiplegia: caused by involvement of hemispheric sensory and motor pathways.
- Worsening headache.
- Papillary changes.
- Dysconjugate gaze and inability to move one eye beyond midposition: caused by involvement of cranial nerves III, IV, and VI.
- Seizures.
- Involvement of other cranial nerves: depends on the severity of neurologic insult.

*If these indicators of increased intracranial pressure are left untreated, the patient will undergo irreversible brain damage or death. If these indicators occur suddenly, there will be displacement of brain substance (herniation), which will progress rapidly to permanent brain damage or death. For additional information about herniation syndromes, see Traumatic Brain Injury (Chapter 3).

Fundoscopic assessment

See Chapter 7 "General Neurologic Assessment."

SCREENING LABWORK

- CSF analysis may be performed to confirm the presence of blood in the CSF in patients with symptoms suggestive of SAH but with no clear abnormalities detected on the CT scan. The presence of xanthochromia (yellow-tinged) CSF is caused by the breakdown of hemoglobin and signals possible hemorrhage. CSF pressure, normally 0 to 15 mm Hg (75 to 180 mm H_2O), may be elevated. The pressure is proportionate to the amount of bleeding. Protein may increase to 80 to 130 mg/dL (normal is 15 to 50 mg/dL). Note: Performance of lumbar puncture in the patient with SAH and increased ICP carries substantial risk of herniation and rebleeding; thus, it is not a routine study in this patient population. In patients with SAH and an external ventricular drain for the management of hydrocephalus, CSF may be sampled as part of a workup of infectious causes of sustained fever.
- Electrolytes and glucose levels should be monitored at least daily to detect hyponatremia and hyperglycemia. Fluid management in SAH after an aneurysm is secured can be associated with hypokalemia, hypomagnesemia, and hypophosphatemia, thus these electrolytes should also be monitored on at least a daily basis.
- ABG analysis: To detect hypoxemia and hypercapnia and to determine appropriate respiratory therapy.

DIAGNOSTIC TESTING

Refer to Neurologic Diagnostic Testing, Chapter 7.

COLLABORATIVE MANAGEMENT

CARE PRIORITIES

1. Pharmacotherapy

- **Calcium channel blocker:** Nimodipine (Nimotop) inhibits calcium influx across the cell membrane of vascular smooth muscles. The resulting decrease in peripheral vascular resistance and vasodilation is believed to increase perfusion in cerebral vessels. Although nimodipine does not prevent vasospasm, its use has been shown to be associated with improved long-term outcomes in patients who experience vasospasm. Nimodipine is given within 96 hours after hemorrhage as 60 mg enterally every 4 hours for 21 days (the recommended course of therapy). Some patients experience significant decreases in BP with nimodipine and may require a dosage schedule of 30 mg every 2 hours. IV administration of calcium antagonists is not recommended at this time.
- **Antihypertensives:** Antihypertensive therapy is used cautiously in this patient population because allowing hypertension is a significant element of standard therapeutic management in aneurysmal SAH. Hydralazine hydrochloride (Apresoline), labetalol (Normodyne), or nicardipine (Cardene) may be administered to control BP both before definitive securing of the ruptured aneurysm and after clipping or coiling to maintain BP in desired measurements. Maintaining BP at less than 200 mm Hg has been recommended.
- **Osmotic diuretics:** Mannitol (Osmitrol), urea (Ureaphil), and glycerin (Glycerol) may be used to reduce ICP and treat cerebral edema via diuresis to remove fluid from the brain. Patients should be monitored for electrolyte imbalances, other systemic side effects, and adverse reactions related to fluid shifting.

HIGH ALERT   With the rapid movement of extracellular fluid from brain tissue to plasma with associated decrease in brain volume, potential for rebleeding may be increased after giving mannitol. Mannitol may cause a rebound increase in intracranial pressure 8 to 12 hours after administration, while fluid shifts from cells into the vascular compartment. Furosemide (Lasix) is often used to decrease the rebound effect of mannitol.

- **Loop diuretics:** Furosemide (Lasix) is often used as a sole agent to decrease cerebral edema without causing the rise in intracranial blood volume that occurs with mannitol.

- **Corticosteroids:** Dexamethasone (Decadron) is a controversial medication used to relieve cerebral edema and decrease ICP. Use of dexamethasone is most likely to be seen in the immediate postoperative management of the patient who has undergone surgical intervention to secure the aneurysm. The patient should be monitored carefully for side effects, including gastrointestinal (GI) tract irritation. Medications such as H_2-blockers or proton pump inhibitors may be used to reduce the risk of gastritis and ulceration.
- **Antipyretics:** Acetaminophen is used to control fever, which increases cerebral metabolism. Aspirin is usually avoided, because its platelet action impairs clotting and promotes bleeding. In patients requiring multiple interventions to manage increased ICP, sustained fever can compromise outcome and aggressive measures may be required to control the fever. Clinical trials have been conducted to evaluate conventional treatment (use of acetaminophen and cooling blankets) compared with addition of an intravascular catheter–based heat exchange system for patients with temperatures higher than 38° C and have shown the effect to decrease fever.
- **Anticonvulsants:** Patients with aneurysmal SAH are at high risk for seizures, thus antiepileptic drugs such as phenytoin (Dilantin) or levetiracetam (Keppra) may be used to control or prevent seizures. If phenytoin is used, monitoring of drug levels is required to ensure the optimal dose and avoid toxicity.
- **Analgesics:** Blood in the SAS is very irritating and the headache associated with SAH can be difficult to control. Acetaminophen is commonly used along with a combination of IV and oral narcotic analgesics as necessary. Pain medications should not routinely be withheld solely out of concern for the ability to detect future neurologic deficits. Pain should always be treated. Stress management techniques can be a helpful adjuvant therapy. Photophobia may persist for several days after SAH and contribute to patient discomfort. Maintaining a low light environment even after the aneurysm is secured can be helpful with this issue.
- **Stool softeners:** Restrictions in activity related to hospitalization and narcotic analgesic use can predispose the patient to constipation. Docusate sodium (Colace) is the drug of choice for preventing straining, which can increase ICP.
- **Insulin:** Glucose control particularly intraoperatively. More research is needed to determine specific critical timing of stricter glucose controls for patients with aneurysmal SAH.
- **Statins:** The use of statins is a newer therapy supported by metaanalysis, which has indicated that the initiation of statins after SAH reduces the incidence of vasospasm, delays ischemic deficits, and affects mortality. Liver function tests and creatine kinase should be assessed before initiation of statin therapy and then monitored on a weekly basis during acute management of aneurysmal SAH. Patients who do not otherwise require statin therapy will require it only during hospitalization.
- **Triple H therapy:** Each of the following therapies may be used singly or in combination.

Safety Alert   *Although hypervolemic-hypertensive therapy with hemodilution (triple H therapy) represents standard management in subarachnoid hemorrhage for vasospasm, it carries great risks. The patient's cardiovascular status requires close monitoring, because patients with existing cardiovascular disease may be unable to tolerate the hypervolemia. Additionally, the patient should be very closely monitored to establish whether their neurologic function varies with changes in blood pressure or fluid status. If used before the aneurysm is secured, this modality may precipitate intracranial pressure with rerupture of and rebleeding from the aneurysm. When used after definitive intervention, the patient may experience cerebral edema with cerebral ischemia and subsequent neurologic deficit.*

- **Hypervolemia** (saline, whole blood, packed cells, plasma protein fraction, albumin, or hetastarch): Increases circulating volume to prevent ischemia caused by vasospasm. The patient's neurologic status is often used to gauge the effectiveness of hypervolemic therapy. If concern exists about the patient's ability to tolerate hypervolemia, noninvasive methods of monitoring cardiac output and index can be employed. Use of central venous catheters and central venous pressure (CVP) monitoring is restricted to patients with clinical symptoms of vasospasm. Very rarely, invasive hemodynamic monitoring with a pulmonary artery catheter may be required.

- **Hemodilution (albumin and crystalloid fluids):** Decreases blood viscosity. CVP greater than 8 mm Hg is usually sufficient to maintain hypervolemia and dilute the hematocrit to less than 35%.
- **Hypertension:** By increasing BP, CPP increases and may help prevent ischemia and infarction. Once the ruptured aneurysm is definitively secured, hypertension is allowed up to systolic BPs (SBPs) of 200 to 220 mm Hg. If a patient develops clinical symptoms of vasospasm, continuous IV vasopressors such as phenylephrine or norepinephrine may be used to assess for clinical improvement with elevation of BP to a maximum systolic pressure of 240 mm Hg. Ideally, BP is maintained 60 mm Hg above baseline.

2. Surgical/endovascular intervention

Initial management involves stabilizing the patient and minimizing the risk of rerupture of the aneurysm. The National Institute of Neurological Disorders and Stroke (NINDS), a division of the National Institutes of Health (NIH), is recognized as the leader in research on the brain and nervous system in the United States. The NINDS sponsored the International Study of Unruptured Intracranial Aneurysms, including more than 4000 patients at 61 sites in the United States, Canada, and Europe. Results revealed that the risk of rupture for aneurysms less than 7 mm in size is low. The findings provide a comprehensive evaluation of these vascular defects, offering guidance to both patients and healthcare professionals facing the difficult decision about the best treatment for a cerebral aneurysm.

Advances in imaging, use of microscopes intraoperatively, dedicated neurologic intensive care units, endovascular treatment methods, and aggressive cerebral vasospasm prevention and management have reduced morbidity and mortality. Treatment options depend on assessment of preoperative risk factors, predictive indicators, and location and size of the aneurysm. Successful treatments include endovascular embolization ("gluing"), surgical clipping, and endovascular detachable coiling.

Recent studies confirm improved patient outcomes when the ruptured aneurysm is secured within the first 24 to 72 hours for patients with grade I or II symptoms (Hunt and Hess Scale). Early intervention may prevent rebleeding, an often fatal complication, and allows for the management of vasospasm without risk of rebleeding. Securing of the aneurysm during the time period associated with the highest risk of development of cerebral arterial vasospasm has been shown to be associated with increased morbidity and mortality. If the aneurysm is not secured within 24 to 72 hours of rupture, repair should be delayed until the peak time for vasospasm (7 to 10 days after SAH) has passed. Patients with grades III to V symptoms are generally considered poor interventional risks, especially in the period immediately after SAH. If these patients are clinically unstable, they may be treated medically until they improve or stabilize enough for endovascular or surgical intervention. Surgery is considered for a patient with a large intracranial clot causing life-threatening, intracranial brain shifting. Intervention is delayed for a patient with cerebral vasospasm until the vasospasm subsides.

Although surgical clipping of aneurysms had previously been the only method of intervention available, neurovascular interventionalists can now use an alternative to surgery using Guglielmi detachable coils (GDC coils). The overall size and location of the aneurysm and the aneurysmal neck size are evaluated to decide if this option is feasible. GDC coils are microcoils composed of a soft platinum alloy that are placed with use of a microcatheter through the femoral artery. The catheter is advanced into the cerebral circulation using radiographic imaging. Low-voltage current is applied to the guide wire to detach the coil(s) placed into the sac of the aneurysm. Placement of one or more coils fills the sac, reduces the pressure inside, and isolates the aneurysm from normal circulation. When this is performed for the management of unruptured aneurysm, the patient's hospital stay is very brief (24 to 48 hours) unless the aneurysm ruptures or another complication of angiography occurs. Endovascular treatment complications differ from those associated with surgical clipping and can include arterial dissection, arterial perforation, distal embolization, and groin hematomas. Aneurysmal recurrence has been seen in a small number of cases. However, endovascular methods have become an acceptable alternative to microsurgical clipping in appropriate cases.

Neurovascular interventionalists can also perform cerebral angioplasty for arterial vasospasm to decrease vascular narrowing and reverse ischemia in patients with new-onset vasospasm within 6 to 12 hours of onset. Patient selection for this is limited to those whose vasospasm involves accessible major cerebral vessels; distal cerebral arterial vasospasm is not amenable to angioplasty.

3. Management of hydrocephalus

- External ventricular drainage: Hydrocephalus develops in 20% to 25% of patients with SAH from a ruptured cerebral aneurysm. Patients with symptomatic hydrocephalus generally require placement of an external ventricular drainage system for management of their hydrocephalus. For those with massive hydrocephalus, coma and Hunt and Hess classification of III or IV, placement of an external ventriculostomy drain can decompress the ventricles enough to produce significant improvements in the patient's neurologic function and make the patient a candidate for intervention to secure the ruptured aneurysm.
- Ventricular shunt: Most patients do not develop chronic hydrocephalus following SAH. For those who do develop a chronic problem, the percentage of those who initially require extraventricular drainage who progress to needing a shunt is not clearly reflected in the literature. When a shunt is necessary, one end of a small catheter is positioned into a ventricle, with the other end draining into a body cavity or space (e.g., SAS, cistern, peritoneum, vena cava, pleura). Major complications include infection and malfunction. If the shunt has a valve for the purpose of controlling drainage or preventing reflux of CSF, the surgeon may request that the valve be pumped periodically to ensure proper functioning. For nursing interventions after shunt placement, see Box 7-2.

CARE PLANS FOR CEREBRAL ANEURYSM AND SUBARACHNOID HEMORRHAGE

RISK FOR INEFFECTIVE CEREBRAL TISSUE PERFUSION *related to vasospasm of cerebral vessels and/or decreased intracranial adaptive capacity related to increased ICP.*

Goals/Outcomes: Maintain normal ICP and/or minimize clinical effects on cerebral adaptability through preventive measures, aggressive volume management, regulation of cerebral blood flow, and close hemodynamic monitoring. **NOC** Circulation Status.

Cerebral Perfusion Promotion

1. Bed rest, with aneurysm precautions and prevention of ICP.
2. Subarachnoid precautions are instituted while the patient is awaiting definitive management of a ruptured cerebral aneurysm. Try to keep the patient quiet and calm in a soothing environment, with lowered lights and noise level.

Box 7-2	NURSING INTERVENTIONS AFTER SHUNT PLACEMENT

- After the shunting, assess the patient for indicators of increased ICP (see Box 7-1) caused by either the disease itself or shunt malfunction.
- Position the patient on side opposite the insertion site, either flat or with head elevated slightly (as prescribed) to prevent pressure on shunt mechanism.
- Assess vital signs; LOC (orientation to time, place, and person); papillary light reflex; and motor function.
- Monitor I&O, and limit fluids as prescribed.
- Avoid severe head and neck rotation, flexion, or hyperextension to prevent kinking, compression, or twisting of the shunt catheter, which would impede CSF flow.
- If the shunt has a valve for controlling drainage or preventing reflux of CSF, pump the valve to ensure proper functioning, according to the surgeon's directive. Usually the valve is located behind or above the ear and is the approximate diameter of a fingertip. Pumping involves gentle, serial compressions of the tissue over the shunt. If the valve is working properly, the emptying and refilling of the valve will be felt with palpation.
- Assess for indicators of meningitis including peritonitis and sepsis, caused by presence of shunt mechanism. (See *Peritonitis*, Chapter 9, and Systematic Inflammatory Response Syndrome, Sepsis, Septic Shock, and Multiple Organ Dysfunction Syndrome, Chapter 11.)

CSF, Cerebrospinal fluid; *ICP,* intracranial pressure; *I&O,* intake and output; *LOC,* level of consciousness.

3. Active ROM and isometric exercises are restricted during acute and preoperative stages to prevent increased ICP.
4. Passive ROM is prescribed to prevent formation of thrombi, with subsequent pulmonary emboli.
5. Bowel management program is essential to prevent straining at stool. Instruct the patient to avoid activities using isometric muscle contractions (e.g., pulling or pushing side rails, pushing against the foot board), which raise SBP, with resultant increased ICP.

NIC Instruct the patient to avoid coughing because increased intrathoracic pressure increases ICP.

Intracranial Pressure Monitoring

1. Increased ICP is common after SAH, but its manifestations range from minimal (e.g., persistent headache or drowsiness) to severe (e.g., coma or death). Elevated ICP that does not respond to treatment has been associated with poor patient outcomes.
2. Cerebral perfusion pressure: In patients who require invasive devices to manage their ICP, the critical care nurse strives to maintain normal ICP (0 to 10 mm Hg with an upper limit of 15 mm Hg) and CPP of 60 to 80 mm Hg. Calculate CPP by the formula: CPP − MAP (mean arterial BP) = ICP. CPP of less than 30 mm Hg causes cerebral anoxia.
3. Head-of-the-bed elevation: A 30- to 45-degree angle facilitates venous outflow from the intracranial cavity and lowers ICP. The head should be kept in straight alignment to prevent increased ICP secondary to obstruction of jugular venous outflow. Values of 180 to 220 mm Hg as prescribed end points of management of SBP.

IMPAIRED GAS EXCHANGE OR INEFFECTIVE AIRWAY CLEARANCE *related to altered LOC*

Goals/Outcomes: Effective airway clearance and gas exchange and maintain appropriate $Paco_2$ level, which can affect ICP.

NOC Respiratory Status: Gas Exchange.

Ventilation Assistance

1. Supplemental oxygen, maintenance of patent airway, possible intubation, and ventilation if needed. Serial ABG tests are performed to identify hypoxemia (Pao_2 less than 80 mm Hg) and hypercapnia ($Paco_2$ greater than 45 mm Hg). Carbon dioxide is a potent cerebral vasodilator that can increase ICP in patients who are already at risk. *Note:* Mechanical ventilation may be implemented to manage potential hypoxemia and to control the level of carbon dioxide effectively, without prompting hypocapnia. Hypocapnia has been used in the management of acute brain injury and is life-saving in some situations, but can produce neuronal ischemia, injury, and potentially worsen the outcome. Use should be limited exclusively to emergency management of life-threatening intracranial hypertension while awaiting additional treatment measures. Carbon dioxide level should be normalized as soon as possible when hyperventilation has been used. Improper use of hypocapnia may result in more harm than benefit.

Oxygen Therapy

1. Suctioning: Avoid vigorous, prolonged suctioning, which precipitates hypoxemia and hypercapnia.
   - Preoxygenation using 100% oxygen helps prevent cerebral vasodilation associated with hypercapnia. Adjusting the Fio_2 to 1.0 (100% oxygen) on the ventilator is preferred to bag-valve-tube manual preoxygenation.

RISK FOR INJURY *related to the potential impact of hyperglycemia*

Goals/Outcomes: Glucose levels are controlled within normalized measurements throughout all phases of treatment.

NOC Risk Control.

Risk Identification

1. Hyperglycemia: Studies have shown that admission hyperglycemia or perioperative hyperglycemia is associated with poor outcome after aneurysmal SAH. Daily glucose monitoring is encouraged. More frequent monitoring and intervention are required in patients with persistent hyperglycemia.
2. Further research is underway to determine the critical timing for strict glucose control, effect on neurologic outcome, and how serum glucose levels impact brain glucose concentrations.

RISK FOR IMBALANCED FLUID VOLUME *related to initiation of measures to maintain hypervolemia*

Goals/Outcomes: Adequately managed intake and output with control of fluid volumes affecting systemic and cerebral blood flow and electrolyte levels.
NOC Fluid Balance.

Fluid/Electrolyte Management
1. Fluid balance is maintained based on CVP, weight, and monitoring of intake/output (I&O) balance.
2. Electrolytes should be replaced on the basis of the patient's laboratory values.
3. Hyponatremia is often seen in this patient population. Standard fluid management can make it difficult to determine whether the underlying cause is CSW or SIADH. Regardless of the underlying cause, hyponatremia is treated with salt repletion because the fluid restriction commonly used in other patient populations to manage SIADH is contraindicated in patients with SAH who are still at high risk for vasospasm and cerebral ischemia. In mild hyponatremia, initial repletion is oral (e.g., salt tablets with meals). If hyponatremia does not respond to oral replacement, IV use of hypertonic saline (1.8% or 3%) is initiated. Hyponatremia requires frequent monitoring of laboratory values to assess effectiveness of therapy. Once the patient's sodium normalizes, therapy is slowly tapered to assess the patient's ability to maintain a normal serum sodium level.
4. Triple H therapy may lead to fluid volume overload and must be closely monitored. Multiple electrolyte abnormalities are often seen with triple H therapy, and serum magnesium and phosphorus levels should be monitored regularly along with standard blood chemistries.
5. Maintain adequate nutrition intake using enteral feedings, oral intake, parenteral nutrition, or lipid emulsions as indicated by the patient's neurologic status. Initially patients may have severe nausea and vomiting following aneurysmal rupture, but this generally resolves in the first 24 hours.

ADDITIONAL NURSING DIAGNOSES

As appropriate, see nursing diagnoses and interventions in Nutrition Support (Chapter 1), Mechanical Ventilation (Chapter 1), Alterations in Consciousness (Chapter 1), Prolonged Immobility (Chapter 1), Emotional and Spiritual Support of the Patient and Significant Others (Chapter 2), Diabetes Insipidus (Chapter 8), and Syndrome of Inappropriate Antidiuretic Hormone (Chapter 8).

CARE OF THE PATIENT AFTER INTRACRANIAL SURGERY

Cranial surgery can be performed to remove a space-occupying lesion such as a tumor, to evacuate a hematoma or abscess, or remove a foreign object. A patient may have a surgical repair of a vascular abnormality, such as an aneurysm or arteriovenous malformation (AVM), or to correct skull fractures. The neurosurgeon may elect to perform a procedure as a treatment modality, such as to drain CSF from the ventricular system or to divert CSF to promote dural repair, control seizures or tremors, and reduce pain. Minimally invasive intracranial procedures using stereotactic techniques are used for some biopsies and for implantation of deep brain stimulators for control of essential tremors. Endoscopic and stereotactic aspiration is being performed for noncomatose patients with basal ganglia hemorrhages. The type of surgical approach the neurosurgeon takes depends primarily on the location of the pathologic condition. The supratentorial approach is used to remove or correct problems in the frontal, temporal, or occipital lobes, as well as in the diencephalic area (i.e., pituitary, hypothalamus). Lesions of the cerebellum and brainstem usually require an infratentorial (i.e., suboccipital) approach. The transsphenoidal approach gains access to the pituitary gland to remove a tumor, control bone pain associated with metastatic cancer, or attempt to arrest the progression of diabetic retinopathy in a patient with diabetes mellitus.

NEUROLOGIC ASSESSMENT: POSTOPERATIVE CARE
GOAL OF SYSTEM ASSESSMENT
Evaluate for several key nursing diagnoses requiring emergent intervention:
- Alteration in cerebral tissue perfusion caused by increased ICP or cerebral vasospasm.
- Impaired gas exchange and/or ineffective airway clearance resulting from altered LOC.
- Risk of infection at site or as a result of CSF leak.
- Fluid volume deficit or excess.

- Impaired mobility.
- Altered sensory perception involving trunk, extremities, or cranial nerves.
- Alteration in cardiac output from dysrhythmias.
- Pain.

HISTORY AND RISK FACTORS

The critical care nurse caring for a postoperative neurosurgical patient must have a thorough understanding of the patient's preoperative history and condition requiring surgical intervention and, most importantly, knowledge of the patient's baseline or immediate preoperative neurologic assessment findings. It is essential to note any changes in assessment to evaluate for new postoperative neurologic changes resulting from the surgical intervention. Neurologic assessment data must be closely monitored for new focal changes, noting a trend in assessment data and correlated to the pathophysiologic process to identify appropriate nursing interventions. Three key causes of acute deterioration in a patient's neurologic status in the immediate postoperative period are cerebral edema, hemorrhage into or around the surgical site, and new onset of seizure activity.

VITAL SIGNS

- BP, HR, and RR changes: May further alter cerebral tissue perfusion. Uncontrolled high BP can lead to intracranial hemorrhage (ICH); therefore, close monitoring is important to keep the SBP less than 160 to 200 mm Hg to prevent bleeding. Hypotension reduces cerebral perfusion and may cause cerebral ischemia. Monitor rate, rhythm, and depth of respirations for changes or abnormal breathing patterns.
- Hyperthermia: May be associated with injury or irritation of the hypothalamic temperature-regulating centers, presence of blood in the cerebral spinal fluid (CSF), or infection. Elevated temperature increases the metabolic needs of the brain, potentially leading to increased blood flow to the area, with concomitant cerebral hyperemia.
- Intracranial pressure: If intracranial pressure (ICP) monitoring is used, the critical care nurse must understand the dynamics of cerebral perfusion pressure (CPP). A postoperative increase in the volume of brain tissue (e.g., edema), CSF, or blood or the addition of a hematoma can cause intracranial hypertension. The normal ICP is generally 0 to 10 mm Hg (up to 15 mm Hg). CPP is inversely related to ICP and in pressures less than 50 to 60 mm Hg can lead to cerebral ischemia or infarction: $CPP = MAP - ICP$.

OBSERVATION

- Level of consciousness: The improvement in the degree of LOC depends on preoperative damage to cerebral tissue. Consciousness often improves while anesthesia wears off, or while cerebral edema subsides, and while ICP approaches normal.
- Pupillary changes: Pupillary abnormalities can indicate unilateral or bilateral brain dysfunction, interruption of sympathetic or parasympathetic pathways, damage in the brainstem, cranial nerve damage, and herniation.
- Communicative and cognitive deficits: The ability to communicate and understand spoken or written words after surgery depends on the level of preoperative dysfunction, the site of the lesion, extent of the procedure, and the degree of postoperative cerebral edema.
- Broca (expressive, motor, nonfluent) aphasia: Inability to communicate verbally or in writing. Can understand situations, follow commands.
- Wernicke (receptive, sensory, fluent) aphasia: The patient does not understand the situation and cannot follow commands appropriately.
- Cerebrospinal fluid (CSF) leakage: Assess for CSF leakage from the ear (otorrhea), from the nose (rhinorrhea), which is seen particularly with transsphenoidal surgery, and also from the surgical site. The leakage of CSF indicates an open pathway to the subarachnoid space (SAS), which carries a serious risk of infection. Causes specific to craniotomy include the use of an external ventricular drainage device (used as a treatment modality), which can be a source of entrance of organisms, a remote site infection, and if additional surgery is required. Treatment of a CSF leak depends upon severity, site, and the risk for infection. It may include the use of an external drainage system (e.g., lumbar subarachnoid drain) to divert CSF flow and thus reduce pressure. Keeping the patient flat (if not contraindicated) will allow time for the dural tear to heal. Surgical intervention may be done to seal the dural leak at the site of origin.

OBSERVATION AND FUNCTIONAL ASSESSMENT

1. Assess motor function and sensory responses

Improvement in both motor and sensory perception may occur while cerebral edema subsides.

- Motor: Motor deficits (weakness or paralysis) are caused by injury or edema to the primary motor cortex and corticospinal (pyramidal) tracts.
- Sensory: Sensory deficits occur when the primary sensory cortex, the sensory association areas of the parietal lobe, or the spinothalamic tracts are injured or edematous. Sensory deficits include inability to distinguish objects according to characteristics (e.g., size, shape, weight) and inability to distinguish overall changes in temperature, touch, pressure, and position.

2. Assess for cranial nerve impairment

The degree of cranial nerve deficit(s) depends on site of the lesion, preoperative deficit, degree of postoperative cerebral edema, and surgical approach. Infratentorial surgery for lesions in the posterior fossa (brainstem and cerebellum) involves significant cranial nerve manipulation with high risk of injury to cranial nerves IX, X, and XII, which innervate the pharynx and tongue. Risk of airway obstruction is high. Removal of tumors (i.e., acoustic neuromas) may injure the cranial nerve VII and result in facial paralysis and loss of corneal reflex. The loss of corneal reflex may be caused by surgical trauma to frontal lobe motor pathways or brainstem cranial nerve nuclei. Corneal abrasion, ulceration, and blindness may occur if not recognized and treated promptly. Always prevent corneal abrasion and ir-ritation. Keep cornea moist with prescribed ophthalmic solution and use an eye shield if indicated.

Cranial nerve deficit(s) may improve while cerebral edema resolves or may be permanent. Nursing assessment of cranial nerve dysfunction is important. For more information about the function of all the cranial nerves, see Appendix 3.

SCREENING LABWORK

- Sodium levels and osmolality: Important for management of SIADH and diabetes insipi-dus (DI). Close monitoring during hyperosmolar therapy is important. Hypernatremia may indicate dehydration if associated with DI. Hyponatremia may be associated with SIADH. If sodium level is not managed appropriately, cerebral edema may result.
- Cerebrospinal fluid (CSF) analysis: Evaluates the color, white blood cell (WBC) count, differential, glucose content, and protein level, which are important whenever a CSF leak develops.
- Complete blood count (CBC), electrolytes, and coagulation studies: Evaluates for anemia, hypoglycemia or hyperglycemia; hyponatremia or hypernatremia; potential for hemor-rhage or infection.
- Anticonvulsant medication levels: If the patient is receiving anticonvulsant therapy, monitor for subtherapeutic and supratherapeutic levels.

DIAGNOSTIC TESTING

Refer to Neurologic Diagnostic Testing, Chapter 5.

COLLABORATIVE MANAGEMENT AFTER INTRACRANIAL SURGERY

CARE PRIORITIES

1. Respiratory support

Supplemental oxygen, intubation, and mechanical ventilation as needed. In patients requiring mechanical ventilation who have potential or actual increased ICP, use of hyperven-tilation needs careful monitoring to avoid cerebral vasoconstriction. The Brain Trauma Foundation standard emphasizes that in the absence of increased ICP, prophylactic hyperven-tilation ($Paco_2$ less than 25 mm Hg) is not recommended. $Paco_2$ is maintained within normal limits unless acute elevation in ICP is present with the possibility of imminent cerebral her-niation. A brief period of hyperventilation may be instituted in the setting of imminent her-niation. Use of prophylactic hyperventilation ($Paco_2$ less than 35 mm Hg) should be avoided during the first 24 hours or used only if increased ICP does not respond to other measures such as CSF drainage, sedation, or use of neuromuscular blocking agents.

2. Positioning

The HOB is most often elevated 30 degrees to promote venous drainage, which reduces ICP. The head should be kept in straight alignment with the trunk to prevent increased ICP and to facilitate venous return.

- In posterior fossa surgery (infratentorial approach), the supporting muscles of the neck are altered. Patients should be turned with the neck in alignment with the head and with the head, neck, and shoulders supported.
- After hemicraniectomy, to avoid injury, patients may not be turned to the side from which hemicraniectomy has been removed unless appropriate support is provided to keep the head and neck aligned with the shoulders to keep the weight of the head from directly laying on the flap. Label head dressing, chart, and bed with location of missing bone. A head protective device such as a specially sized helmet should be worn.
- After procedures in which a large intracranial space is left after extensive surgery, to avoid a sudden shift in intracranial contents, with subsequent hemorrhage or herniation, the patient should not be positioned on operative side immediately after surgery.

3. Manage pain

- Analgesics: Clinical trials have shown that the addition of tramadol or nalbuphine to acetaminophen controls pain more adequately in patients who have undergone craniotomy. Patients may also require opiate medications including fentanyl, morphine, hydromorphone, and remifentanil for pain relief.

Note: The effect of morphine and tramadol patient-controlled analgesia (PCA) on arterial carbon dioxide tension is still unknown for patients who have undergone craniotomy.

4. Reduce cerebral edema:

- Corticosteroids (e.g., dexamethasone): To decrease cerebral edema.

Note: Not indicated for patients with traumatic brain injury (TBI). Research is ongoing to determine whether steroids are effective in the treatment of cerebral edema. They are prescribed for the treatment of vasogenic cerebral edema and edema caused by cerebral tumor.

> **Safety Alert** *Steroids can cause a hyperosmolar state and dehydration. Monitor serum osmolality and electrolytes and assess fluid status before and after administration.*

- Osmotic diuretics (e.g., mannitol): To control cerebral edema causing increased ICP. Dose is usually 0.25 to 1 g/kg of 20% solution administered over 20 to 30 minutes, and ICP levels should be measured before, during, and after administration of mannitol. When the ICP reaches a desired fixed reduced level (usually within 15 minutes), the dose of mannitol needs to be gradually reduced.
- Fluid and electrolyte management: Hypertonic saline may be used to prevent or treat increasing cerebral edema. Serum sodium levels should be maintained at less than 155 mEq/L. Patients with serum sodium levels greater than 160 mEq/L are at higher risk for treatment-related renal failure, pulmonary edema, and heart failure. If serum sodium levels are elevated greater than 160 mEq/L for more than 48 hours, the risk for complications, including seizures, increases.

5. Perioperative and postoperative deep venous thrombosis (DVT) prevention

> **Safety Alert** *A systematic review of literature done for the Agency for Healthcare Research and Quality (AHRQ) showed that the risk of neurosurgical patients for deep venous thrombosis (DVT) is 28%. The 5 Million Lives Campaign, National Hospital Quality Measure of The Joint Commission, National Hospital Quality Measure by the Centers for Medicare and Medicaid Services, and the National Quality Forum all endorse aspects of DVT prophylaxis. Craniotomy patients without contraindications for anticoagulation should receive DVT prophylaxis using either a low–molecular-weight heparin or low-dose unfractionated heparin given as an alternative. Pharmacologic agents can be used as an adjunct to mechanical prophylaxis using intermittent pneumatic compression, elastic stockings, or both. Venous imaging techniques such as ultrasonography can be used before discharge to detect thrombosis.*

6. Control seizures

Antiepileptic agents: Phenytoin, fosphenytoin, and levetiracetam should be considered for prophylaxis of provoked or early seizures occurring within 7 days of surgery. Use of other agents such as carbamazepine, phenobarbital, and valproate remains controversial and in some studies has not shown to reduce postoperative seizures.

7. Prevent infection

Antibiotics: Prevent postoperative surgical site infection or respiratory or urinary tract infection. Randomized controlled trials have shown that in patients undergoing craniotomy, the use of prophylactic antibiotics reduces the frequency of postoperative meningitis.

Safety Alert *The American Society of Health System Pharmacists and the Centers for Disease Control and Prevention have recommended that antibiotic administration be via the intravenous route at induction of anesthesia and/or that the bactericidal concentration of the drug be established in the tissues and serum when the incision is made.*

---

8. Nutrition support

The method and type of nutrition support are determined by the patient's condition and may include any of the following: oral feedings, enteral feedings, supplements, or parenteral nutrition (i.e., total parenteral nutrition, fat emulsion therapy). See Nutrition Support (p. 117).

9. Reduce fever

Antipyretics: Treat elevated temperature, which can increase use of oxygen and glucose supplies.

10. Prevent gastric ulcers

Histamine H_2-receptor antagonists/proton pump inhibitors: To inhibit gastric secretions and thus prevent or facilitate healing of gastric ulcers and prevent bleeding.

11. Facilitate mobility and return of functions needed for activities of daily living

Physical medicine consultation: To evaluate the patient and plan for rehabilitation: physical and occupational therapies for planning return of function.

Speech therapy may be important for dysphagia screening, monitoring for meeting communication needs.

12. Implement therapeutic hypothermia

The effects of cooling of the injured brain continues to be studied to evaluate the effects of mild to moderate hypothermia on protection against ischemic and nonischemic brain hypoxia, traumatic brain injury, and anoxic injury with cardiac arrest. Prophylactically induced hypothermia has yet to be shown as having beneficial effects on outcomes of traumatic brain injury.

CARE PLANS: COMPLICATIONS AFTER INTRACRANIAL SURGERY

DECREASED INTRACRANIAL ADAPTIVE CAPACITY *related to possible changes in intracranial fluid or brain tissue volume following surgery.*

- -

Goals/Outcomes: Maintain normal ICP (0 to 10 mm Hg with upper limit of 15 mm Hg) through regulation of cerebral flow and cerebral spinal circulation.

NOC Neurologic Status: Consciousness.

 Cerebral Perfusion Promotion

1. Monitor for increased ICP with potential for herniation: Cerebral edema, hemorrhage, infection, and surgical trauma can all lead to increased ICP with herniation (see Box 7-1). Some cerebral edema is expected after intracranial surgery, and usually peaks approximately 72 hours after surgery (see Traumatic Brain Injury, Chapter 3). Postoperative uncontrolled nausea and vomiting can cause high intraabdominal and also increased intrathoracic pressure (e.g., high positive-end expiratory pressure [PEEP] ventilator settings) leading to high ICP.

2. Monitor for intracranial bleeding: Postoperative bleeding can be related to the surgical site and may be intracerebral, intracerebellar, subarachnoid, subdural, epidural, or intraventricular. Coagulation profiles and platelet counts should be monitored closely. Bleeding may be caused by the lengthy and extensive surgical procedure, high BP, prolonged anesthesia, preexisting medical problems, or medications. Contusions can develop after evacuation of epidural or subdural hematomas and may create a mass effect.
3. Control seizures: Generalized or partial seizures can occur as a result of surgical trauma, irritation of cerebral tissue by the presence of blood, cerebral edema, cerebral hypoxia, hypoglycemia, preexisting seizure disorder, or inadequate anticonvulsant levels. The use of anticonvulsants prophylactically remains controversial.
4. Monitor for hydrocephalus: May appear before surgery or occur after surgery as an acute or chronic complication. Usually it is caused by a slowing or complete stoppage of the flow of CSF through the ventricular system secondary to edema, bleeding, scarring, or obstruction. For further discussion, see Cerebral Aneurysm and Subarachnoid Hemorrhage (p. 629).
5. Assess for tension pneumocephalus: Uncommon but can occur as a result of air entering the subdural, extradural, subarachnoid, intracerebral, or intraventricular spaces and is an emergent situation. May be a complication of infratentorial/posterior fossa craniotomy, burr holes for removal of chronic subdural hematoma, and transsphenoidal hypophysectomy. Rapid decompression is usually required.

INEFFECTIVE BREATHING PATTERN *related to altered level of consciousness (LOC) and inability to maintain adequate airway and respiratory rate (RR)*

Goals/Outcomes: Maintain adequate airway, provide supplemental oxygenation, ventilate the lungs as necessary to maintain $Paco_2$ to 35 mm Hg. Increase in $Paco_2$, hypercapnia, can lead to cerebral vasodilation with a subsequent increase in intracranial volume, and thus increased ICP. A severe drop in $Paco_2$ can lead to cerebral vasoconstriction and cerebral ischemia.
NOC Respiratory Status: Gas Exchange.

Ventilation Assistance
1. Monitor for partial or complete airway obstruction caused by accumulation of secretions, improper positioning, or change in LOC.
2. Assess for increased crackles caused by neurogenic pulmonary edema resulting from a sudden increase in ICP.
3. Assess for changes in LOC caused by cerebral edema that causes compression of brainstem respiratory centers.
4. Discourage vigorous coughing, because it increases ICP.
5. Encourage deep breathing to help prevent atelectasis and pneumonia.
6. Follow institutional protocol for venous thromboembolism (VTE)/DVT prophylaxis to help prevent pulmonary embolism.

RISK FOR INFECTION *related to presence of invasive devices within the cranium.*

Goals/Outcomes: Prevent infection at site or secondary infections, such as meningitis, encephalitis, or ventriculitis, or as a result of invasive procedures.
NOC Risk Control.

Infection Control
1. Monitor for a central nervous system (CNS) infection: Can be caused by a preoperative event such as organisms introduced at the time of injury (e.g., gunshot wound) or a break in sterile technique or as a result of the nature of the surgical procedure involving opening of the dura. (See Meningitis, Chapter 7.)
2. Monitor for a ventriculostomy-related infection: A ventriculostomy may be performed with the introduction of an intraventricular catheter to monitor and manage postoperative ICP or to provide external ventricular drainage for CSF diversion secondary to dural leaks. Extended duration of catheterization has been correlated with increasing risk of CSF infections. Antibiotic coated intraventricular catheters are also available for use.

DEFICIENT FLUID VOLUME OR EXCESS FLUID VOLUME *related to hormonal or electrolyte imbalances*

Goals/Outcomes: Adequately managed I&O, control of fluid imbalances resulting from hormonal or electrolyte disturbances, and prevention of fluid loss.
NOC Fluid Balance.

Fluid Management
1. Monitor for sodium imbalance secondary to diabetes insipidus and SIADH: Results from disturbance of the hypothalamus or posterior lobe of the pituitary gland. ADH is produced in the hypothalamus and stored in the posterior pituitary.
   - Diabetes insipidus results from decreased ADH production, which leads to excessive urinary output, with potentially serious fluid and electrolyte problems (see Diabetes Insipidus, Chapter 8). Diabetes insipidus may result from cerebral edema, gland manipulation, or partial or total removal of the gland.
   - SIADH, a less common problem, results from an increase in the release of ADH, which leads to resorption of large amounts of water via the renal tubules with concurrent loss of large amounts of sodium. Similar to diabetes insipidus, SIADH can cause serious fluid and electrolyte problems (see Syndrome of Inappropriate Antidiuretic Hormone, Chapter 8).
2. Assess for hypovolemic shock: May occur as a result of general fluid loss associated with treatment using osmotic diuretics; therefore, close monitoring is essential. Close observation for the development of diabetes insipidus postoperatively is required because severe dehydration and hypovolemic shock may occur.
3. Monitor for gastrointestinal bleeding: GI bleeding associated with cerebral trauma and the postoperative period after neurosurgery can cause fluid volume deficit. Although the cause is unclear, stress from the trauma or the surgery can produce continuous vagal stimulation leading to a hyperacidic state resulting in gastric erosion, ulceration, and ultimately hemorrhage. These conditions also result from medications, especially corticosteroids (see Acute Gastrointestinal Bleeding, Chapter 9). Other GI conditions may occur, such as constipation, after neurologic surgery. Decreased or absent peristalsis results from prolonged anesthesia, immobility, trauma, electrolyte deficiencies, and mechanical bowel obstruction (e.g., obstipation).

IMPAIRED PHYSICAL MOBILITY *related to prolonged bed rest or motor dysfunction*

Goals/Outcomes: Prevent vascular complications through appropriate pharmacotherapy and mechanical prophylaxis, and prevent atrophy and/or joint contractures through passive exercises, early mobilization, and activity progression. **NOC** Mobility.

Exercise Promotion
1. Thrombophlebitis, DVT, and pulmonary embolism: May result from prolonged bed rest and immobility after intracranial surgery. Other factors such as a prolonged surgical procedure, preexisting hypercoagulable states, and other blood dyscrasias may influence the postoperative complications. VTE is the most frequent complication following craniotomy for removal of brain tumors. Prophylactic management standards have been developed for the prevention of DVT.

DECREASED CARDIAC OUTPUT *related to unstable BP or cardiac dysrhythmias*

Goals/Outcomes: Stabilize BP and HR within normal limits to maintain adequate cardiac output, thereby promoting appropriate cerebral blood flow.
NOC Circulation Status.

Cardiac Precautions
1. Monitor for cardiac dysrhythmias: May occur as a result of cerebral hypoxia or ischemia, manipulation of the brainstem, or the irritating effects of blood in the CSF (see Dysrhythmias and Conduction Disturbances, Chapter 5).

PAIN *related to headache or discomfort secondary to surgical intervention*

Goals/Outcomes: Pain and discomfort are controlled based on the patient's self-reported pain score (if verbal) or appropriate nonverbal pain scale, stable vital signs, and lack of skeletal muscle tension and behavioral signs. Pain and autonomic system stimulation and physical agitation can increase ICP, produce sleep deprivation, and mask neurologic changes and thereby lead to further complications.
NOC Pain Control.

Pain Management
1. Medicate and intervene appropriately to keep the patient's pain controlled and maintain comfort level. Use of an evidence-based pain scale measurement such as a numerical rating scale (1 to 10) or a behavioral pain scale may be appropriate for patients with impaired communication ability.

2. Assess level of sedation appropriately. Overmedication with analgesics or sedatives in postoperative patients with altered LOC can produce impaired gas exchange and compromised airway.

ADDITIONAL NURSING DIAGNOSES

See also nursing diagnoses and interventions in Traumatic Brain Injury (Chapter 3), Sedation and Neuromuscular Blockade (Chapter 1), Cerebral Aneurysm and Subarachnoid Hemorrhage (Chapter 7), Status Epilepticus Chapter 7, Meningitis (Chapter 7), Diabetes Insipidus (Chapter 8), Syndrome of Inappropriate Antidiuretic Hormone (Chapter 8), Nutrition Support (Chapter 1), Prolonged Immobility (Chapter 1), and Emotional and Spiritual Support of the Patient and Significant Others (Chapter 2).

MENINGITIS

PATHOPHYSIOLOGY

Meningitis is an inflammation of the brain and spinal cord, the CNS, affecting the meninges (i.e., dura, arachnoid, pia), brain surface, and cranial nerves. Meningeal infection comes about through environmental exposure or as a result of direct contamination through invasive procedures or surgeries. Meningitis is a reportable disease in all states. There are several types of meningitis, broadly classified as bacterial (pyogenic), viral, aseptic, tuberculous, fungal, and eosinophilic (parasitic). The causative agent travels in the bloodstream from various sources before entering the cerebral spinal fluid (CSF. The CSF is unable to mount an antimicrobial response because it lacks immunoglobulins and complement. Therefore, when contamination of the CSF takes place, phagocytosis and opsonization of the microbes do not occur. Bacterial meningitis, a consequence of bacterial invasion, progresses through four interconnected phases: (1) invasion of host leading to central nervous system (CNS) infection, (2) inflammation of the subarachnoid and ventricular space while bacteria multiply, (3) pathophysiologic changes consistent with progression of inflammation, and (4) neuronal damage.

BACTERIAL MENINGITIS

The most common type of meningitis is bacteria, which can be community-acquired or hospital-acquired. Transmission of bacterial meningitis can occur through environmental exposure or because of an invasive procedure (placement of external ventricular device or craniotomy), injury (e.g., open/penetrating wounds), facial or basilar skull fractures, shunt occlusion/malfunction, otitis media, sinusitis, or bacteremia (e.g., endocarditis, pneumonia). Bacterial types usually appear within 3 to 7 days after exposure. The most common agents associated with bacterial meningitis are discussed as follows.

Streptococcus pneumoniae, a gram-positive cocci, has been the leading cause of adult meningitis in the United States. Pneumococcal meningitis occurs in crowded conditions and is spread seasonally (fall and winter). *S. pneumoniae* is not as prevalent a cause of meningitis since the development of Pneumovax and Prevnar vaccines. Pneumococcal meningitis may occur following an upper respiratory tract infection or nasopharyngeal colonization with a pneumococcal strain, is a complication of conditions associated with CSF leaks, is associated with asplenia, and is more prevalent in immunocompromised persons and in older adults.

Neisseria meningitidis, a gram-negative cocci, is the second leading cause of meningitis in the United States. *N. meningitidis* is endemic in the United States, can cause community epidemics, and has resulted in death in previously healthy young adults. Infection is more likely to occur in young children, persons with immune deficiencies (human immunodeficiency virus [HIV]), or complement component deficiencies (e.g., congenital, associated with nephrotic syndrome, hepatic failure, systemic lupus erythematosus, or multiple myeloma). Other risk factors include nasopharyngeal carrier states and high-risk sexual behaviors. Vaccinations have reduced the number of cases since 2005.

Haemophilus influenzae, a gram-negative bacilli, had been the most common cause of meningitis in children before 1990. Since 1990, the *H. influenzae* vaccine type B (Hib vaccine) has reduced the incidence of bacterial meningitis substantially in infants and children, making it a disease predominantly of adults. Before 1990, *H. influenzae* type B serotype was the leading cause of bacterial meningitis in all age groups. Other serotypes continue to affect children and adults. Predisposing factors include upper respiratory tract infections, diabetes mellitus, hypogammaglobulinemia, alcoholism, and head trauma.

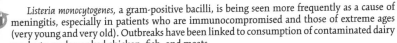

Listeria monocytogenes, a gram-positive bacilli, is being seen more frequently as a cause of meningitis, especially in patients who are immunocompromised and those of extreme ages (very young and very old). Outbreaks have been linked to consumption of contaminated dairy products, undercooked chicken, fish, and meats.

Gram-negative species (*Escherichia coli*, *Klebsiella pneumoniae*, *Proteus mirabilis*, and *Pseudomonas aeruginosa*) are increasing in prevalence as a hospital-acquired cause secondary to trauma or neurosurgical procedures. Spontaneous gram-negative meningitis is found in older adults, the immunocompromised, or persons with underlying conditions such as cirrhosis, diabetes mellitus, malignancy, or splenectomy. The urinary tract is the usual portal of entry of bacteria. Other surgical procedures complicated by gram-negative infections are ventriculoperitoneal shunts, craniofacial repair, ventriculostomy, hypophysectomy, reservoir insertion, and myelography.

Other microbes

Also associated with meningitis are *Mycobacterium pneumoniae*, *Borrelia burgdorferi*, and *Treponema pallidum*.

TUBERCULOUS MENINGITIS

Mycobacterium tuberculosis as a CNS disease and manifested as meningitis is documented in children and adults where tuberculosis has a regional prevalence. In more developed regions, *M. tuberculosis* meningitis is related more to reactivation of the disease. Other risk factors for development of *M. tuberculosis* are older age, alcoholism, malnutrition, and immunocompromised states including HIV and patients with malignancies. Older adults and children living among people with tuberculosis have increased risk.

FUNGAL MENINGITIS

Cryptococcus neoformans, an opportunistic organism seen with acquired immune deficiency syndrome (AIDS), is the leading cause of CNS fungal infection. Other fungi-associated meningitis include *Candida albicans*, and histoplasmosis meningitis is also seen in immunocompromised patients and evolving from progressive disseminated histoplasmosis.

VIRAL MENINGITIS

Enteroviruses are the most common cause of viral meningitis that occurs in the spring and fall seasons. The condition generally lasts 7 to 10 days and, although serious, is rarely fatal in people with normal immune systems. Herpes viruses, including herpes simplex viruses (the cause of chickenpox, Epstein-Barr virus, and shingles), measles, and influenza may lead to viral meningitis. Mosquitoes and other insects spread arboviruses, which cause infections that lead to viral meningitis.

EOSINOPHILIC MENINGITIS

Infestation by *Angiostrongylus cantonensis*, a parasitic nematode, results in severe gastrointestinal (GI) or CNS disease in humans, depending on the species. *A. cantonensis*, also known as the rat lungworm, causes eosinophilic meningitis. Prevalent in Southeast Asia and Tropical Pacific Islands, the nematode resides in rodents and transmission is through larvae found in rat feces. Slugs or mollusks ingest the larvae. Humans are incidental hosts as a result of eating infected slugs, raw vegetables, or vegetable juices contaminated with the slugs or their slime.

ASEPTIC MENINGITIS SYNDROME

In aseptic meningitis, the clinical and laboratory evaluations provide evidence for inflammation, but bacterial culture results are negative. It may be drug-induced, related to infection, or unrelated to infection. Aseptic meningitis has been linked to adverse drug reactions with nonsteroidal antiinflammatory drugs, antimicrobials such as trimethoprim-sulfamethoxazole, antiepileptics, and immunoglobulin. The syndrome is also associated with oncologic diagnoses (hematologic malignancies, lymphomas, leukemias, breast, lung, melanomas, and GI), systemic lupus erythematosus, and brain surgery or brain trauma.

NONINFECTIOUS CAUSES

Sarcoidosis, leptomeningeal carcinomatosis, systemic lupus erythematosus, Wegener granulomatosis, and Behçet disease.

> **Safety Alert**
>
> *Acute meningitis may manifest as a community-acquired illness with a negative Gram stain. The pathogen causing the disease may never be determined. Syphilis, bacteremia, and Borrelia burgdorferi (Lyme disease) have been identified in some cases. Variables affecting diagnosis of meningitis include presentation in winter months, age older than 60 years, and comorbid disease, especially immunodeficiency.*

NEUROLOGIC ASSESSMENT: MENINGITIS

GOAL OF SYSTEM ASSESSMENT

A complete neurologic examination should be performed to establish the patient's baseline neurologic function. Examination of associated systems (head, eye, ear, nose, and throat [HEENT] and respiratory) provides additional data. When diagnosed one or more signs of meningitis are positive (Table 7-2).

Bacterial meningitis presents with classic symptoms of fever, altered mental status, headache, photophobia, nuchal rigidity, and nausea and vomiting. Immediate diagnosis and isolation of the organisms are paramount in this life-threatening disease. Delay in obtaining the necessary information needed to diagnosis and treat the underlying organism will increase morbidity and mortality.

HISTORY AND RISK FACTORS

- Age
- Community setting
  - College dormitories, military barracks
  - Exposure to insects or rodents
- Recent surgery or medical problems
  - Cochlear implants, brain surgery, or traumatic brain injury
  - Antibiotic use
- Tuberculosis risk
- Work exposure (healthcare workers)
- Lifestyle
  - Recent travel
  - High-risk sexual activity
  - IV drug use
- Immunocompromised
  - Splenectomy
  - HIV
  - Hepatitis
  - Chemotherapy
- History of present illness
  - Time course for symptom development
  - Recent infection (respiratory/ear)
  - Recent trauma to the head
  - Exposure to meningitis

Table 7-2	POSITIVE MENINGEAL SIGNS	
Test/Description	**Positive Findings**
Stiff neck sign (nuchal rigidity): Raise the patient's head by flexing the neck and attempting to make the patient's chin touch the sternum.	Pain and resistance to neck motion.
Brudzinski sign: Assess for nuchal rigidity.	Flexion of the hips and knees when the examiner flexes the patient's neck.
Kernig sign: Flex the patient's leg at the knee and hip when the patient is supine, and then attempt to straighten the leg.	Pain in the lower back and resistance to straightening the leg.

- Use of antibiotics
- Petechial or ecchymotic rash
- Ear or nose drainage
- Medical/social history
  - Drug allergies
  - Past medical history
  - Recent surgical procedure
  - Immunocompromising condition
  - IV drug use
  - HIV status or risk behavior
  - Travel to endemic meningococcal area

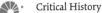

- Critical History
  - Exposure
  - Drug allergies

VITAL SIGNS

- BP, HR, and RR changes: May further alter cerebral tissue perfusion. Monitor rate, rhythm, and depth of respirations for changes or abnormal breathing patterns. Use of pulse oximetry and electrocardiographic (ECG) monitoring is recommended.
- Hyperthermia: May be associated with injury or irritation of the hypothalamic temperature-regulating centers, presence of blood in the CSF, or infection. Elevated temperature increases the metabolic needs of the brain, potentially leading to increased blood flow to the area, with concomitant cerebral hyperemia and ischemia.

OBSERVATION

A constellation of early symptoms is associated with most types of meningitis and includes headache, fever, neck stiffness, and altered mental status. At least one of these symptoms is found in most types of meningitis. Other symptoms such as papilledema, seizures, focal deficits (cranial nerve palsies), and coma may be seen early or late in the development of meningitis. Meningitis is associated with cerebral infarction and arthritis in some cases. The clinical features of specific types of meningitis are described as follows. Common meningeal signs demonstrated in meningitis are found in Table 7-2.

Level of consciousness

When assessing LOC it is important not to use subjective terms such as "stupor or lethargy" but rather to assess and communicate clearly the description of the patient's spontaneous activity, response to verbal stimuli and reaction to painful stimuli, and how this differs from previous assessment. Assess for an acute change in mental status or fluctuation in mental status; various scales can be used that include LOC and other key indicators. Examples are the Richmond Agitation and Sedation Score (RASS) and Glasgow Coma Scale (GCS).

Pupillary changes

Examine pupils for size (in mm), shape, symmetry, reactivity to light, constriction, consensual response, and accommodation. Pupillary abnormalities can indicate unilateral or bilateral brain dysfunction, interruption of sympathetic or parasympathetic pathways, damage in the brainstem, cranial nerve damage, and herniation.

Clinical presentation

- *S. pneumoniae:* The classic presentation of pneumococcal meningitis is fever, headache, meningismus (meningeal irritation), and altered mental status that progresses quickly to coma. Nuchal rigidity and Kernig or Brudzinski sign are present. Nausea, vomiting, profuse sweats, weakness, myalgia, seizures, and cranial nerve palsies may also be present.
- *N. meningitidis:* Patients may quickly deteriorate, beginning with fever and early macular erythematous rash that progresses rapidly to petechial and purpuric states, conjunctival petechiae, and aggressive behavior. Dysfunctions of cranial nerves VI, VII, and VIII (see Appendix 4) and aphasia, ventriculitis, subdural empyema, cerebral venous thrombosis, arthritis with positive joint cultures, and disseminated intravascular coagulation may occur. Age-phasic patterns are noted with increases in patients younger than 1 year old, increasing in ages 18 to 24 years old, and increasing again in those older than 65 years old.

- *H. influenzae:* The most distinguishing sign is early development of deafness, which can occur within 24 to 36 hours after onset. A morbilliform or petechial rash may be present.
- *L. monocytogenes:* Seizures may occur and rhombencephalitis may be present. Rhomben-cephalitis seen early in the course of infection is characterized by focal deficits such as ataxia, cranial nerve palsies, and nystagmus. Conclusive diagnosis may require serology testing.
- Gram-negative species: In older adults, fever may be absent or low grade and headache may not be reported. Meningeal signs may be subtle, but confusion, severe mental status changes, and pneumonia are commonly reported. Nuchal rigidity in older adults must be differentiated from degenerative changes of the cervical spine.
- *B. burgdorferi:* The symptoms of meningitis may be preceded by symptoms of Lyme disease, which occur in three stages. The first stage is a "bull's eye" rash within a few days of the tick bite followed by headache, stiff neck, lethargy, irritability, and changes in mental status, especially memory loss. Stage two, weeks to months after the tick bite, causes persistent headache, nausea, vomiting, malaise, irritability, cranial nerve deficits, mental status changes, peripheral neuropathies, and myalgias. In the last or third stage, arthritic types of symptoms and brain parenchymal changes are apparent.
- *A. cantonensis or Angiostrongylus costaricensis:* Presence of these parasites is difficult to detect because there is no specific blood test or method to identify the larvae. Symptoms include severe headache, stiff neck, paresthesias, and facial nerve palsy. Symptoms of meningitis may be preceded by GI impairment. A high blood or CSF eosinophil level indicates the presence of parasites. History of ingesting raw vegetables, undercooked snails, slugs or other transport hosts may provide clues to the diagnoses.
- *M. tuberculosis:* A slow-onset process that causes neurologic damage before treatment is sought. Three stages are identified: (1) prodromal occurs over 2 to 3 weeks associated with general malaise, headache, and low-grade fever; (2) meningitis phase with common signs and symptoms; and (3) paralytic phase with coma, seizures, and hemiparalysis. Common symptoms include headache, lethargy, confusion, nuchal rigidity, cranial nerve abnormalities, SIADH, weight loss, and night sweats. Kernig and Brudzinski sign are present. The chest radiographic results may be clear, and purified protein derivative may be nonreactive. Maintain a high index of suspicion in tuberculosis-prevalent regions, persons with history of tuberculosis (reactivation infection in adults), and those with active tuberculosis in other systems.
- *C. neoformans:* Because the infection is subacute, fever and headache may have a subtle pattern lasting for weeks while other symptoms of meningitis occur, including positive meningeal signs (Table 7-2), alterations in mental status (e.g., hyperactivity, bizarre behavior, emotional lability, poor judgment), photophobia, focal cranial nerve deficits, nausea, vomiting, and (rarely) seizures.
- *C. albicans:* Same clinical manifestations as bacterial meningitis. In patients with neutropenia only fever may be present.
- Aseptic meningitis syndrome: Fever, headache, stiff neck, fatigue, anorexia, and altered LOC are seen several hours after ingestion of causative drug. Severity varies with amount of drug taken and previous exposures. CSF glucose may be slightly elevated.
- Acute meningitis with negative Gram stain: Fever and neck stiffness are the most frequent findings. The Gram stain for bacteria is negative, but CSF WBC count is elevated. Symptoms are similar to those for other types of meningitis.
- Other associated clinical signs: Asymmetrical facial weakness, oropharyngeal thrush, cervical lymphadenopathy, maculopapular rash, parotitis, and vesicular/ulcerated genitals may be present with viral or bacterial causes of meningitis.

FUNCTIONAL ASSESSMENT
1. Assess motor function and sensory responses
- Motor: Assess bilateral muscle strength, symmetry of movement, and coordination. Assess for abnormal motor movements unilaterally and bilaterally, such as decorticate posturing (abnormal flexion), decerebrate posturing (abnormal extension), or flaccidity. Motor deficits (weakness or paralysis) are caused by injury or edema to the primary motor cortex in the precentral gyrus and corticospinal (pyramidal) tracts.
    - Babinski sign, Kernig sign, and Brudzinski sign: See Chapter 7 General Neurologic Assessment.

- Sensory: Assess perception of touch, proprioception, pain, temperature, and vibration (if possible). Superficial and deep reflexes are tested on symmetrical sides of the body and compared noting the strength of contraction. Sensory deficits occur when the primary sensory cortex, the sensory association areas of the parietal lobe, or the spinothalamic tracts are injured or edematous. Sensory deficits include the inability to distinguish objects according to characteristics (e.g., size, shape, weight) and inability to distinguish overall changes in temperature, touch, pressure, and position. Improvement in both motor and sensory perception may be seen while cerebral edema subsides.

2. Assess for cranial nerve impairment

Cranial nerve deficit(s) may improve while cerebral edema resolves or may be permanent. Nursing assessment of cranial nerve dysfunction is important. For more information about the function and testing of all the cranial nerves, see Appendix 3.

SCREENING LABWORK

- CSF analysis: Evaluates the color, WBC count, differential, glucose content, and protein level.
- CBC including differential, electrolytes, blood cultures, and coagulation studies: Evaluate for anemia, hypoglycemia, or hyperglycemia; potential for hemorrhage or infection.
- Specimen analysis: Nasopharyngeal and rectal swaps, and stool cultures to identify causative agents.
- Viral assays, cultures, and serology testing: Venereal Disease Research Laboratory test (VDRL), HIV, lymphocytic choriomeningitis virus, polymerase chain reaction, Lyme serology, and other viral testing including mumps and measles.

DIAGNOSTIC TESTS

Bacterial meningitis presents with classic symptoms of fever, altered mental status, headache, and nuchal rigidity. Immediate diagnosis and isolation of the organisms are paramount in this life-threatening disease. Delay in obtaining the necessary information needed to diagnosis and treat the underlying organism will increase morbidity and mortality.

Diagnostic Tests for Meningitis

Test	Purpose	Abnormal Findings
Imaging		
Computed tomography (CT) of brain — Do not delay lumbar puncture or administration of antibiotics for the CT scan, especially if the history does not support a traumatic injury or an expanding intracranial lesion.	Provides details of structures of bone, tissue, and fluid-filled spaces. Detects exudate, abscesses, and intracranial pathology (e.g., tumors, brain injury), and hydrocephalus.	Shift of structures caused by masses (tumors), edema (brain injury), exudate, abscesses, hemorrhage, hematomas, infarction, hydrocephalus, facial fractures, and soft tissue injuries.
Magnetic resonance imaging (MRI) of the brain	Provides more detailed image of tissue through minute oscillations of hydrogen atoms in the brain that create graphic image of bone, fluid, and soft tissue.	Masses, exudate, abscesses, and intracranial pathology (e.g., tumors, brain injury).
Laboratory Testing		
Serum complete blood count (CBC) with white blood cell (WBC) count, and differential (monitor eosinophils)	Assesses for presence of infection or parasites.	Elevated WBCs. Elevated eosinophils.
Bacterial culture and Gram stains (cerebrospinal fluid [CSF] and blood)	Identifies bacteria.	Positive or negative gram stains identify organisms. Blood culture with organism identification.

Diagnostic Tests for Meningitis—cont'd

Test	Purpose	Abnormal Findings
CSF analysis A lumbar puncture (LP) should not be done following head injury, if focal neurologic deficits or papilledema are present, because these signs indicate increased intracranial pressure (ICP) (see Box 7-1). Antibiotic therapy should not be delayed if CSF samples cannot be obtained. Polymerase chain reaction (PCR) assays antibody titers A DNA-based CSF test to check for the presence of causes of meningitis including herpes simplex virus 1 (HSV1), HSV2, varicella zoster (VZV), human immunodeficiency virus (HIV), Epstein-Barr virus (EBV), West Nile virus, cytomegalovirus (CMV), human herpesvirus 6 (HHV-6). Other CSF studies Venereal Disease Research Laboratory test Fluorescent treponemal antibody-absorption (evaluates for syphilis) Eosinophils	Most important laboratory test for diagnosing meningitis. CSF may be obtained through an intraventricular catheter, ventriculostomy, reservoir via cervical approach, or LP. Note: Clinical signs of improvement rather than repeat CSF analysis are a better indicator of treatment response. However, repeat LP if: (1) there is no clinical improvement within 24 to 72 hours after antibiotic treatment is initiated; (2) it is performed 2 to 3 days after initiation of treatment if microorganisms are resistant to standard therapy; and (3) fever persists for greater than 8 days.	The CSF is analyzed for cell count with white cell differential, glucose, eosinophils, protein, Gram stain, acid-fast stain, culture, and sensitivity (Table 7-3). CSF studies include the following: Cultures: Bacterial, viral, fungal, *Mycobacterium tuberculosis* cultures with sensitivities, and aerobic and anaerobic cultures. *Latex agglutination:* For bacterial antigens of *Neisseria meningitidis, Streptococcus pneumoniae, Escherichia coli,* influenza type B (Hib), group B strep. Antigen: Cryptococcal and histoplasma polysaccharide antigen (bacterial antigen testing rarely useful). Antibodies: *Coccidioides immitis* complement fixation antibodies, HSV, and VZV antibodies.
Blood, urine, and sputum cultures	Identifies infecting organisms and determines bacteremia, urinary tract infection, or respiratory tract infection.	Presence of infecting organisms in the bloodstream, urinary tract, or lungs/upper airways.

Table 7-3	MENINGITIS: TYPICAL CEREBROSPINAL FLUID FINDINGS		
Findings	**White Cell Count**	**Glucose**	**Protein**
Normal	0 to 5/mm^3 lymphocytes	40 to 80 mg/dL	15 to 50 mg/dL
Bacterial	Predominantly polycytes: 1000 to 10,000	Greater than 40 mg/dL (two thirds of serum glucose)	100 to 500 mg/dL
Viral	Predominantly lymphocytes (may see polycytes initially)	Normal	Slightly elevated
Tuberculous	Elevated lymphocytes: 100 to 400; lymphocyte elevation minimal or absent in patients who are immunocompromised	Greater than 40 mg/dL or 50% of blood glucose drawn simultaneously	100 to 500 mg/dL; may increase gradually with progression of disease
Fungal	Predominantly elevated lymphocytes	Slightly decreased	Elevated
Lyme disease	Mildly elevated lymphocytes	Normal	Mildly elevated
Aseptic (nonbacterial)	Elevated lymphocytes	Normal	50 to 100 mg/dL

COLLABORATIVE MANAGEMENT

CARE PRIORITIES

1. Control infection

- Antibiotic therapy: There are three major caveats to treating bacterial meningitis. First, the bactericidal agent must be effective against the organism; second, the agent must achieve a bactericidal effect within the CSF, only IV antibiotics should be used, except for rifampin that is useful as a synergistic agent; and third, the drug has optimal pharmacodynamics.
- Rapid sterilization of CSF via appropriate pharmacologic therapy (Table 7-4): Prophylaxis, using appropriate antimicrobials for people exposed to *N. meningitidis* (rifampin or spiramycin) or *H. influenzae* meningitis, is recommended.

> **Safety Alert**
> *If mechanical ventilation is already in place, ventilator settings will vary, depending on the patient's size and arterial blood gas results. Check ventilator settings at set intervals. Consult with an intensivist, pulmonologist, associated advanced practice provider, and/or respiratory therapy staff members regarding setting changes as the patient's needs change.*

2. Reduce inflammation with adjunctive pharmacologic therapies

Dexamethasone may decrease inflammation by reducing cytokines produced by bacterial products. In recent studies, improvement in outcome, decrease in neurologic sequelae, and reduction in mortality with the use of dexamethasone have been reported. Recommended dosage is 0.15 mg/kg every 6 hours for 4 days. Start dose with or just before first antibiotic dose. Given if suspected bacterial meningitis occurs in a developed country; NOT recommended for bacterial meningitis in undeveloped countries.

3. Monitor

It is important to monitor neurologic status, vital signs, and respiratory status. The patient may need to be intubated and placed on a ventilator. Watch for signs of increased ICP or hydrocephalus.

4. Maintain fluid and electrolyte balance

Overhydration and underhydration can lead to adverse effects. Research supports the use of IV maintenance fluids over fluid restriction during the first 48 hours of treatment of bacterial meningitis. Electrolyte imbalances should be corrected. Monitor urine output and serum osmolality and watch for signs and symptoms of SIADH.

5. Provide adequate nutrition

Oral feeding should be encouraged when possible. Enteral or parenteral feeding may be initiated. Parenteral nutrition is used if enteral feeding is not tolerated. Hydration should be maintained.

6. Control seizures with antiepileptic therapy

Used prophylactically or if seizures occur as a result of neuronal irritability. Seizures increase metabolic rate and cerebral blood flow, which may cause deterioration in patients with cerebral edema and intracranial hypertension. Use seizure precautions and protect from injury if seizures occur.

7. Maintain normothermia/control fever

Keep normothermic to decrease oxygen demand. Normothermia helps to prevent intracranial hypertension associated with increased metabolic rate. Fever should be controlled by antipyretics such as acetaminophen or use of other noninvasive or invasive cooling measures.

8. Prevent infection

Vaccines are currently available for meningitis prophylaxis. These include the following: (1) influenza type B (Hib), given as a childhood immunization; (2) bacillus Calmette-Guérin (BCG), used for tuberculosis, also prevents tuberculosis meningitis; (3) pneumococcal vaccine

Table 7-4	COMMON DRUG THERAPY FOR THE MANAGEMENT OF MENINGITIS*	

Causative Agent	Characteristic	Age/Therapy
Bacterial Meningitis		
Streptococcus pneumoniae	Gram-positive cocci	2 to 50 years: Vancomycin with third-generation cephalosporin (cefotaxime or ceftriaxone) Older than 50 years: Vancomycin with third-generation cephalosporin (cefotaxime or ceftriaxone) plus ampicillin Consider rifampin if dexamethasone is given
Haemophilus influenzae	Gram-negative bacilli	Cefotaxime or ceftriaxone, add rifampin if pharyngeal colonization
Neisseria meningitidis	Gram-negative cocci	2 to 50 years: Vancomycin with third-generation cephalosporin (cefotaxime or ceftriaxone) Older than 50 years: Vancomycin with third-generation cephalosporin (cefotaxime or ceftriaxone) plus ampicillin Consider rifampin if dexamethasone is given
Listeria monocytogenes	Gram-positive bacilli	Vancomycin with third-generation cephalosporin (cefotaxime or ceftriaxone) plus ampicillin or Ampicillin or penicillin G (Infectious Diseases Society of America)
Mycobacterium tuberculosis	Acid-fast bacteria	Isoniazid, rifampin, ethambutol, pyrazinamide
Borrelia burgdorferi	Spirochete	Ceftriaxone or penicillin G
Fungal		
Cryptococcus neoformans	Fungus	Amphotericin B, flucytosine, fluconazole, or itraconazole
Bacilli		
	Gram-negative, aerobic	Older than 50 years: Vancomycin with third-generation cephalosporin plus ampicillin
Pseudomonas aeruginosa, Klebsiella pneumonia, Escherichia coli, Citrobacter, Acinetobacter, Enterobacter, Serratia marcescens	Gram-negative	High doses of third-generation cephalosporins, aminoglycosides

Adapted from Tunkel A: Initial therapy and prognosis of bacterial meningitis in adults. In Calderwood S, editor: *UpToDate*, Waltham, 2014, Wolters Kluwer. Retrieved from www.uptodate.com/contents/initial-therapy-and-prognosis-of-bacterial-meningitis-in-adults; Friedman N, Sexton D: Gram-negative bacillary meningitis: epidemiology, clinical features, and diagnosis. In Sexton D, editor: *UpToDate*, Waltham, 2014, Wolters Kluwer. Retrieved from www.uptodate.com/contents/gram-negative-bacillary-meningitis-epidemiology-clinical-features-and-diagnosis?source=see_link; Tunkel A, Hartman B, Kaplan S, et al: Practice guidelines for the management of bacterial meningitis. *Clin Infect Dis* 39:1267-1284, 2004.
*These therapies are subject to change based on the Centers for Disease Control and Prevention recommendations and new studies.

recommended for those who are chronically ill and adults older than 65 years of age; and (4) *N. meningitides* vaccines for specific or combined prophylaxis for five investigational subgroups. The Centers for Disease Control and Prevention (CDC) guidelines recommend that "Transmission-Based Precautions" be implemented until effectiveness of antimicrobial treatment is established.

9. Facilitate mobility

Physical therapy, occupational therapy, and speech therapy should be initiated as soon as the patient is stable, to minimize physical (contractures and muscle atrophy) and cognitive complications. Prevent pressure ulcers, pneumonia, or DVTs related to immobility. Initiate DVT prophylaxis including sequential stockings and prophylactic anticoagulants as indicated.

10. Evaluate the need for support services
Evaluate the need for home healthcare, support groups, and social services.

CARE PLANS: MENINGITIS

DECREASED INTRACRANIAL ADAPTIVE CAPACITY *related to altered fluid dynamics secondary to brain and spinal cord inflammation.*

Goals/Outcomes: Within 72 hours of initiation of antimicrobial therapy, the patient's ICP returns to normal range (less than 15 mm Hg), as evidenced by improved neurologic status that may include orientation to time, place, and person; bilaterally equal and normoreactive pupils; bilaterally equal strength and tone of extremities; absence of cranial nerve palsies; RR 12 to 20 breaths/min with normal depth and pattern; cardiopulmonary improvement: HR 60 to 100 beats/min (bpm), and BP within the patient's normal range; and abatement of clinical signs and symptoms of increased ICP: absence of headache, vomiting, papilledema, and other clinical indicators of increased ICP. After instruction, the patient verbalizes knowledge of the importance of avoiding Valsalva-like activities.
NOC Neurologic Status.

Neurologic Monitoring
1. Assess neurologic status at least hourly. Monitor pupils, LOC, and motor activity; perform cranial nerve assessments (see Appendix 3). Early indicators of increased ICP and possible herniation include decreased LOC, changes in pupillary size and reaction, a decreased motor function (weakness, posturing), and cranial nerve palsies.
2. Monitor the patient and report physical indicators of increased ICP (see Box 7-2) to the advanced practice provider. If no ICP monitor is inserted, then monitor neurologic status as discussed in point 1.
3. Monitor vital signs at least every 15 minutes if the patient has signs of increased ICP. Be alert to changes in respiratory pattern, fluctuations in BP and pulse, widening pulse pressure, and slow HR.
4. Optimize cerebral oxygenation. Keep the patient's head in neutral alignment, maintain a patent airway, and provide supplemental oxygen as prescribed. Ensure that the patient's neck is not constricted by the endotracheal (ET) tube securement device, tracheotomy ties, and oxygen tubing.
5. Avoid overhydration, which increases cerebral edema. Ensure precise delivery of IV fluids and timely delivery of medications prescribed for the prevention of sudden increases or decreases in ICP, BP, HR, or RR. Do not use IV fluids that contain dextrose.
6. Teach the patient to avoid activities that increase ICP: coughing, straining, and bending over.
7. If the patient shows evidence of increased ICP, implement measures to decrease ICP.

NIC Cerebral Edema Management; Cerebral Perfusion Promotion; Intracranial Pressure Monitoring: Neurologic Monitoring.

ACUTE PAIN *related to headache, photophobia, and fever secondary to meningeal irritation*

Goals/Outcomes: Within 2 hours of initiating interventions to relieve pain, the patient reports pain relief, as documented by a pain scale.
NOC Comfort Level.

Pain Management
1. Monitor the patient for pain and discomfort. Devise a pain rating scale with the patient. Administer analgesics as prescribed. (See Pain, Chapter 1.)
2. Monitor temperature every 2 hours and as needed. Implement external or internal cooling or warming methods and prescribed antipyretics/antibiotics to keep temperature within prescribed limits.
3. Maintain an environment of comfort for each individual patient.
4. Provide care and visiting hours to allow for uninterrupted periods (at least 90 minutes) of rest. If ICP is elevated, clustering care is contraindicated.
5. Darken the patient's room or provide blindfold to minimize the discomfort of photophobia.

RISK FOR INFECTION *related to possible cross-contamination secondary to communicable bacterial and aseptic meningitis*

Goals/Outcomes: Other patients, staff members, and patient's significant others do not exhibit evidence of having acquired meningitis: diminished LOC, confusion, fever, headache, nuchal rigidity, and other signs (see previous sections for Meningitis on Neurologic Assessment, Chapter 7, and Diagnostic Tests for Meningitis, Chapter 7).
NOC Infection Severity.

For patients with bacterial meningitis
Infection Control
1. Some forms of bacterial meningitis are transmitted via droplet contact. Provide the patient with a private room.
2. Initiate "Transmission-Based Precautions": Droplet, on admission, and maintain them for at least 24 hours after start of antimicrobial therapy.
   - Standard precautions should be instituted to provide safety and protection regardless if infection is bacterial, fungal, or viral. Be alert for airborne pathogens and those in stool or oral secretions.
   - Contact (fecal and oral) precautions should be initiated for enteroviral causes of meningitis.

ADDITIONAL NURSING DIAGNOSES

See Risk for Trauma (Oral and Musculoskeletal) in Status Epilepticus (Chapter 7). Because these patients are at risk for SIADH, see Syndrome of Inappropriate Antidiuretic Hormone (Chapter 8). See SIRS, Sepsis, and MODS (Chapter 11), because these patients are at risk for septic shock; Nutrition Support (Chapter 1), Prolonged Immobility (Chapter 1), and Emotional and Spiritual Support of the Patient and Significant Others (Chapter 2).

NEURODEGENERATIVE AND NEUROMUSCULAR DISORDERS
PATHOPHYSIOLOGY

Neurodegenerative diseases are conditions wherein the neurons, or the myelin sheath of the neurons of the brain and spinal cord, are destroyed. Cells of the brain and spinal cord do not effectively regenerate in large numbers, thus profound destruction is sometimes devastating. Over time, the progressive destruction leads to dysfunction and disabilities. The disorders are divided into two groups: conditions affecting movements (e.g., ataxia) and conditions affecting memory (e.g., dementia), which are not mutually exclusive. Alzheimer, Pick, Parkinson, Huntington, and Lou Gehrig (amyotrophic lateral sclerosis[ALS]) diseases, prion diseases (Creutzfeldt-Jakob[CJD]), and multiple sclerosis are a few of the more commonly recognized conditions. Some of the diseases are genetic, whereas alcoholism, cancer, and vascular disease are associated with other conditions. Environmental toxins, chemicals, or viruses may cause other disorders. Neurodegeneration often begins long before the patient manifests symptoms. Treatments vary with each disorder.

Neuromuscular disorders include the neurodegenerative diseases, which affect voluntary movements. Communication between the nervous system and muscles is not possible when nerves are destroyed. Muscles weaken and atrophy as a result of disuse. Weakness may also be associated with muscle twitching, cramps, and pain, along with joint and movement deficits. These disorders may affect the heart and respiratory muscles. Many neuromuscular disorders are genetic, whereas others are immune-mediated (associated with an immunologic disorder). Myasthenia gravis (MG), Guillain-Barré syndrome (GBS), and muscular dystrophy are several of the more commonly recognized conditions. Most of the diseases are incurable. The goal of treatment is to improve symptoms, increase mobility, and lengthen life. Patients with MG may experience difficulties with medication management resulting in a crisis, which is rather easily corrected with the proper medication adjustment. Patients with other neuromuscular disorders may require more elaborate treatments including high-dose corticosteroids, plasmapheresis, and more prolonged hospitalization.

Diagnosis of neuromuscular diseases depends on the identification of a specific defect of neuromuscular function. The functional defect can sometimes be inferred by a physical examination done by a physician or advanced practice provider coupled with laboratory testing of blood and possibly CSF. A more extensive diagnostic process evaluates the function of nerves, muscles, and the connections between them by using two complementary techniques—nerve conduction velocity (NCV) testing and electromyography (EMG).

Care of patients who are critically ill may involve managing patients with respiratory failure and cardiovascular instability related to exacerbations of neuromuscular disorders. Patients at this stage of instability may be terminally ill. Patients with either MG or GBS may be treated and fully recover. This chapter will focus on MG and GBS; however, the nursing diagnoses, interventions, and outcomes are common to most neurodegenerative and neuromuscular disorders.

MYASTHENIA GRAVIS
PATHOPHYSIOLOGY
Myasthenia gravis (MG) is a chronic, progressive autoimmune disorder causing weakness and abnormal fatigability of the voluntary striated skeletal muscles. MG usually affects women between 20 and 40 years of age and men after age 40 years; the peak incidence for women is during the second and third decades and for men during the sixth decade. The overall ratio of affected women to men is 3:2. Of patients with MG, 85% to 90% have an anti–acetylcholine receptor (anti-AChR) antibody (immunoglobulin). MG is associated with other autoimmune disorders. The thymus gland undergoes pathologic changes in 80% of patients with MG and may produce anti-AChR antibodies when exposed to inflammation. The course of the disease depends on the muscle groups involved and the degree of their involvement.

MG causes changes in the structural integrity of the postsynaptic membrane at the neuromuscular junction by markedly reducing the number of AChRs. Acetylcholine (ACh), a neurotransmitter, is synthesized and stored in the terminal expansion of motor nerve axons. ACh is released into the synaptic cleft. The attachment of ACh to AChR on the postsynaptic membrane activates muscle action potential, resulting in muscle contraction. Contraction terminates when ACh is deactivated by acetylcholinesterase in the neuromuscular junction.

Patients may experience remissions and exacerbations. Many medications can increase the weakness associated with MG, including several commonly administered antibiotics (erythromycin, aminoglycosides, and azithromycin) and cardiac medications such as magnesium or antidysrhythmic agents including procainamide, beta-adrenergic–blocking agents, and quinidine. Paradoxical weakness may occur when a patient receives an excessive dose of anticholinesterase medications (cholinesterase inhibitors such as physostigmine or neostigmine), which are used to treat MG. Distinguishing worsening MG from side effects from prescribed medication effects can be difficult. Exacerbations can be profound, and thus are called crises.

A myasthenic *or* cholinergic crisis may occur rapidly or incipiently. Myasthenic crisis can occur as part of the natural course of MG or may result from other factors, including infection, tapering of immunosuppressive medications, administration of various other medications, pregnancy, childbirth, or following a surgical procedure, ultimately resulting in respiratory failure from weakness of the respiratory muscles. Severe weakness of the oropharyngeal muscles (bulbar signs) is often associated with respiratory muscle weakness, resulting in dysphagia and aspiration. Endotracheal (ET) intubation with mechanical ventilation may be needed. A *cholinergic crisis* results from excessive doses of anticholinesterase medications and rarely occurs if the dose of medications remains within the normally prescribed range. The patient is acutely aware of all sensations. Crisis is dramatic and frightening.

ASSESSMENT
GOAL OF ASSESSMENT
The assessment differentiates between acute and chronic neurologic assessment findings. Signs of myasthenic and cholinergic crises may be subtle. Increasing anxiety, apprehension, or insomnia may indicate the onset of crisis.

HISTORY AND RISK FACTORS
History of rheumatoid arthritis, systemic lupus erythematosus, thyrotoxicosis, Sjögren syndrome, polymyositis, ulcerative colitis, Hashimoto thyroiditis, and pernicious anemia. Recent infection, trauma, surgery, temperature extremes, stress, endocrine imbalance, or intake of medications with neuromuscular-blocking properties, such as sedatives, tranquilizers, opiates, or antibiotics (e.g., neomycin, kanamycin, gentamicin, streptomycin, tetracycline), may prompt crisis.

VITAL SIGNS
· Findings vary significantly, depending on whether the patient is experiencing a crisis.
· RR may be normal or slightly tachypneic.
· Tachycardia may be present with impending respiratory failure.

OBSERVATION
· Patients may be asymptomatic or have mild symptoms if crisis develops slowly.
· Weakness and abnormal fatigability of skeletal muscles, which worsens with sustained efforts.

SYMPTOM PROGRESSION
Ocular muscle group
First muscle group to be affected in 65% of patients. During course of disease, 90% will have ocular involvement. Eye signs include ptosis (drooping of one or both eyelids), diplopia (double vision), and inability to maintain upward gaze.

Muscles of face, neck, and oropharynx with bulbar signs
Second area of involvement. Bulbar signs are present, with increased risk of aspiration as a result of difficulty chewing, dysphagia, dysarthria, inability to close mouth, nasal regurgitation of fluids, mushy and nasal tone to voice, neck-muscle weakness with head bob, inability to raise chin off chest, and loss of facial expression.

Muscles of limbs and trunk
Weakness is greater in proximal muscles than distal. Strength is decreased in all extremities, with inability to maintain position without support. Diaphragmatic and intercostal weakness, dyspnea, ineffective cough, and accumulation of secretions are present, which increases the risk for respiratory arrest.

Myasthenic and cholinergic crises
Increasing anxiety, apprehension, or insomnia may indicate the onset. ABG values may be normal. Note subtle decreases in chest expansion and air movement and increased dysphagia, dysarthria, and dysphonia. Accumulation of oropharyngeal secretions increases the risk of aspiration.
· Myasthenic crisis: Occurs when the patient needs increased medication as a result of drug tolerance or an exacerbation of the disease. Signs and symptoms: Increasing muscle weakness despite normal or increased drug dose, increasing anxiety and apprehension, severe ocular and bulbar weakness, with rapid onset of respiratory muscle weakness, which can lead to respiratory arrest.
· Cholinergic crisis: Results from an overdose of anticholinesterase medication, causing a depolarizing neuromuscular blockade. Signs and symptoms: Increasing muscle weakness, increasing anxiety and apprehension, fasciculations (twitching) around the eyes and mouth, diarrhea and cramping, sweating, pupillary constriction, sialorrhea (excessive salivation), and difficulty breathing and swallowing.

AUSCULTATION
· Breath sounds may reflect reduced movement of air or shallow breaths.

Diagnosis of Myasthenic or Cholinergic Crisis		
Test	**Purpose**	**Abnormal Findings**
Tensilon (edrophonium) test With myasthenia gravis (MG), weakness and muscle fatigue will improve within 30 to 60 seconds of receiving intravenous Tensilon injection (2 to 10 mg), and improvement will last up to 5 minutes.	Identifies the type of crisis. Tensilon is a short-acting anticholinesterase agent that delays hydrolysis of acetylcholine, permitting the acetylcholine released by the nerve to act repeatedly over a longer period.	Myasthenic crisis: Weakness improves with edrophonium chloride (Tensilon) versus Cholinergic crisis: Symptoms worsen with Tensilon. Test is done by a neurologist who assesses the patient's immediate response.

Continued

Diagnosis of Myasthenic or Cholinergic Crisis—cont'd

Test	Purpose	Abnormal Findings
Caution: Have atropine sulfate at the bedside during Tensilon test to reverse the effects of Tensilon if the patient is in cholinergic crisis.		
Serum antibody titer Correlation between titer and disease severity and course has not been proven.	Assesses for the presence of serum antibodies against acetylcholine receptors.	Elevated serum antibodies against acetylcholine receptors are present in 80% to 90% of cases of generalized MG.
Electromyography Muscle action potentials are recorded from selected skeletal muscles.	Tests muscle action potentials, reflective of ability to contract.	The amplitude of the evoked muscle action potentials falls rapidly in persons with MG.
Mediastinal magnetic resonance imaging of the thymus gland or mediastinoscopy.	To evaluate for thymic abnormalities, present in 80% of patients with MG.	65% to 90% have thymic hyperplasia, whereas 10% to 15% have gross or microscopic thymomas.
Thyroid studies Thyroid abnormalities are often present in young women.	To evaluate for hyperthyroidism.	MG is associated with Hashimoto thyroiditis, an autoimmune thyroid disorder.
Other laboratory tests: Creatine phosphokinase, erythrocyte sedimentation rate, and antinuclear antibody levels. There is a frequent concurrence of other immunologic disorders with MG.		

COLLABORATIVE MANAGEMENT

CARE PRIORITIES FOR PATIENTS WITH MYASTHENIA GRAVIS

1. Manage respiratory failure

ET intubation with mechanical ventilation may be necessary, depending on the degree of involvement of the respiratory muscles. (See Mechanical Ventilation, Chapter 1.) Bilevel positive-pressure ventilation (BiPAP) may also be used effectively in a subset of patients, if able to breathe somewhat effectively.

2. Provide emergency interventions for myasthenic or cholinergic crisis

Once the patient is stabilized in the intensive care unit (ICU), the type of crisis is identified, and specific treatment is begun. Anticholinesterase medications may be withheld or reduced temporarily. A "drug holiday" will improve subsequent patient responsiveness to medication. With the resumption of anticholinesterase medications, dose, timing, and combinations of medications will need readjustment. In severe MG, plasmapheresis (see later) may hasten improvement of signs and symptoms.

3. Initiate nutrition support

If the patient has dysphagia, enteral or parenteral feedings may be needed. (See Nutrition Support, Chapter 1.)

4. Manage pharmacotherapy during noncrisis periods

Medications must be given on time to maintain therapeutic effects. Drug combinations are patient-specific.

- Cholinesterase inhibitors: Pyridostigmine bromide (Mestinon), neostigmine bromide (Prostigmin), and ambenonium chloride (Mytelase) are used to inhibit the hydrolysis of ACh by acetylcholinesterase at the neuromuscular junction. Pyridostigmine is often used, because it has fewer side effects and is longer acting. The patient is given a dose every 3 hours during the day, and the dose is adjusted based on effects. Sustained-release preparations usually are given at bedtime to maintain the patient's strength throughout the night and early morning hours.
- Immunosuppression: Glucocorticosteroids (e.g., adrenocorticotropic hormone and prednisone) and other immunosuppressive agents: Glucocorticosteroids are used alone or in conjunction with anticholinesterase drugs. They provide clinical improvement for 70% to 100% of patients with MG who refuse thymectomy and have weakness uncontrolled by

anticholinesterase drugs. Although the mechanism of action of steroids is uncertain, studies indicate that they directly influence neuromuscular transmission, suppress the action of the immune system by decreasing the size of the thymus gland and lymphatic tissue, decrease circulating lymphocytes, and decrease antireceptor reactivity of peripheral lymphocytes. Treatment is continued indefinitely. Glucocorticosteroids produce favorable results in all patients with muscle involvement, from ocular to severe respiratory impairment. Azathioprine (Imuran) may be used alone or in combination with other therapies in situations in which response to steroids is poor. Side effects of azathioprine include toxic hepatitis, thrombocytopenia, leukopenia, leukemia, lymphoma, infections, vomiting, and teratogenic effects.

- Immune globulin: Routine use of human immunoglobulin (IG) is not recommended, but administration of IV immunoglobulin (IVIG) may be considered in patients with severe MG for whom other treatments have been unsuccessful or are contraindicated.

5. Consider plasmapheresis

A complete exchange of plasma with removal of abnormal circulating antibodies that interfere with AChRs. Box 7-3 describes potential complications, nursing assessments, and interventions. (For additional information, see Fluid and Electrolyte Disturbances, Chapter 1.)

6. Carefully consider thymectomy

Removal of the thymus gland may prompt clinical improvement in 70% of patients, particularly newly diagnosed females with hyperplasia of thymic tissue. A suprasternal approach, a transsternal approach with sternal splitting, or the minimally invasive technique called video-assisted thoracic surgery may be used. Plasmapheresis is sometimes used before surgery to increase strength and allow for a decrease in medication dose.

CARE PLANS FOR MYASTHENIA GRAVIS

IMPAIRED GAS EXCHANGE *related to altered oxygen supply associated with decreases in chest expansion and air movement secondary to weakness and abnormal fatigability of pharyngeal, diaphragmatic, intercostal, and accessory muscles of respiration.*

Goals/Outcomes: Within 12 to 24 hours of initiation of treatment, the patient has adequate gas exchange, as evidenced by orientation to time, place, and person; RR less than 20 breaths/min with normal depth and pattern (eupnea); PaO_2 greater than 80 mm Hg; $PaCO_2$ less than 45 mm Hg; and oxygen saturation greater than 95%.
NOC Respiratory Status: Gas Exchange; Respiratory Status: Ventilation; Mechanical Ventilation Response: Adult.

 Respiratory Monitoring

1. Assess the patient for indicators of impending respiratory failure or hypoxia: diminished or adventitious breath sounds; changes in rate, rhythm, or depth of respirations; pallor; nasal flaring; use of accessory muscles; and restlessness, irritability, confusion, or somnolence.

2. Monitor ventilatory capability via pulmonary function tests. Vital capacity less than 75% of predicted value, tidal volume less than 1000 mL (or the patient's normal/baseline volume), and RR greater than 34 breaths/min are signals of need for assisted ventilation.

3. Monitor ABG and pulse oximetry results. Falling PaO_2 (less than 60 mm Hg), rising $PaCO_2$ (greater than 50 mm Hg), and falling oxygen saturation, coupled with changes in vital capacity, tidal volume, and increasing RR, indicate the need for additional respiratory support.

4. Provide pulmonary toilet every 2 hours when the patient is awake and as needed. In addition, turn the patient after each physiotherapy session to facilitate lung expansion, decrease risk of atelectasis, and prevent consolidation of secretions.

Safety Alert *To prevent aspiration of secretions, always suction secretions from the trachea and mouth before deflating endotracheal or tracheostomy cuff. Consider use of endotracheal tube with continuous supraglottic suction, if available. This is especially important because of the increase in saliva.*

NIC Airway Management; Coping Enhancement; Acid-Base Monitoring; Oxygen Therapy; Mechanical Ventilation Response: Adult.

Box 7-3 **NURSING INTERVENTIONS FOR COMPLICATIONS OF PLASMAPHERESIS**

Hypovolemia

Can result from rapid removal of up to 3 L of body fluid during plasmapheresis with volume replacement that is too slow during the procedure.

- Perform a baseline assessment of the patient's weight, skin turgor, and VS before the procedure is begun. During plasmapheresis, monitor the patient for thirst, poor skin turgor, dizziness, confusion, nausea, and flattened neck veins. Assess VS continuously for evidence of hypovolemia, including decreased BP and increased HR. Monitor Hct for elevation, which occurs with hypovolemia. Weigh the patient after procedure. Remember that liter of fluid equals 1 kg; thus, hypovolemia can be reflected readily in weight changes.
- Provide fluids during plasmapheresis as prescribed, via oral, enteral, or IV access.
- Monitor and record I&O throughout the procedure. Be alert to oliguria (urinary output less than 30 mL/h for 2 consecutive hours).
- Protect patients who are dizzy or confused by keeping side rails up and the bed in its lowest position.

Clotting Abnormalities

Can result from removal of clotting factors during plasmapheresis.

- Assess PT, PTT, and platelet count before and after procedure. Be alert to PT and PTT greater than those of control values and to increased platelet count. Normal ranges are as follows: PT 11 to 15 seconds, PTT 30 to 40 seconds, and platelet count 150,000 to 400,000/mm^3.
- Be alert to signs of impaired clotting, such as oozing from arterial puncture, venous access, or IV sites. Monitor the patient for epistaxis or other signs of hemorrhage, such as elevated pulse rate, decreased BP, or changes in the patient's mental status.
- Apply firm, continuous (e.g., for 10 minutes) pressure to the arterial puncture site once the catheter or needle is removed. A pressure dressing is recommended.
- Check gastric aspirate and stools for occult blood.
- Instruct the patient to alert staff to the presence of bleeding from puncture and other sites.

Hypokalemia*

Can result from removal of potassium during the plasma exchange.

- Assess serum potassium before, during, and after plasma exchange. Be alert to decreasing levels (less than 3.5 mEq/L).
- Monitor for physical signs of hypokalemia, including bradycardia, fatigue, leg cramps, nausea, and paresthesias.
- Observe cardiac monitor for signs of cardiac dysrhythmias: ST segment depression, flattened T wave, presence of U wave, and ventricular dysrhythmias. Report abnormal cardiac rhythms to the physician.
- During reinfusion of blood, administer potassium as prescribed to prevent hypokalemia and dangerous dysrhythmias. If prescribed, administer antidysrhythmic agents.

Hypocalcemia

Can result from binding of calcium to ACD, the anticoagulant used during plasmapheresis.

- Assess serum calcium levels before, during, and after plasmapheresis. Be alert to decreasing levels (less than 8.5 mg/dL).
- Monitor the patient for signs of hypocalcemia, such as numbness with tingling of fingers and circumoral area, hyperactive reflexes, muscle cramps, tetany, paresthesia, Chvostek sign, diffuse irritability, emotional instability, impaired memory, and confusion.
- Observe cardiac monitor for evidence of hypocalcemia: prolonged QT interval caused by elongation of ST segment.
- Encourage the patient to drink milk before and during the plasma exchange.
- As prescribed, administer calcium gluconate during plasmapheresis if indicators of hypocalcemia occur.

Box 7-3	NURSING INTERVENTIONS FOR COMPLICATIONS OF PLASMAPHERESIS—cont'd

Myasthenic Crisis
Can result from removal of circulating anticholinesterase drugs during plasmapheresis.

Cholinergic Crisis
Can result from removal of antibodies and decreased need for anticholinesterase drugs after plasmapheresis.

- In the event of either crisis, have the following available: IV infusion apparatus, medications (edrophonium chloride [Tensilon], neostigmine bromide, atropine, and pralidoxime chloride [Protopam Chloride]), manual resuscitator bag, automatic external defibrillator (antiepileptic drug), oxygen, suction equipment, and intubation tray if intubation is not already in place.
- Monitor the patient for evidence of crisis, such as decreased vital capacity (less than 1 L), inability to swallow, ptosis, diplopia, dysarthria, dysphonia, dyspnea, muscle weakness, and nasal flaring. Stay with the patient if these signs appear and notify the physician promptly.

*Caution: Patients on prednisone or digitalis therapy are at increased risk for hypokalemia and should be monitored closely for its occurrence.
ACD, Acid-citrate-dextrose; *BP,* blood pressure; *Hct,* hematocrit; *HR,* heart rate; *I&O,* intake and output; *IV,* intravenous; *PT,* prothrombin time; *PTT,* partial thromboplastin time; *VS,* vital signs.

INEFFECTIVE AIRWAY CLEARANCE *related to ineffective cough; decreased energy; abnormal fatigability of diaphragmatic, intercostal, pharyngeal, and accessory muscles of respiration.*

Goals/Outcomes: Within 24 to 48 hours of intervention/treatment, the patient's airway is clear, as evidenced by absence of adventitious breath sounds.
NOC Aspiration Prevention; Respiratory Status: Airway Patency.

Airway Management
1. Assess breath sounds, effectiveness of the patient's cough, and the quality, amount, and color of sputum. Consult the physician or advanced practice provider for significant findings, including the patient's inability to raise secretions; for secretions that are tenacious, thick, or voluminous.
2. Suction secretions as indicated, using hyperoxygenation before and after procedure.

> **Safety Alert** *Range of motion is done gently during the acute phase. Overly aggressive exercise may exacerbate weakness and accelerate the demyelinating process.*

3. Place the patient in semi-Fowler to high Fowler position to facilitate chest excursion and decrease risk of aspiration. Fully elevate HOB during feedings.
4. Assess vital signs for indicators of atelectasis and upper respiratory tract infection (see Risk for Infection, which follows). Report significant findings to the advanced practice provider.
5. Increase activity as tolerated to minimize stasis of secretions and to facilitate lung expansion.
6. Administer or assist with noninvasive BiPAP as needed.
7. Keep a tracheostomy tube and obturator at the bedside in the event of inadvertent extubation.

NIC Artificial Airway Management; Cough Enhancement: Oxygen Therapy; Ventilation Assistance.

RISK FOR INFECTION *related to inadequate primary defenses (stasis of secretions); inadequate secondary defenses (suppressed inflammatory response); invasive procedures (e.g., insertion of ET tube); chronic disease.*

Goals/Outcomes: The patient is free of infection, as evidenced by normothermia; HR 60 to 100 bpm; pulmonary secretions that are clear, thin in consistency, and odorless; and WBC count less than 11,000/mm³.
NOC Immune Status.

Health Screening

1. Monitor for temperature greater than 37.7° C (100° F), tachycardia, and diaphoresis.
2. Assess color, consistency, amount, and odor of secretions. Report changes in sputum color to the provider. Obtain sputum specimens for culture as indicated.
3. Monitor CBC results for elevation of WBC count (greater than 11,000/mm^3).
4. Administer antibiotics as prescribed.
5. Protect the patient from persons with infection, particularly upper respiratory tract infection.
6. Turn and reposition the patient at least every 2 hours to prevent stasis of secretions.

IMPAIRED SWALLOWING *related to decreased or absent gag reflex; decreased strength or excursion of muscles involved in mastication; facial paralysis; mechanical obstruction (tracheostomy tube).*

Goals/Outcomes: Before oral foods and fluids are given or reintroduced, the patient demonstrates capability for safe and effective swallowing, as evidenced by the presence of gag reflex and adequate strength and excursion of muscles involved in mastication.
NOC Aspiration Prevention; Swallowing Status.

Aspiration Precautions

1. Assess the patient for the presence of the gag reflex, ability to swallow, and strength and excursion of muscles involved in mastication. As indicated, consult with a speech therapist to determine the patient's ability to swallow.
2. If the patient cannot swallow, confer with the provider regarding alternate method of nutrition support, such as enteral or parenteral nutrition (see Nutrition Support, Chapter 1).
3. After the patient's gag reflex and ability to swallow return, begin oral feedings cautiously.
   - When reinstating oral intake, offer a few ice chips to help stimulate the swallowing reflex, progress to semisolid foods (e.g., textured food, applesauce) and then to solid foods. Confer with the speech/swallowing therapist regarding a dysphagia diet and teaching swallowing techniques.
   - Elevate the HOB greater than 70 degrees to facilitate gravity flow through the pylorus and to minimize regurgitation and aspiration.
   - Provide small feedings at frequent intervals (e.g., every 4 hours while the patient is awake).
   - Avoid cold foods and beverages, which cause bloating and upward pressure on the diaphragm.
   - Keep suction equipment at the bedside; suction excess secretions as necessary after each feeding. Inspect the mouth for residual food after meals. Provide for oral hygiene after every meal.
4. If the patient begins oral feedings with a tracheostomy tube in place, elevate the HOB greater than 70 degrees. Inflate tracheostomy tube cuff for 30 minutes before and after feeding to prevent aspiration. Progress the diet slowly, as described in the previous intervention.
5. If the patient is unable to communicate verbally, be alert to signs of severe aspiration: dyspnea, tachypnea, restlessness, agitation, pallor, and presence of adventitious breath sounds. If these signs occur, discontinue feeding immediately; elevate the HOB; and provide oxygen. If a tracheostomy tube is in place, suction to remove food or secretions obstructing the airway.

NIC Swallowing Therapy; Positioning; Nutrition Management.

DISTURBED SENSORY PERCEPTION (VISUAL) *related to altered sensory perception associated with diplopia or ptosis.*

Goals/Outcomes: Within 48 to 72 hours of this diagnosis, the patient relates that vision is adequate to perform activities of daily living (ADLs).
NOC Neurologic Status: Cranial/Sensory/Motor Function.

Environmental Management: Safety

1. Assess for and document signs of weakness of the ocular muscles (i.e., diplopia, ptosis, incomplete closure of the eye).
2. Provide an eye patch or frosted lens for the patient with diplopia; alternate the patch or lens to the opposite eye every 2 to 3 hours during the patient's waking hours.
3. Provide eyelid crutches for the patient with ptosis, or loosely tape eyelids open but only when providing direct care.
4. Administer artificial tears in each eye at least every 4 to 6 hours to lubricate and protect corneal tissue.

5. As indicated, provide assistance with ADLs and ambulation to protect the patient from injury.
6. Keep the patient's environment consistent to facilitate location of desired objects.

NIC Communication Enhancement: Visual Deficit; Environmental Management; Fall Prevention; Surveillance: Safety.

DEFICIENT KNOWLEDGE *related to thymectomy procedure, including preoperative and postoperative care.*

Goals/Outcomes: Before surgery, the patient verbalizes understanding of the surgical procedure, including preoperative and postoperative care.
NOC Knowledge: Treatment Procedure(s).

Teaching: Procedure/Treatment
1. Explain thymectomy and its relationship to MG.
2. Provide information about preoperative routine. Discuss medications, application of antiembolic hose, the potential for postoperative discomfort, and the availability of analgesic agents. Advise the patient that medications may change after surgery, because the patient may improve. With a thoracotomy approach, explain postoperative chest tubes. With a transcervical approach, a wound drainage system (e.g., Hemovac) is used.
3. Teach coughing and deep-breathing techniques used after surgery.
4. Explain that plasmapheresis may be performed preoperatively to improve the patient's clinical state. (See Deficient Knowledge: Purpose and Procedure for Plasmapheresis, which follows.)
5. Explain that pulmonary function and ABG tests will be performed preoperatively and postoperatively to assist in determining the patient's respiratory status.
6. Explain the possibility of tracheostomy with assisted ventilation to prevent respiratory problems that can occur from stresses of surgery or myasthenic or cholinergic crisis.
7. Explain that results of a thymectomy vary and may not be apparent for several months to years.

DEFICIENT KNOWLEDGE *related to purpose and procedure for plasmapheresis*

Goals/Outcomes: Before the first plasma exchange, the patient verbalizes knowledge of the purpose and procedure for plasmapheresis.
NOC Knowledge: Treatment Procedure(s).

Teaching: Procedure/Treatment
1. Assess the patient's previous experience with and knowledge of plasmapheresis.
2. As appropriate, teach the patient the following about plasmapheresis: (1) blood is withdrawn via an arterial catheter, anticoagulated, and then passed through a cell separator; (2) the plasma portion of the blood that contains the AChR antibodies is removed; (3) red blood cells (RBCs), WBCs, and platelets are mixed with saline, potassium, and plasma protein fraction and then are returned to the body.
3. Advise the patient that plasmapheresis is generally performed to control severe symptoms until other modalities (i.e., medications, thymectomy) take effect, when other treatments have failed, or to increase the patient's strength and improve general status before surgery.
4. Explain that the nurse will make assessments before, during, and after plasmapheresis (see Box 7-3).
5. Advise the patient that the procedure takes several hours and may be performed daily.
6. Explain that the degree of weakness may increase during and after the procedure because of the removal of plasma-bound medications (corticosteroids, anticholinesterase agents). Reassure the patient that he or she will be monitored closely during the procedure and will receive appropriate medication after plasmapheresis.

DEFICIENT KNOWLEDGE *related to signs and symptoms of myasthenic and cholinergic crises.*

Goals/Outcomes: Within 24 hours of stabilization of respiratory status, the patient and significant others verbalize the signs and symptoms of impending myasthenic and cholinergic crises.
NOC Knowledge: Disease Process.

Teaching: Disease Process
1. Assess the patient's/family's knowledge of myasthenic and cholinergic crises.

2. Explain the differences between myasthenic crisis: an exacerbation of the myasthenic symptoms, frequently triggered by an infection; and cholinergic crisis: an episode triggered by toxic levels of anticholinesterase medication. The crisis, regardless of type, may manifest similar symptoms, including abdominal cramping, diarrhea, generalized weakness, increased pulmonary secretions, and impaired respiratory function.

3. Advise the patient/family to immediately report signs and symptoms of crisis.

4. Prepare the patient for potential discharge when stabilized and consider the use of home health services for follow-up after discharge.

5. Teach the patient and significant others how to use emergency respiratory support equipment (manual resuscitator bag and suction apparatus) and facilitate it being available in the home if the patient has a history of crisis events.

6. Advise the patient to carry an identification card with diagnosis, medications, medication contraindications, advanced practice provider and/or physician's name and phone number.

7. Provide contact information for Myasthenia Gravis Foundation of America, Inc., 355 Lexington Avenue, 15th Fl., New York, NY 10017; Tel: 800-541-5454; fax: 212-370-9047; website: www. myasthenia.org.

ADDITIONAL NURSING DIAGNOSES

See also Nutrition Support (Chapter 1), Mechanical Ventilation (Chapter 1), and Emotional and Spiritual Support of the Patient and Significant Others (Chapter 2).

GUILLAIN-BARRÉ SYNDROME

PATHOPHYSIOLOGY

Guillain-Barré syndrome (GBS) is a disorder wherein the immune system mistakenly attacks the peripheral nervous system, causing weakness and paresthesias of the lower extremities. Symptoms can intensify and ascend toward the head, resulting in loss of ability to use all muscles. When severe, the patient is totally paralyzed and the disorder is life threatening, with impending respiratory muscle paralysis and cardiovascular instability. GBS is not considered a classic neuromuscular or neurodegenerative disorder, because the onset is sudden, with rapid progression, and once peaked, patients have the potential for a complete recovery.

This disorder is an acute inflammatory, immune-mediated, demyelinating polyneuropathy of the peripheral nervous system, affecting 1.5 to 2 individuals per 100,000 population.

GBS affects mainly the Schwann cell, which synthesizes and maintains the peripheral nerve myelin sheath. Studies suggest that macrophages penetrate the basement membrane and strip apparently normal myelin from intact peripheral nerve axons, causing the characteristic signs and symptoms of GBS. The ventral (motor) root axons of the anterior horn cells, which innervate voluntary skeletal muscles, are primarily involved. Dorsal (sensory) root axons of the posterior horn are not as affected. Recovery of neurologic function depends on proliferation of Schwann cells and remyelination of axons. Recovery can be expected in 80% to 90% of cases, with minor residual deficits in less than half of the patients, and 2% to 5% experiencing recurrence after complete recovery.

ASSESSMENT: GUILLAIN-BARRÉ SYNDROME

GOAL OF ASSESSMENT

Identify the extent of current neurologic deficits, compared with the baseline, and intervene in profound deterioration. There are several clinical variations of signs and symptoms: ascending, descending, the Miller Fisher variant, or pure motor. The disease generally has three phases: (1) acute phase of 1 to 3 weeks after onset of the first symptom; (2) plateau phase beginning with no further clinical deterioration and lasting several days to weeks; and (3) recovery phase, which can last 4 months up to 2 years and correlates with the remyelination and axonal regrowth process.

HISTORY AND RISK FACTORS

Respiratory or GI illness 10 to 14 days before onset of the neurologic symptoms, in which (1) a viral agent such as parainfluenza 2 virus, measles, mumps, rubella, varicella, or herpes zoster is present (50% of cases); (2) recent vaccination (15% of cases), such as for influenza; and (3) recent surgical procedure (5% of cases). Miller Fisher syndrome, an acute axonal variant of GBS, has been shown to follow infection with *Campylobacter jejuni*.

VITAL SIGNS

- Autonomic nervous system involvement (a type of autonomic dysreflexia): Occurs in most patients with GBS: sinus tachycardia, bradycardia, orthostatic hypotension, hypertension, excessive diaphoresis, bowel and bladder dysfunction, loss of sphincter control, increased pulmonary secretions, SIADH, and cardiac dysrhythmias (a common cause of death).

OBSERVATION

- Ascending flaccid motor paralysis is the most common presenting sign and is associated with the early loss of deep tendon reflexes.
- Symmetric motor weakness, decreased or absent deep tendon reflexes, hypotonia or flaccidity of affected muscles, presence of respiratory abnormalities (e.g., nasal flaring, hypoventilation), facial paralysis.
- Weakness, usually preceding the paralysis, is symmetrical, begins in distal muscle groups, and ascends to involve more proximal muscles.
- Muscles of respiration (intercostals and diaphragm) are frequently involved. Approximately half of all patients will require mechanical ventilation.
- Complaints of distal paresthesias are common. In more serious or prolonged cases, proprioceptive and vibratory dysfunctions are present. Sensory complaints usually appear first, with muscle weakness developing rapidly over 24 to 72 hours. Approximately 90% of patients reach the peak of dysfunction within 2 weeks.
- Loss of pain and temperature sensations in a glove-and-stocking distribution has been reported.
- Cranial nerve involvement: All cranial nerves except I and II may be involved. See Appendix 3.

Diagnosis of Guillain-Barré Syndrome

The diagnosis for Guillain-Barré syndrome (GBS) is based on clinical presentation, history of antecedent illness, and cerebrospinal fluid (CSF) findings. A detailed neurologic examination must be done as a baseline to assess for any changes as the disease progresses.

Test	Purpose	Abnormal Findings
Lumbar puncture (LP) and CSF analysis The CSF findings may be attributable to deposits of immunoglobulins IgG, IgM, and IgA localized to the nerve roots.	Assesses for abnormalities in CSF that distinguish GBS from other neurodegenerative disorders. CSF protein, normally between 15 and 45 mg/dL, may peak 4 to 6 weeks after onset of GBS to levels of several hundred mg/dL.	CSF analysis usually shows albuminocytologic dissociation: an elevated protein, without increase in white blood cells (WBCs). This dissociation may be noted during the course of GBS and is helpful in differentiating GBS from other central nervous system (CNS) disorders.
Electromyography (EMG) or nerve conduction velocity (NCV)	Assesses NCV deficit as a result of the demyelination of peripheral nerves.	EMG and NCV demonstrate profound slowing of motor conduction velocities and conduction blocks several weeks into the illness.
Pulmonary function studies	Assesses for respiratory insufficiency during initial diagnostic evaluation.	Vital capacity (VC) of less than 1 L indicates a possible need for assisted ventilation and should be assessed every 2 to 4 hours during the early acute phase.
Arterial blood gas analysis	Assesses for respiratory failure. Performed if VC drops below 1 L or if the patient is dyspneic, confused, restless, has nasal flaring, use of accessory muscles of respiration, or is breathless.	A decrease in Pao_2 greater than 10 to 15 mm Hg or an increase in $Paco_2$ of 10 to 15 mm Hg over baseline or normal value signals the need for immediate intubation or tracheostomy.

COLLABORATIVE MANAGEMENT

CARE PRIORITIES

1. Provide respiratory support
ET intubation with assisted mechanical ventilation, as necessary.

2. Perform plasmapheresis
Involves a complete exchange of plasma with the removal of abnormal circulating antibodies that affect the peripheral nerve myelin sheath. Removal of these autoantibodies may lessen the duration and severity of GBS. For nursing interventions for complications of plasmapheresis, see Box 7-3.

3. Administer IVIG (IV immunoglobulin G or IVIG)
IVIG given at 0.4 mg/kg/body weight/day for 5 days has been recommended as an alternative to plasma exchange in children and adults with GBS.

4. Support cardiovascular function and carefully monitor for dysrhythmias
Continuous cardiac monitoring may be initiated to assess for dysrhythmias, which are a common cause of death; arterial pressure monitoring may be used to evaluate hypertension or hypotension; and antihypertensive agents or vasopressors may be administered to maintain BP within normal levels.

5. Manage bowel and bladder dysfunction
Some patients may experience a paralytic ileus. Nasogastric suction and parenteral infusion may be started; stool softeners and laxatives may be given for constipation. A urinary catheter may be inserted in patients with urinary retention.

6. Provide nutrition support
Parenteral feedings are given until return of peristalsis. Tube feedings or gastrostomy feedings are used for patients with severe dysphagia. With recovery of gag reflex and swallowing ability, the diet will progress to semisolid and solid foods, which are more readily swallowed than are liquids.

7. Rehabilitation
Active and passive ROM exercises are performed at frequent intervals during all phases of GBS. Activity must be balanced with caloric intake to prevent muscle wasting. When the patient's condition stabilizes, a physiatrist consultation to plan rehabilitation with physical and occupational therapy should be done while the patient is in critical care. The primary goal is to pace recovery to obtain maximum mobility, promote self-care, and adapt to changes in body image. Rehabilitation does not improve nerve regeneration.

> **Safety Alert** *Because of the risk of fatal cardiac dysrhythmias in Guillain-Barré syndrome, continuous cardiac monitoring is recommended for the first 10 to 14 days of hospitalization.*

CARE PLANS FOR GUILLAIN-BARRÉ SYNDROME

IMPAIRED GAS EXCHANGE *related to altered oxygen supply associated with decreased lung expansion secondary to weakness or paralysis of intercostal and diaphragmatic muscles.*

Goals/Outcomes: Within 12 to 24 hours of this diagnosis, the patient has adequate gas exchange, as evidenced by orientation to time, place, and person; RR 12 to 20 breaths/min with normal pattern and depth; HR less than 100 bpm; BP within the patient's normal range; PaO_2 greater than 80 mm Hg; $PaCO_2$ less than 45 mm Hg; and oxygen saturation greater than 94%.

NOC Respiratory Status: Gas Exchange; Respiratory Status: Ventilation; Mechanical Ventilation Response: Adult.

 Respiratory Monitoring

1. Monitor for respiratory distress. Report adventitious breath sounds (crackles, rhonchi); decreased or absent breath sounds; temperature greater than 37.7° C (100° F); increased HR and BP; tidal volume or vital capacity

decreased from baseline; decreased Pao_2 or $Paco_2$ increased by greater than 10 to 15 mm Hg from baseline; abnormal RR or rhythm; increasing restlessness, anxiety, or confusion.
2. Assess for weakness hourly, or as often as needed. Ascending motor and sensory dysfunctions usually occur rapidly (over 24 to 72 hours) and can lead to respiratory arrest.
3. Prepare to assist with intubation for respiratory failure.
4. Maintain mechanical ventilation as indicated. (See Mechanical Ventilation, Chapter 1.)
5. Monitor ABG results and pulse oximetry. Consult the advanced practice provider for continued abnormalities.

NIC Airway Management; Acid-Base Monitoring; Oxygen Therapy; Mechanical Ventilation, Respiratory Status: Ventilation.

INEFFECTIVE AIRWAY CLEARANCE *related to ineffective cough; decreased energy; increasing paralysis of respiratory, pharyngeal, and facial muscles; absence of the gag reflex.*

Goals/Outcomes: Within 12 to 24 hours of this diagnosis, the patient's airway is clear, as evidenced by absence of adventitious breath sounds; HR 60 to 100 bpm; BP within the patient's baseline range; RR 12 to 20 breaths/min with normal depth and pattern; tidal volume within baseline measurements; Pao_2 greater than 80 mm Hg; $Paco_2$ less than 45 mm Hg.
NOC Aspiration Prevention; Respiratory Status: Airway Patency.

Airway Management
1. Monitor for crackles, rhonchi, and decreased or absent breath sounds; increased HR and BP; tidal volume or vital capacity decreased from baseline; abnormal RR or rhythm; decrease in Pao_2 or increase in $Paco_2$; and increasing restlessness or anxiety.
2. Suction the airway as needed is determined by auscultation findings. When the paresis or paralysis subsides (usually after 2 to 4 weeks) cranial nerve function will begin to return (i.e., gag reflex, swallowing, coughing). Evaluate the patient's ability to cough, whether or not he or she has been placed on mechanical ventilation. Assess for the presence of adventitious sounds to determine effectiveness of the patient's cough.
3. Deliver oxygen and humidification as prescribed.
4. Maintain mechanical ventilation as prescribed. (See Mechanical Ventilation, Chapter 1.)
5. Maintain adequate hydration to minimize thickening of pulmonary secretions.
6. Turn and reposition the patient at least every 2 hours to prevent stasis of secretions.

NIC Positioning; Airway Suctioning; Respiratory Monitoring; Cough Enhancement; Aspiration Precautions: Positioning.

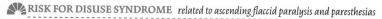

RISK FOR DISUSE SYNDROME *related to ascending flaccid paralysis and paresthesias*

Goals/Outcomes: The patient maintains baseline/optimal ROM of all joints and baseline muscle size and strength; no evidence of DVT.
NOC Endurance.

Energy Management
1. Assess neurologic function hourly or as often as indicated. Ascending motor and sensory dysfunction usually occurs rapidly (over 24 to 72 hours). When neurologic dysfunction is progressing in GBS crisis, assess motor and sensory deficits by starting with the lower extremities and working upward.
   - Assess muscle symmetry by using a side-to-side comparison.
   - Assess for DVT. Monitor for fever and calf tenderness. Apply antiembolic stockings as prescribed to help promote tissue perfusion.
   - Assess muscle strength. For lower extremities: Have the patient pull heel of foot toward the buttocks as you provide resistance by holding onto the foot. For upper extremities: Have the patient extend and flex the wrists and arms against your resistance.
   - Assess deep tendon reflexes of the Achilles, patellae, biceps, triceps, and brachioradialis. Normal response is $+2$; report decreased $(+1)$ or absent (0) response.
   - Assess for paresthesia, including the location, degree, and whether it is ascending.
   - Assess position sense by moving the patient's big toe or thumb up and down while patient's eyes are closed. Note vibratory sense by placing a vibrating tuning fork over bony prominences.

- Assess response to light touch or pinprick by starting at the feet and working upward to determine the level of dysfunction. *Note:* Sensory symptoms are usually milder than motor complaints, with vibration and position sensations affected most often. However, approximately 25% of affected patients will experience pain, requiring analgesia. When light touch, pinprick, and temperature sensations are affected, they most often are found in a glove-and-stocking distribution. Patients frequently experience muscle tenderness and sensitivity to pressure.
- Assess for cranial nerve dysfunction (see Appendix 3).
2. Turn and record and report sensorimotor deficit, including degree of involvement.
3. Reposition the patient in correct anatomic alignment every 2 hours or more often if requested by the patient. Support the patient's position with pillows and other positioning aids.

Activity Therapy
1. To maintain the patient's muscle function and prevent contractures, ensure that active or passive ROM exercises are performed every 2 hours during all phases of GBS. Involve significant others in exercises, if appropriate.
2. Obtain a physical therapy referral, and begin rehabilitation planning process during the early stages of the disorder.
3. As indicated, apply splints to hands-arms and feet-legs to help prevent contracture; alternate splints so that they are on for 2 hours and off for 2 hours.
4. Specialty beds may be used to manage the respiratory, integumentary, autonomic, and musculoskeletal problems.

NIC Neurologic Monitoring; Exercise Therapy (All); Exercise Promotion; Positioning.

AUTONOMIC DYSREFLEXIA (AD) (OR RISK FOR SAME) *related to excessive or inadequate activity of the sympathetic or parasympathetic nervous system.*

Goals/Outcomes: The patient has no symptoms of AD, as evidenced by normal T wave configuration on ECG, HR 60 to 100 bpm, BP within the patient's normal range, cool and dry skin, patient's normal strength, and absence of headache and chest and abdominal tightness.
NOC Neurologic Status: Autonomic; Symptom Severity; Vital Signs.

Dysreflexia Management
1. Assess for signs of AD: cardiac dysrhythmias; HR less than 60 bpm or greater than 100 bpm; elevated and sustained BP (greater than 250 to 300/150 mm Hg); facial flushing; increased sweating, possibly caused by loss of thermal regulation; extreme generalized warmth; profound weakness; and complaints of severe headache or tightening in the chest and abdomen.
2. Place the patient on cardiac monitor as prescribed.

Safety Alert	*Care must be taken to avoid stimulation of autonomic dysreflexia by using generous amounts of anesthetic ointment and ensuring gentle insertion when giving suppository or enema.*

3. Monitor the patient carefully during activities that are known to precipitate AD: position changes, vigorous coughing, and suctioning. The patient should be taught to avoid straining with bowel movements.
4. Be aware of and implement measures to prevent and intervene immediately to remove causes that may precipitate AD such as the following:
   - Bladder stimuli: urinary tract infection, cystoscopy, urinary catheter insertion, clogged urinary catheter, urinary calculi.
   - Bowel stimuli: fecal impaction, rectal examination, enemas, suppositories. Ensure that the patient is well hydrated and has stool softeners and laxatives prescribed to reduce the chance of constipation.
   - Sensory stimuli: pressure caused by tight clothing, dressings, bed covers, thigh straps on urinary drainage bags; prolonged pressure on skin surface or over bony prominences; temperature changes, such as exposure to a cool breeze or draft.
5. If indicators of AD are present, implement the following:
   a. Elevate the HOB or place the patient in a sitting position to promote decrease in BP.
   b. Monitor BP and HR every 3 to 5 minutes until the patient's condition stabilizes.
   c. Determine and remove offending stimulus:
      - For example, if the patient's bladder is distended, catheterize cautiously, using sufficient lubricant.

- If the patient has an indwelling urinary catheter, check for obstruction such as granulation in catheter or kinking of tubing. As indicated, irrigate catheter, using no greater than 30 mL normal saline. If infection is suspected, obtain a urine specimen for culture and sensitivity testing once crisis stage has passed.
- Carefully check for fecal impaction. Perform the rectal examination gently, using an ointment that contains a local anesthetic (e.g., Nupercainal).
- Check for sensory stimuli, loosen clothing, bed covers, or other constricting fabric as indicated.

6. Consult the advanced practice provider if symptoms do not abate within 15 to 30 minutes, especially elevated BP. This may lead to seizures, subarachnoid (SAH) or intracerebral hemorrhage (ICH), or other stroke.
7. As prescribed, administer antihypertensive agents and monitor effectiveness.

NIC Neurologic Monitoring; Vital Signs Monitoring; Urinary Elimination Management.

DECREASED CARDIAC OUTPUT (OR RISK FOR SAME) *related to decreased afterload secondary to reduced peripheral vascular tone. Normovolemic patients may have a decreased cardiac output as a result of vasodilation. This is similar to the vascular response seen in distributive (e.g., anaphylactic, septic) shock.*

Goals/Outcomes: The patient has adequate cardiac output, as evidenced by BP within the patient's normal range; HR 60 to 100 bpm; urinary output greater than 0.5 mL/kg/h; peripheral pulses greater than 2 + on a 0-to-4 + scale; orientation to time, place, and person; CVP 4 to 6 mm Hg; pulmonary artery wedge pressure 6 to 12 mm Hg; systemic vascular resistance 900 to 1200 dynes/s/cm^{-5}; cardiac output 4 to 7 L/min; and normal sinus rhythm.
NOC Tissue Perfusion: Peripheral; Tissue Perfusion: Cerebral.

Hemodynamic Regulation
1. Monitor the patient for indicators of decreased cardiac output: drop in SBP greater than 20 mm Hg from baseline, SBP less than 80 mm Hg, or a continuing drop in SBP of 5 to 10 mm Hg with every assessment; HR greater than 100 bpm; irregular HR; restlessness, confusion, and dizziness; warm and flushed skin; edema; and decreased urinary output less than 0.5 mL/kg/h for 2 consecutive hours. Monitor hemodynamic pressures, particularly pulmonary artery wedge pressure, cardiac output, and systemic vascular resistance.
2. Assess and report changes in cardiac rate and rhythm.
3. Implement measures to prevent decreased cardiac output caused by orthostatic hypotension:
   - Change the patient's position slowly.
   - Perform ROM exercises every 2 hours to prevent venous pooling.
   - Apply elastic antiembolic stockings as prescribed to promote venous return.
   - Keep the patient's legs straight. Do not use pillows or "gatch" the knees on the bed.
   - Collaborate with the physical therapist to use a tilt table to help stand the patient.
4. As prescribed, administer fluids to treat hypotension.
5. Administer a vasopressor (e.g., norepinephrine) to counteract peripheral vasodilation.

NIC Cardiac Care: Acute; Circulatory Precautions; Resuscitation; Shock Prevention.

SENSORY/PERCEPTUAL ALTERATIONS (OR RISK FOR SAME) *related to altered sensory transmission secondary to cranial nerve involvement with GBS.*

Goals/Outcomes: The patient reports normal vision and exhibits normal pupillary and gag reflexes, intact corneas, ability to masticate, and full ROM of head and shoulders.
NOC Neurologic Status: Cranial/Sensory/Motor Function.

Environmental Management: Safety
1. Assess cranial nerve function (see Appendix 3).
   - If the patient experiences a deficit, place objects where the patient can see them and assist with ADLs.
   - Cover one eye with a patch or frosted lens if the patient has diplopia; alternate patch or lens every 2 to 3 hours during patient's waking hours.
   - Use eyelid crutches for patients with ptosis.
   - Assess the patient for corneal irritation or abrasion. Apply artificial tear drops or ointments as prescribed. Secure the eyelid in a closed position if corneal reflex is diminished or absent.

- Suction during oral hygiene. Do not feed the patient an oral diet until the gag reflex returns.
- Position the patient's head in a position of comfort and proper anatomic alignment.

NIC Neurologic Monitoring; Peripheral Sensation Management; Surveillance: Safety.

CONSTIPATION *related to hypoperistalsis or paralytic ileus associated with neuromuscular impairment.*

Goals/Outcomes: Within 3 to 5 days of this diagnosis, the patient has a bowel movement.
NOC Bowel Elimination; Hydration.

Bowel Management

1. Assess the patient's GI status: bowel sounds, abdominal distension, nausea, vomiting, and abdominal discomfort. In the presence of hypoperistalsis or paralytic ileus, the patient will exhibit (1) high-pitched, tinkling sounds that will be heard early in obstruction or ileus or (2) a decrease or absence of sounds occurring with complete obstruction or paralytic ileus.
2. If the patient is having bowel movements, determine the amount, consistency, and frequency. Question the patient about his or her usual pattern of bowel elimination.
3. Provide 2 to 3 L/day of fluid to prevent dehydration and constipation. This may be contraindicated for the patient with impaired renal or cardiac status.
4. Begin bowel training program based on the patient's needs and status of dietary intake:
   - Provide a high-fiber diet if the patient is able to chew and swallow without difficulty.
   - If the patient is bedbound, bulk-forming laxatives should be avoided.
   - Give the patient prune juice every evening.
   - Establish a regular time for elimination and have a bedpan readily available.
   - Facilitate the patient's normal bowel habits; ensure privacy.
   - Administer stool softeners (e.g., docusate sodium).
   - Carefully administer prescribed medicated suppositories.

 Safety Alert *High doses of phenytoin can cause seizure activity; therefore, greater than 30 mg/kg is not recommended. If seizures persist after 20 mg/kg dose, an additional 5 to 10 mg/kg may be given, up to a maximum total dose of 30 mg/kg.*

---

5. See Risk for Disuse Syndrome (p. 664), for neuroassessment measurements. Also see Box 7-3 for the following complications: hypovolemia, clotting abnormalities, hypokalemia, and hypocalcemia.

NIC Constipation/Impaction Management; Fluid Monitoring; Nutrition Management.

Resources for education
GBS/CIDP Foundation International
Address: The Holly Building 104 1/2 Forrest Ave, Narberth, PA 19072
E-mail: info@gbs-cidp.com
Website: www.gbs-cidp.org
Tel: 610-667-0131; 866-224-3301
Fax: 610-667-7036

For more information on neurologic disorders or research programs funded by the National Institute of Neurological Disorders and Stroke, contact the Institute's Brain Resources and Information Network (BRAIN) at:
Brain Resources and Information Network (BRAIN)
P.O. Box 5801
Bethesda, MD 20824
Tel: 800-352-9424
Fax: 301-402-2186
Email: braininfo@ninds.nih.gov
http://www.ninds.nih.gov

ADDITIONAL NURSING DIAGNOSES

See also Urinary Retention in Acute Spinal Cord Injury (Chapter 3). See Deficient Knowledge: Related to Postorgan Transplant Care (Chapter 11). For other nursing diagnoses and interventions, see the following as appropriate: Nutrition Support (Chapter 1), Mechanical Ventilation (Chapter 1), Prolonged Immobility (Chapter 1), and Emotional and Spiritual Support of the Patient and Significant Others (Chapter 2).

STATUS EPILEPTICUS

PATHOPHYSIOLOGY

Status epilepticus (SE) is a state of recurring or continuous seizures of at least 30 minutes' duration, in which the patient does not return to full consciousness from the postictal state before another seizure occurs. A practical definition of SE may be revised to include seizures of only 5 minutes' duration, because of a high likelihood that they will continue. If possible, treatment should be initiated immediately to prevent neuronal injury, which may begin within 20 to 30 minutes of the onset of SE. The mortality rate for SE is estimated to be from 12% to 25%.

There are two major types of SE: convulsive and nonconvulsive. Another classification is based on Gastaut and used by Engel in which generalized SE includes convulsive SE (generalized tonic-clonic seizures) and partial SE. Convulsive SE is more common and is considered a life-threatening medical emergency, because the hypoxia and metabolic exhaustion of neuronal tissue may cause neuronal death. Partial SE includes simple partial SE (focal motor or epilepsia partialis continua) and complex partial SE (temporal or nontemporal seizures). The term "nonconvulsive status" may also be used to describe absence, complex partial SE, and simple partial SE. Clinical diagnosis of the type of nonconvulsive seizure activity is difficult, and thus requires continuous video-electroencephalographic (video-EEG) monitoring to validate that the condition is present.

Refractory SE is present when the seizures, either convulsive or nonconvulsive, continue despite treatment with a therapeutic dose of a benzodiazepine and an initial loading dose of an anticonvulsant.

SE in persons with epilepsy is often as a result of nonadherence with medications or a drop in anticonvulsant serum levels caused by alcohol abuse or infection. Other causes for individuals with and without preexisting epilepsy include acute metabolic disturbances (e.g., hypoglycemia, hyponatremia, hypocalcemia), stroke, CNS infection (e.g., meningitis, encephalitis), CNS trauma or tumors, sepsis, hypoxia, and alcohol or drug abuse. Prompt treatment may prevent complications including cardiac dysrhythmias, hyperthermia, aspiration, hypertension or hypotension, anoxia, hyperglycemia or hypoglycemia, dehydration, rhabdomyolysis, myoglobinuria, and oral and/or musculoskeletal injuries. The prognosis of SE is thought to be related to the etiology and how fast treatment is initiated.

ASSESSMENT

GOAL OF SYSTEM ASSESSMENT

Evaluate for cessation of seizures, return to baseline neurologic function, injury, and to determine cause of seizures.

HISTORY AND RISK FACTORS

Epilepsy, drug or alcohol abuse, recent head injury, stroke or brain tumor, CNS infection, headaches; if patient is in critical care or hospital: sepsis and metabolic disturbance. If the patient is taking anticonvulsant medications, note the following: drug name, dosage, time last taken, length of time drug has been taken, and any recent medication changes. Determine if the patient is taking any other medications, including name, dosage, and time last taken. Some medications may lower the seizure threshold.

VITAL SIGNS

Changes resulting from the massive sympathetic nervous system response to continuous, generalized seizures include hypertension, tachycardia, dysrhythmias, tachypnea, and hyperthermia.

OBSERVATION AND SEIZURE ASSESSMENT

Evaluate for ongoing seizures.

- Changes or fluctuations in mental status such as confusion, dreamy state, stupor, or changes in behavior.
- Automatisms.
- Lip smacking, chewing, swallowing.
- Speech difficulty.
- Twitching of the face, hand, arm, leg (focal motor seizures).
- Mild clonic movements (e.g., fluttering of the eyelids).
- Eye deviation or nystagmus.
- Tonic-clonic activity of all extremities.

SCREENING LABWORK

Blood tests can reveal causes of seizures.

- Blood chemistries: Electrolyte imbalance or metabolic disturbance.
- CBC: Elevated WBCs may indicate infection as cause.
- Anticonvulsant blood levels: Decreased or low levels may be cause of return of seizures.
- Serum drug screen: Rule out drug or alcohol intoxication.
- ABGs: Obtain baseline levels and state of oxygenation.

ELECTROENCEPHALOGRAPHY

Continuous EEG monitoring is used to determine whether the patient is still in SE even though there are no clinical signs or very subtle clinical signs and for those patients who are placed in a medication-induced coma for refractory SE.

Diagnostic Tests for Status Epilepticus

Test	Purpose	Abnormal Findings
Electrolytes Sodium Calcium Magnesium Glucose	Assesses for possible causes of status epilepticus (SE)	Hyponatremia, hypocalcemia, hypoglycemia
Complete blood count	Assesses for infection	Infection may be a precipitant for SE
Serum drug screen	Assesses for drug and/or alcohol intoxication	May be a precipitant for SE
Antiepileptic drug levels	Determines amount of drugs in the system	Low levels may be cause of SE
Arterial blood gases	Obtains baseline levels and determines oxygen saturation	Acidosis: Respiratory and lactic; decreased oxygen saturation attributable to convulsive SE and medication administration
Continuous electrocardiographic monitoring	Evaluates cardiovascular status, especially during medication administration	Phenytoin and other antiepileptic drugs can cause dysrhythmias and hypotension
Continuous electroencephalographic monitoring	Evaluates electrical activity of the brain for ongoing seizures even if there are no clinical signs of seizures	Epileptiform discharges and seizure activity
Computed tomography brain scan Lumbar puncture	Evaluates for any brain abnormalities responsible for SE Assesses for abnormalities in the central nervous system that may indicate infection as a reason for refractory status	Space-occupying lesions See meningitis section

COLLABORATIVE MANAGEMENT

CARE PRIORITIES

1. Support of ventilation and perfusion

Cardiopulmonary function and vital signs are closely monitored. Measures should be initiated to maintain a patent airway, including intubation, as well as ventilatory and cardiovascular support. The metabolic rate and oxygen demands are high during constant seizures, which prompt tachycardia to try to meet the demand. The patient may need support to try to augment cardiac output if the response is insufficient to meet the demand. Cardiac dysrhythmias, hypertension or hypotension, and dehydration are common complications of SE. More extensive evaluation for muscle damage should be done if lengthy tonic-clonic seizures continue or occur frequently. Patients can develop rhabdomyolysis, which may lead to acute kidney injury if not appropriately managed.

2. Establish IV access

For medication administration, fluid resuscitation, and to draw blood for needed labwork.

3. Pharmacotherapy

Prevention of Wernicke-Korsakoff syndrome: 100 mg IV thiamine and 50 mL of 50% glucose are administered if chronic alcohol ingestion or hypoglycemia is suspected.

First-line or emergent therapies

Administration of fast-acting anticonvulsant: Given to quickly achieve high serum and brain concentrations. Not used as long-acting anticonvulsant. First-line agents are benzodiazepines. Treatment is most effective when started promptly.

- **Lorazepam (Ativan)**
  - Preferred by most epileptologists because therapeutic effect is longer lasting.
  - 0.1 mg/kg, up to 4 mg per dose, given IV, may repeat in 5 to 10 minutes. Do not infuse faster than 2 mg/min.
  - Monitor respiratory and cardiovascular status continuously.

OR

- **Diazepam (Valium)**
  - 0.15 mg/kg, up to 10 mg per dose, given IV, may repeat in 5 minutes.
  - Do not infuse faster than 5 mg/min to avoid respiratory depression and hypotension, which may occur with faster infusion rate.

OR

- **Midazolam (Versed)**
  - 0.2 mg/kg intramuscularly up to maximum of 10 mg.
  - Short duration of action, usually used in the field before hospitalization or when IV access is not available.
  - Monitor respiratory and cardiovascular status.

Second-line or urgent therapy

It is recommended to immediately start a second antiepileptic drug after benzodiazepines. The drug of choice depends on several factors, including etiology, comorbidities, and side effects. Several trials have suggested that IV valproate may be as effective as phenytoin. Phenobarbital is not used as frequently because of its side effects and long half-life.

Administration of a long-acting anticonvulsant:

- Fosphenytoin (Cerebyx)
  - Usual IV loading dose is 20 mg/kg PE (phenytoin equivalents). Infusion rate is 100 to 150 mg PE/min. Most IV solutions are compatible with fosphenytoin, including dextrose solutions. Phlebitis and soft tissue damage at IV site are not seen as frequently with fosphenytoin.
  - Monitor vital signs closely. Hypotension and cardiac dysrhythmias may develop.
  - If SE persists after 20 mg/kg, an additional 5 mg/kg may be given 10 minutes after loading infusion.

OR (if fosphenytoin is not used)

- Phenytoin (Dilantin)
  - Usual loading dose is 20 mg/kg given IV. Do not infuse faster than 50 mg/min to avoid serious dysrhythmias, including asystole.
  - Phlebitis and soft tissue damage at IV site may occur.

- Flush line with normal saline only. Microcrystallization, which occurs when phenytoin is used with dextrose, may also occur when it is used in saline as a continuous drip.
- Monitor closely for hypotension and dysrhythmias, and purple glove syndrome.

 Safety Alert *If given simultaneously with or after lorazepam or diazepam, respiratory depression and hypotension can occur, possibly necessitating ventilatory support.*

Administration of IV valproate (Depacon)
- Usual dose is 20 to 40 mg/kg IV, an additional 20 mg/kg may be given 10 minutes after initial dose.
- Infuse at 3 to 6 mg/kg/min.
- Monitor for hyperammonemia, pancreatitis, thrombocytopenia, hepatotoxicity.

Administration of IV levetiracetam (Keppra)
- Usual dose is 1000 to 3000 mg IV.
- Infused at 2 to 5 mg/kg/min IV.

Administration of IV phenobarbital: Used if the patient is allergic to phenytoin.
- Usual dose is 20 mg/kg. Do not infuse faster than 50 to 100 mg/min. May give additional 5 to 10 mg/kg, 10 minutes after loading dose.

 Safety Alert *Neuromuscular blockade stops only movements (not brain electrical activity) and should be administered only when continuous electroencephalographic monitoring is available.*

4. Treatment of refractory status

Aggressive treatment is required for refractory SE that continues despite administration of benzodiazepines, phenytoin or fosphenytoin, valproate, levetiracetam, and phenobarbital.

Consider deep sedation/general anesthesia using propofol, midazolam, or pentobarbital.
- Consider use of additional IV boluses of antiepileptic drugs, IV lacosamide, or topiramate by nasogastric tube.
- Continuous EEG monitoring is required for patients in refractory SE to determine effectiveness of treatment.
- There are no current studies comparing these agents to help determine which is the most effective in the treatment of refractory SE.

Pentobarbital coma
- Loading dose is 5 to 15 mg/kg, may give additional 5 to 10 mg/kg; administer at an infusion rate less than 50 mg/min. Maintenance dosage is 0.5 to 5 mg/kg/h to stop seizures.
- Monitor respiratory and cardiovascular activity continuously.
- Mechanical ventilation required; vasopressors are usually required.
- Periodic tapering of pentobarbital is done to see if seizures have remitted.
- The patient may be in a coma for days to weeks.

Propofol
- Start at 20 μg/kg/min, with a loading dose of 1 to 2 mg/kg given IV. Initial maintenance dosage of 30 to 200 μg/kg/min to stop seizure activity. Adjust dose according to EEG findings.
- Monitor respiratory and cardiovascular activity continuously.
- Mechanical ventilation required; vasopressors are usually required.
- Periodic tapering of propofol is done to see if seizures have remitted.

Midazolam
- Loading dose is 0.2 mg/kg given by IV, administer at an infusion rate of 2 mg/min. Maintenance dosage of 0.05 to 2 μg/kg/h to stop seizure activity.
- Monitor respiratory and cardiovascular activity continuously.
- Mechanical ventilation required; vasopressors are usually required.
- Periodic tapering of midazolam is done to see if seizures have remitted.

Other pharmacologic agents being used and studied in the treatment of refractory status include ketamine, corticosteroids, inhaled anesthetics, and IVIG and plasmapheresis.

Nonpharmacologic treatments that are being studied are vagus nerve stimulation, ketogenic diet, hypothermia, electroconvulsive therapy, transcranial magnetic stimulation, and emergency surgical management. These are typically being done in patients in whom all of the therapies discussed in this section have been ineffective in controlling the status.

There is much to be gained in more research studies looking at the best treatment for status that are based on better evidence than is in the current literature.

Safety Alert *Use of Sedation*

A thorough neurologic evaluation to rule out organic causes of agitation is indicated. Sedation may be used as adjunctive therapy for patients with increased intracranial pressure (ICP) to reduce the risk of extending the stroke, which in the worst case scenario may result in permanent loss of ability to interact with the environment or death. Benzodiazepines, fentanyl (Sublimaze), or morphine sulfate are effective. Propofol (Diprivan) is a short-acting, intravenous hypnotic agent that is also cautiously used for sedation. Pentobarbital coma is occasionally used for patients who experience high ICP that does not respond to other forms of therapy. (See Sedation and Neuromuscular Blockade, Chapter 1.)

---

5. Nutrition support

Enteral or parenteral nutrition may be necessary, depending on the duration of the SE and the patient's underlying nutritional state.

CARE PLANS FOR STATUS EPILEPTICUS

IMPAIRED GAS EXCHANGE *related to altered oxygen supply associated with hypoventilation and bradypnea secondary to depressant effect of seizures and medications on respiratory center.*

Goals/Outcomes: Within 1 hour of treatment/intervention, the patient has adequate gas exchange, as evidenced by PaO_2 greater than 80 mm Hg, $PaCO_2$ 35 to 45 mm Hg, pH 7.35 to 7.45, and RR 12 to 20 breaths/min with normal depth and pattern.

NOC Respiratory Status: Ventilation.

Respiratory Monitoring
1. Monitor for respiratory distress. Note RR, depth, and rhythm and skin color. Report use of accessory muscles, rapid or labored respirations, and cyanosis.
2. Monitor ABG values to assess oxygenation. Be alert to hypoxemia (PaO_2 less than 80 mm Hg) and respiratory acidosis ($PaCO_2$ greater than 45 mm Hg; pH less than 7.35).
3. Keep intubation equipment ready for airway and ventilation assistance.
4. Position an oral airway to help maintain open airway. Suction as necessary.
5. Keep the patient turned to the side to allow secretions to drain.
6. Administer oxygen as prescribed.
7. Administer antiepileptic medications within prescribed criteria to avoid further depression of respiratory center.

NIC Airway Management; Oxygen Therapy; Aspiration Precautions.

ALTERED TISSUE PERFUSION: CEREBRAL AND CARDIOPULMONARY *related to altered blood flow during continuous seizure activity or vasodilatory effects of specific antiepileptic medications. Note: metabolic demands of the brain and heart are increased greatly during seizure activity; adequate cerebral perfusion is essential to maintain brain function.*

Goals/Outcomes: Within 1 hour of treatment/intervention, the patient has adequate cerebral and cardiopulmonary perfusion, as evidenced by orientation to time, place, and person; normal sinus rhythm on ECG; BP within the patient's normal range; RR 12 to 20 breaths/min with normal depth and pattern (eupnea); and absence of headache, papilledema, and other clinical indicators of increased ICP.

NOC Tissue Perfusion: Cerebral; Tissue Perfusion: Cardiac.

Cerebral Perfusion Promotion
1. Support ventilation and perfusion for maximal delivery of oxygen to the brain. Monitor vital signs every 2 to 5 minutes. Respiratory depression, decreased BP, and dysrhythmias can occur with rapid infusion of diazepam and phenytoin. BP must be maintained within normal limits for optimal brain perfusion.

2. Monitor for dysrhythmias, especially during medication administration.
3. Ensure safe administration of antiepileptic drugs: diazepam at 5 mg/min; lorazepam at 2 mg/min; phenobarbital at 50 to 100 mg/min; or phenytoin at 50 mg/min.
4. Perform baseline and serial neurologic assessments to determine the presence of focal findings that suggest an expanding lesion.

NIC Cerebral Perfusion Promotion; Neurologic Monitoring; Seizure Management; Cardiac Care: Acute.

RISK FOR TRAUMA (ORAL AND MUSCULOSKELETAL) *related to seizure activity*

Goals/Outcomes: The patient's mouth and extremities are not injured during the seizure.
NOC Tissue Integrity: Skin and Mucous Membranes.

Environmental Management: Safety
1. Keep side rails padded and up at all times, with bed in the lowest position.
2. Perform protective measures during the seizures:
   - Put a soft object such as a flat pillow under the patient's head.
   - Move sharp or potentially dangerous objects away from the patient.
   - Loosen any tight clothing.
   - Avoid restraining the patient. The force of tonic-clonic movements may cause strains and fractures of extremities if thrashing occurs with restraints in place.
   - Avoid forcing airway into the patient's mouth when jaws are clenched. Force could break teeth, and the patient could swallow or aspirate them.
   - Avoid use of tongue blade, which could splinter and cut the mouth.
   - Stay with the patient; assess and record seizure type and duration. Record any automatic behavior (e.g., lip smacking, chewing movements), motor activity, incontinence, tongue biting, and postictal state.
3. After seizure, reorient and reassure the patient.

NIC Environmental Management: Safety; Positioning; Seizure Precautions; Seizure Management.

NONCOMPLIANCE WITH PRESCRIBED MEDICATION REGIMEN *related to misunderstanding of healthcare recommendations, not understanding importance of following medication schedule, running out of medication, stopping medication intentionally.*

Goals/Outcomes: Within the 24-hour period before discharge from the critical care unit, the patient verbalizes understanding of the rationale and importance of taking the medication as prescribed, as well as the consequence of noncompliance.
NOC Compliance Behavior.

Mutual Goal Setting
1. Once a diagnosis of noncompliance with the medication regimen has been established, determine the patient's reason for noncompliance.
2. Assess patient's understanding of epilepsy and its treatment.
3. Ensure that the patient is aware that stopping the antiepileptic medication can result in serious problems, including SE. If the patient plans to stop the medication for any reason, he or she should consult with the physician.
4. Evaluate the effect epilepsy has on the patient's lifestyle.
5. Once the cause of noncompliance is identified, work to find a solution. If the patient has side effects from the medication, such as gastric upset, suggest that the patient try taking the medication after meals. If the gastric upset is a result of increasing the medication, advise the patient to increase the dose more slowly.
6. Refer the patient to regional epilepsy support groups and the Epilepsy Foundation of America (EFA), including regional affiliate and national headquarters.
7. As appropriate, refer the patient to a nurse specialist or social worker at a regional center for individual counseling.

NIC Teaching: Prescribed Medication; Decision-Making Support; Coping Enhancement; Values Clarification.

DEFICIENT KNOWLEDGE *related to disease process, treatment, and lifestyle changes that epilepsy necessitates.*

Goals/Outcomes: Within the 24-hour period before discharge from the critical care unit, the patient verbalizes understanding of epilepsy, including its etiology and pathophysiology and seizure classification, as well as its treatment and the lifestyle changes it necessitates.

NOC Knowledge: Disease Process.

Teaching: Disease Process
1. Assess knowledge level and provide necessary information about epilepsy.
2. Ask the patient to describe seizure(s) in detail, including warning signals (aura) at the beginning of seizures. Explain that the aura or warning signals onset of seizures and that the patient should lie down or get into a safe position to prevent injury.
3. Assess the patient's knowledge of antiepileptic medications, including name(s), purpose, schedule, dosage, precautions, and side effects. Reinforce importance of maintaining a constant blood level of medication by taking it as prescribed. Reinforce importance of keeping appointments for labwork. Explain if the medication is missed or taken erratically, he or she cannot attain the blood level needed to prevent seizure breakthrough. If a dosage of medication is missed, instruct the patient to notify the physician and/or advanced practice provider.
4. Emphasize to the patient that a normal life is possible.
5. Ensure that the patient knows that sleep deprivation can precipitate SE. Every patient must know his or her own limits. Having epilepsy does not mean it is necessary to get more sleep than do persons who do not have epilepsy.
6. Teach the patient/significant others the importance of safety measures used during a seizure. Emphasize how to ease the patient to the floor and turn him or her to a side-lying position.
7. Inform the patient of local driving regulations/laws for persons with epilepsy.
8. Teach the patient the importance of avoiding dangerous machinery and heights if his or her seizures are not being controlled adequately by medications.

NIC Teaching: Individual; Support Group.

INEFFECTIVE COPING *related to frustration related to unpredictable nature of the disease.*

Goals/Outcomes: Within 24 to 48 hours of this diagnosis, the patient verbalizes feelings, identifies strengths and ineffective coping behaviors, and understands responsibility for self-care.

NOC Coping.

Coping Enhancement
1. Assess the patient's knowledge of the disease and its treatment.
2. Encourage the patient to express feelings so that areas of major concern are known.
3. Involve the patient in decisions regarding care so that he or she has more sense of control over life (e.g., encourage the patient to participate in the decision for scheduling the medications). Problem solve for major concerns.
4. Help the patient set realistic goals for employment and living arrangements. Refer the patient to regional or local EFA as appropriate.
5. Encourage the patient to educate others in what to do should a seizure occur.
6. Encourage involvement in support groups; coping strategies can be learned from other persons with seizures.

NIC Coping Enhancement; Crisis Intervention; Emotional Support; Support System Enhancement.

ADDITIONAL NURSING DIAGNOSES

For other nursing diagnoses and interventions, see the following as appropriate: Mechanical Ventilation (Chapter 1) and Emotional and Spiritual Support of the Patient and Significant Others (Chapter 2).

STROKE: ACUTE ISCHEMIC AND HEMORRHAGIC

PATHOPHYSIOLOGY

The term stroke refers to a neurologic deficit caused by an acute focal injury of the central nervous system (CNS) of vascular cause, including cerebral infarction, intracerebral hemorrhage (ICH), and subarachnoid hemorrhage. Stroke, previously termed cerebrovascular accident (CVA), is the fourth-leading cause of death in the United States. The American Heart Association (AHA) estimates that approximately 795,000 people will have a new or recurrent stroke annually of which 610,000 will be first-time strokes and 185,000 will be recurrent strokes. Stroke was the underlying cause of death in 129,476 cases in 2010. Stroke is the leading cause of long-term disability in the United States. Cost to treat stroke may increase from $71.55 billion in 2010 to $183.13 billion in 2030 per year, according to the American Heart Association/American Stroke Association (AHA/ASA). One third of patients with stroke do not survive, one third suffer with long-term disability, and one third with no or minimal disability. Although men have a higher incidence of stroke at younger ages, the incidence is reversed and higher for women by age 75 years and older. Women experience 55,000 more strokes each year than do men. In addition, the risk of stroke varies with ethnicity and age. Blacks and Hispanics are at increased risk compared with whites. The risk of stroke increases with age; however, in 2009 34% of hospitalized patients with stroke were younger than 65 years of age.

The classification of stroke depends on the preceding pathophysiologic event. Eighty-seven percent are ischemic strokes, 10% are ICHs, and the remaining 3% are SAHs. Subcategories are shown in Figure 7-1. Acute ischemic stroke (AIS) and ICH are discussed here. Subarachnoid hemorrhage (SAH) from cerebral aneurysmal rupture was discussed in an earlier section of this chapter (see Cerebral Aneurysm and Subarachnoid Hemorrhage, Chapter 7).

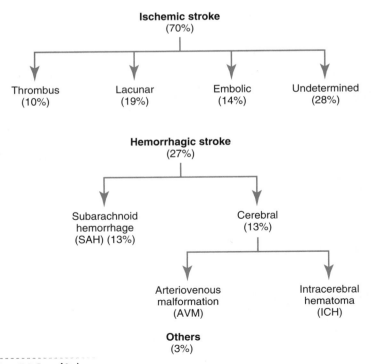

Figure 7-1 Types of Stroke.

A transient ischemic attack (TIA) is a temporary episode of neurologic dysfunction, caused by focal brain, spinal cord, or retinal ischemia, without acute infarction. Although not considered a stroke, TIAs presage 15% of all strokes, and 12% of patients with a TIA will die within 1 year. A TIA may precede an AIS by hours to years. Studies of patients in Northern California showed that 5% had strokes within 2 days, 11% within 3 months, and 33% within 1 year of having a TIA. Atherosclerosis of the arteries supplying the brain is the most common cause of TIA. TIAs generally last less than 24 hours, with most episodes persisting less than 1 hour.

Before the introduction of thrombolytic therapy, a stroke was not always considered a medical emergency, because there was little to offer patients to stop the process. While therapies evolved, an AIS became an emergency because treatment with thrombolytics must be provided within 3 to 4.5 hours after symptom onset (also known as "Time Last Known Well [TLKW]" or "Last Known Normal [LKN]") to be effective. The U.S. Food and Drug Administration (FDA) has approved thrombolytic therapy within the first 3 hours of TLKW. However, in one randomized clinical trial, IV thrombolytics were shown to be beneficial when administered 3 to 4.5 hours after TLKW. Although not FDA-approved for use after 3 hours, the AHA/ASA guidelines do recommend initiation for patients who meet the criteria. Exclusion criteria for thrombolytic therapy 3 to 4.5 hours after TLKW include further criteria in addition to those included in the 3-hour time window: persons older than 80 year of age, a history of previous stroke and diabetes, any anticoagulant use before admission (even if international normalized ratio [INR] is less than 1.7), NIH Stroke Scale greater than 25, and CT findings involving more than one third of the middle cerebral artery (MCA) territory (as evidenced by hypodensity, sulcal effacement, or mass effect estimated by visual inspection or use of the ABC/2 formula (ellipsoid) revealing a mass of greater than 100 mL). Ideally, thrombolytics should be administered within the first hour of arrival in a hospital/stroke center. In many states, emergency medical services (EMS) have been instructed to bypass noncertified primary stroke centers, and take patients with stroke to advanced primary stroke centers or comprehensive stroke centers for evidence-based care and best possible outcomes. Patieents with hemorrhagic strokes may require immediate treatment intervention to reduce intracranial pressure (ICP), such as inserting a ventriculostomy to drain cerebral spinal fluid (CSF). Regardless of the type of stroke, early assessment and intervention is crucial in minimizing complications.

AIS most commonly results from atherosclerosis of blood vessels perfusing the brain. Approximately 20% of AIS results from large artery atherosclerotic disease (extracranial or intracranial), most often associated with thrombus formation related to an unstable plaque. A thrombus is a clot formed in the artery, usually in branches with low flow resulting from plaque. Thrombotic strokes are usually caused by local atherosclerosis of cerebral arteries. Characteristic deficits are produced depending on the artery involved (Table 7-5). Another 25% of AIS results from thrombosis of small perforating intracranial arteries that result in lacunar or subcortical strokes. An additional 20% of AIS results from low to absent cerebral perfusion caused by cardiogenic emboli, most often resulting from atrial fibrillation. Cerebral emboli may be formed in the heart, in the carotid, or other cerebral arteries, and migrate to occlude an artery in the brain. The remaining 30% are cryptogenic and can include critically ill patients in shock experiencing systemic hypoperfusion.

Cerebral ischemia disrupts the sodium/potassium (Na^+/K^+) pump, leading to neuronal depolarization and neurotransmitter release, followed by a massive flux of ions and water resulting in brain cell edema, extracellular K1, and intracellular calcium (Ca^{2+}) increase. Brain cells deprived of oxygen begin anaerobic metabolism, and the resulting lactic acidosis and high concentration of intracellular Ca^{2+} lead to cellular death. Lactic acidosis prompts the *CNS ischemic response*: The vasomotor center is stimulated, which causes vasoconstriction with marked elevation in BP. Systolic BPs (SBPs) less than 220 mm Hg and diastolic BPs (DBPs) less than 120 mm Hg are not treated, because this is a natural response to perfuse the ischemic brain. EMS is encouraged not to treat hypertension in the field so as to maintain perfusion to the penumbra. If thrombolytic therapy is to be initiated, the BP is lowered to less than 185/110 mm Hg. This CNS ischemic response is seen during the acute phase of stroke.

ICH can occur anywhere in the brain (Table 7-6). Although various pathophysiologic events can result in ICH, the most common cause is hypertension, usually resulting in the rupture of a small penetrating artery in the subcortical region. Other causes include bleeding disorders from anticoagulants, abnormal vasculature, alcohol abuse, and liver disease. Damage occurs because accumulated blood destroys and displaces the brain tissue. Disrupted tissue

Table 7-5	CEREBRAL PERFUSION NEUROANATOMY RELATED TO NEUROLOGIC DEFICIT	
Vessel	**Area Supplied**	**Deficit**
Internal carotid artery	Right or left hemisphere	Contralateral motor or sensory deficit, aphasia with dominant hemisphere, neglect with non-dominant hemisphere, contralateral visual field deficit (hemianopia), contralateral eye deviation
Middle cerebral artery	Right or left convex surface of the brain, most of the basal ganglia, internal capsule, putamen, and globus pallidus	Contralateral hemiplegia (arm and face and leg), sensory involvement, aphasia of dominant hemisphere, neglect of nondominant hemisphere (denial of weakness), homonymous hemianopsia
Anterior cerebral artery	Right or left frontal lobe, corpus callosum, caudate nucleus, internal capsule	Weakness or sensory loss of contralateral leg and proximal arm; behavior disturbance: abulia, confusion, memory loss, urinary incontinence
Posterior cerebral artery	Midbrain thalamus, choroid plexus, occipital lobe, and medial temporal lobe	Contralateral visual field deficit, color blindness, impaired depth perception, occasional sparing of central vision, memory loss, sensory loss, nystagmus, pupillary abnormalities, ataxia
Vertebral artery	Medulla and/or cerebellum	Face, nose, or eye ipsilateral numbness with contralateral body numbness, facial weakness, vertigo, ataxia, nystagmus, dysphagia, dysarthria
Basilar artery cerebellum	Pons, midbrain, and/or locked-in syndrome (pons)	Quadriplegia or hemiplegia/paresis, dysarthria, dysphagia, ataxia, nystagmus, vertigo, coma

Table 7-6	HEMORRHAGIC LOCATIONS AND SYNDROMES
Area	**Syndrome**
Putamen	Contralateral hemiplegia, hemisensory loss, hemianopsia, slurred speech
Thalamic	Contralateral hemiplegia; hemisensory loss; small, poorly reactive pupils; decreased level of consciousness
Pontine	Locked-in syndrome (awake, aware, unable to verbally communicate, quadriplegia), coma
Cerebellar	Occipital headache, ataxia, dizziness, headache, nausea, vomiting
Lobar	Mimics cerebral infarct (e.g., contralateral motor and sensory signs)

and the ruptured vessel reduce normal blood flow to the area that surrounds the already injured brain tissue, resulting in some ischemic injury. Intracerebral blood may rupture into the ventricles, creating risk for communicating hydrocephalus. Lobar hemorrhages are less common and most often occur in older adults with cerebral amyloid angiopathy. Other common causes of hemorrhage include vascular anomalies such as arterial venous malformations (AVMs), arterial venous fistulas (AVFs), vasculitis, neoplasms, hematologic disorders, and stimulant abuse (e.g., cocaine, amphetamines). Tighter BP control in the setting of acute ICH to less than 160/90 mm Hg can limit the increase in ICH size during the acute period.

ASSESSMENT OF STROKE: ACUTE ISCHEMIC STROKE AND INTRACRANIAL HEMORRHAGE

GOAL OF SYSTEM ASSESSMENT

During the hyperacute phase, determine stroke type, cause, location, and eligibility for thrombolytic therapy. Then, evaluate for risk factors of stroke extension or secondary neurologic injury.

HISTORY AND RISK FACTORS

Evaluation can provide valuable clues that help facilitate the diagnosis of stroke. Important aspects of a patient's history include the time a patient was last witnessed to be in their normal state (TLKW or LKN), current anticoagulant use, history of previous stroke with residual disability, and history of recent surgeries, bleeding, or any previous history of ICH.

- Risk factors commonly associated with AIS include the following: Hypertension, smoking, diabetes mellitus, hypercholesterolemia, atrial fibrillation, hormone replacement therapy, oral contraceptives, dilated cardiomyopathy, ventricular thrombus after acute MI, valvular disease, sedentary lifestyle, aging, obesity, previous history of TIA or stroke, ethnicity including Native American, Alaska Native, African American, or Hispanic origin, previous MI, or family history of stroke or TIA. Risk factors specific to women include pregnancy-associated hypertension and preeclampsia. Additionally, the metabolic syndrome, a combination of insulin resistance, abdominal adiposity, hypercholesterolemia, and hypertension, contributes to significantly more strokes in women than men.
- Risk factors commonly associated with ICH include hypertension, smoking, African-American ethnicity, aging, excessive alcohol consumption, bleeding disorders, and liver dysfunction, in addition to known underlying vascular anomalies.

VITAL SIGN ASSESSMENT

- Measure BP according to stroke classification, and guidelines pretherapy and posttherapy.
- Document mean arterial pressure (MAP) and track trends; titrate medications to maintain measurements.
- Respiratory status: Rate, rhythm quality, and breath sounds; proper positioning and turning to maintain adequate oxygenation.
  - Maintain Pao_2 greater than 94% for adequate oxygenation to the brain.
  - A Glasgow Coma Scale (GCS) score of 8 or less, rapidly decreasing GCS scores, or compromised ventilation require emergent airway control via rapid sequence intubation.
  - Implement continuous cardiac monitoring: Observe for dysrhythmias including QT prolongation, ST segment depression, T wave inversion, U waves, and ventricular ectopy.
  - Dysrhythmias after stroke may be caused by the release of catecholamines, resulting in hypertension, cardiac irritability, and/or muscle damage.
  - ECG monitoring for the first 24 to 72 hours is recommended. Individuals with new ECG changes have a less favorable prognosis.
  - Monitor for hyperthermia and hypothermia: Maintain normal thermal temperature.
- Monitor blood glucose throughout hospitalization. Typically, it is measured four times a day before meals and at bedtime, although it varies depending on the level.
  - Severe hyperglycemia is associated with decreased reperfusion after thrombolytic therapy, expansion of the infarcted area, and a poor prognosis. Therefore, it must be measured before administration of tissue plasminogen activator (tPA) therapy.
  - Blood glucose should be maintained with a goal of normoglycemia (less than 180 mg/dL). Normoglycemic patients should not be given IV fluids with excessive glucose, to avoid exacerbation of ischemic injury resulting from hyperglycemia.

NEUROLOGIC EVALUATION: OBSERVATION

General presentation: Acute ischemic stroke and intracranial hemorrhage

Signs and symptoms of stroke include sudden onset of weakness or numbness of the face, arm, and/or leg, one-sided facial droop, blurred or loss of vision in one eye, inability to produce or understand speech, fixed gaze to the right or left side, change in level of consciousness (LOC), neglect or ignoring of one side, ataxia, and possible headache.

- Use a recognized Stroke Assessment Scale to identify deficits and the time of onset: Several stroke assessment scales are available, including the FAST (Face, Arm, Speech, Time), the Cincinnati Prehospital Stroke Scale (CPSS), the Los Angeles Prehospital Stroke Scale (LAPSS), Miami Emergency Neurologic Deficit (MEND) examination, the Recognition of Stroke in the Emergency Room Scale (ROSIER), and the Melbourne Ambulance Stroke Scale (MASS). EMS is encouraged to do a MEND assessment in the field, which is a combination of the CPSS and NIH Stroke Scale (NIHSS). The MEND examination is reproducible in the hospital setting.
- Rate stroke severity: Use the NIHSS, the shortened prehospital version (sNIHSS), the Los Angeles Motor Scale, the European Stroke Scale, or the Canadian Neurological Scale.
- Perform a complete neurologic assessment to establish baseline status (see Neurological Assessment, Chapter 7).
- Obtain information regarding baseline neurologic function (e.g., dementia, previous stroke, and neuropathy) and *identify* risk factors associated with stroke.

Clinical presentation: Acute ischemic stroke (Table 7-5)

- Sudden or acute onset of symptoms. Although both thrombotic and embolic strokes can begin abruptly, the former are more likely to evolve over several hours and may fluctuate over several hours or days.
- Those with AIS do not usually experience pain other than a headache, nor do they have altered LOC unless the stroke causes mass effects as a result of swelling or involves the brainstem or thalamic regions bilaterally.
- Women more often report stroke symptoms such as face and limb pain, hiccups, nausea, general weakness, chest pain, palpitations, fainting, shortness of breath, and seizures. Further research is being conducted to better understand the gender differences related to stroke.
- Embolic stroke: The deficit caused is usually maximal at onset and often occurs during activity.
- Ischemic stroke caused by MCA occlusion: In the dominant hemisphere, patients are usually awake with hemiparesis, aphasia, visual field cut, and sensory loss. In the nondominant hemisphere, patients are usually awake with hemiparesis, neglect including denial of their own weakness and denial of their own contralateral limbs, visual field cut, and sensory loss.
- Acute hemispheric infarction: People have elevated arterial BP and often appear drowsy even in the absence of swelling.

Clinical presentation: Intracranial hemorrhage (Table 7-6)

- Severe headache, altered LOC, vomiting, very high BP, and increased ICP.
- Symptoms of ICH depend on the size and location of the hematoma. A relatively small hemorrhage into the brainstem may produce quadriplegia and coma, whereas a hematoma of similar size in the basal ganglia may produce hemiparesis without altered LOC. A larger hematoma (as measured by CT brain scan) may indicate a poorer prognosis.
- The neurologic deficit may evolve over minutes to a few hours.

SCREENING NEUROLOGIC IMAGING

CT imaging of the head without contrast is diagnostic for ICH and guides decision-making for treatment.

- Prepare to transfer the patient to radiology for immediate acute imaging of the brain.
- Continue aggressive monitoring of vital signs and neurologic status while maintaining safety of the patient during transport.

SCREENING LABWORK

- Biochemical profile: Evaluates for abnormal glucose and electrolyte imbalances.
  - On admission, screening for hypoglycemia is the only mandatory laboratory test, although other tests may be performed.
- Coagulation profile: To determine risk for bleeding and/or clotting.
- Complete blood count: Evaluates for abnormal platelets, sepsis, and anemia.
- Cardiac biomarkers: Troponin may be used to evaluate for cardiac ischemia.
- Toxicology: May be used to determine if intoxication is related to neurologic changes.

Diagnosis of Acute Ischemic Stroke versus Hemorrhagic Stroke

Test	Purpose	Abnormal Findings
Imaging		
Computed tomography (CT) brain scan without contrast	Performed emergently, is the gold standard for differentiating ischemic from hemorrhagic stroke; may be done at intervals to monitor progress.	Within the first few hours after acute ischemic stroke, the scan may appear normal. Intracranial hemorrhagic (ICH) is easily diagnosed on CT—blood appears as a bright white signal.
CT angiogram	To visualize the vascular system of the brain	Vascular anomalies, narrowing, or occlusion.
CT perfusion	Provides information related to cerebral blood flow and volume; used to guide clinical decision-making regarding the use of thrombolysis or interventional procedures.	Compromised blood flow; determines volume of brain at risk for infarction.
Magnetic resonance imaging (MRI) and magnetic resonance arteriogram (MRA)	MRI is most useful for patients with ischemia in identifying the cause and area involved. Provides detailed information regarding the area of injury or its vascular supply (MRA).	Infarcts, areas at risk or ischemic areas, vascular defects, stenosis, and occlusion. Diffusion-weighted imaging is a measurement of cytotoxic edema. Perfusion-weighted imaging can identify brain tissue at risk for infarction.
Positron emission tomography and single-photon emission computed tomography	To evaluate brain metabolism and blood flow using three-dimensional imaging produced using a radioactive tracer.	Demonstrates abnormal function of the brain by revealing abnormal structures, metabolism, and perfusion.
Cerebral angiography	The gold standard for evaluating cerebral vasculature; invasive procedure with minimal risk used to visualize the cerebral blood vessels.	Provides specific information on the cause of stroke by identifying the blood vessel involved.
Doppler Testing		
Transthoracic echocardiogram or transesophageal echocardiogram	Evaluates heart structure and function.	Extremely useful in detecting blood clots, masses, and tumors that are located inside the heart; determines severity of certain valve problems and helps detect infection of heart valves, atrial septal defect, or patent foramen ovale. All can contribute to clot formation and emboli causing thromboembolic stroke.
Carotid Doppler or duplex	Evaluates blood flow and presence or degree of stenosis in the extracranial carotid arteries.	Carotid stenosis or clot formation in the carotid artery.
Transcranial Doppler	Evaluates the intracranial vessels and assesses the velocity of blood flow in the anterior and posterior cerebral circulation; also used to evaluate vasospasm, to determine brain death via detection of cerebral circulatory arrest, for intraoperative monitoring, and to identify microemboli.	Vasospasm, cerebral circulatory arrest, and emboli.

Continued

Diagnosis of Acute Ischemic Stroke versus Hemorrhagic Stroke—cont'd

Test	Purpose	Abnormal Findings
Laboratory Testing		
Hematology profile or complete blood count	Screens for anemia (may alter cerebral blood flow), determines status of platelets. 2010 ICH guidelines recommend replacement of platelets as soon as possible in those with thrombocytopenia.	If the number of platelets is too low, excessive bleeding can occur. If the number of platelets is too high, blood clots can form. Anemia decreases oxygen-carrying capacity and increases cerebral velocities.
Biochemical profile	Helps determine fluid and electrolyte balance.	Hyponatremia, hyperosmolality, hyperglycemia, or hypoglycemia.
Coagulation profile	Detects hypercoagulable or hypocoagulable blood. May include levels of homocysteine, proteins C and S. Warfarin may prolong international normalized ratio.	Anticoagulant proteins may be deficient in the young (<45 years) patient with stroke. Deficient coagulation factors may prompt ICH.
Less Commonly Done Tests		
Lupus anticoagulant, anticardiolipin antibody, and hemoglobin (Hgb) electrophoresis	Screens for possible causes of stroke and to assess presence of sickle cell disease (Hgb electrophoresis).	Outside normal range indicating possible risk factor or cause.
Syphilis (e.g., Venereal Disease Research Laboratory test, rapid plasma reagin, fluorescent treponemal antibody); sedimentation rate	To assess for syphilis infection.	Positive results.
Drug screen (e.g., cocaine, amphetamine)	Assesses for presence of drugs that may alter level of consciousness.	Positive results, indicating that the patient has drugs in the bloodstream and/or urine.
Lumbar puncture	Measures cerebrospinal fluid (CSF) pressures and obtains CSF specimen when infections such as meningitis or neurosyphilis are suspected; may be performed when subarachnoid hemorrhage is suspected and CT is normal.	Elevated protein, low glucose, elevated white blood cell count, and elevated CSF pressure.
Electroencephalography	Measures brain activity or seizure activity, although rarely done.	Possible slowing or low voltage over the infarct, except in lacunar infarcts, where results are usually normal.

COLLABORATIVE MANAGEMENT

AMERICAN HEART ASSOCIATION/AMERICAN STROKE ASSOCIATION GUIDELINES FOR ACUTE ISCHEMIC STROKE AND HEMORRHAGIC STROKE MANAGEMENT ARE THE MOST REFERENCED PUBLICATIONS FOR SETTING THE STANDARDS OF PRACTICE

The Joint Commission (TJC) developed its program on the basis of these guidelines. Effective January 1, 2014, all organizations seeking Joint Commission Disease-Specific Care (DSC) certification for stroke must use a set of eight standardized performance measures. Detailed information on TJC's DSC stroke measure set is available in the Specifications Manual for National Inpatient Hospital Quality Measures, version 4.3b, updated April 2014.

Website: www.jointcommission.org/specifications_manual_for_national_hospital_inpatient_quality_measures.aspx

TJC quality indicators for acute ischemic stroke are:

1. *Deep Venous Thrombosis Prophylaxis
2. Discharged on Antithrombotics
3. Anticoagulation Therapy for Atrial Fibrillation/Flutter
4. Thrombolytic Therapy Administered (in eligible patients)
5. Antithrombotic Therapy by End of Hospital Day 2
6. Discharged on Statin Medication
7. *Stroke Education
8. *Assessed for Rehabilitation

TJC quality indicators for intracranial hemorrhage are:

1. *Deep Venous Thrombosis Prophylaxis
2. Dysphagia Screening
3. *Stroke Education
4. Smoking Cessation/Advice Counseling
5. *Assessed for Rehabilitation

*Indicators for both acute ischemic stroke and intracranial hemorrhage.

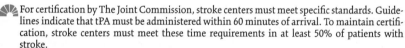 For certification by The Joint Commission, stroke centers must meet specific standards. Guidelines indicate that tPA must be administered within 60 minutes of arrival. To maintain certification, stroke centers must meet these time requirements in at least 50% of patients with stroke.

1. Door to physician time (less than 10 minutes).
2. Door to laboratory time (less than 10 minutes).
3. Door to CT (less than 25 minutes).
4. Door to laboratory results (less than 45 minutes).
5. Door to needle time (less than 60 minutes).

CARE PRIORITIES

Goals of management are to prevent secondary neurologic damage, secondary complications, and to promote optimal functional outcome. Early detection via accurate neurologic examination and immediate medical or surgical intervention help prevent stroke extension, increased brain edema, and hydrocephalus. Physical examination findings guide medical and nursing interventions. The Joint Commission requires the following list of interventions for certified stroke centers: initiation of DVT prophylaxis, discharge on antithrombotic medications, anticoagulation therapy for patients with atrial fibrillation/flutter, administration of thrombolytic therapy, initiation of antithrombotic therapy by the end of the second hospital day, stroke education, and assessment for rehabilitation.

1. Rapidly evaluate patients for type of stroke and minimize brain damage

Medical Therapies:

- Oxygen therapy: Maintain oxygen saturation of at least 94% using 2 to 3 L nasal cannula oxygen. Maximizing oxygenation is of paramount importance for all patients with stroke.
- Hydration: IV fluids (initially without dextrose) help maintain adequate circulating blood volume.

- For intracranial hemorrhage: Replace platelets or coagulation factors if needed. If INR is elevated, hold warfarin and treat with prothrombin complex concentrate, fresh-frozen plasma, and/or vitamin K.

Acute Ischemic Stroke:

- Thrombolysis: Clots are "dissolved" using IV recombinant tissue plasminogen activator (rtPA). The window of treatment for ischemic stroke has been extended from 3 hours to 4.5 hours after onset of symptoms. Stroke centers strive to provide rtPA within 1 hour of arrival. Vital signs and neurologic assessments should be performed every 15 minutes after rtPA initiation for a total of 2 hours. Following these 2 hours, monitor vital signs and perform neurologic examinations every 30 minutes for 6 hours and then every hour for 16 hours. Heparin, aspirin, clopidogrel, dipyridamole, or warfarin should NOT be given for the initial 24 hours, after which these antithrombotic agents should be started as prescribed. During and following infusion, monitor for major and minor bleeding complications. Continuous cardiac monitoring should remain in place for at least 72 hours.

HIGH ALERT   If the patient experiences profound deterioration in neurologic status during recombinant tissue plasminogen activator (rtPA) infusion, a hemorrhagic complication may have ensued. If suspected, the rtPA infusion should be discontinued immediately. Subsequent measurements include vital signs and neurologic assessments every 15 minutes, and consideration of hyperventilation, mannitol infusion, administration of blood products (cryoprecipitate, fresh-frozen plasma, platelets, factor VIIa, and packed red blood cells), possible initiation of hemodynamic monitoring, and further neurodiagnostic testing and laboratory tests to evaluate the potential for further bleeding.

Antithrombotic Therapy: Antithrombotics should be ordered within the first 24 hours of admission for those who are ineligible for thrombolysis. Continuous cardiac monitoring should be provided for up to 48 hours for patients ineligible for thrombolysis.

- Antiplatelet therapy: Used to reduce risk of ischemic stroke and decrease frequency of TIAs. Aspirin (50 to 325 mg/day dosage range) is the most common agent, usually given once daily. Aspirin/extended-release dipyridamole 25/200 mg (Aggrenox) is given twice daily, but more than 30% of patients who take it have headaches. However, the dose may be titrated to reduce this side effect. Clopidogrel (Plavix) 300 mg may be given as a loading dose followed by 75 mg daily.
- Anticoagulation: If long-term anticoagulation is planned, the patient is converted to oral warfarin (Coumadin) therapy or newer anticoagulants, including direct thrombin inhibitors.

Interventional approaches for acute ischemic stroke

- Intraarterial thrombolysis using rtPA has a 6-hour window in which to implement the therapy directly into the cerebral vasculature. This approach is much more successful with strokes secondary to large vessel occlusion.
- Mechanical disruption of the clot using stent retrievers have been shown to be most effective as revascularization tools and consist of deploying a stent into the clot and subsequently pulling the stent and associated clot out. The Penumbra Stroke System is a suction device that breaks down and sucks the clot back through the catheter. Both devices may dislodge the clot and cause it to migrate distally.
- Carotid stenting: Stents may be used for carotid stenosis. Patients who meet criteria include those who are not surgical candidates and are symptomatic from their carotid stenosis.

Endovascular surgery: Interventional approaches for intracranial hemorrhage

- Patients may have an AVM or AVF as an underlying cause for hemorrhage. These lesions are embolized using a single therapy or an adjunctive therapy before surgical removal of the vascular anomaly or use of radiosurgery. Embolization may be achieved using either a polymer or "glue," or GDC coils, which are placed to occlude the malformation (see Cerebral Aneurysm and Subarachnoid Hemorrhage, Chapter 7).

2. Manage hypertension and stabilize vital signs

Antihypertensives are frequently used in the stroke population to control hypertension. If IV thrombolysis is administered, SBP must remain less than 185 mm Hg and DBP less than

110 mm Hg during and following therapy, to reduce risk of symptomatic ICH. For long-term management, antihypertensive agents are selected based on the individual's medical history. Long-term therapy may be prescribed based on the Eighth Joint National Committee (JNC 8) guidelines (Table 7-7). SBP is often elevated in the acute phase and requires vasoactive IV medications such as nicardipine (Cardene IV) or labetalol (Normodyne). Hypotension is a concern, especially in the patient with ICH, because MAP is decreased. If MAP is decreased in the presence of normal or elevated ICP, a decrease in CPP results, further compromising neurologic status. Vasopressors and/or inotropes may be titrated to keep MAP high enough to maintain CPP greater than 60 mm Hg.

Acute Ischemic Stroke:

- Patients eligible for a reperfusion strategy (including tPA) with SBP of greater than 185 mm Hg or DBP greater than 110 mm Hg should have BP reduced to less than 185 mm Hg and DBP to less than 110 mm Hg before beginning the reperfusion strategy. tPA is contraindicated if BP cannot be reduced to these measurements. For at least 24 hours after reperfusion, SBP for those who were initially hypertensive should be maintained at less than 180 mm Hg with DBP less than 105 mm Hg. The advanced practice provider should be notified of an SBP greater than 180 mm Hg or less than 110 mm Hg, DBP greater than 105 mm Hg or less than 60 mm Hg, HR less than 50 bpm or greater than 110 bpm, RR greater than 24 breaths/min, temperature greater than 37.5° C (99.6° F), or a deterioration in neurologic status.
- Patients who have concomitant medical problems that require management of hypertension should be provided with aggressive BP reduction.
- Patients who are not eligible for thrombolytic therapy should have BP reduced to less than 220 mm Hg, with DBP reduced to less than 120 mm Hg. The advanced practice provider should be called if the SBP is greater than 220 mm Hg or less than 110 mm Hg, the DBP is greater than 120 mm Hg or less than 60 mm Hg, HR is less than 50 bpm or greater than 110 bpm, RR is greater than 24 breaths/min, temperature is greater than 37.5° C (99.6° F), or if there is a deterioration in neurologic status.

Intracranial Hemorrhage:

The AHA/ASA guidelines recommend the following for management of BP in patients with ICH/acute cerebral hemorrhage:

- If SBP is greater than 200 mm Hg or MAP is greater than 150 mm Hg, aggressive BP reduction should be considered with continuous IV infusion; BP should be monitored every 5 minutes.
- If SBP is greater than 180 mm Hg or MAP is greater than 130 mm Hg with possibly elevated ICP, reduction of BP with concurrent ICP monitoring should be considered to assist in keeping CPP at 60 to 80 mm Hg.

Table 7-7	**CLASSIFICATION AND MANAGEMENT OF BLOOD PRESSURE FOR ADULTS**		
Population	**Goal Blood Pressure,* mm Hg**	**Lifestyle Modification**	**Initial Drug Therapy**
Younger than 60 years	Less than 140/90	Yes	Nonblack: thiazide-type diuretic, ACEI, ARB, or CCB (alone or in combination*,†)
Older than 60 years	Less than 150/90		
Older than 18 years with diabetes	Less than 140/90	Yes	Black: thiazide-type diuretic or CCB (alone or in combination†)
Older than 18 years with chronic kidney disease	Less than 140/90	Yes	ACEI or ARB (alone or in combination with other drug classes*,†)

From Dennison-Himmelfarb C, Handler J, Lackland DT, et al: 2014 evidence-based guideline for the management of high blood pressure in adults report from the panel members appointed to the Eighth Joint National Committee (JNC 8). *JAMA* 311:507-520, 2014.

*ACEIs and ARBs should not be used in combination. Beta-blockers, aldosterone antagonists, or other antihypertensives may be added if initial therapy combination is ineffective.

†Initial combined therapy should be used cautiously in those at risk for orthostatic hypotension.

ACEI, Angiotensin-converting enzyme inhibitor; *ARB*, angiotensin receptor blocker; *BP*, blood pressure; *CCB*, calcium channel blocker.

- If SBP is greater than 180 mm Hg or MAP is greater than 130 mm Hg and there is no indication of increased ICP, reduction of MAP to less than 110 mm Hg or 160/90 mm Hg (a moderate reduction) should be considered.
- Patients with hypotension should be evaluated and treated using standard therapy with aggressive fluid resuscitation, and determination of the etiology of low BP, including hypovolemia and dysrhythmias. Vasopressors may be used if absolutely necessary to raise BP to improve cerebral blood flow.

3. Monitor ICP and manage CPP

CPP − MAP = ICP (keep CPP greater than 60 mm Hg). Invasive monitoring may be necessary for patients with increased infarct size, increased edema, and hydrocephalus. Patients with increased ICP may receive mannitol or hypertonic saline, which lowers ICP by reducing water within brain cells. Careful monitoring of ICP for rebound effect is necessary after mannitol infusion. Patients should remain on bed rest until stabilized. Serum osmolality should be assessed to prevent excessive dehydration. Patients with hydrocephalus often require a ventriculostomy. For more information about ICP monitoring and CPP management, see Traumatic Brain Injury, Chapter 3.

- Invasive monitoring: Assessment and maintenance of neurologic monitors is an essential part of the neurologic assessment.
- ICP monitoring: Ensure an adequate wave form, zero balance equipment, and patency of tubing (if applicable), and maintain sterility of system. Increased ICP is attributable to extension of the infarct or hematoma and its associated edema. May cause midline shift and herniation; increased ICP is associated with hydrocephalus after ICH; seizures generally occur within the first 24 hours but may present at any time.
- Extraventricular drainage: Maintain sterility of system and proper positioning for drainage. Maintain patency. Observe/document color, consistency, and amount of CSF.

4. Prevent stroke extension

The opportunity to prevent further stroke depends on adequate perfusion of the penumbra, which is the ischemic brain tissue surrounding the initial infarct that is at immediate risk of infarction. Perfusing the penumbra decreases the potential infarct size and optimizes patient outcome. A "normal" BP may be too low, causing further ischemia and infarct by decreasing cerebral perfusion. Arterial BP should not be lowered abruptly in patients with AIS. At times, maintenance of a somewhat elevated BP may be warranted, depending on the underlying vascular and brain pathology. In contrast, with ICH many practitioners believe that an elevated BP should be reduced aggressively. The best approach is unclear, and therefore the treatment of increased BP in ICH requires individual consideration (Table 7-7).

Choose evidence-based tools for monitoring neurologic changes:

- NIH Stroke Scale (NIHSS) (Table 7-8): Provides a better measurement of deficits and is easy to use. It also guides the examiner in evaluating cognitive, language, and motor deficits that are unique to stroke. A comprehensive neurologic assessment assists the critical care nurse in detecting changes in neurologic status and the response to interventions.
- Glasgow Coma Scale (GCS) (see Appendix 2): Used to measure changes in LOC in those who cannot participate in NIHSS.

5. Prevention of recurrent stroke

- Target BP should be individualized to each patient. Patients with moderate hypertension may benefit from a drop of 10 mm Hg SBP and 5 mm Hg DBP.
- Lifestyle changes should be part of all stroke prevention programs.
- The JNC 8 report should be used to guide the choice of antihypertensive medications. Ideal choices remain uncertain. A diuretic coupled with an angiotensin-converting enzyme inhibitor (ACEI) is acceptable. For some patients, the choice of a specific class of antihypertensive medication is clearer (see Table 7-7).

6. Manage agitation

Safety Alert *Antibiotics are given immediately after lumbar puncture or CT and after blood cultures.*

Table 7-8	NATIONAL INSTITUTES OF HEALTH STROKE SCALE (NIHSS)

Patient Identification ___ __.__ __ __ __
Pt. Date of Birth ___ __/__ __/__ __
Hospital _____(__ __.__ __)
Date of Exam ___ __/__ __/__ __

Interval: [ ] Baseline   [ ] 2 hours post treatment   [ ] 24 hours post onset of symptoms ±20 minutes
[ ] 7-10 days   [ ] 3 months   [ ] Other _____(___ ___)
Time: ___ ___:___ ___ [ ]am [ ]pm
Person Administering Scale _____

Administer stroke scale items in the order listed. Record performance in each category after each subscale exam. Do not go back and change scores. Follow directions provided for each exam technique. Scores should reflect what the patient does, not what the clinician thinks the patient can do. The clinician should record answers while administering the exam and work quickly. Except where indicated, the patient should not be coached (i.e., repeated requests to patient to make a special effort).

Instructions	Scale Definition	Score
1a. Level of Consciousness (LOC): The investigator must choose a response if a full evaluation is prevented by such obstacles as an endotracheal tube, language barrier, orotracheal trauma/bandages. A 3 is scored only if the patient makes no movement (other than reflexive posturing) in response to noxious stimulation.	0 Alert; keenly responsive. 1 Not alert; but arousable by minor stimulation to obey, answer, or respond. 2 Not alert; requires repeated stimulation to attend, or is obtunded and requires strong or painful stimulation to make movements (not stereotyped). 3 Responds only with reflex motor or autonomic effects or totally unresponsive, flaccid, and flexic.	_____
1b. LOC Questions: The patient is asked the month and his/her age. The answer must be correct; there is no partial credit for being close. Aphasic and stuporous patients who do not comprehend the questions will score 2. Patients unable to speak because of endotracheal intubation, orotracheal trauma, severe dysarthria from any cause, language barrier, or any other problem not secondary to aphasia are given a 1. It is important that only the initial answer be graded and that the examiner not "help" the patient with verbal or nonverbal cues.	0 Answers both questions correctly. 1 Answers one question correctly. 2 Answers neither question correctly.	_____
1c. LOC Commands: The patient is asked to open and close the eyes and then to grip and release the non-paretic hand. Substitute another one-step command if the hands cannot be used. Credit is given if an unequivocal attempt is made but not completed as a result of weakness. If the patient does not respond to command, the task should be demonstrated to him or her (pantomime), and the result scored (i.e., follows none, one, or two commands). Patients with trauma, amputation, or other physical impediments should be given suitable one-step commands. Only the first attempt is scored.	0 Performs both tasks correctly. 1 Performs one task correctly. 2 Performs neither task correctly.	_____

Continued

Table 7-8	**NATIONAL INSTITUTES OF HEALTH STROKE SCALE (NIHSS) — (cont'd)**

Instructions	*Scale Definition*	*Score*
2. Best Gaze: Only horizontal eye movements will be tested. Voluntary or reflexive (oculocephalic) eye movements will be scored, but caloric testing is not done. If the patient has a conjugate deviation of the eyes that can be overcome by voluntary or reflexive activity, the score will be 1. If a patient has an isolated peripheral nerve paresis (cranial nerves III, IV, or VI), score a 1. Gaze is testable in all aphasic patients. Patients with ocular trauma, bandages, pre-existing blindness, or other disorder of visual acuity or fields should be tested with reflexive movements, and a choice made by the investigator. Establishing eye contact and then moving about the patient from side to side will occasionally clarify the presence of a partial gaze palsy.	0 Normal. 1 Partial gaze palsy; gaze is abnormal in one or both eyes, but forced deviation or total gaze paresis is not present. 2 Forced deviation, or total gaze paresis not overcome by the oculocephalic maneuver.	_____
3. Visual: Visual fields (upper and lower quadrants) are tested by confrontation, using finger counting or visual threat, as appropriate. Patients may be encouraged, but if they look at the side of the moving fingers appropriately, this can be scored as normal. If there is unilateral blindness or enucleation, visual fields in the remaining eye are scored. Score 1 only if a clear-cut asymmetry, including quadrantanopia, is found. If the patient is blind from any cause, score 3. Double simultaneous stimulation is performed at this point. If there is extinction, the patient receives a 1, and the results are used to respond to item 11.	0 No visual loss. 1 Partial hemianopia. 2 Complete hemianopia. 3 Bilateral hemianopia (blind including cortical blindness).	
4. Facial Palsy: Ask or use pantomime to encourage the patient to show teeth or raise eyebrows and close eyes. Score symmetry of grimace in response to noxious stimuli in the poorly responsive or noncomprehending patient. If facial trauma/bandages, orotracheal tube, tape, or other physical barriers obscure the face, these should be removed to the extent possible.	0 Normal symmetrical movements. 1 Minor paralysis (flattened nasolabial fold, asymmetry on smiling). 2 Partial paralysis (total or near-total paralysis of lower face). 3 Complete paralysis of one or both sides (absence of facial movement in the upper and lower face).	
5. Motor Arm: The limb is placed in the appropriate position: extend the arms (palms down) 90 degrees (if sitting) or 45 degrees (if supine). Drift is scored if the arm falls before 10 seconds. The aphasic patient is encouraged using urgency in the voice and pantomime, but not noxious stimulation. Each limb is tested in turn, beginning with the nonparetic arm. Only in the case of amputation or joint fusion at the shoulder, the examiner should record the score as untestable (UN), and clearly write the explanation for this choice.	0 No drift; limb holds 90 (or 45) degrees for full 10 seconds. 1 Drift; limb holds 90 (or 45) degrees, but drifts down before full 10 seconds; does not hit bed or other support. 2 Some effort against gravity; limb cannot get to or maintain (if cued) 90 (or 45) degrees, drifts down to bed, but has some effort against gravity. 3 No effort against gravity; limb falls. 4 No movement. UN Amputation or joint fusion, explain: 5a. Left Arm 5b. Right Arm	

Table 7-8	**NATIONAL INSTITUTES OF HEALTH STROKE SCALE (NIHSS) — (cont'd)**

Instructions	*Scale Definition*
6. Motor Leg: The limb is placed in the appropriate position: hold the leg at 30 degrees (always tested supine). Drift is scored if the leg falls before 5 seconds. The aphasic patient is encouraged using urgency in the voice and pantomime, but not noxious stimulation. Each limb is tested in turn, beginning with the nonparetic leg. Only in the case of amputation or joint fusion at the hip, the examiner should record the score as untestable (UN), and clearly write the explanation for this choice.	0 No drift; leg holds 30-degree position for full 5 seconds. 1 Drift; leg falls by the end of the 5-second period but does not hit bed. 2 Some effort against gravity; leg falls to bed by 5 seconds, but has some effort against gravity. 3 No effort against gravity; leg falls to bed immediately. 4 No movement. UN Amputation or joint fusion, explain: _____ 6a. Left Leg 6b. Right Leg
7. Limb Ataxia: This item is aimed at finding evidence of a unilateral cerebellar lesion. Test with eyes open. In case of visual defect, ensure testing is done in intact visual field. The finger-nose-finger and heel-shin tests are performed on both sides, and ataxia is scored only if present out of proportion to weakness. Ataxia is absent in the patient who cannot understand or is paralyzed. Only in the case of amputation or joint fusion, the examiner should record the score as untestable (UN), and clearly write the explanation for this choice. In case of blindness, test by having the patient touch nose from extended arm position.	0 Absent. 1 Present in one limb. 2 Present in two limbs. UN Amputation or joint fusion, explain: _____
8. Sensory: Sensation or grimace to pinprick when tested, or withdrawal from noxious stimulus in the obtunded or aphasic patient. Only sensory loss attributed to stroke is scored as abnormal, and the examiner should test as many body areas (arms [not hands], legs, trunk, face) as needed to accurately check for hemisensory loss. A score of 2, "severe or total sensory loss," should only be given when a severe or total loss of sensation can be clearly demonstrated. Stuporous and aphasic patients will, therefore, probably score 1 or 0. The patient with brainstem stroke who has bilateral loss of sensation is scored 2. If the patient does not respond and is quadriplegic, score 2. Patients in a coma (item 1a = 3) are automatically given a 2 on this item.	0 Normal; no sensory loss. 1 Mild-to-moderate sensory loss; the patient feels pinprick is less sharp or is dull on the affected side; or there is a loss of superficial pain with pinprick, but the patient is aware of being touched. 2 Severe-to-total sensory loss; the patient is not aware of being touched in the face, arm, and leg.

Continued

Table 7-8	NATIONAL INSTITUTES OF HEALTH STROKE SCALE (NIHSS) — (cont'd)
Instructions	**Scale Definition**
9. Best Language: A great deal of information about comprehension will be obtained during the preceding sections of the examination. For this scale item, the patient is asked to describe what is happening in the attached picture, to name the items on the attached naming sheet, and to read from the attached list of sentences. Comprehension is judged from responses here, as well as to all of the commands in the preceding general neurologic exam. If visual loss interferes with the tests, ask the patient to identify objects placed in the hand, repeat, and produce speech. The intubated patient should be asked to write. The patient in a coma (item 1a = 3) will automatically score 3 on this item. The examiner must choose a score for the patient with stupor or limited cooperation, but a score of 3 should be used only if the patient is mute and follows no one-step commands.	0 No aphasia; normal. 1 Mild-to-moderate aphasia; some obvious loss of fluency or facility of comprehension, without significant limitation on ideas expressed or form of expression. Reduction of speech and/or comprehension, however, makes conversation about provided materials difficult or impossible. For example, in conversation about provided materials, the examiner can identify picture or naming card content from the patient's response. 2 Severe aphasia; all communication is through fragmentary expression; great need for inference, questioning, and guessing by the listener. Range of information that can be exchanged is limited; listener carries burden of communication. The examiner cannot identify materials provided from the patient response. 3 Mute, global aphasia; no usable speech or auditory comprehension.
10. Dysarthria: If the patient is thought to be normal, an adequate sample of speech must be obtained by asking the patient to read or repeat words from the attached list. If the patient has severe aphasia, the clarity of articulation of spontaneous speech can be rated. Only if the patient is intubated or has other physical barriers to producing speech, the examiner should record the score as untestable (UN), and clearly write an explanation for this choice. Do not tell the patient why he or she is being tested.	0 Normal. 1 Mild-to-moderate dysarthria; the patient slurs at least some words and, at worst, can be understood with some difficulty. 2 Severe dysarthria; the patient's speech is so slurred as to be unintelligible in the absence of or out of proportion to any dysphasia, or is mute/anarthric. Intubated or other physical barrier, explain:
11. Extinction and Inattention (formerly Neglect): Sufficient information to identify neglect may be obtained during the previous test. If the patient has a severe visual loss preventing visual double simultaneous stimulation, and the cutaneous stimuli are normal, the score is normal. If the patient has aphasia but does appear to attend to both sides, the score is normal. The presence of visual spatial neglect or anosognosia may also be taken as evidence of abnormality. Because the abnormality is scored only if present, the item is never untestable.	0 No abnormality. 1 Visual, tactile, auditory, spatial, or personal inattention or extinction to bilateral simultaneous stimulation in one of the sensory modalities. 2 Profound hemiinattention or extinction to more than one modality; does not recognize own hand or orients to only one side of space. —————

7. Optimize regulatory functions

To prevent secondary complications, see Table 7-9. In general, patients with stroke need adequate cerebral blood flow and perfusion with adequate glucose and oxygenation. Nursing interventions help facilitate optimal cerebral perfusion.

8. Provide rehabilitation

Should begin immediately once stabilized. Consults to a physiatrist, physical therapist, occupational therapist, and speech therapist should be made within the first 24 hours. Death within the first month after stroke is commonly caused by acute MI, pneumonia, and sepsis, which can result from inactivity. Pulmonary embolism, DVT, skin breakdown, and depression are also common.

Table 7-9	MAINTENANCE OF NORMAL REGULATORY FUNCTIONS IN STROKE	
Function	**Goal/Rationale**	**Intervention(s)**
Optimal body position	Facilitate cerebral blood flow: An ideal position has not been determined. Patient response determines the best position. Arterial perfusion improves with head down, whereas venous drainage improves with head elevated.	Keep HOB elevated 25 to 30 degrees. Lower HOB to flat to increase cerebral perfusion. HOB should be elevated to decrease ICP in patients with hemorrhagic strokes. Keep neck neutral; avoid bending at the waist.
Temperature	Maintain normothermia: Decreases metabolic demands and ICP.	Temperature greater than 38° C (100.4° F) should be treated with acetaminophen.
Breathing and patent airway	Maximize oxygenation: Optimizes O_2 delivery to the brain, prevents atelectasis and pneumonia; reducing intrathoracic and intraabdominal pressures helps to prevent increased ICP; the patient may be unable to protect his or her airway, resulting in aspiration of secretions.	Administer O_2, individualize positioning, pulmonary toilet; Suctioning: No longer than 10 seconds in duration; preoxygenate with 100% for full 2 minutes between each attempt; his or her do not provide overly aggressive manual ventilation when suctioning.
Circulation	Control dysrhythmias and promote electrolyte balance: Normal sinus rhythm optimizes CO to promote perfusion to the brain; hemorrhagic strokes are more likely to cause dysrhythmias. Promote hydration: Helps maintain normal circulating blood volume.	Monitor dysrhythmias for at least 24 hours; cardiac monitoring should be continued for 72 hours if thrombolytics were used. Manage fluid and electrolyte imbalances. Administer IV fluids at 75 mL/h during the first 1 to 3 days, depending on the patient's initial hydration status.
Digestion and bowel elimination	Prevent aspiration pneumonia: Swallowing dysfunction may be present. Reduce incidence of stress ulcers and constipation: Straining with bowel movements increases ICP.	NPO until ability to swallow has been evaluated within the 24 hours of hospitalization. Bedside swallow may precede modified barium swallow. Initiate proton pump inhibitors or H_2-blockers and a bowel program. H_2-blockers may cause delirium.
Cellular glucose supply	Maintain a normal blood glucose level: Optimizes brain cell function by ensuring adequate intracellular supply of glucose.	Aggressively manage blood glucose to control hyperglycemia and prevent/treat hypoglycemia; avoid glucose-containing IV solutions in the emergency department.
Nourishment	Maintain an anabolic state; prevent catabolism: Promote optimal healing opportunity and prevent recurrent stroke by controlling CVD/ASHD risk factors.	Initiate nutrition as soon as possible; enteral feeding, then long-term diet to meet caloric needs; low-Na^+, low-fat, weight reduction if needed.
Urinary continence	Prevent urinary tract infection and skin breakdown: Removal of Foley catheter may prompt skin breakdown if the patient is incontinent.	Prevent unnecessary use of urinary Foley catheter; remove within 48 hours if possible; bladder training as soon as possible.
Mobility and endurance	Promote proper body alignment and muscle strengthening: Prevents contractures, DVT, and complications of immobility.	Perform ROM exercises, regular repositioning; increase activity as tolerated; use mobility beds if needed. Initiate DVT prophylaxis.
Skin integrity	Prevent skin breakdown and dependent edema	Keep skin clean and dry; use pressure relief surfaces.

Continued

Table 7-9	**MAINTENANCE OF NORMAL REGULATORY FUNCTIONS IN STROKE—(cont'd)**	
Function	**Goal/Rationale**	**Intervention(s)**
Communication	Develop appropriate communication techniques; promotes sense of well-being; facilitates more timely response to patient needs when requests are understood.	Provide pictorial board so that the patient can point at needs, ask yes and no questions that do not require long answers, provide pencil and paper for those who can write; ensure glasses and hearing aides are in place for those who use them.

CO, Cardiac output; *CVD/ASHD*, cardiovascular disease/atherosclerotic heart disease; *DVT*, deep venous thrombosis; *HOB*, head of the bed; *ICP*, intracranial pressure; *IV*, intravenous; *Na1*, sodium; *NPO*, nothing by mouth; *O₂*, oxygen; *ROM*, range of motion.

9. Manage seizures

Anticonvulsant therapy is used for seizures in the acute phase. Generally, the patient is given a loading dose of phenytoin (Dilantin) or fosphenytoin (Cerebyx), followed by a maintenance dosage. Benzodiazepines (e.g., Ativan) may be used initially. Patients with ICH are given seizure prophylaxis, whereas patients with AIS are managed only when active seizures are present. Temperature greater than 38° C (100.4° F) should be treated with acetaminophen.

10. Surgical management

- Carotid endarterectomy: Surgical removal of plaque in the obstructed carotid artery to promote blood supply to the brain should be performed within 2 weeks following a minor, nondisabling stroke. Carotid endarterectomy is the treatment of choice for patients with greater than 70% symptomatic carotid stenosis.
- Craniotomy: Often young patients with AIS need to be watched carefully for signs of increased ICP and pending herniation as a result of the lack of space in the cranium. A hemicraniectomy may be considered as a preventative measure for patients younger than 60 years of age with large MCA infarcts who have limited comorbidities. Hematoma evacuation may be performed by aspiration through a burr hole or clot evacuation by craniotomy for patients who have expanding clot, uncontrolled ICP, edema, or mass effect.

NURSING CARE PLANS: ACUTE ISCHEMIC STROKE AND INTRACRANIAL HEMORRHAGE

DECREASED INTRACRANIAL ADAPTIVE CAPACITY *related to interrupted blood flow secondary to thrombus or embolus.*

Goals/Outcomes: Within 72 hours of diagnosis, the patient has adequate cerebral tissue perfusion, as evidenced by no decrease in LOC; no deterioration in motor function on affected side; and no new or further deterioration of language, cognition, or visual field per NIHSS (see Table 7-8).
NOC Neurologic Status.

Neurologic Monitoring

1. Assess for neurologic changes hourly in the acute phase. Use NIHSS to record and monitor neurologic changes after stroke.
2. Maintain ICP less than 15 mm Hg and CPP greater than 60 mm Hg: CPP − MAP = ICP.
3. Position the patient to maintain adequate cerebral perfusion. Keep the HOB at 25 to 30 degrees or less as tolerated for patients with ischemic stroke. Keep the HOB raised at 30 degrees as tolerated for patients with hemorrhagic stroke. Avoid extreme hip flexion. When positioning, monitor tolerance to position change.
4. Maintain SpO₂ of at least 94%. Consider ICP effects of respiratory care. Suction only if needed. Assess breath sounds frequently. Avoid activities that can increase ICP (e.g., excessive coughing). Avoid hypercapnia and hypoxia.
5. Maintain adequate SBP. Higher pressures (140 to 180 mm Hg) may be necessary to perfuse an area of brain at risk of infarction if ischemia is present. For patients with hemorrhagic stroke, maintain adequate BP. Use vasodilators or vasopressors as necessary to optimize BP and maintain CPP at greater than 60 mm Hg for all patients with stroke. For patients with AIS, lower the HOB to flat to promote cerebral perfusion.

6. Notify the advanced practice provider of deterioration in neurologic status or the vital sign changes as described in Collaborative Management.
7. Use sedation as prescribed and monitor response: Effects of sedation and changes in ICP.

NIC Cerebral Perfusion Promotion; Positioning: Neurologic; Neurologic Monitoring.

IMPAIRED PHYSICAL MOBILITY *related to decreased motor function of upper and/or lower extremities and trunk after stroke.*

Goals/Outcomes: At time of discharge from ICU, the patient has no complications of immobility such as skin breakdown, contracture formation, pneumonia, or constipation.
NOC Mobility Level.

Exercise Promotion: Strength Training
1. Turn and position frequently as tolerated. Transfer toward unaffected side.
2. Teach methods for turning and moving using stronger extremity to move weaker extremity.
3. Position weaker extremities to avoid contracture formation, frozen shoulder, or foot drop.
4. Begin passive ROM within 24 hours of admission. Modify exercises if BP or ICP increases.
5. Obtain physical therapy and occupational therapy referrals as soon as possible to establish appropriate therapy.
6. Have the patient cough and breathe deeply as tolerated at scheduled intervals.

NIC Positioning; Exercise Therapy: Joint Mobility; Self-Care Assistance.

IMPAIRED VERBAL COMMUNICATION *related to aphasia secondary to cerebrovascular insult.*

Goals/Outcomes: At a minimum of 24 hours before discharge from ICU, the patient demonstrates improved self-expression and relates decrease in frustration with communication.
NOC Communication Ability.

Communication Enhancement: Speech Deficit
1. Evaluate for aphasia: Partial or complete inability to use or comprehend language and symbols. Assess nature and severity of aphasia: Ability to point to and name specific objects, follow simple directions, understand "yes/no" and complex questions, repeat simple and complex words and sentences, relate purpose or action of the objects, fulfill written request, write request, and read. May occur with dominant (typically left) hemisphere damage.
   - Receptive aphasia (e.g., Wernicke, sensory): Inability to comprehend spoken words. The patient may respond to nonverbal cues.
   - Expressive aphasia (e.g., Broca, motor): Difficulty expressing words or naming objects. Gesture, groans, swearing, or nonsense words may be used. Use of a picture or word board may be helpful.
2. Assess for dysarthria, which signals risk for aspiration resulting from ineffective swallowing and gag reflexes. Consult with the speech therapist to assess ways to promote independence and facilitate swallowing.
3. Decrease environmental distractions, such as television or others' conversations. Fatigue affects ability to communicate; plan adequate sleep/rest.
4. Communicate frequently as follows: Face the patient, establish eye contact, speak slowly and clearly, give the patient time to process information and give answer, keep messages short and simple, stay with one clearly defined subject, avoid questions with multiple choices, and instead phrase questions that can be answered "yes" or "no," and use the same words each time when repeating a statement or question. If the patient does not understand after repetition, try different words. Use gesture, facial expressions, and pantomime to supplement and reinforce message.
5. Help patients regain use of symbolic language: Start with nouns and progress to more complex statements. Keep a record at the bedside of words to be used (e.g., "pill" rather than "medication"). Treat the patient as an adult. Do not speak louder unless the patient is hard of hearing. Be respectful.
6. Facilitate verbal expression and naming objects: Encourage the patient to repeat words after you say them to practice verbal expression. Expect labile emotions, because patients are frustrated and emotional about impaired speech. Patients who cannot monitor their speech may not speak sensible language but may think they are making sense.

7. Avoid labeling the patient "belligerent" or "confused" when the problem is aphasia and frustration. Patients with nondominant (right) hemisphere damage may speak well, but may give overly detailed information, or go off on tangents. Redirect by saying, "Let's go back to what we were talking about."
8. Ensure that call light is available and the patient knows how to use it. If the patient is unable to use call light, check frequently and anticipate needs to ensure safety and trust.

NIC Communication Enhancement: Speech, Visual, Hearing Deficits; Active Listening: Anxiety Reduction; Touch.

ADDITIONAL NURSING DIAGNOSES

See care of the patient after Intracranial Surgery (Chapter 7), Cerebral Aneurysm and Subarachnoid Hemorrhage (Chapter 7), Risk for Trauma (Oral and Musculoskeletal) in Status Epilepticus (Chapter 7), Traumatic Brain Injury (Chapter 3), and Prolonged Immobility (Chapter 1).

SELECTED REFERENCES

Adams HP Jr, del Zoppo G, Alberts MJ, et al: Guidelines for the early management of adults with ischemic stroke: a guideline from the American Heart Association/American Stroke Association Stroke Council, Clinical Cardiology Council, Cardiovascular Radiology and Intervention Council, and the Atherosclerotic Peripheral Vascular Disease and Quality of Care Outcomes in Research Interdisciplinary Working Groups: the American Academy of Neurology affirms the value of this guideline as an educational tool for neurologists, *Stroke* 38:1655–1711, 2007, (published corrections appear in Stroke 38:e38, 2007, and 38:e96, 2007).

Albers GW, Amarenco P, Easton JD, et al: Antithrombotic and thrombolytic therapy for ischemic stroke: American College of Chest Physicians evidence based guidelines, *Chest*, ed 8, 133(Suppl 6): 630S–669S, 2008.

Alexander S, Gallek M, Presciutti M, Zrelak P: *Care of the patient following subarachnoid hemorrhage. AANN clinical practice guidelines series,* Glenview, 2012, American Association of Neurological Nurses.

Alshekhlee A, Miles JD, Katirji B, et al: Incidence and mortality rates of myasthenia gravis and myasthenic crisis in US hospitals, *Neurology* 72:1548, 2009.

American Academy of Neurology: Practice parameters: determining brain death in adults (summary statement). Report of the Quality Standards Subcommittee of the American Academy of Neurology, *Neurology* 45:1012–1014, 1995.

Aranda A, Foucart G, Ducassé JL, Grolleau S, et al: Generalized convulsive status epilepticus management in adults: a cohort study with evaluation of professional practice, *Epilepsia* 51(10):2159–2167, 2010.

Arif H, Hirsch LJ: Treatment of status epilepticus, *Semin Neurol* 28:342–354, 2008.

Australasian Transplant Coordinators Association Inc: *National guidelines for organ and tissue donation,* ed 4, Adelaide, 2008, Australasian Transplant Coordinators Association Inc.

Awada R, Parimisetty A, Lefebvre d'Hellencourt C: *Influence of obesity on neurogenerative diseases,* Rijeka, 2013, InTech. http://www.dx.doi.org/10.5772/53671.

Baird TA, Parsons MW, Phanh T, et al: Persistent poststroke hyperglycemia is independently associated with infarct expansion and worse clinical outcome, *Stroke* 34:2208–2214, 2003.

Barker FG II: Efficacy of prophylactic antibiotics against meningitis after craniotomy: a meta-analysis, *Neurosurgery* 60:887–894, 2007.

Barr J, Fraser GL, Puntillo K, et al: American College of Critical Care Medicine: clinical practice guidelines for the management of pain, agitation, and delirium in adult patients in the intensive care unit, *Crit Care Med* 41:263–306, 2013.

Bederson JB, Connolly ES, Batjer HH, et al: Guidelines for the management of aneurysmal subarachnoid hemorrhage: a statement for healthcare professionals from a special writing group of the Stroke Council, American Heart Association, *Stroke* 40:994–1025, 2009.

Bickley L: *Bates' guide to physical examination and history taking,* ed 11, Philadelphia, 2013, Wolters Kluwer Health/Lippincott Williams & Wilkins.

Bleck TP: Intensive care unit management of patients with status epilepticus, *Epilepsia* 48(Suppl 8):59–60, 2007.

Brain Trauma Foundation: *TBI guidelines.* http://www.braintrauma.org/coma-guidelines/searchable-guidelines/.

Brophy G, Bell R, Claassen J, et al: Guidelines for the evaluation and management of status epilepticus, *Neurocrit Care* 17:3–23, 2012.

Bruno A, Levine SR, Frankel MR, et al: Admission glucose level and clinical outcomes in the NINDS rt-PA Stroke Trial, *Neurology* 59:669-674, 2002.

Caplan LR: Transient ischemic attack: definition and natural history, *Curr Atheroscler Rep* 8:276-280, 2006.

Carter BL, Rogers M, Daly J, et al: The potency of team-based care interventions for hypertension: a meta-analysis, *Arch Intern Med* 169:1748-1755, 2009.

Castillo J, Leira R, Garc√≠a MM, et al: Blood pressure decrease during the acute phase of ischemic stroke is associated with brain injury and poor stroke outcome, *Stroke* 35:520-526, 2004.

Centers for Disease Control and Prevention: *Physical activity for everyone*, Atlanta, 2015, Centers for Disease Control and Prevention. http://www.cdc.gov/physicalactivity/everyone/measuring/index.html.

Chobanian V: Impact of nonadherence to antihypertensive therapy, *Circulation* 120:1558-1560, 2009.

Choi EK, Fredl V, Zachodni C, et al: Brain death revisited: the case for a national standard, *J Law Med Ethics* 36:824-836, 2008.

Claassen J, Hirsch LJ, Emerson RG, et al: Treatment of refractory status epilepticus with pentobarbital, propofol, or midazolam: a systematic review, *Epilepsia* 43:146-153, 2002.

Claassen J, Lokin JK, Fitzsimmons BF, et al: Predictors of functional disability and mortality after status epilepticus, *Neurology* 58:139-142, 2002.

Cummings B, Noviski N, Moreland MP, et al: Circulatory arrest in a brain-dead organ donor: is the use of cardiac compression permissible? *J Intens Care Med* 24:389-392, 2009.

Curley G, Kavanagh BP, Laffey JG: Hypocapnia and the injured brain: more harm than benefit, *Crit Care Med* 38:1348-1359, 2010.

Dennison-Himmelfarb C, Handler J, Lackland DT, et al: 2014 evidence-based guideline for the management of high blood pressure in adults report from the panel members appointed to the Eighth Joint National Committee (JNC 8), *JAMA* 311:507-520, 2014.

Diringer MN, Bleck TP, Claude Hemphill J, et al: Critical care management of patients following aneurysmal subarachnoid hemorrhage: recommendations from the Neurocritical Care Society's Multidisciplinary Consensus Conference, *Neurocrit Care* 15:211-240, 2011.

Dorhout Mees SM, Luitse MJ, van den Bergh WM, et al: Fever after aneurismal subarachnoid hemorrhage: relation with extent of hydrocephalus and amount of extravasated blood, *Stroke* 39:2141-2143, 2008.

Easton JD, Saver JL, Albers GW, et al: Definition and evaluation of transient ischemic attack: a scientific statement for healthcare professionals from the American Heart Association/American Stroke Association Stroke Council; Council on Cardiovascular Surgery and Anesthesia; Council on Cardiovascular Radiology and Intervention; Council on Cardiovascular Nursing; and the Interdisciplinary Council on Peripheral Vascular Disease, *Stroke* 40:2276-2293, 2009.

Edlow JA, Samuels O, Smith WS, Weingart SD: Emergency neurological life support: subarachnoid hemorrhage, *Neurocrit Care* 17(Suppl 1):S47-S53, 2012.

FitzMaurice E, Wendell L, Snider R, et al: Effect of statins on intracerebral hemorrhage outcome and recurrence, *Stroke* 39:2151-2154, 2008.

Fountas KN, Kapsalaki EZ, Lee GP, et al: Terson hemorrhage in patients suffering aneurismal subarachnoid hemorrhage: predisposing factors and prognostic significance, *J Neurosurg* 109:439-444, 2008.

Friedman N, Sexton D: *Gram-negative bacillary meningitis: epidemiology, clinical features, and diagnosis.* In Sexton D, editor: *UpToDate*, Waltham, 2014, Wolters Kluwer. http://www.uptodate.com/contents/gram-negative-bacillary-meningitis-epidemiology-clinical-features-and-diagnosis?source=see_link.

Gastaut H: Classification of status epilepticus, *Adv Neurol* 34:15-35, 1983.

Go AS, Mozaffarian D, Roger VL, et al: Heart disease and stroke statistics—2014 update: a report from the American Heart Association, *Circulation* 129:e28-e292, 2014.

Greer DM, Varelas PN, Hague S, et al: Variability of brain death determination guidelines in leading US neurologic institutions, *Neurology* 70:284-289, 2008.

Guo J, Wang S, Li R, et al: Cognitive impairment and whole brain diffusion in patients with carotid artery disease and ipsilateral transient ischemic attack, *Neurol Res* 36:41-46, 2014.

Hall MJ, Levant S, DeFrances CJ: *Hospitalization for stroke in U.S. hospitals, 1989-2009. In NCHS Data Brief, No. 95*, Hyattsville, 2012, National Center for Health Statistics.

Hankey GJ: Impact of treatment of people with transient ischemic attacks on stroke incidence and public health, *Cerebrovasc Dis* 6(Suppl 1):26-33, 1996.

Heurer GG, Smith MJ, Elliott JP, et al: Relationship between intracranial pressure and other clinical variables in patients with aneurismal subarachnoid hemorrhage, *J Neurosurg* 101:408-416, 2004.

Honda H, Warren DK: Central nervous system infections: meningitis and brain abscesses, *Infect Dis Clin North Am* 23:609-623, 2009.

Hsieh ST, Wijdicks EFM: Brain death worldwide: accepted fact but no global consensus in diagnostic criteria, *Neurology* 67:919, 2006.

Hughes RA, Wijdicks EFM, Barohn R, et al: Practice parameter: immunotherapy for Guillain-Barré syndrome: report of the Quality Standards Subcommittee of the American Academy of Neurology, *Neurology* 61:736–740, 2003.

Johnson R: Aseptic meningitis in adults. In Hirsch M, editor: *UpToDate*, Waltham, 2012, Wolters Kluwer. http://www.uptodate.com/contents/aseptic-meningitis-in-adults.

Juel VC: Myasthenia gravis: management of myasthenic crisis and perioperative care, *Semin Neurol* 24:75, 2004.

Kleindorfer DO, Khoury J, Moomaw CJ, et al: Stroke incidence is decreasing in whites but not in blacks a population-based estimate of temporal trends in stroke incidence from the Greater Cincinnati/Northern Kentucky Stroke Study, *Stroke* 41:1326–1331, 2010.

Knake S, Gruener J, Hattemer K, et al: Intravenous levetiracetam in the treatment of benzodiazepine refractory status epilepticus, *J Neurol Neurosurg Psychiatry* 79:588–589, 2008.

Lee GD, Issenberg SB, Gordon MS, et al: Stroke training of prehospital providers: an example of simulation-enhanced blended learning and evaluation, *Med Teach* 27:114–121, 2005.

Leonard J: *Central nervous system tuberculosis*. In von Reyn CF, Edwards M, editors: *UpToDate*, Waltham, 2014, Wolters Kluwer. http://www.uptodate.com/contents/central-nervous-system-tuberculosis.

Long T, Sque M, Addington-Hall J: What does a diagnosis of brain death mean to family members approached about organ donation? A review of the literature, *Progr Transplant* 18:118–126, 2008.

Lozier AP, Sciacca RR, Romagnoli MF, et al: Ventriculostomy-related infections: a critical review of the literature, *Neurosurgery* 51:170–181, 2002.

Machado C, Lin KC, Kuo JR, et al: Variability of brain death determination guidelines in leading US neurologic institutions, *Neurology* 71:1125–1126, 2008.

McGirt MJ, Woodworth GF, Ali M, et al: Persistent perioperative hyperglycemia as an independent predictor of poor outcome after aneurismal subarachnoid hemorrhage, *J Neurosurg* 107:1080–1085, 2007.

McKeown DW, Bonser RS, Kellum JA: Management of the heartbeating brain-dead organ donor, *Br J Anaesth* 108(Suppl 1):i96–i107, 2012.

Meierkord H, Boon P, Engelsen, et al: EFNS guidelines on the management of status epilepticus in adults, *Eur J Neurol* 17:348–355, 2010.

Milhaud D, Popp J, Thouvenot E, et al: Mechanical ventilation in ischemic stroke, *J Stroke Cerebrovasc Dis* 13:183–188, 2004.

Misra UK, Kalita J, Patel R: Sodium valproate versus phenytoin in status epilepticus: a pilot study, *Neurology* 67:340–342, 2006.

Mocco J, Ransom ER, Komotar RJ, et al: Preoperative prediction of long-term outcome in poor-grade aneurismal subarachnoid hemorrhage, *Neurosurgery* 59:529–538, 2006.

Mortimer DS, Jancik J: Administering hypertonic saline to patients with severe traumatic brain injury, *J Neurosci Nurs* 38:142–146, 2006.

Naidech AM, Levasseur K, Liebling S, et al: Moderate hypoglycemia is associated with vasospasm, cerebral infarction, and 3-month disability after subarachnoid hemorrhage, *Neurocrit Care* 12:181–187, 2010.

Nor AM, Davis J, Sen B, et al: The Recognition of Stroke in the Emergency Room (ROSIER) Scale: development and validation of a stroke recognition instrument, *Lancet Neurol* 4:727–734, 2005.

Pieracci FM, Barle PS, Pomp A: Critical care of the bariatric patient, *Crit Care Med* 34:1796–1804, 2006.

Qui W, Zhang Y, Sheng H, et al: Effects of mild hypothermia on patients with severe traumatic brain injury after craniotomy, *J Crit Care* 22:229–235, 2007.

Rahman S, Hanna MG: Diagnosis and therapy in neuromuscular disorders: diagnosis and new treatments in mitochondrial diseases, *J Neurol Neurosurg Psychiatry* 80:943–953, 2009.

Rhoney D, Peacock WF: Intravenous therapy for hypertensive emergencies, part 1, *Am J Health Syst Pharm* 66:1343–1352, 2009.

Rinkel GH, Feigin VL, Algra A, et al: Calcium antagonists for aneurismal subarachnoid hemorrhage, *Cochrane Database Syst Rev* 4:CD00027, 2002.

Rosamond W, Flegal K, Furie K, et al: Heart disease and stroke statistics: 2008 update: a report from the American Heart Association Statistics Committee and Stroke Statistics Subcommittee, *Circulation* 117:e25–e146, 2008.

Rosen DS, Macdonald RL: Subarachnoid hemorrhage grading scales: a systematic review, *Neurocrit Care* 2:110, 2005.

Sacco RL, Kasner S, Broderick JP, et al: An updated definition of stroke for the 21st century: a statement for healthcare professionals from the American Heart Association/American Stroke Association, *Stroke* 44:2064–2089, 2013.

Seif-Eddeine H, Treiman DM: Problems and controversies in status epilepticus: a review and recommendations, *Expert Rev Neurother* 11(12):1747–1758, 2011.

Seneviratne J, Mandrekar J, Wijdicks EF, Rabinstein AA: Predictors of extubation failure in myasthenic crisis, *Arch Neurol* 65:929–933, 2008.

Sexton D: Dexamethasone to prevent neurological complications of bacterial meningitis in adults. In Calderwood S, editor: *UpToDate*, Waltham, 2014, Wolters Kluwer. http://www.uptodate.com/contents/dexamethasone-to-prevent-neurologic-complications-of-bacterial-meningitis-in-adults.

Sharar E: Current therapeutic options in severe Guillain-Barré syndrome, *Clin Neuropharmacol* 29:45–51, 2006.

Shorvon S, Ferlisi M: The outcome of therapies in refractory and super-refractory convulsive status epilepticus and recommendations for therapy, *Brain* 135:2314–2328, 2012.

Souter J: Bacterial meningitis: vaccines and prophylaxis, *Professional Nurs Today* 16:10–15, 2012.

Stecker MM, Kramer TH, Raps EC, et al: Treatment of refractory status epilepticus with propofol: clinical and pharmacokinetic findings, *Epilepsia* 39:18–26, 1998.

Steinbrook R: Organ donation after cardiac death, *N Engl J Med* 357:209, 2007.

Summers D, Leonard A, Wentworth D, et al; on behalf of the American Heart Association Council on Cardiovascular Nursing and the Stroke Council: Comprehensive overview of nursing and interdisciplinary care of the acute ischemic stroke patient: a scientific statement from the American Heart Association, *Stroke* 40:2911–2944, 2009.

Sutter R, Marsch S, Ruegg S: Safety and efficacy of intravenous lacosamide for adjunctive treatment of refractory status epilepticus: a comparative cohort study, *CNS Drugs* 27:321–329, 2013.

Towfighi A, Saver JL: Stroke declines from third to fourth leading cause of death in the United States historical perspective and challenges ahead, *Stroke* 42:2351–2355, 2011.

Treiman DM, Meyers PD, Walton NY, et al: A comparison of four treatments for generalized convulsive status epilepticus. Veterans Affairs Status Epilepticus Cooperative Study Group, *N Engl J Med* 339:792–798, 1998.

Truog RD, Miller FG: The meaning of brain death. A different view, *JAMA Intern Med* 174:1215–1216, 2014.

Tunkel A: Clinical features and diagnosis of acute bacterial meningitis. In Calderwood S, editor: *UpToDate*, Waltham, 2014, Wolters Kluwer. http://www.uptodate.com/contents/clinical-features-and-diagnosis-of-acute-bacterial-meningitis-in-adults.

Tunkel A: Initial therapy and prognosis of bacterial meningitis in adults. In Calderwood S, editor: *UpToDate*, Waltham, 2014, Wolters Kluwer. http://www.uptodate.com/contents/initial-therapy-and-prognosis-of-bacterial-meningitis-in-adults?source=see_link.

Tunkel A, Hartman B, Kaplan S, et al: Practice guidelines for the management of bacterial meningitis, *Clin Infect Dis* 39:1267–1284, 2004.

Verchere E, Grenier G, Mesli A, et al: Postoperative pain management after supratentorial craniotomy, *J Neurosurg Anesthesiol* 14:96–101, 2002.

Walker MC: Status epilepticus on the intensive care unit, *J Neurol* 250:401–406, 2003.

White H, Boden-Albala B, Wang C, et al: Ischemic stroke subtype incidence among whites, blacks, and Hispanics: the northern Manhattan study, *Circulation* 111:1327–1331, 2005.

Wijdicks EFM: The diagnosis of brain death, *N Engl J Med* 344:1215–1221, 2001.

Wijdicks EFM, Rabinstein AA, Manno EM, et al: Pronouncing brain death: contemporary practice and safety of the apnea test, *Neurology* 71:1240–1244, 2008.

Wijdicks EFM, Varelas PN, Gronseth GS, Greer DM: Evidence-based guideline update: determining brain death in adults: report of the Quality Standards Subcommittee of the American Academy of Neurology, *Neurology* 74:1911–1918, 2010.

Working Group on Status Epilepticus: Treatment of convulsive status epilepticus: recommendations of the Working Group on Status Epilepticus, *JAMA* 270:854–859, 1993.

8   Endocrinologic Disorders

ENDOCRINE ASSESSMENT

Assessment of the endocrine system is complex when assessing the system as a whole because it regulates all body functions in conjunction with the nervous system. Focusing on assessment appropriate to critically ill patients, the following principles should be considered:

1. Critical illness initiates the stress response.
2. The stress response increases the metabolic rate.
3. The hypothalamic-pituitary axis (Figure 8-1) regulates the metabolic rate. The thyroid and adrenal glands are extremely stressed by the stimulus of critical illness to maintain the increased metabolic rate, along with meeting the energy demands at the cellular level. Hypofunction of the thyroid and adrenal glands requires assessment of not only those (the primary) glands but also the hypothalamus (produces releasing factors) and anterior pituitary (produces stimulating hormones.) The hypothalamic-pituitary-target organ feedback loop must be fully intact to maintain normal metabolism.
4. The stress response markedly increases endogenous glucocorticoids, which increase blood glucose. The pancreas may not be able to produce sufficient insulin to manage the glucose level, resulting in hyperglycemia. Insulin may be required to manage hyperglycemia until the stress of illness resolves. People with diabetes mellitus are always challenged with hyperglycemia and, with additional illness, can experience the crisis states of diabetic ketoacidosis (DKA) and hyperosmolar hyperglycemic syndrome (HHS).
5. Under prolonged extreme stress, both the adrenal glands and thyroid may be unable to sustain hormone production to support the stress level. Supplemental glucocorticoids (corticosteroids) and thyroid hormones may be needed.
6. The assessment of the patient who is critically ill should focus on the signs of failure of the endocrine system to support the stress response. Signs of hypofunction are explained the sections on hyperglycemia, adrenal crisis, and myxedema coma. Patients with adequate function of the pancreas, thyroid, and adrenal glands under normal conditions may not be able to maintain balance when exposed to the stress of critical illness. Those with underlying hypofunction are more likely to experience crises.
7. Hyperthermia and cardiac symptoms can make diagnosis of thyroid storm difficult, as the crisis mimics other cardiac crises and infection. Thyroid storm results from underlying Graves disease/hyperthyroidism rather than being a complication of critical illness. Some patients with Graves disease are undiagnosed when critical illness manifests from any cause.
8. Assessment of the causes of unusual fluid and electrolyte imbalances should include evaluation of posterior pituitary function in addition to screening for renal dysfunction. Posterior pituitary dysfunction may result in abnormal levels of antidiuretic hormone (ADH) and may be a complication of critical illness or may result from hypothalamic or pituitary disease. Posterior pituitary hypofunction results in diabetes insipidus (DI), which produces dehydration. Posterior pituitary hyperfunction results in syndrome of inappropriate antidiuretic hormone (SIADH), which results in hyponatremia that can reach critical states if not properly addressed. Nephrogenic DI results from failure of the kidneys to respond to ADH. The elderly are at higher risk of complications with DI as a result of age-related changes to the thirst mechanism and renal function.
9. Medication noncompliance for management of existing endocrine disease must be assessed. People with lower income are at higher risk of crisis because of an inability to purchase medications, and teenagers may not practice meticulous management,

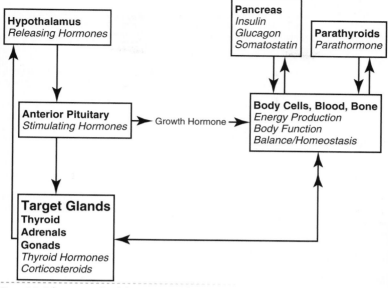

Figure 8-1 Endocrine system: hypothalamic-pituitary axis feedback loop.

particularly those with diabetes mellitus. Elders may not take medications appropriately because of a lack of understanding or misdosing caused by deteriorating short-term memory. Poor historians or those with undiagnosed endocrine disease must be carefully assessed to discover underlying glandular dysfunction. Occasionally, patients referred to as "failure to thrive" are found to have underlying endocrine dysfunction.

Considerations for the bariatric patient: Postoperative bariatric (weight loss) surgery patients require frequent blood glucose monitoring to avoid hypoglycemia. Response to the surgery is individual. Conversely, if the patient is hyperglycemic, insulin resistance is often the cause. All patients should have a baseline glycated hemoglobin (HbA1c) test to determine glucose control preoperatively, given that Type 2 diabetes is extremely common in the overweight population. Manage all patients according to serial laboratory results and assessment.

ACUTE ADRENAL INSUFFICIENCY (ADRENAL CRISIS)
PATHOPHYSIOLOGY

Acute adrenocortical insufficiency, also known as adrenal crisis and Addisonian crisis, is a life-threatening condition that manifests as shock with profound, refractory hypotension and may be induced by hypothalamic-pituitary axis dysfunction. The function of the adrenal cortex is dependent on the hypothalamic-pituitary axis, consisting of a cascade of events beginning with the hypothalamus secreting releasing factors, which:

1. Stimulate the pituitary to secrete stimulating hormones (adrenocorticotropic hormone [corticotropin, or ACTH]), which
2. Stimulates the cortex of the adrenal glands to secrete glucocorticoids (cortisol), mineralocorticoids (aldosterone), and androgens, which
3. Facilitates cellular functions throughout the body (metabolism), which
4. Creates signals back to the hypothalamus from the cells to increase or decrease releasing hormones (see Figure 8-1).

The most common disease process associated with adrenal insufficiency is severe sepsis with pituitary suppression. Inappropriately rapid withdrawal of pharmacologic steroids can also result in a crisis during critical illness or may cause critical illness. Adrenal crisis is also associated with acute exacerbation of chronic adrenocortical insufficiency in patients who become stressed by sepsis, surgery, adrenal hemorrhage (septicemia-induced Waterhouse-Friderichsen syndrome from meningococcemia), and anticoagulation complications. There are approximately 50 total hormones produced by the adrenal glands, with cortisol and aldosterone being by far the most abundant.

If primary adrenal insufficiency is the cause of the crisis, the adrenal glands are the root cause of the problem. Addison disease manifests when the entire adrenal cortex is destroyed, which stops the production of glucocorticoids (cortisol) and mineralocorticoids (aldosterone). Glucocorticoids are essential hormones produced by the adrenal cortex that help maintain vascular tone and cardiac contractility, facilitate wound healing, and support immunity. Cortisol deficiency intensifies the clinical effects of hypovolemia by promoting a decrease in vascular tone, which is partially related to unopposed endothelial production of nitric oxide, and a decreased vascular response to the catecholamine hormones epinephrine and norepinephrine. Relative hypoglycemia may be present, as the breakdown of stored glycogen is not possible without cortisol. Mineralocorticoid hormones are primary regulators of fluid and electrolyte balance, and, when unavailable, patients experience hyponatremia, hypovolemia, hyperkalemia, and metabolic acidosis. Large amounts of sodium and water are excreted in the urine. Severe hypotension, shock, and eventually death may occur without intravenous (IV) adrenocortical hormone and fluid replacement. In patients with chronic primary adrenocortical insufficiency or Addison disease, physical stress or trauma may exacerbate a crisis. Acute crises may be prevented by tripling hormone replacement doses during periods of stress.

Primary adrenal insufficiency is relatively rare, can be acute or chronic, and is most often caused by autoimmune-mediated, idiopathic atrophy. Other causes include tuberculosis, fungal infection, hemorrhage, congenital adrenal hyperplasia, enzyme inhibitors (e.g., metyrapone), cytotoxic agents (e.g., mitotane), and other diseases infiltrating the adrenal glands.

Secondary adrenal insufficiency results from any process that involves the hypothalamus and/or pituitary gland which reduces corticotropin secretion. Inflammatory mediators or trauma may suppress or damage the hypothalamus or pituitary. Pituitary or other tumors may impair pituitary function or, in rarer cases, produce glucocorticoids, which suppress the hypothalamic-pituitary axis.

Exogenous or pharmacologic glucocorticoids (e.g., hydrocortisone) elevate the circulating level of the hormones, which results in hypothalamic-pituitary-adrenal axis dysfunction. With higher levels of circulating glucocorticoids, the adrenal glands do not receive signals to produce endogenous cortisol. When glucocorticoid therapy is abruptly discontinued or weaned too quickly, the adrenal gland cannot immediately respond, given the axis has been "turned off" during pharmacologic therapy and the patient experiences adrenal crisis.

Critical Illness Induced Adrenal Insufficiency

Adrenal insufficiency is common in patients who are critically ill and is increasingly reported in sepsis, severe pneumonia, adult respiratory stress syndrome, trauma, HIV infection, or after treatment with etomidate (anesthetic agent used for rapid sequence endotracheal intubation). A large body of evidence demonstrates significant neuroendocrine dysfunction in the anterior and posterior hypothalamic-pituitary-adrenal axis in adults who are critically ill, including abnormalities in adrenal gland modulation, vasopressin release, and thyroid hormone metabolism. During critical illnesses such as sepsis, adrenal hypofunction can result from overwhelming destruction of adrenal glands themselves (bleeding/ischemic necrosis or Waterhouse-Friderichsen syndrome). The neuroendocrine response to critical illness is varied and complex. Stress-induced increase in the output of cortisol results in marked changes in substrate mobilization, resulting in a ready supply of energy sources for use by vital organs. A surge in ADH results in water retention to maintain operating ranges of volume and osmolality. Glucose mobilization and synthesis provide energy and result in osmotic changes that temporarily recruit volume from the intracellular fluid. Catecholamines not only augment vascular tone but also liberate free fatty acids to fuel the heart and skeletal muscles and hepatic gluconeogenesis and to serve as substrates for hepatic ketone body production. If sustained, however, these profound responses come with substantial costs. Substrate mobilization via proteolysis results in unsustainable losses of structural and muscle proteins that manifest as atrophy and wasting. Unbalanced stress metabolism leads to hyperglycemia with far-reaching effects on immune competence and neurologic morbidities. Often the presenting signs are hemodynamic instability and persistent hypotension, as well as a petechial/purpuric rash. This syndrome is complicated by hypoglycemia, hyponatremia, and hyperkalemia. It is a medical emergency and needs to be treated urgently with antibiotics and hydrocortisone. Critical illness-induced adrenal insufficiency is not readily identified by all practitioners. Patients with pituitary dysfunction generally do not require mineralocorticoid replacement, because the release of aldosterone is dependent on release of angiotensin II rather than ACTH from the pituitary.

RESEARCH BRIEF 8-1

Sprung and colleagues published a multicenter, double-blind, randomized clinical trial in 2008. Fifty-two ICUs enrolled 500 patients who were older than 18 years of age with onset of septic shock within the previous 72 hours (SBP less than 90 mm Hg systolic despite fluids or need for vasopressors for longer than 1 hour). An ACTH 250 μg stimulation test was performed on all patients meeting criteria. Nonresponders were those patients whose serum cortisol level rose less than 9 μg/dL after stimulation. All of these patients then received hydrocortisone dosing or placebo. Hydrocortisone was administered in the following pattern of deceleration:

1. 50 mg IV every 6 hours for 5 days
2. 50 mg IV every 12 hours on Days 6 to 8
3. 50 mg IV every 24 hours on Days 9 to 11 and then stopped

The results were dismal in terms of mortality reduction because there was little difference from placebo. Of note, however, was that the group receiving hydrocortisone spent less time in shock by the prior mentioned definition.

From Sprung CL, Annane D, Keh D, et al: Hydrocortisone therapy for patients in septic shock. *N Engl J Med* 358:111–124, 2008.

ENDOCRINE ASSESSMENT ADRENAL GLANDS

GOAL OF SYSTEM ASSESSMENT

The goal of system assessment is to evaluate for severe hypotension refractory to volume and vasopressor administration.

HISTORY AND RISK FACTORS

- Hypotension, refractory to volume and vasopressors. Glucocorticoids (steroids) have been abruptly withdrawn and patients are not given sufficient steroids to manage additional stress
- Adrenalectomy, hypophysectomy, sepsis, HIV
- Other medications: β-adrenergic blockers, diuretics, angiotensin-converting enzyme (ACE) inhibitors, angiotensin release blockers (ARBs), nitrates, aspirin, and other platelet inhibitors

OBSERVATION AND VITAL SIGNS: PRIMARY (FIRST-DEGREE) AND SECONDARY (SECOND-DEGREE) INSUFFICIENCY

- Severe hypotension resulting from vascular collapse
- Acute abdomen assessment findings: abdominal pain, distention, tachypnea

OBSERVATION AND VITAL SIGNS: PRIMARY (FIRST-DEGREE) INSUFFICIENCY ONLY

- Prominent nausea and vomiting, weight loss
- Bronze hue to the skin secondary to excess production of ACTH

SCREENING LAB WORK
For Suspected Acute Adrenal Crisis

The gold standard for assessing adrenal insufficiency is the use of the insulin tolerance test, which involves the IV injection of insulin. Insulin injections are intended to cause extreme hypoglycemia (<2.2 mmol/L [40 mg/dL]). Normally, ACTH and growth hormone (GH) are released during the stress response. ACTH elevation causes the adrenal cortex to release cortisol. Cortisol and GH serve as counterregulatory hormones, counteracting the action of insulin, which should abate hypoglycemia. Plasma glucose and cortisol (and sometimes ACTH) are measured before injection and again at 15, 30, 45, 60, 75, and 90 minutes. If the stress response is abnormal, the patient will become hypoglycemic. This test is not typically performed in patients who are critically ill, because it is considered unsafe in unstable or unconscious patients and contraindicated in patients with coronary heart disease or seizures.

- Random plasma cortisol level: Drawn before initiating hydrocortisone replacement, but must be interpreted with caution in critically ill patients because greater than 90% of circulating cortisol is protein-bound. When patients are hypoproteinemic, with serum albumin less than 2.5 g/dL, low values may be gleaned from *all* cortisol testing in patients who have normal adrenal function. A random plasma cortisol level of greater than 25 μg/dL excludes both primary and secondary adrenal insufficiency.
- Free cortisol level: Done in the setting of hypoproteinemia to better determine the cortisol level. An abnormal test may require a complete endocrinology assessment when the patient stabilizes. At this time, free cortisol is the most reliable test.

For Noncritical Adrenocortical Insufficiency

- Corticotropin (ACTH) stimulation test: The goal is to differentiate primary from secondary adrenocortical insufficiency or to assess if the adrenal cortex is capable of producing cortisol. Testing of the hypothalamic-pituitary-adrenal axis using this test can differentiate primary from secondary insufficiency. Baseline plasma cortisol level is drawn immediately before ACTH administration.
  1. A dose of 250 μg of synthetic ACTH is given by IM or IV injection.
- Low-dose protocol: Doses as low as 1 μg/kg of ACTH have been used to more closely mimic the amount of normal physiologic ACTH released.
  2. Within 15 to 30 minutes of receiving ACTH, the normal adrenal cortex releases two to five times the baseline or basal plasma cortisol level.
  3. Thirty or 60 minutes following the ACTH injection, another cortisol level is measured. If the low-dose protocol was used, only the 30-minute cortisol level is accurate.
  4. If evaluating for primary adrenal insufficiency, aldosterone levels are drawn with the cortisol levels. The 30-minute aldosterone level is more accurate than the 60-minute level.
- Cortisol level: Does not increase at least a total of 9 mg/dL at 30 or 60 minutes following ACTH administration. Typically will rise to above 20–30 mg/dL.
- Aldosterone level (if testing specifically for primary insufficiency): An initial value of less than 5 ng/100 mL that fails to double or increase by at least 4 ng/100 mL at 30 minutes following ACTH administration.

The 2012 Surviving Sepsis Campaign Guidelines recommend an evidence-based protocol approach to possible adrenal insufficiency in severe sepsis:
1. IV hydrocortisone should not be used to treat adult septic shock patients if adequate fluid resuscitation and vasopressor therapy are able to restore hemodynamic stability, as defined by capillary refill of ≤2 seconds, normal blood pressure (BP) for age, normal pulses with no differential between peripheral and central pulses, warm extremities, and urine output more than 1 mL/kg/h; and are able to hemodynamic stability, as defined by achievable, dose hydrocortisone alone at 200 mg/d (evidence grade 2C).
2. When hydrocortisone is given, a continuous infusion should be used rather than repetitive bolus injections (evidence grade 2D).
3. The ACTH stimulation test should not be used to identify which adults with septic shock should receive hydrocortisone (evidence grade 2B).
4. Corticosteroids should not be administered for the treatment of sepsis in the absence of shock (evidence grade 1D).
5. Clinicians should taper the treated patient from steroid therapy when vasopressors are no longer required (evidence grade 2D).

Diagnostic Tests for Acute Adrenal Insufficiency

Test	Purpose	Abnormal Findings
Noninvasive		
Chest radiograph	Assess for heart size and presence of opportunistic infections (primary)	The chest radiogram may be normal but often reveals a small heart. Stigmata of earlier infection or current evidence of tuberculosis (TB) or fungal infection may be present when this is the cause of Addison disease.
Computed tomography (CT) scan of abdomen	Assess abdominal organs, size, presence of blood (primary)	Abdominal CT scan may be normal but may show bilateral enlargement of the adrenal glands in patients with Addison disease because of TB, fungal infections, adrenal hemorrhage, or infiltrating diseases involving the adrenal glands. In Addison disease caused by TB or histoplasmosis, evidence of calcification involving both adrenal glands may be present. In idiopathic autoimmune Addison disease, the adrenal glands usually are atrophic.
Blood Studies		
Complete blood count (CBC) Hemoglobin (Hb) Hematocrit (Hct) RBC count (RBCs) WBC count (WBCs)	Assess for anemia, inflammation and infection (primary and secondary)	CBC may reveal a normocytic normochromic anemia, which, upon initial presentation, may be masked by dehydration and hemoconcentration. Relative lymphocytosis and eosinophilia may be present.
Electrolytes Potassium (K^+) Sodium (Na^+)	Assess for abnormalities of aldosterone (primary)	Elevation in K^+ may cause dysrhythmias; decrease of Na^{2+} may indicate fluid retention and/or concomitant heart failure.
Serum glucose	Assess for relative hypoglycemia (primary and secondary)	Hypoglycemia may be present in fasted patients, or it may occur spontaneously. It is caused by the increased peripheral utilization of glucose and increased insulin sensitivity. It is more prominent in children and in patients with secondary adrenocortical insufficiency.
Thyroid-stimulating hormone	Assess for thyroid dysfunction (primary and secondary)	Increased thyroid-stimulating hormone, with or without low thyroxine, with or without associated thyroid autoantibodies, and with or without symptoms of hypothyroidism, may occur in patients with Addison disease and in patients with secondary adrenocortical insufficiency caused by isolated ACTH deficiency. These findings may be reversible with cortisol replacement.

Acute Adrenal Insufficiency (Adrenal Crisis)

COLLABORATIVE MANAGEMENT

DIAGNOSIS AND MANAGEMENT OF CORTICOSTEROID INSUFFICIENCY IN CRITICALLY ILL PATIENTS

Recommendations for the diagnosis and management of corticosteroid insufficiency in critically ill adult patients: consensus statements from an international task force by the American College of Critical Care Medicine.

In 2008, an interdisciplinary, multispecialty task force of experts in critical care medicine from the membership of the Society of Critical Care Medicine and the European Society of Intensive Care Medicine was convened. In addition, international experts in endocrinology were invited to participate. The goal was to develop a strategic tool for defining and treating critical illness acute adrenal insufficiency.

Treatment	Rationale
Moderate dose of hydrocortisone (200 to 300 mg/d) for critically ill patients with septic shock.	Six randomized control trials demonstrate significant and greater shock reversal in patients who received hydrocortisone, although there was no difference in mortality.

Continued

DIAGNOSIS AND MANAGEMENT OF CORTICOSTEROID INSUFFICIENCY IN CRITICALLY ILL PATIENTS — cont'd

Treatment	Rationale
Moderate dose of hydrocortisone in the management of severe early ARDS (PF ratio >200) instituted before Day 14.	Five randomized studies evaluated moderate hydrocortisone administration in ARDS from various origins. Consistent improvement was reported in the PF ratio, inflammatory markers were reduced, and both ventilator days and ICU length of stay were reduced.
In patients with septic shock, intravenous hydrocortisone should be given in a dose of 200 mg/d in four divided doses or as a bolus of 100 mg followed by a continuous infusion at 10 mg/h (240 mg/d). The optimal initial dosing regimen in patients with early severe ARDS is 1 mg/kg/d methylprednisolone as a continuous infusion.	Multiple clinical trials, both randomized and not, as well as prospective and retrospective of patients in severe sepsis and ARDS.
Glucocorticoid (GC) treatment should be tapered slowly and not stopped abruptly.	Abruptly stopping hydrocortisone will likely result in a rebound of proinflammatory mediators, with recurrence of the features of shock (and tissue injury).
Treatment with dexamethasone has previously been suggested in patients with septic shock until an ACTH stimulation test is performed. This approach can no longer be endorsed.	Physiologic and pathologic understanding that dexamethasone leads to immediate and prolonged suppression of ACTH.

From Marik PE, Pastores SM, Annane D, et al: *Crit Care Med* 36:1937–1949, 2008.

CARE PRIORITIES

1. Correct hypovolemia

Initiate replacement of intravascular fluid volume. Rapid volume replacement is essential, using normal saline crystalloid IV solution. Administer 1 L over the first hour, followed by an additional 1 to 2 L over the next 6 to 8 hours. If hypovolemia persists, colloid/volume-expanding IV solutions may be necessary.

2. Manage hypotension

Use vasopressors if intravascular volume replacement fails to effectively increase BP (see Appendix 6). Response to catecholamine infusions (epinephrine, norepinephrine, dopamine) is reduced in adrenal insufficiency; higher-than-normal doses may be needed to manage refractory hypotension.

3. Replace cortisol

During stressful situations, the normal adrenal gland output of cortisol is approximately 250 to 300 mg over 24 hours. IV hydrocortisone should be given only to adult patients with septic shock after it has been confirmed their BP is poorly responsive to fluid resuscitation and vasopressor therapy.

- Hydrocortisone 100 mg in 100 mL of normal saline solution by continuous IV infusion at a rate of 12 mL/h. Infusion may be initiated with 100 mg of hydrocortisone as an IV bolus.
- The infusion method maintains plasma cortisol levels more adequately at steady stress levels, especially in the small percentage of patients who are rapid metabolizers and who may have low plasma cortisol levels between the IV boluses. Rapid metabolizers have a greater likelihood of having low plasma cortisol levels between IV boluses.
- As the patient improves and as the clinical situation allows, the hydrocortisone infusion can be gradually tapered over the next 4 to 5 days to daily replacement doses of approximately 3 mg/h (72 to 75 mg over 24 h) and eventually to daily oral replacement doses when oral intake is possible.
- An alternative method of hydrocortisone administration is 50 to 75 mg IV every 4 to 6 hours for 5 days.
- After 2 to 3 days, the stress hydrocortisone dose should be reduced to 100 to 150 mg, administered over a 24-hour period, regardless of the patient's clinical status. In addition

to helping with adrenal recovery, lower doses may help abate gastrointestinal (GI) bleeding.
- If the patient receives at least 100 mg of hydrocortisone in 24 hours, no mineralocorticoid replacement is necessary, because the mineralocorticoid activity of hydrocortisone in this dosage is sufficient.
- As the hydrocortisone dose continues to be weaned, mineralocorticoid replacement should begin in doses equivalent to the daily adrenal gland aldosterone output of 0.05 to 0.1 mg daily or every other day.

4. Maintain normal blood glucose level

If the patient is initially hypoglycemic, 50% dextrose may be needed to correct hypoglycemia. When hydrocortisone or other cortisol replacement is initiated, hyperglycemia may result. An insulin infusion may be needed to control the blood glucose (see Hyperglycemia, Chapter 8).

 Safety Alert *The need for aggressive insulin titration is reduced if the patient is managed using a continuous (24-hour) infusion of cortisol replacement rather than bolus doses every 6 hours.*

CARE PLANS FOR ADRENAL INSUFFICIENCY

 DEFICIENT FLUID VOLUME *related to failure of regulatory mechanisms secondary to impaired secretion of aldosterone, causing increased sodium excretion with resultant diuresis.*

Goals/Outcomes: Within 12 hours of initiating treatment, the patient is moving toward normovolemia as evidenced by BP approaching normal range; heart rate (HR) 60 to 100 beats/min (bpm); respiratory rate (RR) 12 to 20 breaths/min with normal pattern and depth, or, if on the ventilator, weaning from the ventilator; central venous pressure (CVP) 2 to 6 mm Hg; if hemodynamic monitoring is in place, pulmonary artery wedge pressure (PAWP) approaching 6 to 12 mm Hg; normal sinus rhythm on electrocardiogram (ECG); and improvement in level of consciousness (LOC).
NOC Fluid Balance

Fluid and Electrolyte Management
1. Monitor vital signs and hemodynamic measurements every 15 minutes until stabilized for 1 hour. Consult advanced practice provider promptly for deterioration in vital signs or hemodynamics.
2. Administer IV fluids to replace fluid volume. Initially, rapid fluid replacement is essential.
3. Maintain accurate input and output (I&O) record. Weigh the patient daily.
4. Monitor for electrolyte imbalance. Imbalances associated with adrenal insufficiency include the following:
   - Hyponatremia: Headache, malaise, muscle weakness, abdominal cramps
   - Hyperkalemia: Lethargy, nausea, hyperactive bowel sounds with diarrhea, numbness or tingling in extremities, muscle weakness. Be aware that hyperkalemia will worsen in the presence of metabolic acidosis.
5. Monitor ECG continuously; observe for potassium-related changes. Increased ventricular irritability may signal hypokalemia. (See Fluid and Electrolyte Disturbances, Hypokalemia, Chapter 1.)
6. Monitor laboratory results. With appropriate treatment, serum sodium levels should rise to normal and serum potassium levels should fall to normal. Prevent rapid correction or overcorrection of hyponatremia. Serum sodium levels should not be allowed to increase by more than 12 mEq/L during the first 24 hours of treatment because of the risk of neurologic damage. (See Fluid and Electrolyte Disturbances, Hyponatremia, Chapter 1, or Syndrome of Inappropriate ADH, Chapter 8.)
7. Assess mental and respiratory status at frequent intervals. Institute safety measures as indicated. Reorient and reassure the patient as needed.
8. Encourage oral fluid intake as the patient's condition stabilizes. Add sodium-rich foods (see Box 8-1) as tolerated. Begin oral glucocorticoid replacement therapy as prescribed.
9. Consult advanced practice provider if signs and symptoms of fluid and/or electrolyte imbalance persist or worsen.

NIC Fluid Monitoring; Neurologic Monitoring; Hypovolemia Management; Electrolyte Management: Hyponatremia; Electrolyte Management: Hyperkalemia

RISK FOR INJURY *related to potential for acute regulatory dysfunction (cortisol and aldosterone deficiency) secondary to increased psychological, emotional, or physical stressors with increased hormonal demand and inadequate adrenal reserves.*

Acute Adrenal Insufficiency (Adrenal Crisis)

| Box 8-1 | PATIENT AND FAMILY EDUCATION CONCERNING GLUCOCORTICOID AND MINERALOCORTICOID REPLACEMENT |

Glucocorticoids (e.g., Cortisone Acetate, Prednisone)

Glucocorticoids (e.g., Cortisone Acetate, Prednisone) and mineralocorticoids: two-thirds of dose in the morning and one-third of dose in the afternoon).

Glucocorticoids (e.g., cortisone acetate, prednisone): Be alert for indicators of infection (e.g., fever, nausea, diarrhea, malaise).

Glucocorticoids: Take with food to decrease gastric irritation.

Glucocorticoid overreplacement: Weight gain (moon face, truncal obesity); edema; thin, fragile skin (striae, easy bruising); slow wound healing; chronic fatigue; emotional lability

Glucocorticoid underreplacement: Weight loss, hyperpigmentation, skin creases, anorexia, nausea, abdominal discomfort, chronic fatigue, depression, irritability

Mineralocorticoids (e.g., Fludrocortisone, Desoxycorticosterone Acetate)

- Weigh self regularly, and report to provider: Sudden gains or losses >2 lb/wk, chronic fatigue, depression, and irritability.
- Mineralocorticoid overreplacement: Edema, muscle weakness, hypertension
- Mineralocorticoid under-replacement: Excessive urination, weight loss, decreased skin turgor

---

Goals/Outcomes: The patient does not manifest symptoms of sepsis; is able to verbalize orientation to time, place, and person, has stable weight, urine output less than 80 to 125 mL/h, HR 60 to 100 bpm, BP within the patient's normal range, and normothermia.

NOC Immune Status; Infection Status; Energy Conservation

Energy Management

1. Monitor and report signs of increasing crisis: urinary output increased from usual amount, changes in LOC, orthostatic hypotension, nausea, vomiting, and tachycardia.
2. Provide a quiet, nonstressful environment. Adjust lighting to meet needs of individual activities, avoiding direct light in the eyes. Control noise when possible. Prevent unnecessary interruptions, and allow for rest periods. Limit the number of visitors and the length of time they spend with patient. Speak softly and reassuringly to patient.
3. Monitor for and manage hyperthermia using tepid baths, antipyretics, and cooling blankets.
4. Maintain a cool environmental temperature. Maintain strict environmental asepsis, and monitor the patient carefully for signs of infection. Avoid exposing the patient to staff members or visitors who have colds or infections.

NIC Fluid Monitoring; Environmental Management; Infection Protection

DEFICIENT KNOWLEDGE: ILLNESS CARE *related to prevention of adrenal crisis in patients with chronic adrenal insufficiency or those undergoing steroid therapy.*

Goals/Outcomes: Before discharge from the intensive care unit (ICU), the patient understands factors that increase the risk of adrenal crisis, how to avoid adrenal crisis, precautions that must be taken, and when to notify advanced practice provider.

NOC Knowledge: Disease Process; Knowledge: Energy Conservation; Knowledge: Medication

Teaching: Disease Process

1. Teach the patient about prescribed medications, including purpose, dosage, route of administration, and potential side effects (Box 8-1). Medication administration should mimic normal diurnal pattern of plasma cortisol levels (e.g., two-thirds in the morning and one-third in late afternoon).
2. Provide dietary instruction: dietary sodium and potassium may need to be adjusted on the basis of the patient's clinical condition and drug therapy (see discussions of sodium and potassium in Fluid and Electrolyte Disturbances, Chapter 1).
3. Explain the importance of controlling stress, both emotional and physiologic, which increases adrenal demand. Teach the patient to seek medical intervention during times of increased stress (e.g., fever, infection). Medication dosages may need to be increased.

4. Teach indicators of overreplacement and underreplacement of steroids, which require prompt medical attention (see Box 8-1).
5. Stress the importance of never abruptly discontinuing use of any steroid preparation. Use must be tapered to avoid precipitation of crisis.
6. Remind the patient of the importance of continued medical follow-up.
7. Explain the procedure for obtaining a medical alert bracelet or card.

NIC Teaching: Prescribed Medication; Emotional Support

DIABETES INSIPIDUS
PATHOPHYSIOLOGY

Diabetes insipidus (DI) is a metabolic disorder that affects total body free water regulation, resulting in an abnormally high output of extremely dilute urine, increased fluid intake, and constant thirst. The volume of hypotonic urine excreted is 3 to 20 L per day. Vasopressin (antidiuretic hormone [ADH]) is a key component in the regulation of fluid and electrolyte balance through direct effects on renal water regulation. Vasopressin is produced in the hypothalamus, is stored in the posterior pituitary gland, and exerts action in the kidneys for water regulation. Three subtypes of receptors respond to the effects of vasopressin (Table 8-1).

When any aspect of water regulation fails, if free water is lost, the extracellular fluid volume rapidly decreases, causing plasma osmolality and serum sodium to rise. Plasma osmolality is the main determinant of vasopressin secretion from the posterior pituitary. The osmoregulatory systems for thirst and vasopressin secretion, and the actions of ADH on renal water excretion, maintain plasma osmolality between 284 and 295 mOsmol/kg. Thirst and drinking are key processes in the maintenance of fluid and electrolyte balance. Thirst perception and the regulation of water ingestion involve complex neural and neurohormonal pathways. Thirst occurs when plasma osmolality rises above 281 mOsmol/kg, similar to the threshold for ADH release. The osmoreceptors regulating thirst are located in the hypothalamus.

Situations that alter the balance between plasma osmolality and vasopressin concentration include:

- Rapid changes of plasma osmolality: Rapid increases in plasma osmolality result in an abnormal increase in ADH/vasopressin release.
- Drinking fluids: Oral fluid consumption rapidly suppresses the release of ADH, through afferent pathways originating in the oropharynx.
- Pregnancy: The osmotic threshold for ADH release is lowered in pregnancy.
- Aging: Plasma vasopressin concentrations increase with age, together with enhanced ADH responses to osmotic stimulation. Age-related changes in ADH production can result in blunting of the thirst response, decreased fluid intake, impaired ability to excrete a free water load, and reduced ability of the kidneys to concentrate urine. These changes predispose the elderly to both hypernatremia and hyponatremia.

Table 8-1	LOCATIONS AND ACTIONS OF VASOPRESSIN RECEPTORS		
	V_{1a}	V_{1b}	V_2
Location	Central nervous system Vascular smooth muscle Liver Platelets	Anterior pituitary gland	Distal nephron
Physiologic effects	Neurotransmitter and autonomic neuroregulation Smooth muscle contraction Stimulation of glycogenolysis Increased platelet adhesion	Increased ACTH release	Increased production and action of aquaporin-2

Diabetes Insipidus

Table 8-2	FOUR MAJOR SUBTYPES OF DIABETES INSIPIDUS	
Subtypes of DI	**Pathophysiology**	**Common Etiology**
Central	Lack of ADH production by the posterior pituitary gland	Head injury, pituitary tumor and postpituitary tumor resection, cerebral ischemia, intracerebral hemorrhage, CNS infection, brain death, idiopathic
Nephrogenic	Inability of the kidneys to respond to normal amounts of ADH	Medications, ethanol abuse, chronic hypercalcemia, hypokalemia osmotic diuresis, congenital disorder, polycystic kidney disease, pyelonephritis, Sjögren syndrome, sickle cell anemia
Gestational	Blunted thirst response related to pregnancy, and placenta increases the action of vasopressinase, which results in decreased circulating ADH	Last trimester of pregnancy in women who have oligohydramnios, preeclampsia, and/or hepatic dysfunction
Dipsogenic	ADH suppression Caused by increased fluid intake	Unquenchable thirst, massive water intake; psychogenic causes may be associated with mental illness

There are four major subtypes of DI, based on which mechanism involved with concentrating urine has failed (Table 8-2):

- Central, hypothalamic, or pituitary DI (neurogenic DI) is the most common type and is caused by lack of vasopressin (ADH) production by a diseased or destroyed posterior pituitary gland. The lack of ADH results in massive diuresis because ADH normally prompts the kidney to concentrate the urine. Approximately 50% of central DI is idiopathic, as diagnostic testing does not reveal a cause. Central DI is usually permanent, but the signs and symptoms (i.e., thirst, drinking fluids, and urination) are controlled by daily use of synthetic vasopressin.
- Nephrogenic DI (NDI) is caused by inability of the kidneys to respond to normal amounts of ADH, resulting from a variety of drugs or kidney diseases, including genetic predisposition. The collecting tubules have decreased permeability to water caused by decreased response to vasopressin by the nephrons. NDI does not improve with synthetic vasopressin and may not improve when probable causes are managed. Familial NDI requires lifelong management. Treatments partially relieve the signs and symptoms. Medications, including lithium, amphotericin B, and demeclocycline can induce NDI. Hypercalcemia can sometimes prompt NDI.
- Gestational or gestogenic DI results from a lack of vasopressin that develops during the third trimester of pregnancy if the pregnant woman's thirst center is abnormal, causing a blunted thirst response, and/or the placenta destroys vasopressin too rapidly. The placenta may increase the action of vasopressinase, the enzyme that breaks down vasopressin. The condition is controlled using synthetic vasopressin until the DI resolves. Vasopressin can generally be discontinued 4 to 6 weeks after delivery. Signs and symptoms of DI will recur with subsequent pregnancies.
- Dipsogenic DI or primary polydipsia results from vasopressin suppression caused by excessive fluid intake. Primary polydipsia is most often caused by an abnormality in the thirst center of the brain. Unquenchable thirst results in water intoxication. Dipsogenic DI is differentiated from central (pituitary) DI using the water deprivation test. There is no cure for dipsogenic DI at present, but symptoms can be safely relieved. Psychogenic polydipsia is another subtype; it is because of psychosomatic causes and has no treatment that is recognized as consistently effective.

The most common presentation of DI is following head trauma or intracranial surgery. When a person cannot adequately respond to stimulation of the thirst center by drinking fluids, extracellular and intracellular dehydration may result. Electrolyte imbalance, primarily hypernatremia, may produce neurologic symptoms ranging from confusion, restlessness, and irritability to seizures and coma. DI sometimes occurs in brain-dead organ donors and must be managed to effectively preserve organs.

In normal individuals, a more concentrated circulating volume stimulates ADH release through activation of osmoreceptors that monitor serum osmolality. ADH is also released as part of the renin-angiotensin-aldosterone mechanism as a result of hypotension sensed by the juxtomedullary apparatus located outside the glomerulus of the kidney. A 5% to 10% decrease in arterial BP is necessary to increase circulating vasopressin concentrations. Progressive hypotension in individuals who are healthy results in an exponential increase in plasma ADH via baroreceptor stimulation, whereas osmoregulated ADH release in response to dehydration is more linear. If the hypothalamus is damaged, production of ADH may not be possible and both the ability to regulate circulating volume and vascular tone may be affected. Baroregulated (pressure response) release of vasopressin is a key physiologic mediator in an integrated hemodynamic response to volume depletion.

ENDOCRINE ASSESSMENT: DIABETES INSIPIDUS

GOAL OF ASSESSMENT

The clinical presentation of DI is dependent on the overall health of the patient and the primary cause. Evaluate for degree of dehydration and its effects on overall hemodynamics, heart rate/rhythm, and mental status. Generally, DI is recognized and managed before resulting in serious complications. Practitioners working with brain-dead organ donors must be particularly alert to the occurrence of DI. Severe, unmanaged, or undermanaged dehydration in cases of DI may cause hemoconcentration, which may predispose the patient to thrombosis. Dehydration and electrolyte imbalance must be prevented or managed immediately to avoid possible organ damage.

HISTORY AND RISK FACTORS

Central/Hypothalamic/Pituitary Diabetes Insipidus

Brain tumors, especially in the hypothalamus or pituitary region; neoplasms such as leukemia or breast cancer; surgery in the area of the pituitary gland; intracranial hemorrhage; brain death; head injury, especially to the base of the brain; meningitis or encephalitis; any disorder that causes increased intracranial pressure; cerebral hypoxia; and various inheritable defects. Those with genetic defects have the onset in early childhood. Genetic predisposition is revealed by family history.

Nephrogenic Diabetes Insipidus

From medications (e.g., lithium, demeclocycline, glyburide, phenytoin), insufficient dose prescribed of ADH, ethanol abuse, chronic hypercalcemia, hypokalemia, osmotic diuresis, congenital disorder of defective expression of renal vasopressin 2 (V_2) receptors, or patients with polycystic kidney disease, pyelonephritis, renal amyloidosis, myeloma, Sjögren syndrome, or sickle cell anemia.

Gestational Diabetes Insipidus

Seen in patients during the last trimester of pregnancy who have oligohydramnios, preeclampsia, and/or hepatic dysfunction. In addition to the blunted thirst response associated with pregnancy, these patients break down only endogenous vasopressin (ADH) and can be managed with synthetic vasopressin (desmopressin).

Dipsogenic Diabetes Insipidus

Unquenchable thirst with massive water intake; psychogenic causes may be associated with patients with a history of mental illness. Water intoxication from massive fluid intake presents with headache, loss of appetite, lethargy, and nausea and signs such as an abnormally large decrease in the plasma sodium concentration (hyponatremia).

VITAL SIGNS

- Tachycardia and tachypnea are present with dehydration.
- Diuresis alone may have no effect on vital signs if the patient is able to drink enough fluids.
- Orthostatic hypotension if dehydration is present.

OBSERVATION

- Polyuria with dilute urine; 3 to 20 Ld of urine may be excreted, with specific gravity of 1.000 to 1.005.

- History may include nocturia (getting up frequently at night to urinate) and/or enuresis (bed-wetting).
- Extreme thirst
- Dehydration: Poor skin turgor, dry mucous membranes, sunken eyes, slow capillary refill
  1. Electrolyte imbalance: Generalized weakness, possible exhaustion, nausea and vomiting, impaired vision and leg cramps may be present; patients may become unable to get out of bed.
  2. Urine output: More than 200 mL/h for 2 consecutive hours or greater than 500 mL/h, especially if risk factors are present.
  3. Hemodynamics: CVP less than 2 mm Hg; PAWP less than 6 mm Hg. It is not routine practice to use hemodynamic monitoring solely to manage DI, but if DI develops in a critically ill patient, readings typically reflect hypovolemia.
- Altered mental status: Serum hyperosmolality and hypernatremia affect consciousness and behavior. Changes may also be related to the underlying disease.
  1. Cranial nerve examination may be abnormal, with nerve palsies present.
  2. Altered level of consciousness (confusion, disorientation, agitation) is more common with older adults; in extreme unmanaged cases, coma and seizures are possible.

AUSCULTATION
- In rare cases, bowel sounds may be lessened if hypovolemic shock has reduced abdominal vessel perfusion.

SCREENING LAB WORK
- Point-of-care (POC) capillary blood glucose to rule out hyperglycemia as the cause of diuresis
- Fluid and electrolyte imbalance screening:
  a. Electrolyte panel: To assess for hypernatremia and concentrations of other electrolytes associated with hemoconcentration
  b. Urinalysis/specific gravity: Assesses for dilute, poorly concentrated urine
  c. Urinary and serum osmolality: Values may become similar. When kidneys properly concentrate urine, urine osmolality is generally four times the value of serum osmolality.

Diagnostic Testing for Diabetes Insipidus

Test	Purpose	Normal Values	Abnormal Findings
Urine osmolality	Assesses for decreased concentration or dilute urine	24-h specimen: 300–900 mOsmol/kg of H_2O Random specimen: 50–1200 mOsmol/kg of H_2O Urine to serum ratio: 1:1 to 3:1	Decreased to <200 mOsmol/kg; may be higher if volume depletion is present
Urine specific gravity	Assesses for dilute urine	1.010 to 1.025	Specific gravity: <1.005
Serum osmolality	Assesses for concentrated blood/hemoconcentration	278 to 300 mOsmol/kg	Increased to >290 mOsmol/kg
Serum sodium	Monitors for hypernatremia	134 to 142 mEq/L	Increased to >147 mEq/L
Plasma ADH level (vasopressin level)	Assesses if vasopressin is elevated or decreased	<2.5 pg/mL or <2.3 pmol/L	Central DI: Decreased Nephrogenic DI: Normal or increased Gestational DI: Decreased Dipsogenic DI: Decreased

Diagnostic Testing for Diabetes Insipidus — cont'd

Test	Purpose	Normal Values	Abnormal Findings
Water deprivation test (Miller-Moses test) Dehydration should prompt the kidneys to concentrate urine.	To distinguish between the types of DI. Assesses for changes in weight, serum and urine osmolality, and specific gravity when fluid intake is prohibited.		Differentiates psychogenic polydipsia from DI. Central DI and NDI are unaffected by this test.
ADH (Vasopressin) test ADH administration will correct the problem if ADH was lacking.	Assesses if the kidneys begin to concentrate urine when ADH is administered. Distinguishes NDI from other types of DI.		Corrects central/neurogenic DI, wherein ADH is lacking. NDI is unaffected by ADH administration, since the problem is unrelated to lack of ADH.
Brain or pituitary magnetic resonance imaging (MRI)	MRI scan used to identify pituitary lesions that may have caused the DI.		If the patient has the "bright spot" or hyperintense emission from the posterior pituitary gland, the patient likely has primary polydipsia. If the "bright spot" is small or absent, the patient likely has central DI.

COLLABORATIVE MANAGEMENT

CARE PRIORITIES

1. Rehydrate if Dehydration and/or Hypovolemia are Present

- Place at least two large-bore IV lines, or have a central line inserted.
- Administer hypotonic IV fluids (5% dextrose solution, 0.45% saline). Hyperglycemia and volume overload should be avoided.
- In the geriatric population, be aware of individual comorbidities such as diabetes and congestive heart failure during rehydration.
- Avoid overly aggressive correction of hypernatremia. Do not decrease sodium level by more than 5mEq/L/h or more than 12 mEq/L within 24 hours.
- The patient may be allowed to drink fluids, with the volume accurately recorded.
- Monitor urine output every 1 to 2 hours. Fluid can be replaced milliliter for milliliter. Total water deficit may be estimated by assuming body water composes approximately 60% of total body weight in kilograms.
- Formula for calculating body water deficit: (0.6 [weight in kilograms]) × (serum sodium − 140)/140 = body water deficit (in liters)
- Monitor continuous ECG for tachycardia and dysrhythmias.
- Evaluate basic ABCs (airway, breathing, and circulation) if the patient becomes hypotensive.
- Monitor daily weights.

2. Administer Exogenous ADH (Vasopressin) (for Central DI and Gestational DI)

- Use of desmopressin acetate (DDAVP) is popular because it produces fewer side effects (Table 8-3).
- Several preparations are available, and dosage is adjusted to the patient's response to DI management. Vasopressin's potential vasoconstrictive effects occur rarely with appropriate dosing for management of DI. Excessive dosing of ADH may cause hypertension and cardiac symptoms; other side effects include abdominal cramping and increased peristalsis.

3. Manage Electrolyte Imbalances, Focusing on Hypernatremia

- Before rehydration, patients are hypernatremic. Hypernatremia should resolve with aggressive hydration.
- Serum osmolality, electrolyte levels (sodium and potassium) should be measured at least daily. They should be monitored more frequently if the patient has hemodynamic instability.

Table 8-3	VASOPRESSIN PREPARATIONS					
Generic Name	**Trade Name**	**Route**	**Onset**	**Duration**	**Total Daily Dose**	**Comments**
Desmopressin acetate	DDAVP Stimate Minirin	Intranasal	1 to 2 hours	8 to 12 hours	10 to 40 µg daily	Administered by nasal spray or rhinal tube applicator Action decreased by nasal congestion/discharge or atrophy of nasal mucosa Stored in refrigerator Drug of choice for chronic CDI
		Subcutaneous	Within ½ hour	1.5 to 4 hours	0.1 to 2 µg daily in two divided doses	Keep refrigerated More potent than intranasal route
		Intravenous	Within ½ hours	1.5 to 4 hours	0.1 to 2 µg daily in two divided doses	Keep refrigerated More potent than intranasal route
		Oral tablets	1 to 2 hours	8 to 12 hours	100 to 1000 µg daily in two or three divided doses	Simple to use More consistent absorption and few side effects
Vasopressin	Pitressin	Subcutaneous	1 to 2 hours	2 to 8 hours	5 to 10 units (20 U/mL)	Used primarily to confirm the diagnosis, differentiate between CDI and NDI, and treat acute situations.
		Intramuscular	1 to 2 hours	2 to 8 h	5 to 60 U daily given in two to four divided doses	
		Continuous intravenous infusion	Within ½ hour		0.2 U/min and titrated to a maximum dose of 0.9 U/min	Titrate for Urine <200 mL/h
Lysine vasopressin	Diapid	Intranasal	Within 1 hour	3 to 8 hours	7 to 14 µg in four doses (every 6 hours)	Lower cost than DDAVP for patients with partial CDI who require one or two daily doses.

CDI, Central diabetes insipidus; NDI, nephrogenic diabetes insipidus.

4. Identify and Manage the Precipitating Cause

- As dehydration is managed, efforts should be underway to identify the cause of DI, if not initially known, using the water deprivation test and ADH test. A thorough history and physical examination may help identify possible causes. Consider NDI in the elderly patients using polypharmacy. Consider NDI in patients with a history of mental illness. NDI can occur in patients with a remote history of lithium use.
- Subsequent diagnostics may be needed to identify additional disease processes that may have resulted in DI.

5. Manage NDI (ADH-insensitive) with pharmacotherapy

- Thiazide diuretics (e.g., hydrochlorothiazide [HCTZ]) in combination with a low-sodium diet are the major form of therapy for NDI to reduce the loss of free water in the urine.
- Chlorpropamide stimulates the release of ADH and facilitates the renal response to ADH.
- Amiloride hydrochloride (a potassium-sparing diuretic) is the medication of choice for the treatment of lithium-induced NDI.
- Nonsteroidal antiinflammatory drugs (NSAIDs) such as indomethacin have been used as adjunctive therapy in NDI.

CARE PLANS FOR DIABETES INSIPIDUS

DEFICIENT FLUID VOLUME *related to diuresis secondary to ADH deficiency or altered ADH action.*

Goals/Outcomes: Within 12 hours of initiating treatment, the patient is euvolemic, reflected by BP 90/60 mm Hg or greater (or within patient's normal range), mean arterial pressure (MAP) 70 mm Hg or greater, HR 60 to 100 bpm, CVP 2 to 6 mm Hg, urinary output 0.5 to 1.5 mL/kg/h, intake equal to output plus insensible losses, firm skin turgor, pink and moist mucous membranes, and stable weight. ECG exhibits normal sinus rhythm. Electrolyte values are serum sodium 137 to 147 mEq/L, serum osmolality 275 to 300 mOsmol/kg, urine osmolality 300 to 900 mOsmol/24 h, and urine specific gravity 1.010–1.030.

NOC Fluid Balance, Electrolyte and Acid-Base Balance, Hydration

Hypovolemia Management

1. Monitor vital signs every 15 minutes until the patient is stable for 1 hour. Monitor CVP, MAP, and, if hemodynamic monitoring was in place, pulmonary artery pressure (PAP), and pulmonary capillary wedge pressure (PCWP), if ordered. Consult advanced practice provider for the following: HR greater than 140 bpm or BP less than 90/60 mm Hg or decreased more than 20 mm Hg from baseline, or MAP decreased more than 10 mm Hg from baseline, CVP less than 2 mm Hg, and PAWP less than 6 mm Hg. Manage judiciously in all patients, including organ donors who are brain-dead.
2. Monitor hydration status: mucous membranes, pulse rate and quality, and BP. Excessive water intake may result in fluid overload, particularly in elders and children.
3. Administer hypotonic solutions (e.g., D_5W, $D_50.25$, or 0.45 NaCl) for intracellular rehydration. Usually, fluids are administered as follows: 1 mL IV fluid for each 1 mL of urine output. In patients with brain injury, moderate diuresis may be permitted to avoid the need for administering osmotic diuretics. Hypernatremia, if present, must be corrected slowly (at a rate no greater than 0.5 mEq/L/h or 12 mEq/L/d) to prevent cerebral edema, seizures, permanent neurologic damage, or death.
4. Administer exogenous ADH as ordered. Observe for a reduction in urine output. Monitor for side effects: hypertension, cardiac ischemia, and hyponatremia.
5. Weigh the patient daily, at the same time and using the same scale and while the patient is wearing the same garments to prevent error. Consult an advanced practice provider for weight loss greater than 1 kg/d.
6. Observe for indications of dehydration (e.g., poor skin turgor, delayed capillary refill, weak/thready pulse, dry mucous membranes, hypotension).
7. Monitor for fluid overload, which can occur as a result of rapid infusion of fluid or excessive fluid intake in patients with heart failure: jugular vein distention, dyspnea, crackles (rales), and CVP greater than 12 mm Hg.
8. If urinary catheter has been removed, observe for resolution of nocturia (waking up at night to urinate) and enuresis (bed-wetting) as treatment progresses.

Fluid/Electrolyte Management

1. Monitor laboratory studies, observing for an appropriate response to treatment, including a decrease in serum sodium, increase in serum and urine osmolality, and increase in urine specific gravity.

2. Monitor urine specific gravity hourly to evaluate response to therapy. Patients may be allowed to develop hypotonic polyuria between doses of vasopressin to demonstrate persistence of DI when transient DI is suspected.
3. Report lack of improvement or deterioration to the advanced practice provider. Urine output greater than 200 mL/h for 2 consecutive hours, or 500 mL/h in the presence of risk factors, should be reported.
4. Instruct patients with permanent DI to wear a medical alert bracelet labeled with DI. Immediate family members should be familiar with the patient's current treatment plan in case they are contacted in an emergency.

NIC Fluid Monitoring; Intravenous (IV) Therapy; Invasive Hemodynamic Monitoring; Electrolyte Management: Hypernatremia

DISTURBED SENSORY PERCEPTION (VISUAL AND AUDITORY) *related to hyperosmolality, dehydration, or hypernatremia.*

Goals/Outcomes: The patient verbalizes orientation to time, place, and person; the patient is protected from unnecessary complications and bodily injury.
NOC Cognitive Orientation

Surveillance
1. Monitor neurologic status frequently. Notify advanced practice provider of deterioration.
2. Keep bed in lowest position with side rails raised if the patient is confused.
3. Consider nasogastric tube with suction for comatose or brain-dead organ donor patients to decrease likelihood of aspiration.
4. Elevate head of the bed (HOB) to 30 degrees to minimize the risk of aspiration.

NIC Neurologic Monitoring

RISK FOR INFECTION *related to inadequate primary defenses secondary to incisional opening into sella turcica for patients who have undergone transphenoidal hypophysectomy.*

Goals/Outcomes: The patient is free of infection as evidenced by normothermia; verbalization of orientation to time, place, and person; and absence of cerebrospinal fluid (CSF) leakage or nuchal rigidity. HR 100 bpm or less, BP within patient's normal range, white blood cell (WBC) count $11,000/mm^3$ or less, and negative culture results.
NOC Infection Severity, Immune Status

Infection Protection
1. For patients who have undergone transphenoidal hypophysectomy, inspect nasal packing often for frank bleeding or evidence of CSF leak. If glucose is detected in clear nasal drainage (tested using a glucose reagent stick), CSF is leaking, which indicates a flaw in cranial bone integrity. (See Care of the Patient After Intracranial Surgery, Chapter 7.)
2. Elevate the HOB to minimize the chance of bacterial migration into the brain if CSF leak is suspected. Consult advanced practice provider promptly.
3. Monitor for infection, including elevated temperature, nuchal rigidity, and altered LOC.
4. Monitor for increased WBC count, which initially may reflect dehydration or the stress response.
5. Because the patient is at higher risk for bacterial infection, invasive lines should be managed carefully to avoid bloodstream infection (BSI). Central lines should be removed as soon as possible.
6. To prevent injury and contamination of operative site, patients should not brush their teeth until instructed to do so by the physician. Provide sponge-tipped applicators for oral hygiene.

NIC Incision Site Care; Infection Protection; Neurologic Monitoring

DEFICIENT KNOWLEDGE: ILLNESS CARE *related to the need to manage transient to permanent DI and possible management of additional hormonal imbalance if anterior pituitary was damaged or removed; care after transphenoidal hypophysectomy.*

Goals/Outcomes: Before discharge from ICU, the patient verbalizes understanding of the basics of DI management and care after transphenoidal hypophysectomy, if appropriate.
NOC Knowledge: Illness Care; Knowledge: Medication; Knowledge: Treatment Regimen

Teaching: Procedure/Treatment
1. Teach the patient appropriate administration of exogenous vasopressin and its side effects.
2. Explain exogenous hormone replacement if the anterior pituitary gland was damaged or removed during surgery. If the patient is also experiencing anterior pituitary dysfunction (panhypopituitarism), teach the indicators of hormone replacement excess or deficiency.
   - Adrenal hormone excess: weight gain, moon face, easy bruising, fatigue, polyuria, polydipsia
   - Adrenal hormone deficiency: weight loss, easy fatigability, abdominal pain, excess pigmentation
   - Thyroid hormone excess: heat intolerance, irritability, tachycardia, weight loss, diaphoresis
   - Thyroid hormone deficiency: bradycardia, cold intolerance, weight gain, slowed mentation
   - Androgen replacement deficiency: some degree of sexual dysfunction, ranging from menstrual irregularities to infertility and impotence
3. Demonstrate the method for accurate measurement of urine specific gravity and the importance of keeping accurate records of test results.
4. Teach when to seek medical attention, including signs of dehydration (hypernatremia) and water intoxication (hyponatremia).
5. Explain the importance of obtaining a medical alert bracelet and identification (ID) card.
6. Stress the importance of continued medical follow-up.
7. For patients with permanent need for hormone replacement, explain the method for obtaining a medical alert bracelet and ID card outlining diagnosis and appropriate treatment in the event of an emergency.

NIC Teaching: Disease Process; Teaching: Prescribed Medication; Emotional Support

ADDITIONAL NURSING DIAGNOSES

If the patient has developed DI following a transphenoidal hypophysectomy, see Decreased intracranial adaptive capacity, Ineffective breathing pattern, Risk for infection, and Pain in Care of the Patient after Intracranial Surgery, Chapter 7; also see Hypernatremia and Hyponatremia in Fluid and Electrolyte Disturbances, Chapter 1.

HYPERGLYCEMIA

PATHOPHYSIOLOGY

Over the last several decades, the incidence of diabetes mellitus has risen. According to the 2014 National Diabetes Statistics Report, 29.1 million Americans, or 9.3% of the U.S. population, have diabetes. Of these, 8.1 million people are undiagnosed. The disease is associated with serious complications, including heart disease, stroke, kidney disease, various eye diseases, and nerve damage, which contribute to increased medical costs. Direct costs of care are about $176 billion dollars; 2.3 times higher than for people without diabetes.

Type 1 and type 2 diabetes result from separate causes. People with type 1 diabetes are genetically predisposed to a trigger, often a viral illness, which results in destruction of the insulin-producing beta cells in the pancreas, leading to an abrupt, permanent loss of insulin production. Insulin is the hormone that attaches cells, allowing passage of glucose from the bloodstream into the cell. People with type 1 diabetes require daily insulin injections to support their basal metabolic needs and to manage hyperglycemia resulting from food ingestion.

People with type 2 diabetes are initially insulin-resistant and subsequently have a gradual decline in insulin production and secretion over years of time. T-defective cellular insulin receptors do not allow transport of glucose into the cell by insulin. The lack of receptor insulin sensitivity is associated with increased hepatic glucose production, given cells "signal" that the intracellular environment lacks glucose needed to produce sufficient energy for effective cellular function of all organs and body systems. Additional hepatic glucose production further increases blood glucose levels. Type 2 diabetes is initially treated with oral agents and is likely to require insulin as the disease progresses.

The importance of managing hyperglycemia in hospitalized patients came to the forefront in 2001 with a landmark study by Van den Berghe and colleagues. The study revealed dramatic improvement in outcomes of postoperative cardiovascular surgical intensive care patients when glucose was maintained at 80 to 110 mg/dL using IV insulin as opposed to a conventional treatment goal of 180 to 200 mg/dL. With this goal for "tight control," patients with no previous history of diabetes often required treatment as well because, postoperatively, the stress response elevated blood glucose. After 12 months of study, intensive insulin therapy reduced ICU mortality to 4.6% from 8.0% with conventional therapy ($P < 0.04$ with adjustment for sequential analyses). For patients who remained in the unit longer than 5 days, mortality using intensive insulin therapy was reduced to 10.6% from 20.2% using conventional therapy. Total in-hospital mortality was reduced 34%, BSIs by 46%, acute renal failure requiring dialysis or hemofiltration by 41%, the median number of red blood cell transfusions by 50%, and critical illness polyneuropathy by 44%. The greatest reduction in mortality involved deaths caused by multiple organ failure with a proven sepsis focus. Many hospitals found this target unachievable, given that the risk of hypoglycemia was too high, unless there was a knowledgeable champion to oversee safe, effective, and efficient methods of insulin administration.

The Van den Berghe study raised awareness of the importance of glycemic control. In early 2009, the NICE SUGAR study improved practice by providing a more realistic, safer, and achievable target glucose range. The trial highlighted the unacceptably high incidence of hypoglycemia seen with tight control and recommended hypoglycemia could be avoided while maintaining glucose control using a less stringent target. On the basis of this study, the American Diabetes Association (ADA) and American Association of Clinical Endocrinologists (AACE) now recommend patients who are critically ill be controlled to glucose values of 140 to 180 mg/dL. For more stable hospitalized patients who are eating meals, the recommendation is for premeal blood glucose values be less than 140 mg/dL. There are patients who may benefit from a lower target, but, given the nature of critical illness, the target glucose range should not be lower than 110 mg/dL for patients who are critically ill. The Society of Thoracic Surgeons recognizes use of IV insulin for cardiac surgery patients to maintain a target of 110 to 140 mg/dL as a class I treatment recommendation.

No "best" method for dosing and delivery of IV insulin has been established. Evidence revealed insulin binds to IV tubing, and therefore 20 to 50 ml must be flushed through the tubing into an external receptacle before initiating the insulin infusion. Binding sites within the wall of the tubing are "saturated" with insulin by this procedure, allowing for all insulin within the infusion to be delivered to the patient. There are no guidelines for standardization of a "loading dose" or initial IV bolus, at what rate to begin the infusion, or titration to the patient's response. Thus, glucose management targets have been set without a "road map" for how to safely achieve them. Institutions are best served to have an interprofessional committee decide the type of dosing and monitoring regimen that is both safe and feasible. The patient population, available infusion pumps, nurse and physician expertise with evidence-based hyperglycemia management practices, nurse staffing, and physician support must be considered to both control blood glucose and protect patients from hypoglycemia. Many published protocols require hourly glucose monitoring and dosage adjustment. Given the workload associated with hourly monitoring, several computerized insulin-dosing systems are available to assist nurses with ongoing infusion management.

Despite quality organizations and insurers' familiarity with the challenges of glycemic control, in October 2009, occurrences of hypoglycemia, diabetic ketoacidosis (DKA), and hyperglycemic hyperosmolar syndrome (HHS) were deemed "never events" for hospitalized patients. If patients can be harmed by the occurrence of a problem acquired in the hospital, insurers are not required to pay for care associated with a selection of those events considered preventable. If patients are admitted with a history of the selected condition, hospitals are paid if the problem reoccurs during hospitalization. Careful admission screening of all patients related to past experience with both hyperglycemia and hypoglycemia is of paramount importance to realize payment for treatment of the patients.

DIABETIC KETOACIDOSIS
PATHOPHYSIOLOGY

DKA is a life-threatening complication of diabetes mellitus characterized by hyperglycemic crisis, ketosis, acidosis, hypovolemic shock caused by dehydration, and electrolyte imbalance involving potassium. Progressive hyperglycemia occurs because of inadequate circulating insulin, preventing cellular uptake of glucose and resulting in a state of starvation at the cellular level. Without glucose available inside the cells, the cells are unable to perform their work effectively. Starvation prompts glucagon secretion from the pancreas and release of other stress hormones, including catecholamines, cortisol, and GH, which facilitate glycogenolysis and gluconeogenesis, further raising plasma glucose. Intracellular hypoglycemia continues to prompt a series of responses in an effort to produce glucose to "feed" the "starving cell." Proteolysis and lipolysis ensue, forming free fatty acids, which are converted to ketoacids (acetoacetate, β-hydroxybutyrate, and acetone), caused by lack of intracellular glucose required for normal metabolic conversion of the acids.

Accumulation of ketones creates a metabolic acidosis. The excessive glucose and ketones in the blood cause severe osmotic diuresis as intracellular fluids move into the vascular compartment to dilute the blood; however, the excess fluid is eliminated by the kidneys, which also lose the ability to effectively eliminate excess glucose. A vicious cycle of progressive metabolic disruption begins and will continue until hydration, insulin, and additional management of acidosis/fluid and electrolyte imbalance are provided. Osmotic diuresis causes loss of sodium, potassium, phosphorus, magnesium, and body water, which leads to dehydration and, possibly, hypovolemic shock. Increased blood viscosity and platelet aggregation can result in thromboembolism.

Despite significant loss of potassium in the urine, the patient may initially manifest normal or elevated plasma potassium because of the dramatic shift of potassium out of the cells secondary to insulin deficiency, acidosis, and tissue catabolism. Dehydration lowers BP and decreases tissue perfusion. Because of a lack of oxygen delivery, cells begin anaerobic metabolism. The resulting lactic acid waste products worsen acidosis. Low pH stimulates the respiratory center, producing deep, rapid Kussmaul respirations. Abundant plasma ketones cause fruity or acetone breath. If not managed, elevated serum osmolality, acidosis, and dehydration depress consciousness to a coma state. Death can result.

The cause of death in patients with DKA and the other hyperglycemic emergency, HHS, is rarely caused by the metabolic complications of hyperglycemia or metabolic acidosis. Death is related to the underlying medical illness that caused the metabolic decompensation. Successful treatment depends on a prompt and careful evaluation for the precipitating cause(s). The clinical symptoms of DKA generally appear within 24 hours of failure to manage hyperglycemia.

HYPERGLYCEMIC HYPEROSMOLAR SYNDROME

PATHOPHYSIOLOGY

Hyperglycemic hyperosmolar syndrome (HHS) is a life-threatening emergency created by a relative insulin deficiency and significant insulin resistance, resulting in severe hyperglycemia with profound osmotic diuresis, leading to life-threatening dehydration and hyperosmolality. HHS is also known as hyperosmolar hyperglycemic state, hyperosmolar nonketotic syndrome (HONK), hyperosmolar nonketotic state (HNS), hyperglycemia hyperosmolar nonketotic syndrome (HHNS), and, traditionally, hyperosmolar hyperglycemic nonketotic coma (HHNK). HHNK, HHNS, HNS, and HONK are somewhat incorrect titles for the syndrome, as recent evidence reveals a mild degree of ketosis is often present with HHS, and true coma is uncommon. The mortality rate of HHS ranges from 10% to 50%, higher than that for DKA (1.2% to 9%). Mortality data are difficult to interpret because of the high incidence of coexisting diseases or comorbidities.

Historically, HHS and DKA were described as distinct syndromes, but one-third of patients exhibit findings of both conditions. HHS and DKA may be at opposite ends of a range of decompensated diabetes, differing in time of onset, degree of dehydration, and severity of ketosis. HHS occurs most commonly in older people with type 2 diabetes, but with the recent obesity epidemic, occasionally obese children and teenagers with both diagnosed and undiagnosed type 2 diabetes manifest HHS. The cascade of events in HHS begins with osmotic diuresis. Glycosuria impairs the ability of the kidney to concentrate urine, which exacerbates the water loss. Normally, the kidneys eliminate glucose above a certain threshold and prevent a subsequent rise in blood glucose level. In HHS, the decreased intravascular volume or possible underlying renal disease decreases the glomerular filtration rate, causing the glucose level to increase. More water is lost than sodium, resulting in hyperosmolarity. Insulin is present, but not in adequate amounts to decrease blood glucose levels, and with type 2 diabetes, significant insulin resistance is present. DKA and HHS are compared in Table 8-4.

Primary causes of HHS include infections, noncompliance with a diabetes management regimen, undiagnosed diabetes, medications, substance abuse, and coexisting diseases. Infections

Table 8-4	COMPARISON OF DIABETIC KETOACIDOSIS (DKA) AND HYPERGLYCEMIC HYPEROSMOLAR SYNDROME (HHS)	
Criterion	**DKA**	**HHS**
Diabetes type	Type 1	Type 2; rarely, Type 1
Typical age group	More common in young children and adolescents than adults	57 to 69 years with average age 60 years
Signs and symptoms	Polyuria, polydipsia, polyphagia, weakness, orthostatic hypotension, lethargy, changes in LOC, fatigue, nausea, vomiting, abdominal pain	Same as DKA, but slower onset Also, very commonly, neurologic symptoms predominate
Physical assessment	Dry and flushed skin, poor skin turgor, dry mucous membranes, decreased BP, tachycardia, altered LOC (irritability, lethargy, coma), Kussmaul respirations, fruity odor to the breath	Same as DKA, but no Kussmaul respirations or fruity odor to the breath; instead, occurrence of tachypnea with shallow respirations
History and risk factors	Recent stressors such as surgery, trauma, infection, MI; insufficient exogenous insulin; undiagnosed type 1 diabetes mellitus	Undiagnosed type 2 diabetes mellitus; recent stressors such as surgery, trauma, pancreatitis, MI, infection; high-calorie enteral or parenteral feedings in a compromised patient; use of diabetogenic drugs (e.g., phenytoin, thiazide diuretics, thyroid preparations, mannitol, corticosteroids, sympathomimetics)
Monitoring parameters	*ECG:* Dysrhythmias associated with hyperkalemia: peaked T waves, widened QRS complex, prolonged PR interval, flattened or absent P wave. Hypokalemia (K^+ <3 mEq/L), which may produce depressed ST segments, flat or inverted T waves, or increased ventricular dysrhythmias	ECG evidence of hypokalemia as listed with DKA Hemodynamic measurements: CVP <3 mm Hg below patient's baseline; PADP and PAWP <4 mm Hg below patient's baseline
Diagnostic tests	Serum glucose: >250 mg/dL	>600 mg/dL
	Serum ketones: Large presence	Usually absent to mild presence because of dehydration
	Urine glucose: Positive	Positive
	Urine acetone: "Large"	Usually negative
	Serum osmolality: >290 mOsmol/L	>320 mOsmol/L
	Bicarbonate: <15 mEq/L	>15 mEq/L
	Serum pH: <7.2	Normal or mildly acidotic (pH ≤7.4)
	Anion Gap: Elevated >13	Normal
	Serum potassium: normal or elevated >5.0 mEq/L initially and then decreased	Normal or >3.5 mEq/L
	Serum sodium: elevated, normal, or low	Elevated, normal, or low
	Serum Hct: elevated because of osmotic diuresis with hemoconcentration	Elevated because of hemoconcentration
	BUN: elevated >20 mg/dL	Elevated
	Serum creatinine: >1.5 mg/dL	Elevated
	Serum phosphorus, magnesium, chloride: decreased	Elevated
	WBC: elevated, even in the absence of infection	Normal unless infection present

Table 8-4	COMPARISON OF DIABETIC KETOACIDOSIS (DKA) AND HYPERGLYCEMIC HYPEROSMOLAR SYNDROME (HHS)—cont'd	
Criterion	**DKA**	**HHS**
Onset	A few days	Days to weeks
Mortality	1 to 10%	14 to 58% because of age group and complications such as stroke, thrombosis, renal failure

BP, Blood pressure; *BUN*, blood urea nitrogen; *CVP*, central venous pressure; *DKA*, diabetic ketoacidosis; *ECG*, electrocardiogram; *Hct*, hematocrit; *HHS*, hyperglycemic hyperosmolar syndrome; *LOC*, level of consciousness; *MI*, myocardial infarction; *PADP*, pulmonary artery diastolic pressure; *PAWP*, pulmonary artery wedge pressure; *WBC*, white blood cell count.

are the leading cause (57% of patients); pneumonia (often Gram-negative) is the most common, followed by urinary tract infection (UTI) and sepsis. Lack of compliance with diabetic medications or other aspects of diabetes management may be a frequent cause (21%). Undiagnosed diabetes prompts a failure to recognize early symptoms of the complications of unmanaged hyperglycemia. Acute coronary syndrome (myocardial infarction [MI]), stroke, pulmonary embolus, and mesenteric thrombosis have caused HHS. At least one study revealed that, in urban populations, the three leading causes are lack of compliance with medications, drinking alcohol, and using cocaine. Chronic use of steroids and gastroenteritis are commonly associated with HHS in children.

The blood glucose level is higher with HHS than with DKA. A global electrolyte loss is present. Sodium and potassium levels vary at diagnosis, but deficiencies of both are present. Magnesium, calcium, phosphate, and chloride deficiencies evolve. Patients may lose from 15% to 25% of total body water, or approximately 100 to 200 mL/kg. Fluids are drawn from cells to dilute the concentrated bloodstream, resulting in significant intracellular dehydration. Neurologic deficits occur in response to severe dehydration and hyperosmolality. The blood is highly viscous and flow slows, increasing risk for the formation of thromboemboli. Increased cardiac workload and decreased renal and cerebral blood flow may result in MI, renal failure, and stroke.

Unlike DKA, wherein acidosis produces severe symptoms, HHS develops slowly, and frequently symptoms are nonspecific. Polyuria and polydipsia occur but may be ignored. Neurologic deficits may be mistaken for dementia. Similarity of symptoms to other disease processes in older adults may delay diagnosis and treatment, allowing the process to progress.

METABOLIC ASSESSMENT: HYPERGLYCEMIA

GOAL OF METABOLIC ASSESSMENT

Evaluate for degree of hyperglycemia and its effects on overall hemodynamics, respiratory rate/pattern, and mental status. Hyperglycemia may be asymptomatic or, with DKA, result in hypotension causing decreased perfusion, increased work of breathing with Kussmaul respirations, ineffective breathing patterns, abdominal pain, and neurologic deficits, including coma and/or stroke-like symptoms. HHS findings are similar but are more likely to result in neurologic changes, cause abdominal pain less often, and almost never cause compensatory Kussmaul respirations, because acidosis is mild, if present at all. Dehydration, hyperglycemia, and acidosis must be managed immediately. Associated electrolyte imbalances may be managed as the patient's glucose level normalizes and hydration is provided.

HISTORY AND RISK FACTORS

Hyperglycemia manifests more commonly in hospitalized patients with diabetes mellitus or impaired glucose tolerance than in hospitalized patients without diabetes who experience an exaggerated response to stress. Patients who are obese are more likely to have insulin resistance associated with metabolic syndrome, impaired tolerance for glucose, or undiagnosed type 2 diabetes mellitus. Type 2 diabetic patients generally manifest HHS when hyperglycemia is ineffectively managed. Rarely, a patient with type 2 diabetes will manifest DKA. The

Hyperglycemia

majority of patients with DKA have type 1 diabetes mellitus. The patient with type 1 diabetes will die without adequate insulin administration.

Recent stressors that prompt DKA in patients with diabetes mellitus infection (20% to 55%)

This may be overestimated because DKA may prompt leukocytosis and vasodilation, which mimic sepsis.

Inadequate insulin/noncompliance (15% to 40%)

Teenagers may be at higher risk for noncompliance; all illnesses increase stress, which increases the need for insulin. Patients with type 1 diabetes are totally reliant on administration of exogenous insulin to control hyperglycemia, because without functional beta islet cells in the pancreas, they have no ability to produce insulin.

Undiagnosed diabetes (10% to 25%)

Onset of type 1 diabetes is generally preceded by a significant illness; often a viral infection or childhood disease.

Other medical illness (10% to 15%)

Pneumonia, UTI, ischemic bowel, pregnancy, hypothyroidism, pancreatitis, pulmonary embolism, surgery, and new medications (notably corticosteroids, sympathomimetics, alpha- and beta-blockers, fluoroquinolone antibiotics [Levaquin; Janssen Pharmaceuticals, Titusville, NJ], and diuretics)

Cardiovascular disease (3% to 10%)

Significant cardiovascular disease may be the result of diabetes mellitus, and thus unstable patients may experience variable stress levels, making control of hyperglycemia difficult. Vascular events such as MI, cerebrovascular accident (CVA), or ischemic bowel may precipitate or worsen DKA.

Cause unknown (5% to 35%)

Any physiologically stressing illness or event has the potential to cause the condition. Certain women are more likely to go into DKA at the time of menstruation. Severe emotional stress is associated with onset of DKA.

Recent stressors that prompt HHS in patients with diabetes mellitus

Diabetes: First symptomatic presentation of undiagnosed hyperglycemia; poor control of hyperglycemia (noncompliance, inadequate resources, abuse or neglect of the patient by caregivers or self-inflicted, accidental omission of medication, or ingestion of excessive carbohydrates)

Associated medical conditions

1. Infection: Urinary tract, pneumonia, cellulitis, sepsis, dental infection/abscess
2. Cardiovascular disease: MI or other acute coronary syndromes
3. Cerebral vascular disease: Stroke or intracranial hemorrhage
4. Temperature alteration: Hyperthermia or hypothermia
5. Mesenteric ischemia: Intestinal/bowel ischemia or bowel infarction
6. Pancreatitis
7. Pulmonary embolism
8. Acute abdomen
9. Acute renal failure or decompensated chronic renal failure ("acute on chronic")
10. Burns
11. Hyperthyroidism
12. GI bleeding
13. Cushing syndrome or other ACTH-secreting tumor

Medication-related

1. Beta-blockers: Metoprolol, atenolol, propranolol
2. Carbonic anhydrase inhibitors: Diazoxide

3. Calcium channel blockers: Diltiazem, verapamil
4. Antipsychotics: Chlorpromazine, olanzepine
5. Loop and thiazide diuretics: Furosemide, bumetanide, HCTZ
6. Glucose-containing fluids: Total parenteral nutrition, tube feedings, dialysis solutions
7. Glucocorticoids/steroids: Cortisone, hydrocortisone, prednisone, methylprednisolone
8. H_2-receptor antagonists: Ranitidine, cimetidine, famotidine
9. Anticonvulsants: Phenytoin
10. Substance abuse: Alcohol, amphetamines, cocaine, 3,4-methylenedioxy-methamphetamine, popularly known as "ecstasy")

VITAL SIGNS
- Findings vary significantly, depending on patient's situation. Mild to moderate hyperglycemia generally has no effect on vital signs.
- Tachycardia and tachypnea are present if a hyperglycemic crisis (DKA, HHS) is present or if hypoglycemia is present. Hypovolemia alone may prompt tachycardia and possibly associated tachypnea.
- Hypotension is present with DKA and HHS or if hypoglycemia is present.

OBSERVATION
- Mild to moderate hyperglycemia alone may not cause overt physical assessment changes.
- Skin should be examined for lesions, rashes, cellulitis, and other signs of possible infection.
- If the patient presents to the emergency department, observe for signs of recent alcohol consumption.
- DKA: Kussmaul respirations (rapid, deep) are present to exhale CO_2 as a compensatory response to relieve metabolic acidosis; may appear fatigued, with or without diaphoresis from Kussmaul breathing.
- DKA and HHS:
  1. Significant abdominal pain: Present in at least 40% of patients; paralytic ileus or gastroparesis may be present but will resolve when hyperglycemia and dehydration are managed.
  2. Hypoperfusion: Ashen, pale, or grayish blue facial color, lip color, or nail beds caused by severe hypotension and decreased blood volume because of dehydration
  3. Dehydration: Poor skin turgor, dry mouth and/or lips, sunken eyes, slow capillary refill
  4. Malaise: Generalized weakness, possible exhaustion, nausea and vomiting, impaired vision, and leg cramps may be present; patients may become unable to get out of bed.
  5. Cranial nerve dysfunction: Examination may be abnormal with nerve palsies present.
  6. Altered mental status: Confusion, disorientation and agitation are more common with older adults. Stroke-like symptoms may be present. Coma is present in about 10% of patients presenting with HHS. Seizures are present in 25% of HHS patients.
  7. Severe shock: If severe shock has ensued, agitation is more commonly associated with hypoxemia; somnolence is associated with hypercarbia (elevated CO_2 level) and acidosis.
  8. Associated findings: Heart failure, pneumonia, and other risk factors if hyperglycemic crisis is present.

AUSCULTATION
- Hyperglycemia does not change baseline physical assessment, unless it has progressed to crisis level (DKA, HHS).
- Clear breath sounds with DKA and HHS because dehydration is present.
- Bowel sounds may be absent if paralytic ileus and gastroparesis are present with DKA and HHS.
- Heart sounds may reflect heart failure with DKA and HHS.

PALPATION
- DKA: Abdomen may be palpated if abdominal pain is present.

PERCUSSION

- DKA and HHS: Lung percussion may reveal presence of consolidation or fluid (dullness) indicative of a pulmonary infection.

SCREENING LAB WORK

- POC capillary blood glucose: Bedside glucose monitoring using a glucose meter for immediate evaluation of capillary glucose level.
  - If POC glucose is elevated, a plasma glucose sample should be drawn.
  - In addition, if DKA or HHS is suspected:
- Arterial blood gas (ABG) analysis: Done promptly to evaluate for acidosis, hypoxemia, and hypercapnia
- Complete blood count (CBC): Evaluate for elevated WBCs indicative of infection
- Sputum and urine culture and sensitivity: Identifies infecting organism
- Blood culture and sensitivity: If positive, indicates organism has migrated into the bloodstream to cause a systemic infection

Diagnostic Tests for Hyperglycemia and Hyperglycemic Emergencies

Test	Purpose	Abnormal Findings
Hemoglobin A1c (HbA1c) or glycosylated hemoglobin: Performing this test more frequently than every 6 to 8 weeks does not yield useful information about blood glucose control	Assesses for control of blood glucose for the 6 to 8 weeks preceding the test. Recommended screening for a ll hospitalized patients so poorly controlled blood glucose readings can be addressed immediately to avoid development of DKA (diabetic keto-acidosis) or HHS (hyperglycemia hyperosmolar syndrome)	HbA1C target: <6.5–7 for most people. A less stringent target of 7 to 8% may be appropriate for patients with limited life expectancy, advanced complications, sever hypoglycemic unawareness or extensive comorbidities. An abnormal HbA1C result may be used to help determine if a change in the previous home plan is required. If a patient without diabetes has an elevated value, the patient should undergo a full evaluation for presence of undiagnosed diabetes.
Fasting blood glucose (FBG): Test is performed in the morning after fasting all night and before consuming breakfast.	Evaluates the effectiveness of basal insulin dosage by assessing for presence of hyperglycemia or hypoglycemia; used for daily screening of blood glucose control during hospitalization	≤40 mg/dL: Severe hypoglycemia 41 to 69 mg/dL: Hypoglycemia 70 to 110 mg/dL: Normoglycemia 111 to 125 mg/dL: Borderline hyperglycemia 126 to 180 mg/dL: Hyperglycemia 181 to 220 mg/dL: Significant hyperglycemia >220 mg/dL: Possible impending DKA or HHNS if glucose is not managed
Mealtime blood glucose: Generally, a point-of-care (POC) reading is done either 15 to 30 minutes before a meal or as the meal begins.	Assesses blood glucose control with existing hyperglycemia management program	Premeal glucose: < 110 mg/dL. If <140 mg/dL, no change in premeal dose of short-acting insulin is required. Once >140 mg/dL a supplemental dose of short-acting insulin may be necessary.
Postprandial blood glucose: May be done 1 to 2 hours following meals using serum glucose or point of care capillary glucose readings	Evaluates ability of glucose to normalize following a meal. Readings may be done 1–2 hours following the meal.	180 mg/dL: If glucose is >180 mg//dL at 1 hour following a meal, the patient is unable to produce enough insulin, or has not received enough mealtime insulin, or may be insulin-resistant, or may require initiation of mealtime insulin. 140 mg/dL: If glucose is >140 mg/dL at 2 hours following a meal, the patient is unable to produce enough insulin or may be insulin-resistant.

Diagnostic Tests for Hyperglycemia and Hyperglycemic Emergencies—cont'd

Test	Purpose	Abnormal Findings
Oral glucose tolerance test: Following at least 8 hours of fasting, oral glucose is consumed by the patient to determine how quickly it is cleared from the blood.	Used to test for diabetes, insulin resistance, and reactive hypoglycemia. Fasting blood glucose (FBG) is used at the beginning of the test. Additional readings are done 2 hours later. Fasting readings are compared to 2 hours after glucose ingestion to determine extent of glucose intolerance.	FBG 126 mg/dL with 2-hour reading 200 mg/dL: Confirms diagnosis of diabetes mellitus (DM) FBG 111 to 125 mg/dL with 2-hour reading >140 mg/dL: Patient has impaired glucose tolerance (IGT) FBG 111< to 125 mg/dL with 2-hour reading >140 mg/dL: Patient has impaired fasting glucose (IFT)
Arterial blood gas analysis (ABG): Done promptly, following confirmation of hyperglycemia to assess for DKA and HHS.	Assess for abnormal gas exchange or compensation for metabolic derangements in patients in hyperglycemic crisis; profound acidosis can indicate DKA is present, since HHS typically presents with minimal to mild acidosis unless prolonged, severe hypovolemic shock is present.	pH changes: With DKA, may be 6.8 to 7.2; acidosis results from ketosis or lactic acidosis Carbon dioxide: With DKA, decreased CO_2 reflects tachypnea and Kussmaul respirations Hypoxemia: With DKA or HHS, P_{AO_2} <80 mm Hg may indicate pneumonia precipitated the crisis Oxygen saturation: If pneumonia or heart failure is present, S_{AO_2} may be <92% Bicarbonate: HHS: $HCO_3$2 15 to 22 mEq/L; DKA: $HCO_3$2 may be <15 mEq/L Base deficit: HHS at or above −2; DKA, above −10
Complete blood count (CBC)	Evaluates for presence of infection	Increased WBC count: >11,000/mm^3 is seen with bacterial pneumonias, urinary tract infections and other infections.
Sputum Gram stain, culture, and sensitivity	Screens for pneumonia, a common underlying cause of hyperglycemic crisis; identifies infecting organism	Gram stain-positive: Indicates organism is present Culture: Identifies organism Sensitivity: Reflects effectiveness of drugs on identified organism
Blood culture and sensitivity	Screens for sepsis, a common underlying cause of hyperglycemic crisis Identifies whether an organism has become systemic	Secondary bacteremia: A frequent finding; patients with bacteremia are at higher risk for developing respiratory failure.
Blood chemistry	Screens for electrolyte imbalances; potassium imbalances may create potentially dangerous dysrhythmias	DKA and HHS: Hypernatremia is present: BUN, creatinine, and K1 may be elevated, normal, or low. Anion gap DKA: >13 Anion gap HHS: 10 to 12
Plasma osmolality	Screens for elevated osmolality associated with severe hyperglycemia	Osmolality is increased more with HHS than with DKA. DKA: 290 to 320 mmol/L HHS: >320 mmol/L
Urine ketones	Screens for the presence of ketones to confirm diagnosis of DKA; HHS does not cause ketonuria.	DKA: Ketones strongly positive HHS: Ketones negative, or mildly positive
12-Lead ECG	Used to rule out myocardial infarction as the cause of HHS or DKA	Hyperkalemia: Tall, peaked T waves if increased K^+ is present before management of hyperglycemia, hypovolemia and acidosis; PVCs/ventricular irritability is seen with decreased K^+ seen as insulin normalizes glucose.

Hyperglycemia

Continued

Diagnostic Tests for Hyperglycemia and Hyperglycemic Emergencies—cont'd		
Test	**Purpose**	**Abnormal Findings**
Chest radiograph	Screens for pneumonia and acute respiratory distress syndrome, which may prompt DKA and HHS	"Fluffy whiteness" may not initially be present caused by dehydration, but may appear as patient is rehydrated if patient has underlying pneumonia or ARDS
Computed tomography (CT) brain scan to altered mental status or "stroke-like" symptoms	Screens for ischemic and hemorrhagic stroke, which may prompt DKA and HHS	Generally not done until patient has had at least 1 hour of rehydration and insulin therapy to see if symptoms resolve spontaneously.

COLLABORATIVE MANAGEMENT

When managing hyperglycemia in hospitalized patients, the following key elements should be considered in evaluating current management blood glucose control strategies:

1. Oral hypoglycemic agents are not recommended for use in acutely ill or unstable hospitalized patients, because the response to therapy is unpredictable
2. Guidelines should be evidence-based and parallel the recommendations of the recognized expert organizations (ADA and AACE).
3. Protocols and/or order sets must be "user-friendly" and clearly written with minimal abbreviations and strive to keep mathematical calculations to a minimum.
4. A system should be in place to identify patients who need insulin or adjustment in an existing insulin regimen.
5. Variations in nutritional requirements and/or nutritional support should be identified, recognized, and included in the planning of any insulin-dosing regimen for patients with varying levels of stability as they move through the hospital.
6. Requirements for safe insulin administration, including availability of POC testing, IV pumps that can deliver volumes less than 1 mL accurately, and staffing with competent nurses must be considered before implementation of a glycemic control program.
7. Expert nurse consultants and/or certified diabetes educators who can provide education should be available to both patients and staff nurses.
8. An interdisciplinary team should be formed to address the following questions about the hospital's hyperglycemia management practices:
   A. Does the current insulin dosing regimen:
      1. Assume all patients can be placed into one of a few subgroups for dosage adjustment?
      2. Take into consideration the patient's insulin sensitivity and/or insulin resistance when titrating toward the target level?
      3. Provide small, incremental dosage changes to keep the patient safely within the target range without causing extreme fluctuations in glucose (hypoglycemia, when treated, resulting in hyperglycemia)?
      4. Have equipment/infusion reconstitution available for insulin dosage adjustments of 0.1 U/h, which several best practice dosing regimens require?
   B. Has the total hyperglycemia management approach been proved to be effective and safe and meet current evidence-based guidelines? Have data been gathered on the patients to measure both glucose control and incidence of hypoglycemia?
   C. Can nurses throughout the hospital safely implement the insulin-dosing regimen? During IV insulin infusions and when patients are transitioned from IV to subcutaneous insulin, nurses must be appropriately educated and have sufficient staffing to safely manage the patients.

CARE PRIORITIES

1. Resuscitate patients with severe dehydration in hypovolemic shock

- Evaluate basic ABCs: airway, breathing, and circulation.
- Intubate and ventilate patients with hypoxemia/decreasing oxygen saturation.
- Place at least two large-bore IV lines or have a central line inserted.
- Monitor continuous ECG, pulse oximetry, and frequent, if not constant, BP.

- Apply oxygen, or set oxygen appropriately if mechanical ventilation is used.
- Monitor urine output judiciously.
- Consider inserting a nasogastric tube if high risk for aspiration.

2. Provide aggressive rehydration to replace fluid loss from polyuria

HHS:

- Large amounts of isotonic IV fluids (normal saline, sometimes greater than 9 L) may be required to rehydrate the patient. Half-normal saline is sometimes used. Osmotic diuresis causes a 100 to 200 mL/kg fluid loss. At least 1 L of saline should be administered during the first hour of therapy. The remaining 8 L should ideally be infused within the next 24 hours.
- Once the blood sugar falls below 300 mg/dL, change the IV fluid to 5% dextrose with 45% NaCl at 150 to 250 ml/h.
- Hemodynamic or CVP monitoring may be needed to provide aggressive rehydration, as large amounts of fluids may not be well tolerated in older adults. Highly viscous blood is prone to thrombosis. Patients, particularly elders, are at risk of developing thrombotic complications before, during, and after a severe hyperglycemic crisis.

DKA:

- Large amounts of nondextrose, isotonic IV fluids are needed. Half-normal saline is sometimes used. From 1 to 2 L may be needed over the first 60 to 90 minutes. Approximately 4 L should be infused over the first 5 hours, and then the patient should be reevaluated for need for further hydration.
- Once the blood sugar falls below 300 mg/dL, change the IV fluid to 5% dextrose with 45% NaCl at 150–250 ml/h.
- Older patients or those with comorbidities that complicate therapy may require hemodynamic or CVP monitoring to guide fluid replacement. Rehydration improves perfusion, which improves oxygen delivery and thus helps to reestablish aerobic metabolism.
- As cellular metabolism normalizes, lactic and ketotic acidosis resolve.

3. Support hemodynamics/perfusion

Hemodynamic monitoring may be useful in guiding fluid replacement tolerance and efficacy and may help recognize the patient's response to the effects of other comorbidities. Although hypovolemic shock is the primary problem associated with hyperglycemia, cardiogenic shock may ensue if the patient has had an MI, or septic shock is possible if severe infection is present. Use of catecholamine infusions and steroids should be avoided, if possible, until hyperglycemia is resolved.

4. Control hyperglycemia

Continuous IV insulin infusion via infusion pump is the preferred method for delivering insulin. An initial IV insulin bolus may be administered at 0.1 U/kg. Many institutions use a concentration of 1 U of insulin in 1 mL of IV fluid to simplify rate and dosage calculations. The IV insulin infusion dose may be initiated at up to 0.1 U/kg/h during crisis states. It is imperative to perform hourly glucose monitoring for drip titration to ensure effectiveness of the dosage regimen. If the blood glucose does not decreased by 10%, or 50 mg/dL in the first hour, the infusion dose may need to be increased by 0.05–0.1 U/kg/h. Titrate the infusion to achieve a gradual blood glucose decrease of 50–70 mg/dL/h. Once the blood glucose is below 200 mg/dL for DKA and 300 mg/dL for HHS, decrease the insulin infusion rate by 50% to very gradually decrease blood glucose to achieve a target range of 140 to 180 mg/dL. For blood sugar less than 80 mg/dL, the insulin infusion can be held (paused) for 1 hour, then restarted at a lower rate. Achievement of target range or overshooting target range does not mean the insulin infusion can be permanently discontinued. The rationale is similar to the use of BP control medications. Achievement of the target is only the first step to sustained control. The transition from the insulin drip to a subcutaneous basal/bolus insulin regimen can occur when the patient can tolerate eating, the blood glucose falls is 200 mg/dL, $HCO_3$2 is above 18 mEq/L, pH is higher than 7.3, and anion gap is normal.

5. Manage electrolyte imbalances, focusing on potassium imbalances

Before rehydration, patients are hypernatremic and may be hyperkalemic. Those with DKA are more likely to be hyperkalemic because of the presence of metabolic acidosis, during which hydrogen ions force K1 (potassium ions) out of the cells into the bloodstream. As hydration progresses, perfusion improves, acidosis resolves, and potassium moves back into the cells, with a high probability of creating hypokalemia. Electrolytes should be measured every 2 hours. Begin adding 20 to 30 mEq/L potassium to the IV solution when the level falls below 5.2 mEq/L, with the aim of keeping the potassium level between 4–5 mEq/L. Should the potassium level fall below 3.3 mEq/L during the process of controlling the hyperglycemic crisis, immediately hold (pause) the IV insulin to slow movement of potassium out of the blood stream and into the cell, to avoid life-threatening dysrhythmias. Replacement of calcium, magnesium, and phosphates may be done as needed. Chlorides are replaced by the normal saline IV solutions. Use of bicarbonate for management of acidosis is not recommended, unless the acidosis does not respond to hydration and insulin or when essential medications needed for support of hemodynamics fail to work in the acidotic environment (e.g., if catecholamines are needed to support BP).

6. Identify and manage the precipitating cause

As hyperglycemia is managed, further efforts should be underway to identify the cause of the hyperglycemic crisis. A robust listing of risk factors and probable causes was included in the beginning of the hyperglycemia section with infections and cardiac and vascular occlusive events as the most likely precipitating events for the hyperglycemic crisis. If the pH and anion gap fail to improve with hydration and insulin, other causes of shock and acidosis should be evaluated and managed accordingly.

CARE PLANS FOR HYPERGLYCEMIA

GLUCOSE, RISK FOR UNSTABLE BLOOD *related to hyperglycemia resulting from the stress response associated with critical illness, and in those who have or may be at risk for diabetes mellitus.*

Goals/Outcomes: The patient is free of hyperglycemia reflected by normoglycemia and normovolemia; pH and serum osmolality are within normal limits.

NOC Blood Glucose Level, Hydration

Hyperglycemia Management
1. Monitor blood glucose levels as ordered or according to protocol.
2. Facilitate the patient having HbA1c measured to assess for glycemic control before hospitalization. If the patient has received transfusions, HbA1c is no longer a reliable measure of blood glucose control, because the patient is circulating blood that includes another person's glycohemoglobin.
3. Assess for signs and symptoms of hyperglycemia, including polyuria, polyphagia, blurred vision, headache, change in LOC, weakness, and lethargy.
4. Monitor for urine ketones if the patient has type 1 diabetes, is prone to ketosis because of type 2 diabetes, or manifests severe hyperglycemia.
5. Monitor ABGs in severely hyperglycemic patients to assess if acidosis is present.
6. Identify possible causes of hyperglycemia and work with physicians to construct an individualized management plan.
7. Evaluate hydration status if the patient has been hyperglycemic with polyuria caused by osmotic diuresis.
8. Encourage oral noncaloric fluid/water intake.
9. Monitor for potassium imbalance, with awareness that hyperglycemic patients can experience wide variation in potassium when IV insulin therapy is used to control hyperglycemia. As glucose normalizes, hypokalemia may be present and should be managed with careful potassium replacement.
10. Instruct the patient and significant others on how to prevent, recognize, and manage hyperglycemia.
11. Encourage the patient to participate in POC testing to assist in refining testing techniques if needed.
12. Discuss the need to count and control ingested carbohydrates to provide the best opportunity for glycemic control. Explain the difference in simple (bad) and complex (good) carbohydrates and how they are metabolized.
13. Ensure the patient understands the need for adherence to the prescribed diet and exercise regimen.
14. Assess whether or not the patient has the financial means to procure the proper food and medications to control hyperglycemia following discharge from the hospital.

Hypoglycemia Management
1. Identify patients at increased risk for hypoglycemia.
2. Monitor blood glucose levels carefully as ordered, especially if insulin is used to manage hyperglycemia.

3. Assess for signs and symptoms of hypoglycemia, including changes in personality, irritability, shakiness or tremors, sweating, nervousness, palpitations, tachycardia, nausea, headache, dizziness, weakness, faintness, blurred vision, difficulty concentrating, confusion, coma, or seizures.
4. Maintain IV access for more precise management of hypoglycemia using IV 50% dextrose rather than glucagon for instances of severe hypoglycemia that render the patient unable to take glucose tablets, juice, or milk.
5. Ensure the patient is given IV fluids containing 5% dextrose when glucose approaches 250 mg/dL if receiving an IV insulin infusion for management of severe hyperglycemia.
6. Keep the patient off oral food and fluids or on a no-calorie liquid diet while receiving an insulin infusion. If patients receive meals while insulin is infusing, additional mealtime subcutaneous insulin should be given, rather than adjusting IV insulin to cover glucose increases resulting from meals. If the IV insulin infusion is titrated upward throughout the day for meals, the probability of hypoglycemia is high when the patient stops eating meals at night.
7. Instruct the patient and significant others regarding the signs, symptoms, and management of hypoglycemia.
8. Collaborate with the patient and care team members to make changes in the insulin regimen if hypoglycemic episodes occur more than occasionally.

FLUID VOLUME, DEFICIENT *related to hyperglycemia-induced dehydration and osmotic diuresis.*

Goals/Outcomes: Within 12 hours of initiating treatment, the patient is euvolemic as evidenced by BP 90/60 mm Hg or greater (or within patient's normal range), MAP 70 mm Hg or greater, HR 60 to 100 bpm, CVP 2 to 6 mm Hg, balanced I&O, urinary output 0.5 mL/kg/h or greater, firm skin turgor, and pink and moist mucous membranes. ECG exhibits normal sinus rhythm.
NOC Fluid Balance, Electrolyte and Acid–Base Balance, Hydration

Hypovolemia Management
1. Monitor vital signs every 15 minutes until the patient is stable for 1 hour. Monitor CVP, MAP, and possibly PAP and PCWP, if ordered. Consult advanced practice provider for the following: HR greater than 140 bpm or BP less than 90/60 or decreased 20 mm Hg or greater, or MAP decreased 10 mm Hg or greater from baseline, CVP less than 4 mm Hg, and PAWP less than 6 mm Hg.
2. Monitor hydration status: mucous membranes, pulse rate and quality, and BP.
3. Monitor I&O. Decreased urine output may indicate inadequate fluid volume or impending renal failure. Consult physician for urine output less than 0.5 mL/kg/h for 2 consecutive hours.
4. Replace volume with IV fluids. Monitor for fluid overload, which can occur as a result of rapid infusion of fluids: jugular vein distention, dyspnea, crackles (rales), and CVP greater than 6 mm Hg.

Fluid/Electrolyte Management
1. Monitor for abnormal electrolyte levels as ordered.
2. Note an increase in anion gap (greater than 14 mEq/L), signaling increased production or decreased excretion of acids. Anion gap should decrease steadily with successful treatment of DKA.
3. Monitor for symptomatic cardiac dysrhythmias. (See Fluid and Electrolyte Disturbances, Chapter 1.)
4. Observe for clinical signs of electrolyte imbalance associated with DKA and its treatment:
   • Hypokalemia: Ventricular dysrhythmias, muscle weakness, anorexia, and hypoactive bowel sounds
   • Hypophosphatemia: Muscle weakness, malaise, confusion, respiratory failure, decreased oxygen delivery, and decreased cardiac function
   • Hypomagnesemia: Anorexia, nausea, vomiting, lethargy, weakness, personality changes, tetany, tremor or muscle fasciculations, seizures, confusion, and difficulty managing hypokalemia
5. Weigh the patient daily, and monitor trends.

NIC Fluid Monitoring; Invasive Hemodynamic Monitoring; Acid-Base Management: Metabolic Acidosis; Electrolyte Management: Hypokalemia

RISK FOR INFECTION *related to inadequate secondary defenses (suppressed inflammatory response) caused by protein depletion and hyperglycemia.*

Goals/Outcomes: The patient is free of infection as evidenced by normothermia; HR 100 bpm or less, BP within patient's normal range, WBC count 11,000/mm^3 or less, and negative culture results.
NOC Infection Severity, Immune Status

Hyperglycemia

Infection Protection
1. Monitor for signs of infection. Fever may be suppressed secondary to acidosis. Monitor for increased WBC count, which initially may reflect dehydration or the stress response.
2. Because the patient is at higher risk for bacterial infection, invasive lines should be managed carefully to avoid BSI. Central lines should be removed as soon as possible.
3. Manage urinary catheters meticulously to prevent UTI.
4. Maintain skin integrity. Assess for areas of decreased sensation.

NIC Skin Surveillance

CONFUSION, ACUTE *related to hyperosmolality, dehydration, or hypoglycemia*

Goals/Outcomes: The patient verbalizes orientation to time, place, and person; the patient is protected from unnecessary complications and bodily injury.
NOC Cognitive orientation

Neurologic Monitoring
1. Monitor neurologic status frequently. Notify advanced practice provider of deterioration.
2. Keep bed in lowest position with side rails raised, if the patient is confused.
3. Consider nasogastric tube with suction for comatose patients to decrease likelihood of aspiration.
4. Elevate HOB to 30 degrees to minimize the risk of aspiration.
5. Monitor blood glucose hourly while the patient is receiving insulin infusion. Consult advanced practice provider if blood glucose drops faster than 100 mg/dL/h or if it drops to less than 250 mg/dL. Obtain prescription for glucose-containing IV solution to prevent hypoglycemia and allow the continued administration of insulin necessary to correct acidosis.

NIC Hyperglycemia Management; Hypoglycemia Management

DEFICIENT KNOWLEDGE *related to new-onset diabetes or misunderstanding of the causes and prevention of DKA or HHS.*

Goals/Outcomes: By discharge from the hospital, the patient will be able to explain causes, symptoms, and prevention of DKA or hyperglycemic crisis.
NOC Hyperglycemia management, hypoglycemia management

Teaching, Disease Process
1. Consider referral to a diabetes educator for new onset of diabetes or new to insulin, poor understanding of sick day management, poor control as evidenced by elevated HbA1C.
2. Explain relationship of illness and stress to DKA or HHS.
3. Review symptoms of hyperglycemia, such as polyuria, polydipsia, blurred vision, lethargy, weakness, and headache. GI symptoms such as nausea, vomiting, and abdominal pain are more common with DKA, whereas confusion, change in mentation, and neurologic symptoms similar to stroke are more common with HHS.
4. Review diabetes sick day management guidelines:
   • Patients should continue their insulin or other medication. During illness, sometimes additional insulin is required.
   • Monitoring of blood sugar should be done more frequently. If not eating, the patient should monitor it every 2 to 4 hours or more.
   • People with type 1 diabetes should monitor for ketones every 4 hours. Notify the advanced practice provider if moderate to large amounts of ketones are present.
   • The patient should drink large amounts of clear liquids not containing caffeine. If unable to eat solid food, the patient should increase intake of nutritious caloric liquids as tolerated
   • Patients must understand the need to contact the advanced practice provider or seek care in a hospital emergency room if symptoms of hyperglycemia worsen, vomiting persists, unable to tolerate liquids, urine testing reveals moderate to large amounts of ketones, or unable to control blood sugar.
5. Ensure the patient has follow-up physician and/or advanced practice provider appointment before discharge.
6. Provide community resources for outpatient education. The American Diabetes Association (ADA) website is another option for patients who have limited access to community resources.

7. Provide the address and websites for the ADA: American Diabetes Association, 18 East 48th Street, New York, NY 10017; www.ada.org and www.diabetes.org

NIC Teaching: Prescribed Diet; Teaching: Prescribed Medication; Teaching: Prescribed Activity/Exercise; Emotional Support

ADDITIONAL NURSING DIAGNOSES

See also nursing diagnoses and interventions in Hyperkalemia, Hypokalemia, and Hypovolemia in Fluid and Electrolyte Disturbances, Chapter 1; Alterations in Consciousness, Chapter 1; Prolonged Immobility, Chapter 1; and Emotional and Spiritual Support of the Patient and Significant Others, Chapter 2.

MYXEDEMA COMA
PATHOPHYSIOLOGY

Myxedema coma is a life-threatening condition that occurs when hypothyroidism is untreated or when a stressor such as infection affects an individual with known or unknown hypothyroidism. The clinical picture of myxedema coma includes exaggerated hypothyroidism, with decreased mental status or coma, hypoventilation, hypothermia, hypotension, seizures, and shock. Myxedema coma usually develops slowly, has a greater than 50% mortality rate, and requires prompt, aggressive treatment. Even with early diagnosis and treatment, mortality is nearly 45%.

Hypothyroidism is a common endocrine disorder reflecting inadequacy of production or uptake of the thyroid hormone. Localized disease of the thyroid gland that results in decreased thyroid hormone production is the most common cause of hypothyroidism. Normally, the thyroid gland releases 100 to 125 nmol of thyroxine (T_4) daily and only small amounts of triiodothyronine (T_3). T_4 is a prohormone that functions as a reservoir for the more metabolically active form of the thyroid hormone, T_3. Primary conversion occurs in the peripheral tissues via 5'-deiodination. Decreased production of T_4 and failure of deiodinization to T_3 causes an increase in the secretion of thyroid-stimulating hormone (TSH) by the functional pituitary gland. TSH stimulates hypertrophy and hyperplasia of the thyroid gland and an increase in thyroid T_4–5'-deiodinase activity. Early in the disease process, compensatory mechanisms maintain T_3 levels; however, this compensatory mechanism may be short-lived.

Individuals who are acutely or critically ill may have an extreme disruption of the normal hypothalamic–anterior pituitary–thyroid axis, particularly related to the nocturnal surge that is normally seen with thyrotropin. These patients will have a low T_3 level even after the TSH is restored to normal, and they are commonly referred to as presenting with low T_3 syndrome. Patients with poor heart function or more intense inflammatory reaction show more pronounced downregulation of the thyroid system. During sepsis, the pituitary gland is activated via blood-borne proinflammatory cytokines and through a complex interaction between the autonomic nervous system and the immune cells. Sepsis elicits a pattern of pituitary hormone dysfunction that may cause a significant decrease in the secretion of TSH.

Hypothyroidism results in inadequate amount of circulating thyroid hormone, causing a decrease in metabolic rate that affects all body systems.

Primary hypothyroidism, the most common presenting form of thyroidal disorders, is caused by thyroid suppression for any direct reason (i.e., cancer, radiation, autoimmune dysfunction).

1. Autoimmune: The most frequent cause of acquired hypothyroidism is autoimmune thyroiditis (Hashimoto thyroiditis). The body recognizes the thyroid antigens as foreign, and a chronic immune reaction ensues, resulting in lymphocytic infiltration of the gland and progressive destruction of functional thyroid tissue. Most affected individuals have circulating antibodies to thyroid tissue.
2. Postpartum thyroiditis: Ten percent of postpartum women develop lymphocytic thyroiditis 2 to 10 months after delivery. The frequency may be 5% in women with type 1 diabetes mellitus. The condition may only last 2 to 4 months but usually requires treatment with levothyroxine; however, postpartum patients with lymphocytic thyroiditis are at increased risk of permanent hypothyroidism. The hypothyroid state may be preceded by a short thyrotoxic state.

3. Subacute granulomatous thyroiditis: Inflammatory conditions or viral syndromes may be associated with transient hyperthyroidism followed by transient hypothyroidism. This presentation is linked to fever, malaise, and a painful and tender gland.

Secondary hypothyroidism results from inadequate secretion of TSH from the anterior pituitary gland. The cause of the deficiency is not always clear, but it is often associated with surgery, trauma, or radiation therapy. If TSH level is inadequate, the thyroid lacks the proper stimulus to produce T_4.

Tertiary hypothyroidism is related to hypothalamic dysfunction and is diagnosed by the release of thyrotropin-releasing hormone (TRH). Other causes are listed in Box 8-2.

Because all metabolically active cells require thyroid hormone, the effects of hormone deficiency vary. Systemic effects are caused by either derangements in metabolic processes or direct effects by myxedematous infiltration in the tissues. The patient's presentation may vary from asymptomatic to, rarely, coma with multisystem organ failure (myxedema coma). The incidence of hypothyroidism is 0.1–2% in the general population and is eight times more likely to occur in women than in men. It frequently presents in the later years of life. Older women are the most likely candidates to present with myxedema.

 Safety Alert *Euthyroid sick syndrome (ESS) may manifest as a low T_3, low T_4, low TSH, or all three. ESS results from inactivation of 5′-deiodinase, resulting in conversion of FT_4 to rT_3 (a reverse form of T_3 that is not metabolically active). ESS may occur in critically ill patients without any known cause but may also present in patients who have diabetes mellitus, malnutrition, or iodine loads or as the result of medications (amiodarone, PTU, glucocorticoids).*

Euthyroid sick syndrome (ESS) should be considered when TSH and/or T_4 are normal, T_3 is low, and the patient presents with symptoms that suggest hypothyroidism.

ENDOCRINE ASSESSMENT: MYXEDEMA COMA

GOAL OF SYSTEM ASSESSMENT

Evaluate for end-organ effects of hypothyroidism, including altered mental status, hypothermia, hypoglycemia, hypotension, bradycardia, and hypoventilation. Not all patients have noticeable myxedema (polysaccharide accumulation).

HISTORY AND RISK FACTORS

Signs and symptoms may be life-threatening in a patient with history of hypothyroidism who has experienced a recent stressful event. Undiagnosed patients may report early fatigue, weight gain, anorexia, lethargy, cold intolerance, menstrual irregularities, constipation,

Box 8-2	COMMON CAUSES OF ACUTE HYPOTHYROIDISM

Primary hypothyroidism
- Hashimoto thyroiditis (autoimmune)
- Surgical removal of thyroid gland
- Ablation with radioactive iodine
- External irradiation
- Defective iodine organification
- Thyroid tumor
- Drug related
- Lithium
- Interferon
- Amiodarone

Secondary hypothyroidism
- Pituitary or hypothalamic disease

depression, and muscle cramps. Family may report depression, psychosis, cognitive dysfunction, or poor memory.

> **Safety Alert** *A change in mental status may be the most compelling sign to assist in making the diagnosis.*

VITAL SIGNS

Cardinal signs and symptoms of myxedema coma include hypothermia (may be less than 26.6° C, 80° F), hypoventilation, hypotension, and bradycardia, as well as hyponatremia and hypoglycemia. The presentation of any three of these signs and symptoms together should be considered in differential diagnosis as signs of acute hypothyroidism until proven otherwise.

> **Safety Alert** *The presence of a normal temperature in a patient who appears to present with acute hypothyroid dysfunction is abnormal and should be considered an indicator of infection.*

OBSERVATION

Cardiac: Nonspecific ECG changes, prolonged conduction times, prolonged QT syndrome. Cardiac enlargement, possible effusion, or low cardiac output. If hypotensive, may be refractory to volume and vasopressors until thyroid hormone given.

Respiratory: Respiratory depression from reduced hypoxic drive and decreased ventilatory response and increasing CO_2. The increase in CO_2 is a major factor in the induction of coma. May also have edema of the conducting airways.

Gastrointestinal: Anorexia, nausea, abdominal pain, and constipation. Quiet abdomen, ileus, and megacolon are not uncommon.

HYPOTHYROIDISM

- Possible presence of obesity and/or weight gain from fluid retention
- The skin may be dry, cool, and coarse, and the hair may be thin, coarse, and brittle. The tongue may be enlarged (macroglossia), and the reflexes may be slowed. Periorbital edema may be noted.
- There may be a surgical scar or a goiter when evaluating the neck. Nodules may be palpated.
- The patient may have muscle weakness, memory and mental impairment, and constipation.
- Polysaccharide substances may be deposited beneath the skin (myxedema), which may prompt hypovolemia.

> **Safety Alert** *A change in mental status may be the most important sign. It is commonly noted first to be lethargy, then stupor, and ultimately coma.*

SCREENING LAB WORK

Blood studies may reveal the presence of thyroid dysfunction. Expected abnormalities include (see also Figure 8-2):

- TSH increased or normal (chronic thyroiditis)
- T_4 decreased
- Hypercholesterolemia
- Elevated serum lactate
- Hypoglycemia
- Hyponatremia
- Hypoxemia
- Hypercapnia

Common Diagnostic Tests for Hypothyroid Crisis: Myxedema Coma

Test	Purpose	Abnormal Findings
Blood Studies		
Thyroid-stimulating hormone (TSH): Standard normal: 0.4 to 4.5 mIU/L Revised normal: 0.4 to 2.5 mIU/L TSH >2.5 mIU/L from the NHANES III study indicated hypothyroidism.	Measures TSH output from the anterior pituitary. Completes a negative feedback loop with the thyroid. When thyroid hormone level decreases, TSH level should increase.	Elevated unless hypothyroidism is longstanding or severe. When TSH is higher than 2.5 mIU/L in the presence of clinical symptoms, the diagnosis of hypothyroidism will be considered positive until proved otherwise. Always beneficial to also evaluate T_4 at the same time. If TSH is higher than 4.5 mIU/L, the diagnosis of hypothyroidism is considered positive.
Thyroperoxidase antibodies	Assesses for thyroid antibodies	Positive test signals chronic autoimmune thyroiditis.
Free T_4 or free thyroxine index (FTI): Normal: 60 to 170 nmol/L	Measures the level of primary thyroid hormone May be unreliable in the face of critical illness	Decreased. When levels are below normal, diagnosis of hypothyroidism is made. If the TSH is high, diagnosis will be a primary hypothyroidism. If TSH is normal or low and T_4 is low, the problem is in the hypothalamic-pituitary response to elevated circulating thyroid levels (secondary hypothyroidism). However, if the T_3 is also low, this may signify euthyroid sick syndrome.
T_3 (triiodothyronine) Normal: 0.8 to 2.7 nmol/L	Measures the more metabolically active form of the thyroid hormone.	Controversial regarding value of treatment of low levels because it has a higher frequency of adverse cardiac events and is generally reserved for patients who are not improving clinically on LT_4.
Thyroid-binding globulin (TBG)	To measure the level of the protein that binds with circulating thyroid hormones. Abnormal T_4 or T_3 measurements are often caused by binding protein abnormalities rather than to abnormal thyroid function.	Total T_4 or T_3 must be evaluated with a measure of thyroid hormone binding such as T_3 resin uptake or assay of thyroid-binding globulin. These methods are known as free T_4 or free T_3, even though they do not measure free hormone directly.
Electrolytes: Potassium (K^+) Magnesium (Mg^{2+}) Calcium (Ca^{2+}) Sodium (Na^+)	Assess for possible abnormalities	Frequently, abnormalities of calcium are related to parathyroid disorders exist concurrently with thyroid dysfunction.
Radiology/Imaging		
Thyroid scan with radioactive iodine uptake ^{123}I or ^{99m}Tc pertechnetate	To identify thyroid nodules	Not beneficial in hypothyroidism as uptake of radioactive iodine may not occur
Thyroid scan ^{131}I and radioactive iodine uptake	To identify thyroid nodules by assessing the uptake of this isotope.	In primary hypothyroidism, will be <10% in a 24-hour period. In secondary hypothyroidism, uptake increases with administration of exogenous TSH.
Chest radiograph	Assess size of heart, and presence of pericardial or pleural effusion	Cardiac enlargement or fluid around the heart is common with myxedema
Ultrasound	Assess size and presence of nodules and goiter	Abnormal thyroid is unusual in Hashimoto disease.
Fine-needle biopsy	Evaluate suspicious nodes	Cancerous cells indicate thyroid cancer

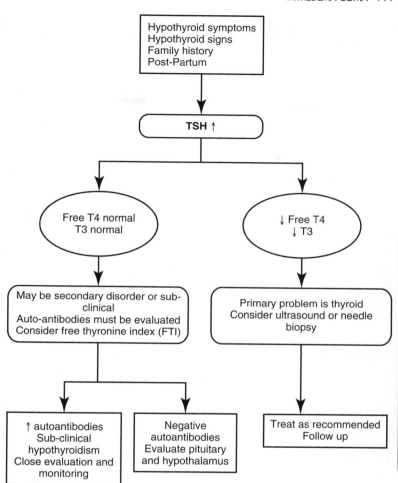

Figure 8-2 Diagnosing hypothyroidism.

Myxedema Coma

COLLABORATIVE MANAGEMENT

CARE PRIORITIES

1. Stabilize the patient

- Perform emergent endotracheal intubation and provide mechanical ventilation support: Required to relieve or prevent profound hypoxemia and CO_2 narcosis detected by SpO_2 and $ETCO_2$ monitoring. ABG monitoring is done periodically to validate SpO_2 and $ETCO_2$ and to monitor pH.
- Treat hypothermia: Although the hypothermia will be addressed ultimately by the institution of thyroid hormone, it may take several days. Extreme caution must be taken when rewarming (only passive techniques should be used) to avoid uncompensated vasodilation and profound hypotension.
- Treat hypotension: Before institution of even passive rewarming, careful volume resuscitation should occur. Administer of IV isotonic fluids (normal saline and lactated Ringer's solution). Hypotonic solutions, such as 5% dextrose in water (D_5W), are contraindicated

because they decrease serum Na1 levels further. These patients respond poorly to vasopressors because of alteration in sympathetic response. Consider IV vasopressin or IV corticosteroids.

 2. Administer IV thyroid hormone as soon as possible: Patients may die without prompt treatment

The best dose or approach to rapidly returning the circulating and active hormones to normal is uncertain, and therefore recommendations tend to be empiric at best. Practitioners often initially administer T_4 (levothyronine). An effective approach is to use IV LT_4 at a dose of 4 µg/kg of lean body weight, or approximately 200–250 µg as a bolus in a single or divided dose, depending on the patient's risk of cardiac disease (if at risk, give one-half the dose), followed by 100 µg 24 hours later for stabilization, then 50 µg IV or by mouth (PO) daily, given with IV or PO glucocorticoids.

Thyroid Hormone Supplementation   Use of IV triiodothyronine (LT_3): Controversial therapy because it has a higher frequency of adverse cardiac events and is generally reserved for patients who are not improving clinically on LT_4. Oral thyroid hormone (i.e., levothyroxine): This is not the avenue of choice in myxedema coma. It is given early in treatment for primary hypothyroidism. To prevent hyperthyroidism caused by too much exogenous hormone, patients are started on low doses that are increased gradually based on serial laboratory tests (TSH and T_4) and adjusted until the TSH is in a normal range. This therapy is continued for the patient's lifetime. For patients with secondary hypothyroidism, thyroid supplements can promote acute symptoms and therefore are contraindicated.

> **Safety Alert**   *Rapid IV administration of thyroid hormone should be done with careful monitoring, as this may cause hyperadrenalism. Concomitant administration of IV hydrocortisone helps prevent adrenal problems but may cause hypoadrenalism if not carefully monitored.*

3. Manage hyponatremia
If serum Na1 is greater than 120 mEq/L, fluids are restricted. If serum Na1 is less than 120 mEq/L, consider administration hypertonic (3%) saline followed by water diuresis.

4. Manage hypoglycemia
IV solutions containing glucose or 50% dextrose (D_{50}).

5. Manage associated illnesses such as infections

6. Administer stool softeners
To minimize constipation caused by decreased gastric secretions and peristalsis.

7. Avoid barbiturates
Because of alterations in metabolism, patients with hypothyroidism do not tolerate barbiturates and sedatives, and therefore central nervous system (CNS) depressants are contraindicated.

CARE PLANS FOR MYXEDEMA COMA

INEFFECTIVE PROTECTION (MYXEDEMA COMA) *related to inadequate response to treatment of hypothyroidism or stressors such as infection.*

Goals/Outcomes: The patient is free of symptoms of myxedema coma as evidenced by HR greater than 60 bpm, BP greater than 90/60 mm Hg (or within patient's normal range), RR greater than 12 breaths/min with normal depth and pattern, and orientation to person, place, and time.

NOC Risk Control

Risk Identification
1. Monitor vital signs frequently and note bradycardia, hypotension, or decrease in RR. Report systolic BP greater than 90 mm Hg, HR less than 60 bpm, or RR less than 12 breaths/min.

2. Monitor the patient for hypoxia. Report significant findings to advanced practice provider.
3. Monitor serum electrolytes and glucose levels. Note decreasing Na1 (less than 137 mEq/L) and glucose (less than 60 mg/dL).
   - Restrict fluids or administer hypertonic saline as prescribed to correct hyponatremia. Do not correct too rapidly, to avoid central pontine myelinolysis.
   - In chronic, severe symptomatic hyponatremia, the rate of correction should not exceed 0.5–1 mEq/L/h, with a total increase not to exceed 12 mEq/L/d. It is necessary to correct the hyponatremia to a safe range (usually to no greater than 120 mEq/L) rather than to a normal value.
4. Administer IV thyroid replacement hormones with IV hydrocortisone and IV glucose to treat hypoglycemia.
5. Monitor for heart failure: jugular vein distention, crackles (rales), shortness of breath (SOB), peripheral edema, weakening peripheral pulses, and hypotension. Notify advanced practice provider of any significant findings.
6. Keep an oral airway and manual resuscitator at the bedside in the event of seizure, coma, or the need for ventilatory assistance.

NIC Vital Signs Monitoring; Respiratory Monitoring; Shock Prevention; Cardiac Care: Acute

INEFFECTIVE BREATHING PATTERN *related to enlarged thyroid gland and/or decreased ventilatory drive caused by greatly decreased metabolism.*

Goals/Outcomes: The patient maintains effective breathing pattern as evidenced by RR 12 to 20 breaths/min with normal depth and pattern, normal skin color, oxygen saturation greater than 95%, and absence of adventitious breath sounds. If ineffective breathing pattern occurs, it is reported and treated promptly.
NOC Respiratory Status: Ventilation; Vital Signs

Respiratory Monitoring
1. Assess rate, depth, and quality of breath sounds. Monitor for inadequate ventilation: changes in respiratory rate or pattern, falling SpO_2, pallor, or cyanosis. Report findings to advanced practice provider promptly, including presence of adventitious sounds (e.g., from developing pleural effusion) or decreasing or crowing sounds (e.g., from swollen tongue or glottis).
2. Measure $ECTO_2$ and SpO_2 intermittently or continuously in patients with decreased ventilatory drive.
3. Teach the patient coughing, deep breathing, and use of incentive spirometer. For respiratory distress, assist provider with intubation or tracheostomy and maintenance of mechanical ventilatory assistance. Suction upper airway as needed.

NIC Airway Management

EXCESS FLUID VOLUME *related to compromised regulatory mechanisms occurring with associated adrenal insufficiency.*

Goals/Outcomes: By a minimum of 24 hours before hospital discharge, the patient is normovolemic as evidenced by urinary output greater than 0.5 mL/kg/h, stable weight, nondistended jugular veins, presence of eupnea, and peripheral pulse amplitude $\geq 2+$ on a 0 to $4+$ scale.
NOC Fluid Balance

Hypervolemia Management
1. Monitor I&O hourly for evidence of decreasing output.
2. Weigh the patient at the same time every day, using the same scale. Monitor for the following indicators of heart failure: jugular vein distention, crackles (rales), SOB, dependent edema of extremities, and decreased pulse amplitude. Report significant findings to provider.
3. Restrict fluid and Na1 intake as prescribed.

NIC Fluid Management; Electrolyte Monitoring

ACTIVITY INTOLERANCE *related to weakness and fatigue secondary to slowed metabolism and decreased cardiac output caused by pericardial effusions, atherosclerosis, and decreased adrenergic stimulation.*

Myxedema Coma

Goals/Outcomes: During activity patient rates perceived exertion at 3 or less on a 0 to 10 scale and exhibits cardiac tolerance to activity as evidenced by HR 20 bpm or less over resting HR, systolic BP 20 mm Hg or less over or under resting systolic BP, warm and dry skin, and absence of crackles (rales), murmurs, chest pain, and new dysrhythmias.

NOC Activity Tolerance; Endurance; Energy Conservation

Energy Management
1. Monitor vital signs frequently for hypotension, slow pulse, dysrhythmias, complaints of chest pain or discomfort, decreasing urine output, and changes in mentation. Promptly report significant changes to provider
2. Balance activity with adequate rest to decrease workload of the heart.
3. Administer IV isotonic solutions such as normal saline to help prevent hypotension.

NOC Activity Therapy; Exercise Promotion: Strength Training

RISK FOR INFECTION *related to compromised immunologic status secondary to alterations in adrenal function.*

Goals/Outcome: The patient is free of infection as evidenced by normothermia, absence of adventitious breath sounds, normal urinary pattern and characteristics, and well-healing wounds.

NOC Status; Infection Severity

Infection Protection
1. Monitor for infection: fever, erythema, swelling, or discharge from wounds or IV sites; urinary frequency, urgency, or dysuria; cloudy or malodorous urine; presence of adventitious sounds on auscultation of lung fields; and changes in color, consistency, and amount of sputum. Minimize risk of UTI by providing care of catheters.
2. Provide care to maintain skin integrity and prevent pressure ulcers.
3. Advise visitors who have contracted or been exposed to a communicable disease not to enter patient's room without appropriate infection control precautions.

NIC Identification; Infection Protection

RISK FOR IMBALANCED NUTRITION: MORE THAN BODY REQUIREMENTS *related to slowed metabolism*

Goals/Outcomes: The patient does not gain weight. Within the 24-hour period before hospital discharge, the patient verbalizes understanding of the rationale and measures for the dietary regimen.

NOC Status: Food and Fluid Intake; Weight Control

Nutritional Management
1. Provide a diet that is high in protein and low in calories and sodium.
2. Encourage foods that are high in fiber content (e.g., fruits with skins, vegetables, whole-grain breads and cereals, nuts) to improve gastric motility and elimination.
3. Administer vitamin supplements as prescribed.

NIC Counseling; Weight Management

CONSTIPATION *related to inadequate dietary intake of roughage and fluids, bed rest, and/or decreased peristalsis secondary to slowed metabolism.*

Goals/Outcomes: Within 48 to 72 hours of admission, the patient resumes normal pattern of bowel elimination.

NOC Elimination

Bowel Management
1. Monitor bowel function; report problems to the physician. Note decreasing bowel sounds, distention, and increased abdominal girth (may indicate ileus or an obstruction).

2. Encourage the patient to maintain a diet with adequate roughage and fluids. Ensure that fluid intake in persons without underlying cardiac or renal disease is at least 2 to 3 L/d.
3. Administer stool softeners and laxatives as prescribed.

 Safety Alert   *Suppositories may be contraindicated because of the risk of stimulating the vagus nerve (decreases HR and BP).*

NIC Constipation/Impaction Management; Fluid Management

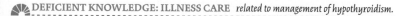

DEFICIENT KNOWLEDGE: ILLNESS CARE *related to management of hypothyroidism.*

Goals/Outcomes: Within the 24-hour period before hospital discharge, the patient verbalizes knowledge of potential side effects of prescribed medications, dietary guidelines, signs and symptoms that require medical attention, and importance of following the prescribed medical regimen.
NOC Knowledge: Disease Process

Teaching: Disease Process
1. Provide teaching about medications, including drug name, purpose, dosage, schedule, precautions, drug–drug and food–drug interactions, and potential side effects. Remind the patient that thioamides, iodides, and lithium are contraindicated because they decrease thyroid activity. Be sure the patient is aware that thyroid replacement medications are to be taken for life.
2. Review dietary requirements and restrictions, which may change as hormone replacement therapy takes effect.
3. Explain expected changes with hormone replacement therapy: increased energy level, weight loss, and decreased peripheral edema. Neuromuscular problems should improve.
4. Stress the importance of continued, frequent medical follow-up.
5. Discuss the importance of avoiding physical and emotional stress, and ways for the patient to maximize coping mechanisms for dealing with stress.
6. Review signs and symptoms that require medical attention: fever or other symptoms of upper respiratory, urinary, or oral infections and signs and symptoms of hyperthyroidism, which may result from excessive hormone replacement.
7. Women trying to become pregnant, who have subclinical hypothyroid, may require an increase in levothyroxine to increase the chance of conception.

NIC Management; Exercise Promotion; Teaching: Prescribed Diet; Teaching: Disease Process; Anxiety Reduction

SYNDROME OF INAPPROPRIATE ANTIDIURETIC HORMONE

Syndrome of inappropriate antidiuretic hormone (SIADH), also known as syndrome of inappropriate antidiuresis (SIAD), is a potentially lethal condition that involves an alteration in sodium and water balance. It is associated with water retention caused by a failure to suppress ADH secretion. SIADH is one of the most common etiologies of hyponatremia in hospitalized patients, including those in the ICU. The syndrome occurs in the absence of renal dysfunction or recognized stimuli that would typically induce release of ADH. Patients with SIADH have hypoosmolality and hyponatremia, but are euvolemic. The sodium level is normal, but there is an increase in total body water in the intravascular space.

SIADH is considered a paraneoplastic syndrome as it can be caused by an alteration in the immune system caused by the presence of tumor cells. Several other etiologies, including those that are pulmonary, neurologic, or hormonal in nature, as well as several medications, have been implicated in its development. Prompt and accurate diagnosis and initiation of therapies to correct serum sodium levels are essential. Management depends on the degree of hyponatremia, associated manifestations, and how rapidly it occurred. Meticulous critical care nursing care is pivotal to avoid life-threatening sequelae in the acute phase of this condition.

PATHOPHYSIOLOGY

ADH (the type in humans is termed arginine vasopressin [AVP]) is a hormone composed of nine amino acids. It is therefore considered a peptide hormone (as opposed to a steroid hormone). Its two main functions are to control levels of body water and BP. For the purposes of this chapter, the focus is on ADH's role in control of body water.

ADH is synthesized by the supraoptic nucleus (a collection of nerve cell bodies) in the hypothalamus and is secreted from the posterior pituitary gland (neurohypophysis). When triggered, the nerve cells release ADH. Production of ADH triggers absorption of free water in the distal convoluted tubules and collecting duct of the kidneys. This occurs because of binding of ADH to the V_2 receptor.

The primary trigger of the supraoptic nucleus to release ADH is an elevated serum osmolality. Other significant triggers include a decrease in circulating blood volume, hypotension, and angiotensin II (part of the renin-angiotensin-aldosterone system). Pain, other sources of stress, nausea, pregnancy, hypoglycemia, nicotine, and some drugs (e.g., morphine sulfate) are also implicated as stimuli affecting ADH release. Cancer cells may also secrete ADH; this is especially true of small cell lung cancer. Conversely, the two main inhibitors of ADH secretion are hypoosmolality and hypervolemia.

Normally, ADH is secreted by the posterior pituitary when triggered by an increase in serum osmolality; changes in serum osmolality are detected by osmoreceptors in the hypothalamus. ADH secretion is also stimulated by decreased circulating blood volume or BP. These pressure changes are sensed by baroreceptors located in the aortic arch, carotid sinus, and right atrium. ADH then stimulates V_2 receptors in the collecting duct cells of the kidney, causing reabsorption of water, which lowers serum osmolality.

Secretion of ADH results in urine concentration and decreased urine output. There is a direct relationship between serum ADH levels and concentration of urine, meaning that as serum ADH levels increase, the concentration of urine increases.

In SIADH, the amount of ADH release is higher than expected, given the patient's serum osmolality. AVP secretion remains increased despite a serum osmolality that normalizes. Further, in patients with SIADH, increasing water intake does not decrease ADH secretion and concentrated urine persists. When the body produces excess ADH, the kidneys are unable to eliminate the excess water. This results in an increase in total body water, despite the absence of renal dysfunction. As fluid accumulates, sodium levels are diluted; this results in hypotonic hyponatremia.

Four types of SIADH have been identified based on the impairment in patterns of AVP secretion. These are delineated in Table 8-5.

RESEARCH BRIEF 8-2

The incidence of SIADH-induced hyponatremia is up to 15% in patients with small cell lung cancer (SCLC). This condition has high morbidity and mortality rates and frequently delays initiation of antineoplastic therapies. This prospective case series describes management of hyponatremia with tolvaptan in 10 patients with SCLC. Treatment with tolvaptan led to an improved performance status on all patients, allowing them to begin chemotherapy in time. Rapid and effective correction of symptoms and serum sodium levels were achieved. There were no prolonged hospitalizations associated with the patient's condition or therapies.

From: Petereit C, Zaba O, Teber I, et al: A rapid and efficient way to manage hyponatremia in patients with SIADH and small cell lung cancer: treatment with tolvaptan. *BMC Pulm Med* 13:55, 2013.

ASSESSMENT

HISTORY AND RISK FACTORS

A number of etiologic factors for the development of SIADH have been identified. These factors can cause release of ADH but are not directly related to serum osmolality or fluid volume status. These factors are listed in Table 8-6.

Table 8-5   TYPES OF SIADH

Type	Description	Common Cause(s)	Prevalence
A	Exemplified by unpredictable, unregulated AVP release. AVP release does not correspond with plasma osmolality. Most common type of SIADH.	Lung cancer Nasopharyngeal tumors	40%
B	Characterized by a low and consistent secretion of AVP. The osmotic threshold for secretion of AVP is decreased. This means that secretion of AVP will occur at lower than normal plasma osmolality levels ("reset osmostat")	Tumors	20 to 40%
C	Absence of suppression of AVP despite plasma osmolality levels below the osmotic threshold. Serum AVP levels are elevated despite low plasma osmolality levels. Low levels of persistent AVP secretion occur.	Dysfunction of hypothalamic inhibitory neurons	Rare
D	Low or untraceable levels of AVP with no irregularity in AVP response	Nephrogenic SIADH caused by a genetic mutation	Rare

Table 8-6   ETIOLOGIC FACTORS OF SYNDROME OF INAPPROPRIATE ANTIDIURETIC HORMONE AND HYPONATREMIA

Pulmonary-related	Medication-related
Abscess Acute respiratory failure Asthma Atelectasis Pneumonia (e.g., Legionella, Mycoplasma) Pneumothorax Tuberculosis Vasculitis	Amantadine Amiodarone Amitriptyline Angiotensin-converting enzyme inhibitors Bromocriptine Carbamazepine Carboplatin Chlorpropamide Ciprofloxacin Cisplatin Cyclophosphamide (high-dose) Haloperidol Ifosfamide Imatinib (high-dose) Interferon-α Interferon-γ Lamotrigine Levetiracetam Lorcainide Melphalan Methotrexate Monoamine oxidase inhibitors Moxifloxacin Nonsteroidal anti-inflammatory drugs Opiates Oxcarbazepine Phenothiazines Prostaglandins Quinolones Serotonin and norepinephrine reuptake inhibitors (e.g., venlafaxine) Selective serotonin reuptake inhibitors

Syndrome of Inappropriate Antidiuretic Hormone

Continued

Table 8-6	ETIOLOGIC FACTORS OF SYNDROME OF INAPPROPRIATE ANTIDIURETIC HORMONE AND HYPONATREMIA — cont'd
Pulmonary-related	**Medication-related**
	Sodium valproate Tacrolimus Thioridazine Thiothixene Tolbutamide Tolterodine Tricyclic antidepressants Vinblastine Vincristine Vinorelbine
Neurology-related	**Hormone-related**
Brain trauma CNS infection (e.g., meningitis, meningoencephalitis) Guillain-Barré syndrome Intracranial bleeding/hemorrhage (e.g., subdural or subarachnoid hemorrhage) Lambert-Eaton myasthenic syndrome Multiple sclerosis Psychosis Stroke	Hypopituitarism Hypothyroidism Exogenous hormone administration (e.g., vasopressin, desmopressin, oxytocin)
Cancer-related	**Other**
Adrenal tumors Brain tumors Breast cancer Endometrial cancer Extrapulmonary small cell carcinomas Gastric cancer Genitourinary tract malignancy (e.g., bladder, ureteral) Head and neck cancer (e.g., oropharyngeal, nasopharyngeal) Lymphoma Mesothelioma Multiple myeloma Olfactory neuroblastoma Pancreatic cancer Prostate (poorly differentiated acinar adenocarcinoma) Sarcoma (Ewing) Small cell lung cancer Thymoma	Chemotherapy-induced nausea "Ecstasy" (3,4-methylenedioxymethamphetamine) Exercise (prolonged, strenuous) Genetic abnormalities (i.e., gene for renal vasopressin-2 (V_2) receptor, gene affecting hypothalamic osmolality sensing) Graft-versus-host disease (acute) HIV infection (symptomatic) or AIDS Idiopathic Interventional procedures (e.g., cardiac catheterization) Porphyria (acute intermittent) Positive pressure ventilation Stem cell transplant Surgical procedures (e.g., transphenoidal pituitary, surgery on bones and joints, carotid endarterectomy, cardiac, open and laparoscopic abdominal) Vasculitis

VITAL SIGNS

In the absence of comorbidities (e.g., heart failure, hypokalemia), as patients with SIADH are euvolemic, they will not have orthostatic BP changes. HR and CVP values will be within the expected range for the patient.

OBSERVATION

The manifestations of SIADH depend on the degree of hyponatremia and how rapidly it developed. Patients are more likely to be symptomatic if sodium levels decline rapidly and may be asymptomatic if serum sodium levels are 130 mEq/L or above. Manifestations based on degree of hyponatremia appear in Table 8-7.

Patients with SIADH are euvolemic. As such, there will be absence of edema.

LAB WORK

Blood and urine test results are evaluated concomitantly with assessment of extracellular fluid volume status. Evaluation of volume status is essential for accurate interpretation of laboratory results. Results of blood and urine tests in SIADH are as follows:

- Serum sodium level decreased: Less than 134 mEq/L
- Serum osmolality decreased: Less than 280 mOsmol/kg
- Urine sodium level increased: Greater than 40 mmol/L with normal dietary intake of sodium and water (no fluid restriction in progress) (spot or 24-hour urine sample)
- Urine osmolality: Greater than 100 mOsmol/kg (spot or 24-hour urine sample)
- Serum uric acid level low or within range: Less than 4 mg/dL
- Blood urea nitrogen decreased: Less than 10 mg/dL
- Plasma vasopressin level: Inappropriately elevated in relation to plasma osmolality
- Serum potassium: Within appropriate range for patient

Table 8-7	MANIFESTATIONS OF SIADH BASED ON DEGREE OF HYPONATREMIA
Degree of Hyponatremia	**Associated Symptoms**
Mild: sodium 130 to 134 mEq/L	Weakness Headache Memory difficulties Malaise Gait disturbances Falls Apathy Fatigue Myalgia Irritability Restlessness
Moderate: sodium 125 to 129 mEq/L	Headache Trouble thinking clearly Nausea Vomiting Confusion Seizures Hyporeflexia Muscle weakness, spasms, or cramps Hypotension Oliguria Lethargy Anorexia Abdominal pain
Severe: sodium <125 mEq/L	Altered mental status (e.g., lethargy, delirium) Seizures Decreased deep tendon reflexes Agitation Hallucinations Incontinence Pseudobulbar palsy Coma Respiratory collapse Death

Syndrome of Inappropriate Antidiuretic Hormone

- Absence of acid–base imbalance
- Serum glucose level: Within appropriate range for the patient (to validate that hyperglycemia is not causing a false hyponatremia)

DIFFERENTIAL DIAGNOSIS

When attempting to diagnose a patient with SIADH, the following conditions associated with hyponatremia and euvolemic hyponatremia should be ruled out:

- Hypothyroidism
- Hypocortisolism
- Adrenal insufficiency
- Glucocorticoid deficiency (especially in patients with neurosurgical disorders)
- "Reset osmostat" (may be seen in pregnancy, chronic malnutrition, epilepsy, and paraplegia)
- Illnesses causing diarrhea
- Inappropriate volume repletion following exercise
- Extreme intake of water
- Very low protein intake
- Primary polydipsia

COLLABORATIVE MANAGEMENT

The management of patients with SIADH varies, depending on the patient symptomatology and associated degree of hyponatremia. It is essential for patients with severe hyponatremia that developed within the past 48 hours to be treated to avoid life-threatening neurologic complications. Mainstays of treatment for all patients include eliminating the underlying cause of SIADH and correction of serum sodium levels. The latter may be accomplished in a number of different ways, including fluid restriction, administration of sodium, vasopressin receptor antagonist administration, or combinations of these therapies. Each of these treatment modalities has associated drawbacks. Hyponatremia is the primary complication associated with SIADH. The suggested treatment goal for patients with SIADH is serum sodium of at least 130 mEq/L. This will help mitigate neurologic symptoms associated with lower sodium levels.

CARE PRIORITIES

1. Correct acute, symptomatic hyponatremia

- **Hypertonic saline**

  Patients with severe symptomatic hyponatremia (presence of seizures or intracranial conditions) may receive hypertonic (3%) saline. Infusion via a central venous catheter is recommended. The suggested bolus dose is 100 mL. This may be repeated once or twice more in 10-minute intervals if the patient's neurologic symptoms worsen or do not improve. Administration of hypertonic saline is the most effective way to correct severe hyponatremia and improve associated neurologic function. It is essential that serum sodium levels be corrected by no more than 0.5 to 1 mEq/L/h to avoid central pontine myelinolysis.

  Patients with a serum sodium less than 120 mEq/L that developed over more than 48 hours who have less severe neurologic symptoms should receive hypertonic saline to raise serum sodium levels by 1 mEq/L for 3 to 4 hours. Subsequent infusion rates should be titrated so that serum sodium levels correct less than 10 mEq/L in 24 hours and no more than 18 mEq/L in 48 hours.

- **Fluid restriction**

  Fluid restriction is indicated for patients who have mild symptoms associated with hyponatremia (e.g., gait disturbances, forgetfulness). The purpose of fluid restriction is to attain a negative water balance. Fluid restriction entails limiting total intake to no more than 1000 mL/d. In some cases, if the patient does not respond adequately, total intake may be limited to no more than 500 mL/d. It may take several days before appreciable increases in serum sodium levels are realized. Fluid restriction is indicated primarily for chronic hyponatremia associated with SIADH. Difficulties with the patient compliance with prolonged fluid restriction are reported. Fluid restriction is contraindicated in patients who recently had a subarachnoid hemorrhage; in these patients, fluid restriction may cause cerebral vasospasm, which may be fatal.

- *Isotonic saline infusions with diuretics*

  Serum sodium levels may also be corrected with infusions of isotonic saline (0.9%) with administration of IV loop diuretics (e.g., furosemide). Isotonic saline may be administered to patients with SIADH who are hyponatremic but asymptomatic. It is not recommended in patients who are symptomatic. Loop diuretic administration results in an increase in free water excretion. Loop diuretics are typically indicated for patients with a urine osmolality two times greater than serum osmolality. Administration results in decreased concentration of urine and increased water excretion. Loop diuretics are reported not to be useful in long-term therapy. Monitoring for hypokalemia and hypovolemia is essential with loop diuretic therapy as the diuretic effect is more significant in patients with SIADH and normal renal function.

  It is possible for serum osmolality and serum sodium levels to decrease further when patients receive isotonic saline. This is caused by the osmolality of isotonic sodium being lower than urine osmolality. In this case, the isotonic saline serves as a source of free water. This usually occurs in patients with a urine osmolality greater than 530 mOsmol/kg. Salt tablets administered orally may also be used to correct hyponatremia in patients with mild symptoms associated with hyponatremia.

2. Vasopressin-receptor antagonist therapy

Of the three vasopressin receptors in the body, the V_2 receptors have implications for the treatment of SIADH. The V_2 receptors are responsible for regulating the antidiuretic response. The other two receptors, V_{1a} and V_{1b}, produce vasoconstriction and release of ACTH, respectively.

As their name connotes, vasopressin receptor antagonists block AVP from binding to receptors in the collecting ducts, thereby inhibiting the actions of vasopressin. Administration of a vasopressin receptor antagonist results in an increase of free water excretion by the kidneys (aquaresis); sodium and potassium excretion are not affected. This results in an increased sodium level and decreased urine osmolality. Mental status improvement has also been reported in patients with SIADH who have a serum sodium level less than 130 mEq/L. Vasopressin receptor antagonists are not indicated in patients who are hyponatremic but asymptomatic.

Vasopressin receptor antagonists are available in oral and IV formulations. As it may be challenging to predict the rate of sodium correction with vasopressin receptor antagonists, their use is generally reserved for when fluid restriction has not been successful.

Tolvaptan is the oral agent and conivaptan is an IV formulation of this class of drugs that are approved by the Food and Drug Administration (FDA). Dosing of tolvaptan starts at 15 mg/d; up to 60 mg/d may be given. It is FDA-approved for patients with hypervolemic or euvolemic hyponatremia (serum sodium 125 mEq/L or less.). Patients with less severe hyponatremia who have not been successfully treated with fluid restriction may also be given tolvaptan. Side effects of tolvaptan include liver toxicity, dry mouth, constipation, and excess thirst. Because of the risk of hepatotoxicity, administration of tolvaptan is typically limited to no more than 30 days and is contraindicated in patients with liver dysfunction, as an increase in liver enzymes was reported in clinical trials. Tolvaptan is also contraindicated in patients with hypovolemic hyponatremia or anuria and in those with inability to recognize and respond to thirst.

Conivaptan, because it is an IV formulation, requires hospital admission. However, its administration will increase sodium levels more quickly than fluid restriction and salt tablets (for patients with mild to moderate levels of hyponatremia and who have few or no related symptoms). Patients with more severe levels of hyponatremia or with mild or moderate symptoms may receive conivaptan with or without hypertonic saline. The initial dose of conivaptan is 20 mg over 30 minutes; this is followed by another infusion of 20 mg over 24 hours. Side effects include nausea, vomiting, diarrhea, and infusion site reactions.

3. Manage chronic hyponatremia

Patients with chronic hyponatremia may be treated in the ambulatory setting. These patients may receive demeclocycline, a derivative of tetracycline (Declomycin®; Wyeth Ayerst Pharmaceuticals, Collegeville, PA) administered at 600 to 1200 mg/d in divided doses. Demeclocycline causes a decrease in ADH response by the distal convoluted tubules; this results in an increase in free water excretion. Concomitant fluid restriction is not required. Typically, patients with malignancy are treated with demeclocycline. It takes 2 to 3 days for treatment to start to become effective; response rates as long as weeks in duration have also been reported. Notable side effects include skin photosensitivity, nephrotoxicity (mainly in patients with actual or potential renal dysfunction), nausea, diarrhea, and anorexia. Patients with baseline renal dysfunction may also develop renal toxicity from demeclocycline. Patients receiving demeclocycline should be monitored for polyuria. They should have their sodium levels monitored while on therapy, as hypernatremia may develop in the face on ongoing fluid restriction.

Lithium has been used in the past in the management of chronic SIADH. Some preclinical studies have suggested that lithium may increase the efficacy of aquaretic agents. Like demeclocycline, lithium causes a decrease in ADH response by the distal convoluted tubules. Administration results in polyuria and polydipsia by causing nephrogenic DI. It takes 4 days for the drug to take effect. Because of the potential to cause nephrotoxicity and neuropsychiatric side effects, use of lithium has mostly ended. Other side effects are GI and hypothyroidism. Lithium also is effective in fewer patients than demeclocycline is.

Oral urea administration causes an osmotic diuresis. It increases excretion of water and fosters promotes sodium retention. Because of its associated bitter taste, its use is not widely accepted. Side effects include hypersensitivity, azotemia, and liver failure. Some data suggest that urea may have some favorable results in the long-term setting. Data on patients in the ICU suggest that urea may be useful in patients in the ICU with hyponatremia associated with SIADH. Its use seems limited to patients who have a moderate increase in urine osmolality. Urea administration is rarely used in the United States because of its lack of availability in pharmacies.

Correction of chronic hyponatremia should not exceed 10 mEq/L over 24 hours and 18 mEq/L over 48 hours. Monitoring of serum sodium should be conducted initially every 2 to 3 hours and then every 3 to 4 hours until the patient's condition stabilizes.

4. Identify and manage underlying cause

A number of the underlying causes of SIADH can be managed successfully. These include discontinuation of medications that may be causing the syndrome, treatment of the underlying infection, or managing any hormone-related etiologies. Other causes, such as small cell lung cancer and other malignancies, may pose challenges in treating SIADH.

5. Monitor for complications

Nursing care during therapy for SIADH includes monitoring for complications, monitoring serum electrolyte results daily, obtaining daily weights, and monitoring intake and output.

While serum sodium levels are being addressed, it is pivotal to ensure that these levels do not correct too rapidly. Some patients in clinical trials with vasopressin receptor antagonist therapy had too rapid a correction of sodium. Sodium correction in the acute setting should not exceed 0.5 to 1mEq/L/h. Such can result in severe neurologic complications such as central pontine myelinolysis, which is shrinkage of brainstem cells causing quadriparesis, pseudobulbar palsy, coma, and death. Meticulous monitoring of sodium levels is required.

Patients receiving demeclocycline or lithium should have renal function monitoring because of the potential for nephrotoxicity associated with these agents. Patients receiving tolvaptan therapy must be monitored for liver dysfunction. Symptoms that should be reported include jaundice, fatigue, anorexia, discomfort in the area of the right upper quadrant of the abdomen, and dark urine.

Patients with hyponatremia are at risk for the development of seizures. Monitoring and implementation of seizure precautions are recommended to protect the patient from harm.

Patients with severe SIADH and chronic hyponatremia are at risk for the development of alterations in bone metabolism that can lead to osteoporosis. Bone protection therapy and monitoring of bone density is recommended in these patients.

CARE PLANS FOR SYNDROME OF INAPPROPRIATE ANTIDIURETIC HORMONE

IMPAIRED NEUROLOGIC FUNCTIONING *related to hyponatremia*

Goals/Outcomes: Patient's neurologic function will improve as serum sodium level normalizes. The patient will not develop complications related to too rapid a correction of serum sodium level. Vital signs will remain within range appropriate for the patient.

NOC Neurological Status: Consciousness; Fluid Balance

Electrolyte Management: Hyponatremia
1. Minimize stimuli that can increase ADH release (e.g., pain, stress).
2. Ensure medications prescribed for other comorbid conditions do not trigger ADH release
3. Monitor for changes in neurologic status, vital signs, intake and output, and daily weight.
4. Monitor for symptoms associated with hyponatremia.
5. Monitor trends in laboratory values (serum sodium, serum osmolality, urine sodium).
6. Administer hypertonic saline to initiate correction of acute hyponatremia. Carefully titrate infusion to avoid central pontine myelinolysis.
7. Administer pharmacotherapy to increase sodium levels, as prescribed. Note and document efficacy.
8. Monitor for signs and symptoms of fluid overload (e.g., elevated CVP, tachycardia, edema, SOB when lying flat, crackles, jugular vein distention).
9. Implement seizure precautions (e.g., functioning suction equipment, appropriately sized oropharyngeal airway, avoiding restraint use, side rails raised and appropriately padded.)

NIC See Fluid and Electrolyte Imbalances, Hyponatremia. Chapter 1

THYROTOXICOSIS CRISIS (THYROID STORM)
PATHOPHYSIOLOGY

Thyroid storm is a medical emergency caused by uncontrolled hyperthyroidism. Patients occasionally present with cardiovascular collapse and shock. Hyperthyroidism or thyrotoxicosis is a condition of increased circulating thyroid hormone. The crisis results from a surge of thyroid hormones into the bloodstream, which results in profound stimulation of the sympathetic nervous system (SNS), with marked increases in body metabolism. The hypothalamus, anterior pituitary, and thyroid normally work together to balance the level of circulating thyroid hormone. Hyperthyroidism may be caused by an increased synthesis and secretion of thyroid hormones (thyroxine and triiodothyronine) from the thyroid or from increased secretion of TSH from the anterior pituitary, possibly by an increase in TRH from the hypothalamus or by autonomous thyroid hyperfunction. Symptoms of hyperthyroidism can also result from excessive release of thyroid hormone from the thyroid without increased synthesis. Such release is commonly caused by the destructive changes of various types of thyroiditis. Thyrotoxicosis crisis may also follow subtotal thyroidectomy because of manipulation of the gland during surgery. Various clinical syndromes also produce hyperthyroidism, but thyroid storm is most often associated with Graves disease, also known as diffuse toxic goiter. Causes of acute hyperthyroid states are listed in Box 8-3. Not all conditions listed are associated with thyroid storm.

  Safety Alert *Treatment with amiodarone (a common K+ antagonist used for dysrhythmia management) may cause either hyperthyroidism OR hypothyroidism and must be considered when evaluating either condition.*

 Safety Alert *Low TSH may also indicate euthyroid sick syndrome (ESS). When serum thyrotropin is decreased or suppressed by severe or critical illness or by medications, particularly high doses of glucocorticoids and dopamine, this abnormality may be the diagnosis.*

 Safety Alert *Life-threatening illness in patients with preexisting thyroid disorders may be precipitated by extremes of the primary disorder. These conditions present with exaggerated nonspecific signs and symptoms of the underlying thyroid dysfunction.*

 Safety Alert *Exacerbated hyperthyroidism occurs in 1 in 500 pregnancies and is second in frequency only to diabetes as an endocrine disorder of pregnancy. During pregnancy, thyroid storm is seen most often in patients with undertreated or undiagnosed hyperthyroidism. As many as 20% to 30% of cases may result in maternal and fetal mortality.*

Thyrotoxicosis Crisis (Thyroid Storm)

| Box 8-3 | COMMON CAUSES OF ACUTE HYPERTHYROID STATES |

- Graves disease
- Toxic multinodular goiter
- Solitary hyperfunctioning nodules
- Autoimmune and subacute postpartum thyroiditis
- Thyrotropin-secreting tumors
- Iodine-induced hyperthyroidism
- Excessive pituitary thyroid-stimulating hormone or trophoblastic disease
- Excessive ingestion of thyroid hormone

Abnormal laboratory analysis of thyroid function provides a relatively definitive diagnosis. Initial serum measurements should include free T_4 and TSH, but concerns regarding thyroid dysfunction should be referred to an endocrinology specialist for a more thorough and evaluative diagnostic panel. Calcium regulation may also be affected by thyroid disease if there is a problem with the level of thyrocalcitonin, a third thyroid hormone that is stimulated by increased calcium levels to help lower the calcium level. Recent diagnostic tests have isolated a long-acting thyroid stimulator, suggesting the disease is an autoimmune response. An acute decrease in thyroxine-binding globulin (inactivating or binding thyroid hormone) facilitates high levels of free and metabolically active hormone. The increased circulating levels of active thyroid hormone increase the response of β-adrenergic receptors (sympathetic stimulation increase) and also increase the system responsiveness to catecholamines.

ENDOCRINE ASSESSMENT: HYPERTHYROIDISM

GOAL OF SYSTEM ASSESSMENT
Evaluate for end-organ effects of hyperthyroidism. Thyroid hormones work with adrenal glucocorticoid hormones to facilitate carbohydrate, fat, and protein metabolism; work with insulin and GH to promote growth; increase HR and the force of contraction; help to regulate respiratory drive; help increase production of red blood cells; and increase metabolism.

HISTORY AND RISK FACTORS
A patient with a history of hyperthyroidism resulting from Graves disease, thyroid nodules, or toxic goiter who has undergone a recent stressful experience, including severe infection, trauma, major surgery, thromboembolism, DKA, or preeclampsia, pregnancy, labor, and/or delivery. Complaints include night sweats, unexplained weight loss, rapid gastric turnover with increased bowel movements or diarrhea, feelings of impending doom, rapid HR, and sleep disturbances. (See SIRS, Sepsis, and MODS, Chapter 11, Hyperglycemia, Chapter 8, High-Risk Obstetrics, Chapter 11.)

VITAL SIGNS
- May have hyperpyrexia (fever)
- Acute exacerbation of tachycardia, palpitations, or new-onset atrial fibrillation with chest discomfort in a patient with enlargement of the thyroid gland
- Both hypertension and widened pulse pressure are common.

OBSERVATION
- Confused, possibly psychotic, disoriented person with CNS irritability
- Hyperreflexia and fine tremor may be present.
- Coma, heart failure, and generalized muscle weakness may be present.
- Possible recent weight loss
- Patients with Graves disease (only in this form of thyrotoxicosis) have significant immune system components that may express as soft tissue swelling around the eye orbit, causing the protrusion of the eyes (exophthalmos), stare, and/or lid lag.
- Males often have gynecomastia. Many patients have fine hair and thin skin.
- Dependent lower-extremity edema, alteration in appetite, change in vision, and fertility or menstrual dysfunctions are possible.

PALPATION
- The thyroid gland in Graves disease will usually be enlarged, soft, and symmetrical, although occasionally it may be firm and irregular.
- Older patients may not have enlarged thyroid glands, which may lead to dismissal of the diagnosis.
- Palpation is not the definitive method to evaluate thyroid dysfunction.

SCREENING LAB WORK
- TSH level: Any type or cause of hyperthyroid disease (except when the cause is secondary excessive TSH production) will create a suppression of TSH. The development of TSH-sensitive testing has made the diagnosis of thyroid dysfunction much simpler.
- T_4 level: Unstable patients who have been diagnosed previously and/or are treated for thyroid disorders require a serum thyroxine (T_4) assessment, which will be significantly more valuable in diagnosis. See Figure 8-1 for diagnostic principles.

Common Diagnostic Tests for Thyrotoxic Crisis

Test	Purpose	Abnormal Findings
Blood Studies		
Thyroid-stimulating hormone (TSH): TSH is produced by the anterior pituitary gland in response to decreased T_4 level. The hypothalamus, anterior pituitary gland and thyroid are connected in an "axis" of function. Normal/standard: 0.4 and 4.5 mIU/L	To assess if TSH level is normal. TSH is decreased when T_4 level is increased. If T_4 is constantly increased, the TSH level is suppressed (low or decreased) by the high level of T_4. Normally, TSH release is needed to stimulate the thyroid to produce additional T_4.	When TSH is low in a patient with symptoms of thyroid storm, the diagnosis of hyperthyroidism will be considered positive until proven otherwise. If TSH is not prompting the increase in T_4, the thyroid has started generating T_4 abnormally. It is always beneficial to also evaluate T_4 at the same time. If the TSH is low while the T_4 is high, the patient is diagnosed with primary hyperthyroidism.
Free T_4 (thyroxine) Normal: 60 to 170 nmol/L	Measures the primary thyroid hormone	When levels are above normal, diagnosis of hyperthyroidism is made. If TSH and T_4 are both high, the problem is in the hypothalamic-pituitary response to elevated circulating thyroid levels (secondary hyperthyroidism).
T_3 (triiodothyronine) Normal: 0.8 to 2.7 nmol/L	Measures the more metabolically active form of the thyroid hormone.	Controversial
Thyroid-binding globulin (TBG)	To measure the level of the protein that binds with circulating thyroid hormones. Abnormal T_4 or T_3 measurements are often caused by binding protein abnormalities rather than to abnormal thyroid function.	Total T_4 or T_3 must be evaluated with a measure of thyroid hormone binding such as T_3 resin uptake or assay of thyroid-binding globulin. These methods are known as free T_4 or free T_3, even though they do not measure free hormone directly.
Radioactive iodine uptake	Differentiates the cause of thyroid disorder	May identify "hot" or "cold" nodules
Cholesterol analysis	Routine screening in biochemical profile	Hypercholesterolemia
Glucose	Routine screening in biochemical profile	Hyperglycemia; patients also have an impaired glucose tolerance test.

Continued

Common Diagnostic Tests for Thyrotoxic Crisis — cont'd		
Test	**Purpose**	**Abnormal Findings**
Electrolytes: Potassium (K^+) Magnesium (Mg^{2+}) Calcium (Ca^{2+}) Sodium (Na^+)	Assess for possible abnormalities	Frequently, abnormalities of calcium are related to parathyroid disorders that exist concurrently with thyroid dysfunction.
Radiology		
Thyroid scan ^{123}I (preferably) or ^{99m}Tc pertechnetate	Assesses the uptake of this isotope in the thyroid. Assess size of heart, thoracic cage (for fractures), thoracic aorta (for aneurysm), and lungs (pneumonia, pneumothorax) Assists with differential diagnosis of chest pain	Scan is done to help determine the cause of the hyperthyroidism. The scan may also be useful in assessing the functional status of any palpable thyroid irregularities or nodules associated with a toxic goiter.

COLLABORATIVE MANAGEMENT

CARE PRIORITIES

1. Stabilize the patient
- Reduce the stress response with β-adrenergic–blocking agents (e.g., esmolol, metoprolol, propranolol): Control tachycardia, manage atrial fibrillation if present, anxiety, heat intolerance, and tremor. Does not decrease the metabolic rate and has a mild effect on global oxygen consumption. Do not assume improvement in the thyroid disorder itself, only its symptoms. Calcium channel blockers may be used if β-blockers are contraindicated.
- Oxygen: Used per nasal cannula or mask as needed to maintain Spo_2 greater than 95%.
- Control fever: Antipyretic medications (i.e., acetaminophen) or hypothermia blanket is used. Aspirin is contraindicated, as it worsens thyroid crisis.
- Rehydrate using IV fluids: Fever and rapid metabolism can lead to dehydration.
- Correct electrolyte imbalance: Various imbalances may occur. Replace electrolytes as appropriate.
- Glucocorticoids: Administered to help inhibit conversion of thyroxine (T_4) to T_3 and prevent adrenal insufficiency.
- Minimize anxiety with mild tranquilizers: Also promote rest.

2. Treat the thyroid with antithyroid agents (thioamides)
Noninvasive, relatively cost-effective therapy with low risk of permanent hypothyroidism and a low cure rate.
- Propylthiouracil (PTU) has been the first line of treatment and is more effective in thyroid storm than methimazole. Can be used in pregnant patients. If the patient is unable to swallow, the medication is given using a nasogastric tube. Iodides (potassium iodide or Lugol solution) are given several hours after PTU to avoid a buildup of hormones stored in the thyroid gland.
- Methimazole may also be used. Both thioamides may cause leukopenia, rash, urticaria, fever, arthralgias, and, rarely, agranulocytosis. Methimazole may have a lower rate of these effects. Agranulocytosis (complete lack of granulocytes) causes fever and sore throat. If agranulocytosis is confirmed by CBC, the thioamide should be stopped.
- Iodides (SSKI): Sodium or potassium iodide drops may be given to help inhibit the release of thyroid hormone or to help abate accumulation of hormones stored in the thyroid. May stain the teeth.

3. Cure the thyroid with radioactive iodine
It is the most cost-effective and commonly used agent. Use usually results in hypothyroidism, requiring replacement therapy. Cannot be used for the pregnant patient, as the

thyroid gland of the fetus may also be destroyed. Usually reserved for the following indications:

- Failure to respond to antithyroid drugs
- Relapse after 1 to 2 years of therapy
- Toxic multinodular goiter
- Solitary toxic nodules
- Noncompliant patients

4. Perform a subtotal thyroidectomy to provide a rapid, effective, curative therapy

Most invasive and expensive therapy; hypothyroidism is inevitable. Surgical removal of part of the gland often is the best treatment for patients with extremely enlarged glands or multinodular goiter. Surgery is avoided in the pregnant patient because of risk of miscarriage or preterm delivery. The patient is prepared with antithyroid agents until normal thyroid function is achieved (usually 6 to 8 weeks). The most frequent postoperative complication is hemorrhage at the operative site. The following complications are rare but can be extremely serious: hypoparathyroidism, laryngeal nerve injury, and tetany from damage to the parathyroid glands.

CARE PLANS FOR THYROID STORM

 INEFFECTIVE PROTECTION *related to potential for thyrotoxic crisis (thyroid storm) secondary to emotional stress, trauma, infection, pregnancy (especially labor and delivery), or surgical manipulation of the gland.*

Goals/Outcomes: The patient is free of symptoms of thyroid storm as evidenced by normothermia, BP 90/60 mm Hg or greater (or within patient's baseline range), HR 100 bpm or less, and orientation to person, place, and time. If thyroid storm occurs, it is noted promptly and reported immediately.

NOC Immune Hypersensitivity Response

Risk Identification

1. Measure and report rectal or core temperature greater than 38.3° C (101° F): often the first sign of impending thyroid storm.
2. Monitor vital signs hourly for evidence of hypotension and increasing tachycardia and fever.
3. Monitor the patient for signs of congestive heart failure, which occurs as an effect of thyroid storm: jugular vein distention, crackles (rales), decreased amplitude of peripheral pulses, peripheral edema, and hypotension. Immediately report any significant findings to physician, and prepare to transfer the patient to ICU if they are noted. Maternal and fetal monitoring is initiated on pregnant patients.
4. Provide a cool, calm, protected environment to minimize emotional stress if possible. Reassure patient, and explain all procedures. Limit the number of visitors.
5. Ensure good handwashing and meticulous aseptic technique for dressing changes and all procedures. Advise visitors who have contracted or been exposed to a communicable disease either not to enter patient's room or to use appropriate infection control precautions.
6. Administer acetaminophen to decrease temperature.

> **Safety Alert**   *Aspirin is contraindicated because it releases thyroxine from protein-binding sites and increases free thyroxine levels.*

7. Provide cool sponge baths or apply ice packs to patient's axilla and groin areas to decrease fever. If high temperature continues, obtain a prescription for a hypothermia blanket.
8. Administer PTU as prescribed to prevent further synthesis and release of thyroid hormones.
9. Administer β-blockers as prescribed to block SNS effects.
10. Administer IV fluids as prescribed to provide adequate hydration and prevent vascular collapse. Fluid volume deficit may occur because of increased fluid excretion by the kidneys or excessive diaphoresis. Carefully monitor I&O hourly to prevent fluid overload or inadequate fluid replacement. Decreasing output with normal specific gravity may indicate decreased cardiac output, whereas decreasing output with increased specific gravity can signal dehydration.
11. Administer iodides as prescribed, 1 hour after administering PTU.

> **Safety Alert**   *If given before PTU, iodides can exacerbate symptoms in susceptible persons.*

Thyrotoxicosis Crisis (Thyroid Storm)

12. Administer small doses of insulin as prescribed to control hyperglycemia. Hyperglycemia can occur as an effect of thyroid storm because of the hypermetabolic state.
13. Administer prescribed supplemental oxygen to support increased metabolism. Monitor with pulse oximetry to maintain oxygen saturation of 95% or more.

NIC Cardiac Care: Acute; Surveillance: Late Pregnancy; Fluid/Electrolyte Management; Hyperglycemia Management; Energy Management; Nutritional Monitoring; Vital Signs Monitoring

IMPAIRED SWALLOWING (OR RISK FOR SAME) *related to edema or laryngeal nerve damage resulting from surgical procedure.*

Goals/Outcomes: The patient reports swallowing with minimal difficulty, has minimal or absent hoarseness, and is free of symptoms of respiratory dysfunction as evidenced by RR 12 to 20 breaths/min with normal depth and pattern and absence of inspiratory stridor. Laryngeal nerve damage, if it occurs, is detected promptly and reported immediately.
NOC Aspiration Prevention, Swallowing Status

Aspiration Precautions
1. Monitor respiratory status for signs of edema (i.e., dyspnea, choking, inspiratory stridor, inability to swallow). Assess patient's voice. Slight hoarseness is normal after surgery. Persistent hoarseness indicates laryngeal nerve damage. If bilateral nerve damage is present, upper airway obstruction can occur. Report findings to advanced practice provider promptly.
2. Elevate HOB 30 to 45 degrees to minimize edema and incisional stress. Support patient's head with flat or cervical pillows so that it is in a neutral position.
3. Keep tracheostomy set and oxygen equipment at the bedside at all times. Suction upper airway as needed, using gentle suction to avoid stimulating laryngospasm.
4. To minimize pain and anxiety and enhance patient's ability to swallow, administer analgesics promptly and as prescribed.

NIC Management; Nutrition Therapy; Respiratory Monitoring; Swallowing Therapy

ANXIETY *related to SNS stimulation*

Goals/Outcomes: Within 24 hours of hospital admission, the patient is free of harmful anxiety as evidenced by a HR 100 bpm or less, RR 12–20 breaths/min with normal depth and pattern, and absence of or decreases in irritability and restlessness. The patient and significant others verbalize knowledge about the causes of the patient's behavior.
NOC Anxiety Level, Anxiety Self-control

Anxiety Reduction
1. Assess for anxiety; administer short-acting sedatives (e.g., lorazepam) as prescribed.
2. Provide a quiet, stress-free environment away from loud noises or excessive activity.
3. Limit number of visitors and the amount of time they spend with patient. Advise significant others to avoid discussing stressful topics and to refrain from arguing with the patient.
4. Administer β-blockers as prescribed to reduce anxiety, tachycardia, and heat intolerance.
5. Reassure the patient that anxiety is related to the disease and that treatment decreases severity.
6. Inform significant others that the patient's agitated behavior should not be taken personally.

NIC Coping Enhancement; High-Risk Pregnancy Care

IMBALANCED NUTRITION: LESS THAN BODY REQUIREMENTS *related to hypermetabolic state and/or inadequate nutrient absorption.*

Goals/Outcomes: By a minimum of 24 hours before hospital discharge, the patient has adequate nutrition as evidenced by stable weight and a positive nitrogen balance.
NOC Nutritional Status

Nutrition Therapy
1. Provide foods high in calories, protein, carbohydrates, and vitamins.
2. Administer vitamin supplements as prescribed, and explain their importance to patient.
3. Administer prescribed antidiarrheal medications, which increase absorption of nutrients from the GI tract.
4. Weigh the patient daily, and report significant losses to advanced practice provider.

NIC Weight Management; Weight Gain Assistance; Nutritional Counseling

DISTURBED SLEEP PATTERN *related to accelerated metabolism*

Goals/Outcomes: Within 48 hours of hospital admission, the patient relates the attainment of sufficient rest and sleep.

Sleep Enhancement
1. Adjust care activities to patient's tolerance.
2. Provide frequent rest periods of at least 90-minute duration. If possible, arrange for the patient to have bed rest in a quiet, cool room.
3. Administer short-acting sedatives (e.g., lorazepam) as prescribed to promote rest.

NIC Anxiety Reduction; Meditation Facilitation

IMPAIRED TISSUE INTEGRITY OF THE CORNEA *related to dryness that can occur with exophthalmos in persons with Graves disease.*

Goals/Outcomes: Within 24 hours of admission, patient's corneas are moist and intact.
NIC Tissue Integrity: Skin and Mucous Membranes

Eye Care
1. Teach the patient to wear dark glasses in the sun or for highly lit areas to protect the cornea.
2. Administer lubricating eye drops as prescribed to supplement lubrication and decrease SNS stimulation, which can cause lid retraction.
3. If appropriate, apply eye shields or tape the eyes shut at bedtime.
4. Administer thioamides as prescribed to maintain normal metabolic state and halt progression of exophthalmos.

NIC Skin Care: Topical Treatments

DEFICIENT KNOWLEDGE: MEDICATIONS *related to the potential for side effects from iodides and thioamides or stopping thioamides abruptly.*

Goals/Outcomes: Within the 24-hour period before hospital discharge, the patient verbalizes knowledge about potential side effects of prescribed medications, signs and symptoms of hypothyroidism and hyperthyroidism, and the importance of following the prescribed medical regimen. The patient understands that he or she must be seen within 4 months for endocrine follow-up.
NOC Knowledge: Medications; Knowledge: Illness Care

Teaching: Individual
1. Explain importance of taking antithyroid medications daily, as prescribed.
2. Teach indicators of hypothyroidism (e.g., early fatigue, weight gain, anorexia, constipation, menstrual irregularities, muscle cramps, lethargy, inability to concentrate, hair loss, cold intolerance, and hoarseness), which may occur from excessive antithyroid medication, and the signs and symptoms that necessitate medical attention, including cold intolerance, fatigue, lethargy, and peripheral or periorbital edema.
3. Teach side effects of thioamides and symptoms that require medical attention: appearance of a rash, fever, or pharyngitis, which can occur in the presence of agranulocytosis and require prompt medical intervention.
4. Discuss signs of worsening hyperthyroidism, including high body temperature, palpitations, rapid HR, irritability, anxiety, and feelings of restlessness or panic.
5. Explain importance of continued and frequent medical follow-up.

6. Indicators that require medical attention: fever, rash, or sore throat (side effects of thioamides), and symptoms of hypothyroidism or worsening hyperthyroidism.
7. For patients receiving radioactive iodine, explain the importance of not holding children to the chest for 72 hours following therapy, because children are more susceptible to the effects of radiation. Explain that there is negligible risk for adults.
8. Stress the importance of avoiding physical and emotional stress early in the recuperative stage and maximizing coping mechanisms for dealing with stress.
9. For patients at risk for heart failure with or without hypothyroidism or hyperthyroidism may have an exacerbation of heart failure symptoms.

NIC Learning Facilitation; Health Education; Teaching: Disease Process; Teaching: Prescribed Medication; Teaching: Activity/Exercise

ADDITIONAL NURSING DIAGNOSES

See Compromised Family Coping, in Oncologic Emergencies, Chapter 11; Nutritional Support, Chapter 1; Alterations in Consciousness, Chapter 1; Emotional and Spiritual Support of the Patient and Significant Others, Chapter 2; Dysrhythmias and Conduction Disturbances, Chapter 5; Heart Failure, Chapter 5.

SELECTED REFERENCES

Abraham A, Shafi F, Iqbal M, et al: Syndrome of inappropriate antidiuretic hormone due to multiple myeloma, *Mo Med* 108:377–379, 2011.

Afshinnia F, Sheth N, Perlman R: Syndrome of inappropriate antidiuretic hormone in association with amiodarone therapy: a case report and review of literature, *Ren Fail* 33:456–468, 2011.

Agha A, Thornton E, O'Kelly P, et al: Posterior pituitary dysfunction after traumatic brain injury, *J Clin Endocrinol Metab* 89:5987–5992, 2004.

Ahmed M, Pattar J: SIADH following laparoscopic (totally extraperitoneal) inguinal hernia repair, *Ann R Coll Surg Engl* 94:e166–e167, 2012.

Albright TN, Zimmerman MA, Selzman CH: Vasopressin in the cardiac surgery intensive care unit, *Am J Crit Care* 11:326–330, 2002. [Erratum to Vasopressin in the cardiac surgery intensive care unit *Am J Crit Care* 11:503, 2002.].

Aperis G, Alivanis P: Tolvaptan: a new therapeutic agent, *Rev Recent Clin Trials* 6:177–188, 2011.

Bahn RS, Burch HB, Cooper DS, et al: Hyperthyroidism and other causes of thyrotoxicosis: management guidelines of the American Thyroid Association and American Association of Clinical Endocrinologists, *Endocr Pract* 17:456–520, 2011.

Bornstein SR: Predisposing factors for adrenal insufficiency, *N Engl J Med* 360:2328–2339, 2009.

Brent GA, editor: *Thyroid function testing: Springer Series Vol. 28: Endocrine updates*, ed 1, New York, 2010, Springer.

Bryan MK, Nguyen MT, Hilas O: Syndrome of inappropriate antidiuretic hormone associated with tolterodine therapy, *Consult Pharm* 25:320–322, 2010.

Castillo JJ, Vincent M, Justice E: Diagnosis and management of hyponatremia in cancer patients, *Oncologist* 17:756–765, 2012.

Centers for Disease Control and Prevention (CDC): *National diabetes statistics report, 2014: Estimates of diabetes and its burden in the United States*, Atlanta, GA, 2014, National Center for Chronic Disease Prevention and Health Promotion, CDC. http://www.cdc.gov/diabetes/pubs/statsreport14/national-diabetes-report-web.pdf.

Chaker AJ, Vaidya B: Addison disease in adults: diagnosis and management, *Am J Med* 123:409–413, 2010.

Charmandari E, Nicolaides NC, Chrousos GP: Adrenal insufficiency, *Lancet* 383:2152–2167, 2014.

Cini G, Carpi A, Mechanick J, et al: Thyroid hormones and the cardiovascular system: pathophysiology and interventions, *Biomed Pharmacother* 63:742–753, 2009.

Cohen J, Venkatesh B: Relative adrenal insufficiency in the intensive care population; background and critical appraisal of the evidence, *Anaesth Intensive Care* 38:425–436, 2010.

COIITSS Study Investigators: Corticosteroid treatment and intensive insulin therapy for septic shock in adults: a randomized controlled trial, *JAMA* 303:341–348, 2010.

Cooper DS, Doherty GM, Haugen BR, et al: Revised American Thyroid Association management guidelines for patients with thyroid nodules and differentiated thyroid cancer, *Thyroid* 19:1167–1214, 2009.

Coussement J, Danguy C, Zouaoui-Boudjeltia K, et al: Treatment of the syndrome of inappropriate secretion of antidiuretic hormone with urea in critically ill patients, *Am J Nephrol* 35:265–270, 2012.

Crawford K: Guidelines for care of the hospitalized patient with hyperglycemia and diabetes, *Crit Care Nurs Clin North Am* 25:1–6, 2013.

Decaux G, Andres C, Gankam Kengne F, Soupart A: Treatment of euvolemic hyponatremia in the intensive care unit by urea, *Crit Care* 14:R184, 2010.

Decaux G, Musch W: Clinical laboratory evaluation of the syndrome of inappropriate secretion of antidiuretic hormone, *Clin J Am Soc Nephrol* 3:1175–1184, 2008.

Decaux G: The syndrome of inappropriate secretion of antidiuretic hormone (SIADH), *Semin Nephrol* 29:239–256, 2009.

Dellinger RP, Levy MM, Rhodes A, et al: Surviving Sepsis Campaign: International Guidelines for Management of Severe Sepsis and Septic Shock: 2012, *Crit Care Med* 41:580–637, 2013.

Ebner FH, Hauser TK, Honegger J: SIADH following pituitary adenoma apoplexy, *Neurol Sci* 31:217–218, 2010.

Edmunds MW, Mayhew MS, Bridgers C: Thyroid medications. In Edmunds MW, Mayhew MS: *Pharmacology for the primary care provider*, ed 3, St Louis, 2009, Mosby, pp 559–567.

Ellison DH, Berl T: The syndrome of inappropriate antidiuresis, *N Engl J Med* 356:2064–2072, 2007.

Eskes SA, Wiersinga WM: Amiodarone and thyroid, *Best Pract Res Clin Endocrinol Metab* 23:735–751, 2009.

Esposito P, Piotti G, Bianzina S, et al: The syndrome of inappropriate antidiuresis: pathophysiology, clinical management and new therapeutic options, *Nephron Clin Pract* 119:c62–c73, 2011.

Fenske W, Allolio B: The syndrome of inappropriate secretion of antidiuretic hormone: diagnostic and therapeutic advances, *Horm Metab Res* 42:691–702, 2010.

Garber JR, Cobin RH, Gharib H, et al: Clinical practice guidelines for hypothyroidism in adults: cosponsored by the American Association of Clinical Endocrinologists and the American Thyroid Association, *Endocr Pract* 18:988–1028, 2012.

Gharib H, Papini E, Paschke R, et al: American Association of Clinical Endocrinologists, Associazione Medici Endocrinologi, and European Thyroid Association Medical Guidelines for Clinical Practice for the Diagnosis and Management of Thyroid Nodules, *Endocr Pract* 16(Suppl 1):1–43, 2010.

Gilbar PJ, Richmond J, Wood J, Sullivan A: Syndrome of inappropriate antidiuretic hormone secretion induced by a single dose of oral cyclophosphamide, *Ann Pharmacother* 46:e23, 2012.

Goldberg PA, Kedves A, Walter K, et al: "Waste not want not": determining optimum priming volumes for intravenous insulin infusions, *Diabetes Technol Ther* 8:598–601, 2006.

Grant JF, Cho D, Nichani S: How is SIADH diagnosed and managed? *Hospitalist*, July 1, 2011. http://www.the-hospitalist.org/article/how-is-siadh-diagnosed-and-managed/.

Gray ST, Holbrook EH, Najm MH, et al: Syndrome of inappropriate antidiuretic hormone secretion in patients with olfactory neuroblastoma, *Otolaryngol Head Neck Surg* 147:147–151, 2012.

Graziani G, Cucchiari D, Aroldi A, et al: Syndrome of inappropriate secretion of antidiuretic hormone in traumatic brain injury: when tolvaptan becomes a life saving drug, *J Neurol Neurosurg Psychiatry* 83:510–512, 2012.

Hamdy O: *Diabetic ketoacidosis treatment & management*. Diseases/conditions, Oct 29, 2014. http://emedicine.medscape.com/article/118361-treatment.

Hamdy O: *Diabetic ketoacidosis Diseases/conditions Oct 29,2014*. http://emedicine.medscape.com/article/118361-overview.

Handelsman Y, Mechanick JI, Blonde L, et al: American Association of Clinical Endocrinologists Medical Guidelines for Clinical Practice for developing a diabetes mellitus comprehensive care plan, *Endocr Pract* 17(Suppl 2):1–53, 2011.

Hannon MJ, Thompson CJ: The syndrome of inappropriate antidiuretic hormone: prevalence, causes, and consequences, *Eur J Endocrinol* 162(Suppl 1):S5–S12, 2010.

Hollowell J, Staehling N, Flanders D, et al: Serum TSH, T4, and Thyroid Antibodies in the United States Population (1988 to 1994): National Health and Nutrition Examination Survey (NHANES III), *The Journal of Clinical Endocrinology & Metabolism* 87(2):489–499.

Holm EA, Bie P, Ottesen M, et al: Diagnosis of the syndrome of inappropriate secretion of antidiuretic hormone. *South Med J* 102:380–384, 2009.

John CA, Day MW: Central neurogenic diabetes insipidus, syndrome of inappropriate secretion of antidiuretic hormone, and cerebral salt-wasting in traumatic brain injury, *Crit Care Nurse* 32:e1–e8, 2012.

Juul KV, Bichet DG, Nørgaard JP: Desmopressin duration of antidiuretic action in patients with central diabetes insipidus, *Endocrine* 40:67–74, 2011.

Katsilambros N, Kanaka-Gantenbein C, Liatis S, et al: Diabetic ketoacidosis in adults. In *Diabetic emergencies: diagnosis and clinical management*, ed 2, Hoboken, NJ, 2011, Wiley-Blackwell.

Kazama I, Arata T, Michimata M, et al: Lithium effectively complements vasopressin V2 receptor antagonist in the treatment of hyponatraemia of SIADH rats, *Nephrol Dial Transplant* 22:68–76, 2007.

Khardori R, Castillo D: Endocrine and metabolic changes during sepsis: an update, *Med Clin North Am* 96:1095–1105, 2012.

Kitabchi AE, Umpierrez GE, Miles JM, Fisher JN: Hyperglycemic crisis in adult patients with diabetes, *Diabetes Care* 32:1335–1343, 2009.

Kittisupamongkol W: Hyperthyroidism or thyrotoxicosis? *Cleve Clin J Med* 76:152, 2009.

Ku E, Nobakht N, Campese VM: Lixivaptan: a novel vasopressin receptor antagonist, *Expert Opin Investig Drugs* 18:657–662, 2009.

Lam SW, Bauer SR, Guzman JA: Septic shock: the initial moments and beyond, *Cleve Clin J Med* 80:175–184, 2013.

Langouche L, Van den Berghe G: The dynamic neuroendocrine response to critical illness, *Endocrinol Metab Clin North Am* 35:777–791, 2006.

LeBeau SO, Mandel SJ: Thyroid disorders during pregnancy, *Endocrinol Metab Clin North Am* 35:117–136, 2006.

Lehrich RW, Greenberg A: Hyponatremia and the use of vasopressin receptor antagonists in critically ill patients, *J Intensive Care Med* 27:207–218, 2012.

Lewis MA, Hendrickson AW, Moynihan TJ: Oncologic emergencies: pathophysiology, presentation, diagnosis, and treatment, *CA Cancer J Clin* 61:287–314, 2011.

Luber SD, Fischer DR, Venkat A: Care of the bariatric surgery patient in the emergency department, *J Emerg Med* 34:13–20, 2008.

McCance KL, Huether SE, Brashers VL, Rote NS: Unit VI: The endocrine system. In *Pathophysiology: the biologic basis for disease in adults and children*, ed 6, St Louis, 2010, Mosby, pp 696–780.

Mechanick JI, Youdim A, Jones DB, et al: Clinical practice guidelines for the perioperative nutritional, metabolic, and nonsurgical support of the bariatric surgery patient–2013 update: cosponsored by American Association of Clinical Endocrinologists, the Obesity Society, and American Society for Metabolic & Bariatric Surgery, *Endocr Pract* 19:337–372, 2013.

Molitch ME: Anterior pituitary. In Goldman L, Ausiello DA, editors: *Cecil Medicine*, ed 23, Philadelphia, PA, 2008, Saunders, pp 1674–1691.

Molitch ME: Neuroendocrinology and the neuroendocrine system. In Goldman L, Ausiello DA, editors: *Cecil Medicine*, ed 23, Philadelphia, PA, 2007, Saunders Elsevier, pp 1664–1674.

O'Connor KJ, Wood KE, Lord K: Intensive management of organ donors to maximize transplantation, *Crit Care Nurse* 26:94–100, 2006.

Pelosof LC, Gerber DE: Paraneoplastic syndromes: an approach to diagnosis and treatment, *Mayo Clin Proc* 85:838–854, 2010. [Erratum to Paraneoplastic syndromes: an approach to diagnosis and treatment, *Mayo Clin Proc* 86:364, 2011.].

Peri A, Combe C: Considerations regarding the management of hyponatraemia secondary to SIADH, *Best Pract Res Clin Endocrinol Metab* 26(Suppl 1):S16–S26, 2012.

Peri A, Pirozzi N, Parenti G, et al: Hyponatremia and the syndrome of inappropriate secretion of antidiuretic hormone (SIADH), *J Endocrinol Invest* 33:671–682, 2010.

Peters S, Kuhn R, Gardner B, Bernard P: Use of conivaptan for refractory syndrome of inappropriate secretion of antidiuretic hormone in a pediatric patient, *Pediatr Emerg Care* 29:230–232, 2013.

Pieracci FM, Barie PS, Pomp A: Critical care of the bariatric patient, *Crit Care Med* 34:1796–1804, 2006.

Pollock F, Funk DC: Acute diabetes management: adult patients with hyperglycemic crises and hypoglycemia, *AACN Adv Crit Care* 24:314–324, 2013.

Robertson GL: Vaptans for the treatment of hyponatremia, *Nat Rev Endocrinol* 7:151–161, 2011.

Ross DS: Radioiodine therapy for hyperthyroidism, *N Engl J Med* 364:542–550, 2011.

Santacroce L: *Paraneoplastic syndromes*. Aug 3, 2014. http://emedicine.medscape.com/article/280744-overview.

Schrier RW, Gross P, Gheorghiade M, et al: Tolvaptan, a selective oral vasopressin V2-receptor antagonist, for hyponatremia, *N Engl J Med* 355:2099–2112, 2006.

Sejling AS, Pedersen-Bjergaard U, Eiken P: Syndrome of inappropriate ADH secretion and severe osteoporosis, *J Clin Endocrinol Metab* 97:4306–4310, 2012.

Shaaban H, Thomas D, Guron G: A rare case of metastatic ductal type prostate adenocarcinoma presenting with syndrome of inappropriate secretion of antidiuretic hormone: a case report and review, *J Cancer Res Ther* 8:308–310, 2012.

Siani A, Gabrielli R, Accrocca F, Marcucci G: SIADH after carotid endarterectomy, *Ann Vasc Surg* 26:859.e7–e8, 2012.

Siegenthaler W: Disorders of sodium and water homeostasis. In *Siegenthaler's differential diagnosis in internal medicine: from symptom to diagnosis*, New York, 2007, Thieme, pp 895–944.

Siraj ES: Update on the diagnosis and treatment of hyperthyroidism, *J Clin Outcomes Manag* 15:298–307, 2008.

Soupart A, Coffernils M, Couturier B, et al: Efficacy and tolerance of urea compared with vaptans for long-term treatment of patients with SIADH, *Clin J Am Soc Nephrol* 7:742–747, 2012.

Sterns RH: *Pathophysiology and etiology of the syndrome of inappropriate antidiuretic hormone secretion (SIADH)*, July 15, 2014. http://www.uptodate.com/contents/pathophysiology-and-etiology-of-the-syndrome-of-inappropriate-antidiuretic-hormone-secretion-siadh.

Sterns RH: *Treatment of hyponatremia: syndrome of inappropriate antidiuretic hormone secretion (SIADH) and reset osmostat.* UpToDate. http://www.uptodate.com/contents/treatment-of-hyponatremia-syndrome-of-inappropriate-antidiuretic-hormone-secretion-siadh-and-reset-osmostat?source=search_result&search=Treatment+of+hyponatremia%3A+syndrome+of+inappropriate+antidiuretic+hormone+secretion+%28SIADH%29+and+reset+osmostat&selectedTitle=1~150.

Stewart PM, Krone NP: The adrenal cortex. In Melmed S, Polonsky KS, Larsen PR, Kronenberg HM, editors: *Williams textbook of endocrinology*, ed 12, Philadelphia, PA, 2011, Saunders, pp 479–544.

Suemori K, Hasegawa H, Nanba C, et al: Syndrome of inappropriate secretion of antidiuretic hormone induced by tacrolimus in a patient with systemic lupus erythematosus, *Mod Rheumatol* 21:97–100, 2011.

Tantisattamo E, Ng RC: Dual paraneoplastic syndromes: small cell lung carcinoma-related oncogenic osteomalacia, and syndrome of inappropriate antidiuretic hormone secretion: report of a case and review of the literature, *Hawaii Med J* 70:139–143, 2011.

Torgersen C, Luckner G, Schröder DC, et al: Concomitant arginine vasopressin and hydrocortisone therapy in severe septic shock: association with mortality, *Intensive Care Med* 37:1432–1437, 2011.

Venkatesh B, Cohen J: Adrenocortical (dys)function in septic shock—a sick euadrenal state, *Best Pract Res Clin Endocrinol Metab* 25:719–733, 2011.

Wartofsky L: Myxedema coma, *Endocrinol Metab Clin North Am* 35:687–698, 2006.

Webster Marketon JI, Sternberg EM: The glucocorticoid receptor: a revisited target for toxins, *Toxins (Basel)* 2:1359–1380, 2010.

Wei J, Xiao Y, Yu X, et al: Early onset of syndrome of inappropriate antidiuretic hormone secretion (SIADH) after allogeneic haematopoietic stem cell transplantation: case report and review of the literature, *J Int Med Res* 38:705–710, 2010.

Wesche D, Deen PMT, Knoers NVAM: Congenital nephrogenic diabetes insipidus: the current state of affairs, *Pediatr Nephrol* 27:2183–2204, 2012.

Yam FK, Eraly SA: Syndrome of inappropriate antidiuretic hormone associated with moxifloxacin, *Am J Health Syst Pharm* 69:217–220, 2012.

Zietse R, van der Lubbe N, Hoorn EJ: Current and future treatment options in SIADH, *NDT Plus* 2(Suppl 3):iii12–iii19, 2009.

Thyrotoxicosis Crisis (Thyroid Storm)

GASTROINTESTINAL ASSESSMENT: GENERAL

GOAL OF SYSTEM ASSESSMENT

Evaluate for dysfunctional ingestion and digestion of food and elimination of waste products. When assessing the surgical bariatric patient (person of size), assess the type of gastric bypass performed, the number of days that have elapsed since surgery, and the amount of weight lost as a result of the surgical procedure.

VITAL SIGN ASSESSMENT

- Heart rate (HR), blood pressure (BP), and peripheral pulses to identify volume status, because significant fluid losses can occur with gastrointestinal (GI) bleeding or diarrhea.
- Note temperature, because infections of the GI tract are common.
- Considerations for the surgical bariatric patient: HR greater than 110 beats/min (bpm), BP decrease of greater than 10% from baseline, and temperature elevated greater than 38.6° C (101.5° F) are signs of anastomotic leak and is a surgical/medical emergency that can lead to death.

OBSERVATION

Observe the abdomen for distension and skin color changes, which may be signs of other system disorders.

- Cullen sign (bluish umbilicus) may indicate intraabdominal hemorrhage.
- Turner sign (bruising on the flanks) may indicate retroperitoneal hemorrhage.
- Visible, torturous, dilated abdominal veins may indicate inferior vena cava obstruction.
- Cutaneous abdominal angiomas may indicate liver disease.
- Considerations for the bariatric patient: Assess for abdominal hernias around the umbilicus or anywhere along the abdominal wall resulting from the pressure the excess abdominal fat exerts on the musculature during movement.
- Assess urine output to help determine hydration status.

AUSCULTATION

Evaluate bowel sounds in each of the quadrants in a systemic manner.

- Hyperactive bowel sounds may indicate diarrhea or early intestinal obstruction.
- Hypoactive to absent bowel sounds may indicate paralytic ileus or peritonitis.
- High-pitched rushing sounds may indicate intestinal obstruction.
- Considerations for the bariatric patient: Query the patient and assess for what is the normal bowel pattern.
  - Assess for constipation and diarrhea.

Evaluate for systolic bruits (humming, swishing, or blowing sounds) over:

- Abdominal aorta: partial arterial obstruction.
- Renal artery: renal artery stenosis.
- Iliac artery: hepatomegaly.

PALPATION

The normal abdomen should be soft and nontender to palpation. Palpate for liver enlargement and tenderness. The spleen is not normally palpable. If found palpable, the spleen is enlarged. Further palpation must be discontinued, because it may cause splenic rupture.

Safety Alert	*If the abdomen is rigid, do not palpate; it is a sign of peritoneal inflammation. Palpation could cause rupture of the inflamed organ.*

NUTRITION ASSESSMENT

Evaluate for risk factors and indications of malnutrition for which patients who are critically ill are at risk. Malnutrition may occur resulting from negative caloric intake with concomitant GI obstruction, malabsorption syndromes, infectious diseases, certain medications, and surgical treatment. Additionally, caloric needs are greatly increased in the critically ill as a result of hypermetabolic states produced by trauma, fever, sepsis, and wound healing.

- Evaluate for general signs of malnutrition (Table 9-1).
- Considerations for the surgical bariatric patient: Never insert a nasogastric (NG) or any type of feeding tube, because the gastric bypass   surgery has altered the anatomy of the stomach.
- Considerations for the surgical bariatric patient: Pills must be crushed. Find alternative medications for extended or sustained release, because they will not be absorbed.
- Considerations for the bariatric patient (person of size): Malnutrition is common in the person of size. When critically ill, the person of size will need the appropriate calories to support metabolic demands resulting from the state of illness. A critical illness is not the appropriate time to place a person of size on a diet.
- Evaluate weight for increases and decreases.
- Laboratory identification of malnutrition:
    - Serum albumin less than 3 g/dL.
    - Serum transferrin less than 200 mg/dL.
    - Serum prealbumin less than 16.0 mg/dL.
    - Total lymphocyte count between 15% and 40% of the WBC with an absolute lymphocyte count of 1000-3500/cm^3
    - Triglycerides less than 150mg/dL.

Table 9-1	GENERAL SIGNS OF MALNUTRITION	
Body System	**Signs**	**Deficiency**
Skin, nails	Dry skin Brittle nails; spooned-shaped nails Considerations for the surgical bariatric patient: Will have vitamin deficiencies if not on multivitamins	Vitamin deficiency Iron deficiency
Mouth	Cracks; beefy, red tongue	Vitamin deficiency
Stomach	Decreased gastric acidity Delayed gastric emptying	Protein deficiency
Intestines	Decreased motility and absorption Diarrhea Considerations for the surgical bariatric patient: Will have protein deficiency unless on high protein diet	Protein deficiency Altered normal flora
Liver/biliary	Hepatomegaly Ascites	Decreased absorption of fat-soluble vitamins Protein deficiency
Cardiovascular	Edema Tachycardia; hypotension	Protein deficiency Fluid volume deficiency
Musculoskeletal	Decreased muscle mass Subcutaneous tissue loss	Protein, carbohydrate, and fat deficiency

Gastrointestinal Assessment: General

SCREENING LABWORK

- Serum electrolyte levels.
- Complete blood count (CBC).
- Serum amylase.
- Serum lipase.
- Liver function tests (LFTs).

ACUTE GASTROINTESTINAL BLEEDING

PATHOPHYSIOLOGY

Bleeding can occur at any point along the upper (esophagus, stomach, and duodenum) and lower (small intestine, large intestine/colon, rectum) portions of the alimentary tract, but is more prevalent in the upper segment. Both upper and lower GI bleeding account for significant morbidity, with a mortality rate of 3% to 14%. Mortality may reach 40% in the presence of hemodynamic instability. The occurrence of acute GI bleeding is decreasing in the United States resulting from a reduced incidence of *Helicobacter pylori* infection and advances in ulcer-prevention strategies including consistent use of prophylactic medications in nonsteroidal antiinflammatory drug (NSAID) users. The following overview presents common GI bleeding sites and occurrences.

UPPER GASTROINTESTINAL BLEEDING

Esophagus

Esophageal varices (EVs) are the most common cause of massive and persistent esophageal hemorrhage. EVs are caused by significant portal hypertension causing bleeding to occur under high pressure. Acute variceal bleeding is severe, difficult to control, and rarely resolves spontaneously. Less frequent causes of EV bleeding include esophagitis, esophageal ulcers, and tumors. Maneuvers that increase intraabdominal pressure (IAP) (e.g., retching, vomiting, straining, coughing, blunt abdominal trauma) can lead to a Mallory-Weiss (MW) tear (a laceration at the esophagogastric junction), which can result in massive bleeding. MW tears are commonly found in patients with hiatal hernia.

Stomach and Duodenum

The most common cause of upper GI bleeding (UGIB) is peptic ulcer disease (PUD), accounting for greater than 50% of UGIB disorders. Peptic ulcers are chronic lesions that are most prevalent in the stomach and duodenum. These lesions extend from the protective mucosa of the GI tract into the submucosa, exposing tissue to gastric acids with eventual autodigestion. Bleeding occurs when the ulcer erodes into a blood vessel. *H. pylori* and NSAID use account for the majority of PUD cases. *H. pylori* infection is more strongly associated with the pathogenesis of peptic ulceration than gastric hyperacidity. The toxins and enzymes released by the *H. pylori* organism are believed to cause mucosal injury through proinflammatory processes and by decreasing duodenal mucosal bicarbonate production resulting in ulceration.

Stress ulceration is a common and potentially life-threatening phenomenon that occurs in patients who are critically ill, with higher incidence in those who are mechanically ventilated. Stress ulcers comprise multiple lesions, generally confined to the gastric fundus. Ulcers primarily result from stress-related hyperacidity of critical illness and gastric mucosal ischemia secondary to diversion of blood away from the GI tract during the stress response. Curling ulcers occur in the proximal duodenum and are seen in patients with major burn injuries or major trauma. Ischemia and necrosis of the mucosa results from decreased plasma volume. Cushing ulcers are a related condition associated with high gastric acid output and prone to perforation that occurs in patients with increased intracranial pressure. These patients have sustained a serious head injury or are experiencing a critical central nervous system (CNS) disorder. PUD resulting from a hypersecretory state is observed in Zöllinger-Ellison syndrome (ZES). In ZES, ulcerations occur in the stomach, duodenum, and jejunum resulting from excessive gastrin secretion by a tumor, resulting in hyperacidity with mucosal erosion. Benign or malignant GI neoplasms may initiate severe bleeding episodes, especially tumors located in the vascular system that supplies the GI tract.

Ulcer bleeding from the upper GI (UGI) tract is usually self-limiting, most often ceasing spontaneously with the exception of EVs. Recurrent bleeding arises in a substantial proportion of patients and is associated with a poor prognosis. The need for accurate diagnosis and effective therapy is crucial.

LOWER GASTROINTESTINAL BLEEDING
Small Intestine
The structures distal to the ligament of Treitz (a thin muscular band that wraps around the small intestine where the duodenum and jejunum meet) are affected by conditions including arteriovenous malformation, intussusception of the small bowel, acute superior mesenteric artery occlusion, and Crohn disease.

Large Intestine
The most common cause of significant lower GI bleeding (LGIB) is colonic diverticulosis, accounting for up to 50% of all cases. Arteriovenous malformation of the ascending colon and the cecum is also a usual cause of massive colonic bleeding. Inflammatory bowel diseases such as ulcerative colitis and Crohn disease result in friable intestinal mucosa, which can lead to massive hemorrhage and other serious complications, including bowel obstruction and perforation. Other causes include colonic polyps, benign or malignant neoplasms and congenital malformation such as hemangioma or telangiectasia.

Rectum
Hemorrhoids and neoplasms frequently cause LGIB but are usually hemodynamically insignificant.

NEIGHBORING ORGANS
Pancreas and Vascular Grafts
Acute pancreatitis (discussed later in this chapter) and pancreatic pseudocyst are disorders associated with hemorrhage. Patients with intraabdominal vascular grafts are at risk for the development of aortoenteric fistulas with massive GI hemorrhage.

Systemic Organ Diseases
Hypoperfusion associated with decreased cardiac output (CO) or volume depletion can lead to GI ischemia, resulting in necrosis and hemorrhage. A high incidence of GI bleeding is associated with uremia in patients with kidney failure because of platelet dysfunction from abnormal adhesiveness, resulting in prolonged bleeding time. Collagen vascular diseases such as systemic lupus erythematosus can result in thrombosis of small vessels in the small intestine, eventually leading to ulceration. Coagulopathic conditions (e.g., disseminated intravascular coagulation [DIC], thrombocytopenia) are associated with hematemesis and melena caused by decreased clotting ability.

MEDICATIONS
Long-standing use of aspirin, corticosteroids, or anticoagulants is associated with serious GI bleeding. Ethanol may cause or potentiate ulcer bleeding because it induces gastric mucosal injury. NSAIDs cause increased risk of serious GI bleeding, ulceration, and perforation of the stomach and intestines. Traditional NSAIDs are nonselective inhibitors of both cyclooxygenase-1 (COX-1) and cyclooxygenase-2 (COX-2) enzymes. COX-1 enzymes regulate gastroduodenal mucosal protective mechanisms. COX-2 enzymes are involved in inflammatory and pain responses. The newer COX-2 selective inhibitors were believed to block pain and inflammation while leaving protective mucosal mechanisms intact, thereby significantly lowering the incidence of GI ulceration and bleeding compared with traditional NSAIDs. However, the COX-2 inhibitors were shown to increase the risk of cardiovascular disease, especially in older adults, resulting in the removal of two of three COX-2 agents from the market. Currently, celecoxib (celebrex) is the only COX-2 selective inhibitor available in the United States. This COX-2 inhibitor is still associated with an increased risk for GI bleeding, while to a lesser degree than traditional NSAIDS; additionally, it does not appear to pose any greater risk for cardiovascular disease than traditional NSAIDs.

OTHER
Obscure GI bleeding is bleeding from an unknown site despite endoscopic and colonoscopy evaluation. These patients are believed to have a source in the small intestine that cannot be pinpointed. These patients may present with visible or occult bleeding (iron deficiency

anemia and/or positive for fecal occult blood). Bleeding as a result of minor trauma: In addition to major abdominal trauma (Chapter 3), foreign bodies such as razors, screws, or nails may lacerate gastric or intestinal mucosa, causing bleeding.

GASTROINTESTINAL ASSESSMENT: ACUTE GASTROINTESTINAL BLEEDING

GOAL OF ASSESSMENT
Evaluate patients for severity of active bleeding, shock states, or risk of rebleeding.

HISTORY AND RISK FACTORS
History and risk factors include critical illness, especially that caused by major injury, surgery, CNS disorder, or burns; prolonged shock or hypoperfusion; organ failure; EVs, excessive alcohol, NSAIDs, or corticosteroid ingestion; inflammatory bowel disease; foreign body ingestion; hiatal hernia; hepatic, pancreatic, or biliary tract disease; blood dyscrasias; penetrating or blunt trauma; familial cancer; recent abdominal surgery; and the presence of *H. pylori*. Identification of those at risk for recurrent bleeding is essential to guide therapy and prevent recurrence. Risk factors associated with rebleeding are listed in Box 9-1.

VITAL SIGN ASSESSMENT
- Systolic BP less than 90 to 100 mm Hg with an HR greater than 100 bpm in a previously normotensive individual signals a 20% or greater reduction in blood volume.
- Orthostatic hypotension signs will be positive revealing a decrease in systolic BP greater than 10 mm Hg with an increase in HR of 10 bpm. Orthostatic hypotension is indicative of recent blood loss of 500 to 1000 mL in the adult.
- Respiratory rate (RR) will be mildly elevated as a response to the diminished oxygen-carrying capacity of the blood. If abdominal pain is present, ventilatory excursion may be limited.
- Urine output will be decreased as a result of volume depletion.

BLOOD LOSS
- The amount of blood lost and rate of bleeding will have varying effects on cardiovascular and other body systems.
- Blood loss of 1000 mL within 15 minutes usually produces tachycardia, hypotension, nausea, weakness, and diaphoresis. Adults can lose up to 500 mL of blood in 15 minutes and remain free of associated symptoms.
- Massive hemorrhage, which is generally defined as loss of greater than 50% of total blood volume within 3 hours.
- Syncope associated with hypotension may also occur.
- Sequestration of fluid into the peritoneum and interstitium further depletes intravascular volume.
- Severe hypovolemic shock and decreased CO can lead to ischemia of various organs, especially the brain and kidneys.

Box 9-1	RISK FACTORS TO PREDICT RECURRENT BLEEDING

- Large-volume blood loss on admission with transfusion of greater than 6 units
- Shock
- Age greater than 60 years
- Hematemesis as the initial sign of hemorrhage
- Stigmata of ulcer bleeding as identified endoscopically (see Box 9-2)
- Bleeding that occurs while hospitalized for another problem

ABDOMINAL PAIN
* Mild to severe epigastric pain is often associated with gastroduodenal ulcerative or erosive disease. The pain is described as dull or gnawing.
* Pain may diminish when blood covers and protects the eroded tissue.
* Blood can irritate the bowels, thereby increasing transit time in the lower GI tract, causing diarrhea.

OBSERVATION
* Extremities are cool and diaphoretic.
* Pallor or cyanosis may be present.
* Alterations in level of consciousness (LOC) with restlessness and confusion.
* Emesis or gastric aspirate contains obvious whole blood or old blood that resembles coffee grounds.
* Hematemesis usually occurs with UGIB from above the ligament of Treitz. Bleeding originating below the level of the duodenum is not usually associated with hematemesis. Emesis of bright red blood is suggestive of recent or ongoing bleeding, and dark, coffee-ground emesis suggests that the bleeding stopped some time ago.
* Abnormal stool:
    * Melena (black, tarry, shiny, stools containing blood, with a distinctive fetid odor) is usually present with UGIB. May also be present with bleeding from the small intestine or proximal large intestine.
    * Hematochezia refers to bright red blood per rectum that is usually caused by a colonic or anorectal source. If the patient is acutely hypotensive however, hematochezia would indicate a severe, brisk UGI bleed with rapid transport through the GI tract.
    * Massive LGIB is associated with dark red "currant jelly" stools or passing fresh blood with clots.
* Jaundice, vascular spiders, ascites, and hepatosplenomegaly are suggestive of liver disease.

AUSCULTATION
* Abdominal auscultation may reveal hyperactive bowel sounds caused by mucosal irritation by blood.
* A silent abdomen suggests serious complications such as ileus, perforation, or vascular occlusion.

PALPATION
* Palpation may reveal epigastric tenderness, which is expected in peptic ulceration.
* An epigastric mass or enlarged lymph nodes may indicate gastric malignancy.
* Decreased peripheral pulses, delayed capillary refill (greater than 2 seconds).

NUTRITION ASSESSMENT
* Evidence of malnutrition will be noted in the presence of chronic liver disease or active, excessive alcohol use.

SCREENING LABWORK
* CBC: May identify decreased hemoglobin (Hgb) and decreased hematocrit (Hct).
* LFTs: May be elevated if advanced liver disease is present.
* Serum chemistry: May identify increased blood urea nitrogen (BUN).

HEMODYNAMIC MEASUREMENTS
* Decreased central venous pressure (CVP).
* Decreased mean arterial pressure (MAP).
* Increased stroke volume variation (SVV).

Diagnostic Tests for Acute Gastrointestinal Bleeding

Test	Purpose	Abnormal Findings
Blood Studies		
Complete blood count (CBC) with differential Hemoglobin (Hgb) Hematocrit (Hct) Red blood cell (RBC) count White blood cell count Platelet count	Serial Hgb and Hct values monitor the amount of blood lost. Total counts monitor hematologic function, except for platelets, which may be nonfunctional despite normal number present.	Initiate blood transfusions for Hgb <7 g/dL. The first Hct value may be near normal 45% because the ratio of blood cells to plasma remains unchanged initially. However, Hct is expected to fall dramatically ≤27% while volume is restored and extravascular fluid mobilizes into the vascular space (hemodilution). Hct <21% generally requires transfusion. Platelet count rises within 1 hour of acute hemorrhage. Leukocytosis occurs frequently following acute hemorrhage.
Serum chemistry: Blood urea nitrogen (BUN) Creatinine BUN:creatinine (Cr) ratio Serum chloride Serum potassium Serum glucose Liver function tests (LFTs): Total bilirubin Ammonia	To assess fluid and electrolyte status. LFTs monitor for hepatic involvement.	BUN will be elevated as a result of dehydration. Cr may be mildly elevated as a result of ↓ glomerular filtration rate secondary to hypovolemia. BUN:Cr ratio ≥25:1 mg/dL suggests upper gastrointestinal (GI) bleed. Hypochloremia, hypokalemia and ↑ serum bicarbonate will be noted with excessive vomiting or gastric suction. Mild hyperglycemia is the result of the body's compensatory response to a stressful stimulus. Hyperbilirubinemia is caused by the breakdown of reabsorbed RBCs and blood pigments. Ammonia levels are often elevated in patients with hepatic disease. Plasma protein levels may rise in response to increased hepatic production.
Arterial blood gas (ABG)	Assesses acid-base status. Lactic acid levels may be drawn separately and may be available on certain ABG analyzers.	Severe shock states produces lactic acidosis reflected by low arterial pH and serum bicarbonate levels and the presence of an anion gap. Hypoxemia may be present with low perfusion states.
Coagulation studies	To assess for preexisting risk factors for bleeding: liver disease; anticoagulant or antiplatelet therapy for cardiac disease. Large blood volume transfusions may lead to the development of coagulopathies.	Elevation of fibrinogen levels, fibrin split products/fibrin degradation products, prothrombin time, partial thromboplastin time, international normalized ratio may be seen.
12-Lead electrocardiogram	Monitor for severe cardiac ischemia findings as a result of hypoperfusion.	Ischemic changes include ST depression and T wave inversion.

Diagnostic Tests for Acute Gastrointestinal Bleeding—cont'd

Test	Purpose	Abnormal Findings
Radiologic Procedures		
Esophagogastroduodenoscopy	To accurately assess the source of upper GI ulcer bleeding. To locate the ulcer, visualize and implement endoscopic therapy, such as sclerosing bleeding vessels.	Endoscopic ulcer findings (endoscopic stigmata) include: Clean ulcer base Adherent clot Visible vessel Active bleeding
Plain films: Abdominal radiograph Chest radiograph	To identify the presence of dilated bowel or free air. A chest x-ray is taken to establish baseline pulmonary status.	Free air seen under the diaphragm suggests perforation.
Barium studies	Usually reserved for nonemergent situations to verify the presence of tumors or other large GI lesions.	Not usually used for acute GI bleeding, because this procedure does not allow for the provision of endoscopic therapy.
Colonoscopy	Direct visualization of the rectum and sigmoid colon through an endoscope for diagnosis and triage of lower GI bleeding.	Mucosal bleeding, polyps, hemorrhoids, and other lesions may be identified. Biopsy specimen may be obtained. Emergent colonoscopy is difficult as a result of length of time for adequate bowel preparation.
Angiography	The visualization of active bleeding from an arterial site or from a large vein in the lower GI tract. Bleeding flow rate must be at least 0.5 to 1.0 mL/min to be visualized by this test.	Clearly identifies bleeding GI arterial systems. Therapeutic arterial embolization or vasopressin infusion may be performed to stop the bleeding during angiography. Complications include dye-induced renal failure, arterial dissection and occlusion, bowel infarction, and myocardial infarction with vasopressin infusion.
Nuclear medicine: Technetium-labeled red blood cell scan	To detect low-flow rate bleeding in the lower GI tract. Usefulness is controversial.	Identifies low-flow bleeding rates of 0.1 to 0.5 mL/min in the lower GI tract. Accuracy remains questionable.

BLOOD UREA NITROGEN–TO–CREATININE RATIO

Elevated BUN:creatinine ratio up to 36:1 mg/dL reflects a disproportionate increase in BUN compared with a mild increase in serum creatinine with UGIB resulting from red blood cells (RBCs) that have bled and pooled in the UGI tract being consumed and digested by duodenal/proximal small intestinal bacteria. The resulting urea is absorbed. BUN increases without a corresponding increase in creatinine. BUN increases are NOT seen with bleeding from the colon or the lower portion of the small intestine. Dehydration contributes to the increased BUN and total protein levels. Mild reduction in glomerular filtration rate from volume depletion causes a mild creatinine elevation.

ESOPHAGOGASTRODUODENOSCOPY

Esophagogastroduodenoscopy is the most accurate means of determining the source of UGI ulcer bleeding. Visualization of the esophagus, stomach, and duodenum using a fiber optic endoscope passed through the mouth is usually performed within the first 12 hours after admission of the patient to identify the exact source of bleeding and characteristics of ulcers, if present. Endoscopic ulcer findings are referred to as endoscopic stigmata. Stigmata indicative of bleeding ulcers, bleeding EVs, or ulcers at risk for rebleeding are identified in Box 9-2,

Box 9-2 STIGMATA OF ACTIVE OR RECENT HEMORRHAGE

Endoscopic Ulcer Findings From Active or Recent Upper Gastrointestinal Hemorrhage:

Diagnostic Endoscopic Findings (Prevalence)	Rebleeding Rate Without Treatment (%)	Rebleeding Rate With Treatment (%)
• Active arterial spurting (12%)	90	15-30
• Nonbleeding visible vessel (22%)	50	15-30
• Active oozing of blood (14%)	10	
• Adherent or overlying clot without oozing (10%)	33	5
• Flat, pigmented slough or spot on the ulcer base (10%)	7	
• Clean ulcer base (32%)	3	

Endoscopic findings in descending order are indicative of high risk for continued bleeding or rebleeding, requiring more aggressive therapy. For patients who do not exhibit these findings, the risk of rebleeding is significantly lower.

Adapted from Wilkins T, Khan N, Nabh A, et al: Diagnosis and management of upper gastrointestinal bleeding. *Am Fam Phys* 85:469-476, 2012.

Stigmata of Active or Recent Hemorrhage (SARH). SARH findings are helpful in determining the course of direct therapy as well as providing prognostic information. Antacids and sucralfate should be withheld until after the procedure, because they can alter the appearance of lesions. Gastric biopsy is usually obtained with endoscopy for *H. pylori* diagnosis as well as to exclude gastric malignancy.

Electrocoagulation, injection therapy (epinephrine), laser, hemoclips, and other therapeutic techniques such as scleral therapy and variceal ligation (banding) may be used during this procedure to stop current bleeding or prevent further bleeding.

COLONOSCOPY
Colonoscopy is diagnostic for patients with LGIB for identification of bleeding through visualization. Colonoscopy is usually performed within 12 to 24 hours of presentation. If a visible vessel or adherent clot is noted, direct therapy can be provided. Direct therapy includes laser therapy, heater probes, electrocoagulation, injection, and argon plasma coagulation. Bleeding from colonic diverticula is usually from multiple sites and intermittent, therefore, direct intervention is frequently limited.

COLLABORATIVE MANAGEMENT
Acute GI bleeding can occur from various lesions or sites in the GI tract. The amount of blood loss can vary from minor to massive (Table 9-2) depending on the cause, resulting in hypovolemic shock with significant associated mortality. The patients requiring intensive care management are those with severe bleeding, advanced age, and significant comorbidities such as end-stage renal disease, hepatic disease, or cardiovascular disease. Severe gastrointestinal bleeding is defined as GI bleeding:
- Identified by documented hematemesis, melena, hematochezia, or positive NG lavage;
- Accompanied by shock or orthostatic hypotension;
- Causing a decrease in the hematocrit value by at least 6% (or a decrease in the hemoglobin level of at least 2 g/dL), or requiring transfusion of at least 2 units of packed RBCs (pRBCs).

Collaborative management focuses on cessation of active bleeding, identification and treatment of the underlying pathophysiology, and the prevention of rebleeding. Some patients develop GI bleeding during hospitalization for another reason as in the case of

Table 9-2	SEVERITY OF BLOOD LOSS	
Severity of Bleed	**Percent of Intravascular Blood Loss**	**Blood Pressure (BP, bpm) and Heart Rate (HR, mm Hg) Findings**
Massive	20% to 25%	Systolic BP < 90 mm Hg HR >100 bpm
Moderate	10% to 20%	Orthostatic hypotension HR ≥100 bpm
Minor	<10%	Normal BP HR ≤100 bpm

Adapted from Rockey DC: Gastrointestinal bleeding. In Sleisenger MH, Feldman M, Fordtran JS, et al, editors: *Sleisenger & Fordtran's gastrointestinal and liver disease: pathophysiology, diagnosis, management*, ed 8, Philadelphia, 2006, Saunders.

stress ulceration. Stress ulcer prophylaxis has been included in the management of patients who are critically ill and mechanically ventilated.

CARE PRIORITIES

Assessing the bleeding severity and restoration of hemodynamic stability of the patient are immediate priorities in the acute phase of GI bleeding. Intensive care unit monitoring is necessary to reduce morbidity and mortality. Once stabilized, care priorities will shift to the identification and management of the bleeding source.

1. Fluid and electrolyte management

Volume replacement in acute GI bleeding must be a priority. Large-bore intravenous (IV) lines should be placed and rapid fluid resuscitation initiated. Volume replacement should include a combination of crystalloid and blood products. Unstable patients with poor tissue perfusion may require blood products. Packed cells and fresh-frozen plasma should be balanced to provide for both the replacement of cells and clotting components. Large transfusions will cause Ca^{2+} to bind with the citrate (the preservative in stored blood) and deplete free Ca^{2+} levels. In addition, large-volume blood transfusions can lead to coagulation disorders. Vasopressors and inotropic agents should be used *only* if tissue perfusion remains compromised despite adequate intravascular volume replacement. Hemodynamic monitoring is essential for continuous evaluation of the patient's volume status, especially in patients older than 50 years or those with chronic illnesses such as cardiovascular, pulmonary, renal, or hepatic disease. Overaggressive volume resuscitation may result in fluid volume excess with complications of cardiac failure and pulmonary edema. Electrolyte levels should be closely monitored, especially in patients with renal or hepatic disease.

2. Respiratory support

Provide oxygen therapy by nasal cannula or face mask. Supplemental oxygen is necessary as a result of blood loss, which reduces the number of RBCs available for oxygen-carrying capacity. Continuous or frequent pulse oximetry monitoring is recommended in patients who are actively bleeding to monitor oxygen saturation, but arterial blood gas (ABG) analysis may be needed to check Sao_2 if the patient is markedly anemic. More aggressive ventilatory support may be required for patients with persistent hypoxemia, evidence of early respiratory failure, or impending acute respiratory distress syndrome (ARDS), as well as for patients who were aggressively volume resuscitated.

3. Nutrition support

As soon as the hemodynamic status of the patient stabilizes, nutrition support must be considered. Patients with active bleeding, visible vessels, or clots may receive clear liquids following successful endoscopic hemostasis. Patients with clean-based ulcers may receive a regular diet following endoscopy.

4. Gastric intubation

Gastric intubation may be performed but is not required for patients with UGIB for diagnosis, prognosis, visualization, or therapeutic effect. Gastric lavage is performed using room temperature normal saline or water to clear blood and clots from the stomach and to allow for estimation of ongoing blood loss. A lavage free of blood suggests a lower GI source of bleeding. There is no evidence that lavage stops the bleeding. Gastric intubation is avoided if EVs are the suspected bleeding source. Balloon tamponade may be necessary for the patient with variceal bleeding refractory to medical and endoscopic therapy.

5. Endoscopic therapies

Coagulopathy and thrombocytopenia should be corrected before endoscopy. In cases of respiratory insufficiency, altered mental status, with ongoing bleeding, endotracheal intubation is indicated before endoscopy to stabilize the patient and protect the airway. Early endoscopy, within the first 24 hours of admission increases diagnostic accuracy, reduces the risk of rebleeding, and decreases the length of hospitalization. Endoscopy should be performed within 12 hours of admission for the patient with suspected varices. Endoscopic modalities for the achievement of hemostasis include: thermal therapy (electrocoagulation or heater probe and injection of sclerosant), epinephrine injection therapy (should be used in conjunction with second modality), and the application of hemoclips (clips that serve to apply mechanical pressure to the bleeding site) are generally effective in stopping bleeding for both UGIB and LGIB. Complications of endoscopy include perforation and MW tears.

6. Pharmacotherapy

Pharmacotherapy including vasopressin and nitroglycerin is only available for the management of UGIB. No pharmacologic therapies for LGIB are currently available. In the upper GI tract, increased gastric acidity is believed to impede blood clotting, although gastric alkalinization may facilitate platelet aggregation, thus promoting acid-lowering pharmacotherapies. Pharmacologic agents involved in ulcer treatment include antacids, H$_2$-receptor antagonists, proton-pump inhibitors (PPIs), prostaglandin analogues, somatostatin, and octreotide.

Antacids (aluminum hydroxide, calcium carbonate, citrocarbonate, magaldrate, magnesium hydroxide, simethicone): Oral antacids raise gastric pH levels and decrease the corrosiveness of gastric acid. They may relieve dyspepsia but have no effect on bleeding ulcers.

Histamine H$_2$-receptor antagonists (e.g., famotidine, ranitidine, cimetidine, nizatidine): Inhibit gastric acid and pepsin secretion, and are useful in the treatment of ulcerative disease and for stress ulcer prophylaxis. The usefulness in an active bleeding ulcer is unsupported. They provide inferior acid inhibition to PPIs. Cimetidine is avoided in patients who are critically ill because it inhibits certain liver enzymes, resulting in potential drug interactions.

Proton-pump inhibitors (e.g., esomeprazole, lansoprazole, omeprazole, pantoprazole, rabeprazole): PPIs deactivate the enzyme system that pumps hydrogen ions from parietal cells, thereby inhibiting gastric acid secretion. PPIs have become the preferred agent for erosive ulcer disease with bleeding. Acid-inhibitory effects of PPIs are significantly stronger than H$_2$-receptor antagonists. IV PPIs or high-dose oral PPIs following a bleeding episode are effective in reducing the incidence of rebleeding, the number of transfusions, and the need for further endoscopic therapy. Preendoscopic IV PPIs may reduce high-risk stigmata in patients with UGIB and is recommended. IV PPIs are additionally recommended in patients for whom endoscopy must be delayed or cannot be tolerated.

Prostaglandin analogues (e.g., misoprostol [Cytotec]): Synthetic prostaglandin E$_1$ enhances the body's normal mucosal protective mechanisms by stimulating mucosal blood flow and bicarbonate secretion, and reducing mucosal cell turnover. They are useful in reducing the incidence of ulcer development in patients taking NSAIDs.

Vasoconstrictors: Vasopressin may help slow variceal bleeding.

Octreotide, a somatostatin analogue: Causes splanchnic vasoconstriction and reduced portal pressure. In combination with endoscopic therapies, it has been shown to control variceal bleeding and reduce the risk of recurrence. No improvement in mortality has been shown with its use in this population.

Sucralfate (Carafate): Oral sucralfate may be prescribed for patients with gastric erosions. Sucralfate combines with gastric acid and forms an adhesive-protective coating over damaged mucosa and does not alter gastric pH. Sucralfate frequently causes constipation and should be avoided in patients with chronic renal insufficiency.

Pharmacotherapy for H. pylori: Eradication of *H. pylori* is effective with combination therapies, monotherapy is useless. "Triple therapy" includes two antibiotics (clarithromycin and amoxicillin or metronidazole) and a PPI. "Quadruple therapy" includes bismuth salicylate, metronidazole, tetracycline, and a PPI or H_2-blocker. There are several triple therapy combination preparations available to allow the patient to receive the combination in one pill.

7. Surgical management

Many surgical techniques are used for both acute UGIB and LGIB, depending on the location and severity of the lesion. EVs are best managed with endoscopic ligation (banding) or sclerotherapy. Band ligation involves wrapping elastic bands over the varices in the distal esophagus; sclerotherapy involves the injection of a sclerosing agent. Ulcerative disease requires surgery if the lesion continues to bleed despite aggressive medical and endoscopic therapy or if complications such as perforation or obstruction develop. Oversewing of the bleeding vessel is usually followed by an acid-reducing procedure such as antrectomy, which removes acid-secreting cells, or vagotomy, which denervates the acid-producing fundic mucosa. Pyloroplasty is performed if there is impairment of gastric emptying. In the patient whose condition is unstable, both vagotomy and pyloroplasty are performed. Antrectomy and vagotomy may be performed in patients whose condition is more stable with anastomosis of the stomach to the duodenum (Billroth I procedure). Also common is the Billroth II procedure for duodenal ulcers involving antrectomy with gastrojejunostomy. Massive LGIB is difficult to control and may require aggressive surgical procedures such as a colectomy with the creation of a permanent ileostomy or internal ileal pouch.

CARE PLANS FOR ACUTE GASTROINTESTINAL BLEEDING

DEFICIENT FLUID VOLUME *related to active loss secondary to hemorrhage from the GI tract.*

Goals/Outcomes: Within 8 hours of diagnosis, the patient will be normovolemic, as evidenced by systolic BP greater than 100 mm Hg, HR less than 100 bpm, CVP 2 to 6 mm Hg, urinary output greater than 0.5 mL/kg/h, Hct greater than 24%, platelet count greater than 50,000/mm³, and prothrombin time (PT) less than 15 seconds.
NOC Electrolyte and Acid-Base Balance; Fluid Balance.

Fluid Management

1. Monitor BP continuously with an arterial catheter for the patient with severe GI bleeding. Be alert to MAP decreases of greater than 10 mm Hg.
2. Monitor postural vital signs for the patient with mild to moderate GI bleeding on admission, every 4 to 8 hours, and more frequently if recurrence of active bleeding is suspected: measure BP and HR with the patient in a supine position, followed immediately by measurement of BP and HR with the patient in a sitting position (as tolerated). A decrease in systolic BP greater than 10 mm Hg or an increase in HR of 10 bpm with the patient in a sitting position suggests a significant intravascular volume deficit, with approximately 15% to 20% loss of volume.
3. Monitor HR, electrocardiogram (ECG), and cardiovascular status hourly, or more frequently in the presence of active bleeding or unstable vital signs. Be alert to a sudden increase in HR, which suggests hypovolemia.
4. Continuously monitor SVV and stroke index (SI) in patients who are mechanically ventilated whose volume status is unstable when available. Assist-control mode is recommended for patients undergoing SVV monitoring. Be alert to low or decreasing CVP. CVP less than 2 mm Hg, SI less than 33, and SVV greater than 13% to 15% are suggestive of hypovolemia and the need for volume restoration.
5. Measure urinary output hourly. Be alert to output less than 0.5 mL/kg/h for 2 consecutive hours. Increase fluid intake or consider fluid bolus if decreased output is caused by hypovolemia and hypoperfusion.

Fluid Resuscitation

1. Obtain two large-bore IV lines (16- or 18-gauge) and/or central venous access.
2. Initiate crystalloid replacement therapy with a combination of normal saline and Lactated Ringer (LR) solution. Fluid may be warmed to prevent hypothermia.
3. Administer pRBCs for persistently low Hct of less than 21% to 24%. Anticipate that Hct will increase by 3% following 1 unit of pRBCs.
4. Fresh-frozen plasma may be administered after 3 units of pRBCs are transfused.
5. Monitor PT and activated partial thromboplastin time (aPTT); administer fresh-frozen plasma if PT is greater than 1.5 times normal or aPTT is greater than 2 times normal.

6. Monitor ionized calcium levels closely because of the tendency of calcium to bind with citrate. Administer calcium gluconate for ionized calcium based on institutional protocol.
7. Prepare for platelet transfusion before endoscopy if platelets fall below 50,000/dL with normal function or 100,000/dL if dysfunction is suspected.

Shock Management
1. Initiate fluid replacement (see Fluid and Electrolyte Disturbances, Chapter 1).
2. Collaborate with the physician or nurse practitioner to administer vasoactive medication if shock persists with volume resuscitation.
3. Monitor for cerebral ischemia or indications of insufficient cerebral blood flow.
4. Monitor renal function (BUN and creatinine levels for elevations), because intravascular volume depletion can lead to prerenal acute kidney injury.
5. Monitor tissue oxygenation using ABG, central venous oxygen saturation (Scvo$_2$), and serum lactate measurements as ordered.
6. Monitor ECG for ST segment depression and T wave inversion, which may be seen as a result of the shock state.

Bleeding Reduction: Gastrointestinal
1. Administer PPIs IV as ordered before endoscopy. Vasopressin (Pitressin) may help slow variceal bleeding.
2. Measure and record all GI blood losses from hematemesis, hematochezia, and melena.
3. Check all stools and gastric contents for occult blood.
4. Ensure proper function and patency of NG tubes. Do not occlude the air vent because this may result in vacuum occlusion. Confirm placement of gastric tube by x-ray, capnography or colorimetric capnometry, and reposition as necessary.
5. Balloon tamponade may be necessary as a temporizing measure for the patient with bleeding EVs. Balloons should be inflated for no more than 12 hours.
6. Teach the patient signs and symptoms of actual or impending GI hemorrhage: pain, nausea, vomiting of blood, dark stools, lightheadedness, and passage of frank blood in stools. Reinforce the importance of seeking medical attention promptly if signs of bleeding occur.
7. Teach the patient the importance of avoiding medications/agents with the potential for gastric irritation: aspirin, NSAIDs, and ethanol.

NIC Blood Products Administration; Hemodynamic Regulation; Gastrointestinal Intubation; Bleeding Precautions; Teaching: Individual; Surgical Preparation.

DECREASED CARDIAC OUTPUT *related to decreased preload secondary to acute blood loss.*

Goals/Outcomes: Within 8 hours of diagnosis, CO approaches normal limits with adequate tissue perfusion, as evidenced by cardiac index (CI) greater than 2.5 L/min/m^2, MAP greater than 65 mm Hg, CVP 2 to 6 mm Hg, urinary output greater than 0.5 mL/kg/h, normal sinus rhythm on ECG, distal pulses greater than 2+ on a 0-to-4+ scale, and brisk capillary refill (less than 2 seconds).
NOC Blood Loss Severity.

Hemodynamic Regulation
1. Administer vasopressors and inotropic agents as prescribed if tissue perfusion remains inadequate following intravascular volume replacement.
2. Monitor ECG for evidence of myocardial ischemia (i.e., ST segment depression, T wave inversion, and ventricular dysrhythmias).
3. Monitor for physical indicators of diminished CO, including pallor, cool extremities, capillary refill greater than 2 to 3 seconds, and decreased or absent amplitude of distal pulses.
4. Monitor vital signs and CO, and replace volume as indicated (see Fluid and Electrolyte Disturbances, Chapter 1).
5. Monitor for oliguria hourly; report urine output less than 0.5 mL/kg/h for 2 consecutive hours.

Respiratory Monitoring
1. Administer oxygen via nasal cannula or facemask to facilitate maximal oxygen delivery.
2. Monitor pulse oximetry and ABG values for hypoxemia. Report arterial Pao$_2$ less than 80 mm Hg and oxygen saturation below 92%, demonstrates altered mental status with severe bleeding.

3. Prepare for endotracheal intubation and mechanical ventilation if the patient is distressed with oxygen saturation less than 90% with supplemental oxygen.
4. Monitor for respiratory crackles, which can result from overaggressive fluid resuscitation.

NIC Cardiac Care: Acute; Oxygen Therapy; Invasive Hemodynamic Monitoring; Dysrhythmia Management.

ACUTE PAIN *related to chemical or physical injury of GI mucosal surfaces caused by digestive juices and enzymes or tissue trauma.*

Goals/Outcomes: Within 2 hours of diagnosis, the patient's subjective evaluation of discomfort improves, as demonstrated by a decreased reported pain level. Nonverbal indicators of discomfort, such as grimacing, are absent.
NOC Comfort Level; Pain Control.

Pain Management
1. Monitor and document presence of abdominal pain or discomfort. Utilize appropriate pain scale. Pain may disappear during a bleeding episode because blood covers and protects eroded tissue.
2. Administer opiate analgesics with caution to patients who are hypovolemic to avoid hypotension and respiratory depression.
3. Supplement analgesics with nonpharmacologic maneuvers to aid in pain reduction. Head of bed (HOB) elevation may be useful in reducing the discomfort of gastric reflux, as long as it does not compromise hemodynamic status. Reflux may prompt variceal bleeding.

NIC Analgesic Administration; Distraction; Environmental Management; Vital Signs Monitoring.

DIARRHEA *related to irritation and increased motility secondary to the presence of blood in the GI tract.*

Goals/Outcomes: By hospital discharge, the patient's stools are normal in consistency and frequency, and results are negative for occult blood.
NOC Fluid Balance; Bowel Elimination; Electrolyte and Acid-Base Balance.

Diarrhea Management
1. Monitor and record the amount, frequency, and characteristics of the patient's stools.
2. Provide bedpan or bedside commode (only for patients who are hemodynamically stable). Consider use of a contained bowel management system device such as Flexiseal or Actiflo. Use with caution in patients who may be anticoagulated.
3. Minimize embarrassing odor by removing stool promptly and using room deodorizers.
4. Use matter-of-fact approach when assisting the patient with frequent bowel elimination. Reassure the patient that frequent elimination is a common problem for most patients with GI bleeding.
5. Evaluate bowel sounds every 4 hours. Anticipate normal to hyperdynamic bowel sounds. Absence of bowel sounds (especially in association with severe pain or abdominal distension) may signal serious complications such as ileus or perforation.
6. Report abnormal serum sodium, potassium, and calcium levels to the physician or nurse practitioner.

NIC Electrolyte Monitoring; Fluid/Electrolyte Management.

IMBALANCED NUTRITION: LESS THAN BODY REQUIREMENTS *related to inability to ingest or digest food secondary to vomiting, mucosal ulceration, ileus, or active GI bleeding.*

Goals/Outcomes: Within 7 days of diagnosis (or by hospital discharge), the patient has adequate nutrition, as evidenced by stable weight, prealbumin 20 to 30 mg/dL, and a state of nitrogen balance on nitrogen studies.
NOC Nutrition Status.

Nutrition Management
1. Collaborate with intraprofessional team to estimate the patient's individual metabolic needs on the basis of activity level, underlying disease process, and nutrition status before hospitalization.

2. Provide clear liquid diet (for high-risk stigmata) or regular diet (for patients with a clean ulcer base) following endoscopic hemostasis as prescribed.
3. Monitor prealbumin and report decreasing levels.
4. Weigh the patient daily at the same time of day, using the same scale. Weight can be a practical indicator of nutrition status if the patient's weight changes are interpreted on the basis of the following factors: fluid shifts (edema, diuresis, third spacing), surgical resection, and weight of dressings and equipment.

NIC Nutrition Monitoring; Aspiration Precautions.
For additional information, see Nutrition Support, Chapter 1.

ADDITIONAL NURSING DIAGNOSES

See other nursing diagnoses and interventions as appropriate: Hemodynamic Monitoring (Chapter 1), Prolonged Immobility (Chapter 1), and Emotional and Spiritual Support of the Patient and Significant Others (Chapter 2).

ACUTE PANCREATITIS

PATHOPHYSIOLOGY

Acute pancreatitis (AP) is an autodigestive process of the pancreas and surrounding tissue by pancreatic enzymes, resulting in the most common cause of GI disease–related hospitalizations in the United States. Normally, pancreatic acinar cells produce and secrete inactive proteolytic enzymes. These proenzymes travel through the pancreatic duct safely until reaching the duodenum, where they are activated by other enzymes found in the intestinal brush border. In AP, the proenzyme trypsinogen is prematurely activated to the proteolytic enzyme trypsin within the acinar cells of the pancreas. Once secreted into the pancreatic duct, trypsin activates other proenzymes, resulting in enzymatic autodigestion of the pancreas. The exact mechanisms prompting trypsin to be prematurely activated remains unanswered. AP is created by a series of events. Initially, the activated digestive enzymes within the pancreas digest pancreatic tissue, leading to inflammation and capillary leakage. Eventually, these enzymes may also digest elastin in blood vessel walls, causing vascular injury that sometimes leads to hemorrhage. The spread of inflammatory mediators (kinins, complement, coagulation factors) released at the site of tissue and vessel injury cause further edema, inflammation, thrombosis, and result in systemic inflammatory response syndrome (SIRS). Significant pancreatic edema leads to rupture of the pancreatic ducts and spillage of pancreatic enzymes into the peripancreatic tissue, resulting in injury. Pancreatic necrosis develops when the pancreatic blood supply is significantly disrupted. Pancreatic necrosis along with organ failure are defining features of severe disease. Shock, distant organ dysfunction, and/or multiple organ dysfunction syndrome (MODS) can ensue.

AP is clinically classified as mild or severe. In cases of mild AP, there is local inflammation, interstitial edema identified by imaging, and the absence of pancreatic necrosis and/or organ failure. The pancreatic blood supply is preserved. Patients usually improve in 48 to 72 hours with supportive management. Mild AP accounts for the majority of cases with a mortality rate of less than 1%. The incidence of progression from mild to severe AP may be increasing. Approximately, 15% to 20% of patients with mild AP will develop severe disease. Severe acute pancreatitis (SAP) is a life-threatening condition currently described in two distinct phases: early (within the first week) and late (after the first week). Early disease is characterized by persistent organ failure and/or SIRS lasting longer than 48 hours. Organ failure may be identified by two or more of the following: shock (systolic BP less than 90 mm Hg), pulmonary insufficiency ($PaO_2 \leq 60$ mm Hg), kidney failure (serum creatinine greater than 2 mg/dL), or GI bleeding (greater than 500 mL/24 h). Late SAP involves the development of one or more local complications that include sterile or infected pancreatic/peripancreatic necrosis, acute pseudocyst, acute peripancreatic fluid collection, and walled-off pancreatic necrosis (WOPN) (see Complications).

Alcoholism and gallstones account for 80% of all AP cases. Alcohol sometimes has a direct toxic effect on the pancreatic acinar cells or may cause inflammation of the sphincter of Oddi, resulting in the retention of enzymes in the pancreatic duct. In patients with gallstones, AP may be caused by obstruction of the pancreatic duct by gallstones lodged at the shared outlet of the pancreatic duct and common bile duct into the duodenum. When the outlet is blocked, bile can reflux into the pancreatic duct. Once AP ensues, hypercalcemia, hyperlipidemia, and hypertriglyceridemia are often found to be present and may cause AP. AP is often associated with a recent endoscopic retrograde cholangiopancreatography (ERCP) procedure: the most common iatrogenic cause. Other causative factors include blunt or penetrating trauma, metabolic factors, infectious agents, and certain drugs (Box 9-3). Despite the capacity for thorough investigation, the cause of AP is idiopathic in approximately 15% to 20% of cases.

RISK STRATIFICATION

Timely identification of patients at risk for developing SAP is crucial to planning appropriate care to achieve the best outcomes. Predicting severity early is crucial in preventing complications and mortality. It is difficult to distinguish mild from severe disease in the early stages. Several classification systems have been developed to determine severity. Ranson's criteria for non–gallstone AP provide a scale of severity for AP based on age, blood gas, hematologic, and biochemical changes. Pancreatitis is classified as severe when three or more of Ranson's 11 criteria are met during the first 48 hours following presentation (Box 9-4). The Acute Physiology and Chronic Health Evaluation (APACHE) II scoring system (Table 9-3) is another tool to determine severity. An APACHE II score of less than 8 points within the first 48 hours is directly related to better survival. Higher scores during this time interval are associated with increased morbidity and mortality rates. Scoring systems are often cumbersome and should be used in conjunction with ongoing clinical findings and other laboratory data. The less cumbersome Bedside Index of Severity in Acute Pancreatitis (BISAP) was recently developed for risk stratification during the first 12 hours of admission. The index includes five commonly available clinical variables that are each assigned 1 point. A simple score of 3 points or greater is associated with increased risk of complications and mortality (Box 9-5).

COMPLICATIONS

The inflammation associated with AP is nonbacterial. Pancreatic necrosis is usually sterile but can become infected. In SAP, the inflammatory process results in extensive pancreatic and peripancreatic necrosis of mesenteric and retroperitoneal fat tissue that prompts late-phase local complications, which increase mortality and significantly lengthen the clinical course of disease. Infected pancreatic necrosis should be suspected when worsening of pain, fever, and leukocytosis manifest between 7 and 10 days after admission. Infective necrosis often leads to

Box 9-3	PRECIPITATING FACTORS FOR ACUTE PANCREATITIS

Mechanical blockage of pancreatic ducts
- Biliary tract disease (e.g., gallstones)
- Structural abnormalities (e.g., pancreas divisum)
- Post-ERCP
- Tumors

Toxic/metabolic factors
- Ethyl alcohol
- Hyperlipidemia
- Hypertriglyceridemia (may cause up to 5% of cases)
- Hypercalcemia
- Pregnancy

Infection
- Viral (e.g., mumps, Coxsackie virus B, hepatitis B, HIV, CMV)
- Bacterial (e.g., *Mycoplasma pneumoniae, Salmonella typhi*)

Trauma
- External
- Surgical

Ischemia
- Prolonged/severe shock
- Vasculitis

Drugs
- Corticosteroids
- Estrogens
- NSAIDs
- Sulfonamides
- Thiazides
- Tetracycline

CMV, Cytomegalovirus; *ERCP*, endoscopic retrograde cholangiopancreatography; *HIV*, human immunodeficiency virus; *NSAIDs*, nonsteroidal antiinflammatory drugs.

Box 9-4 | RANSON CRITERIA FOR CLASSIFYING THE SEVERITY OF PANCREATITIS

At presentation
- Age ≥55 years
- WBCs ≥16,000/mm³
- Glucose ≥200 mg/dL
- AST ≥250 units/L
- LDH ≥350 units/L

After initial 48 hours
- Base deficit ≥4 mEq/L
- BUN increased ≥5 mg/dL

- Fluid sequestration ≥6 L
- Serum Ca²⁺ >8 mg/dL
- Hematocrit decrease >10%
- Po₂ (from ABG) >60 mm Hg

Ranson criteria scoring mechanism
Score 0 to 2—minimal mortality rate
Score 3 to 5—10% to 20% mortality rate
Score >5—50% mortality rate

ABG, Arterial blood gas; *AST*, aspartate aminotransferase; *BUN*, blood urea nitrogen; *Ca²⁺*, calcium; *LDH*, lactate dehydrogenase; *Po₂*, partial pressure of oxygen; *WBCs*, white blood cells.

sepsis and MODS as a result of translocation of bacteria from the poorly functioning gut. Pancreatic pseudocysts can form, comprising encapsulated fluid collections with high enzyme concentration and variable amounts of tissue debris. Although the majority of pseudocysts are sterile, some become infected resulting in hemorrhage or rupture, which prompts pancreatic ascites. Pseudocysts usually form within or adjacent to the pancreas but can migrate into the chest or other locations. Other unencapsulated acute peripancreatic fluid collections form in the peripancreatic area in approximately 30% of AP cases. WOPN defines a collection of pancreatic and peripancreatic debris and liquefied dead tissue encased in a fibrous tissue wall. WOPN develops over a 4-week period in patients with necrotizing pancreatitis.

A major initial complication of SAP is hypovolemia resulting from plasma volume fluid sequestration into the interstitium, retroperitoneum, and the gut. Massive, life-threatening hemorrhage from rupture of necrotic tissue results in severe anemia and hypotension. SIRS ensues, wherein inflammatory mediators trigger vasodilation and increased capillary permeability, which further contributes to severe hypovolemia and hypotension. Hypoalbuminemia is frequently present, which prompts intravascular fluids to move through the permeable capillaries more rapidly, because oncotic pressure is reduced. Severe hypotension may persist despite volume repletion given there is too little protein to hold the volume within the blood vessels. If hypovolemia is not adequately corrected promptly, acute kidney injury and MODS may develop (see Systemic Inflammatory Response Syndrome, Sepsis, Septic Shock, and Multiple Organ Dysfunction Syndrome, Chapter 11).

Mild to severe respiratory failure with hypoxemia is common in AP patients with SIRS. Respiratory complications are related to right-to-left vascular shunting within the lung and alveolar-capillary leakage caused by the circulating inflammatory mediators resulting in ARDS (see Acute Lung Injury and Acute Respiratory Distress Syndrome, Chapter 4). In addition, elevation of the diaphragm, atelectasis, and pleural effusion caused by subdiaphragmatic inflammation of the pancreas and surrounding tissues, and/or pancreatic ascites, can compromise ventilation further. Inflammatory mediators and vascular injury may lead to intravascular coagulopathy or DIC, resulting in life-threatening complications such as major thrombus formation and pulmonary emboli. The circulatory and respiratory failures that ensue are often the cause of death in these patients.

ASSESSMENT

GOAL OF SYSTEM ASSESSMENT: ACUTE PANCREATITIS
Evaluate for organ and systemic involvement of dysfunctional pancreatic secretions.

HISTORY AND RISK FACTORS
- Excessive alcohol ingestion; biliary tract disease; recent ERCP; hypertriglyceridemia greater than 1000 mg/dL; use of drugs such as steroids, furosemide, thiazides, and certain NSAIDs; viral infections (human immunodeficiency virus [HIV]); penetrating and blunt injuries to the pancreas; pregnancy; primary hyperparathyroidism; uremia.

Table 9-3	THE ACUTE PHYSIOLOGY AND CHRONIC HEALTH EVALUATION (APACHE) II SCORING SYSTEM								
Feature					**Acute Physiology Score (APS)**				
Physiologic variable	+4	+3	+2	+1	0	+1	+2	+3	+4
Temperature	≥41	39-40.9		38.5-38.9	36-38.4	34-35.9	32-33.9	30-31.9	≤29.9
Mean arterial blood pressure	≥160	130-159	110-129		70-109		50-69		≤49
Heart rate	≥180	140-179	110-139		70-109		55-69	40-54	≤39
Respiratory rate	≥50	35-49		25-34	12-24	10-11	6-9		≤5
AaDO₂*	≥500	350-499	200-349		100	61-70		55-60	<55
Pao₂†					>70				
Arterial pH	≥7.7	7.6-7.69		7.5-7.59	7.33-7.49		7.25-7.32	7.15-7.24	<7.15
Serum bicarbonate‡	≥52	41-51.9		32-40.9	23-31.9		18-21.9	15-17.9	<15
Serum sodium	≥180	160-179	155-159	150-154	130-149		120-129	111-119	≤110
Serum potassium	≥7	6-6.9		5.5-5.9	3.5-5.4	3-3.4	2.5-2.9		<2.5
Serum creatinine	≥3.5	2-3.4	1.5-1.9		0.6-1.4		<0.6		
Hematocrit	≥60		50-59.9	46-49.9	30-45.9		20-29.9		<20
White blood cell count	≥40		20-39.9	15-19.9	3-14.9		1-2.9		<1

Continued

Table 9-3	THE ACUTE PHYSIOLOGY AND CHRONIC HEALTH EVALUATION (APACHE) II SCORING SYSTEM—cont'd		
Feature		**Acute Physiology Score (APS)**	
Age Points (AP)		**Chronic Health Problems (CHP)**	**Scoring**
Age (years)	Points	For patients with history of severe organ system insufficiency or immunocompromise, assign points as follows:	APS + AP + CHP = total score[§]
≤44	0	Nonoperative patients 5 points	
45-54	2	Emergency postoperative patients 5 points	
55-64	3	Elective postoperative patients 2 points	
65-74	5		
≥75	6		

From Knaus WA, Draper EA, Wagner DP, Zimmerman JE: APACHE II: a severity of disease classification system. *Crit Care Med* 13:818-829, 1985.
*Use if F_{IO2} <50%.
†Use if percentage of inspired oxygen (F_{IO2}) >50%.
‡Use only if no arterial blood gas measurements are available.
§APACHE II score ≥ 8 identifies severe acute pancreatitis and the need for intensive care.
A-a_{PO2}, alveolar-arterial oxygen pressure; P_{aO2}, partial pressure of oxygen in arterial blood.

Box 9-5   BEDSIDE INDEX OF SEVERITY IN ACUTE PANCREATITIS (BISAP) SCORE

Clinical Variables	Point Allocation
BUN (blood urea nitrogen) >25 mg/dL	1
Impaired mental status	1
SIRS (systemic inflammatory response syndrome) 2 or more of the following: • Temperature <36° C or >38° C • Pulse >90bpm • Respiratory rate >20 breaths/min or Pao$_2$ <32 mm Hg • White blood cell count <4000 or >12,000 or 10% bands	1
Age >60 years	1
Pleural effusion	1

A score of 3 is associated with 5% to 8% mortality; 4 is associated with 13% to 19% mortality; 5 is associated with 22% to 27% mortality.

VITAL SIGN ASSESSMENT
- Tachycardia and hypotension result from massive intravascular losses.
- Increased temperature greater than 38.5° C (101.3 F) and tachycardia are associated with an inflammatory response.

ABDOMINAL PAIN
- Sudden onset of epigastric pain (often after excessive food or alcohol ingestion) lasting 12 to 48 hours, described as mild discomfort to severe distress, and located from the midepigastrium to the right upper quadrant (RUQ). Occasionally pain is reported in the left upper quadrant.
- Pain is typically described as boring and deep.
- Pain may radiate to the back.
- Nausea, vomiting, hematemesis, and restlessness typically accompany the pain; diarrhea and melena may also be present.

OBSERVATION
- Mild to moderate ascites may be present.
- Dyspnea and cyanosis may be observed if ARDS is present (see Acute Lung Injury and Acute Respiratory Distress Syndrome, Chapter 4).
- Jaundice may be present with biliary tract disease.
- Grey Turner sign (flank ecchymosis) and Cullen sign (umbilical ecchymosis) occur in approximately 1% of cases and are associated with a poor prognosis.
- Severe hypocalcemia may elicit Chvostek sign (facial twitching after a facial tap) or Trousseau sign (hand spasms when BP cuff inflates). Hypocalcemia causes numbness or tingling in the extremities that progresses to tetany if calcium is severely depleted.
- Abdominal distension is often present in SAP resulting from gastric, small bowel, or colonic ileus.

AUSCULTATION
- Diminished, sluggish, or absent bowel sounds reflective of GI dysfunction and paralytic ileus.
- Breath sounds may be decreased or absent, suggesting focal atelectasis or pleural effusion. Effusions are usually left-sided but can be bilateral. Auscultation of crackles reflects hypoventilation caused by pain, early ARDS, or microemboli.

PALPATION

- Abdominal tenderness is common.
- Abdominal palpation will reveal localized tenderness in the RUQ or diffuse discomfort over the upper portion of the abdomen without rigidity or rebound.
- An upper abdominal mass may be palpated as a result of the inflamed pancreas or a pseudocyst.
- In the presence of hemorrhage or severe hypovolemia, the hands are cool and sweaty to touch.
- Peripheral pulses will be diminished and capillary refill delayed with hemorrhage or severe hypovolemia.

NUTRITION ASSESSMENT

- Malnutrition may be present, especially if there is a history of alcoholism (see Table 9-1).

SCREENING LABWORK

- Serum electrolyte levels: Hypercalcemia.
- CBC: Leukocytosis.
- Serum amylase: ↑↑↑.
- Serum lipase: ↑↑↑.
- LFTs: Elevated with alcoholic or biliary involvement.
- Serum triglycerides: Elevated to greater than 1000 mg/dL (hypertriglyceridemia may cause up to 5% of cases of AP).

HEMODYNAMIC MEASUREMENTS FOR COMPLICATIONS OF SAP

- Hypovolemic shock: Decreased CVP and CO from hemorrhage or dehydration.
- SIRS: CO may be elevated and systemic vascular resistance (SVR) decreased initially. Urine output decreases while the body attempts to conserve intravascular volume.
- ARDS or pulmonary emboli: Increase in pulmonary vascular resistance.

Diagnostic Tests for Acute Pancreatitis

The diagnosis of acute pancreatitis (AP) is based on the presence of two of the following three criteria:
(1) Abdominal pain characteristic of AP;
(2) Characteristic radiographic evidence of AP on imaging (abdominal ultrasonography);
(3) Elevation of amylase and/or lipase ≥ three times upper limit of normal.
The following tests are used to support the diagnosis and trend the progression of the disease.

Test	Purpose	Abnormal Findings
Blood Studies		
Complete blood count (CBC): White blood cell (WBC) count Red blood cell (RBC) count Hemoglobin (Hgb) Hematocrit (Hct) Platelets	Assesses for inflammation and infection. Platelets may be consumed if inflammation is severe enough to prompt disseminated intravascular coagulation (DIC). Reflective of volume status and oxygen-carrying capacity.	Leukocytosis with a WBC count of 11,000 to 20,000/mm³ is reflective of the acute inflammatory process and not bacterial infection. Bacterial infection may ensue in a small percentage of patients reflecting a WBC count ≥20,000/mm³. Hct and Hgb levels vary, depending on the presence of hemorrhage (decreased) or dehydration (increased).
Serum amylase	Cardinal finding consistent with AP but only supports, does not confirm the diagnosis of AP. Amylase rises almost immediately with onset of pain but returns to normal within 3 to 5 days.	Serum elevations in amylase levels ≥3 times the upper normal limit, in the absence of kidney failure is consistent with AP. This level does not trend with the severity of AP.

Diagnostic Tests for Acute Pancreatitis—cont'd

Test	Purpose	Abnormal Findings
Serum lipase	To assist with the diagnosis of AP. Lipase remains elevated for 14 days, thereby providing greater sensitivity than amylase.	Serum elevations in lipase levels ≥3 times the upper normal limit, in the absence of kidney failure, is most consistent with AP. Serum lipase is more specific for AP and is preferred over amylase where available.
Serum calcium	Assesses for hypercalcemia and hypocalcemia. Some calcium is protein-bound; serum levels depend on albumin levels. While serum albumin levels decrease with intravascular fluid losses, reductions in serum calcium levels will follow.	Hypercalcemia caused by hyperparathyroidism has been associated with AP as a cause. Serum calcium levels may decrease dramatically (≤8 mg/dL) in severe AP, because calcium binds with free fatty acids released during lipolysis of peripancreatic fat tissue predisposing the patient to tetany and other complications of hypocalcemia.
Serum glucose	Assesses for hyperglycemia as a determinant of injury to pancreatic islet cells.	Blood glucose values are commonly ≥200 mg/dL.
Serum triglyceride	Assesses for possible cause of AP.	Serum triglyceride levels ≥1000 mg/dL are found to be a causative factor in up to 5% of all AP cases.
Serum creatinine	Evaluates renal function.	Levels ≥1.5 mg/dL are seen in patients with acute kidney injury.
Electrolytes: Serum potassium Serum magnesium Serum bicarbonate	Assesses levels closely during fluid resuscitation.	Hyperkalemia is present initially resulting from significant cellular damage releasing large amounts of K^+ into circulation and increases with acidosis associated with shock. Increased serum bicarbonate and hypokalemia values reflect metabolic alkalosis later, usually the result of fluid therapy, vomiting, or gastric suctioning. Hyponatremia and hypomagnesemia will be seen with vomiting and fluid sequestration.
Liver function tests (LFTs): Serum bilirubin Alkaline phosphatase (ALP) Aspartate aminotransferase (AST)	To assess liver involvement and distinguish between alcohol-induced and gallstone-induced disease.	Persistent elevation of liver enzymes suggests hepatic inflammation caused by alcohol ingestion or viral hepatitis. Elevated total bilirubin levels and ALP value ≥150 International Unit/L are suggestive of biliary disease.
C-Reactive protein (CRP)	Assesses for severe inflammation. CRP is a nonspecific acute phase reactant of inflammation that is suggestive of severe AP.	A CRP level ≥150 mg/L at 48 hours after disease onset is suggestive of pancreatic necrosis.

Acute Pancreatitis

Continued

Diagnostic Tests for Acute Pancreatitis — cont'd

Test	Purpose	Abnormal Findings
Coagulation studies	Assesses the extent of coagulopathic involvement, because inflammatory mediators trigger the coagulation cascade. In severe AP, DIC may develop.	Decreases in platelets and fibrinogen will be present, because they are rapidly consumed. Elevations in circulating levels of fibrin are associated with microthrombi in the pancreas and other tissues.
Arterial blood gas (ABG)	Assesses oxygenation status and acid-base balance	Decreased arterial oxygen tension is a common finding and may be present without other symptoms of pulmonary insufficiency. Early hypoxia produces a mild respiratory alkalosis. Arterial oxygen saturation may be diminished.
Nutrition profile: Serum albumin Serum transferrin Serum prealbumin Total lymphocyte count (TLC)	Assesses nutrition status to identify preexisting malnutrition and to guide nutrition replacement therapy.	Decreased albumin, transferrin, and TLC are indicative of malnutrition and seen in patients with alcoholic disease. Prealbumin levels will rise with effective therapy.

Noninvasive Cardiology

Electrocardiogram	Assesses and monitors for cardiac rhythm disturbances.	ST segment depression and T wave inversion may be seen as a result of the shock state, the severe pain that causes coronary artery spasm, or the effect of trypsin and bradykinins on the myocardium. Hypocalcemia results in widening of the QT interval.

Radiology

Radiography: Abdominal radiograph Chest radiograph	Abdominal x-rays: assess for bowel dilation. Chest x-rays: identify pulmonary involvement.	Abdominal radiograph identifies dilation of the bowel and ileus. Chest radiograph distinguishes effusions from atelectasis and identifies characteristic infiltrates consistent with acute respiratory distress syndrome.
Computed tomography (CT) scan of the abdomen Contrast-enhanced CT	Estimates size of the pancreas; identifies fluid collection, cystic lesions, areas of necrosis, and masses; visualizes biliary tract abnormalities; and monitors inflammatory swelling of the pancreas. It can determine the presence or extent of necrosis, and thus serves as an indicator of disease severity.	Enlarged pancreas, dilation of the common bile duct, and evidence of gallstones. Confirms the diagnosis of AP. Multiloculated gas within the pancreas and surrounding tissue confirms the presence of infected pancreatic necrosis.
Transabdominal ultrasonography	Initial radiographic test to rule out a biliary source. Supports the diagnosis of AP.	Detects gallstones, biliary sludge, and biliary dilation.
Magnetic resonance imaging	Assessment of the severity of AP. Reserved for patients in whom the diagnosis of AP is unclear.	Detects the presence of pancreatic necrosis and complications without the use of intravenous contrast.

Diagnostic Tests for Acute Pancreatitis — cont'd

Test	Purpose	Abnormal Findings
Magnetic resonance cholangiopancreatography	Assessment of the biliary tree and pancreatic parenchyma; detection of stones in the common bile duct.	Confirms the presence of choledocholithiasis. Identifies rare morphologic abnormalities.
Endoscopic ultrasonography	Used to visualize the opening to the pancreas when a biliary cause of AP is suspected, to observe for swelling, ductal abnormalities, and presence of tumors or gallstones.	Confirms the presence of choledocholithiasis and occult microlithiasis.
Endoscopic retrograde cholangiopancreatography	Indicated for patients with biliary pancreatitis with cholangitis. Used to relieve obstruction caused by stone impaction.	Not indicated for diagnosis of severe AP, because it may aggravate inflammation.

SERUM LIPASE AND AMYLASE

Serum lipase has become a primary diagnostic marker for AP. Serum amylase is not sensitive diagnostically in cases of delayed clinical presentation; pancreatitis caused by hypertriglyceridemia; and in patients with chronic pancreatitis experiencing an acute attack. Prolonged clamp time with coronary artery bypass grafting or valve replacement can lead to AP in which only amylase is elevated.

COLLABORATIVE MANAGEMENT

Management includes risk stratification, monitored supportive care, efforts to prevent, limit and treat complications, and recurrences. The American College of Gastroenterology (ACG) guidelines "Management of Acute Pancreatitis" frame the management priorities. Because AP is a disease of significant variability, there is a paucity of large randomized controlled trials. The ACG practice guidelines (Box 9-6) present recommendations based on: scientific studies and best evidence of new understandings and developments in the diagnosis, etiology, and management of AP.

CARE PRIORITIES FOR SEVERE ACUTE PANCREATITIS

A team approach is necessary to optimize the management of the patient with SAP. Care priorities reflect adequate fluid resuscitation, the correction of electrolyte and metabolic abnormalities, effective pain control, provision of nutrition, and the prevention of complications and recurrences.

1. Aggressive fluid resuscitation

The inflammatory process results in fluid sequestration and extensive intravascular volume loss into the pancreas and abdomen leading to hypovolemia and hemoconcentration. Vomiting, gastric suctioning, and hemorrhage contribute to the hypovolemic state. The hypovolemia and hemoconcentration lead to shock wherein the capillary beds are poorly perfused. Colloids and crystalloids are administered to replace volume losses and minimize interstitial edema. Crystalloids reduce hemoconcentration and improve perfusion. LR solution is recommended for initial fluid resuscitation. LR appears to be more beneficial as the initial IV solution resulting in fewer patients developing SIRS as compared with patients receiving normal saline. Albumin may be considered for serum albumin less than 2 g/dL, but the proteins may leak from capillaries and increase interstitial edema. pRBCs may be transfused for Hct less than 24%. Fresh-frozen plasma may be needed for evidence of coagulopathy. Peritoneal and interstitial fluid sequestration continues throughout the acute phase. Volume replacement is essential. CVP monitoring may assist fluid management. Pulmonary artery pressure, CI, stroke volume index, and $ScvO_2$ monitoring and vasopressors may be needed. Fluid overload is a concern, especially in patients with cardiovascular dysfunction and/or ARDS.

2. Support ventilation and oxygenation

In SAP-related pulmonary congestion, pleural effusion and atelectasis result in respiratory insufficiency or failure. Abdominal distension and retroperitoneal fluid sequestration cause

| Box 9-6 | AMERICAN GASTROENTEROLOGY ASSOCIATION RECOMMENDATIONS FOR ACUTE PANCREATITIS |

Diagnosis
- Established by the presence of two out of three of the following criteria: abdominal pain consistent with the disease, serum amylase and/or lipase greater than three times the upper normal limit, and/or characteristic findings from abdominal imaging.
- Contrast-enhanced computed tomography and/or magnetic resonance imaging should be reserved for patients in whom the diagnosis is unclear or who fail to improve in the first 48 to 72 hours.

Determination of etiology
- Transabdominal ultrasound should be performed on all patients.
- In the absence of gallstones and significant history of alcohol use, serum triglycerides should be obtained and considered the etiology if greater than 1000 mg/dL.
- A pancreatic tumor should be considered in patients older than 40 years.
- Patients with idiopathic pancreatitis should be referred to centers of expertise.

Assessment of severity
- Assess hemodynamic status on presentation and begin resuscitative measures.
- Risk assessment should be performed for appropriate triage.
- Patients with organ failure should be admitted to an intensive care unit.

Management
- Aggressive fluid resuscitation is most beneficial in the first 12 to 24 hours.
- Fluid requirements should be reassessed at frequent intervals for the next 24 to 48 hours.
- Endoscopic retrograde cholangiopancreatography should be performed within 24 hours of admission in patients with acute pancreatitis and concurrent acute cholangitis.
- Antibiotics should be administered for extrapancreatic infections.
- Routine use of prophylactic antibiotics in patients with severe acute pancreatitis is NOT recommended.
- The use of antibiotics in patients with sterile necrosis to prevent the development of infected necrosis is not recommended.

Data from the American College of Gastroenterology Guideline: Management of acute pancreatitis. *Am J Gastroenterol* 108:1400-1415, 2013.

diaphragmatic elevation and ventilatory restriction. Oxygen administration is initiated if hypoxemia is present. Early respiratory failure is detected by a decrease in Pao_2 with increase in $Paco_2$. If severe pulmonary insufficiency develops, intubation and positive-pressure ventilation is required. Mechanical ventilation is frequently necessary for the patient with SAP. ARDS is a complication found in 20% of patients with SAP. IV fluids are given cautiously to prevent fluid overload resulting in cardiopulmonary compromise.

3. Correct electrolyte and metabolic abnormalities
Hypocalcemia commonly occurs in patients with SAP and is a marker of poor prognosis. Ionized levels should be monitored, because with low albumin levels the amount of measured protein-bound calcium is falsely low. If levels are low or if the patient develops signs of neuromuscular instability, replace with calcium chloride. Because hypercalcemia is a cause of AP, calcium replacement is prescribed cautiously. Ensure magnesium and albumin levels are adequate. Magnesium can be lost caused by vomiting, urinary loss, or resulting from deposition in areas of fat necrosis.

Hyperglycemia is also included as a poor prognostic marker. Hyperglycemia and glycosuria are consequences of glucagon release in the patient with SAP as a response to stress. Hyperglycemia is also related to the decreased release of insulin by impaired pancreatic islet cells.

Hyperglycemia can worsen neutrophil function, increasing the risk of pancreatic infection. Insulin should be administered IV and titrated to keep glucose less than 180 mg/dL. Meticulous serum glucose control management facilitates control of serum triglycerides.

4. Provide effective pain control

Acute abdominal pain is caused by peritoneal irritation from the inflamed pancreas. Opioid analgesics are administered for relief of severe pain. Continuous or intermittent IV therapy is used, depending on the severity of the pain. Patient-controlled analgesia (PCA) is a helpful mode of delivery. Morphine has been implicated in the past as causing spasm of the sphincter of Oddi, thus worsening the pancreatitis. However, no evidence has been found to demonstrate this in humans. Its use in AP has not been shown to adversely affect outcomes. Meperidine was the analgesic of choice but has an active neurotoxic metabolite that accumulates with long-term use, causing agitation, seizures, and muscle fibrosis. Because of these side effects, many hospitals have limited the availability of IV meperidine. Hydromorphone or sublimaze are alternatives.

 Safety Alert *Although short-term meperidine can be used safely, use of longer than a few days, at doses exceeding 100 mg every 3 hours, must be avoided.*

5. Initiate nutrition support

Nutrition supplementation should be considered early to promote tissue repair in patients with SAP, because they are unable to tolerate eating for several days. Enteral feedings should be the primary therapy in patients with or predicted SAP and should be started within the first 48 hours of admission. Enteral nutrition has been shown to assist in maintaining the mucosal barrier of the gut, and preventing the translocation of gut bacteria that seed pancreatic necrosis. Although the nasojejunal (NJ) route has been preferred to avoid stimulation of gastric secretions, NG enteral nutrition also appears to be safe. Either elemental or polymeric enteral nutrition formulations can be used. Weighted NJ tubes should be positioned beyond the ligament of Treitz. The ligament of Treitz is a musculofibrous band that extends from the ascending part of the duodenum and jejunum to the right crus of the diaphragm and tissue around the celiac artery. NG enteral nutrition requires the patient to be placed on aspiration precautions. Enteral nutrition can therefore be administered either by the NJ or NG route. Enteral feedings are tolerated in most patients with meticulous attention to feeding tolerance and consulting with dieticians and nutrition support pharmacists regarding elemental or polymeric feedings (see Nutrition Support, Chapter 1). If enteral feedings are not tolerated, total parenteral nutrition (TPN) can be administered as second-line therapy, necessitating insertion of a central IV catheter. TPN continues to be associated with significant complications from the catheter, ranging from catheter-related sepsis, local abscess, localized hematomas, pneumothorax, venous thrombosis, venous air embolism, and metabolic complications such as hyperglycemia and electrolyte imbalance. Low-fat oral feedings are begun after the initial episode subsides and bowel function returns.

6. Suppress pancreatic secretions

The assumption that the inflamed pancreas requires rest by fasting until complete resolution of AP no longer appears to be supported by laboratory and clinical observations. Bowel rest is associated with intestinal mucosal atrophy and increased infectious complications. Enteral tube feeding should be primary therapy for patients with SAP either by the NJ or NG route and should be started within 48 hours of hospitalization.

Aspiration of gastric secretions via NG suction demonstrated no benefit in patients with mild to moderate AP and is therefore not recommended in these cases. NG suction is only useful for cases of SAP with unremitting vomiting, abdominal distension, or pain not relieved by analgesia. Reducing gastric acidity by administering histamine H_2-receptor antagonists or PPIs may help to prevent stress ulceration. Agents that suppress pancreatic secretions such as somatostatin and octreotide have generally produced disappointing results in human studies and are no longer recommended. Peritoneal lavage has been used in the past to remove toxic necrotic compounds present in peritoneal exudates. This procedure has not been shown to reduce mortality or morbidity in patients with SAP and is no longer recommended.

7. Manage medically versus surgically

In patients with gallstone AP, cholecystectomy should be performed upon recovery to prevent recurrence. SAP is generally managed medically. Surgical intervention is no longer indicated for patients with asymptomatic pseudocysts and sterile necrosis regardless of size or location. Minimally invasive necrosectomy by laparoscopic, radiologic, or endoscopic approach is indicated for stable patients with infected necrosis or pseudocysts, but should be delayed for more than 4 weeks after initial presentation to allow liquefaction of the contents and for the development of a fibrous wall. Any type of invasive intervention before the 4-week period is associated with increased mortality.

8. Prevent infection; the role of antibiotics

The routine use of prophylactic antibiotics to prevent the development of infected pancreatic necrosis in patients with SAP is no longer recommended. Patients with suspected or proven infected necrosis should receive antibiotics. Choice of antibiotic should be determined by initial computed tomography (CT)-guided fine needle aspiration (FNA) for Gram stain and culture. If FNA is unattainable, empirical antibiotics should be used. Antibiotic choice must provide adequate penetration of necrotic tissue, such as carbapenems, quinolones, and metronidazole. These have been shown to delay or sometimes totally avoid the need for surgical intervention.

9. Intraabdominal pressure monitoring

The measurement of IAP for intraabdominal hypertension (IAH) should be considered in patients with SAP who are mechanically ventilated when signs of deterioration are present (2012 International Association of Pancreatology/American Pancreatic Association [IAP/APA] guidelines). Patients with AP who have not yet developed SAP may benefit from IAP monitoring before mechanical ventilation has been initiated. IAH is defined by a repeated pathologic increase in IAP greater than 12 mm Hg and is reported to occur in 60% to 80% of patients with SAP. A subset of these patients will develop abdominal compartment syndrome, which is defined as a sustained IAP greater than 20 mm Hg that is associated with new-onset organ failure. Medical treatment should target hollow viscera volume reduction, intravascular/extravascular fluid correction, and abdominal wall expansion. Invasive management should only be considered in patients with sustained IAP greater than 25 mm Hg refractory to medical therapy (see Abdominal Hypertension and Abdominal Compartment Syndrome, Chapter 11).

10. Prevent recurrence

Patients with alcohol-related pancreatitis should be referred for substance abuse counseling services despite alcohol cessation not always preventing further attacks. Patients with gallbladder-related pancreatitis should undergo cholecystectomy and endoscopic sphincterotomy if medically cleared for these procedures to prevent recurrence. Avoid the use of ERCP as an initial diagnostic tool for unexplained abdominal pain to reduce the risk of post-ERCP pancreatitis, given that pancreatitis is the most common complication of ERCP.

CARE PLANS FOR ACUTE PANCREATITIS

DEFICIENT FLUID VOLUME *related to decreased intake, vomiting, NG suction, fluid loss into the pancreas and abdomen or with SAP, massive fluid sequestration within the peritoneum and retroperitoneal space; hemorrhage associated with tissue necrosis; and systemic vasodilation and increased capillary permeability from inflammatory mediators.*

Goals/Outcomes: Within 24 hours of diagnosis, the patient becomes normovolemic, as evidenced by MAP 65 to 85 mm Hg, HR less than 120 bpm, sinus rhythm on ECG, CVP 2 to 6 mm Hg, CO 4 to 6 L/min, brisk capillary refill (less than 2 seconds), peripheral pulses at least 2+ on a 0-to-4+ scale; urinary output greater than 0.5 to 1 mL/kg/h; Hct 35% to 44%.

NOC Electrolyte and Acid-Base Balance; Fluid Balance.

Fluid Resuscitation
1. Obtain and maintain large-bore IV, central venous access, and CVP monitoring.
2. Administer IV fluids; LR is recommended for initial fluid resuscitation; 5 to 10 mL/kg/h initially until goals are met.

3. Aggressive IV hydration with volumes of 250 to 500 mL/h may be necessary in patients with no cardiac or renal comorbidities and is of most benefit the first 12 to 24 hours.
4. Consider administering pRBCs for Hct less than 30%. Anticipate an increase in Hct of 3% following 1 unit of pRBCs.
5. Consider administering albumin for serum albumin less than 2 g/dL, but observe for worsening of edema if capillary leak is severe.
6. Monitor coagulation studies and CBC.
7. Administer fresh-frozen plasma for coagulopathy and to replace lost circulating proteins.
8. Monitor BUN for appropriate reductions.
9. Assess for signs of overaggressive fluid resuscitation (see Fluid Volume Excess).

Fluid Management
1. Administer crystalloids, colloids, or a combination of both as prescribed.
2. Monitor BP every 1 to 2 hours if losses are caused by fluid sequestration, inadequate intake, or slow bleeding. Monitor BP continuously with arterial line, or hourly and increase to every 15 minutes if the patient has active blood loss or massive fluid sequestration.
3. Monitor cardiovascular status at least every 1 to 2 hours, and more often with SAP.
4. Measure urinary output hourly. Report output less than 0.5 mL/kg/h for 2 consecutive hours. Evaluate intravascular volume and cardiovascular function, and increase fluid intake promptly if decreased urinary output is caused by hypovolemia and hypoperfusion.
5. Monitor for indicators of hypovolemia, including cool extremities, delayed capillary refill (greater than 2 seconds), and decreased amplitude of or absent distal pulses.
6. Estimate ongoing fluid losses. Measure all drainage from tubes, catheters, and drains. Note the frequency of dressing changes because of saturation with fluid or blood. Compare 24-hour urine output with 24-hour fluid intake, and record the difference.
7. Administer room temperature IV fluids.
8. Continuously monitor HR and ECG. Be alert to increases in HR, which suggest hypovolemia.
9. Monitor cardiovascular status hourly including CVP.
10. Measure hemodynamic measurements every 1 to 4 hours: CVP, CI, stroke volume index or continuously using an arterial-based system, SVV when appropriately available. Be alert to low or decreasing values in patients with borderline cardiac function or respiratory function. An elevated HR, decreased CVP, decreased CI less than 2.5 L/min/m^2, stroke volume index less than 33 mL/m^2/beat, and SVV greater than 15% (on assist-control mode mechanical ventilation) are suggestive of hypovolemia.
11. Consider fluid bolus for urine output less than 0.5 mL/kg/h for 2 consecutive hours. If SAP is present, initiate fluid resuscitation and shock management.
12. Weigh the patient daily, using the same scales and method. Weight may increase as a result of significant capillary leak and anasarca with intravascular volume depletion.
13. Evaluate characteristics of all fluids lost. Note color and odor. Be alert to the presence of particulate matter, fibrin, and clots. Test GI aspirate, drainage, and excretions (including stool) for the presence of occult blood.

Shock Management
1. Monitor fluid status (see Fluid Management, Fluid Resuscitation).
2. Collaborate with the physician or advanced practice provider to administer vasoactive medication if shock persists with volume resuscitation.
3. Monitor for cerebral ischemia or indications of insufficient cerebral blood flow.
4. Monitor renal function (BUN and creatinine levels for elevations), because intravascular volume depletion can lead to prerenal azotemia.
5. Monitor tissue oxygenation using ABG, SvO$_2$ or ScvO$_2$ monitoring, and serum lactate measurements.
6. Monitor ECG for ST segment depression and T wave inversion, which may be seen as a result of the shock state.

Electrolyte Management
1. Monitor for manifestations of electrolyte imbalance. Calcium, sodium, magnesium, and potassium are lost with fluid sequestration and vomiting.
2. Maintain IV solutions containing electrolytes at a constant rate.
3. Continuously monitor ECG for alterations related to electrolyte imbalances.
4. Monitor ionized calcium. Widening of the QT interval is suggestive of severe hypocalcemia. Hypocalcemia may produce numbness or tingling in the extremities that can progress to tetany.
5. Administer calcium gluconate or calcium chloride for low ionized calcium. Calcium chloride will provide a higher level of calcium replacement given the strength and chemical composition.
6. Monitor T wave as a sign of alterations in serum potassium levels.

NIC Fluid/Electrolyte Management; Fluid Monitoring; Hemodynamic Regulation; Hypovolemia Management; Invasive Hemodynamic Monitoring; Shock Prevention; Bleeding Precautions; Bleeding Reduction; Hypervolemia Management.

DECREASED CARDIAC OUTPUT *related to myocardial depression secondary to circulating vasoactive amines or hypocalcemia with SAP; decreased preload secondary to hypovolemia.*

Goals/Outcomes: Within 12 hours of diagnosis, CO becomes adequate, as evidenced by CI greater than 2.5 L/min/m², brisk capillary refill (less than 2 seconds), peripheral pulses greater than 2+ on a 0-to-4+ scale, urinary output greater than 0.5 mL/kg/h, and warm skin.
NOC Circulation Status.

Hemodynamic Regulation
1. Restore acceptable preload by correcting hypovolemia (see preceding nursing diagnosis, Fluid Volume Deficit).
2. Administer inotropic agents. Consider dobutamine for myocardial contractile support. Monitor hemodynamic measurements carefully to observe for vasodilation if dose of dobutamine is low.
3. Space out procedures and treatments to allow long periods (at least 90 minutes) of uninterrupted rest.
4. Minimize anxiety-producing situations and assist the patient with reducing anxiety.

NIC Care: Acute; Shock Management; Cardiac: Dysrhythmia Management; Anxiety Reduction; Energy Management.

ACUTE PAIN *related to chemical injury to the pancreas and peripancreatic tissue secondary to release of pancreatic enzymes.*

Goals/Outcomes: Within 2 to 4 hours of diagnosis, the patient's subjective evaluation of discomfort improves, as documented by a pain scale. Ventilation and hemodynamic status are uncompromised, as evidenced by MAP greater than 70 mm Hg, HR 60 to 100 bpm, and RR 12 to 20 breaths/min with normal depth and pattern (eupnea).
NOC Pain Control; Pain Level; Comfort Level.

Analgesia Administration
1. As prescribed, administer IV opiate analgesic before pain becomes severe.
2. Meperidine may be used initially for up to 3 days, but should not be administered long-term because of metabolite accumulation, which can cause neurologic adverse effects. Meperidine is avoided in patients with SAP, because analgesia is needed for more than 3 days. Hydromorphone may be a better alternative.
3. Monitor HR and BP at least every 1 to 2 hours in patients with SAP. Opiates cause vasodilation and can add to the serious hypotension of the patient who has SAP with volume depletion. Monitor every 15 minutes if severe pain is uncontrolled. Consult with the physician or advanced practice provider for changes in analgesic medications and dosages.
4. Evaluate effectiveness of medication and consult the physician or advanced practice provider for dose and drug manipulation.
5. Consider continuous infusion or PCA for more effective pain control.
6. Consider epidural route if IV route is ineffective.
7. If medications are not effective, prepare the patient for splanchnic block or other pain-relieving procedure.
8. Assess for anxiety and consider sedatives in conjunction with analgesia.

Safety Alert	*Opioid analgesics decrease intestinal motility and delay return to normal bowel function.*

9. Monitor respiratory pattern and LOC closely because both may be depressed by the large amounts of opiate analgesics usually required to control pain.

Pain Management
1. Pancreatitis can be very painful. Prepare significant others for personality changes and behavioral alterations associated with extreme pain and opiate analgesia. Family members sometimes misinterpret the patient's lethargy or unpleasant disposition and may even blame themselves. Reassure them that these are normal responses.
2. Supplement analgesics with nonpharmacologic maneuvers to aid in pain reduction. Modify the patient's body position to optimize comfort. Many patients with abdominal pain find a dorsal recumbent or lateral decubitus bent-knee position most comfortable.

3. Consider cultural influences on pain response.
4. Anxiety reduction contributes to pain relief, ensure consistency and promptness in delivering analgesic.
5. Provide continual reassurance to both patients and their families that all possible measures are being implemented to relieve pain.

NIC Patient-Controlled Analgesia (PCA) Assistance; Environmental Management: Comfort; Coping Enhancement;
Teaching: Prescribed Medication; Simple Guided Imagery; Respiratory Monitoring.

IMPAIRED GAS EXCHANGE *related to atelectasis and ARDS; elevation of the diaphragm and
pleural effusion caused by subdiaphragmatic inflammation of the pancreas, and with SAP, alveolar-
capillary membrane changes secondary to microatelectasis, inflammatory mediators, and pulmonary
fluid accumulation.*

Goals/Outcomes: Within 4 hours of diagnosis, the patient has adequate gas exchange, as evidenced by SaO_2
greater than 92%; PaO_2 greater than 80 mm Hg; $PaCO_2$ 35 to 45 mm Hg; RR 12 to 20 breaths/min with normal depth
and pattern; orientation to time, place, and person; and clear and audible breath sounds.
NOC Respiratory Status: Gas Exchange; Respiratory Status: Ventilation.

Airway Management
1. Administer oxygen via nasal cannula to maintain oxygen saturation greater than 92%. Check oxygen delivery
system at frequent intervals to ensure proper delivery.
2. Monitor and document RR every 1 to 2 hours as indicated. Note pattern, degree of excursion, and whether
the patient uses accessory muscles of respiration. Consult the physician for significant deviations from
baseline.
3. Auscultate both lung fields every 4 hours. Note presence of abnormal sounds (crackles, rhonchi, wheezes) or
diminished sounds.
4. Be alert to early signs of hypoxia, such as restlessness, agitation, and alterations in mentation.
5. Monitor SpO_2 via continuous pulse oximetry or frequent SaO_2 by ABG values during the first 48 hours. Many patients with pancreatitis do not have obvious clinical symptoms of respiratory failure, and a decreased arterial oxygen tension may be the first sign of ARDS or failure. Consult the physician or advanced practice provider if
PaO_2 is less than 60 to 70 mm Hg or if oxygen saturation falls below 92%.
6. Maintain a body position that optimizes ventilation and oxygenation. Elevate HOB 30 degrees or higher, depending on the patient's comfort. If pleural effusion or other defect is present on one side, position the patient
with the unaffected lung dependent to maximize the ventilation-perfusion relationship.
7. If the patient fails to stabilize, prepare for endotracheal intubation and mechanical ventilation.
8. Hypoxemia in the absence of preexisting pulmonary disease may be an early sign of ARDS.
9. Monitor pulmonary artery pressures, because pulmonary hypertension is anticipated in patients
with ARDS.
10. Avoid overaggressive fluid resuscitation (see Excess Fluid Volume in the following section).

NIC Acid-Base Management; Airway Management; Oxygen Therapy; Respiratory Monitoring; Positioning; Fluid
Monitoring; Hypervolemia Management.
See Acute Lung Injury and Acute Respiratory Distress Syndrome, Chapter 4, for additional information.

EXCESS FLUID VOLUME *related to excessive intake secondary to overaggressive fluid
resuscitation.*

Goals/Outcomes: Within 24 hours of diagnosis, the patient will be normovolemic, as evidenced by MAP 65 to
85 mm Hg, HR 60 to 100 bpm, RR 12 to 20 breaths/min with normal pattern and depth, and absence of adventitious
breath sounds and S3 gallop.
NOC Fluid Overload Severity; Fluid Balance; Electrolyte and Acid-Base Balance.

Hypervolemia Management
1. Evaluate the patient every 1 to 2 hours for clinical indicators of fluid volume excess: dyspnea, orthopnea,
increased RR and effort, S3 gallop, or crackles. Document new findings and report changes.
2. Consider administering furosemide (Lasix) or other diuretic as prescribed to promote diuresis, after volume
status has been evaluated. Patients may be intravascularly hypovolemic despite significant weight gain

resulting from third spacing of fluids. Diuresis may not prove to be beneficial. Document response to diuretic therapy.

NIC Fluid/Electrolyte Management; Fluid Monitoring; Hemodynamic Regulation.

RISK FOR INFECTION *related to tissue destruction and loss of protective barriers.*

Goals/Outcomes: The patient remains free of infection, as evidenced by core or rectal temperature less than 38° C (100.4° F), negative culture results, HR 60 to 100 bpm, RR 12 to 20 breaths/min, BP within the patient's normal range, CVP 2 to 6 mm Hg, and orientation to time, place, and person. See Chapter 11 for additional information on Sepsis.
NOC Infection Severity; Immune Status.

Infection Protection
1. Check temperature every 4 hours. Be aware that hypothermia may precede hyperthermia in some patients.
2. Temperature may be slightly elevated resulting from the inflammatory process. If temperature remains elevated for longer than 1 week, suspect that the patient may have developed bacterial (infected) pancreatic necrosis.
3. If temperature suddenly rises, obtain specimens for culture of blood, sputum, urine, and other sites as prescribed. Monitor culture reports and report positive findings promptly.
4. Evaluate orientation and LOC every 2 to 4 hours. Report significant deviations from baseline.
5. Monitor BP, HR, RR, CO/CI, and CVP every 1 to 4 hours. An elevated CO/CI and decreased CVP may suggest systemic inflammatory response or sepsis. Be alert to increases in HR and RR associated with temperature elevations.
6. Monitor white blood cell (WBC) count and anticipate a mild leukocytosis of 11,000 to 20,000/mm^3 as a result of the inflammatory response of SAP. If WBC count is greater than 20,000/mm^3, suspect infected pancreatitis. If total WBC count is elevated, monitor WBC differential for an elevation of bands (immature neutrophils).
7. Prophylactic antibiotics are NOT recommended for sterile pancreatitis unless the pancreas is greater than 30% necrosed, as evidenced by CT scan.
8. If prescribed, administer parenteral antibiotics in a timely manner. Reschedule antibiotics if a dose is delayed for greater than 1 hour. Recognize that failure to administer antibiotics on schedule can result in inadequate blood levels and treatment failure.
9. Do not administer prophylactic antibiotics for SAP.
10. Patients with infected pancreatitis evidenced by FNA-positive result for bacteria on Gram stain or culture require antibiotic therapy and may require laparoscopic, endoscopic, or radiologic intervention.

NIC Medication Management; Vital Signs Monitoring; Temperature Regulation; Intravenous (IV) Therapy.

IMBALANCED NUTRITION: LESS THAN BODY REQUIREMENTS *related to decreased oral intake secondary to nausea, vomiting, and nothing-by-mouth (NPO) status; increased need secondary to tissue destruction.*

Goals/Outcomes: The patient maintains baseline body weight and demonstrates a positive nitrogen balance.
NOC Nutrition Status; Nutrition Status: Food and Fluid Intake.

Nutrition Management
1. Collaborate with the advanced practice provider, dietitian, and pharmacist to estimate the patient's individual metabolic needs, based on activity level, presence of infection or other stressor, and nutrition status before hospitalization. Overuse of calcium supplements can cause AP; this mechanism should be added as noted earlier. Develop a plan of care accordingly.
2. Determine preexisting malnutrition with a nutrition assessment.
3. If the patient's condition improves after 48 hours of resting the bowel, oral intake of clear liquids can be slowly started. Mild to moderate increases in serum amylase and lipase may be noted. Feedings should continue unless these elevations are threefold above normal range.
4. If the patient's condition does not improve after 48 hours of bowel rest, administer elemental enteral feedings via NJ feeding tube or jejunostomy as prescribed. Pancreatic secretions are not stimulated with the delivery of enteral elemental nutrition into the mid- or distal jejunum. Ensure tube placement beyond the ligament of Treitz.

5. Monitor bowel sounds every 4 hours. Document and report deviations from baseline. Withhold jejunal feedings if bowel sounds are absent unless elemental feedings are used.
6. Monitor blood glucose levels every 4 to 8 hours or as prescribed. Treat blood glucose levels greater than 180 mg/dL with exogenous insulin.
7. If enteral feedings are not tolerated, begin TPN as prescribed. Monitor closely for evidence of hyperglycemia (e.g., Kussmaul's respirations; rapid respirations; fruity, acetone breath odor; flushed, dry skin; deteriorating LOC), which is commonly associated with pancreatitis. Administer insulin as prescribed.
8. Begin low-fat oral feedings when acute episode has subsided and bowel function has returned. This may take several weeks in some patients.

NIC Enteral Tube Feeding; Aspiration Precautions; Total Parenteral Nutrition (TPN) Administration; Venous Access Device (VAD) Maintenance; Hyperglycemia Management; Hypoglycemia Management.
For additional details, see Nutrition Support, Chapter 1.

DEFICIENT KNOWLEDGE *related to lack of exposure to healthcare information*

Goals/Outcomes: Before hospital discharge, the patient verbalizes knowledge regarding availability of alcohol rehabilitation programs, prescribed medications, importance of a low-fat diet, indicators of actual or impending GI hemorrhage, indicators of infection, and the importance of seeking medical attention promptly if signs of recurring pancreatitis appear.
NOC Knowledge: Disease Process; Knowledge Treatment: Regimen.

Teaching: Disease Process
1. Inform patients whose pancreatitis is caused by excessive alcohol intake about the availability of alcohol rehabilitation programs.
2. Teach the patient about prescribed medications including drug name, dosage, purpose, schedule, precautions, and side effects.
3. Advise the patient about the importance of adhering to a low-fat diet if prescribed.
4. Instruct the patient about the indicators of actual or impending GI hemorrhage: nausea, vomiting blood, dark stools, lightheadedness, and passing frank blood in stools.
5. Teach the indicators of infection: fever, unusual drainage from surgical incisions or peritoneal lavage site, warmth or erythema surrounding surgical sites, and abdominal pain. Have the patient demonstrate oral temperature-taking technique using the type of thermometer that will be used at home.
6. Stress the importance of seeking medical attention promptly if signs of recurrent pancreatitis (i.e., pain, change in bowel habits, passing blood in the stools, or vomiting blood) or infection (see Risk for Infection) appear.

NIC Prescribed Activity Exercise; Prescribed Diet; Prescribed Procedure/Treatment; Prescribed Medication; Behavior Modification.

ADDITIONAL NURSING DIAGNOSES

As appropriate, see nursing diagnoses and interventions in the following: Acute Respiratory Distress Syndrome (Chapter 4), Acute Renal Failure (Chapter 6), and Systemic Inflammatory Response Syndrome, Sepsis, Septic Shock, and Multiple Organ Dysfunction Syndrome (Chapter 11). Also see Prolonged Immobility (Chapter 1) and Emotional and Spiritual Support of the Patient and Significant Others (Chapter 2).

ENTEROCUTANEOUS FISTULA
PATHOPHYSIOLOGY

Enterocutaneous fistulas (ECFs) are formed when trauma, surgery, infection, neoplastic disease, or other pathologic condition results in a GI-cutaneous communication. Classifications include spontaneous (15% to 25%) or postoperative (75% to 85%) (. Spontaneous fistulas occur in patients with inflammatory bowel disease (IBD) (Crohn disease > indeterminate colitis > ulcerative colitis), cancer, diverticular disease, appendicitis, perforated bowel disease, radiation enteritis, or ischemic bowel. Postoperative fistulas account for the majority of ECFs and are observed following abdominal surgery for IBD, intestinal malignancy, recurrent explorations, or after extensive lysis of adhesions for conditions such as small bowel obstruction. For patients with severe abdominal trauma, severe intraabdominal sepsis, or complex surgical pathologies, open abdominal (OA) management has become a recurrent treatment option. In OA management, the peritoneal cavity is left open and abdominal contents are protected with a temporary dressing until bowel edema reduces or washouts are no longer required and the peritoneum can be closed. A new type of ECF has emerged as a complication of OA management called enteroatmospheric fistula (EAF). EAFs develop from edematous loops of bowel within the wound bed of an open abdomen that became injured.

Fistulas can be classified as high output (greater than 500 mL/d), moderate output (200 to 500 mL/d), and low output (less than 200 mL/d). High-output proximal small bowel fistulas are the most difficult to manage with losses as high as 2 L in 24 hours. Drainage from proximal fistulas is hypertonic; rich in enzymes, electrolytes, and proteins; thin in consistency and tends to be copious. Extensive skin and tissue breakdown often occur because of the presence of activated pancreatic enzymes in fistula drainage. Electrolyte and protein loss is great with high-output proximal fistulas. Drainage from distal sites, such as the ileum and colon, is thick and of less volume than is proximal fistula drainage.

Three factors are associated with mortality in patients with ECFs: (1) fluid and electrolyte imbalance, (2) malnutrition, and (3) sepsis. Fluid, potassium, sodium, proteins, and bicarbonate may be lost in great quantities. Replacement by enteral nutrition or parenteral nutrition (TPN) is complex, and proper balance is often difficult to achieve. Sepsis is frequently associated with bowel fistulization caused by anastomotic breakdown, local wound contamination, or inadequate drainage. Hypercatabolism and malnutrition are associated with both sepsis and fistulization, creating a great demand for calories and protein. Aggressive nutrition support and meticulous local wound management are crucial to patient survival. Mortality rates for ECF have declined overall because of advances in nutrition, wound care, and surgical technique to 5% to 15%.

GASTROINTESTINAL ASSESSMENT: ENTEROCUTANEOUS FISTULA

GOAL OF ASSESSMENT: ENTEROCUTANEOUS FISTULA
Evaluate the functional integrity of the intestinal tract.

HISTORY AND RISK FACTORS
- Direct trauma to the GI system, especially the bowel.
- Infection of surgical wound, drainage tract, or peritoneum.
- Prolonged catabolic state in association with bowel injury, GI neoplasm, GI abscess, or severe inflammatory bowel disease.
- Complex GI surgical procedures, such as extensive lysis of adhesions for intestinal obstruction or complicated intestinal anastomosis.
- Trauma surgery with missed injuries; emergency surgery with inadequate bowel preparation; damage control operations, where the abdomen is left open as a result of packing, or edematous bowel unable to be closed.
- History of IBD, especially Crohn disease. ECFs affect approximately 30% of people with Crohn disease.

VITAL SIGN ASSESSMENT
- Increased temperature and tachycardia resulting from infection or dehydration.
- Irregular HR as a result of fluid loss and hypokalemia.
- Decreased urinary output with increased specific gravity caused by excessive fluid loss.

ABDOMINAL PAIN
- Tenderness, erythema, and possibly pain at the incision/fistula site caused by irritation from fistula output or infection.
- Muscle weakness from hypokalemia.

ABDOMINAL DRAINAGE
- Discharge of bile, enteric contents, or gas through a surgical incision.
- Sudden increase in the amount of drainage from a surgical incision or drainage catheter.

- Change in the nature of drainage from serous or serosanguineous to yellow, green, brown, or foul-smelling.
- Change in pancreatic drainage to milky white suggests a pancreatic fistula.

OBSERVATION
- Mental confusion is often present as a result of electrolyte imbalance, dehydration, or early sepsis.
- Sunken eyes, poor skin turgor, and dry oral mucosa are associated with dehydration.
- Peripheral edema and muscle wasting related to protein loss.
- Erythema, maceration, and edema may be present on the abdomen because of irritating fistula drainage.

AUSCULTATION
- Diminished or absent bowel sounds if peritonitis or ileus is present.

PALPATION
- Discomfort and guarding on abdominal palpation over an abdominal mass (abscess) or near a drain site or surgical incision.

NUTRITION ASSESSMENT
- Weight loss and loss of muscle mass resulting from protein losses and hypercatabolism.
- Decreased serum albumin and transferrin both indicate malnutrition.

SCREENING LABWORK
- Serum electrolyte levels: Depleted as a result of external losses through the fistula.
- Fistula fluid can be analyzed for electrolyte determination. Electrolyte replacement can be formulated on the basis of the results.
- CBC: Anemia may be present reducing oxygen-carrying capacity.

HEMODYNAMIC MEASUREMENTS
- Decreased BP, MAP, and CVP if severe dehydration is present.
- If early sepsis is present, expect elevated CO and decreased SVR.
- Oxygen demand is increased and may exceed supply. Svo_2, $Scvo_2$ will fall without aggressive pulmonary and cardiovascular support.
- The patient will exhibit general hemodynamic instability until fluid balance, inflammation, and infection are controlled.

Diagnostic Tests for Enterocutaneous Fistula		
Test	**Purpose**	**Abnormal Findings**
Blood Studies		
Complete blood count (CBC): White blood cell (WBC) count	Assesses for inflammation, infection, and sepsis.	Leukocytosis with WBC count >12,000/mm^3. Leukopenia with WBC count <4000/mm^3. Normal WBC with >10% bands.
Red blood cell (RBC) count: Hemoglobin (Hgb) Hematocrit (Hct)	Reflective of blood volume status and oxygen-carrying capacity.	Hct and Hgb levels will be elevated as a result of the presence of significant dehydration. Anemia will develop as a result of the prolonged period of illness.
Electrolytes: (Serum) potassium Magnesium Calcium Bicarbonate	Determines accurate electrolyte levels to dictate appropriate replacement, because large quantities may be lost through fistula drainage.	Hypokalemia Hypocalcemia Hypomagnesemia Metabolic acidosis

Enterocutaneous Fistula

Continued

Diagnostic Tests for Enterocutaneous Fistula—cont'd		
Test	**Purpose**	**Abnormal Findings**
Nutrition profile: Serum albumin, transferrin, prealbumin	Evaluates nutrition status and initiates aggressive nutrition support early.	These laboratory tests will vary in individual patients. Serum transferrin levels >140 mg/dL have been shown to correlate with the spontaneous closure of enterocutaneous fistulas, thereby reducing mortality among these patients. Levels <140 is a poor prognostic finding. Serum albumin 3 g/dL or less at the time of fistula presentation is a poor prognostic indicator. Prealbumin levels will rise with effective nutrition therapy.
Noninvasive Cardiology		
Electrocardiogram	Assesses and monitors for cardiac rhythm disturbances related to hypokalemia, hypocalcemia, and hypomagnesemia.	Hypokalemia may result in flattening of T wave or U wave development. Hypocalcemia, hypokalemia, and hypomagnesemia can result in widening of the QT interval.
Radiology		
Fistulogram: Water-soluble contrast medium injected into the suspected fistula	To identify the anatomy and characteristics of the fistula tract.	Radiographs will confirm anatomic site of origin and fistula tract.
Computed tomography (CT) scan	CT may be used to identify abscesses associated with fistulization.	Confirmation of intraperitoneal abscess is made. Percutaneous drainage may be performed.
Upper gastrointestinal (GI) series	An upper GI series may be indicated if the suspected fistula is proximal to the intestines.	Upper GI series may reveal esophageal, gastric, or duodenal fistulas.

NONRADIOGRAPHIC EVALUATION

Bedside maneuver: An external fistula can be simply confirmed without radiology by the oral administration of charcoal. The visible presence of dye in the drainage confirms the presence of a fistula.

Biopsy: In patients with neoplastic disease, a biopsy specimen of the fistula tract may be obtained to determine the presence of malignancy within the tract.

Culture: Fistula effluent from the stomach, duodenum, biliary tree, and pancreas may be cultured for evidence of infection. Small and large bowel fistulas are generally not cultured because of the expected presence of bacteria.

COLLABORATIVE MANAGEMENT

Early management of ECF presents a considerable challenge requiring advanced support of a multidisciplinary team in a surgical intensive care unit setting. The patient with ECF is typically malnourished with a recent history of malignancy, inflammatory or infectious disease, postoperative or traumatic bowel injury, dehiscence, or inadvertent enterotomy. Their physiologic and nutrition reserves are significantly compromised. Treatment is usually complicated by sepsis and the metabolic and fluid derangements caused by the fistula. Early fistula identification is imperative to implement appropriate management strategies, including patient stabilization, investigation of the fistula, evaluation of surgical need, and the promotion of healing.

CARE PRIORITIES

Once the fistula is diagnosed, immediate management should focus on fluid restoration and the correction of electrolyte abnormalities. The control of sepsis and septic complications, nutrition support, and fistula management are key components to positive outcomes and should be addressed concurrently.

1. Fluid and Electrolyte Replacement

Crystalloid resuscitation with normal saline or LR solution. Often, the amount to be delivered is prescribed in direct relation to fistula output, especially when the output is widely variable. Effluent from each fistula is measured separately for accurate estimation of specific electrolyte and fluid losses. In general, fistulas more proximal result in greater fluid, electrolyte, and protein losses.

2. Control of Sepsis

Sepsis is often seen in the patient with postoperative ECF following a bowel procedure where bowel contents escape into the peritoneum. All team members should participate in the evaluation of a septic foci. Blood, wound, fistula drainage, sputum, and venous catheter tips should be cultured. Empirical antibiotic therapy is indicated with diagnosis of sepsis followed by specific therapy. Intraperitoneal abscesses should be drained cautiously, because manipulation of the septic foci may lead to its spread. If no evidence of sepsis is observed, antibiotic therapy should be withheld in the postoperative period. In patients with ECF, indiscriminate antibiotic use will lead to the emergence of highly resistant bacteria. (See Sepsis, Chapter 11.)

3. Nutrition Support

Patients with a fistula are typically malnourished because of their postoperative NPO status, the hypercatabolism of sepsis, and the protein- and mineral-rich intestinal fluid loss from the fistula. Both TPN and enteral nutrition can be used to manage patients with ECF based on a thorough nutrition assessment.

Enteral nutrition is currently advocated over TPN, because enteral nutrition enhances mucosal proliferation, promotes villus growth, improves hepatic protein synthesis, and stimulates the enterocyte, whereas TPN has been shown to cause intestinal mucosal atrophy. However, TPN remains a valuable therapeutic modality for patients who cannot tolerate enteral nutrition and in combination with enteral nutrition for patients who are unable to absorb sufficient calories from enteral feedings alone. Enteral feedings can be initiated by a weighted nasoduodenal intestinal feeding tube if there is sufficient (approximately 4 feet) functioning small bowel length between the ligament of Treitz (a thin muscle that wraps around the small intestine where the duodenum and jejunum meet) and the fistula. Enteral feedings can be optimized in patients with a feeding jejunostomy (placed at the time of their surgery) distal to the fistula, as is the case of many postoperative ECFs. In some cases, enteral feedings may be infused into the fistula itself. The volume and concentration of enteral feedings are started low and increased incrementally; supplementation with TPN is necessary to meet caloric and protein requirements during this time. For some patients, TPN supplementation is needed throughout the duration of care. Enteral feedings are slowed or discontinued if fistula output increases after initiation of feedings.

Patients with proximal small bowel fistulas, prolonged ileus, or extensive intraabdominal sepsis usually require TPN. Optimizing nutrition status will enhance the immune system, preserve lean cell mass, and promote wound healing. Improved nutrition status correlates with spontaneous fistula closure.

4. Fistula Management

Ideally, drainage from each fistula is collected separately to assess individual fistula activity and healing. Individualized systems of gravity or gentle suction drainage and barrier skin protection are devised for each patient. Good local management reduces the incidence of wound-related bacteremias and increases the rate of wound healing. EAFs are managed with negative pressure wound management therapy (NPWT) devices previously referred to as vacuum-assisted closure (VAC) systems. The system consists of a porous foam pad that connects to subatmospheric suction under an occlusive dressing. NPWT devices divert fistula drainage away from the wound by providing continuous negative pressure suction to the wound surface. NPWTs protect the skin and reduce patient discomfort from multiple dressing changes, because they require changes only once every 2 to 3 days. This system effectively promotes wound healing by increasing the rate of tissue granulation and augmenting wound contracture.

Somatostatin analogues: Somatostatin analogues such as octreotide have been shown to inhibit gastric secretions and should decrease fistula output. However, studies showed no significant improvement in fistula closure rate or improvement in mortality rates. Somatostatin is associated with a frequent incidence of hyperglycemia and can cause increased nausea. Therefore, somatostatin analogs are not indicated for routine use in patients with ECF. Octreotide has been shown to provide improved healing time in patients with high-output fistulas, perhaps by decreasing a high-output fistula to a low-output fistula. The role of octreotide is currently limited for use with high-output fistulas.

Surgery: Spontaneous fistula closure occurs in approximately 30% of patients with ECF with adequate nutrition support and successful treatment of sepsis. If spontaneous closure does not occur after 4 to 6 weeks of management, surgical resection is considered. Surgery is indicated in the following instances: (1) to close fistulas that continue to drain significant amounts despite absence of infection and appropriate nutrition support; (2) to explore and drain fistula tracts that could not be identified or drained by less invasive techniques; and (3) if overwhelming sepsis fails to respond to antibiotics and supportive therapy. Persistently draining fistulas are surgically closed with a procedure involving resection with end-to-end anastomosis. Postoperatively, parenteral nutrition and antibiotic coverage are continued. A gastrostomy is usually created to allow for prolonged intestinal decompression and drainage. The patient may remain NPO for greater than 1 to 2 weeks after surgery, depending on the rate of healing and the return of bowel function. An alternate feeding strategy is initiated during this time.

CARE PLANS FOR ENTEROCUTANEOUS FISTULA

DEFICIENT FLUID VOLUME *related to the active loss of intestinal fluids rich in electrolytes, minerals, and protein through fistula output.*

Goals/Outcomes: Within 8 hours of diagnosis, the patient's volume status is stabilized, as evidenced by balanced daily input and output, urinary output $\geq$0.5 mL/kg/h, HR less than 100 bpm, CVP 2 to 8 mm Hg, and MAP $\geq$ 60 mm Hg; moist mucous membranes, good skin turgor, warm extremities, peripheral pulses greater than 2+ on a 0-to-4+ scale, brisk capillary refill (less than 2 seconds); orientation to time, place, and person; and stable weight. The goals of improvement for patients who are extremely ill are adjusted according to the predicted best values the patient can achieve with their level of organ impairment.

NOC Fluid Balance.

Fluid/Electrolyte Management

1. Evaluate the fluid balance by calculating and comparing daily intake and output. In patients with high-output fistulas, evaluate total intake and output every 8 hours. Record all sources of output, including drainage from each fistula.
2. Administer IV crystalloids to replace fistula output. Generally, fistula output is isosmotic with high potassium content. Thus, normal saline with a potassium supplement should be administered.
3. Measure and evaluate vital signs, every 1 to 2 hours, depending on hemodynamic stability. Be alert to increasing HR, decreasing CVP, and decreasing MAP, which indicate inadequate intravascular volume.
4. Monitor fluid responsiveness measurements such as systolic pressure variation (SPV), pulse pressure variation (PPV), and SVV when available. If SPV greater than 5 mm Hg, PPV greater than 13% to 15%, and SVV greater than 13% to 15%, the patient is deemed fluid responsive.
5. Consider administering pRBCs for Hct less than 21%. Transfusion should be based on the symptoms of the patient. Transfusion of pRBCs will improve oxygen-carrying capacity. Anticipate an Hct increase of 3% following 1 unit of pRBCs.
6. Measure urine output every 1 to 2 hours. Consult the advanced practice provider if urine output is less than 0.5 mL/kg/h or if specific gravity increases and urine volume decreases.
7. Assess and document condition of mucous membranes and skin turgor. Dry membranes and inelastic skin indicate inadequate fluid volume and the need for increase in fluid intake (per os [PO] or IV route).
8. Control sources of insensible fluid loss by humidifying oxygen, maintaining comfortable environment, and controlling fever (if present) with antipyretics such as acetaminophen.
9. Monitor for manifestations of electrolyte imbalance, most commonly hypokalemia, hypocalcemia, and hypomagnesemia that are lost through fistula output.

10. Monitor ECG for T wave flattening or the presence of a U wave, indicative of hypokalemia.
11. Monitor ECG for prolongation of the QT interval, a result of hypokalemia, hypocalcemia, and hypomagnesemia.

NIC Fluid Monitoring; Hemodynamic Regulation; Hypovolemia Management; Invasive Hemodynamic Monitoring; Shock Prevention.

INFECTION, RISK FOR AND ACTUAL *related to inadequate primary defenses (altered integumentary system, disruption in continuity of GI system), hypercatabolic state, presence of invasive lines, protein loss/malnutrition, and gut contamination of bowel contents.*

Goals/Outcomes: The patient remains free of infection, as evidenced by core or rectal temperature less than 37.8° C (100° F), negative culture results, HR 60 to 100 bpm, RR 12 to 20 breaths/min, BP within the patient's normal range, and orientation to time, place, and person.
NOC Wound Healing: Secondary Intention.

Infection Control
1. Use standard precautions if contact with drainage is possible. Effective handwashing is essential.
2. Check rectal or core temperature every 4 hours for increases or decreases. If temperature suddenly rises, assess the patient for potential sources, noting presence of purulent secretions; erythema around wound, drain, or fistula site; and pain, tenderness, or masses with abdominal palpation. Consult the advanced practice provider for temperature elevation and assessment findings. Obtain specimens for culture of likely sites for infection as prescribed by the physician or unit protocol.
3. Evaluate mental status every 1 to 2 hours. Document and report significant deviations from baseline values.
4. Monitor BP, HR, RR every 1 to 2 hours. Be alert to increases in HR and RR associated with temperature elevations.
5. Administer IV antibiotics in a timely manner. Reschedule antibiotics if a dose is delayed for greater than 1 hour. Recognize that failure to administer antibiotics on schedule can result in inadequate blood levels and treatment failure.
6. Optimize gravity drainage of fistula by prone or upright positioning as tolerated by the patient.
See Systemic Inflammatory Response Syndrome, Sepsis, Septic Shock, and Multiple Organ Dysfunction Syndrome care plans, Chapter 11.

NIC Medication Management; Hemodynamic Regulation; Vital Signs Monitoring; Temperature Regulation; Intravenous (IV) Therapy; Wound Care.

IMBALANCED NUTRITION: LESS THAN BODY REQUIREMENTS *related to decreased intake, protein loss via fistula output, disruption of GI tract continuity, and the hypercatabolism of sepsis.*

Goals/Outcomes: By the time of hospital discharge, the patient has adequate nutrition, as evidenced by food intake that increases to his or her recommended daily allowance, and body weight that returns to baseline or within 10% of the patient's ideal weight.
NOC Nutrition Status: Nutrient Intake.

Nutrition Management
1. Collaborate with the physician or advanced practice provider, dietitian, and pharmacist to estimate the patient's metabolic needs on the basis of activity level, estimated metabolic rate, and baseline nutrition status.
2. Determine preexisting malnutrition status.
3. Monitor nutrition laboratories. Serum albumin and transferrin are good prognostic indicators for mortality, morbidity, and spontaneous fistula closure.
4. Monitor for the presence of bowel sounds every 2 hours. If bowel sounds are absent, consider duodenal or jejunal elemental feedings.
5. If fistula output increases in response to enteral feedings, slow the rate of infusion or reduce the strength of the feeding. If the patient tolerates oral feedings but they increase fistula output, increase the frequency of the feedings and decrease the amount consumed at each feeding.
6. Elemental feeding formulas may be more readily absorbed when the entire intestine is not available for normal absorption.

7. Prepare the patient for parenteral feedings if enteral feedings are inadequate for the patient's requirements.
8. Apply NG suction only in the presence of obstruction or prolonged ileus. In their absence, NG drainage shows little benefit. They may inappropriately contribute to complications such as patient discomfort, sinusitis, pulmonary aspiration, and gastroesophageal reflux.

NIC Nutrition Monitoring; Fluid/Electrolyte Management; Total Parenteral Nutrition (TPN) Administration; Enteral Tube Feeding.
For additional information, see Nutrition Support, Chapter 1.

IMPAIRED TISSUE INTEGRITY *related to chemical trauma, infection, and malnutrition*
- -
Goals/Outcomes: Within 72 hours of diagnosis, the patient's tissue adjacent to the fistula is free of erythema, excoriation, and edema.
NOC Wound Healing: Secondary Intention; Tissue Integrity: Skin and Mucous Membranes.

Wound Care
1. Assess the extent of the local problem (Box 9-7). Consult the physician for signs of extensive damage to the tissue adjacent to the fistula (i.e., severe local erythema, excoriation, edema, maceration).
2. Establish drainage and collection system for each fistula (Box 9-8). Consult the advanced practice provider regarding use of device(s).

Box 9-7 NURSING ASSESSMENT OF ENTEROCUTANEOUS FISTULA

- Evaluate size, shape, and location of the fistula. Reposition or lift skin folds as necessary.
- Identify any potential leakage tracks created by skin folds or body hollows.
- Examine the condition of adjacent skin and tissue. Note the presence and spread of both erythema and excoriation, which suggest leakage tracks.
- Note the consistency and characteristic of fistula output.
- Assess each fistula separately.
  Document all findings and compare them with baseline assessment made at the time of initial evaluation.

Box 9-8 RECOMMENDATIONS FOR CONTAINING FISTULA DRAINAGE

- Clean the intact skin surrounding the fistula with a nonirritating antibacterial cleanser.
- Clip body hair (if present) around the fistula.
- Remove pooled drainage from the wound and surrounding area by using sterile absorbent pads or gentle suction. The help of an assistant may be necessary to maintain a dry field during application of the collection device.
- Apply a barrier powder (e.g., karaya or Orahesive) to excoriated skin. A flexible transparent dressing (e.g., Op-Site) can be used to protect intact skin.
- Use a skin paste (e.g., Stomahesive or karaya) to fill in any grooves surrounding recessed fistulas.
- Apply a sized barrier sheet (e.g., Stomahesive, HolliHesive) to the surrounding skin, being careful not to overlap the fistula.
- Attach a collecting bag to the barrier sheet base. For high-output fistulas, a urostomy bag and collecting system may be necessary. Transparent appliances enable observation of drainage. Devices that have a drainage opening permit emptying and measurement of output.
  Reposition the patient frequently to optimize gravity of fistula output.

3. Note characteristic, color, odor, and volume of output from each fistula. Consult the advanced practice provider for significant changes in these indicators.
4. If increased fistula output results from oral or enteral feedings, eliminate or modify the feedings as prescribed.
5. Consult the wound ostomy continence nursing (WOCN) services for recommendations in pouching complex or multiple fistulas.
6. Consider wound management with an NPWT device; currently used to effectively divert intestinal output from the wound and increase blood flow to the area.
7. NPWT dressing is changed approximately every 3 to 7 days by a WOCN. With this frequency of dressing change, the surrounding skin is protected and patient discomfort is reduced.

NIC Ostomy Care; Tube Care; Fluid/Electrolyte Management.

DISTURBED BODY IMAGE *related to biophysical change secondary to presence of external fistula.*

Goals/Outcomes: By hospital discharge, the patient acknowledges body changes, as evidenced by viewing fistula and not exhibiting preoccupation with or depersonalization of fistula.
NOC Body Image.

Body Image Enhancement
1. Evaluate the patient's reaction to the fistula by observing and noting evidence of body image disturbance.
2. Anticipate feelings of shock and repulsion initially. Be aware that the development of an external fistula is usually an unanticipated complication and patients are not emotionally prepared for the disfigurement.
3. Anticipate and acknowledge normalcy of feelings of rejection, isolation, and uncleanliness (because of odor and possible presence of feces).
4. Offer the patient an opportunity to view fistula/wound as desired. Use mirrors if necessary.
5. Encourage the patient and significant others to verbalize feelings regarding fistula/wound.
6. If possible, offer the patient an opportunity to participate in wound care. The patient may be able to perform simple tasks, such as holding the bag into which you will deposit the soiled dressing or applying the pouch that collects drainage.
7. Convey an accepting attitude toward the patient. Many fistulas that require critical care involve open and infected wounds. If the attending nurse is inexperienced in dressing these complex wounds, another, more experienced nurse should be present during the initial dressing change.
8. Reassure the patient that the fistula is not permanent. Acknowledge that a scar will be visible but the fistula will close with appropriate care.

NIC Coping Enhancement; Self-Care Assistance; Support System Enhancement.

IMPAIRED ORAL MUCOUS MEMBRANE *related to prolonged NPO status*

Goals/Outcomes: Within 24 hours of diagnosis, the patient's oral mucosa is intact, moist, and free of pain and oral lesions.
NOC Oral Hygiene; Tissue Integrity: Skin and Mucous Membranes.

Oral Health Maintenance
1. Inspect the patient's oral cavity, noting the degree of moisture, inflammation, bleeding, or lesions. Consult the physician for open lesions and bleeding.
2. Assist the patient with brushing teeth with a soft-bristle toothbrush. Provide mouth care every 4 hours.
3. For patients with altered LOC, massage gums and teeth with saline-moistened, sponge-tipped applicator and brush teeth gently if there is no evidence of bleeding. Carefully suction the solution from the oral cavity throughout the procedure with a tonsil suction device.
4. Keep the lips moist with emollients such as lanolin. Take care to apply emollient to external tissue only. Oil-containing emollients are harmful if aspirated or otherwise introduced into the respiratory tract.

NIC Oral Health Promotion.

ADDITIONAL NURSING DIAGNOSES

See Nutrition Support (Chapter 1) for additional information about the patient with extra nutrition needs. See Emotional and Spiritual Support of the Patient and Significant Others (Chapter 2) for psychosocial nursing diagnoses and interventions. Also see nursing diagnoses and interventions related to sepsis under Systemic Inflammatory Response Syndrome, Sepsis, Septic Shock, and Multiple Organ Dysfunction Syndrome (Chapter 11).

HEPATIC FAILURE

PATHOPHYSIOLOGY

There are various manifestations of acute and chronic liver failure. Fluid retention, edema, and ascites are common to acute and chronic hepatic failure and are attributed to: (1) intrahepatic vascular obstruction with transudation of fluid into the peritoneum; (2) defective albumin synthesis, resulting in decreased colloid osmotic pressure with failure to retain intravascular fluid; and (3) disturbances of various hormones, including renin, aldosterone, and renal prostaglandins, resulting in sodium and water retention. Massive ascites is usually the result of cirrhosis.

Hepatic encephalopathy occurs in both acute and chronic liver failure. A state of decreased mentation, neuromuscular function, and consciousness are the hallmarks of hepatic encephalopathy. Patients with stage one (mild) hepatic encephalopathy have problems concentrating, difficulty writing, memory loss, subtle personality changes, mood swings, and sleep alteration that may result in loss of awareness of time of day or night; often switching daytime activities into night activities. Patients with stage two (moderate) hepatic encephalopathy have less energy, have slurred speech, behave strangely, forget more frequently, and have problems with basic math. Patients with stage three (severe) hepatic encephalopathy are somnolent, may have syncopal episodes, and exhibit extreme changes in behavior. Monitoring patients for seizures and dementia is crucial. These patients are often poorly functional at home and are reported to be jumpy, fearful, and have absolutely no basic math skills. Patients in stage four (hepatic coma) are admitted directly to the ICU, usually arriving unconscious or semiconscious. Patients with stage one and two are usually ambulatory and receive outpatient treatment for hepatic encephalopathy with oral medications. Patients with stage three are often bordering on critical illness, whereas patients with stage four generally require mechanical ventilation and sedation in the ICU. Complications of hepatic encephalopathy include brain swelling with herniation, coma, and death.

Both acute and chronic hepatic failure affect the physiologic status of all organs. Key differences between the two include progression rate of liver failure, previous history of liver disease, type of treatments required, and prognosis.

ACUTE LIVER FAILURE

Acute liver failure (ALF) is defined as a severe, sudden loss of hepatocytes resulting in failure of hepatic function, accompanied by encephalopathy and coagulation disorder. ALF occurs without a previous history of liver disease. Although there are approximately 2000 cases per year in the United States, ALF is more common in less developed countries with 50% mortality. In the United States, acetaminophen overdose is the leading etiology, whether intentional overingestion (suicide) or through inappropriate self-medication or "therapeutic misadventure." Other common causes of ALF in the United States include misuse of medications and herbal supplements (prescription, over-the-counter, and complementary/alternative), viral hepatitis, autoimmune liver disease, shock, mushroom poisoning (commonly *Amanita phalloides*), hypoperfusion of the liver (i.e., Budd-Chiari syndrome), Wilson disease, acute fatty liver of pregnancy, herpes viruses, and malignant infiltration. Outcomes have improved considerably in the past decade, resulting from more timely admission of patients to specialty ICUs of liver transplant centers. Transplant centers are familiar with appropriate crisis management, including palliative, non–disease-specific treatments (i.e., N-acetylcysteine [NAC]). The outcomes of the Acute Liver Failure Study Group revealed that patients with slowly evolving etiologies have a poorer prognosis than when ALF developed hyperacutely (within less than 1 week). For those who fail to show signs of spontaneous recovery, liver transplantation using a whole cadaver graft is considered standard of care. Survival rates for the first year of transplant in patients with ALF are lower than those patients transplanted for chronic liver failure (CLF). After the first year, survival rates are essentially the same.

Heart failure may occur in worsening ALF. While the condition progresses, dysrhythmias result from reduced beta-adrenergic receptor signal transduction, defective cardiac excitation-contraction coupling, and conduction abnormalities. Right ventricular failure ensues and causes venous engorgement resulting in hepatic congestion. The decreased forward flow of blood from the failing right-to-left heart circulation results in reduced CO. Decreased hepatic blood flow, with congestion of the vena cava from blood "backing up" from the failing right side of the heart, impedes the emptying of the portal vein into the vena cava.

Heart failure progressively damages the hepatocytes attributable to hypoxia resulting from circulatory impairment. The portal vein supplies up to 83% of the blood flow to the liver, with the hepatic artery supplying up to 34% (varies from person to person by approximately ±17%). In the final stages of ALF, profound peripheral vasodilation results in severe vascular congestion and third spacing of intravascular fluids including ascites, which causes hemodynamic collapse. Hypotension, tachycardia, heart murmur, warm extremities, an exaggerated precordial impulse, palmar erythema, and/or spider angiomas are present.

CHRONIC LIVER FAILURE

Loss of hepatocytes, abnormal microcirculation, and impaired hepatic function of 6 months or longer duration are hallmarks of chronic liver failure (CLF), eventually requiring transplant resulting from end-stage liver disease (ESLD). Chronic liver disease is associated with slowly progressing, widespread tissue necrosis, fibrosis, liver nodule formation, and cirrhosis, ultimately resulting in hepatic failure. The usual causes are long-term alcohol ingestion, chronic viral hepatitis, prolonged cholestasis, long-term use of certain medications, alpha$_1$-antitrypsin deficiency, diabetes, hemochromatosis, malnutrition, glycogen storage disease, and cystic fibrosis. CLF is a leading cause of morbidity and mortality in the United States with alcohol consumption and chronic viral hepatitis being responsible for the majority of ESLD cases necessitating liver transplantation. Most patients with cirrhosis remain asymptomatic for years until hepatic decompensation ensues. Approximately 40% of liver transplants performed in the United States are attributable to ESLD secondary to hepatitis C. The U.S. Food and Drug Administration (FDA) has recently approved direct-acting antivirals for hepatitis C that will profoundly change the face of ESLD and liver transplantation in the future. Nonalcoholic fatty liver disease attributable to risk factors such as lipidemia (hypertriglyceridemia), obesity, and diabetes is quickly becoming a more prevalent liver disease and in the near future will be responsible for more cases of ESLD. In the great majority of cases, CLF takes decades to manifest itself with symptoms requiring treatment and eventual referral to a liver transplant center.

In patients with cirrhosis, portal hypertension creates hyperdynamic circulation, reflected by decreased SVR, hypotension, increased CO, tachycardia, and bounding pulses. Progression to advanced liver disease correlates with worsening hyperdynamic circulation.

Patients with chronic liver disease may have hepatopulmonary syndrome (HPS) that results from intrapulmonary microvascular dilation that may or may not be coupled with portal hypertension. There may be diffuse or localized dilated pulmonary capillaries. Less common are the presence of pleural and pulmonary arteriovenous communications. Arterial hypoxemia, commonly present in chronic liver disease, is attributable to multiple coexisting causes such as ascites, hepatic hydrothorax, and/or chronic obstructive pulmonary disease. Dyspnea (shortness of breath) may be present at rest or during exertion and is the main symptom, particularly after long-standing liver disease. Upon examination, spider angioma, digital clubbing, cyanosis, and platypnea (shortness of breath relieved when lying down) are common findings. Liver transplantation can reverse HPS if the patient survives longer than 6 months posttransplant and can improve to the point that supplemental oxygen may no longer be needed.

As defined by the National Institutes of Health Patient Registry for the Characterization of Primary Pulmonary Hypertension, a patient has portopulmonary hypertension (POPH) in the presence of portal hypertension with a mean pulmonary artery pressure ≥25 mm Hg and pulmonary capillary wedge pressure less than 15 mm Hg. Symptoms include fatigue, dyspnea, peripheral edema, syncope, chest pain, and a systolic murmur. ECG in 90% of patients reflects right bundle branch block, right-axis deviation, or a right ventricular hypertrophy. According to the American Association for the Study of Liver Diseases (AASLD) practice guidelines, POPH can potentially improve with liver transplantation and has acceptable short-term outcomes. In some patients, vasodilator therapy can even be discontinued posttransplant. Transjugular intrahepatic portosystemic shunting (TIPS) is useful for treating portal hypertension associated with refractory ascites and esophageal varices in the patient with cirrhosis who has ESLD. In over 90% of patients, TIPS procedures decompress the portal vein. Studies have shown that the rate of new or worsening hepatic encephalopathy after TIPS is 20% to 31%.

Spontaneous bacterial peritonitis is a spontaneous infection that affects up to one third of patients with ESLD. The most common organism found in the peritoneal fluid of patients with spontaneous bacterial peritonitis is *Escherichia coli*, believed to be attributable to translocation of the bacteria from the intestinal lumen. Prevention of spontaneous bacterial peritonitis is key with the use of oral antibiotics.

Hepatorenal syndrome (HRS) is defined by the International Club of Ascites as renal impairment or failure that occurs in patients with advanced chronic liver disease, liver failure, and portal hypertension. Patients have marked abnormalities in the arterial circulation and activity of the endogenous vasoactive systems. There are two types of HRS defined by the International Club of Ascites: type 1 is rapidly progressive, with baseline creatinine level doubling in less than 2 weeks to a value greater than 2.5 mg/dL. Type 2 is a slower disease that consists of moderate renal failure and is commonly associated with refractory ascites. The vast majority of patients have no intrinsic renal disease. Significant renal vasoconstriction results in low glomerular filtration rate, whereas arterial vasodilation in the extrarenal circulation results in reduction of SVR and hypotension. Factors that reduce renal perfusion in patients with chronic liver disease are dehydration, lactulose therapy, use of NSAIDs, hemorrhage, and paracentesis. For patients with cirrhosis who develop renal dysfunction, the risk of death increases sevenfold and 50% of patients die within a month of onset.

BENEFITS OF CARE IN A TRANSPLANT CENTER

Regardless if liver failure is acute or chronic, expert interdisciplinary collaboration provides rapid evaluation for etiology and timely access to appropriate treatment. Severity of liver damage is accurately assessed for possible listing as a liver transplantation candidate. Failure of other organs is often linked to liver dysfunction. Highly specialized evaluation is needed to identify and vigilantly manage these complex patients.

HEPATIC ASSESSMENT

GOAL OF SYSTEM ASSESSMENT

A thorough physical assessment along with an accurate history should produce a correct liver disease diagnosis in the majority of cases. Evaluate for cause of and subsequent hepatic and multisystem effects of ALF, because severe liver damage has already occurred upon presentation for care.

HISTORY AND RISK FACTORS

Evaluate for family/personal history of liver disease, exposure to toxins, exposure to complementary and alternative medications, street or prescription drug use, acetaminophen use and abuse, alcohol use and abuse, exposure to *Bacillus cereus* toxin (through food ingestion), and *Amanita phalloides* mushroom poisoning.

- Enquire about adherence with taking antibiotics for spontaneous bacterial peritonitis prophylaxis, diuretics, beta-blockers (for control of portal hypertension), lactulose (to keep ammonia level from rising, thereby preventing hepatic encephalopathy), and any nonprescribed or non–physician-recommended over-the-counter medications.
- Enquire about depression, recent travel abroad, and prescription, over-the-counter, and street drug use.

VITAL SIGN ASSESSMENT

- Neurologic assessment, including Glasgow Coma Scale score, in some cases an intracranial pressure (ICP) monitor, and an arterial line may be needed for patients who are severely ill.
- HR (preferably apical), heart rhythm, and BP to evaluate if liver disease is affecting CO and perfusion; risk of hemorrhage is also a complication.
- Normal to bounding pulses, low normal BP, elevated CO associated with decreased peripheral vascular resistance and expanded total blood volume.
- Take BP while the patient is lying down, sitting up, and standing (if able)—this also helps to observe for platypnea.

- Take temperature; if elevated may be attributable to an acute bacterial, viral, or fungal process that may be affecting the liver.
- If the temperature is low, hypothermia may herald the onset of hepatic encephalopathy.

OBSERVATION

- Evaluate for pallor, jaundice, and scleral icterus and signs of coagulopathies.
- Note spider angioma, skin excoriation (from scratching as a result of increased bilirubin), ecchymosis, petechiae, prominent abdominal collateral veins, palmar erythema, gynecomastia, testicular atrophy, jugular vein distension, needle marks, loss of body hair, loss of muscle mass, peripheral edema, obvious ascites, eye signs mimicking hyperthyroidism, exertional dyspnea, digital clubbing, cyanosis of the nail beds, and umbilical hernias.
- Note muscle weakness and tenderness; a common finding in ESLD from alcohol (EtOH). Measure abdominal girth.
- Note if asterixis (brief periods of "flapping" or irregular flexion of the hands at the wrist) is present.
- Observe for signs of respiratory distress, impaired renal function, and bacterial, viral, and fungal infections.
- Note if questions are answered appropriately and if the patient is awake, alert, and oriented; disoriented or confused.
- Fetor hepaticus may be present (pungent breath odor in some patients with cirrhosis).
- In the presence of tense ascites (which increases intraabdominal pressure), impaired right ventricular filling with decreased stroke volume and decreased CO may be evident.
- If the patient has had a massive variceal hemorrhage or is in septic shock, pulses will be diminished and BP will be low, reflecting circulatory collapse.

PALPATION

Liver palpation can aid in the diagnosis of liver disease etiology and confirm cirrhosis.

- Examine the abdomen; palpate all nine sections of the abdomen, palpate the liver and spleen, and assess for abdominal masses.
- Palpate the liver and other abdominal organs (i.e., spleen). Note liver firmness, size, edges, and possible pain with palpation. Hepatomegaly may be evident. Many times in liver disease, splenomegaly is also appreciated. Gallbladder (if not previously removed) may be palpated (and if palpable and/or painful may be attributable to stones or infection); also assess for the presence of any abdominal masses.
- Note pulse quality and regularity bilaterally (scale 0 to 4+), because bilateral lower extremity edema is common in ESLD and can obscure pulses.
- Ascites can be diagnosed if not obvious with palpation and observation of an abdominal fluid wave upon palpation.
- Assess for lymphadenopathy.

AUSCULTATION

- Listen to the heart, carotid artery, lungs, and abdomen.
- Listen to abdominal sounds in all nine sections of the abdomen.
- Bruits and/or rubs may be present (liver disease–related abdominal bruits can be caused by hepatocellular carcinoma, portosystemic shunt, hepatic artery aneurysm, or alcoholic hepatitis).
- Abdominal friction rub, although rare, is reflective of peritoneal inflammation and may be diagnostic for infection (liver abscess), infarction of the liver, or tumor (hepatocellular carcinoma/liver metastasis).
- Listen for inspiratory crackles in the lungs, particularly at the bases, and end-expiratory wheezing and egophony (if effusions are present). Egophony is tested by asking the patient to say "e" repeatedly as all lung fields are auscultated. The "e" sounds the same over all healthy tissue. Over consolidated areas the "e" sounds like "ay".
- Note if second heart sound and right ventricular heave are present together.

SCREENING LABWORK

Blood testing may differentiate between ALF and chronic liver disease, as well as aid in diagnosing the severity of liver injury and degree of liver function/dysfunction.

Hepatic Failure

- Elevated liver function tests: alanine aminotransferase (ALT), aspartate aminotransferase (AST), gamma-glutamyl transpeptidase (GGT), bilirubin, alkaline phosphatase, with decreased albumin to check for hepatocyte injury, or a cholestatic cause for liver disease (see chart).
- Viral hepatitis studies, drug panel to check for drug-induced liver injury, EtOH level to screen for alcoholic liver disease.
- Coagulation studies: elevated international normalized ratio (INR), prothrombin time (PT), and partial thromboplastin time (PTT) herald a failing liver (see chart).
- Alpha-fetoprotein (AFP): nonspecific cancer marker to screen for hepatocellular carcinoma as a potential cause of liver disease (see chart).
- Electrolytes to monitor for hyponatremia and hypokalemia (see chart).
- Chemistry profile to monitor glucose (because it is often seen) and creatinine/BUN (renal function tests [see chart]).
- Street and therapeutic drug levels.
- Acetaminophen levels and adducts of the main metabolite of acetaminophen (the adducts are detectable even when the acetaminophen is not).
- Arterial ammonia levels.

LIVER BIOPSY
Once thought of as a diagnostic tool, liver biopsy now serves three important roles according to the AASLD liver biopsy position paper: (1) for diagnosis, (2) for assessment of prognosis (disease staging), and/or (3) to assist in making therapeutic management decisions. Liver biopsy is invaluable in patients that present with atypical clinical features, coexisting disorders, and "overlap" syndrome of two liver diseases (such as primary biliary cirrhosis and autoimmune hepatitis).

OTHER STUDIES
Chest radiography, Doppler echocardiography, and ABGs are useful in the diagnoses of HPS and POPH.

Diagnostic Tests for Acute and Chronic Hepatic Failure		
Test	Purpose	Abnormal Findings
Noninvasive Testing		
Electrocardiogram (ECG): 12-Lead ECG: Must be obtained upon admission to the intensive care unit	To assess for cardiac dysrhythmias related to end-stage liver disease.	Hypokalemia, acidosis, or hypoxia may cause cardiac dysrhythmias. Abnormal rate, rhythm may be part of hepatopulmonary syndrome, or portopulmonary hypertension.
Electroencephalogram (EEG)	For the diagnosis and quantification of hepatic encephalopathy.	Often abnormal if hepatic encephalopathy is present. Some correlation with ammonia levels and stage of encephalopathy has been reported.
Neuropsychological testing	To establish a baseline at admission (if the patient is not in a hepatic coma).	A battery of six tests, called the psychometric hepatic encephalopathy score (PHES). A normal score is 0.5 ± 1.83. Those scoring >4 are considered abnormal.
Blood Studies		
Liver function tests	Assesses for enzyme changes indicative of hepatic damage.	Elevated enzymes reflect liver damage.
Alanine aminotransferase (ALT) Aspartate	ALT is useful in determining whether jaundice is caused by liver disease or has a hemolytic cause.	Values >300 units/L are present with acute liver failure. Found primarily in the liver, ALT is the primary marker of hepatic damage.

Diagnostic Tests for Acute and Chronic Hepatic Failure—cont'd

Test	Purpose	Abnormal Findings
Aminotransferase (AST)		AST: Present in organs with high metabolic activity. Damage to the hepatocytes will cause a rise in AST 12 hours after injury and levels will remain elevated for 4 to 6 days. Levels 10 to 100 times normal are not unusual in liver disease.
Alkaline phosphatase (Alk Phos)		Alk Phos: Found in almost all tissue, but most elevations can be localized to the liver or bone. Alk Phos is elevated to varying degrees in various liver diseases.
Bilirubin (TBili or Bili)	To assess the ability of the liver to process bilirubin, which helps with differential diagnosis, and to predict the prognosis.	Bilirubin: Total bilirubin is a byproduct of hemolysis. Elevations occur with excessive red blood cell destruction or when the liver is unable to process normal amounts of bilirubin. Elevations commonly occur in viral hepatitis and cirrhosis. Consistently elevated levels are a poor prognostic sign.
Gamma-glutamyl transpeptidase (GGT)	To assist with diagnosing that liver disease is present.	Present in numerous tissues, but highest in liver disorders. This test can be used to confirm that Alk Phos is elevated resulting from a hepatic-related condition. Usually elevated in cholestatic liver disease, cirrhosis, alcoholic liver disease, and metastasis to the liver.
Albumin	To assess the ability of the liver to synthesize albumin, which helps predict the prognosis.	Synthesized in the liver, maintains blood oncotic pressure, and coagulation proteins needed to form a fibrin clot. Low levels are found in altered synthetic liver function. Decreased levels are seen with ascites and severe liver function, and persistently low levels suggest a poor prognosis.
Glucose	To assess possible cause for altered mentation and lethargy.	Impaired gluconeogenesis and glycogen depletion in the cirrhotic liver cause hypoglycemia, which is usually present in severe or terminal liver dysfunction, causing altered mentation and/or lethargy.
Blood urea nitrogen (BUN) and serum creatinine (Cr)	To assess kidney function/presence of hepatorenal syndrome.	In liver failure, BUN is decreased. However, if the patient has bleeding or has renal insufficiency (impending or actual hepatorenal syndrome), BUN:Cr is elevated.

Continued

Diagnostic Tests for Acute and Chronic Hepatic Failure—cont'd

Test	Purpose	Abnormal Findings
Arterial ammonia	To rule out hepatic encephalopathy or other causes of altered mentation.	Increased as a result of the inability of the failing liver to clear nitrogenous and other waste products. Gastrointestinal (GI) bleeding or an increase in intestinal protein from dietary intake can increase ammonia levels. Elevated levels may herald the development of intracranial hemorrhage.
Electrolytes		
Sodium (Na$^+$)	To differentiate between potential diagnoses.	Decrease in sodium seen in patients with cirrhosis, tense ascites, hepatorenal syndrome.
Potassium (K$^+$)		Decreased potassium observed in those with liver disease accompanied by ascites and in those with alcoholic liver disease. In hepatorenal syndrome, hyperkalemia is observed.
Hematologic Tests		
Hemoglobin (Hgb) Hematocrit (Hct)	To assess if anemia is present.	GI bleeding may be present with decreased Hgb/Hct. Anemia seen in hepatic failure is termed macrocytic (attributable to increase in mean corpuscular volume) and normochromic (normal Hgb).
Platelets	To evaluate for the possibility of bleeding.	Low as a result of platelet destruction and malfunctioning hepatic synthesis of platelets.
White blood count (WBC)	To evaluate for possible infection and inflammation.	Elevated if sepsis is present.
Coagulation Profile		
Prothrombin time (PT) with international normalized ratio (INR) Partial thromboplastin time (PTT)	Useful prognostic indicators in liver disease.	A prolonged PT/INR/PTT is an ominous sign in patients with liver failure, particularly in acetaminophen overdose, or unknown causes of liver failure. King's College Hospital criteria (Box 9-9) is a useful prognostic tool for predicting survival of patients with acute liver failure (ALF).
Other		
Urinalysis	Monitors for development of hepatorenal syndrome (HRS).	Decreased urine sodium excretion, with normal urinary sediment is a sign of HRS. In the presence of ascites, the 24-hour urine volume will be decreased and the 23-hour sodium value will be reduced sometimes to <5 mEq/d in severe cases.

Diagnostic Tests for Acute and Chronic Hepatic Failure—cont'd

Test	Purpose	Abnormal Findings
Alpha-fetoprotein (AFP)	A major plasma protein that is a nonspecific marker in hepatocellular carcinoma monitoring and treatment. Also elevated in patients with chronic hepatitis C virus and in patients with cirrhosis.	Normal levels are < 20 ng/mL.
Acetaminophen level	Useful in patients with ALF upon presentation to rule out other causes of ALF.	Time from ingestion to peak levels approximately 4 hours. Therapeutic levels 10 to 25 μg/mL.
Acetaminophen adducts	When acetaminophen overdose is suspected and no longer detectable, the adducts are specific biomarkers of drug-related toxicity.	Levels $\geq$1.0 mmol/L is a positive result. However, a serum bilirubin >10 mg/dL may cause a false-positive result.
Polymorphonuclear leukocyte count (PMN) _Note:_ A dipstick specifically designed for ascitic fluid is available to give bedside results in 2 to 3 minutes	Useful to quickly diagnose if spontaneous bacterial peritonitis is present. Can initiate empirical antibiotic treatment for spontaneous bacterial peritonitis if PMN count is $\geq$250 cells/mm³ while awaiting culture and sensitivity results.	PMN $\geq$250 cells/mm³.
Radiology		
Chest x-ray	Assesses for any pathology in the lungs and chest cavity, confirms diagnosis of portopulmonary hypertension and hepatopulmonary syndrome.	Tumors, lymph nodes, atelectasis, cardiomegaly, infiltrates, tortuous cardiac vessels, and diaphragm elevation (bilateral or unilateral).
Magnetic resonance imaging (MRI): Hepatic MRI	Assesses liver size, morphology, function, presence of cirrhosis, steatosis, and lesions. Used to characterize known lesions and status of hepatic circulation. Can produce a sharp contrast between tissues and water and/or fat. Can image in transverse, longitudinal, coronal, or oblique planes.	Enlarged liver, cirrhosis, tumors, cysts, hemangiomas, steatosis, macronodular lesions, hemochromatosis (if large iron stores are present), sarcoid nodules, biliary cystadenomas, adenomas, focal nodular hyperplastic nodules, cholangiocarcinoma, abscesses, thromboses, and hepatic congestion.
Computed tomography (CT): Hepatic CT scan	Assesses liver size, presence of cirrhosis, looks for the presence of lesions to characterize known lesions and status of hepatic circulation. Oral or intravenous contrast can be administered to help distinguish the bowel lumen and blood vessels and tissue, respectively.	Enlarged liver, cirrhosis, tumors, cysts, hemangiomas, steatosis, macronodular lesions, hemochromatosis (if large iron stores are present), sarcoid nodules, biliary cystadenomas, adenomas, focal nodular hyperplastic nodules, cholangiocarcinoma, abscesses, thromboses, and hepatic congestion.

Continued

Diagnostic Tests for Acute and Chronic Hepatic Failure—cont'd

Test	Purpose	Abnormal Findings
Ultrasound: Hepatic ultrasound	Assesses for fluid-filled lesions and vascular abnormalities. Also used to "mark the spot" before liver biopsy. Note: Ultrasound is best suited to thinner patients.	Main anatomic features of the liver can be identified, as well as cysts, infections, abscesses, steatosis, hemangiomas, malignant neoplasms, adenomas, hyperplastic lesions, lymphomas, increased echogenicity, hydatid cysts, amebiasis (caused by *Entamoeba histolytica* that can spread to the liver causing liver abscesses), and fungal disease.
Cerebral CT	Used for diagnosis when a subdural hematoma or doubt about etiology of altered consciousness in the patient with end-stage liver disease is in question.	Cortical and subcortical atrophy; benign, neoplastic, and metastatic lesions; hemorrhaging; aneurysms; and hematomas.
Brain flow studies: Technetium scan of the brain	To confirm brain death when the patient is in a hepatic coma when EEG is not confirmatory.	Brain death, as evidenced by lack of blood flow into the brain.
Radioisotope liver scan Injection with radioactive compound and scanned with a scintillation camera or radiography	To determine the presence of three-dimensional lesions in the liver.	Hepatocellular carcinoma, melanoma, Hodgkin and non–Hodgkin lymphoma.
Invasive Testing		
Liver biopsy (can be percutaneous at the bedside or transvenous in interventional radiology) Note: Even when platelets are low, this test can still be performed in interventional radiology transjugularly after platelet infusions, desmopressin (DDAVP), or recombinant factor VIIa, according to local practice.	Used as a diagnostic and prognostic tool. Can grade and stage liver disease. Can differentiate between various liver diseases. Can be used to follow the progression of liver diseases.	Inflammation, fibrosis, cirrhosis, hepatocellular carcinoma, regenerative changes, apoptosis, necrosis, iron, complex carbohydrates, steatosis, copper, granulomas, hepatitis B surface antigen, Mallory bodies, talc crystals, inflammatory cells, microabscesses, Cowdry type A inclusions, etc.

LIVER FUNCTION TESTS

LFTs are nonspecific for diagnosing types of liver disease or measuring efficacy of liver function but rather identify hepatocyte damage or biliary abnormalities (e.g., cholestasis). Once liver dysfunction is established, tests monitor the progression, stabilization, or improvement of liver damage. In treatable liver diseases, such as hepatitis, the tests monitor effectiveness of treatment. Testing is often done serially to increase specificity and sensitivity.

Alanine aminotransferase (ALT) and aspartate aminotransferas (AST)

These enzymes are the most frequently measured indicators of liver dysfunction, because values are elevated in all liver disorders. Although the enzymes are also present in the brain, kidneys, skeletal and cardiac muscles, the concentration is highest in the liver. Values elevate most markedly in acute hepatitis and liver injury from exposure to hepatotoxins. ALT seems to be the more sensitive enzyme specific to hepatocyte damage.

Serum bilirubin (bili)

Bilirubin in the urine is usually diagnostic for biliary liver disease. Up to 80% of bilirubin comes from the breakdown of hemoglobin, whereas the other 20% comes from prematurely

Box 9-9 | KING'S COLLEGE HOSPITAL CRITERIA

ALF from acetaminophen

- pH <7.30 (24 hours after ingestion and after adequate fluid resuscitation)—irrespective of coma grade
- PT* >100 seconds or INR >6.5 with
- Serum creatinine >3.4 mg/dL in grade 3 or 4 encephalopathy

ALF from other causes

- PT >100 seconds (INR >6.5)—regardless of coma grade or any three of the following regardless of encephalopathy grade:
    1. Age <10 years
    2. Age >40 years
    3. Drug toxicity, indeterminate cause of ALF
    4. Duration of jaundice before onset of coma of >7 days
    5. PT >50 seconds (INR ≥3.5)
- Serum bilirubin >17.5 mg/dL

*PT is the most sensitive prognostic marker.
ALF, Acute liver failure; *INR*, international normalized ratio; *PT*, prothrombin time.

destroyed cells found in bone marrow and from hemoproteins throughout the body. Bilirubin alone is not diagnostic for determining the cause of jaundice in a patient. Usually, bilirubin levels are higher in a neoplastic process in the liver than in other causes of liver disease.

Alkaline phosphatase

Similar to the other "liver function" tests, alkaline phosphatase is found in many parts of the body. The liver and bone appear to be the main sources of this enzyme. Elevation of this enzyme is usually seen in hepatobiliary diseases.

Serum albumin

Albumin levels tend to be normal regardless of the cause of liver disease. Hypoalbuminemia is usually found in patients with ESLD and/or cirrhosis where decreased albumin synthesis, ascites, and severe liver damage are present.

Prothrombin time (PT)

The liver synthesizes at least seven blood coagulation proteins. Although a prolonged PT is not specific in diagnosing diseases of the liver, it is prognostic in outcomes in acetaminophen overdose and in patients with alcoholic steatonecrosis, fulminant hepatic necrosis, and acute hepatocellular disease.

LIVER BIOPSY

Liver biopsy is the "gold standard" of testing used to diagnose the type of liver disease, screen for familial disease, monitor and stage the disease, evaluate the degree of hepatocellular injury, evaluate effectiveness of treatment, and confirm rejection episodes in the transplanted liver.

> **HIGH ALERT!**   Risk of death from a liver biopsy complication is estimated to be 1 in 10,000. The patient MUST be adequately prepared for the liver biopsy procedure and the aftercare to minimize potential complications and prevent mortality. The patient and their vital signs must be monitored very closely for signs and symptoms of complications from a biopsy if they are in a hepatic coma or induced coma. If platelets are less than 60,000, the biopsy can still be performed transjugularly in interventional radiology after administration of a platelet transfusion, desmopressin (DDAVP), or administration of recombinant factor VIIa.

Hepatic Failure

Before Biopsy

- Explain the procedure to the patient and significant others. The patient must be able to demonstrate they can exhale and hold their breath during needle insertion, if biopsy is to be performed percutaneously at the bedside.
- The patient should sign informed consent for the procedure before sedation is administered.
- PT, INR, and platelet count values should be done immediately before the biopsy in patients with ALF. If the patient has CLF and is not in decompensation, values should be less than 30 days old.
- Ensure that the patient has not had salicylates (e.g., aspirin or bismuth) or NSAIDs (e.g., ibuprofen, naproxen) for 7 days before the biopsy.
- All anticoagulants must be stopped 72 hours before the biopsy, unless the biopsy is being done emergently for ALF.
- The patient should not have eaten for 4 to 8 hours before the procedure.

During Biopsy

- Assist the patient with proper positioning and with remaining motionless during the procedure.
- Coach the alert patient to exhale and hold their breath during the procedure (or manually ventilate the intubated patient to prevent lung inflation during puncture) to avoid movement of the lung and possible resulting pneumothorax.

After Biopsy

- Apply direct pressure to the biopsy site for 15 minutes followed by a pressure dressing.
- Auscultate breath sounds immediately after the procedure and at 1- to 2-hour intervals to detect pneumothorax or hemothorax (unlikely but serious complications). Diminished sounds on the right side and tachypnea suggest one of these conditions.
- Position the patient on the right side for a minimum of 2 hours after the biopsy to tamponade the puncture site to minimize the risk of hemorrhage.
- Monitor hemoglobin and hematocrit to screen for intraperitoneal bleeding.
- Assess for signs/symptoms of peritonitis and intraperitoneal bleeding: severe abdominal pain, abdominal distension and rigidity, rebound tenderness, nausea, vomiting, tachycardia, tachypnea, pallor, decreased BP, and rising temperature.
- If bleeding is suspected, contact the advanced practice provider to obtain an abdominal/liver ultrasound study.
- Remind the patient that mild shoulder pain may persist for 24 to 48 hours after the biopsy.

COLLABORATIVE MANAGEMENT

HEPATIC FAILURE MANAGEMENT GUIDELINES

Care of patients with end-stage liver disease (ESLD) with acute or chronic liver failure (ALF or CLF) requires a multidisciplinary approach. Although every liver transplant center has its own protocols for the care of these complex patients, all closely follow evidence-based guidelines. ALF is relatively rare, thus attaining an appropriate study sample size has been difficult and prolonged. The Acute Liver Failure Study Group started in 1998, coupled with a study and workshop that were both sponsored by the National Institutes of Health, led by Dr. William H. Lee has produced the largest body of knowledge regarding ALF and is considered the benchmark of care. AASLD practice guidelines and position papers* (authored by Dr. Lee and others) also guide the care of patients pretransplant, and patients with ALF and CLF.

Interventions	Rationale
Head-to-toe assessment, history, transfer to a transplant center, or if at a transplant center, admission to the intensive care unit (ICU)	With a thorough examination, and history, can find cause in the majority of cases. The quicker a diagnosis is made, the sooner treatment can begin.

HEPATIC FAILURE MANAGEMENT GUIDELINES — cont'd

Laboratory evaluations	Need to be extensive to evaluate etiology and severity of liver disease. Key laboratory tests include: alanine aminotransferase, aspartate aminotransferase, bilirubin, gamma-glutamyl transpeptidase, alkaline phosphatase, drugs of abuse profile, acetaminophen level, complete blood count with platelets and differential, comprehensive chemistries to include glucose, blood urea nitrogen/creatinine, alpha-fetoprotein, and arterial ammonia levels.
Liver biopsy	Can confirm a diagnosis, rule out a diagnosis, and may assist in deciding whether to list a patient for transplant.
Use of endoscopy, banding, beta-blockers for bleeding from esophageal varices	Variceal bleeding in patients with cirrhosis has a 30% to 50% mortality rate associated with each bleeding episode. Endoscopy with subsequent banding, or sclerotherapy and use of nonselective beta-blockers can be used to drastically reduce this risk. Beta-blockers should be titrated to decrease resting heart rate by 25% and systolic blood pressure by $\geq$90 mm Hg.
Patient admitted to ICU Head imaging Avoid sedation if possible Ventilator for grade 3/grade 4 encephalopathy Head of bed elevated 30 degrees Consider placement of intracranial pressure (ICP) monitor (according to local practice)	Patients with grade 2 encephalopathy need to be placed in an ICU and monitored closely. Use of short-acting benzodiazepines in small doses for unmanageable agitation. If a ventilator is necessary a nondepolarizing neuromuscular blocking agent such as cisatracurium may be preferable, because they do not cause muscle contractions and therefore do not increase ICP. Although controversial, some transplant centers still use ICP in patients that have grade IV encephalopathy.
Diagnostic imaging; ultrasonography (US), computed tomography (CT) scan, magnetic resonance imaging (MRI), magnetic resonance arthrography (MRA), and endoscopic retrograde cholangiopancreatography (ERCP)	US, CT scan, and/or MRI to assess for tumors, hepatic obstruction, and to grade/stage a liver disease/pathology; MRA to assess hemodynamics; and ERCP to assess biliary status.
Nutrition balance	Protein calorie malnutrition is seen in 60% of patients with CLF and ESLD. It is a predictor for first bleeding episode from varices and is seen in patients with refractory ascites. Patients need to eat 6 to 8 meals per day to improve nitrogen balance and prevent catabolism of muscles. Zinc supplements have been shown to improve encephalopathy.
Controlling ascites	Give prophylactic antibiotics, perform paracentesis, and analyze ascitic fluid; give diuretics and consider a transjugular intrahepatic portosystemic shunting placement procedure.
Monitoring for hepatorenal syndrome (HRS), hepatopulmonary syndrome (HPS), portopulmonary hypertension (POPH) — all of which can complicate care, outcomes, and transplant status	Hemodialysis may be required for HRS, as may a liver-kidney versus a liver transplant; HPS and POPH may improve after a liver transplant over time.

*All guidelines and position papers are available on the AASLD website: www.aasld.org.
AASLD, American Association for the Study of Liver Diseases.

Hepatic Failure

CARE PRIORITIES

Hepatic failure may develop suddenly in a patient with compensated liver disease. Sustained hypoxia or hypotension from any cause can aggravate hepatocellular failure and must be corrected promptly. EtOH, hepatotoxic drugs, and hepatotoxic alternative therapies are eliminated. Minimize use of sedatives and tranquilizers because they may contribute to hepatic encephalopathy.

1. Manage fluid and electrolyte imbalance

When the patient first presents for care, a central line should be inserted. This will assist with restoration of intravascular volume thereby ensuring systemic perfusion, which can help to keep other organs from failing. Maintaining hemodynamics is particularly important if intracranial hemorrhage (ICH) is present or renal function is compromised. The AASLD guidelines recommend that hypotensive patients with ALF be resuscitated with normal saline first. After initial resuscitation, if the patient is acidotic, half-normal saline containing 75 mEq/L sodium bicarbonate should be given. Inotropic or pressors may be needed to maintain an MAP of at least 75 mm Hg or a cerebral perfusion pressure of 60 to 80 mm Hg. Norepinephrine may be used to assist peripheral organ perfusion and preserve splanchnic (hepatic) blood flow. CVP monitoring should be initiated to ensure adequate tissue perfusion without fluid overload. Hypoglycemia is common and a continuous glucose infusion should be used. In addition, potassium, magnesium, and phosphorus move from the intravascular space to the intracellular space, thereby necessitating the need to monitor these electrolytes closely and supplement as needed.

> **HIGH ALERT** Accurate measurements and careful interpretation of hemodynamic measurements are essential because fluid balance is delicate in critically ill patients with hepatic failure. Hemodynamic measurements can be difficult to interpret because circulation is hyperdynamic. Svo_2 or $Scvo_2$ monitoring is helpful in evaluating the adequacy of tissue oxygenation.

2. Provide nutrition therapy

The catabolic rate in ALF increases four times over normal and is associated with negative nitrogen balance. Patients with CLF are usually malnourished and dehydrated upon presentation, because they have increased fat oxidation and gluconeogenesis with protein catabolism. It is imperative that metabolic homeostasis be maintained. AASLD guidelines recommend that enteral or parenteral feedings be initiated early. Restriction of protein should be avoided. It is recommended that 60 g/d be given initially. Sodium is moderately restricted (up to 2000 mg/d) unless significant ascites and peripheral edema are present, wherein a less than 500-mg sodium diet is prescribed. Total caloric intake should be 2500 to 3000 per day.

3. Provide pharmacotherapy that will minimize or avoid further liver dysfunction because all drugs have hepatotoxic potential in a patient with compromised liver function

Some commonly used drugs are hepatotoxic and Box 9-10 lists medications that patients with ALF/their families reported to researchers that were taken before going into ALF. There are numerous medications/classes of medications necessary for the management of liver failure:

- *Sedatives:* May be needed to sedate and paralyze a patient with grade 3 or grade 4 encephalopathy. A nonpolarizing neuromuscular blocking agent, such as cisatracurium, because it does not cause an increase in ICH. After the patient is on a ventilator, propofol can be used because it has a long half-life and therefore smaller doses can be used in the case of inadequate liver function.
- *Histamine H₂-receptor antagonists:* Prophylactic H₂-receptor antagonists are prescribed to block acid secretion and prevent gastric erosions, which are common in patients with chronic or severe hepatic failure. Famotidine, ranitidine hydrochloride, cimetidine, and nizatidine are competitive blockers of histamine and thereby inhibit all phases of gastric acid secretion.
- *Sucralfate (Carafate):* Binds to gastric erosions, aiding in healing established ulcers, and coats the gastric/duodenal mucosa, thereby preventing stress ulcers.

Box 9-10   DRUGS AND SUBSTANCES WITH HEPATOTOXIC POTENTIAL

- Acetaminophen
- Allopurinol
- Amiodarone
- Amoxicillin-clavulanate
- Amphetamines
- Ampicillin
- Antidepressants
- Carbamazepine
- Carbenicillin
- Carbon tetrachloride
- Chloramphenicol
- Chlorpromazine
- Clindamycin
- Cocaine
- Dantrolene
- Dapsone
- Didanosine
- Diclofenac
- Disulfiram
- Efavirenz
- Ethanol
- Etoposide
- 5-Fluorouracil deoxyribonucleoside (FUDR-[intraarterial])
- Flutamide
- Gemtuzumab
- Halothane
- Hydrochlorothiazide
- Imipramine
- Isoflurane
- Isoniazid
- Ketoconazole
- Labetalol
- Lisinopril
- Metformin
- Methotrexate
- Methyldopa
- Monoamine oxidase inhibitors
- Nefazodone
- Nicotinic acid
- Nonsteroidal antiinflammatory drugs
- Ofloxacin
- Oral contraceptives
- Penicillin
- Phenytoin
- Propylthiouracil
- Pyrazinamide
- Quetiapine
- Rifampin
- Rifampin-isoniazid
- Salicylates
- Statins
- Sulfonamides
- Tetracyclines (especially parenteral)
- Tolcapone
- Trimethoprim-sulfamethoxazole
- Troglitazone
- Valproic acid
- Yellow phosphorus
- Numerous complementary and alternative medications

- **Dextrose:** Moderate to severe hypoglycemia can occur because of impaired gluconeogenesis and impaired insulin degradation. Check blood glucose levels every 1 to 2 hours initially upon admission and then every 2 to 4 hours once stabilized. Hypoglycemia should be corrected expeditiously with a bolus of 50% dextrose (D50) or continual infusion of a 10% dextrose solution (D10).
- **N-Acetylcysteine:** Administering NAC protects the liver against free radical injury and is useful in acetaminophen overdose and carbon tetrachloride or trichloroethylene exposure. NAC helps replace glutathione stores in the liver, protecting hepatocytes. It can be administered orally at 140 mg/kg or parenterally 140 mg/kg in 5% dextrose with subsequent doses at 70 mg/kg. Careful observation is necessary during IV administration, because an anaphylaxis-like reaction has been observed.
- **Penicillin/silibinin:** Used commonly as an antidote in Europe for *Amanita phalloides* poisoning; penicillin 300,000 to 1,000,000 units/kg/d and silibinin 20 to 50 mg/kg/d given IV is alleged to be hepatocyte-protective if treatment is started within 24 hours of ingestion. This combination protects as-yet unaffected hepatocytes, thereby preventing further hepatocyte necrosis.
- **Zinc:** In individuals who are malnourished, it is useful not only as a mineral replacement therapy but also to reduce the chance for, or severity of, encephalopathy because it increases hepatic urea synthesis. In other countries, the use of ornithine-aspartate is advocated to improve hepatic and muscular ammonia elimination.

4. Prevent spontaneous bacterial peritonitis

Norfloxacin (400 mg twice a day) is commonly prescribed prophylactically by transplant centers. Other strategies to prevent spontaneous bacterial peritonitis include a single oral

Hepatic Failure

dosage of ciprofloxacin (750 mg) weekly or five dosages of double-strength trimethoprim/sulfamethoxazole per week to prevent infection. Critics argue that not giving a dosage to patients daily may select for resistant bacteria species. Patients with ascites that present to the hospital should have a paracentesis with cultures and sensitivities. Until cultures are available, broad-spectrum third-generation IV cephalosporins (i.e., cefotaxime) that cover up to 95% of flora can be given. PPIs have been associated with the rate of spontaneous bacterial peritonitis in patients with cirrhosis. The majority of patients may have no documented indication for their use.

5. Manage accumulation of ascites

Ascites is the most common complication of cirrhosis. Fluid intake and physical activity are restricted. Dietary restrictions, therapeutic paracentesis, and diuretics are commonly used, while TIPS is usually placed for refractory ascites.

- Sodium: If ascites causes discomfort or dyspnea, sodium is limited to less than 2000 mg/d and diet education is important so that the patient learns to avoid "hidden sodium" in processed and canned foods.
- Diuretics: If more conservative measures are ineffective in controlling ascites, spironolactone (Aldactone), an aldosterone antagonist with weak diuretic action and potassium conservation, or amiloride, another potassium-sparing diuretic, may be used. AASLD guidelines state that if potassium-sparing diuretics alone are ineffective, more potent diuretics such as furosemide (Lasix) or thiazides are added with concurrent use of potassium supplement. For severe ascites, a TIPS may be indicated.
- Paracentesis: Patients with severe ascites are managed with diuretics and large-volume (greater than 5 L) therapeutic paracentesis with or without infusion of albumin or another plasma volume expander (based on local practice). Repeated removal of 4 to 8 L/week of ascitic fluid may be attempted as a temporary measure to relieve refractory ascites. An increase in CO is noted immediately after the procedure. Once discharged from the ICU, if patients cannot make frequent trips to the hospital, a TIPS is indicated, and in some rare instances a peritoneovenous shunt.
- Transjugular intrahepatic portosystemic shunt (TIPS): A nonsurgical, invasive radiology procedure performed that uses a stent to decompress the portal vein and create a new circulatory pathway for blood to flow around the liver back to the heart to help relieve portal hypertension. AASLD guidelines recommend that a polytetrafluoroethylene-covered stent is preferable for TIPS procedures versus bare stents, with studies showing less stent dysfunction, and perhaps improved patient outcomes. In addition, a TIPS can prevent rebleeding from varices and reduce or stop ascites. See Box 9-11 and Fluid Volume Excess, Chapter 9, for nursing implications.
- Peritoneovenous shunt: First introduced in 1974, a peritoneovenous shunt (e.g., LeVeen or Denver shunt) is a long, perforated catheter connected to a pressure-sensitive valve that drains into the superior vena cava. Fluid can flow in only one direction, from the peritoneum into the bloodstream. Because of frequent obstruction, these shunts have fallen out of favor and are usually restricted for patients who (1) live far from a physician or transplant center that can perform paracentesis; (2) the patient is deemed not a candidate for a TIPS; (3) for patients who, as a result of multiple abdominal surgeries/scarring/adhesions, are not candidates for paracentesis; and (4) are used in diuretic-resistant patients who are not transplant candidates. These shunts no longer need to be inserted surgically and can be placed in interventional radiology. See Box 9-11 and *Fluid Volume Excess*, Chapter 9, for nursing implications.

6. Eliminate or correct the precipitating factors of encephalopathy

Up to 80% of patients with cirrhosis and liver failure have cerebral dysfunction or encephalopathy. The causes and precipitating factors include changes in the permeability of the blood-brain barrier, an increase in endogenous benzodiazepines, impairment of neuronal membrane sodium-potassium adenosine triphosphatase (ATPase), abnormal neurotransmitter balance, GI bleed, increased dietary protein, and electrolyte disturbance.

- Restrict physical activity: Permits less stress on all the organs of the body. Less activity reduces the number of metabolites that must be processed by the liver.
- Manage bleeding complications: Factor VIIa, fresh-frozen plasma, and platelets may be given to correct abnormal clotting factors and thrombocytopenia. Vitamin K helps

Box 9-11	NURSING CARE AFTER TRANSJUGULAR INTRAHEPATIC PORTOSYSTEMIC SHUNT OR PERITONEAL VENOUS SHUNT PROCEDURE

Measure urinary output hourly and CVP every 1 to 2 hours.

- Anticipate rapid fluid mobilization, as evidenced by increased CVP and increased urinary output.
- Notify the advanced practice provider of abnormal CVP or lack of diuresis. Failure to mobilize ascitic fluid may signal shunt occlusion or failure.
- Consider use of IAP monitoring to assist with monitoring for IAP increases or intraabdominal hypertension, which can signal a blocked shunt.
- Report lessening of urinary output, because renal function may diminish after this procedure.

Administer IV diuretics as prescribed; monitor K^+ levels; and administer K^+ supplements as prescribed.

- Anticipate prescribed K^+ supplements during the first 24 hours after surgery.
- Be aware that furosemide (Lasix), which is frequently prescribed, may cause K^+ depletion. Likewise, the anticipated diuresis depletes K^+.
- Instruct and coach the patient in the use of an incentive spirometer or similar hyperinflation device.
- Devices that create inspiratory resistance and encourage deep inspiration promote negative inspiratory pressure and facilitate flow of ascitic fluid.
- Encourage the patient to cough hourly.
- Apply elastic abdominal binder.
- This intervention facilitates the flow of ascitic fluid by increasing the pressure gradient externally.

Monitor for evidence of variceal bleeding; report evidence of bleeding to the advanced practice provider.

- Expanded blood volume may increase variceal pressure, resulting in bleeding. Bleeding is evidenced by a sudden decrease in hematocrit (a mild dilutional decrease is anticipated in the immediate postprocedural period), unexplained nausea, lightheadedness, dark stools, or hematemesis.

Monitor for evidence of peritonitis, endocarditis, or other infection.

- Infection occurs frequently. Anticipate antibiotic coverage during the immediate postprocedural period.

Monitor for evidence of postshunt coagulopathy.

- See Ineffective Protection Care Plan in Hepatic Failure, Chapter 9, for details.
- Monitor for other postshunt complications.

Assess for lower extremity edema. After some shunting procedures, none of the venous blood passes through the liver and protein end products are not completely detoxified.

- Monitor for development of hepatic encephalopathy or worsening encephalopathy, because this is the number one side effect from TIPS procedures.

CVP, Central venous pressure; *IAP,* intraabdominal pressure; *IV,* intravenous; K^+, potassium; *PAP,* pulmonary artery pressure; *TIPS,* transjugular intrahepatic portosystemic shunt.

correct bleeding tendencies. Serious coagulopathies require specialized component therapy (see Bleeding and Thrombotic Disorders: Disseminated Intravascular Coagulation, Chapter 10).

- Administer antibiotics: Bacterial translocation is problematic in the patient with chronic hepatic failure as a result of preexisting cirrhosis. Patients who develop infections have a higher mortality rate. A 5- to 7-day course of prophylactic, broad-spectrum antibiotics (i.e., third-generation cephalosporins) is recommended.
- Administer lactulose: A synthetic disaccharide that contains both galactose and lactose decreases the pH of the colon by its conversion into lactic, acetic, and formic acids. The unmetabolized lactulose left in the colon causes osmotic diarrhea and migration of ammonia from the blood to the colon.

> **Safety Alert** *Lactulose use can cause gaseous distension, which may pose technical difficulties for the surgeon should the patient go to transplant.*

- Intracranial pressure monitoring: ICP monitoring is controversial in this patient population with approximately half of 20 U.S. transplant centers polled putting ICP monitoring into practice. ICP monitors are used to monitor for early signs of ICH, which causes fatal uncal herniation. Brain damage may occur quickly and without obvious symptoms when ICP exceeds 20 mm Hg. ICP monitoring may be needed for the most critically ill patients awaiting orthotopic liver transplant to detect cerebral edema and guide pharmacologic management (e.g., mannitol, furosemide) and other therapeutic measures. See discussion in Traumatic Brain Injury, Chapter 3.
- Manage respiratory failure: Intubation or mechanical ventilation may be indicated when gag reflex is impaired by advanced encephalopathy, ventilation is impaired by ascites, or if gastric contents are aspirated. Frequent assessments and continuous pulse oximetry are used to monitor those at high risk for respiratory failure. Adequate tissue oxygenation is crucial because hepatic hypoxia significantly contributes to hepatic failure. Hyperventilation to a $Paco_2$ of 25 to 30 mm Hg restores cerebrovascular autoregulation causing vasoconstriction and reduced ICP.
- Hypertonic saline administration: AASLD guidelines report that prophylactic induction of hypertonic saline in patients with severe encephalopathy (stage four) causes hypernatremia (serum sodium range of 145 to 155 mEq/L), which lowers the incidence of ICH, compared with patients with ALF under normonatremic conditions.

7. Infection control

Whether in acute or chronic liver failure, patients are susceptible to infections. These patients have decreased phagocyte function, decreased complement, and their need for invasive procedures makes them more exposed to various bacteria, viruses, and fungi.

- Monitor laboratory results daily: Daily CBCs with differential should be drawn and monitored for upward trends of WBCs.
- Monitor vitals: Temperature trends, downward trends in BP, rapid RR (if not intubated) can be signs of infection.
- Reverse isolation: Protecting the patient with a reduced ability to fight infection is important. All healthcare providers and visitors should put on a gown, gloves, and wear a mask. Those healthcare providers that have a respiratory infection should not care for this patient.
- Monitor ascitic fluid: Bedside dipsticks are available that will provide a result within 2 to 3 minutes to inform healthcare providers if an infection is present in ascites. This can easily be done at the bedside during a paracentesis. These results can correlate with an upward trend of WBCs.
- Monitor for respiratory infection: Patients that are encephalopathic may not be able to cough, deep breath, or use an incentive spirometer, therefore they should be watched for problems breathing, coughing, shortness of breath, and upward trends in WBCs and temperature. Those patients on a ventilator will also need to be monitored for respiratory infection (i.e., change in color of sputum). Lungs should be auscultated on each shift.

8. Prevent skin breakdown

Patients who are immobile are prone to skin breakdown over bony prominences. Patients with liver failure (particularly those with CLF) are usually malnourished, vitamin-depleted, and dehydrated. In addition, patients with liver failure are not able to fight infections as easily and any damage to skin integrity can cause larger problems such as localized infections, tissue necrosis, bacteremia, and sepsis from bacteria, viruses, and/or fungi entering the compromised skin.

- Assess and manage skin breakdown: Every shift should do a thorough assessment of the patient's skin from head to toe, back and front. Appropriate treatment should be initiated if breakdown is apparent (i.e., pressure-relieving mattress, air mattress, egg crate mattress, etc.). Appropriate dressing to be applied, consult with a wound care nurse if available, and increase frequency of turning and repositioning.

- Worsening edema: While peripheral edema worsens, the chance for "weeping skin" causing a breach in skin integrity can occur. The amount of interstitial fluid exceeds the capillary and the ability of the skin to retain it causing it to weep. The limb may feel cold and wet, blistering may be evident. This can lead to erysipelas and cellulitis. More frequent sheet changes to keep the rest of the skin dry, dressing changes of the area with foam, or a hydrofiber composite dressing material and a compression dressing may help. Severe weeping may call for hourly dressing changes.

9. Pain management

Patients with ascites and edema are uncomfortable as a result of excess fluid compressing internal organs and the skin stretching. In severe cases, skin splitting prompts more significant pain, similar to a burn or ruptured blister. Pain assessments should be done at least every 2 hours and medication for pain administered as needed. Any changes in vital signs must be thoroughly evaluated to discern if fluctuations are attributable to worsening pain or worsening of condition. Nonpharmacologic pain-relief strategies including a change of position, imagery, relaxation exercises, biofeedback, hot or cold compresses, or distraction techniques may be helpful. Spiritual support during a time of suffering may be meaningful, such as having a chaplain or other appropriate religious figure visit the patient. All measures that are effective in relieving pain should be reported to team members and documented in the healthcare record.

- Manage worsening or unrelieved pain: Assess pain level at least hourly; more often if pain is becoming intolerable. Dosage and types of medications should be revised if not effective. Covering open areas of split skin can relieve dermal pain. Ascites pain may be relieved by paracentesis or increased dose of diuretics. Pain associated with worsening edema is sometimes relieved by additional doses of diuretics.
- Monitor for change in location of pain: A change in location of pain can herald disease progression.

10. Hepatic transplantation

The orthotopic liver transplant 1-year survival rate is greater than 90% in patients with CLF and is approximately 65% for patients with ALF. The orthotopic procedure entails a donor organ being placed in the same location as the patient's diseased liver following removal of the native liver. In cases of chronic progressive or acute hepatocyte damage, it is the only treatment available. Because organs are in such limited supply, adult-living donor liver transplantation is being used in recipients whose diagnosis necessitates a liver, but whose "model for end-stage liver disease" (MELD) scores are not high enough to place them at the top of the Organ Procurement Transplant Network/United Network for Organ Sharing transplanted organ waiting list. Hospitalized, critically ill patients are generally eligible to receive a whole liver cadaver graft because their MELD scores place them in the top three on the list. New methods are being sought to extend the life of the native liver until a donor liver becomes available. Auxiliary liver transplantation allows the native liver to remain in the recipient, which will allow it to regenerate. This procedure is only used in potentially reversible conditions. Hepatocyte transplantation, bioartificial liver support, extracorporeal whole-organ perfusion, and other methods such as stem cell transplantation and xenotransplantation are being explored as tools to bridge and increase waiting time to transplantation.

CARE PLANS FOR HEPATIC FAILURE

DEFICIENT FLUID VOLUME *related to intravascular volume depletion resulting from third-spaced fluids.*

Goals/Outcomes: Within 24 hours of this diagnosis, the volume status is improved, as evidenced by MAP greater than 60 mm Hg, HR 60 to 100 bpm, brisk capillary refill, distal pulses greater than 2+ on a 0-to-4+ scale, CVP 2-6 mm Hg, pulmonary artery wedge pressure (PAWP) 6 to 12 mm Hg, CI greater than 5 L/min/m², SVR 900 to 1200 dynes/s/cm⁻⁵, urinary output greater than 0.5 mL/kg/h, and orientation to person, place, time, and situation. The goals of improvement for patients who are extremely ill are adjusted according to the predicted best values the patient can achieve with their level of organ impairment.

NOC Risk Control: Fluid Volume Deficit, Fluid Balance, Fluid Status, Electrolyte, and Acid-Base Balance.

Fluid Management

1. Vital signs and hemodynamics: Assess vital signs and central pressures from hemodynamic monitoring at least hourly. Persistent tachycardia may signal hypovolemia, fever, or decompensation. Fever may be related to infection or cerebral edema.

2. Dysrhythmias: Result from electrolyte imbalances secondary to diarrhea, gastric suctioning, diuretic therapy, or long-standing malnutrition (primarily seen in patients with CLF).

3. Altered vascular responsiveness: Support hyperdynamic circulation, remembering hemodynamic values are deceiving. SVR may not be increased in patients with hypovolemic hepatic failure. A "normal" CO value may actually be too low. Monitor Svo_2 as possible to evaluate the adequacy of tissue oxygenation.

4. Maintain hydration: Be alert to urine output less than 0.5 mL/kg/h for 2 consecutive hours and body weight changes. Weigh daily at the same time, in the same clothing, using the same scale and method. Weight loss should not exceed 0.5 kg/d. If the patient is on a ventilator and/or unable to get out of bed to be weighed, a bed scale should be used. Measure or estimate other sources of fluid loss. Consider cautious increases in fluid intake (e.g., 50 to 100 mL/h). Reevaluate volume status frequently, using extreme caution if administering potent diuretics, which may precipitate encephalopathy or renal insufficiency from rapid fluid and electrolyte changes.

5. Decreasing oncotic pressure: Consult the advanced practice provider if serum albumin and total protein are trending downward.

NIC Cerebral Edema Management; Electrolyte Management; Fluid Management; Electrolyte Management: Hypokalemia; Electrolyte Management: Hyponatremia.

EXCESS FLUID VOLUME *related to significant third-spaced fluids resulting in total body weight gain.*

Goals/Outcomes: Within 48 hours of **this** diagnosis, the patient becomes normovolemic, as evidenced by CVP 2 to 6 mm Hg, PAWP 6 to 12 mm Hg, HR 60 to 100 bpm, RR 12 to 20 breaths/min with normal depth and pattern, decreasing or stable abdominal girth, and absence of crackles, edema, uncomfortable ascites, and other clinical indicators of fluid volume excess. The goals of improvement for patients who are extremely ill are adjusted according to the predicted best values the patient can achieve with their level of organ impairment.

NOC Risk Control: Fluid Volume Deficit, Fluid Balance, Fluid Status, Electrolyte, and Acid-Base Balance.

Hemodynamic Regulation

1. Vital sign and hemodynamics considerations: Monitor and record vital signs and central pressures from hemodynamic monitoring at least hourly. Measure more frequently if the patient is undergoing ultrafiltration or other continuous renal replacement therapy and immediately after ventriculoperitoneal shunt surgery. Consult the advanced practice provider for CVP greater than 8 mm Hg and PAWP greater than 12 mm Hg.

2. Peripheral edema: Note severity and location because this may indicate fluid overload. Jugular vein distension (at a 45-degree HOB elevation) and a CVP greater than 8 mm Hg may indicate fluid overload or decreased CO.

Fluid Management

1. Fluid overload: Consult the advanced practice provider for fluid overload: weight gain, presence of dyspnea, tachypnea, rhonchi, orthopnea, basilar crackles that do not clear with coughing, labored and/or shallow breathing, elevated BP, or S3 heart sound.

2. Restrict fluids: Use minimal amounts of fluids necessary to administer IV medications and maintain IV catheter patency. When fluids are restricted, offer mouth care and/or ice chips (included as part of oral fluid intake measurement).

3. Intraabdominal hypertension: Carefully measure and record abdominal girth daily. Abdominal girth measurements are subject to error. Measure at the widest point with the patient in a tolerable position, and mark this level for subsequent measurements with a permanent marker. Consider using an IAP monitor, via a Foley bladder catheter. Abdominal hypertension is a measurement greater than 12 mm Hg and abdominal compartment syndrome is a measurement greater than 20 mm Hg. Measure IAP hourly. Once a trend is established, measurements can be every 4 hours. If the patient complains of abdominal pain, measurements should revert back to hourly. Measure the patient in the same position each time.

Electrolyte Management: Hypernatremia

1. Hypernatremia and hypokalemia: Consult the advanced practice provider for significantly abnormal serum electrolyte levels, especially sodium and potassium.

2. Malfunctioning TIPS: Ensure proper functioning of TIPS in patients after placement (see Box 9-11).

IMBALANCED NUTRITION: LESS THAN BODY REQUIREMENTS *related to inability to digest food secondary to anorexia, nausea, and medically prescribed dietary restrictions; decreased absorption of nutrients secondary to decreased intestinal motility, altered portal blood flow, decreased intestinal absorption of vitamins and minerals, altered protein metabolism; and the inability of the diseased liver to use nutrients.*

Goals/Outcomes: The patient has adequate nutrition, as evidenced by a state of nitrogen balance as shown by daily fecal excretion of 2 to 3 g of nitrogen and 4 to 20 g of urinary nitrogen, thyroxine-binding prealbumin 200 to 300 μg/mL, and retinol-binding protein 40 to 50 μg/mL. During protein catabolism (proteolysis), nitrogen is excreted in the feces, urine, and blood. If nitrogen balance is negative, the patient is using muscle for protein. At least 5 g of feces needs to be collected with for the test. Urine should be collected for 24 hours. Thyroxine-binding prealbumin (measures protein-calorie malnutrition) and retinol-binding protein (measures visceral protein mass) are serum tests. Blood glucose levels remain within an acceptable range of 100 to 160 mg/dL.
NOC Nutrition Status; Biochemical Measures.

Nutrition Monitoring
1. Comprehensive nutrition assessment: Confer with the advanced practice provider, dietitian, and pharmacist (if parenteral feedings are necessary) to estimate the patient's current nutrition and metabolic needs, based on anthropometric data, creatinine excretion, albumin, and transferrin, as well as presence of encephalopathy, chronic hepatic disease, infection, and nutrition status before hospitalization. For general information, see Nutrition Support, Chapter 1.
2. Appropriate feeding modality: Consult the advanced practice provider regarding administration of parenteral or enteral nutrients. If insertion of a feeding tube becomes necessary, use caution to minimize the risk of rupturing gastroesophageal varices. If parenteral feedings are being administered, monitor IV site for infection and other complications.
3. Food intake: Note, monitor, and record food/fluid ingested and daily caloric intake.
4. Additional vitamins: Administer prescribed vitamin supplements, particularly fat-soluble.
5. Favorite foods: Encourage food to be brought from home if desired by the patient and ensure it meets prescribed dietary restrictions.

Energy Management
1. Balance rest and activity: Encourage bed rest to reduce metabolic demands on the liver and to promote hepatic regeneration. Increase the patient's activity levels gradually while the condition improves.

Hypoglycemia Management
1. Blood glucose management: Monitor blood glucose levels every 1 to 2 hours initially, every 2 to 4 hours when stabilized or as prescribed. Assess for clinical indicators of hypoglycemia: altered mentation, irritability, diaphoresis, anxiety, weakness, and tachycardia. Clinical signs of hypoglycemia can be confused with hepatic encephalopathy. Validate clinical signs with blood glucose levels. Administer D10 or D50 as prescribed for hypoglycemia. Changes in blood glucose are anticipated with chronic liver disease from changes in gluconeogenesis. Administer hypoglycemic agents as prescribed for blood glucose levels greater than 180 mg/dL.

IMPAIRED GAS EXCHANGE *related to altered oxygen supply secondary to arteriovenous shunting, ventilation-perfusion mismatch, and diaphragmatic limitation associated with ascites, hydrothorax, or central respiratory depression occurring with encephalopathy.*

Goals/Outcomes: Within 4 hours of this diagnosis, the patient has adequate gas exchange, as evidenced by Pao$_2$ greater than 80 mm Hg, Paco$_2$ less than 45 mm Hg, RR 12 to 20 breaths/min with normal depth and pattern, oxygen saturation greater than 95% with or without oxygen supplementation or mechanical ventilation, and orientation to person, place, and time. The goals of improvement for patients who are extremely ill are adjusted according to the predicted best values the patient can achieve with their level of organ impairment.
NOC Respiratory Status: Gas Exchange; Respiratory Status: Ventilation.

| **Safety Alert** | *Level of consciousness is difficult to evaluate in the presence of moderate to severe hepatic encephalopathy, and obtaining a baseline level of consciousness is imperative.* |

Hepatic Failure

Oxygen Therapy

1. Respiratory management: Monitor and document RR at least hourly. Note pattern, excursion, depth, and effort. Administer supplemental oxygen as prescribed to enhance cerebral and hepatic oxygenation. Continuous pulse oximetry should be in use. Monitor ABGs and electrolytes to assess acid-base balance as needed.

2. Avoid lying flat: Maintain body positions that optimize ventilation, given the abdomen is enlarged and impairing normal movement of the diaphragm. Elevate HOB 30 degrees or higher, depending on patient comfort and hemodynamic status.

3. Respiratory insufficiency: Consult the advanced practice provider for abnormal Pao_2, $Paco_2$, and oxygen saturation.

Aspiration Precautions

1. Possible aspiration: Assess the patient every 4 hours for atelectasis, hydrothorax (e.g., diminished breath sounds, dullness to percussion), and pulmonary infection. Consult the advanced practice provider if findings suggest respiratory complications.

2. Prevent aspiration: Evaluate the obtunded patient for presence of gag reflex. Consult the speech pathologist for swallowing evaluation. Keep NPO with HOB elevated until the patient's risk for aspiration is fully evaluated. If severe, consult the advanced practice provider regarding the need for endotracheal intubation. Suction secretions from the mouth frequently; offer/assist with frequent mouth care.

DISTURBED SENSORY PERCEPTION *related to endogenous chemical alteration (accumulation of ammonia or other CNS toxins occurring with hepatic dysfunction), therapeutically restricted environment, sleep deprivation, hypoxia, sensory overload (noise, personnel) in ICU, and medication (side effects, toxic levels from the inability of the liver to detoxify appropriately).*

Goals/Outcomes: By the time of hospital discharge, the patient exhibits stable personality patterns, age-appropriate behavior, intact intellect appropriate for level of education, distinct speech, and coordinated gross and fine motor movements. Handwriting is legible, and psychometric test scores are improved from baseline range.
NOC Distorted Thought Self-Control; Information Processing; Neurologic Status: Consciousness.

Fluid and Electrolyte Management

1. Prevent encephalopathy: Avoid or minimize precipitating factors for hepatic encephalopathy (Box 9-12).

    a. Support circadian rhythms: Modify the environment to help keep circadian rhythms in sync (e.g., keep lighting in room appropriate for the time of day, correlate activities of daily living to the correct time of day). Minimize unnecessary noise, lights, and other environmental stimuli.

    b. GI bleeding: Check gastric secretions, vomitus, and stools for occult blood. Evaluate Hct and Hgb for evidence of bleeding. Consult the advanced practice provider for low values that deviate from baseline. Anticipate mild to moderate anemia.

    c. Ammonia: Evaluate serum ammonia levels (normal levels are 40 to 110 mg/dL). Report significant elevations from baseline. Ammonia values and their measurement vary greatly and do not always correlate directly with encephalopathy.

    d. Manage sources of mental confusion:

        (1) Stressing the liver: Avoid use of conventional and alternative drugs that are hepatotoxic (see Box 9-10).
        (2) Correct hypoxemia: Administer supplemental oxygen as necessary (see Impaired Gas Exchange, Chapter 9).
        (3) Electrolyte imbalance: Manage potential sources of electrolyte imbalance (e.g., diarrhea, vomiting, occult bleeding).

    e. Mental status changes: Evaluate patient for CNS effects such as personality changes, childish behavior, intellectual impairment, slurred speech, ataxia, and asterixis.

    f. Testing: Administer daily handwriting or psychometric tests (if appropriate for patient's LOC) to evaluate mild or subclinical encephalopathy. Report significant deterioration in handwriting or in test scores.

    g. Neomycin: Administer neomycin as prescribed to reduce intestinal bacteria, which contribute to the production of cerebral intoxicants. Monitor the patient for evidence of ototoxic effects (i.e., decreased hearing) and nephrotoxic effects (e.g., urinary output less than 0.5 mL/kg/h, increased creatinine levels) of neomycin use. Avoid neomycin administration for patients with renal insufficiency.

    h. Injury protection: Protect the patient who is confused or unconscious from injury.

        a. Tube removal: If the patient is pulling out tubes, discuss with family or significant other to see if someone can stay around the clock, or if a sitter can be provided. As a last resort, apply mittens rather than wrist restraints.

| Box 9-12 | FACTORS THAT CONTRIBUTE TO HEPATIC ENCEPHALOPATHY |

Chronic factors
- Portal-systemic shunting (entry of portal blood into systemic veins without being metabolized by the liver): May occur via damaged liver, collateral vessels, or surgically created portacaval anastomosis
- Dietary protein intake
- Intestinal bacteria
- Acid-base imbalance
- Progressive hepatic insufficiency

Precipitating factors
- Dehydration/electrolyte imbalance: May occur with overdiuresis, diarrhea, vomiting, or other factors
- Excessive paracentesis
- Surgery in a patient with cirrhosis
- Excessive alcohol ingestion
- Sedatives/hypnotics
- Infection
- Constipation
- Extrahepatic bile duct obstruction
- Acute hepatocellular damage
- Viral hepatitis
- Alcoholic hepatitis
- Drug/chemical reactions (see Box 9-10)
- Drug overdose (see Box 9-10)

    b. Call light: Have call light within the patient's reach at all times.
    c. Secure tubes: Tape all catheters and tubes securely to prevent dislodgment.
2. Manage complications of encephalopathy: Consider the possibility of seizures; have airway management equipment readily available.
3. Intracranial pressure management: If ICP monitor is in place, monitor ICP and cerebral perfusion pressure. For patients with increased intracranial pressure (IICP), position carefully (HOB less than 30 degrees) and avoid fluid overload, hypercarbia, and hypoxemia. Administer mannitol and furosemide (Lasix) as prescribed. Sedation or coma induction may be indicated if cerebral edema does not respond to the measures just mentioned.
4. Inform family/significant other(s): Keep family/significant other abreast of all changes, and the possibility of complications and deterioration.

    NIC Environmental Management; Delirium Management; Intracranial Pressure Monitoring.

RISK FOR INFECTION *related to inadequate secondary defenses (impaired reticuloendothelial system phagocytic activity and portal-systemic shunting), multiple invasive procedures, and chronic malnutrition in the patient with cirrhosis.*

Goals/Outcomes: The patient is free of infection, as evidenced by normothermia, HR less than 100 bpm, RR less than 20 breaths/min, negative culture results, WBC count less than 11,000/mm^3, clear urine, and clear, thin sputum. The goals of improvement for patients who are extremely ill are adjusted according to the predicted best values the patient can achieve with their level of organ impairment.
    NOC Immune Status.

Infection Protection
1. Vital signs: Monitor vital signs for evidence of infection (e.g., increases in temperature, heart, and RRs). Avoid measuring temperatures rectally in the patient with rectal varices.
2. Signs of infection: If temperature or WBC elevation is sudden, obtain specimens for blood, sputum, and urine cultures or from other sites as prescribed. Consult the advanced practice provider for positive culture results.

Hepatic Failure

- Underlying leukopenia: Normal or mildly elevated leukocyte count may signify infection in patients with hepatic failure because patients with chronic liver disease often have leukopenia (WBC counts less than 3000/mm³).
- Secretions: Evaluate secretions and drainage for evidence of infection (e.g., sputum changes, cloudy urine).
- Invasive sites: Evaluate IV, central line, and paracentesis site(s) for evidence of infection (erythema, warmth, unusual drainage). It is normal for a paracentesis puncture site to have a small amount of drainage immediately after the procedure. Prolonged or foul-smelling drainage can indicate infection. Use ascitic fluid dipsticks at the bedside to test for infection.

3. Teaching: Teach significant others and visitors proper handwashing technique, use reverse isolation personal protective equipment (gown, mask, and gloves). Restrict visitors with evidence of communicable disease.

INEFFECTIVE PROTECTION *related to clotting anomaly, thrombocytopenia, itching, and disorientation.*

Goals/Outcomes: The patient's bleeding, if it occurs, is not prolonged. The patient's skin is not damaged from scratching. The patient's confusion (if present) and LOC will not lead to injury (see Alterations in Consciousness, Chapter 1).

NOC Blood Coagulation.

Bleeding Precautions
1. Intramuscular injections: Avoid giving intramuscular injections. If they are necessary, use small-gauge needles and maintain firm pressure over injection sites for several minutes. Avoid massaging intramuscular injection sites.
2. Hold pressure: Maintain pressure for several minutes over venipuncture sites. Inform laboratory personnel of the patient's bleeding tendencies.
3. Avoid arterial punctures: If it is necessary to obtain ABG values, consult the advanced practice provider regarding use of an indwelling arterial line. If this is not possible, be certain to maintain pressure over the arterial puncture site and elevation for at least 10 minutes.
4. Blood clotting: Monitor PT/INR levels and platelet counts daily. Consult the physician for significant prolongation of the PT or for significant reduction in the platelet count.
5. Bleeding: Report bleeding to the advanced practice provider. Note oral and nasal mucosal bleeding and ecchymotic areas, and test stools, emesis, urine, and gastric drainage for occult blood.
6. Avoid trauma: Use electric rather than safety razor for patient shaving. Provide soft-bristle toothbrush or sponge-tipped applicator and mouthwash for oral hygiene. Avoid indwelling, large-bore gastric drainage tubes if possible, because they may irritate gastric mucosa or varices, causing bleeding to occur.
7. Manage bleeding: Administer fresh-frozen plasma and platelets as prescribed. Monitor carefully for fluid volume overload (see Excess Fluid Volume, Chapter 9). Administer vitamin K as prescribed.
8. Postshunt coagulopathy: A postshunt coagulopathy may develop in some patients after peritoneal-venous shunt surgery.
9. Disseminated intravascular coagulation: If fibrin degradation products are present in the blood and thrombocytopenia is significant, the patient may have DIC (see Bleeding and Thrombotic Disorders: Disseminated Intravascular Coagulation, Chapter 10).

INEFFECTIVE TISSUE PERFUSION: RENAL *related to risk of diminished arterial flow secondary to increased preglomerular vascular resistance.*

Goals/Outcomes: The patient has adequate renal perfusion, as evidenced by urinary output greater than 0.5 mL/kg/h.

NOC Circulatory Status.

Fluid/Electrolyte Management
1. Hyponatremia: Consult the advanced practice provider for serum sodium less than 120 mEq/L and urine sodium less than 10 mEq/L, associated with the development of HRS.
2. Renal insufficiency: Consult the advanced practice provider for significant increases in creatinine and potassium values. BUN level is not an accurate indicator of renal function, especially in the patient with hepatic failure, because alterations in hepatic function can cause decreased BUN values, and GI bleeding results in increased BUN values.

3. Sodium management: Minimize infusion of sodium-containing fluids because they contribute to ascites and peripheral edema and may potentiate functional renal failure.
4. Phosphates: Report hypophosphatemia (mental confusion, metabolic acidosis, anorexia, cardiac dysrhythmias, hemolytic anemia, lethargy, and bone pain) to the advanced practice provider.
5. Magnesium: Report hypomagnesemia (muscle weakness, nausea, vomiting, tremors, tetany, and lethargy) to the advanced practice provider.
6. For additional information, see nursing diagnoses and interventions in Acute Renal Failure, Chapter 6, and Fluid and Electrolyte Disturbances, Chapter 1.

IMPAIRED TISSUE INTEGRITY *related to chemical irritants (bile salts), impaired mobility, and fluid excess (tissue edema).*

Goals/Outcomes: The patient's tissue remains intact; pruritus is relieved or reduced within 12 hours of this diagnosis.
NOC Comfort.

Skin Surveillance
1. Keep skin smooth: Bathe the patient with a non–soap cleanser. Apply an unscented, non–alcohol-containing lotion while skin is still moist.
2. Prevent scratching: If the patient is confused or obtunded, place the hands in soft gloves or mitts to minimize damage from scratching, and keep nails short.
3. Reduce itching: Administer cholestyramine (e.g., Questran, LoCholest, Colestid) as prescribed to reduce bile acids in the serum and skin, and thereby relieve itching. Avoid administration of other oral medications within 2 hours of cholestyramine administration because they may bind with it in the intestine and reduce its absorption.
4. Initiate pressure ulcer prevention:
    - Use a low-pressure, pressure-reduction, or pressure-redistribution (low air lost) mattress to minimize pressure on fragile tissues.
    - When moving the patient, avoid applying shearing forces to skin. Avoid wrinkled sheets, clothing, and pads under the patient. Keep sheets, clothing, and pads from bunching against the patient's skin. Score the patient's pressure ulcer risk and monitor skin integrity.
5. Prevent skin damage:
    - Dry skin well after morning care. Provide adequate lotion to skin, avoid massaging it in deeply, and rub gently.
    - Use appropriate tape or dressings (i.e., SorbaView, Tegaderm) for skin condition. If possible, use gauze to secure a dressing or IV line, and tape over the gauze to prevent it from unwrapping.

DEFICIENT KNOWLEDGE *related to lack of exposure to healthcare information; cognitive limitation secondary to hepatic encephalopathy.*

Goals/Outcomes: The patient/family/significant other states signs and symptoms of early hepatic encephalopathy, importance of medical follow-up, understanding of disease state, and how to keep it stabilized (i.e., alcohol/drug treatment programs, proper diet, proper infection control methods, taking prescribed medications).
NOC Knowledge: Disease Process; Knowledge: Diet; Knowledge: Medication; Knowledge: Substance Use Control, Risk Control Drug Use, Risk Control Alcohol Use.

Teaching: Disease Process
1. Emphasize the basics: Stress the importance of sufficient rest and adherence to prescribed diet.
2. If hepatic failure is related to hepatitis B virus (HBV) infection:
    a. HBV prophylaxis: Should be considered for sexual partners and household members with possible exposure to HBV (e.g., those who unknowingly shared a toothbrush or razor).
    b. Prevent transmission: Teach the patient and exposure contacts practices that reduce the risk of exposure (e.g., condom use, having own personal grooming items). Prescreening for the presence of hepatitis B (HB) antibodies is encouraged if it does not delay treatment for greater than 14 days after last exposure.
    c. Hepatitis B immune globulin (HBIG): A dose of HBIG is recommended immediately for sexual contacts and household contacts with possible blood and body fluid exposure. A second administration of HBIG vaccine should follow 1 month later.

   d. HB vaccination: The HB vaccine series should be initiated for sexual and household contacts at risk. The first and second vaccines can be given at the same time the two HBIG vaccines are given. Make sure both vaccines are given in separate areas. The HB vaccines are to be given via intramuscular injection in the deltoid muscle only. Stress the importance of not sharing intimate items (e.g., razors, toothbrush, nail clippers).

3. If hepatic failure is related to hepatitis C virus (HCV): No prophylaxis is available to exposed persons. Therefore, baseline hepatitis C (HC) antibodies should be measured, and 1 month later a second sample should be drawn and tested. Based on results, an infectious disease consult may be indicated, along with possible treatment. It is important to note, however, that those with sexual exposure have less than a 5% chance of seroconversion. Those with exposure to blood, particularly through hollow-bore needles, have the greatest chance of seroconversion.

   • HC evolving evidence: The face of HCV treatment is changing. Approximately 40% of transplants in the United States are attributable to ESLD secondary to HCV. The U.S. Centers for Disease Control and Prevention has recommended that all persons born between 1945 and 1965 be tested for HCV given that this group contains the highest number of persons infected. Having medications with minimal side effects, shorter treatment courses make getting more people treated appealing before they reach a point of cirrhosis and declining liver function leading to ESLD, and eventual liver transplantation. HCV is an RNA flavivirus of the *Hepacivirus* genus. There are six confirmed genotypes (1 through 6), with genotype 1 the most difficult to treat and the most prevalent in the United States. In 2011, the FDA approved the first direct-acting HCV antivirals to be used in combination with pegylated interferon (PEG) and ribavirin (RBV). These first-generation direct-acting antivirals (boceprevir and telaprevir) increased treatment response rates when using PEG plus RBV alone from 50% for genotype 1 HCV infection to 75% when boceprevir or telaprevir were added to the PEG plus RBV combination. In 2013, the second generation of direct-acting antivirals was approved by the FDA. Sofosbuvir (SOF) inhibits the HCV NS5B RNA-dependent RNA polymerase. The combination of SOF plus RBV has been shown to be effective against multiple genotypes without PEG use and thereby decreases numerous side effects, including severe effects. Response rates are nearly 100% in patients with genotypes 2 and 3 HCV using an oral regimen, and greater than 90% in patients with genotype 1 HCV. Simeprevir, a second-generation protease inhibitor developed to treat patients with genotype 1, binds to its target differently than boceprevir or telaprevir. Response rates are in the 75% to 80% range in combination with PEG plus RBV. Other treatments are in various stages of development including NS3 protease inhibitors, NS4B inhibitors, NS5A inhibitors, NS5B nucleoside inhibitors, and NS5B nonnucleoside inhibitors. Drugs being developed to attack other host targets include cyclophilin A inhibitors, MiR122 inhibitors, and entry inhibitors.

4. Substance abuse: Inform the patient about the availability of alcohol treatment and drug treatment programs if alcohol- and drug-related hepatic failure has occurred. Explain the availability of support groups (i.e., Alcoholics Anonymous, Al-Anon) for patients and family members when hepatic failure is related to chronic alcohol ingestion.

5. Over-the-counter medications: Caution about the importance of avoiding over-the-counter medications without first consulting a physician. Advise the patient to confer with a physician regarding use of NSAIDs, aspirin, and other medications that contain salicylates for minor aches and pains after hospital discharge.

6. Signs and symptoms of infection: fever; unusual drainage from paracentesis or other invasive procedure sites; warmth and erythema surrounding the invasive sites; or abdominal pain. Have the patient demonstrate the technique for measuring oral temperature with type of thermometer used at home.

7. Signs and symptoms of unusual bleeding: Prolonged mucosal bleeding, very large or painful bruises, and dark stools. Caution that if possible, major dental procedures should be postponed until bleeding times normalize.

8. Sodium and ascites: Inform the patient about sodium restriction if ascites developed during the course of the illness.

9. Protein and encephalopathy: Advise protein restriction if the patient has residual or chronic encephalopathy. Instruct the patient to avoid constipation by increasing bulk in the diet or by using agents prescribed by the physician or advanced practice provider.

10. Alcohol use: Caution about the necessity of alcohol cessation for at least several months after complete recovery from the acute episode. After full recovery, one or two glasses of beer or wine a week are usually allowed if hepatic failure was not related to alcoholism or alcohol ingestion.

11. Weight monitoring: Instruct the patient to weigh himself or herself daily and to report weight loss or gain of greater than 5 lb.

NIC Substance Use Treatment: Drug Withdrawal; Substance Use Treatment: Overdose; Substance Use Treatment: Alcohol Withdrawal, Medication Management, Nutrition Management.

RISK FOR INJURY *related to invasive procedures*

Goals/Outcomes: The patient does not sustain an injury related to liver biopsy, ICP monitoring, or other invasive procedures.

NOC Knowledge Health Promotion; Risk Control: Infection.

Teaching Individual

1. Liver biopsy: Fully prepare the patient emotionally and physically for the procedure.
2. Possible bleeding: Monitor the patient closely after the procedure; observe changes in vital signs that correlate with observations of patient.
   - Monitor dressing over puncture wounds for bleeding. Document amount, frequency of dressing changes, what types of dressings are applied, what the drainage looks like/smells like (if applicable), and what the wound looks like.
3. Infection: Monitor for fever.
4. Encephalopathic patients: Ensure the airway is clear, and reassure the patient someone will accompany and remain with them before, during, and after the procedure.

ADDITIONAL NURSING DIAGNOSES

As appropriate, see the following topics for additional nursing diagnoses and interventions in Chapters 1 and 2: Nutrition Support, Mechanical Ventilation, Prolonged Immobility, and Emotional and Spiritual Support for the Patient and Significant Others.

PERITONITIS
PATHOPHYSIOLOGY

Peritonitis is an inflammation of the peritoneum and can be classified as primary, secondary, or tertiary. Secondary peritonitis, the most common form of peritonitis, is an inflammation of all or part of the peritoneal cavity caused by diffuse microbial proliferation or chemical irritation from leakage of corrosive gastric or intestinal contents into the peritoneum. Ruptured appendix, leaky anastomoses from weight loss surgery (e.g., Roux-en-Y, gastric bypass), perforated peptic ulcer, bowel rupture related to ulcerative colitis or Crohn disease, pancreatitis, abdominal trauma, and ruptured abdominal abscesses are among the many etiologic factors associated with secondary peritonitis. Indwelling tubes and catheters, such as those used for postoperative drainage and peritoneal dialysis, are foreign bodies that compromise peritoneal integrity and permit the entry of infective organisms that can trigger peritonitis. Peritonitis is a leading cause of morbidity in patients with kidney failure who are treated with continuous ambulatory peritoneal dialysis (CAPD). CAPD-associated peritonitis is caused by bacteria (*Staphylococcus epidermidis* and other skin flora) most often, entering the abdominal cavity by the dialysis catheter site.

Primary peritonitis is a bacterial infection of the serous membrane lining the abdominal cavity that occurs spontaneously without any apparent source of contamination, such as bowel perforation. The most common etiology of primary peritonitis is spontaneous bacterial peritonitis, which occurs most commonly in patients with cirrhosis of the liver with ascites. Bacterial seeding of ascitic fluid is believed to result from the translocation of enteric bacteria across the gut wall or mesenteric lymphatic vessels and is associated with a high mortality rate. Tertiary peritonitis represents persistent or recurrent infection following an apparently successfully treated episode of primary spontaneous bacterial peritonitis or secondary peritonitis. Tuberculosis-related peritonitis is rare in the United States with the exception of patients with acquired immunodeficiency syndrome (AIDS), who are frequently infected with multidrug-resistant strains of the bacillus.

Regardless of the initiating factor, the inflammatory process is similar. Initial manifestations are triggered by histamine release and include hyperemia, edema, and vascular congestion. Fluid shifts from intravascular to interstitial spaces creating hypovolemia as a result of increased vascular permeability caused by inflammatory mediators. The circulating blood volume is depleted and hypovolemic shock may ensue. The transudated fluid within the interstitium contains high levels of fibrinogen and thromboplastin. The fibrinogen is converted to fibrin by the thromboplastin. Under normal conditions, the healthy peritoneum is naturally fibrinolytic, and can block fibrin formation. When the peritoneum is weakened or injured, fibrinolysis is hampered and fibrin adheres to the damaged area and forms a barrier that harbors

Peritonitis

and protects bacteria from the normal immune responses, resulting in pockets of infection and abscess formation. In most cases, the fibrin deposits dissolve. The continued presence of fibrin can lead to adhesions and potentially bowel obstruction. With severe inflammation, intraabdominal sepsis may develop.

GASTROINTESTINAL ASSESSMENT: PERITONITIS

GOAL OF SYSTEM ASSESSMENT
Identify early findings of peritoneal irritation.

HISTORY AND RISK FACTORS
Inflammatory processes such as diverticulitis, appendicitis, or Crohn's disease; obstructive events in the small bowel and colon; vascular events such as ischemic colitis, mesenteric thrombosis, or embolic phenomena; blunt or penetrating trauma, especially to hollow viscera; severe hepatobiliary disease; and CAPD. General risk factors include those related to poor tissue healing and infection (e.g., advanced age, diabetes, and vascular disease, advanced liver disease, malignancy, malnutrition, and debilitation). Some patients with severe peritonitis may present in overt septic shock.

VITAL SIGN ASSESSMENT
- Fever of greater than 38° C (100° F to 101° F) is present in most cases.
- Tachypnea and tachycardia result from increased metabolic demands.
- Hypotension may be present resulting from dehydration from vomiting, fever, and third-space losses.
- Hypothermia may be present if the peritonitis advances to severe sepsis.

ABDOMINAL PAIN
- Abdominal pain is the hallmark of peritonitis and may be severe, causing the patient to maintain a fetal position and resist any movement that aggravates the pain. The onset can be sudden or insidious, with the location varying according to the underlying pathology.
- Nausea, vomiting, anorexia, diarrhea, and other changes in bowel habits may also be present and are reflective of GI dysfunction.
- Anorexia and nausea may precede the development of abdominal pain.
- Abdominal pain can be reduced or even absent in older adults resulting in missed diagnosis.

OBSERVATION
- Occasionally, mild to moderate ascites is observed, depending on the cause of the peritonitis.
- RR is rapid and the patient usually has a shallow ventilatory pattern to minimize abdominal movement and pain.
- Restlessness and confusion occur because of impaired cerebral perfusion.

AUSCULTATION
- Auscultation of all four quadrants usually reveals diminished or absent bowel sounds. The complete absence of bowel sounds suggests an ileus—a frequent complication of peritonitis.
- Breath sounds are diminished as a result of shallow respiratory pattern.

PALPATION
- Palpation of the abdomen elicits tympany and tenderness that can be generalized or localized, depending on the nature and extent of infection.
- Rebound tenderness, guarding, and involuntary rigidity may also be present.
- The abdomen may feel firm and boardlike. Occasionally, the abdominal examination reveals an inflammatory mass.
- The abdomen is often distended, a finding that reflects a generalized ileus and may not be present if the infection is well localized.

NUTRITION ASSESSMENT
- Evidence of malnutrition will be noted in the presence of chronic liver or renal disease.

SCREENING LABWORK

- Abdominal paracentesis: Ascitic fluid for cell count, Gram stain, and culture.
- CBC: May reveal anemia and leukocytosis.
- LFTs: Elevated.
- Serum chemistry may indicate kidney dysfunction and electrolyte imbalances.
- Radiologic tests: Abdominal radiograph may reveal free air, abdominal CT of the abdomen.

HEMODYNAMIC MEASUREMENTS

- Hypovolemia with marked tachycardia, hypotension, decreased MAP, and decreased urine output may occur as a result of massive fluid shifts from the intravascular space into the abdominal interstitium and peritoneum and from vasodilation caused by inflammatory mediators.
- Endotoxemic vasodilation is manifested as hypotension with a widened pulse pressure and low CVP, with an initial increase in HR.
- Persistent hypovolemia may result in a dangerously low MAP, thus impairing renal, cardiac, and cerebral perfusion.

Diagnostic Tests for Peritonitis

Test	Purpose	Abnormal Findings
Blood Studies		
Complete blood count with differential: Hemoglobin Hematocrit Red blood cell count White blood cell (WBC) count	Assesses for bacterial infection and anemia.	Leukocytosis ($\geq$11,000 cells/mm^3) with a shift to the left or elevation of immature neutrophils (bands).
Serum chemistry: Blood urea nitrogen (BUN) Creatinine CO_2 Glucose Serum chloride Serum potassium Serum sodium Total bilirubin Serum amylase C-Reactive protein Lactic acid/lactate	Assesses for electrolyte imbalances and organ involvement.	Elevated amylase and lipase with pancreatic involvement (acute pancreatitis). Elevated BUN and creatinine with renal dysfunction. Elevated bilirubin with gallbladder disease. Elevated CO_2 with low Cl$^-$ reflects metabolic alkalosis. Electrolyte losses, especially potassium with vomiting and diarrhea. C-Reactive protein elevation indicates inflammation. Elevated lactate level may indicate sepsis/systemic inflammatory response syndrome.
Diagnostic Paracentesis Peritoneal Fluid Analysis		
Peritoneal neutrophil count	This analysis is useful in confirming the diagnosis of bacterial peritonitis and assists in driving therapy.	WBC count $\geq$250 cells/mm^3 with >50% polymorphonuclear leukocytes is an indication to begin antibiotic therapy.
Peritoneal total protein and lactate dehydrogenase levels	Useful in confirming the diagnosis of bacterial peritonitis.	Total protein >1 g/dL; ascitic low-density lipoprotein greater than serum low-density lipoprotein.

Continued

Peritonitis

Diagnostic Tests for Peritonitis—cont'd

Test	Purpose	Abnormal Findings
Peritoneal glucose level	Useful in confirming the diagnosis of bacterial peritonitis.	Decreased peritoneal fluid glucose level ($<$50 mg/dL).
Gram stain and culture	Identifies causative organism(s) to begin proper empirical or specific antibiotic therapy.	Spontaneous bacterial peritonitis: Monomicrobial infection; *Escherichia coli*, *Klebsiella pneumoniae*, and *Streptococcus pneumoniae* are most common. Secondary peritonitis: Multiple organisms will be present in peritoneal fluid Gram stain and culture.
Radiologic Procedures		
Abdominal radiograph Plain films	Identifies the presence of dilated bowel and free air.	Free air is present in most cases of perforation.
Abdominal computed tomography (CT) scan	Assesses for an intraabdominal source of infection.	Abscess or mass may be identified.
Ultrasonography	Useful in locating small amounts of fluid, as well as in differentiating fluid collections in the abdomen.	Loculated fluid, abscess, bile duct dilation, and pancreatitis may be identified.

HEMATOLOGIC TESTS

Leukocytosis will be present. A low total WBC count may indicate an exhausted bone marrow, with a poor prognosis. Initially, the Hgb and Hct values may be increased because of hemoconcentration, but they will decrease to baseline levels when normal intravascular volume is restored.

BLOOD CHEMISTRY TESTS

Depending on the severity of the patient's condition, blood electrolyte levels may be abnormal. If vomiting is present, metabolic alkalosis is expected. Serum albumin levels are often decreased as a result of increased capillary permeability and leakage. The underlying disease process affects chemistry tests (e.g., patients with pancreatitis, gallbladder disorders, and renal failure). Renal failure is a common complication of peritonitis and a major cause of death.

RADIOLOGIC PROCEDURES

The abdominal radiograph test usually reveals dilation of the large and small bowel, with edema of the small bowel wall. Free air in the abdomen suggests visceral perforation. With abdominal CT, abscesses can be visualized and sometimes drained during the procedure, thus avoiding surgery. Free fluid in the abdomen on ultrasound suggests hemorrhage or ascites.

Nuclear medicine scans

(Gallium, Indium, Technetium) are useful for persistent fever despite adequate antibiotic coverage and negative CT findings.

DIAGNOSTIC PARACENTESIS

Abdominal paracentesis involves the insertion of a catheter or trocar into the abdomen to obtain a specimen. Sterile saline is infused through the catheter, and the return fluid is analyzed for RBC, WBC, and bacteria content. If ascites is present, it may not be necessary to infuse saline because fluid can be removed directly for analysis. Paracentesis may be repeated 48 hours after the initiation of treatment to assess patient response. Multiple organisms on peritoneal or ascitic fluid Gram stain or culture are diagnostic of secondary peritonitis, whereas spontaneous bacterial peritonitis is caused by monomicrobial infection.

COLLABORATIVE MANAGEMENT

Management should be geared toward controlling the infectious source, eliminating bacteria and toxins, modulating the inflammatory process, and preventing organ system failure. Patients should be cared for in an intensive care setting, even if they do not appear critically ill initially.

CARE PRIORITIES

Care priorities begin with volume resuscitation, electrolyte replacement, and empirical antibiotic coverage. Medical, nursing, interventional, and surgical therapies should be complementary involving hemodynamic management, pulmonary support, and renal replacement therapy, and nutrition and metabolic support.

1. Correct fluid and electrolyte imbalances

Significant intravascular volume depletion may occur with peritonitis. In patients who are severely ill, fluid replacement should be guided by invasive hemodynamic monitoring. In most cases, crystalloids are used initially. If there is evidence of decreased intravascular proteins, colloids such as albumin are indicated. The use of IV albumin has also been shown to reduce the incidence of renal failure. If peritonitis is complicated by hemorrhage, pRBCs may be given. Electrolyte replacement, typically potassium, is implemented according to laboratory findings. (See Systemic Inflammatory Response Syndrome, Sepsis, Septic Shock, and Multiple Organ Dysfunction Syndrome, Chapter 11, for additional information.)

2. Control peritoneal infection with antimicrobial therapy

Initiate empirical broad-spectrum parenteral antibiotic therapy early for all suspected cases of peritonitis. Antibiotic therapy should be started as soon as the diagnosis is suspected. Suspicion is identified by clinical findings more so than culture results because a large percentage of patients will exhibit negative culture results. Patients with culture-negative results must also receive antibiotic therapy because without it, severe sepsis and death may follow.

- Third-generation cephalosporins are recommended in cases of spontaneous bacterial peritonitis initially, then, tailor therapy in conformity with cultures. For secondary and tertiary bacterial peritonitis, broad-spectrum gram-negative and anaerobic coverage should be initiated, followed by definitive therapy based on culture sensitivities.
- In severe hospital-acquired cases, imipenem, piperacillin-tazobactam, and a combination of aminoglycoside and metronidazole may be effective. Quinolones are also considered effective therapy.
- The duration of antibiotic therapy must be individualized according to the infectious source, infection severity, underlying disease, and the patient's response to therapy. Therapy for 5 to 10 days is sufficient for most patients.
- The administration of intraperitoneal antibiotics should be considered over parenteral administration for patients with peritoneal dialysis–associated peritonitis. Aminoglycoside therapy should be avoided in patients with chronic liver disease because of an increased risk of nephrotoxicity.
- Antimicrobial prophylaxis should be considered for gastroduodenal procedures involving patients at high risk for postoperative infections including risk factors such as gastroduodenal perforation, decreased gastric motility, gastric outlet obstruction, morbid obesity, and patients receiving acid-suppression therapy. A single dose of cefazolin is recommended.

3. Control peritoneal infection with surgical procedure(s)

Surgical laparotomy is an important therapy in all cases of peritonitis to remove the source of infection and prevent reinfection. Surgical débridement allows for the removal of all intraabdominal foreign material and nonviable tissue. Leaky anastomoses are identified and repaired. If present, bowel perforations and obstructions are corrected and abscesses are drained.

- Laparoscopy: Laparoscopy is currently used for diagnosis and determination of etiology. Laparoscopic procedures have become common for some forms of peritonitis such as for the treatment of peritonitis caused by uncomplicated appendicitis.
- Open wound management of the abdomen with scheduled reoperations is often advocated for severe disease. Open-abdomen technique may reduce the risk of abdominal compartment syndrome, and allow for better management of bowel edema and subsequent

inflammatory changes in the postoperative period. Disadvantages of open-technique include alteration in respiratory mechanics and risk of abdominal contamination with nosocomial pathogens.

- Interventional therapies include percutaneous drainage of abscesses and percutaneous and endoscopic stent placements. Ultrasound- and CT-guided percutaneous drainage has been shown to be efficacious and safe and preferred in some cases, allowing for a delay in surgery until the acute process and sepsis can be resolved.

4. Control pain resulting from peritoneal inflammation

The degree of discomfort caused by peritonitis varies greatly. Opiate analgesics are used parenterally to ensure patient comfort but are given cautiously to avoid compromise of abdominal and respiratory function. These analgesics usually require frequent administration, with the dose titrated for each individual.

5. Provide nutrition support

Nutrition support is crucial for healing and survival. GI function is compromised and motility minimal or absent as a result of inflammatory processes.

- A large-bore NG tube is inserted to reduce or prevent distension caused by obstruction or ileus to reduce IAP. Placement of a small-bore enteric tube (nasoduodenal or NJ tube) is done to provide enteral (tube) feedings and administer medications. Radiographic confirmation of correct placement should be done for all enteric tubes before enteral or medication infusion. Oral intake may be restricted until GI function is regained.
- Jejunal feeding should be initiated as soon as tolerated. Elemental feedings can be administered with or without bowel sounds present. More recent enteral feeding guidelines have challenged the validity of older guidelines for feeding intolerance. Gastric residual volumes exceeding 450 mL and absence of bowel sounds are no longer absolute contraindications for feeding. Newer feeding methods, such as "trickle feedings," may be better tolerated. If enteral feeding is not possible, TPN should be initiated. (See Nutrition Support, Chapter 1.)
- When resumption of bowel sounds or passage of flatus signals the return of GI motility, enteral nutrition with nonelemental (conventional) tube feedings can begin.

6. Intraabdominal pressure monitoring

Peritonitis is a risk factor for IAH. IAH is defined as a pathologic increase in IAP greater than 12 mm Hg and may result in abdominal compartment syndrome. Abdominal compartment syndrome is defined as a sustained IAP greater than 20 mm Hg. If IAH is present, patient management should follow the medical management algorithm of the World Society of the Abdominal Compartment Syndrome (www.wsacs.org). (See Abdominal Hypertension and Abdominal Compartment Syndrome, Chapter 11.)

CARE PLANS FOR PERITONITIS

DEFICIENT FLUID VOLUME *related to active loss secondary to fluid sequestration within the peritoneum.*

Goals/Outcomes: Within 6 hours of diagnosis, the patient becomes normovolemic, as evidenced by the following measurements: MAP $\geq$65 mm Hg; HR 60 to 100 bpm; normal sinus rhythm on ECG; CVP 2-6 mm Hg: superior vena cava oxygenation (Scvo$_2$) or mixed venous oxygen saturation (Svo$_2$) 70% or 65%, respectively; urinary output $\geq$0.5 mL/kg/h; warm extremities, peripheral pulses greater than 2+ on a 0-to-4+ scale, brisk capillary refill (less than 2 seconds); normalization of serum lactate; orientation to time, place, and person; and stable weight. **NOC** Fluid Balance.

Fluid/Electrolyte Management

1. Monitor BP continuously with an arterial catheter. Be alert to MAP decreases of greater than 10 mm Hg, which is indicative of possible sepsis.
2. Monitor HR and ECG every 1 to 2 hours or more often if vital signs are unstable. Be alert to increases in HR, which suggest hypovolemia. Usually, the ECG will show sinus tachycardia. In the presence of hypokalemia caused by prolonged vomiting or gastric suction, ECG may show ventricular ectopy, prominent U wave, and depression of the ST segment.

| **Safety Alert** | *Heart rate increases may be caused by fever, hypovolemia, and vasodilation related to sepsis.* |

3. Maintain crystalloid therapy guided by hemodynamic and fluid responsiveness measurements. Vasopressor therapy should target an MAP of 65 mm Hg.
4. Echocardiography may be used to evaluate CO and ejection fraction. Inotropic therapy may be added to assist CO in conjunction with fluid replacement modalities.
5. Monitor BUN, creatinine, total protein, and albumin levels.
6. Albumin administration at 1 to 1.5 g/kg may be needed to replace losses resulting from capillary leak.
7. Measure urinary output hourly. Be alert to output less than 0.5 mL/kg/h for 2 consecutive hours, which may signal intravascular volume depletion. Consult the advanced practice provider and increase fluid intake promptly if decreased urinary output is caused by hypovolemia and hypoperfusion.
8. Monitor the patient for physical indicators of hypovolemia, including cool extremities, capillary refill greater than 2 seconds, decreased amplitude of peripheral pulses, and neurologic changes such as restlessness and confusion.
9. Estimate ongoing fluid losses. Measure all drainage from tubes, catheters, and drains. Note the frequency of dressing changes as a result of saturation with fluid or blood. Weigh the patient daily, using the same scales and method. Compare 24-hour body fluid output with 24-hour fluid intake, and record the difference.
10. Assess for signs of pulmonary edema resulting from aggressive fluid replacement and increased capillary permeability caused by inflammatory mediators.

NIC Fluid Monitoring; Hemodynamic Regulation; Hypovolemia Management; Invasive Hemodynamic Monitoring; Shock Prevention; Dysrhythmia Management.

RISK FOR INFECTION *related to inadequate primary defenses (traumatized tissue, altered perfusion), tissue destruction, and environmental exposure to pathogens.*

Goals/Outcomes: Severe sepsis does not develop, as evidenced by HR 60 to 100 bpm; RR 12 to 20 breaths/min; CVP 2-6 mm Hg: $ScvO_2$ ≥70% or SvO_2 ≥65%; serum lactate less than 3 mmol/L; urinary output ≥0.5 mL/kg/h; normothermia, negative culture results, and orientation to time, place, and person. (See Sepsis, Chapter 11.)
NOC Infection Severity.

Medication Management
1. Administer empirical broad-spectrum parenteral (IV) antibiotics within 1 hour of recognition of severe sepsis with or without septic shock as recommended by the 2012 Surviving Sepsis Campaign. Reschedule antibiotics if a dose is delayed for greater than 1 hour. Recognize that failure to administer antibiotics on schedule may result in inadequate drug blood levels and treatment failure.
   a. Combination empirical antimicrobial therapy should be administered as ordered.
   b. Intraperitoneal antibiotics should be considered for patients with peritoneal dialysis-associated peritonitis because the peritoneal dialysis catheter provides immediate access to the peritoneum.
2. Administer norepinephrine as the first choice vasopressor to maintain MAP ≥65 mm Hg. Norepinephrine preserves splanchnic blood flow. Vasopressin or epinephrine may be added as ordered. Dopamine is not recommended except in highly selective patients such as those with low risk for tachydysrhythmias or with absolute or relative bradycardia according to the 2012 Surviving Sepsis Campaign guidelines.
3. A trail of antibiotic cessation could be considered for the patient with no defined infectious focus. Continued broad-spectrum antibiotics in these patients may allow resistant organisms to emerge.

Vital Signs Monitoring
1. Monitor for signs of tissue hypoperfusion: CVP less than 8 mm Hg: $ScvO_2$ less than 70% or SvO_2 less than 65%; serum lactate ≥4 mmol/L; MAP less than 65 mmHg; urinary output ≥0.5 mL/kg/h.
2. Monitor fluid responsiveness measurements such as SPV, PPV, and SVV when available. If SPV is greater than 5 mm Hg, PPV greater than 13% to 15%, SVV greater than 13% to 15%, the patient is deemed fluid responsive.
3. Monitor vital signs for evidence of severe sepsis: Increases in HR, RR, and rectal or core temperature every 1 to 2 hours for increases. Be aware that hypothermia may precede hyperthermia in some patients. Hypothermia with leukopenia is a poor prognostic marker.
4. Also note that older adults and those who are immunocompromised may not demonstrate a fever, even with severe sepsis.

5. If the patient has a sudden temperature elevation, obtain culture specimens of blood, sputum, urine, and other sites as prescribed. Monitor culture reports and report positive findings promptly.

Wound Care
1. To minimize microbial growth, facilitate drainage of pus, GI secretions, old blood, necrotic tissue, foreign material such as feces, and other body fluids from wounds.
2. Evaluate wounds for evidence of infection (e.g., erythema, warmth, swelling, unusual drainage). Culture any unusual drainage.
3. Evaluate the patient's orientation to time, place, and person and LOC every 2 to 4 hours. Document and report significant deviations from baseline.

NIC Hemodynamic Regulation; Temperature Regulation; Intravenous (IV) Therapy.
See Systemic Inflammatory Response Syndrome, Sepsis, Septic Shock, and Multiple Organ Dysfunction Syndrome, Chapter 11, for additional information.

HYPERTHERMIA *related to infectious process, increased metabolic rate, and dehydration secondary to peritonitis.*

Goals/Outcomes: The patient's temperature remains within acceptable limits (36° C to 38.9° C [97° F to 102° F]) or returns to acceptable limits within 4 to 6 hours of diagnosis. An open airway is secured in the event of hyperthermic seizures.
NOC Thermoregulation.

Temperature Regulation
1. Monitor rectal or core temperature every 1 to 2 hours.
2. If a hypothermia blanket is required, perform the following interventions for the patient:
   a. Protect skin in contact with the blanket by placing a sheet between the blanket and patient.
   b. Inspect the skin every 2 hours for evidence of tissue damage caused by local vasoconstriction and massage to promote circulation and minimize tissue damage.
   c. Check body temperature at frequent intervals to ensure that shivering does not occur, which increases metabolic demand.
3. If high fever (i.e., greater than 38.9° C [102° F]) ensues, tepid baths may be helpful in reducing the fever.
4. Administer antipyretics as prescribed.
5. An appropriate-size oral airway and suction equipment is kept in the patient's room for use in the event of seizure activity.

NIC Fever Treatment; Vital Signs Monitoring.

IMPAIRED TISSUE INTEGRITY *related to tissue destruction; surgical intervention with exposure to environmental pathogens.*

Goals/Outcomes: By hospital discharge, the patient exhibits no further GI tissue destruction, as evidenced by reduction in pain, return of bowel sounds and bowel function, and wound healing.
NOC Tissue Integrity: Skin and Mucous Membranes.

Infection Control
1. See Medication Management for Risk of Infection.
2. Adjust antibiotic therapy specific to culture sensitivity reports.
3. Monitor renal function for signs of nephrotoxicity secondary to antibiotic therapy.
4. Discuss repeat of paracentesis 48 to 72 hours following the initiation of antibiotic therapy to evaluate effectiveness of therapy.

Wound Care
1. Monitor for surgical site infection (warmth, tenderness, and purulent drainage).
2. If surgical wound is open:
   a. Consider a negative pressure wound device, which applies localized negative pressure directly to the wound. This removes fluid that causes swelling, increases blood flow, and accelerates granulation tissue formation.

b. Maintain dressing membrane, ensure adequacy of drainage, and monitor for granulation tissue formation.
c. Avoid wet-to-dry dressings because they create a lack of a physical barrier to bacterial entry; prompt tissue cooling in wounds, which heal best when kept normothermic; disrupt angiogenesis; and prolong inflammation.
3. Record volume and characteristics of drainage and obtain specimens as needed.
4. Assess for overall improvement within 24 to 72 hours. Failure to progress indicates recurrent, persistent, or new infectious focus.

ACUTE PAIN *related to biological or chemical agents causing injury to the peritoneum and intraperitoneal organs.*

Goals/Outcomes: Within 2 hours of diagnosis, the patient's subjective evaluation of discomfort improves, as documented by a pain scale. Nonverbal indicators of discomfort, such as grimacing, are absent.
NOC Pain Control.

Analgesic Administration
1. Monitor the patient for the presence of discomfort. Use a pain scale to rate discomfort.
2. Administer parenteral analgesics promptly and consistently, before pain becomes severe, to help decrease anxiety, which contributes to the severity of pain. Rate the degree of pain relief using the pain scale.
3. Position the patient to optimize comfort. Many patients with severe abdominal pain find a dorsal recumbent or lateral decubitus bent-knee position more comfortable than other positions.
4. Monitor for diminished RR and depth and decreased LOC hourly if large amounts of opiates are required to control the pain. Many opiates also cause vasodilation and can result in serious hypotension, especially in patients with volume depletion. Opiate analgesics also decrease GI motility and may delay the return of normal bowel function.
5. Monitor HR and BP every 1 to 2 hours or more frequently in patients whose condition is unstable. Consult the advanced practice provider for significant deviations.
6. Evaluate effectiveness of the medication on an ongoing basis. On the basis of the patient's clinical response, discuss dose and drug manipulation with the physician.
7. Avoid administering analgesics to newly admitted patients before they have been fully evaluated by a surgeon, because analgesics can mask important diagnostic clues.

NIC Pain Management; Environmental Management: Comfort; Coping Enhancement; Simple Guided Imagery; Respiratory Monitoring.

IMBALANCED NUTRITION, LESS THAN BODY REQUIREMENTS *related to decreased intake secondary to impaired GI function.*

Goals/Outcomes: The patient maintains baseline body weight, and nitrogen tests show a state of nitrogen balance within 5 to 7 days of this diagnosis.
NOC Nutrition Status: Food and Fluid Intake.

Nutrition Management
1. Monitor bowel sounds every 1 to 4 h; report significant changes (i.e., sudden absence or return).
2. Maintain NPO status during the acute phase of peritonitis with stomach decompression via an NG tube.
3. Initiate postpyloric (jejunal) elemental feedings within the first 24 to 48 hours. Gradually increase enteral intake when gastric motility returns.
4. Consider TPN if jejunal feedings are contraindicated or not tolerated.
5. If abdominal distension is noted, initiate IAP monitoring. Distention can signal complications such as ileus, ascites, or IAH.
6. Administer histamine H_2-receptor antagonists as prescribed to reduce corrosiveness of gastric acid and prevent complications such as stress ulcers.
7. Administer prescribed antiemetic medications as indicated.
8. Ensure that NG and enteral tubes are functioning properly. Evaluate characteristics of the drainage. Irrigate or reposition tubes as necessary.

NIC Nutrition Monitoring; Gastrointestinal Intubation; Total Parenteral Nutrition (TPN) Administration; Enteral Tube Feeding; Aspiration Precautions; Tube Care: Gastrointestinal.
For additional information, see Nutrition Support, Chapter 1.

RISK FOR INTRAABDOMINAL HYPERTENSION *related to intraabdominal inflammation*

Goals/Outcomes: The patient displays no signs of increased IAPs through discharge.

NOC (See Abdominal Hypertension and Abdominal Compartment Syndrome, Chapter 11.)

ADDITIONAL NURSING DIAGNOSES

For other nursing diagnoses and interventions, see the following as appropriate: Hemodynamic Monitoring (Chapter 1), Prolonged Immobility (Chapter 1), Emotional and Spiritual Support of the Patient and Significant Others (Chapter 2), and Systemic Inflammatory Response Syndrome, Sepsis, Septic Shock, and Multiple Organ Dysfunction Syndrome, (Chapter 11).

SELECTED REFERENCES

Ahmed A, Stanley AJ: Acute upper gastrointestinal bleeding in the elderly, *Drugs Aging* 29:933–940, 2012.

Arhi C, El-Gaddai A: Use of silver dressing for management of an open abdominal wound complicated by an enterocutaneous fistula—from hospital to community, *J Wound Ostomy Continence Nurs* 40:101–103, 2013.

Bendis L, Wong F: The hyperdynamic circulation in cirrhosis: an overview, *Pharmacol Ther* 89: 221–231, 2001.

Berlioux P, Robic MA, Poirson H, et al: Pre-transjugular intrahepatic portosystemic shunts (TIPS) prediction of post-TIPS overt hepatic encephalopathy: the critical flicker frequency is more accurate than psychometric tests, *Hepatology* 59:622–629, 2014.

Bernal W, Wendon J: Acute liver failure, *N Engl J Med* 369:2525–2534, 2013.

Blei AT: Brain edema in acute liver failure, *Crit Care Clin* 24:99–114, 2008.

Boyer TD, Haskal ZJ, AASLD: Practice Guidelines Committee: the role of transjugular intrahepatic portosystemic shunt in the management of portal hypertension, *Hepatology* 51:1–16, 2010.

Bradley MJ, DuBose JJ, Scalea TM, et al: Independent predictors of enteric fistula and abdominal sepsis after damage control laparotomy results from the prospective AAST Open Abdomen Registry, *JAMA Surg* 148:947–955, 2013.

Bratzler DW, Dellinger EP, Olsen KM, et al: Clinical practice guidelines for antimicrobial prophylaxis in surgery, *Surg Infect* 14(1):73–128, 2013.

Cobbold JFL, Summerfield JA: The liver in systematic disease. In Friedman LS, Keeffe EB, editors: *Handbook of liver disease*, ed 3, Philadelphia, 2012, Elsevier.

Dasher K, Trotter JF: Intensive care unit management of liver-related coagulation disorders, *Crit Care Clin* 28:389–398, 2012.

Davern TJ, James LP, Hinson JA, et al: Measurement of serum acetaminophen-protein adducts in patients with acute liver failure, *Gastroenterology* 130:687–694, 2006.

Dellinger RP, Levy MM, Rhodes A, et al: Surviving sepsis campaign: international guidelines for management of severe sepsis and septic shock: 2012, *Crit Care Med* 41:580–637, 2012.

Demetriades D, Salim A: Management of the open abdomen, *Surg Clin North Am* 94:131–154, 2013.

Dierdorf-Quatrara BA: Acute pancreatitis and enteral feedings: what is the evidence? *Acad Med Surg Nurses* 20:7–10, 2011.

Dugum M, O'Shea R: Hepatitis C virus: here comes the all-oral treatment, *Cleveland Clin J Med* 81:159–172, 2014.

Dupuis CS, Baptista V, Whaken G, et al: Diagnosis and management of acute pancreatitis and its complications, *Gastrointestinal Intervention* 2:36–46, 2013.

Gagnon LE, Scheff EJK: Outcomes and complications following bariatric surgery, *Am J Nurs* 112:26–36, 2012.

Garcia-Pagan JC, Reverter E, Abraldes JG, et al: Acute variceal bleeding, *Semin Respir Crit Care Med* 33:46–54, 2012.

Garcia-Tsao G, Sanyal AJ, Grace ND, et al; AASLD Practice Guidelines Committee: Management of gastroesophageal varices and variceal hemorrhage in cirrhosis, *Hepatology* 46:922–938, 2007.

Ghany MG, Nelson DR, Strader DB, et al; AASLD Practice Guidelines Committee: An update on treatment of genotype 1 chronic hepatitis C virus infection: 2011 practice guidelines by the American Association for the Study of Liver Diseases, *Hepatology* 54:1433–1444, 2011.

Heidelbaugh JJ, Sherbondy M: Cirrhosis and chronic liver failure: part 1: diagnosis and evaluation, *Am Fam Phys* 74:756–762, 2006.

Heidelbaugh JJ, Sherbondy M: Cirrhosis and chronic liver failure: part 2: complications and treatment, *Am Fam Phys* 74:767–776, 2006.

IAP/APA Working Group: IAP/APA evidence-based guidelines for the management of acute pancreatitis, *Pancreatology* 13(4 Suppl 2):e1–e5, 2013.

Inal MT, Memis D, Sezer YA, et al: Effects of intra-abdominal pressure on liver function assessed with the LiMON in critically ill patients, *Can J Surg* 54:161–166, 2011.

International Club of Ascites: *Criteria for the diagnosis of hepatorenal syndrome*, Padova, 2014, International Club of Ascites. http://www.icascites.org/about/guidelines/.

Jayakumar S, Chowdhury R, Ye C, et al: Fulminant viral hepatitis, *Crit Care Clin* 29:677–697, 2013.

Jensen LL: Guideline: management of patients with ulcer bleeding, *Am J Gastroenterol* 107:345–360, 2012.

Kerlin MP, Tokar JL: Acute gastrointestinal bleed, *Ann Intern Med* 159(3):2–16, 2013.

Kim MY, Baik SK: Hyperdynamic circulation in patients with liver cirrhosis and portal hypertension, *Korean J Gastroenterol* 54:143–148, 2009 (in Korean).

Kuehn BM: Guideline tightens transfusion criteria, *JAMA* 307:1788–1789, 2012.

Kujovich JL: Hemostatic defects in end stage liver disease, *Crit Care Clin* 21:563–587, 2005.

Lee SS, Baik SK: Cardiovascular complications of cirrhosis, In Boyer T, Manns MP, Sanyal AJ, editors: *Zakim and Boyer's hepatology: a textbook of liver disease*, ed 6, Philadelphia, 2012, Saunders Elsevier.

Lee WM, Stravitz T, Larson AM: Introduction to the revised American Association for the Study of Liver Diseases Position Paper on acute liver failure 2011, *Hepatology* 55:965–967, 2012.

Luber S, Fischer D, Venkat A: Care of the bariatric surgery patient in the emergency department, *J Emerg Med* 34:13–20, 2008.

Mandell MS, Tsou MY: Cardiovascular dysfunction in patients with end-stage liver disease, *J Chin Med Assoc* 71:331–335, 2008.

Martin P, DiMartini A, Feng S, et al; AASLD Practice Guidelines Committee: Evaluation for liver transplantation in adults: 2013 practice guideline by the American Association for the Study of Liver Diseases and the American Society of Transplantation, *Hepatology* 59:1144–1165, 2014.

Martindale RG, McClave SA, Vanek VW, et al: Guidelines for the provision and assessment of nutrition support therapy in the adult critically ill patient: Society of Critical Care Medicine and American Society for Parenteral and Enteral Nutrition, *Crit Care Med* 37:1–24, 2009.

McQuaid KR: Gastrointestinal disorders. In McPhee J, Papadakis M, editors: *Current medical diagnosis and treatment*, ed 48, New York, 2009, McGraw-Hill.

Minei J, Champine J: Abdominal abscesses and gastrointestinal fistula, In Feldman M, Friedman L, Brandt J, editors: *Sleisenger and Fordtran's gastrointestinal and liver disease: pathophysiology, diagnosis, management*, ed 9, Philadelphia, 2010, Saunders Elsevier.

Mulhall AM, Jindal SK: Massive gastrointestinal hemorrhage as a complication of the Flexi-Seal fecal management system, *Am J Crit Care* 22:537–543, 2013.

Orangio GR: Enterocutaneous fistula: medical and surgical management including patients with Crohn's disease, *Clin Colon Rectal Surg* 23:169–175, 2010.

O'Shea RS, Dasarathy S, McCullough AJ, et al; AASLD Practice Guidelines Committee: Alcoholic liver disease, *Hepatology* 51:307–328, 2010.

Owen RM, Love TP, Perez, SD, et al: Definitive surgical treatment of enterocutaneous fistula, *JAMA Surg* 148:118–126, 2013.

Parkash O, Hamid S: Are we ready for a new epidemic of under recognized liver disease in South Asia especially in Pakistan? Non-alcoholic fatty liver disease, *J Pak Med Assoc* 63:95–99, 2013.

Parker RI: Coagulopathies in the PICU, *Crit Care Clin* 29:319–333, 2013.

Pieracci F, Barie P, Pomp A: Critical care of the bariatric patient, *Crit Care Med* 34:1796–1804, 2006.

Reuben A, Koch DG, Lee WM: Drug-induced acute liver failure: results of a U.S. multicenter, prospective study, *Hepatology* 52:2065–2076, 2010.

Rockey DC, Caldwell SH, Goodman ZD, et al: AASLD position paper: liver biopsy, *Hepatology* 49:1017–1043, 2009.

Roisin RR, Krowka MJ: Hepatopulmonary syndrome—a liver-induced lung vascular disorder, *N Engl J Med* 358:2378–2387, 2008.

Runyon BA: *AASLD practice guideline: management of adult patients with ascites due to cirrhosis: update 2012*, Virginia, 2012, American Association for the Study of Liver Diseases, March 15, 2014. http://www.aasld.org/sites/default/files/guideline_documents/adultascitesenhanced.pdf.

Savides TJ, Jensen DM: Gastrointestinal bleeding. In Feldman M, Friedman LS, Brant LJ, editors: *Sleisenger and Fordtran's gastrointestinal and liver disease: pathophysiology, diagnosis, management*, ed 9, Philadelphia, 2010, Saunders Elsevier.

Schmidt R: Regulation of hepatic blood flow: the hepatic arterial buffer response revisited, *World J Gastroenterol* 16:6046–6057, 2010.

Schmidt LE, Larsen FS: MELD score as a predictor of liver failure and death in patients with acetaminophen-induced liver injury, *Hepatology* 45:789, 2007.

Shirtliff MD: Necrotizing pancreatitis: halting a harmful progression, *Adv NPs PAs* 2:23–27, 44, 2011.

Slade DA, Carlson GL: Takedown of enterocutaneous fistula and complex abdominal wall reconstruction, *Surg Clin North Am* 93:1163–1183, 2013.

Solomkin JS, Mazuski JE, Bradley JS, et al: Diagnosis and management of complicated intra-abdominal infection in adults and children: guidelines by the Surgical Infection Society and the Infectious Diseases Society of America, *Clin Infect Dis* 50:133–164, 2010.

Stevenson K, Carter CR: Acute pancreatitis, *Surgery* 31:295–303, 2013.

Tenner S, Baillie J, Dewitt J, Vege SS: American College of Gastroenterology Guideline: management of acute pancreatitis, *Am J Gastroenterol* 108:1400–1415, 2013.

Tenner S, Steinberg WM: Acute pancreatitis. In Feldman M, Friedman LS, Brant LJ, editors: *Sleisenger and Fordtran's gastrointestinal and liver disease: pathophysiology, diagnosis, management*, ed 9, Philadelphia, 2010, Saunders Elsevier.

Trevino CM, Verhaalen A, Bruce ML, et al: Conversion of an enterocutaneous fistula associated with an open abdominal wound into a drain-controlled enterocutaneous fistula, *Wounds* 26:43–46, 2014.

Triadafilopoulos G: Management of lower gastrointestinal bleeding in older adults, *Drugs Aging* 29:707–715, 2012.

Wilkins T, Khan N, Nabh A, et al: Diagnosis and management of upper gastrointestinal bleeding, *Am Fam Phys* 85:469–476, 2012.

Younossi Z: *Diabetes, obesity and hypertension increase mortality in HCV patients. Oral presentation at the 44th Annual Meeting of the European Association for the Study of the Liver*, Copenhagen, Denmark, April 22, 2009. http://www.easl.eu/assets/application/files/5b0c67e7cc76a88_file.pdf.

Hematologic/Immunologic Disorders

GENERAL HEMATOLOGY ASSESSMENT

GOAL OF ASSESSMENT

The goal of a basic hematology assessment is to identify assessment and historical factors that correlate with findings on the complete blood count (CBC) to assist in diagnosing a hematologic disorder. Correlation of findings helps with diagnosis and treatment of anemias, allergies, bleeding and clotting disorders, infections, and cancer (especially in patients requiring chemotherapy). The use of many medications and chemotherapy may have a negative effect on the bone marrow, resulting in reduced production of cells reflected on the CBC.

OBSERVATION

Changes in various blood components place patients at higher risk for infection, fatigue, weakness, lethargy, bleeding, and clotting. Patients may report:

- General: Chills, night sweats, altered mental status, confusion, restlessness, vertigo, visual changes.
- Pain: Painful lymph nodes, painful joints, sore throat, sinusitis, headaches, abdominal pain.
- Respiratory: Shortness of breath (SOB), exertional or chronic dyspnea, cough, hemoptysis, orthopnea.
- Cardiovascular: Activity intolerance, dizziness, palpitations, chest discomfort, painful legs, swollen legs.
- Skin: Unusual bruising, itching, paleness, jaundice, grayness, ulcers, difficulty stopping bleeding from small cuts.
- Musculoskeletal: Swollen and/or tender joints, sore muscles, weakness.
- Gastrointestinal: Decreased appetite, feeling of fullness, hematemesis, melena, black stools, "coffee grounds" stomach secretions, weight loss, diarrhea, constipation.
- Genitourinary: Cystitis, hematuria, heavy menstrual periods, enlarged groin lymph nodes.

Considerations for the bariatric patient: Polycythemia may be present as a result of obstructive sleep apnea–associated polycythemia. Hypercoagulability increases the risk for venous thromboembolism. Observing for swelling and tenderness in the lower limbs, and throughout the body if the obese person is not getting out of bed, are of paramount importance. Focusing on early ambulation is a key preventive strategy.

HISTORY

Patients at risk of hematologic or immunologic problems may report having the following disorders:

- Infections: Recent or recurrent; previous blood transfusion.
- Allergies: Foods, beverages, medications, plants, animals, birds, fish, detergents, household cleaners, fragrances, seasonal patterns of respiratory symptoms.
- Immunologic compromise: Cancer, human immunodeficiency virus (HIV), liver or renal disorders; previous splenectomy, diabetes mellitus, rheumatoid arthritis, systemic lupus erythematosus, Sjögren syndrome, Hashimoto thyroiditis.
- Healing: Prolonged bleeding or delayed healing with previous surgeries, including dental procedures.
- Presence of foreign bodies: Prosthetic heart valves, inferior vena cava filter, implantable defibrillators or other cardiac devices, vascular access devices.
- Social history: Multiple sexual partners, excessive alcohol consumption, exposure to chemicals or radiation.

- Medications, including over-the-counter medications: Aspirin, aspirin-containing drugs, nonsteroidal antiinflammatory drugs (NSAIDs); glucocorticoids/steroids, anticoagulants, platelet inhibitors (e.g., clopidogrel), chemotherapy, hormone therapy, oral contraceptives.

Considerations for the bariatric patient: Inflammation and hypercoagulability are present. Adipose tissue produces tumor necrosis factor and interleukin-6. Neutrophils have impaired chemotaxis and activation. Concentrations of fibrinogen and plasminogen activator inhibitor-1 are increased, whereas concentration of antithrombin III (AT-III) and decreased fibrinolysis are decreased in patients who are obese.

COMMONLY REVIEWED COMPONENTS OF THE COMPLETE BLOOD COUNT*

Components	Significance	Normal Values
Hemoglobin (Hgb)	Protein in red blood cells containing iron that carries oxygen to tissues.	14 to 18 g/dL (male) 12 to 16 g/dL (female)
Hematocrit (Hct)	The percentage of red blood cells in the bloodstream. When Hct is too low, those with anemia may experience fatigue.	42% to 52% (male) 37% to 47% (female)
White blood cells (WBCs)	Cells of the immune system that protect the body from bacterial, fungal, and viral infections. Incidence of infection increases when WBCs are decreased.	5000 to 10,000/mm³
Absolute neutrophil count (ANC)	The number of neutrophils (mature white cells) in the blood. Neutrophils are a type of WBC that help fight infection. When ANC decreases, the patient is neutropenic and more prone to infection. Risk of infection increases when the ANC falls below 2000 and the greatest risk is below 500; a "right shift" on the WBC differential.	2000/mm³ and greater
WBC differential	Measures the percentage of each type of WBC in the total WBC count; a "left shift." Indicates that a large percentage of WBCs are neutrophils; indicates that the bone marrow has been stimulated by a severe infection to produce neutrophils to fight the infection. *Bands* are immature neutrophils. "Right shift": Indicates that a small percentage of WBCs are neutrophils, putting the patient at higher risk for an infection; neutropenia. *Eosinophilia:* Increased eosinophils indicate that an allergic reaction is present. *Monocytes and lymphocytes:* Act as "backup" to the neutrophils. Percentages increase during infection when oncology patients begin bone marrow recovery. If levels do not rise and then fall in a normal pattern, this can be an indication that the patient has a poor prognosis for recovery.	Neutrophils: 50% to 62% Bands: 3% to 6% Monocytes: 3% to 7% Basophils: 0% to 1% Eosinophils: 0% to 3% Lymphocytes: 25% to 40%
Platelets (thrombocytes)	Cells that form the matrix on which blood clots are formed.	150,000 to 400,000/mm³

*Information specific to hematologic and/or immunologic findings for each section is presented in disease-specific sections. The basic assessment can be a part of every patient's assessment to determine the risk of development or presence of a hematologic or immunologic disorder.

ANAPHYLACTIC SHOCK
PATHOPHYSIOLOGY

Anaphylaxis (anaphylactic shock) is a potentially life-threatening condition resulting from an exaggerated or hypersensitive response to an antigen or allergen. The typical presentation occurs in a sensitized person (i.e., someone who has been exposed previously to the same antigen) and is within 1 to 30 minutes of exposure to the antigenic substance, although symptoms may not develop for several hours. The most common triggers include drugs, foods, insect stings or bites, antisera, and blood products. Recent studies have found that exercise may induce anaphylaxis. This syndrome may or may not occur independently of food-allergen ingestion. The hypersensitive response results in airway inflammation that causes obstruction and respiratory distress, which can lead to respiratory arrest. In addition, there is a relative hypovolemia caused by massive vasodilation. Fluids shift from the vasculature into interstitial spaces, creating a false hypovolemia or vasogenic (vasodilated) shock, which progresses to end-organ dysfunction secondary to tissue hypoxia from poor perfusion.

The hypersensitivity response occurs primarily on the surface of the mast cells of the lungs, small blood vessels, and connective tissue. The antigen combines with sensitized antibodies from previous exposure (usually immunoglobulin E [IgE] type) and attaches to basophils circulating in the blood. Inflammatory mediators, including histamine, serotonin, kinins, and eosinophil and neutrophil chemotactic factors, are then released from the granules within the cells. Histamine is the primary mediator of an anaphylactic response. Activation of histamine receptors causes increased capillary permeability, increased pulmonary secretions, bronchoconstriction, and systemic vasodilation.

The antigen-antibody complexes activate production of prostaglandins and leukotrienes, which are termed slow-reacting substances of anaphylaxis. These chemical mediators produce systemic effects with potentially deadly results, including profound shock. The leukotrienes produce severe bronchoconstriction and cause venule dilation and increased vascular permeability. The prostaglandins exaggerate bronchoconstriction and potentiate the effects of histamine on vascular permeability and pulmonary secretions. *Kinins* contribute to bronchoconstriction, vasodilation, and increased vascular permeability. Eosinophilic chemotactic factor of anaphylaxis is then released to attract eosinophils, which work to neutralize mediators such as histamine. However, the amount of neutralization is ineffective in reversing the anaphylaxis. (See Figure 10-1 for a depiction of the pathophysiologic process of anaphylaxis.)

Researchers have made a distinction between "true anaphylaxis" and "pseudoanaphylaxis" or an "anaphylactoid reaction." The symptoms, treatment, and mortality risk are identical, but "true" anaphylaxis results directly from degranulation of mast cells or basophils mediated by IgE. Pseudoanaphylaxis results from other causes not directly mediated by antibodies. Differential diagnosis is based on studying the allergic reaction.

RESEARCH BRIEF 10-1

Exercise-induced anaphylaxis (EIA) is a rare and unpredictable form of anaphylaxis that is poorly understood. Between 5% and 10% of anaphylactic episodes are associated with or caused by exercise. EIA may be food-dependent or occur independent of food.

Although the pathophysiology behind EIA is not fully understood, researchers believe that possible causes may include alterations in plasma osmolality and/or pH during exercise, tissue transglutaminase activity, redistribution of blood flow, and changes in gut permeability. Additional research is needed to better understand EIA. Based on current knowledge, if food is contributing to EIA, dietary management is required, and the specific food should be avoided 3 hours before exercise and 1 hour after exercise.

From Robson-Ansley P, Du Toit G: Pathophysiology, diagnosis and management of exercise-induced anaphylaxis. *Curr Opin Allergy Clin Immunol* 10:312-317, 2010.

ASSESSMENT: ANAPHYLACTIC SHOCK

GOAL OF SYSTEM ASSESSMENT

Identify ineffective breathing patterns, altered tissue perfusion, and impaired gas exchange. The clinical presentation will vary in degree, depending on the magnitude of the sensitivity response. History of asthma, previous allergen exposures, and other respiratory diseases should be queried to help optimize the treatment.

- Assess the symptoms: Assess for airway obstruction, ineffective breathing patterns, and impaired gas exchange, along with altered tissue perfusion related to vasodilation and third-spaced intravascular fluids. Symptoms vary with means of antigen entry.
- Classify severity of reaction: Evaluate the severity of the reaction following the initial assessment. Treatment must begin immediately, before diagnostic test results are

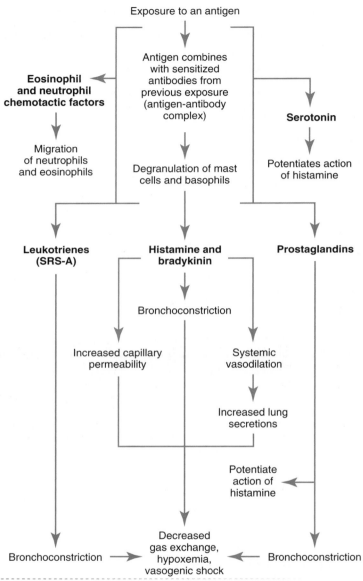

Figure 10-1 Pathophysiologic process of anaphylaxis. (Major chemical mediators are in boldface.)
SRS-A, Slow-reacting substance of anaphylaxis.

available. Shock may progress rapidly to circulatory collapse and cardiopulmonary arrest if improperly managed. The severity of the reaction varies with the means of antigen entry, the amount of antigen absorbed, rate of antigen absorption, and the degree of hypersensitivity. Dramatic symptoms usually develop within minutes and progress rapidly. A more rapid onset correlates with more severe symptoms.

- Evaluate effectiveness of previous treatments: Determine the patient's previous treatment regime if asthmatic, and classify which "step" of treatment has been needed to control symptoms. The patient may need to move to the next step of treatment to maintain control (see Acute Asthma Exacerbation, Chapter 4).

HISTORY AND RISK FACTORS
Recent exposure to:
- Pharmacologic agents: Penicillin, anesthetics, vaccines, contrast media.
- Allergenic foods: Seafood, shellfish, nuts, grains, dairy products.
- Insect bites or stings: Wasps, hornets, bees, fire ants.
- Latex.
- Recent blood transfusion.

VITAL SIGNS
- Severity of all findings varies with the level of sensitivity to the antigen. Patients who are highly sensitive are at risk for impending death if the condition is inappropriately managed.
- Pulse oximetry: Oxygen saturation is decreased from the patient's baseline value.
- Heart rate: Tachycardia (heart rate [HR] greater than 140 beats/min [bpm]).
- Respiratory rate: Tachypnea (respiratory rate [RR] greater than 40 breaths/min).
- Blood pressure: Hypotension may be present. It is exacerbated by underlying vasodilation coupled with increased capillary permeability prompting third spacing of intravascular fluids.

OBSERVATION (see Table 10-1)
- Red to purple discoloration of face and body; "extreme flushing" with swelling of lips, eyelids, and face caused by angioedema.
- Tears coming from eyes with strained facial expression.
- Severe reactions render patients unable to speak resulting from breathlessness.

Table 10-1	SYSTEMIC EFFECTS OF ANAPHYLAXIS	
System	**Effects**	**Cause**
Neurologic	Apprehension; headache; confusion; decreased LOC progressing to coma	Vasodilation; hypoperfusion; cerebral hypoxia or cerebral edema occurring with interstitial fluid shifts
Respiratory	Dyspnea progressing to air hunger and complete respiratory obstruction; hoarseness; noisy breathing; high-pitched, "barking" cough; wheezes; crackles; rhonchi; decreasing breath sounds; pulmonary edema (some patients)	Laryngeal edema; bronchoconstriction; increased pulmonary secretions
Cardiovascular	Decreased BP leading to profound hypotension; increased HR; decreased amplitude of peripheral pulses; palpitations and dysrhythmias (atrial tachycardias, premature atrial beats, atrial fibrillation, premature ventricular beats progressing to ventricular tachycardia, or ventricular fibrillation); lymphadenopathy	Increased vascular permeability; systemic vasodilation; decreased cardiac output with decreased circulating volume; reflex increase in HR; vasogenic shock
Renal	Increased or decreased urine output; incontinence	Decreased renal perfusion; smooth muscle contraction of urinary tract
Gastrointestinal	Nausea, vomiting, diarrhea, abdominal cramping	Smooth muscle contraction of GI tract; increased mucus secretion
Cutaneous	Urticaria; angioedema (hands, lips, face, feet, genitalia); itching; erythema; flushing; cyanosis	Histamine-induced disruption of cutaneous vasculature; vasodilation, increased capillary permeability; decreased oxygen saturation

BP, Blood pressure; *HR*, heart rate; *GI*, gastrointestinal; *LOC*, level of consciousness.

- Use of accessory muscles; fatigued, with or without diaphoresis.
- Chest expansion may be decreased or restricted.
- Altered level of consciousness (LOC) (confusion, disorientation, agitation).
- Agitation is more commonly associated with hypoxemia, whereas somnolence is associated with hypercarbia (elevated carbon dioxide level).
- General early indicators (occurring within seconds to minutes) include uneasiness, lightheadedness, tingling feeling, flushing, and pruritus.
- General late indicators (occurring within minutes to hours) include rapid progression of urticaria involving large areas of skin; angioedema (tissue swelling; more commonly the eyes, lips, tongue, hands, feet, and genitalia); cough, hoarseness, dyspnea, and respiratory distress; lightheadedness or syncope; and abdominal cramps, diarrhea, and vomiting.
- Ingestion of antigen: Cramping, diarrhea, nausea, and vomiting may precede systemic shock symptoms.
- Inhalation of antigen: Cough, hoarseness, wheezing, dyspnea.
- Allergic reaction: Edema, urticaria, itching at the site of a bee sting or drug injection.

AUSCULTATION
- Wheezing bronchial breath sounds.
- Chest may be nearly silent if airflow is severely obstructed.

PALPATION
- Palpate to assess for chest expansion; chest may be hyperinflated if the patient is asthmatic.
- Decreased tactile fremitus may be present if the patient is asthmatic.

PERCUSSION
- May reveal hyperresonance (pneumothorax), a complication of asthma (if present).

Diagnostic Tests for Anaphylaxis

The diagnosis of anaphylaxis is based on presenting signs and symptoms. Treatment should be initiated before laboratory results are available.

Test	Purpose	Abnormal Findings
Arterial blood gas analysis	Assess for abnormal gas exchange or compensation for metabolic derangements. Initially, Pao_2 is normal and then decreases as the ventilation-perfusion mismatch becomes more severe	pH changes: Acidosis may reflect respiratory failure; alkalosis may reflect tachypnea. Carbon dioxide: Elevated CO_2 reflects respiratory failure; decreased CO_2 reflects tachypnea; rising Pco_2 is an ominous sign, because it signals severe hypoventilation, which can lead to respiratory arrest. Hypoxemia: $Pao_2 < 80$ mm Hg. Oxygen saturation: $Sao_2 < 92\%$
Complete blood count with white blood count (WBC) differential	WBC differential evaluates the strength of the immune system's response to the trigger of response	Eosinophils: Increased in patients not receiving corticosteroids; indicative of magnitude of inflammatory response. Hematocrit: May be increased from hypovolemia and hemoconcentration
Tryptase level	Assesses for this chemical mediator released by mast cells following anaphylaxis. May be helpful for confirmation of diagnosis; serial monitoring at the time of presentation, 1 to 2 hours later, and at resolution may increase the sensitivity of the test	Increases within 1 hour following anaphylaxis and remains elevated for 4 to 6 hours; optimally obtained 15 minutes to 3 hours after symptom onset
Immunoglobulin E levels	Used to confirm origin of the reaction is an allergic response	Levels are elevated if allergic response is present
12-Lead electrocardiogram	To detect dysrhythmias reflective of myocardial ischemia	Ischemic changes (ST depression) may be present as shock progresses

COLLABORATIVE MANAGEMENT (see Figure 10-2)

CARE PRIORITIES
Prevention

The goal of management of patients with severe allergies is to quickly identify the offending stimulant and control the allergic response using a stepwise approach to therapies and to prevent exposure to the antigen. Ideally, patients should be educated regarding avoidance of the allergen, but for those with severe allergies, avoidance may not be possible for all substances,

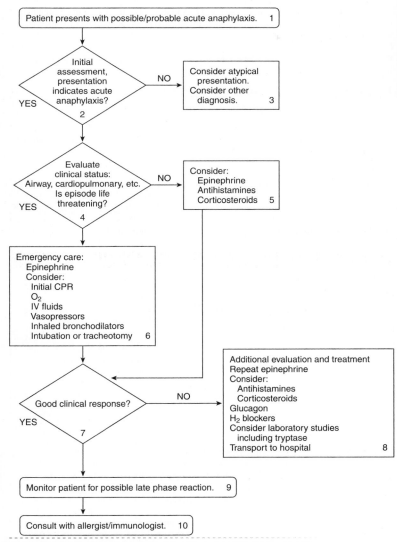

Figure 10-2 Algorithm for the treatment of acute anaphylaxis. (From Nicklas RA, Bernstein I, Li J, et al; Joint Task Force on Practice Parameters for Allergy and Immunology: The diagnosis and management of anaphylaxis. *J Allergy Clin Immunol* 101(6 Pt 2):S465-S528, 1998.)

such as various substances in the air. For patients with asthma, ideal control is attained when patients are free of daytime symptoms, do not awaken breathless or coughing at night, and have few or no limitations on activities. For those with allergies to insects, immunotherapy with hymenoptera venoms is used worldwide as an effective treatment for most patients hypersensitive to stings from bees, wasps, hornets, yellow jackets, or white-faced hornets or bites from fire ants. Food allergy research, including sublingual preparations and vaccines to prevent anaphylaxis from peanuts and other common foods, is underway in leading research centers, including the Johns Hopkins Children's Center. A recent report from the Centers for Disease Control and Prevention revealed that incidence of all food allergies is increasing. Up to 6 million children in the United States, including almost 8% of young children, have at least one food allergy.

When prevention fails, the potential for life-threatening respiratory failure is high during exacerbations unresponsive to treatment within the first hour. Management is directed toward decreasing bronchospasm and increasing ventilation. Other interventions are directed toward treatment of complications. Close monitoring of the patient is necessary after treatment. Biphasic anaphylaxis in which symptoms recur within 1 to 72 hours (usually within 8 to 10 hours) may occur and should be treated as needed.

1. Position the patient and maintain a patent airway

Patients in anaphylactic shock should be placed in supine position with their lower extremities elevated. Early, rapid endotracheal (ET) intubation should be done to manage rapidly progressing laryngeal edema. Severe laryngeal edema may cause complete airway obstruction in minutes. A tracheostomy or an emergency cricothyroidotomy is necessary if ET intubation is not possible.

2. Provide supplemental oxygen

Administered to support ventilation and aerobic metabolism. Amount and method of oxygen administration are guided by arterial blood gas (ABG) results. Supplemental oxygen should be initiated at 6 to 8 L/min via face mask.

3. Manage vasodilation and increased capillary permeability

a. Epinephrine: Epinephrine reverses anaphylaxis by increasing myocardial contractility, dilating bronchioles, constricting blood vessels, inhibiting histamine release, and counteracting histamine. Epinephrine is a first-line medication in anaphylaxis and should be a priority.

Safety Alert *Individuals taking beta-adrenergic–blocking agents such as propranolol may not respond as rapidly as expected to epinephrine and may require higher or additional doses. Glucagon may help to counteract the effects of beta-blocking drugs.*

- Standard adult dose: 0.01 mg/kg (typically 0.2 to 0.5 mg) of a 1:1000 (1 mg/mL) solution, to a maximum of 0.5 mg given intramuscularly (IM) in the mid-anterolateral thigh.
- Repeat dose: May be repeated every 5 to 15 minutes as needed.
- Intravenous (IV) dose: Preferred if the patient is in shock and/or has severe airway obstruction: initial dose of 0.1 to 0.25 mg (1.0 to 2.5 mL of 1:10,000 solution) over 5 to 10 minutes. The dose may be increased to 0.3 to 0.5 mg. Repeat every 5 to 15 minutes as needed.
- IV infusion: After initial dose, an IV drip of epinephrine 1.0 mg in 250 mL 5% dextrose in water (D5W) may be infused at 1 μg/min and increased to 4 μg/min (or more) as needed to achieve desired response.

b. Fluid resuscitation: IV crystalloids (e.g., lactated Ringer, 0.9% normal saline) and/or colloids (e.g., albumin and plasma protein fraction) to increase intravascular volume. Colloids increase colloid osmotic pressure to help retain fluid in the blood vessels. May require rapid infusion of 2 to 3 L of fluids.

c. Vasopressors: Used if fluid replacement does not increase blood pressure (BP). Drugs are titrated for the desired response (see Appendix 6). Usual doses are as follows:

- Dopamine hydrochloride: Effects are dose-dependent. Increases cardiac contractility at 5 to 10 μg/kg/min and systemic vascular resistance at 10 to 20 μg/kg/min. Consider switching to norepinephrine if dose exceeds 20 μg/kg/min.
- Norepinephrine: Initial dose is 2 to 8 μg/min and can be increased to achieve the necessary BP.

- Phenylephrine: Usual dose is 40 to 60 μg/min. Doses exceeding 200 μg/min have been used.

d. Antihistamines: Diphenhydramine: Usual dose is 20 to 50 mg, but 50 to 100 mg may be given IV or IM to relieve urticaria and abdominal cramping. IV H_2-antagonists (e.g., cimetidine, ranitidine) are also used.

e. Corticosteroids: Used to help decrease release of chemical mediators that increase capillary permeability. Hydrocortisone sodium succinate: loading dose is 100 to 1000 mg IV; or methylprednisolone sodium succinate: loading dose is 125 to 250 mg IV, followed by IV or oral (per os [PO]) corticosteroids for several days.

f. Inhaled bronchodilators (e.g., albuterol): May be given for continued bronchospasm (see Acute Asthma Exacerbation, Chapter 4).

g. Glucagon IV bolus: Use is controversial for counteracting effects of beta-blocking drugs or for other patients who have limited response to treatment. Relaxes smooth muscle and increases HR and force of contraction.

4. Electrocardiogram (ECG) monitoring
To detect dysrhythmias.

CARE PLANS FOR ANAPHYLAXIS AND ANAPHYLACTIC SHOCK

INEFFECTIVE AIRWAY CLEARANCE *related to airway obstruction secondary to bronchoconstriction, increased secretions from the histamine response, and presence of leukotrienes and prostaglandins.*

Goals/Outcomes: Within 20 minutes of treatment/intervention, the patient has adequate spontaneous tidal and expiratory volumes, as evidenced by easier breathing; audible breath sounds in expected range, and no adventitious breath sounds.

NOC Respiratory Status: Ventilation; Vital Signs Status; Respiratory Status: Airway Patency; Symptom Control Behavior; Comfort Level; Endurance.

Airway Management

1. Assess continuously for obstructed airway and increased respiratory effort: Note increased pulmonary secretions, cough, expiratory wheezing, SOB, and dyspnea. Suction secretions as needed. Caution: An oral airway provides airway support only as far as the posterior pharynx. If laryngeal edema is present, the oral airway cannot relieve symptoms because the obstruction is below the oral airway. If ET intubation is attempted and is not possible as a result of laryngeal edema, prepare for tracheostomy or cricothyroidotomy.

2. Monitor for decreased breath sounds or changes in wheezing at frequent intervals: Absent breath sounds in the patient who is distressed may indicate impending respiratory arrest. Identify the patient requiring actual/potential airway insertion. Consult the physician and prepare for ET intubation if lingual edema is present and/or respiratory distress continues.

3. Position the patient for comfort and to promote optimal gas exchange: High Fowler position, with the patient leaning forward and elbows propped on the over-the-bed table to promote maximal chest excursion, may reduce use of accessory muscles and diaphoresis resulting from work of breathing. May not be possible with severe hypotension, as further decrease in BP may result.

Ventilation Assistance

1. Monitor for signs of increasing hypoxia at frequent intervals: Restlessness, agitation, and change in mental status are indicative of severe reaction. Cyanosis of the lips (central) and nail beds (peripheral) are late indicators of hypoxia, but may be difficult to see with severe angioedema.

2. Monitor for signs of hypercapnia at frequent intervals: Confusion, listlessness, and somnolence are indicative of respiratory failure.

3. Provide medications to abate allergic response: Administer epinephrine and IV and inhaled bronchodilators as appropriate to attain control of deterioration.

NIC Airway Insertion and Stabilization; Airway Management; Anaphylaxis Management; Medication Administration, Medication Management, Respiratory Monitoring.

IMPAIRED GAS EXCHANGE *related to alveolar-capillary membrane changes secondary to increased capillary permeability associated with histamine response.*

Goals/Outcomes: Within 20 minutes of initiation of treatment/intervention, the patient has adequate alveolar exchange of CO_2 or O_2, as evidenced by easier breathing, PaO_2 80 mm Hg or greater, and SpO_2 90% or greater.

NOC Respiratory Status: Ventilation.

 Anaphylaxis Management

1. Monitor FIO_2 to ensure that oxygen is within prescribed concentrations. If the patient does not retain carbon dioxide, a 100% nonrebreather mask may be used to provide maximal oxygen support. If the patient retains CO_2 and is unrelieved by positioning, lower-dose oxygen, bronchodilators and steroids, intubation, and mechanical ventilation may be necessary sooner than in patients who are able to receive higher doses of oxygen by mask.
2. Monitor ABGs when continuous pulse oximetry values or patient assessment reflects progressive hypoxemia or development of hypercapnia. Monitor and report ABG values with increasing $PaCO_2$ (greater than 50 mm Hg) or decreasing PaO_2 (less than 60 mm Hg) indicative of impending respiratory failure.
3. Administer antihistamines as prescribed.
4. Administer glucocorticoids as prescribed.
5. Position the patient to alleviate dyspnea (assist the patient to sitting position if BP is stable).
6. Stay with the patient to promote safety and reduce fear. Use calm, reassuring approach.

NIC Respiratory Monitoring; Emotional Support; Medication Administration, Medication Management.

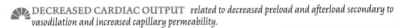 **DECREASED CARDIAC OUTPUT** *related to decreased preload and afterload secondary to vasodilation and increased capillary permeability.*

Goals/Outcomes: Within 4 hours of initiation of treatment, the patient has adequate cardiac output (CO), as evidenced by BP 90/60 mm Hg or greater, strong peripheral pulses, CO 4 L/min or greater, cardiac index (CI) 2.5 L/min/m^2 or greater, systemic vascular resistance (SVR) 900 dynes/s/cm-5 or greater, urinary output 0.5 mL/kg/h or greater, and normal sinus rhythm on ECG.

NOC Circulation Status; Tissue Perfusion: Cardiac; Vital Signs.

Hemodynamic Regulation

1. Assess for physical and hemodynamic indicators of decreased CO:
   - Palpate peripheral pulses for decreasing amplitude, assess the patient for mottling, decreased urine output, or altered mental status.
   - Assess arterial BP or mean arterial pressure (MAP) for any decrease, an indicator of failed compensatory mechanisms.
   - Monitor SVR. A decrease (less than 800 dynes/s/cm-5) is associated with decreased afterload (vasodilation) and may precipitate decreased CO.
   - Monitor CO, $ScvO_2$, and CI if available. A CI of less than 2.0 L/min/m^2 and $ScvO_2$ less than 80% are usually associated with hypoperfusion.
   - Hemodynamic measurements: While vasogenic shock evolves, decreased arterial BP, MAP, CO (less than 4 L/min), CI (less than 2.5 L/min), SVR (less than 800 dynes/s/cm-5), and pulmonary artery wedge pressure (less than 5 mm Hg) are present from worsening vasodilation, progressive shifting of intravascular fluid to interstitial spaces, and decreasing venous return.
2. Monitor for dysrhythmias, such as atrial tachycardias, premature ventricular contractions, ventricular tachycardia, and ventricular fibrillation, which may signal hypoxemia or occur as side effects of drugs such as aminophylline or epinephrine.
3. Monitor for increasing edema.

Safety Alert *Continued swelling, despite treatment, may indicate ineffective treatment, overaggressive fluid therapy, or heart or kidney failure.*

4. Administer epinephrine as prescribed. Observe for therapeutic effects, as evidenced by increased arterial BP and MAP, increased SVR, increased CO/CI, increased $ScvO_2$, stronger peripheral pulses, warming of extremities, and increased urine output.
5. Administer fluid replacement therapy as prescribed, using a large-bore IV catheter. Colloids and crystalloids may be given together.

Safety Alert *During fluid resuscitation, assess the patient for indicators of fluid volume excess, including crackles with chest auscultation, presence of S3 heart sounds, and jugular venous distention. If hemodynamic monitoring lines are present, be alert to increasing pulmonary artery pressure, pulmonary artery wedge pressure, and right atrial pressure.*

6. Prepare for possible vasopressor infusion if hypotension persists after fluid resuscitation and epinephrine administration.

NIC Anaphylaxis Management; Hypovolemia Management; Medication Administration, Medication Management; Cardiac Care: Acute.

ALTERED TISSUE PERFUSION: PERIPHERAL, RENAL, AND CEREBRAL *related to hypovolemia secondary to fluid shift from the vascular space to the interstitial space.*

Goals/Outcomes: Within 4 hours of initiation of treatment, the patient has adequate perfusion, as evidenced by strong proximal peripheral pulses, brisk capillary refill, warm extremities temperature, urinary output 0.5 mL/kg/h or greater, uncompromised neurologic status, and no restlessness, listlessness, and unexplained anxiety.
NOC Tissue Perfusion: Abdominal Organs; Tissue Perfusion: Peripheral; Tissue Perfusion: Cerebral.

Hypovolemia Management
1. Assess peripheral pulses. Report decreased amplitude of pulses.
2. Assess capillary refill. Delayed capillary refill (greater than 2 seconds) is likely with edema and decreased vascular volume.
3. Assess degree of peripheral edema.
4. Assess color and warmth of extremities. Report presence of coolness and pallor.
5. Monitor BP at frequent intervals. Be alert for indicators of hypotension such as BP readings greater than 20 mm Hg below the patient's normal pressure, dizziness, restlessness, altered mentation, and decreased urinary output.
6. Monitor urine output hourly. Continuous CO monitoring using a noninvasive system or a pulmonary artery catheter may be needed to guide fluid resuscitation.
7. Observe for indicators of decreased cerebral perfusion such as anxiety, restlessness, confusion, and decreased LOC.

HIGH ALERT!   Changes in level of consciousness may signal either decreased cerebral perfusion (tissue hypoxia) or increasing intracranial pressure caused by interstitial swelling from capillary permeability. This may be a late sign.

8. Administer fluid and pharmacologic agents as prescribed (see previous nursing diagnosis).

NIC Hemodynamic Regulation; Anaphylaxis Management; Medication Administration, Medication Management.

IMPAIRED SKIN INTEGRITY *related to urticaria and angioedema secondary to allergic response.*

Goals/Outcomes: Within 4 hours of initiation of treatment, the patient states that urticaria is controlled. Skin remains intact.
NOC Tissue Integrity: Skin and Mucous Membranes.

Pruritus Management
1. Assess the patient for urticaria (hives) and itching of hands, feet, neck, and genitalia.
2. Administer antihistamines as prescribed to relieve itching.
3. Discourage the patient from scratching the skin. If unavoidable, teach the patient to use pads of fingertips rather than nails.
4. Apply cool washcloths or covered ice as a soothing measure to irritated and edematous areas.

NIC Environmental Management: Comfort; Medication Administration.

DEFICIENT KNOWLEDGE ILLNESS CARE: SEVERE HYPERSENSITIVITY REACTION, ITS CAUSES, AND ITS SYMPTOMS *related to no previous exposure or incomplete understanding.*

Goals/Outcomes: By the time of discharge from the critical care unit, the patient demonstrates increased knowledge of severe hypersensitivity reactions, as evidenced by verbalization of potential causative factors, symptoms of allergic reaction, need to inform healthcare providers of allergies, importance of wearing medical-alert identification, prescribed treatment modalities when in contact with allergen, and the necessity of informing the primary healthcare provider immediately of any allergic symptoms.

NOC Knowledge: Treatment Regimen; Knowledge: Illness Care; Knowledge: Health Behavior; Knowledge: Disease Process.

Teaching: Disease Process
1. Provide information about the antigenic agent that caused the anaphylaxis, including ways to avoid it in the future.
2. Explain the need for wearing a medical-alert identification tag or bracelet to identify the allergy.
3. Give information about anaphylaxis emergency treatment kits. Teach the patient self-administration technique and the importance of prompt treatment.
4. Stress the importance of seeking treatment immediately if symptoms of allergy occur, including flushing, warmth, itching, anxiety, and hives.
5. Explain the importance of identifying and checking all over-the-counter (OTC) medications for the presence of potential allergens.

NIC Health Education; Risk Identification; Teaching: Prescribed Medication.

ADDITIONAL NURSING DIAGNOSES
Also see nursing diagnoses and interventions in Hemodynamic Monitoring (Chapter 1), Emotional and Spiritual Support of the Patient and Significant Others (Chapter 2), and Mechanical Ventilation (Chapter 1).

PROFOUND ANEMIA AND HEMOLYTIC CRISIS
PATHOPHYSIOLOGY
ANEMIA
Anemia reflects a reduction in total body hemoglobin (Hgb) concentration and is common in patients who are critically ill. By the third day in an intensive care unit, 95% of patients have reduced Hgb concentrations. While Hgb decreases, the oxygen-carrying capacity of the blood is reduced, resulting in tissue hypoxia unless compensatory mechanisms are adequate to assist the body with oxygen delivery. Anemia may be classified under one of three functional classes after initial evaluation of the CBC and reticulocyte index. (See Table 10-2 for functional classification.)

HEMOLYTIC CRISIS
Hemolytic crisis is an acute disorder that frequently accompanies hemolytic anemias. It is characterized by premature pathologic destruction (hemolysis) of red blood cells (RBCs). While RBC destruction accelerates, the oxygen-carrying capacity of the blood decreases, which results in a reduction in the amount of oxygen delivered to the tissues. This hypoxic state produces tissue ischemia and can progress to tissue infarction. Hemolytic episodes can be triggered by both emotional and physiologic states, including stress, trauma, surgery, acute infectious processes, and abnormal immune responses.

ASSESSMENT
GOAL OF SYSTEM ASSESSMENT
Evaluate for decreased oxygen-carrying capacity with subsequent organ dysfunction as a result of decreased production or increased destruction or loss of RBCs.

Table 10-2	**FUNCTIONAL CLASSES OF ANEMIA WITH EXAMPLES**	
Blood Loss/Hemolysis	**Decreased Red Blood Cell Production**	**Maturation Disorders**
Autoimmune diseases: Thrombotic thrombocytopenia purpura, Goodpasture's syndrome, systemic lupus erythematosus, Wegener granulomatosis	Damaged bone marrow: malignancy, lead poisoning, aplastic/hypoplastic anemia, chemotherapy, viruses	Abnormal red blood cell cytoplasm Phenylketonuria, glucose-6-phosphate dehydrogenase
Abnormal hemoglobin: Sickle cell disease, hemoglobin S, C, D, E	Iron deficiency: malignancy, autoimmune disorders	Abnormal red blood cell nucleus
Abnormal red blood cell membranes: Spherocytosis, hemolytic uremic syndrome, paroxysmal nocturnal hematuria	Erythropoietin deficiency: renal failure, malaria, thalassemias	Iron deficiency: dietary, chronic alcoholism
Bleeding/hemorrhage: Physical trauma to blood (bypass, balloon, valves), antibodies (drug-induced antibodies), endotoxins (malaria, clostridia), gastrointestinal bleed, trauma, rupture, excess menstruation	Inflammation/infection: chronic inflammatory disease; critical illness	
Excessive phlebotomies: laboratory sampling	Metabolic disturbance: pernicious anemia, hypothyroidism, megaloblastic anemia	

ANEMIA
Risk factors
Advanced age; environmental exposure to certain chemicals, liver dysfunction, autoimmune or other immunologic disorders, malignancy (and its treatment), drug use (such as aspirin, NSAIDs, warfarin); diets low in protein and iron, iron or folic acid deficiency, B_{12} deficiency, chronic alcoholism, autoimmune disorders.

Clinical presentation (chronic indicators)
- Pallor, melena, hematochezia, fatigue, weight loss, dyspnea on exertion, uremia, sensitivity to cold, intermittent dizziness, excessive menstruation, paresthesias.
- Chronic hemolytic anemia: Jaundice, renal failure, hematuria, arthritis, increased incidence of gallstones, skin ulcers.

Clinical presentation (acute indicators)
- Fever, chest pain, acute heart failure, confusion, irritability, tachycardia, orthostatic hypotension, dyspnea, tachypnea, frank bleeding, critical illness for longer than 3 days.

Vital signs
- Tachypnea, orthopnea, tachycardia, fever.

Observation
- Altered mental status, unusual fatigue or weakness.
- Spider angiomas, unusual bleeding (i.e., stool, urine, emesis).
- ECG changes.
- Monoarticular or polyarticular arthritis.
- Smooth tongue, skin ulcers.

PALPATION
- Bone tenderness (especially rib and sternal areas), joint tenderness.
- Enlargement of the liver and/or spleen.

AUSCULTATION
- Crackles associated with heart failure.

HEMOLYTIC CRISIS

Risk factors

Individuals with mild or chronic hemolytic anemia may be asymptomatic until they are exposed to a severe stressor, such as an acute infectious process, profound emotional upset, critical illness, surgery, or trauma. With added stress, hemolysis can accelerate to a crisis state in which patients experience organ congestion from massive amounts of hemolyzed blood cells, precipitating multiple organ dysfunction syndrome (MODS), and shock.

Clinical presentation (acute)

Fever; abdominal, chest, joint, and back pain; jaundice; headache; dizziness; palpitations; SOB; hemoglobinuria; lymphadenopathy; splenomegaly; and signs of peripheral nerve damage including paresthesias, paralysis, chills, and vomiting.

Clinical presentation (chronic)

Anemia; pallor; fatigue; dyspnea on exertion; mentation changes; icterus; bone infarctions; monoarticular and polyarticular arthritis; hematuria; renal failure; increased gallstone formation; skin ulcers and itching.

Vital signs

- Tachypnea, tachycardia, hypertension.

Observation

- Impaired growth and development, depending on severity and duration of anemia.
- Jaundice; retinal detachment and associated vitreous hemorrhage.
- SOB, with dyspnea on exertion.
- Monoarticular or polyarticular arthritis.
- Hemiplegia, paresthesias.

Palpation

- Splenomegaly, hepatomegaly, lymphadenopathy, or abdominal guarding.
- Chronic skin ulcers, particularly in the ankle area.

Auscultation

- Crackles associated with heart failure.
- Murmurs related to valvular damage.

Diagnostic Tests for Anemias and Hemolytic Crisis

Test	Purpose	Abnormal Findings
Red blood cell (RBC) count	Enumeration of red cells found in each cubic millimeter of blood	Reduced; in hemolytic crisis, an increased number of premature RBCs (nucleated RBCs) will be present
Hemoglobin (Hgb)	Hgb content of RBCs	Decreased
Hematocrit (Hct)	Percentage of RBCs in relation to total blood volume	Decreased
Reticulocyte count, reticulocyte index, corrected reticulocyte	RBC precursors; measures how fast RBCs are produced in the bone marrow	Elevated: Because of increased bone marrow production of RBCs resulting from blood loss or RBC destruction; also a sign of marrow recovery after chemotherapy
Mean corpuscular volume (MCV) (subcategory of red cell indices): Macrocytic: MCV >100 μg^3 Microcytic: MCV <80 μg^3 Normocytic: MCV 80-100 μg^3	Morphologic classification of RBCs: Average size of individual RBCs. Obtained by dividing Hct by total RBC count	Low in microcytic anemia; high in macrocytic anemia

Diagnostic Tests for Anemias and Hemolytic Crisis—cont'd

Test	Purpose	Abnormal Findings
Sickle cell test	Indicative of sickle cell anemia (trait, disease)	Presence of Hgb S
Hgb electrophoresis	Screens for abnormal Hgbs often present in hemolytic anemias. Many hemoglobinopathies are interrelated. Disease expression is based on the degree of genetic abnormalities. Various combinations of abnormal Hgbs are possible	Hgbs A_1, A_2, and F: Normal Hgb Hgb C: Generally benign; may cause joint pain, splenomegaly, and gallstones; may protect against malaria Hgbs D and E: Rarely occur "singly"; sometimes present with sickle cell disease or thalassemias Hgb H: Causes premature destruction of RBCs and abnormal binding of O_2 to RBCs; causes alpha thalassemia Hgb S: Most common abnormal Hgb, occurring in 10% of the African-American population; causes sickle cell disease or sickle cell trait
Erythrocyte sedimentation rate, sedimentation rate or Biernacki's reaction	Rate at which RBCs precipitate in a period of 1 hour: Nonspecific measure of inflammation	Elevated in hemolytic anemia; decreased in sickle cell anemia, polycythemia and congestive heart failure
C_3 proactivator	Proactivator of complement 3 in the alternate pathway of complement activation	Increased in hemolytic anemia
Total iron-binding capacity (TIBC)	Measures the capacity of the blood to bind iron with transferrin; also indirect test of liver function (although rarely used). TIBC is typically measured along with serum iron to evaluate people suspected of having either iron deficiency or iron overload	Normal or reduced, depending on the type of anemia
Ferritin	Iron stores: With damage to organs that contain ferritin (especially the liver, spleen, and bone marrow), ferritin levels can become elevated even though the total amount of iron in the body is normal	Reduced with iron deficiency anemia; normal or elevated with anemia of critical illness; elevated with hemochromatosis
Transferrin	Used to determine the cause of anemia, to examine iron metabolism (e.g., in iron deficiency anemia), and to determine the iron-carrying capacity of the blood	Reduced with anemia of chronic inflammation, anemia of critical illness
Transferrin saturation	The iron concentration divided by TIBC; a more useful indicator of iron status than iron or TIBC alone	Reduced with anemia of chronic inflammation, anemia of critical illness
Folate; folic acid	Measures folic acid in the blood	Reduced with nutrition deficiency leading to megaloblastic anemia
Erythropoietin (EPO)	Measures the amount of a hormone called erythropoietin (EPO) in the blood; acts on stem cells in the bone marrow to increase the production of RBCs; made by cells in the kidney, which release the hormone when oxygen levels are low	Reduced with renal disease and normal in those who are critically ill who should have an elevated level if anemia of any cause is present. Reticulocyte response to EPO has been shown to be reduced in many critically ill patients with elevated EPO levels.
Vitamin B_{12}	Measures the amount of vitamin B_{12} in the blood; used with folic acid test, because a lack of either can cause megaloblastic anemia	Reduced with pernicious or megaloblastic anemia

Continued

Diagnostic Tests for Anemias and Hemolytic Crisis—cont'd

Test	Purpose	Abnormal Findings
Unconjugated bilirubin: Free bilirubin, indirect bilirubin	Measures bilirubin that has not been conjugated in the liver. It gives an indirect reaction to the Van Den Bergh test	Elevated in hemolytic anemia as a result of the inability of the liver to process increasing bilirubin released during hemolysis
Serum lactic dehydrogenase isoenzymes (LDH$_1$ and LDH$_2$)	General indicator of the existence and severity of acute or chronic tissue damage and, sometimes, as a monitor of progressive conditions; monitor damage caused by muscle trauma or injury and to help identify hemolytic anemia	Elevated in hemolytic anemia because of their release when an RBC is destroyed
Haptoglobin level	Used to detect and evaluate hemolytic anemia; not to diagnose cause of the hemolysis. Haptoglobin levels should be drawn before transfusion	Decreased in hemolytic anemia as a result of increased binding of haptoglobin, which facilitates removal of increased Hgb from blood
Peripheral blood smear	Microscopic examination of cells from a drop of blood; investigates hematologic problems or parasites such as malaria and filarial	May reveal abnormally shaped RBCs, such as spherocytes. RBC hyperplasia (abnormal number) is present in nearly all cases of chronic hemolysis with intact bone marrow
Bone marrow aspiration	Evaluates bone marrow status; diagnoses blood disorders and determines if cancer or infection has spread to the bone marrow	May reveal abnormal size, shape, or amounts of RBCs, WBCs, or platelets
Coombs test: Direct antiglobulin test; indirect antiglobulin test	Detects antibodies that may bind to RBCs and cause premature RBC destruction	Positive in antibody-mediated immunologic hemolysis
Immunoglobulin levels	Measures the level of immunoglobulins, also known as antibodies, in the blood.	Elevated: Autoimmune disorders, sickle cell; lower in immunocompromised states
Glucose-6-phosphate dehydrogenase (G6PD) levels	Measures G6PD—enzyme levels are normal in newly produced cells but fall as RBCs age and only deficient cells are destroyed	Decreased in G6PD deficiency, hemolysis. Elevated: myocardial infarction, liver failure, chronic blood loss, hyperthyroidism
Radiologic examinations	x-rays and bone scans Liver/spleen scans	Decreased density, aseptic necrosis of bones Hepatomegaly, splenomegaly, lesions

COLLABORATIVE MANAGEMENT: ANEMIAS
CARE PRIORITIES
1. Oxygen therapy: Administered to relieve SOB or dyspnea
Methods of oxygen delivery range from nasal cannulas, to various face masks, to mechanical ventilation in severe cases.

2. Transfusions/blood component replacement
Packed RBCs may be necessary in the management of profound anemia to help increase the oxygen-carrying capacity of the blood. For patients who refuse blood transfusions, aggressive strategies to augment RBC production such as IV iron therapy and subcutaneous administration of erythropoietin may be implemented. These therapies may take up to 7 days or longer to promote significant improvement in reticulocyte count and Hgb and hematocrit (Hct)

levels. The oxygen-carrying capacity of banked blood is best when used within 14 days of collection. Blood transfused more than 21 days after collection has been linked to increased mortality rates in the critically ill, especially patients who are HIV-positive. Benefits must be weighed against risks, particularly in patients who are immunosuppressed.

RESEARCH BRIEF 10-2

Marik and colleagues conducted a systematic review of 45 cohort studies to determine the correlation between red blood cell transfusion and negative outcome. Outcome measures included mortality, infection, multiorgan dysfunction, and acute respiratory distress syndrome. Forty-two of the 45 studies revealed that risks of transfusion outweighed benefit in treating anemia. Transfusion-related acute lung injury and transfusion-related circulatory overload are some of the most common adverse events. Risks of transfusion must be weighed individually against the risks of anemia, and other treatments such as iron or erythropoiesis-stimulating agents.

From Marik PE, Corwin HL: Efficacy of red blood cell transfusion in the critically ill: a systematic review of the literature. *Crit Care Med* 36:2667-2674, 2008.

---

3. Volume replacement
If the patient is hypovolemic, aggressive fluid and/or blood replacement is mandatory to prevent profound hypotension and shock. Fluid challenges/boluses also assist in prevention of deposition of hemolyzed RBCs in the microvasculature.

4. Elimination of causative factor
Certain drugs and chemicals, cold temperatures, and stress can worsen many anemias, but most profoundly affected are hemolytic and aplastic anemias. Identifying and removing the causative agent can prevent life-threatening crisis. If the patient is bleeding, the cause of the bleeding must be addressed and the bleeding controlled.

5. Folic acid supplement
Necessary for RBC production. Supplements of 1 mg/day are used to treat megaloblastic anemia and, theoretically, to prevent hemolytic crisis in patients with hemolytic anemia. It is not effective in all patients with hemolytic anemia.

6. Iron supplements
Administered for iron-deficiency states to help increase production of normal-size RBCs. May be given IV or enterally. Iron levels must be normal to facilitate the action of erythropoietin injections.

7. Epoetin alfa/erythropoietin, recombinant (Epogen/Procrit)
Stimulates production of RBCs in patients with bone marrow hypofunction/lack of production of RBCs, particularly when related to renal failure. Has been used as an alternative strategy in patients who refuse blood transfusions (in conjunction with IV iron, if needed) and in anemia associated with critical illness. Patients who are critically ill may or may not respond to erythropoietin.

8. Vitamin B$_{12}$
Administered by injections or IV infusion for management of pernicious anemia, a type of megaloblastic anemia caused by failure of the gastric mucosa to absorb vitamin B$_{12}$.

9. Bone marrow transplantation
Recommended for some patients with bone marrow malignancies, sickle cell disease, or aplastic anemia to provide a mechanism for regenerating normal RBC production.

CARE PLANS FOR ANEMIAS

IMPAIRED GAS EXCHANGE *related to lack of RBCs; hemoglobin abnormalities*

Goals/Outcomes: Within 3 to 24 hours of onset of treatment, the patient has adequate gas exchange, as evidenced by HR and RR within 10% of the patient's baseline (or HR 60 to 100 bpm and RR 12 to 20 breaths/min), Hgb and Hct returned to the patient's baseline (or Hgb greater than 12 mg/dL and Hct greater than 37%), oxygen saturation greater than 95%, and BP returned to the patient's baseline (or greater than 90 mm Hg systolic within 24 hours of initiation of treatment).

NOC Respiratory Status: Gas Exchange; Tissue Perfusion: Pulmonary.

Respiratory Monitoring
1. Administer supplemental oxygen, using appropriate device (i.e., nasal cannula, face mask/shield, or mechanical ventilation as necessary). Monitor oxygen liter flow. Provide for oxygen when the patient is transported.
2. Monitor rate, rhythm, and depth of respirations.
3. Monitor for increased restlessness, anxiety, and air hunger.
4. Monitor oxygen saturation using pulse oximetry continuously. Consult the advanced practice provider for persistent values less than 92% or, if oxygen saturation is chronically decreased, a sustained drop of greater than 10% of baseline.
5. Note changes in Sao_2, Svo_2, $Scvo_2$, Sto_2 (if available) and changes in ABG values, as appropriate.
6. Maintain large-bore (18-gauge) IV catheter(s) in case transfusion or rapid volume expansion is necessary. Administer IV fluids to maintain hydration.
7. Transfuse with packed cells (RBCs) (Table 10-3) as prescribed to facilitate oxygen delivery and assist in volume expansion, and/or implement aggressive strategy to augment RBC production.
8. Describe the purpose of blood product transfusion therapy to the patient and significant others.
9. Carefully evaluate dyspnea and chest pain in patients with sickle cell disease because of the possibility of pulmonary infarction.

NIC Airway Management; Oxygen Therapy; Circulatory Precautions; Cardiac Precautions.

ACTIVITY INTOLERANCE *related to anemia/lack of oxygen-carrying capacity of the blood*

Goals/Outcomes: Within 24 hours of onset of treatment, the patient's activity tolerance improves, as evidenced by HR and RR returning to within 10% of baseline (or HR 60 to 100 bpm and RR 12 to 20 breaths/min) and BP returning to within 10% of the patient's baseline (or systolic BP greater than 90% mm Hg). Within 24 hours of initiation of treatment, the patient is able to assist minimally with self-care activities.

NOC Endurance; Activity Tolerance.

Energy Management
1. Alternate periods of rest and activity to avoid stress that increases oxygen demand.
2. Collaborate with occupational therapy, physical therapy, and/or recreational therapy personnel in planning and monitoring an activity program as appropriate.
3. Determine the patient's physical limitations. Focus on what the patient can do rather than on deficits.
4. Reposition the patient slowly while monitoring effects on myocardial and cerebral perfusion.
5. Reduce fear, pain, and anxiety to decrease oxygen demand.
6. Determine causes of fatigue (e.g., treatments, pain, medications).
7. Monitor nutrition intake to ensure adequate energy resources.
8. Teach the patient to avoid stressful situations, which can exacerbate symptoms of anemia and precipitate hemolytic crisis in patients with hemolytic anemia.
9. Teach signs of hypoxemia: altered mental status, activity intolerance, SOB, chest pain, and weakness.
10. Teach the patient and significant others about the specific anemia affecting the patient.
11. See this diagnosis in Prolonged Immobility, Chapter 1.

NIC Activity Therapy; Teaching: Prescribed Activity/Exercise.

RISK FOR IMPAIRED SKIN INTEGRITY *related to impaired oxygen transport secondary to chronic anemia.*

Table 10-3   BLOOD AND BLOOD PRODUCTS*

Product	Volume	Infusion Time	Contents	Possible Complications
Whole blood (rarely used)	500 mL/unit	2 to 4 hours or <1 hour in emergency	All blood components. If fresh, processed with citrate-phosphate-dextrose	Hepatitis, transmission of HIV (human immunodeficiency virus), CMV (cytomegalovirus), EBV (Epstein-Barr virus), and other organisms; transfusion reactions: all types
Packed red blood cells (RBCs)	200-250 mL/unit	1 to 4 hours or <1 hour in emergency	RBCs	See Whole blood
Fresh-frozen plasma	200-250 mL/unit	20 minutes to thaw 0.5 to 1 hour or <0.5 hour in emergency	All clotting factors except platelets	See Whole blood
Platelets	35-50 mL/unit	Direct intravenous push at 30 to 50 mL/min; may combine or "pool" several bags into one; given in multiple units as quickly as possible	Platelets	Transfusion reaction: febrile or mild allergic; may need to premedicate with acetaminophen (Tylenol) or diphenhydramine HCl (Benadryl); rare instance of septic reaction
Cryoprecipitate	10-20 mL/unit	May need 10 to 30 units infused at 1 unit/min or 10-20 mL/min	Factor VIII, factor XIII, and fibrinogen	Small possibility of febrile or mild allergic reaction; rare instance of septic reaction
Granulocytes	300 mL/unit	1 to 2 hours; administer slowly for 5 minutes as test dose	White blood cells (WBCs) extracted from 1 unit of whole blood	Transfusion reactions: all types; often ineffective in elevating WBC count
Leukocyte-poor and washed, frozen RBCs	250-300 mL/unit	2 hours or 1 to 2 hours in emergency	Red cells washed with saline (and possibly irradiated) to remove WBCs and protein from RBCs	Markedly reduced possibility of transfusion reactions: all types
Factor VIII concentrate	10-20 mL/unit	May need >10 units infused at 1 unit/min	Factor VIII (pooled from possibly thousands of donors)	Small possibility of febrile or mild allergic reaction; rare instance of septic reaction
Factor IX concentrate	20-30 mL/unit	May need >10 units infused at 1 unit/min	Factor IX (pooled from possibly thousands of donors)	Small possibility of febrile or mild allergic reaction; rare instance of septic reaction
Volume expanders: Albumin (5% or 25%) Plasma protein fraction Salt-poor albumin	Varies with each product	1 mL/min or as rapidly as tolerated in shock states	Reconstituted from human blood, plasma, or serum	Possible hypervolemia with rapid infusions, particularly with 25% albumin

*Use correct filter with each blood product; most filters can be used to administer 2 to 4 units; either piggyback or flush products with normal saline solution *only.*

Goals/Outcomes: The patient's skin remains intact during hospitalization.

NOC Tissue Integrity: Skin and Mucous Membranes.

Pressure Management
1. Keep extremities warm to promote circulation and help prevent tissue hypoxia.
2. Perform a comprehensive appraisal of peripheral circulation (e.g., check peripheral pulses, edema, capillary refill, color, and temperature of extremity).
3. Monitor for sources of pressure and friction.
4. Monitor for infection, especially of edematous areas.
5. Use a bed cradle to reduce pressure of covers on extremities.
6. Monitor skin and mucous membranes for areas of discoloration and bruising.
7. Monitor skin for rashes, abrasions, excessive dryness, and moisture.
8. Provide adequate nutrition and nutrition supplements as appropriate. Negative nitrogen state or low serum protein or albumin increases the risk for skin breakdown.
9. Teach the patient the signs of skin breakdown, because it can occur at any time with chronic anemia.
10. Instruct the patient on the importance of preventing venous stasis.
11. Teach the patient about appropriate nutrition, as discussed in Nutrition Support, Chapter 1.
12. Apply appropriate skin-saving dressing (e.g., DuoDerm) or initiate aggressive skin care regimen to areas of breakdown.
13. For additional interventions, see Wound and Skin Care, Chapter 1.

NIC Pressure Ulcer Prevention; Skin Surveillance; Nutrition Management; Circulatory Precautions.

COLLABORATIVE MANAGEMENT: HEMOLYTIC CRISIS
CARE PRIORITIES
1. Oxygen therapy
Administered to relieve SOB or dyspnea. Methods of oxygen delivery range from nasal cannulas, to various face masks, to mechanical ventilation in severe cases.

2. Pain management
Aspirin, acetaminophen, NSAIDs, narcotics, and sedatives may be necessary for relief of pain and anxiety associated with hemolytic anemia, particularly during hemolytic crisis.

3. Volume replacement
If the patient is hypovolemic, aggressive fluid and/or blood replacement is mandatory to prevent profound hypotension and shock. Fluid challenges/boluses also assist in the prevention of deposition of hemolyzed RBCs in the microvasculature.

4. Transfusions/blood component replacement
Packed RBCs may be necessary in the management of profound anemia to help increase the oxygen-carrying capacity of the blood. For patients who refuse blood transfusions, aggressive strategies to augment RBC production such as IV iron therapy and subcutaneous administration of erythropoietin may be implemented. These therapies may take up to 7 days or longer to promote significant improvement in reticulocyte count and Hgb and Hct levels. The oxygen-carrying capacity of banked blood is best when used within 14 days of collection. Blood transfused more than 21 days after collection has been linked to increased mortality rates in the critically ill, especially patients who are HIV-positive. Benefits must be weighed against risks, particularly in patients who are immunosuppressed.

5. Red cell exchange therapy for sickle cell crisis
Cytapheresis procedure used to replace sickled RBCs with normal RBCs for patients who are unresponsive to other treatments for sickle cell disease.

6. Thrombocytapheresis
Cytapheresis procedure for patients experiencing symptoms of excessive thrombosis, to attempt rapid platelet reduction to decrease clotting before onset of MODS (see Multiple Organ

Dysfunction Syndrome in Systemic Inflammatory Response Syndrome, Sepsis, and Multiple Organ Dysfunction Syndrome, Chapter 11).

7. Therapeutic phlebotomy

Removal of 200 to 500 mL of whole blood from the patient when iron overload exists.

8. Corticosteroids

Therapy used with limited success in the management of hemolytic anemia.

9. Splenectomy

Removal of the spleen is sometimes recommended for patients suspected of having splenic sequestration crisis related to hemolytic anemia.

CARE PLANS FOR HEMOLYTIC CRISIS

INEFFECTIVE TISSUE PERFUSION: PERIPHERAL, CARDIOPULMONARY, GASTROINTESTINAL, RENAL, AND CEREBRAL *related to interruption of arterial or venous blood flow secondary to formation of microthrombi.*

Goals/Outcomes: Within 24 hours of institution of treatment, the patient has adequate perfusion, as evidenced by warm extremities, pink nail beds; peripheral pulses at least 2+ on a 0-to-4+ scale or the patient's baseline, capillary refill less than 2 seconds, BP within 10% of the patient's normal range (or systolic BP greater than 90 mm Hg), HR and RR within 10% of the patient's baseline (or HR 60 to 100 bpm, RR 12 to 20 breaths/min with a normal depth and pattern), oxygen saturation greater than 95%, urinary output 0.5 mL/kg/h or greater, and orientation to time, place, and person.
NOC Circulation Status.

Circulatory Care: Arterial Insufficiency
1. Initiate aggressive IV fluid volume replacement as prescribed to prevent deposition of hemolyzed RBCs in the microvasculature.
2. Assess extremities for inadequate peripheral perfusion: amplitude of peripheral pulses, coolness, pallor, and prolonged capillary refill. Use Doppler if unable to palpate pulses.
3. Evaluate chest pain. Note cardiac dysrhythmias and symptoms of decreased CO. Monitor respiratory status for symptoms of heart failure.
4. Monitor vital signs frequently for signs of impending shock: increased HR and RR, increased restlessness and anxiety, and cool and clammy skin, followed by a decrease in BP.
5. Monitor abdomen for signs of decreased perfusion.
6. Keep lower extremities elevated slightly to promote venous blood flow.
7. Monitor ventilation and perfusion: assess ABG values for acidosis (i.e., pH less than 7.35, hypercarbia/CO_2 retention [$PaCO_2$ greater than 45 mmHg]), indicating hypoperfusion, and respiratory insufficiency. Assess for hypoxemia using continuous pulse oximetry and $ScvO_2$ or SvO_2 monitoring to detect decreased oxygen saturation. Consult the advanced practice provider for sustained deterioration in status.
8. Monitor urinary output for decrease, which can signal decreased renal perfusion. Consult the advanced practice provider for urine output less than 0.5 mL/kg/h for 2 consecutive hours.
9. Monitor neurologic status every 2 to 4 hours, using the Glasgow Coma Scale (see Appendix 2).
10. Teach the patient and significant others about hemolytic anemia, including the signs of impending hemolytic crisis, rendering information on the following:
    • Indicators of impending hemolytic crisis: Fever, abnormal pain, headache, blurred vision, dizziness, change in mentation, unsteady gait, palpitations, paresthesias, and paralysis.
    • Support groups: Names, telephone numbers, and addresses of other persons/groups that can assist with support of people with hemolytic anemias.
    • Smoking cessation: Support groups and programs that assist in stopping cigarette smoking to decrease vasoconstriction associated with nicotine intake.
    • Medications: Drug name, dosage, frequency, and possible side effects, especially related to steroids: increased appetite, weight gain, "moon face," "buffalo hump," increased possibility of infection, headaches, and increased BP. Explain possible steroid-induced diabetes mellitus.
    • Prevention of infection: Important if the patient is on long-term steroid therapy or had a splenectomy. The patient should obtain an annual flu vaccine; practice good personal hygiene; obtain regular dental check-ups; and get adequate rest, sleep, and relaxation. For splenectomy, patients should have a pneumococcal vaccine and wear a medical-alert identification bracelet.

NIC Cardiac Care: Acute; Circulatory Care: Venous Insufficiency; Respiratory Monitoring; Shock Management: Cardiac; Cerebral Perfusion Promotion; Neurologic Monitoring; Peripheral Sensation Management; Fluid/Electrolyte Management; Fluid Management; Vital Signs Monitoring.

ACUTE PAIN *related to tissue ischemia secondary to vessel occlusion; inflammation/injury secondary to blood within the joints.*

Goals/Outcomes: Within 1 to 2 hours of initiating treatment, the patient's subjective evaluation of discomfort improves, as documented by a pain scale; nonverbal indicators of discomfort are reduced or absent.
NOC Pain Control; Pain Level.

Pain Management

1. Monitor the patient for signs of discomfort, including increases in HR, BP, and RR. Devise a pain scale with the patient, rating discomfort from 0 (no pain) to 10.
2. Perform a comprehensive assessment of pain to include location, characteristics, onset/duration, frequency, quality, intensity or severity of pain, and precipitating factors.
3. Medicate for pain as prescribed. Assess effectiveness of medication using the pain scale. Confer with the advanced practice provider if pain relief is ineffective; devise an alternate plan for analgesia.
4. Recognize that components of chronic and acute pain are present and tolerance may be higher than expected for age and size. During a crisis, exacerbation of pain may be unpredictable as a result of intermittent vessel occlusion, thus both baseline and breakthrough medications will be required to achieve pain relief.
5. If pain medication injections are frequent, consider an IV rather than an IM route, when possible.
6. Administer adjuvant analgesics and/or medications when needed to potentiate analgesia.
7. Consider continuous infusion (alone or with bolus opioids) to maintain serum levels.
8. Collaborate with the advanced practice provider if drug, dose, route of administration, or interval changes are indicated, making specific recommendations based on equianalgesic principles.
9. Consider complementary method of pain control such as relaxation techniques: guided imagery, controlled breathing, meditation, and listening to soft, soothing music. Use therapeutic/healing touch to relieve pain if the practitioner is trained and the patient agrees to participate. Alternatively, consult the trained practitioner.
10. Control environmental factors that may add to discomfort (e.g., room temperature, light, noise).
11. Apply warm compresses to joints to increase circulation and thereby improve tissue oxygenation.
12. Apply elastic stockings to promote venous return and enhance circulation.
13. Teach the patient to perform isometric or range-of-motion exercises to promote circulation.
14. Help allay fears by reassuring the patient that pain will decrease when the crisis subsides.
15. Provide emotional support to the patient during the crisis episode. Reassure the patient that the crisis is time-limited, and enable significant others to be with the patient, if possible, during the crisis.
16. Teach the patient to assess extremities daily for evidence of tissue breakdown or blood sequestration (i.e., swelling, erythema, tenderness) so that early interventions can be implemented in an attempt to prevent severe pain.

NIC Analgesic Administration; Medication Administration; Medication Administration: Intravenous (IV); Heat/Cold Application; Anxiety Reduction; Therapeutic Touch; Music Therapy; Meditation Facilitation.

RISK FOR DEFICIENT FLUID VOLUME *related to failure of renal regulatory mechanisms of fluid and electrolyte balance secondary to microthrombi occluding the nephrons.*

Goals/Outcomes: The patient's volume status returns to normal/baseline, as evidenced by urinary output greater than 0.5 mL/kg/h, stable weight, BP within the patient's normal range, HR 60 to 100 bpm, RR 12 to 20 breaths/min, good skin turgor, moist mucous membranes, urine specific gravity 1.005 to 1.025, and central venous pressure (CVP) 4 to 6 mm Hg.
NOC Fluid Balance; Electrolyte and Acid-Base Balance.

Fluid/Electrolyte Management

1. Monitor intake and output (I&O) hourly. Consult the advanced practice provider for a urinary output less than 0.5 mL/kg/h for 4 consecutive hours. Insert urinary catheter if patient is unable to void.
2. Monitor and document HR, rhythm, pulses, and BP.
3. Evaluate efficacy of volume expansion by closely monitoring CVP. Overzealous volume expansion can lead to heart failure and pulmonary edema, with CVP greater than 20% to 25% of normal values.

4. Administer diuretics as prescribed in the well-hydrated patient with urine output less than 0.5 mL/kg/h.
5. Assess the patient for volume depletion, including poor skin turgor, dry mucous membranes, hypotension, tachycardia, and decreasing urine output and CVP.
6. Monitor electrolytes and serum osmolality. A universal increase in electrolytes and osmolality is indicative of dehydration. A universal decrease signals fluid overload.
7. Assess pH (normal range is 7.35 to 7.45) before replacing electrolytes. Acidosis and alkalosis alter electrolyte values. Replace potassium if the pH is outside the normal range.

NIC Electrolyte Monitoring; Fluid Management; Fluid Monitoring; Intravenous (IV) Therapy; Hypervolemia Management; Shock Management: Volume.

ADDITIONAL NURSING DIAGNOSES

Uncontrolled pain, bleeding, and complications of hemolysis can be terrifying to the patient and significant others, who may fear that the patient will die. Chronic illness with episodic acute exacerbations may require more individualized intervention when handling long-term illness and its sequelae. See Emotional Support of Patient and Significant Others, Chapter 2.

BLEEDING AND THROMBOTIC DISORDERS
PATHOPHYSIOLOGY

Bleeding can result from qualitative (dysfunctional) or quantitative (lack of) abnormalities of platelets and/or coagulation factors, including proteins, in the plasma. Thrombocytopenia is common in the critically ill and, like anemia, necessitates differential diagnosis. The cause of thrombocytopenia, rather than simply the decreased numbers of platelets, poses the greatest threat to the patient who is critically ill. The four main causes of thrombocytopenia are as follows:

1. Hemodilution: Related to administration of large amounts of retained fluids, IV fluids, multiple medications given in 50- to 100-mL "piggybacks," or blood/blood products.
2. Increased platelet destruction or consumption: Includes heparin-induced thrombocytopenia (HIT); antiphospholipid antibody syndrome or lupus anticoagulant syndrome; idiopathic thrombocytopenic purpura (ITP); thrombotic thrombocytopenic purpura (TTP); hemolytic-uremic syndrome; febrile reactions; severe sepsis; and hemolysis, elevated liver enzymes, and low platelet count (HELLP) syndrome. Disseminated intravascular coagulation (DIC) presents with a combined coagulopathy and platelet consumption.
3. Platelet sequestration: Related to hypersplenism and hypothermia.
4. Decreased production of platelets: Caused by alcohol (EtOH) abuse, bone marrow irradiation, bone marrow/stem cell disease, graft-versus-host disease, aplastic anemia, vitamin B_{12} or folate deficiencies, metastatic carcinoma, some renal diseases, leukemia, and myeloproliferative disorders.

Platelet destruction may be mediated by congenital autoimmune or alloimmune disorders, or by acquired immunologic or nonimmunologic mechanisms. Causative or related factors include septicemia, systemic inflammatory response syndrome (SIRS), pulmonary hypertension, extracorporeal circulation, thrombotic disorders, acute transplant rejection, severe allergic reactions, rheumatic disorders, intravascular catheters and prosthetics, fat emboli, acute respiratory distress syndrome, and HIV infection. The most significant diagnostic finding associated with severe thrombocytopenia is the presence of petechiae in dependent areas (i.e., back, ankles, posterior thighs of patients who are bedridden). Larger purpura such as ecchymoses and hematomas may also be present but are nonspecific for diagnosis of platelet disorders. Patients must be assessed for risk of bleeding with thrombocytopenia, considering the severity and cause as well as comorbid factors.

Coagulopathies leading to bleeding (with/without associated thrombi) may be caused by liver disease, vitamin K deficiency, pregnancy-induced hypertension associated with HELLP syndrome, or other defects of blood coagulation factors, such as hemophilia, Von Willebrand disease, and DIC.

Patients prone to thromboembolic conditions include those with platelet abnormalities, including thrombocytosis, diabetes mellitus, hyperlipidemia, heparin-induced thrombocytopenia, systemic lupus erythematosus; blood vessel defects, including venous disease/stasis, roughened surface of vascular endothelium (seen with arteriosclerosis, trauma, severe sepsis, SIRS, or infection), atrial fibrillation, grafts or other devices in place, hyperviscosity, TTP, hemolytic uremic syndrome, vasculitis; and those with systemic illness and conditions, including long bone fractures, orthopedic surgery, abdominal surgery, malignancy, pregnancy or postpartum (risk of venous thromboembolism is five times higher than for nonpregnant women), oral contraceptives, nephrotic syndrome, inflammatory bowel disease, slow/stagnant blood flow through the vessels (e.g., shock states, severe peripheral vascular disease), infusion of prothrombin complex, and sickle cell disease.

When patients are evaluated for a bleeding disorder, the process should include evaluation of platelets, deficiency of a single coagulation factor (factors VII, VIII, IX, X, or XI) or multiple coagulation factors, for endogenous or exogenous antibiotics in the circulation, and consumptive coagulopathy (e.g., ITP, TTP, vasculitis, hemolytic uremic syndrome, paroxysmal nocturnal hematuria, obstetric complication, trauma, liver disease). Adequate levels of calcium and vitamin K are also needed for adequate function of the clotting cascade.

Those suspected of having thromboembolic disease may require evaluation of coagulation factors, circulating antibodies, abnormal proteins (deficient protein C or S), and other endogenous chemicals.

Normal blood coagulation is activated most often as a result of injury to blood vessels, causing the following series of events:

1. Reflex vasoconstriction: Vascular spasm that decreases blood flow to the site of injury.
2. Platelet aggregation: Accumulation of platelets that leads to formation of a platelet plug to help support the repair of the injury. If the damage to the vessel is small, the plug is sufficient to seal the injury. If the hole is large, a blood clot is necessary to stop the bleeding.
3. Activation of plasma clotting factors: Stimulation of factors that leads to the formation of a fibrin clot. The pathways that initiate clotting factors (Figure 10-3) include the following:
   a. Intrinsic system: Initiated by "contact activation" subsequent to an endothelial injury. The problem is "intrinsic" to the circulation, or begins with an injury to the blood or circulatory system.
   b. Extrinsic system: Initiated by tissue thromboplastin released from injured tissue. The problem is "extrinsic" to the circulation, or begins with an injury to tissue rather than within the blood system.
   c. Common pathway: The final part of the coagulation system, which completes the clot formation process begun by either the intrinsic or extrinsic pathway.

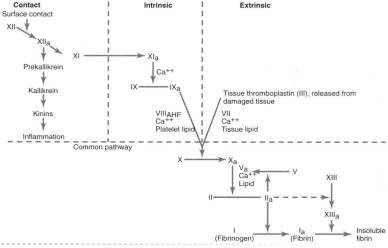

Figure 10-3 Coagulation pathway. (From Janz TG, Hamilton GC: Disorders of hemostasis. In Marx J, Hockberger R, Walls R, editors: *Rosen's emergency medicine: concepts and clinical practice*, ed 7, St Louis, 2009, Mosby.)

d. Clot retraction: Several minutes after its formation, the clot contracts for 30 to 60 minutes to express most of the fluid from within the clot. The expressed fluid is called *serum*, because most of the clotting factors have been used or removed via the clot formation process. Serum is unable to clot. The absence of clotting factors differentiates serum from plasma.

4. Growth of fibrous tissue: Rubbery tissue that completes the clot within approximately 7 to 10 days after injury. This process results in permanent closure of the vessel injury. Both the intrinsic and extrinsic pathways are activated after rupture of a blood vessel. Tissue thromboplastin from the vessel initiates the extrinsic pathway, whereas contact of factor XII and platelets with the injured vessel wall traumatizes the blood and initiates the intrinsic pathway. The extrinsic pathway is able to form clots in as little as 15 seconds with severe trauma, whereas the intrinsic pathway requires 2 to 6 minutes for clot formation. Both are necessary to maintain clot.

HEPARIN-INDUCED THROMBOCYTOPENIA
PATHOPHYSIOLOGY

Heparin is the most widely used IV anticoagulant and one of the most frequently prescribed drugs in the United States. Heparin prevents the conversion of fibrinogen to fibrin. HIT, also called heparin-induced thrombocytopenic thrombosis (HITT), white clot syndrome, or heparin-associated thrombocytopenia (HAT), types I and II, occurs when heparin therapy causes either a mild to moderate (i.e., HAT type I) or severe (i.e., HAT type II) decrease in the number of freely circulating platelets. Platelets in affected patients exhibit unusual aggregation and can result in heparin resistance, arterial and venous thrombosis, and subsequent emboli in extreme cases (Figure 10-4). Depending on the source of the heparin received, HIT is reported in approximately 5% of all patients receiving heparin. Bovine (beef-based) heparin has been associated with HIT more frequently than other heparins. It is estimated that as many as 50% of patients on heparin may be asymptomatic but generate antibodies to heparin-platelet factor 4 (H-PF4), which increases the risk of HIT on their next exposure to heparin. HIT is not related to the heparin dose and has been seen in patients receiving low-dose subcutaneous heparin, as well as in patients receiving simple heparin "flushes" to maintain patency of IV lines.

Two types of HIT have been described:

- Mild to moderate, low morbidity: Generally occurs 1 to 2 days after initiation of heparin. It may resolve within 5 days after symptoms begin. Platelets may decrease to levels as low as 100,000/mm^3 or may remain in the low-normal range. No treatment is required, and heparin therapy may be continued if the patient is asymptomatic.
- High morbidity (immune-mediated): Generally begins 5 to 7 days after initiation of heparin. Symptoms persist until heparin is discontinued. Platelets decrease to less than 100,000/mm^3. Thrombosis with subsequent embolization and bleeding is apparent. Complications may include pulmonary emboli, myocardial infarction, cerebral infarction, and circulatory impairment resulting in limb amputations. Mortality rate is 29%. Overall, 0.6% of all patients receiving heparin therapy develop thromboembolization.

ASSESSMENT
GOAL OF SYSTEM ASSESSMENT

Evaluate for increased risk of inappropriate bleeding or clotting as a result of qualitative or quantitative dysfunction of platelets and clotting factors.

RISK FACTORS
Previous drug-induced or immunologic thrombocytopenia.

VITAL SIGNS
Tachypnea, tachycardia, hypertension.

OBSERVATION
Patients may present with high or low acuity states. Those without clinical symptoms with a slight decrease in platelets are much easier to manage than patients with severe, high

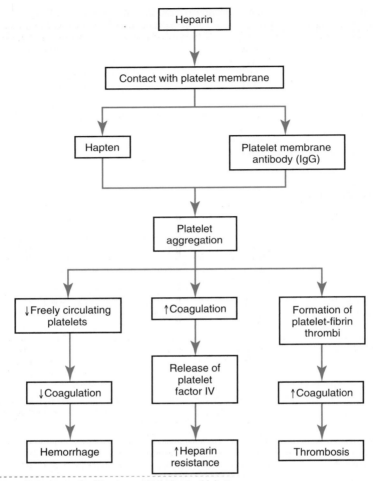

Figure 10-4 Heparin-induced thrombocytopenia. *IgG,* Immunoglobulin G.

morbidity. Extreme cases manifest arterial thrombosis of the distal aorta and proximal lower limb arteries. High morbidity patients present with:

- Petechiae, purpura, ecchymosis, gingival bleeding, hemoptysis, epistaxis, bruising from mucosal surfaces or wounds.
- Signs of arterial occlusion: cold, pulseless extremities.
- Paresthesias; paralysis.
- Severe chest pain and SOB, indicative of myocardial ischemia.
- Diminished LOC, indicative of cerebral ischemia.

PALPATION

- Bone tenderness (especially rib and sternal areas).
- Enlargement of the liver and/or spleen.
- Joint tenderness.
- Enlargement of the liver and/or spleen.
- Abdominal tenderness.

Diagnostic Tests for Heparin-induced Thrombocytopenia

Test	Purpose	Abnormal Findings
Platelet count	Used to diagnose bleeding disorders or bone marrow disease	Mild to moderate: 100,000 to 150,000/mm^3; severe: <100,000/mm^3 caused by severe clumping or aggregation of platelets
Bleeding time	Measures how quickly blood clots, using platelets, coagulation factors, and small vessel vasospasm	Prolonged if platelets are <100,000/mm^3
Platelet antibody screen	Identifies antibodies against platelets	Positive findings because of the presence of immunoglobulin G platelet antibodies
Coagulation screening (prothrombin time [PT]; partial thromboplastin time [PTT], thromboplastin time)	PT: extrinsic pathway (Coumadin) PTT: intrinsic pathway (Heparin)	Normal, because the clotting factors that govern these test results are normal
Fibrinogen	Measures clot formation ability: May be ordered as a follow-up to an abnormal PT or PTT and/or an episode of prolonged or unexplained bleeding	May be low-normal or low as a result of increased consumption. Normal is 200 to 400 mg/dL
Fibrin degradation products (FDPs), fibrin split products (FSP), fibrin breakdown products	Measures fibrin degradation products (which result from clots dissolving) in blood	Elevated to ≥40 µg/mL as a result of fibrinolysis of platelet-fibrin thrombi Normal is <10 µg/mL
Platelet aggregation	Measures the rate and degree to which platelets form a clump	Results will be >100% (or high value of specific laboratory) because of release of platelet membrane antibody leading to "clumping"
Heparin-induced platelet aggregation	Adds patient platelet-poor plasma (as a source of immunoglobulin) to normal platelet-rich plasma in the presence of heparin to induce platelet aggregation	Reflects abnormal aggregation curve with a decrease in the optical density in the aggregometer
Serotonin release testing and ELISA heparin PF4	Detects the presence of antibodies to PF4/heparin/TSP-1 complexes	Helps in the differential diagnosis of heparin-induced thrombocytopenia
Bone marrow aspiration	Evaluates bone marrow status; diagnoses blood disorders and determines if cancer or infection has spread to the bone marrow	Normal or increased number of megakaryocytes (platelet precursors), indicative of normal production of platelets or increased response to need for platelets

COLLABORATIVE MANAGEMENT

CARE PRIORITIES

1. Screen preheparin platelet count, and monitor platelets and amount of heparin needed
A preheparin platelet count is made to establish baseline values. Daily platelet counts should be done for at least the first 4 days of heparin therapy. Subsequent counts are made every 2 days. If increasing amounts of heparin are needed to maintain therapeutic levels (i.e., partial thromboplastin time [PTT] 40 to 60 seconds), heparin resistance should be suspected, which sometimes precedes HIT (see Figure 10-4).

- Consider stopping heparin therapy: If the platelet count is greater than 100,000/mm^3 and the patient is symptom-free, heparin is sometimes continued, but an alternate thrombin inhibitor may be recommended. Oral anticoagulation should begin immediately, if possible. If the platelet count is less than 100,000/mm³ and the patient develops bleeding or thrombosis, heparin must be discontinued immediately (including heparin flushes), alternate anticoagulant initiated, and subsequent complications managed when they occur. Use of low-molecular-weight heparins is contraindicated.

2. Administer defibrinogenating agents if high morbidity symptoms are present
Ancrod (Arvin) may be given to reduce the possibility of thrombosis.

3. Prevent pulmonary emboli with a vena cava filter
If the patient experiences thrombosis with a decrease or loss of perfusion to an extremity, the physician or midlevel practitioner may consider surgical insertion of a vena cava filter to reduce the risk of pulmonary emboli caused by clot migration from an extremity. See Pulmonary Embolus, Chapter 4.
- Warfarin, thrombolytics, and platelet inhibitors: Streptokinase, urokinase, and alteplase (recombinant tissue plasminogen activator [rtPA]) have been used successfully to manage pulmonary emboli in HIT.

4. Maintain anticoagulation, if needed, with a direct thrombin inhibitor
Argatroban and hirudin, direct thrombin inhibitors, block thrombin generation needed for fibrin formation. They may be used alone or in combination with warfarin, as an alternate anticoagulation strategy for patients with HIT. Ximelagatran is the first orally available thrombin inhibitor. Bivalirudin is not licensed for use with HIT but can be used in patients undergoing percutaneous coronary interventions. If the patient needs further anticoagulation, warfarin sodium (Coumadin) should be considered. Platelet inhibitors are contraindicated as a result of current platelet dysfunction.

5. Consider use of newer anticoagulation agents in those who are difficult to manage
New medications using recombinant DNA technology focus on each step of the coagulation process; many are under development. These agents are grouped into three stages of coagulation: initiation, propagation, and fibrin formation. Tissue factor pathway inhibitor, nematode anticoagulant peptide, and factor VIIa target initiation of coagulation. Soluble thrombomodulin, drotrecogin alfa (activated protein C), protein C concentrate, fondaparinux, and idraparinux inhibit clot propagation. Direct thrombin inhibitors (antithrombins) block fibrin formation for clot completion.

6. Provide platelet transfusions for high morbidity patients who continue to bleed
May be initiated after heparin therapy is discontinued if bleeding fails to subside.

7. Provide plasma exchange for high morbidity patients who fail to respond to other therapies
In severe cases, 2 to 3 L of plasma is removed and replaced with albumin, crystalloids, or fresh-frozen plasma to assist in decreasing bleeding by removing bound heparin from the body.

CARE PLANS: HEPARIN-INDUCED THROMBOCYTOPENIA

INEFFECTIVE PROTECTION *related to decreased platelet count with risk of bleeding and thromboembolization.*

Goals/Outcomes: Within 24 hours of discontinuing heparin therapy, the patient exhibits no signs of new bleeding, bruising, or thrombosis, as evidenced by HR 60 to 100 bpm or within 10% of the patient's baseline, RR 12 to 20 breaths/min with normal depth and pattern, systolic BP at least 90 mm Hg, and all peripheral pulses at the patient's baseline or greater than 2+ on a 0-to-4+ scale.
NOC Blood Coagulation.

Bleeding Precautions
1. Assess the patient at least every 2 hours for signs of bleeding, including hemoptysis, ecchymosis, petechiae on dependent areas, gastrointestinal (GI) bleeding, hematuria, and bleeding from invasive procedure sites or

mucous membranes. Monitor the patient closely for hemorrhage. Note Hgb and Hct levels before and after blood loss, and at least daily as indicated.

2. Assess for signs of internal bleeding including tachycardia and dysrhythmias, tachypnea and hypotension. Sustained increase in HR and RR or ECG changes, such as ST segment depression or elevation, may precede hypotension.

3. Protect the patient from trauma that may cause bleeding. Do not use rectal temperatures to monitor for fever. Avoid IM injections and venous and arterial punctures as possible until bleeding time normalizes.

4. Perform a comprehensive assessment of peripheral circulation (e.g., check peripheral pulses, edema, capillary refill, and color and temperature of extremities) at least every 2 hours and assess the patient for signs of thrombosis, including decreased peripheral pulses, altered sensation in extremities (i.e., paresthesias, numbness), pallor, coolness, cyanosis, or capillary refill time more than 2 seconds. Monitor extremities for areas of heat, pain, redness, or swelling.

5. Maintain adequate hydration to prevent increased blood viscosity and to help prevent constipation.

6. Administer stool softeners to help reduce straining with bowel movements, which may prompt rectal bleeding.

7. Monitor platelet count daily for significant changes. Consult the advanced practice provider for values that remain less than 150,000/mm^3 or below the patient's baseline.

8. Monitor heparin dosage carefully. If increasing doses are required to maintain a therapeutic level (PTT 40 to 60 seconds or 2 to 2.5 times the patient's baseline), consult the advanced practice provider regarding possible heparin resistance, an early indicator of HIT. If heparin has been discontinued and new anticoagulants initiated, monitor appropriate values. If a direct thrombin inhibitor (e.g., Argatroban) is used alone, or in combination with warfarin, monitor prothrombin time (PT) and international normalized ratio (INR).

9. Assess the patient's neurologic status hourly if platelet count decreases to less than 30,000.

10. Monitor for signs of MODS secondary to thrombosis or prolonged hypotension, if the patient has hemorrhaged. (See Systemic Inflammatory Response Syndrome, Sepsis, and Multiple Organ Dysfunction Syndrome, SIRS, Chapter 11.)

11. Teach the patient and significant others about the basic pathophysiology of HIT, and instruct them to report this problem to all subsequent healthcare providers. Teach the patient to wear a medical-alert bracelet to alert healthcare providers if the patient becomes unable to speak.

NIC Surveillance: Safety; Vital Signs Monitoring.

DEFICIENT FLUID VOLUME (OR RISK FOR SAME) *related to active blood loss*

Goals/Outcomes: The patient becomes normovolemic within 24 hours of onset of treatment, as evidenced by HR within the patient's normal range or 60 to 100 bpm, RR 12 to 20 breaths/min with normal depth and pattern and urinary output at least 0.5 mL/kg/h, and absence of abdominal discomfort, back pain, or pain from invasive procedure sites.

NOC Fluid Balance.

Hypovolemia Management

1. Monitor the patient for signs of hypovolemia, including increased HR and RR, decreased BP, increased restlessness or fatigue, and decreased urine output.

2. Administer supplemental oxygen if the patient is actively bleeding.

3. Maintain accurate I&O record. Weigh daily and monitor trends.

4. Assess for intraabdominal bleeding: Note any abdominal pain, tenderness, guarding, or back pain.

5. Check excretions for occult blood, and observe for blood in emesis, sputum, feces, urine, nasogastric drainage, and wound drainage as appropriate.

6. Instruct the patient and/or family on the need for blood replacement as appropriate.

7. Replace lost volume with plasma expanders (e.g., albumin, hetastarch) or blood products as indicated. See Table 10-3 for more information.

NIC Electrolyte Management; Fluid Management; Fluid Monitoring; Intravenous (IV) Therapy; Bleeding Reduction: Gastrointestinal; Shock Management: Volume; Blood Products Administration.

ADDITIONAL NURSING DIAGNOSES

Uncontrolled bleeding or thrombotic complications can be terrifying for the patient and significant others, who may fear that the patient will die. See nursing diagnoses and interventions in Emotional and Spiritual Support of the Patient and Significant Others, Chapter 2.

IMMUNE THROMBOCYTOPENIA PURPURA

PATHOPHYSIOLOGY

Immune (often idiopathic) thrombocytopenia purpura (ITP) is a disorder characterized by premature platelet destruction as well as impaired platelet production, resulting in a decrease in the platelet count to below 100,000/mm³. Normal platelet life span averages 1 to 3 weeks, whereas in ITP the platelet life span averages 1 to 3 days because of the presence of antiplatelet IgG and IgM antibodies, which destroy platelets in the reticuloendothelial system of the spleen. The coagulopathy is believed to be an autoimmune response and manifests as both an acute and a chronic problem.

Acute ITP is primarily a childhood disease, characterized by an abrupt onset of severe thrombocytopenia with evident purpura. Usually it occurs within 21 days following a viral infection. At the onset, platelets decrease to less than 20,000/mm³. The chronic form is typically a disease of adults aged 20 to 50 years, but it has occurred in a small percentage of children and older adults. The chronic disease rarely resolves spontaneously, sometimes responds to treatment of the underlying disorder, and usually is not associated with infection but can be related to autoimmune disorders (e.g., systemic lupus erythematosus, rheumatoid arthritis) and neoplastic disorders (e.g., chronic lymphocytic leukemia, lymphoma). Women are affected three times more often than men. Petechiae and purpura are commonly seen on the distal upper and lower extremities. Patients may feel symptom-free until actual bleeding begins. Intracranial hemorrhage is a potential complication. Platelet counts decrease to as low as 5000/mm³ in some patients, but may be as high as 75,000/mm³ in others.

ASSESSMENT

GOAL OF SYSTEM ASSESSMENT

Evaluate for increased risk of inappropriate bleeding or clotting as a result of qualitative or quantitative dysfunction of platelets and clotting factors.

RISK FACTORS

- Acute ITP: History of antecedent viral infection occurring approximately 3 weeks before the hemorrhagic episode.
- Chronic ITP: Insidious and sometimes associated with autoimmune hemolytic anemia, HIV disease, hemophilia, lymphoma, chronic lymphocytic leukemia, systemic lupus erythematosus, sarcoidosis, high-titer anticardiolipin antibodies, pregnancy, malabsorption, and thyrotoxicosis. The cause is often unknown.

VITAL SIGNS

- Tachypnea, tachycardia, hypotension, fever.

OBSERVATION

- Petechiae, purpura, bruising on skin and mucous membranes, prolonged bleeding; intracranial hemorrhage occurs in less than 1% of patients if the thrombocytopenia is severe.
- Diminished LOC, indicative of intracranial hemorrhage.
- Epistaxis, gingival bleeding, GI, genitourinary (GU), gynecologic (GYN) bleeding such as increased menstrual flow.
- Retinal disturbances.

PALPATION

- Enlargement of the liver and/or spleen.
- Lymphadenopathy, hepatomegaly, splenomegaly.
- Joint tenderness.

Diagnostic Tests for Immune Thrombocytopenia Purpura

Test	Purpose	Abnormal Findings
Platelet count	Used to diagnose bleeding disorders or bone marrow disease	Decreased to 5000 to 75,000/mm³ (or lower) because of premature destruction Normal range is 150,000 to 400,000/mm³
Bleeding time	Measures how quickly blood clots, using platelets, coagulation factors, and small vessel vasospasm	Prolonged if platelets are less than 100,000/mm³
Platelet antibody screen	Identifies antibodies against platelets	Positive findings because of the presence of immunoglobulins G and M antiplatelet antibodies
Coagulation screening (prothrombin time [PT]; partial thromboplastin time [PTT]; thromboplastin time)	PT: extrinsic pathway (Coumadin) PTT: intrinsic pathway (Heparin)	Normal, because these tests measure nonplatelet components of the coagulation pathway
Complete blood count with differential	Measures red blood cells, white blood cells (WBCs), platelets, and the WBC differential	Decreased hemoglobin and hematocrit resulting from insidious blood loss or simultaneous hemolytic anemia (Evans syndrome) Normal WBC count: Unless idiopathic thrombocytopenic purpura is associated with another disease impacting differential leukocyte count
Capillary-fragility test: Rumpel-Leede capillary-fragility test	Method to determine a patient's hemorrhagic tendency: Assesses fragility of capillary walls: Used to identify thrombocytopenia. Seldom used in current practice, but may be used to discern from damage as a result of prolonged cuff inflation in patients with blood dyscrasias	Will show >1+, which signals that more than 11 petechiae were present in a 2.5-cm radial area on the skin after prolonged application of a blood pressure cuff Normal is 1+ or <10 petechiae
Bone marrow aspiration	Evaluates bone marrow status; diagnoses blood disorders and determines if cancer or infection has spread to the bone marrow	Biopsy will reveal megakaryocytes (platelet precursors) in normal or increased numbers with a "nonbudding" appearance, possibly indicating defective maturation or failure of platelet production

COLLABORATIVE MANAGEMENT: IMMUNE THROMBOCYTOPENIC PURPURA

CARE PRIORITIES

1. Suppress immune response to reduce platelet destruction

- Corticosteroid therapy: Adrenocorticosteroids (e.g., prednisone 1 to 2 mg/kg/day) are effective in increasing the platelet count in 1 to 3 weeks after initiation of treatment. Effectiveness is attributed to suppression of phagocytic activity of the macrophage system (particularly the spleen), which increases the life span of the antibody-coated platelets. If improvement does not occur within 2 to 3 weeks, excessive doses of steroids are required, or if patient cannot tolerate tapering of steroids, splenectomy should be considered. "Normal" responders are able to have steroid dosage tapered over several weeks until platelets reach a sustained value of 50,000/mm³. Relapse during or after tapering prednisone is a common occurrence.
- IV immunoglobulin (IVIG): Given at 400 mg/kg/day for 2 to 5 consecutive days, resulting in increased platelet count in 60% to 70% of patients. Serum sickness (fever, chills, rash) is not uncommon between 9 and 14 days. It is less effective in patients with long-standing chronic ITP. The platelet level at initiation of treatment and incidence of serum sickness is not necessarily correlated to individual response. Duration of response may be longest in individuals who achieve the highest initial platelet increases.

- Danazol: 400 to 800 mg/day has resulted in complete remission or partial improvement in 60% to 70% of patients in several studies. Use is controversial because other researchers have reported poor results and many untoward side effects.
- Splenectomy: Treatment of choice in cases refractory to corticosteroid therapy. The condition stabilizes in 60% to 70% of patients who undergo splenectomy. The positive results are attributed to the removal of the site of destruction of the antibody-sensitized platelets. Prospective splenectomy candidates should have pneumococcal, meningococcal, and *Haemophilus influenzae* type B vaccinations before a planned splenectomy, to reduce the risk of postoperative infection with these organisms.
- Immunosuppression: Various immunosuppressive drugs, including azathioprine, cyclophosphamide, methotrexate, vincristine, and cyclosporine, given alone or in combination with prednisone, have been used successfully in limited situations. A trial of immunosuppression therapy may be indicated in patients who fail to respond to splenectomy or in those who are too unstable to be surgical candidates.
- Anti-Rh immunoglobulin: Low dose (200 to 1000 μg) given IV for 1 to 5 days has been effective in limited studies. Success of treatment is attributed to sensitization of recipient RBCs, which results in low-grade hemolysis and blockade of the platelet destruction by the reticuloendothelial system.
- Colchicine: A small percentage of patients refractory to other treatments may improve with 1.2 mg colchicine daily for 2 weeks or longer. The drug has been used successfully in limited studies.
- Plasmapheresis: Several days of machine-assisted plasma exchange to remove approximately 1 to 1.5 times the total plasma volume per procedure and replace it with a suitable solution (e.g., colloids, crystalloids, plasma). Therapy is reserved for patients with life-threatening hemorrhage unresponsive to other measures. It is costly and of marginal benefit.

2. Increase platelet count

- Romiplostim: A treatment approved for use in patients with chronic ITP who are refractory to corticosteroids, immunoglobulins, or splenectomy. A thrombopoietin receptor agonist that stimulates bone marrow megakaryocytes to increase platelet production; 1 μg/kg is given as a subcutaneous injection once weekly, titrated to a maximum dose of 10 μg/kg to achieve a platelet count of greater than 50,000. Rare side effects include bone marrow fibrosis and reticulin formation.
- Platelet transfusions: Platelets are given only in cases of life-threatening hemorrhage. The shortened platelet life span renders prophylactic transfusions ineffective.
- Vinca "alkaloid-loaded" platelets: Transfusions of platelets "loaded" with vinblastine may reduce the phagocytic destruction of platelets in patients who fail to respond to other treatments.
- Rituximab: Primary monoclonal antibody used to treat lymphoma, now showing promise in treatment of ITP.

CARE PLANS FOR IMMUNE THROMBOCYTOPENIC PURPURA

INEFFECTIVE PROTECTION *related to decreased platelet count, resulting in increased risk of bleeding.*

- -

Goals/Outcomes: Within 72 hours of onset of treatment, the patient exhibits no clinical signs of new bleeding or bruising episodes. Secretions and excretions are negative for blood, and vital signs are within 10% of the patient's normal range. Within the 24-hour period before discharge from intensive care, the patient and significant others verbalize understanding of the indicators of potential or actual bleeding.

NOC Blood Coagulation.

Bleeding Precautions

1. Monitor the patient for bleeding and hemorrhage, including elevated HR and RR, decreasing BP, oozing from invasive procedure sites, bleeding mucous membranes, hematuria, and GU, GYN, and GI bleeding. Note Hgb and Hct levels before and after blood loss, as indicated.
2. Protect the patient from trauma that may cause bleeding. Avoid taking rectal temperatures.
3. Maintain fluid intake to prevent constipation and administer stool softeners to minimize straining.
4. Monitor skin or mucous membranes for pallor, discoloration, bruising, breakdown, and erythema.

5. Monitor coagulation studies, including PT, PTT, fibrinogen, fibrin degradation products (FDPs), fibrin split products (FSPs), and platelet counts as appropriate.
6. Consult the advanced practice provider for sustained low platelet values (less than 100,000/mm³ or as appropriate for the individual).
7. Avoid administering NSAIDs (e.g., aspirin, ibuprofen). Teach the patient to avoid all medications that potentially decrease platelet aggregation, especially aspirin or aspirin-containing products.
8. For severe menorrhagia, confer with the advanced practice provider regarding the need for progestational hormones for suppression of menses. Assess blood loss by weighing perineal pads or tampons.
9. During the acute (bleeding) phase of ITP, teach the patient to perform oral hygiene using sponge-tipped applicators soaked in water or dilute mouthwash to help prevent gum bleeding. Avoid hydrogen peroxide or lemon-coated swabs.
10. Teach the patient that it is always safer to use an electric razor for shaving.
11. Instruct family member/caregiver about signs of skin breakdown, as appropriate.
12. Teach the patient and significant others to recognize the signs of impending hemorrhage: more rapid pulse and breathing, easy bruising, painful joints, and blood in sputum, urine, or stool.

NIC Skin Surveillance.

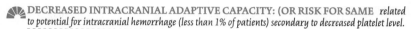 **DECREASED INTRACRANIAL ADAPTIVE CAPACITY: (OR RISK FOR SAME** *related to potential for intracranial hemorrhage (less than 1% of patients) secondary to decreased platelet level.*

Goals/Outcomes: Throughout the hospitalization, the patient remains free of symptoms of intracranial hemorrhage, as evidenced by orientation to time, place, and person; normoreactive pupils and reflexes; the patient's normal visual acuity, motor strength, and coordination; and absence of headache and other clinical indicators of increased intracranial pressure.
NOC Neurologic Status.

Neurologic Monitoring
1. Assess the patient for initial signs of increased intracranial pressure, including diminished LOC, headaches, pupillary responses (e.g., unequal, sluggish/absent response to light), visual disturbances, weakness and paralysis, slow HR, and change in respiratory rate and pattern.
2. Monitor trend of Glasgow Coma Scale (Appendix 2), intracranial pressure, and cerebral perfusion pressure.
3. Increase frequency of neurologic monitoring as appropriate.
4. Avoid activities that increase intracranial pressure (i.e., Valsalva maneuver, hyperthermia, pain, etc.). Administer stool softeners and cough suppressants as prescribed.
5. If initial signs of increased intracranial pressure are noted, consult the physician immediately. Severe intracranial bleeding can lead to herniation. Intracranial pressure can increase rapidly with severe bleeding, sometimes causing death within 1 hour of onset. Signs of impending herniation include unconsciousness, failure to respond to deeply painful stimuli, decorticate or decerebrate posturing, Cushing's triad (i.e., bradycardia, increased systolic BP, widening pulse pressure), nonreactive/fixed pupils, unequal pupils, or fixed and dilated pupils. See Traumatic Brain Injury, Chapter 3 for more information about herniation.
6. Consult with the advanced practice provider regarding management of increased intracranial pressure (see Traumatic Brain Injury, Chapter 3, for collaborative interventions for increased intracranial pressure). For additional interventions for increased intracranial pressure, see Box 3-7.
7. Teach the patient to avoid Valsalva maneuver (e.g., straining at stool or when lifting; forceful and sustained coughing or nose blowing), which could cause intracranial bleeding.
8. Teach the importance of avoiding tobacco products (particularly cigarettes) and excessive caffeine, which may cause vasoconstriction. Constricted vessels may prevent platelets from circulating through portions of the capillary network.

NIC Cerebral Edema Management; Cerebral Perfusion Promotion; Intracranial Pressure Monitoring; Neurologic Monitoring.

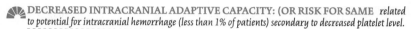 **RISK FOR DEFICIENT FLUID VOLUME** *related to active loss secondary to intraabdominal bleeding or postsplenectomy intraabdominal bleeding.*

Goals/Outcomes: The patient remains normovolemic, as evidenced by HR, RR, and BP within 10% of the patient's normal range (or HR 60 to 100 bpm, RR 12 to 20 breaths/min with normal depth and pattern, systolic BP ≥90 mm Hg); urinary output at least 0.5 mL/kg/h; and absence of abdominal pain or tenderness, back pain, and frank bleeding from the splenectomy incision.
NOC Fluid Balance.

Fluid Management

1. Monitor fluid status, including I&O, and signs of hypovolemia, including increases in HR and RR and decreases in BP, and urinary output, restlessness, fatigue, and orthostatic vital signs.
2. Inspect for bleeding from mucous membranes, bruising after minimal trauma, oozing from puncture sites, and presence of petechiae. Maintain patent IV access.
3. Administer supplemental oxygen as necessary for postoperative status or active bleeding.
4. Replace lost volume with plasma expanders (e.g., albumin, hetastarch) and/or blood products as indicated. See Table 10-3 for information about blood products.
5. Inform the patient of the importance of wearing a medical-alert bracelet and obtaining a pneumococcal vaccination if a splenectomy has been performed.

NIC Bleeding Precautions; Electrolyte Management; Fluid Monitoring; Hypovolemia Management; Intravenous (IV) Therapy; Shock Management: Volume; Blood Products Administration.

ACUTE PAIN *related to joint inflammation and injury secondary to bleeding into the synovial cavity of the joint(s); postsplenectomy pain.*

Goals/Outcomes: Within 4 hours of initiating treatment, the patient's subjective evaluation of discomfort improves, as documented by a pain scale, nonverbal indicators of discomfort are absent or decreased, and HR, RR, and BP are within 10% of the patient's baseline.
NOC Pain Control.

Pain Management

1. Devise a pain scale with the patient, rating discomfort from 0 (no pain) to 10. Perform a comprehensive assessment of pain to include location, characteristics, onset/duration, frequency, quality, intensity or severity, and precipitating factors.
2. Ensure the patient receives appropriate analgesic care. Consult with the advanced practice provider regularly until the patient's pain is controlled. Avoid use of meperidine for pain relief in older adults or individuals with renal compromise; adverse effects are common.
3. Teach the patient causes of the pain, how long it may last, and about discomforts from procedures.
4. Elevate the patient's legs to decrease joint pain in the lower extremities. Avoid knee flexion. Support extremities with pillows, making sure the bed is not "gatched" at the knee.
5. Teach the patient to splint the abdomen when coughing after splenectomy.
6. Evaluate the patient's anxiety level, and provide emotional support to control fear and anxiety. If the patient becomes agitated, evaluate potential causes including hypoxemia, poor pain or anxiety control, fluid and electrolyte imbalance, and alcohol or drug withdrawal, and intervene appropriately.
7. See Pain, Chapter 1, for additional pain interventions. Also see Prolonged Immobility, Chapter 1, for patients who are unable to move or who have limited movement.

NIC Analgesic Administration; Pain Management; Coping Enhancement; Anxiety Reduction.

ADDITIONAL NURSING DIAGNOSES

Uncontrolled bleeding can be terrifying for the patient and significant others, who may fear that the patient will die. Refer to nursing diagnoses in Emotional and Spiritual Support of the Patient and Significant Others, Chapter 2, for appropriate interventions.

DISSEMINATED INTRAVASCULAR COAGULATION
PATHOPHYSIOLOGY

Disseminated intravascular coagulation (DIC) is a syndrome characterized by overstimulation of the normal coagulation cascade, often related to severe sepsis or shock. DIC is a coagulopathy with potential to cause both profuse bleeding and widespread thrombosis leading to MODS. Inherent bodily control of bleeding requires a balance between procoagulants and thrombus formation, along with anticoagulants, inhibitors, and thrombolysis (see Figure 10-3; Table 10-4). The delicate balance may be upset by disease processes (Table 10-5),

Table 10-4	CLOTTING FACTORS: PRIMARY ACTIONS		
Coagulation Factor	**Thrombin-Sensitive/ Promotes Vasoconstriction**	**Vitamin K-Sensitive**	**Sites of Heparin Activity**
I Fibrinogen	✓		
II Prothrombin		✓	✓ IIa
III Tissue thromboplastin (tissue factor)			
IV Calcium			
V Proaccelerin (AC globulin [AC-g])	✓		
VI Not assigned			
VII Proconvertin stable factor (prothrombin accelerator)		✓	
VIII Antihemophilic factor A (antihemophilic factor [AHF], antihemophilic globulin [AHG])	✓		
IX Antihemophilic factor B (plasma thromboplastin component [PTC], Christmas factor)		✓	✓ IXa
X Stuart-Prower factor (Stuart factor)		✓	✓ Xa
XI Plasma thromboplastin antecedent (antihemophilic factor C)			✓ XIa
XII Hageman factor (contact factor)			
XIII Fibrin stabilizing factor	✓		
Other Factors			
Prekallikrein (Fletcher factor)			
High–molecular-weight kininogen (HMWK-Fitzgerald factor)			
Platelets			

resulting in a cascade of uncontrolled coagulation and fibrinolysis. The abnormal clotting cascade that develops during DIC is as follows:

- Platelets and coagulation factors are activated by a disease stimulus and are rapidly consumed, particularly factors V and XIII and fibrinogen.
- Thrombin is formed very rapidly, and inherent inhibitors cannot stop the formation of the vast amounts of thrombin generated. Thrombin directly activates fibrinogen.
- Fibrin is deposited throughout the capillary beds of organs and tissues.
- The fibrinolytic system lyses fibrin and impairs thrombin formation.
- FDPs (or FSPs) result from fibrinolysis, which changes platelet aggregation and inhibits fibrin polymerization. See Figure 10-3 for the normal coagulation pathway.

A predisposing event that damages the vascular endothelium initiates the clotting cascade. Studies reflect that both the intrinsic and extrinsic pathways are activated initially, resulting in an abnormal acceleration of the clotting process. Thrombocytopenia occurs because of thrombin production and microvascular thrombus formation.

ASSESSMENT

GOAL OF SYSTEM ASSESSMENT

Evaluate for increased risk of inappropriate bleeding or clotting as a result of qualitative or quantitative dysfunction of platelets and clotting factors.

Table 10-5	DISSEMINATED INTRAVASCULAR COAGULATION: PREDISPOSING CONDITIONS					
Obstetrics	**Gastrointestinal Disorders**	**Tissue Damage**	**Infections**	**Hemolytic Processes**	**Vascular Disorders**	**Miscellaneous**
Abruption placentae	Cirrhosis	Surgery	Viral	Transfusion reaction	Shock	Fat or pulmonary embolism
Toxemia	Hepatic necrosis	Trauma	Bacterial	Acute hemolysis secondary to infection or immunologic disorder	Aneurysm	Snake bite
Amniotic fluid embolism	Acute fulminant hepatitis	Burns	Rickettsial		Giant hemangioma	Neoplastic disorders (especially prostate, acute promyelocytic leukemia, lymphoma) Acute anoxia
Septic abortion	Pancreatitis	Prolonged extracorporeal circulation	Protozoal			
Retained dead fetus	Peritoneovenous shunts	Transplant rejection	Fungal			
Hydatidiform mole	Necrotizing enterocolitis	Heat stroke				

RISK FACTORS

Any clinical state or pharmacologic therapy (e.g., chemotherapy) that inhibits the removal of activated clotting factors, FDPs, and thromboplastin by the reticuloendothelial system. Any patient is at high risk following severe trauma or with SIRS, a severe infection, sepsis, severe sepsis, septic shock, or invasive procedures. Obstetrics patients with abruptio placentae, amniotic fluid embolism, or eclampsia release procoagulation factors, placing them at risk. DIC can occur as a paraneoplastic syndrome or oncologic emergency related to certain malignancies such as acute promyelocytic leukemia (APL), multiple myeloma, and some solid tumors. DIC may manifest as a profound bleeding/clotting disorder in the acute phase or as a less symptomatic chronic disorder.

In chronic (compensated) DIC, activation of coagulation and fibrinolysis does not occur rapidly enough to exceed the rate of production of clotting factors or inhibitors. The course of DIC depends on the intensity of the stimulus, coupled with the status of the liver, bone marrow, and vascular endothelium. Whether DIC leads to bleeding or to thrombosis is profoundly affected by the underlying disease process.

VITAL SIGNS

- Tachypnea, tachycardia, hypotension.

OBSERVATION

- Bleeding with abrupt onset: From invasive procedure sites and mucosal surfaces (e.g., oral, nasal, tracheal, gastric, urethral, vaginal, rectal); may include hematuria, petechiae, stools or gastric aspirate positive for occult blood, pallor, tachycardia, tachypnea, vertigo, hypotension, ecchymoses (e.g., on palate, gums, skin, conjunctivae), lethargy, irritability, or feeling of impending doom, and possible back pain and abdominal tenderness.
- Anxiety, restlessness.
- Petechiae, purpura, ecchymoses, oozing blood, mottling.
- Conjunctival hemorrhage and periorbital petechiae.
- Acrocyanosis.
- Joint pain, weakness.
- SOB, ST segment elevation/depression, T wave inversion.
- Grey Turner sign (flank ecchymoses).
- Hemoptysis, tarry stools, melena.
- Decreased responsiveness, confusion, altered mentation, headaches.
- Abnormal thrombosis may manifest with extremity pain, diminished pulses, oliguria or anuria, diminished or absent bowel sounds, severe chest pain with SOB (indicative of either myocardial infarction or pulmonary embolism), or paresis or paralysis (indicative of cerebral thrombus).

PALPATION

- Hepatosplenomegaly.
- Abdominal tenderness.

AUSCULTATION

- Diminished or absent bowel sounds.
- Weakened or absent peripheral pulses.

Diagnostic Tests for Disseminated Intravascular Coagulation		
Test	**Purpose**	**Abnormal Findings**
Fibrin degradation products (FDPs), fibrin split products (FSP), fibrin breakdown products	Measures fibrin degradation products (which result from clots dissolving) in blood	Increased (>10 μg/mL) as a result of widespread fibrinolysis, which produces FDPs as the end product of clot lysis Critical value: >40 ng/mL

Continued

Diagnostic Tests for Disseminated Intravascular Coagulation—cont'd

Test	Purpose	Abnormal Findings
D-Dimer assay	Measures cleavage products of fibrin	Increased to >500 as a result of increased thrombin and plasmin generation. This is a rapid measurement technique, less sensitive than FDPs, and not recommended as a substitute for FDPs and fibrinogen determinations
Fibrinogen	Measures clot formation ability: May be ordered as a follow-up to an abnormal prothrombin time (PT) or partial thromboplastin time (PTT), and/or an episode of prolonged or unexplained bleeding	May remain normal or decrease in the early acute phase. As the process continues, fibrinogen levels will decrease. Normal range is 150 to 400 mg/dL
PTT or activated partial thromboplastin time (aPTT)	Measure of the integrity of the intrinsic and common pathways of the coagulation cascade. The aPTT is the time, in seconds, for patient plasma to clot after the addition of an intrinsic pathway activator, phospholipid, and calcium	Prolonged (>40 seconds) because of activation of the intrinsic pathway, causing consumption of coagulation factors. Critical value: >70 seconds. In chronic disseminated intravascular coagulation (DIC), the value may be normal (25 to 35 seconds) or less than normal
PT, international normalized ratio (INR)	Measure of the integrity of the extrinsic pathway of the coagulation cascade	Prolonged (>15 seconds) because of activation of the extrinsic pathway, causing consumption of the extrinsic clotting factors. Critical value: >40 seconds
Thrombin time, thrombin clotting time	Test of the time it takes for a clot to form, measuring the conversion of fibrinogen to fibrin	Prolonged (>1.5 times the control value or >2 seconds in excess of a 9- to 13-second control value) because of rapid conversion of fibrinogen into fibrin
Antithrombin III (AT-III), functional antithrombin III, antithrombin, activity, and antigen	Evaluates whether the total amount of functional antithrombin is normal. Activity will be decreased with both type 1 and type 2 antithrombin deficiencies, thus this test can be used as an initial screen for both. If the antithrombin activity is low, then the antithrombin antigen test is performed to determine the quantity of antithrombin present	Decreased (<50% of control value using a plasma sample, or <80% using functional values) because of rapid consumption of this thrombin inhibitor. The action of AT-III is catalyzed by heparin
Euglobulin clot lysis time	Measures overall fibrinolysis; measures fibrinogen activity via measurement of plasminogen and plasminogen activator, which assist in prevention of fibrin clot formations	Decreased time is seen with DIC. Normal: Lysis in 2 to 4 hours. Critical value: 100% lysis in 1 hour
Platelet count	Used to diagnose bleeding disorders or bone marrow disease	Decreased (<140,000/mm^3) because of rapid rate of platelet aggregation to form clots during DIC. Aggregation decreases the freely circulating platelets
Alpha$_2$-antiplasmin	Measures alpha$_2$-antiplasmin, which is an inhibitor that regulates the fibrinolytic system primarily by blocking the enzymatic activity of plasmin	Decreased because of rapid consumption resulting from large amounts of plasmin generated. When all alpha$_2$-antiplasmin is depleted, excessive hyperfibrinolysis (massive, rapid clot lysis) occurs
Protamine sulfate test	Associated with the formation of excessive amounts of thrombin and secondary fibrinolysis	Results are positive (normal: negative), indicative of presence of fibrin strands
Peripheral blood smear	Microscopic examination of cells from a drop of blood; investigates hematologic problems or parasites such as malaria and filarial	For visualization during microscopic examination of schistocytes and burr cells, which indicate the deposition of fibrin in the small blood vessels

COLLABORATIVE MANAGEMENT: DISSEMINATED INTRAVASCULAR COAGULATION

CARE PRIORITIES

 1. Treat the primary cause of the disease

Aggressively treat the underlying cause. A primary disease promotes the development of DIC. If treatment of the disease fails, the mortality rate of DIC is high. When DIC occurs without apparent cause, the possibility of undiagnosed malignancy (e.g., prostate cancer or APL), a large abdominal aortic aneurysm, a progressive gram-negative bacterial infection, or hepatic cirrhosis should be explored. If the diagnosis is by laboratory tests alone, conservative management is appropriate. Other conditions and medication side effects should be considered (see Table 10-5).

2. Manage abnormal clotting with continuous IV heparin therapy

There are three conditions associated with DIC in which heparin may be effective:
- Underlying malignancy/carcinoma.
- Acute promyelocytic leukemia (APL): A leukemia most often seen in young adults with acute myelocytic anemia, which may also be linked to patients who received radiotherapy for prostate cancer.
- Purpura fulminans/extreme purpura, often seen with severe sepsis.

If used, the patient should have clinically obvious thrombosis. Low-dose therapy (5 to 10 units/kg/h) is considered. Heparin binds to antithrombin, resulting in a strong anticoagulant effect. Use of higher-dose heparin in DIC is associated with a high risk of bleeding, and greater efficacy has not been documented. Heparin may be considered for serious bleeding or clotting when the condition underlying the DIC is not rapidly reversible and the patient's vascular system is surgically intact.

> **Safety Alert** *Patients who have acute promyelocytic leukemia with disseminated intravascular coagulation often experience accelerated symptoms of fibrinolysis (declotting) when receiving chemotherapy. If these individuals receive heparin, an antifibrinolytic agent such as epsilon- (ε-)aminocaproic acid (Amicar) may be added to decrease bleeding.*

3. Manage abnormal bleeding resulting from fibrinolysis with antifibrinolytics

ε-Aminocaproic acid (Amicar) and tranexamic acid (Cyklokapron) are used to inhibit fibrinolysis in patients who are bleeding as a result of a variety of causes. In patients with DIC, these agents should be used with extreme caution because they may convert a bleeding disorder into a thrombotic problem. When used in DIC, these agents are used in combination with heparin to minimize the potential for thrombosis. Failure rates with use are high.

4. Consider use of thrombolytic agents for abnormal clotting

Use of streptokinase, urokinase, and rtPA is not indicated for patients with thrombosis because these agents may facilitate excessive bleeding.

5. Provide replacement of necessary blood components

Clotting factors and inhibitors are replaced in the form of fresh-frozen plasma. The PT/INR may be the most accurate measurement(s) for guiding plasma replacement. Patients with markedly decreased fibrinogen levels may be given cryoprecipitate, which contains 5 to 10 times more fibrinogen than plasma contains. Thrombocytopenia in DIC may not be severe. The platelet count is usually greater than 50,000/mm³. General replacement therapy guidelines indicate that approximately 10 units of cryoprecipitate should be given for every 2 to 3 units of plasma. Platelet transfusions are used if the patient has impaired platelet production and profuse bleeding. Antithrombin III (AT-III) concentrate has been used on a limited basis (see Table 10-3). More recently, DIC is being managed with antithrombin concentrate, activated protein C (drotrecogin alfa), tissue factor pathway inhibitor, and synthetic serine protease inhibitors (e.g., aprotinin).
- RBC replacement: Packed RBCs may be administered to increase oxygen-carrying capacity to maintain a Hgb value 7 to 9 mg/dL or greater than 20% below the patient's baseline if the patient is chronically anemic and symptomatic.

6. Supplement vitamin K₁ (phytonadione) and folate

Patients with DIC are at high risk for deficiency of these substances, and administration of both vitamins is recommended for most patients.

7. Prevent viral infections resulting from immunosuppression with protease inhibitors

Gabexate, nafamostat, and trasylol have been used.

8. Manage hypotension related to heart failure, as appropriate

If the patient becomes severely hypotensive resulting from heart failure, the following drugs may be considered: milrinone, dobutamine, dopamine, epinephrine, and nitroprusside (see Appendix 6).

CARE PLANS: DISSEMINATED INTRAVASCULAR COAGULATION

INEFFECTIVE PROTECTION *related to bleeding resulting from overstimulation of the clotting cascade and rapid consumption of clotting factors.*

Goals/Outcomes: Within 48 to 72 hours of initiation of treatment, the patient is free of symptoms of bleeding, as evidenced by absence of frank bleeding from invasive procedure sites and mucosal surfaces; secretions and excretions that are negative for blood; absence of large or increasing ecchymoses; decreasing purpura; and HR, RR, and BP within 10% of the patient's baseline (or HR 60 to 100 bpm, RR 12 to 20 breaths/min, systolic BP greater than 90 mm Hg).

NOC Blood Coagulation.

Bleeding Precautions

1. Discuss bleeding history with the patient or significant others. Assess previous incidences of bleeding from gums, skin, or urine; tarry/bloody stools; bleeding from muscles or into joints; hemoptysis, vomiting of blood, epistaxis, or prolonged bleeding from small wounds or after tooth extraction; or unusual bruising or tendency to bruise easily. Provide soft tooth brush.
2. Question patients about current medications, including over-the-counter preparations, because many medications promote bleeding (Table 10-6).
3. Monitor coagulation tests daily. Consult the advanced practice provider for abnormal values (Table 10-7).
4. Monitor closely for increased bleeding, bruising, petechiae, and purpura. Assess for internal bleeding by testing suspicious secretions (i.e., sputum, urine, stool, emesis, gastric drainage) for the presence of blood. Monitor for hemorrhage.
5. Monitor neurologic status (see Glasgow Coma Scale, Appendix 2) every 2 hours by assessing LOC, orientation, pupillary reaction, and movement and strength of extremities. Changes in status can indicate intracranial bleeding.
6. Use alcohol-free mouthwash and swabs for oral care to minimize gingival/gum injury. Use normal saline solution (NSS) or solution of NSS and sodium bicarbonate (500 mL NSS with 15 mL bicarbonate) to irrigate the oral cavity if irritated. Massage gums gently with a sponge-tipped applicator to help remove debris. Do not attempt to remove large clots from the mouth, to avoid profuse bleeding.
7. Use electric rather than safety razor for shaving the patient.
8. Refrain from inserting objects into a bleeding orifice. Avoid taking rectal temperatures.
9. Protect the patient from trauma. Avoid unnecessary venipunctures and IM injections.
10. If the patient undergoes an invasive procedure, manually hold pressure over the insertion site for 3 to 5 minutes for IV catheters and 10 to 15 minutes for arterial catheters or until bleeding subsides.
11. Instruct the patient and/or family on signs of bleeding and appropriate actions.
12. Teach the patient the importance of avoiding vitamin K–inhibiting and platelet aggregation–inhibiting medications or vitamin and dietary supplements (see Table 10-6), which promote bleeding.

NIC Infection Control; Infection Protection; Surveillance: Safety.

RISK FOR DEFICIENT FLUID VOLUME *related to bleeding/hemorrhage*

Goals/Outcomes: The patient remains normovolemic, as evidenced by HR and RR within 10% of the patient's baseline (or HR 60 to 100 bpm) and RR 12 to 20 breaths/min with normal depth and pattern; BP within the patient's baseline (or systolic BP greater than 90 mm Hg), warm extremities, distal pulses at least 2+ on a 0-to-4+ scale,

Table 10-6 MEDICATIONS THAT MAY PROMOTE BLEEDING

Medications that Inhibit Platelets or Cause Thrombocytopenia

Analgesics:	Diuretic Agents:	Other:
Nonsteroidal antiinflammatory agents	Sulfonamide derivatives	Antihistamines
Aspirin (acetylsalicylic acid)	Acetazolamide	Ethanol
Acetaminophen	Chlorpropamide	Heparin
Antipyrine	Chlorothiazide	Beta-adrenergic–blocking agents
Ibuprofen	Chlorthalidone	General anesthetics
Indomethacin	Clopamide	Local anesthetics
Fenoprofen	Diazoxide	Chemotherapeutic agents
Sodium salicylate	Furosemide	Vitamin E
Antirheumatic agents	Bumetanide	Estrogens
Oxyphenbutazone	Hydrochlorothiazide	Digitoxin
Phenylbutazone	Tolbutamide	Cimetidine
Hydroxychloroquine	Spironolactone	Levodopa
Gold salts	Mercurial diuretics	Propylthiouracil
Antimicrobials	Glycoprotein IIb/IIIa inhibitors	
Ampicillin	Abciximab	
Cephalothin	Eptifibatide	
Methicillin	Tirofiban	
Penicillin	Phenothiazines	
Pentamidine	Chlorpromazine	
Streptomycin	Promethazine	
Sulfonamides (antibiotics)	Trifluoperazine	
Chloramphenicol	Phosphodiesterase inhibitors	
Isoniazid	Caffeine	
Nitrofurantoin	Dipyridamole	
Rifampin	Theophyllines	
Trimethoprim	Antiplatelet drugs	
Anticoagulants	Aspirin (acetylsalicylic acid)	
Heparin	Ticlopidine	
Enoxaparin	Clopidogrel	
Dalteparin	Prostaglandin I_2	
Thrombolytics	Prostaglandin D_2	
Alteplase	Prostaglandin E	
Reteplase	Sedative-hypnotics	
Streptokinase	Benzodiazepines	
Urokinase	Clonazepam	
Anisoylated plasminogen streptokinase	Diazepam	
Tenecteplase	Vasodilators	
	Nitroglycerin	
	Nitroprusside	

Medications that Inhibit Vitamin K

Salicylates:	Broad-Spectrum Antibiotics:	Vitamins:
Aspirin and aspirin-combination drugs	Sulfonamides	A
Other salicylates	Triple sulfa	E
Coumarins	Sulfamethoxazole	
Anisindione	Sulfasalazine	
Dicumarol	Sulfisoxazole	
Warfarin	Sulfamethoxazole-trimethoprim	
	Clindamycin	
	Gentamicin	
	Neomycin	
	Tobramycin	
	Vancomycin	
	Imipenem	
	Cefamandole	
	Cefoxitin	

Table 10-7	DISSEMINATED INTRAVASCULAR COAGULATION: LABORATORY VALUES		
Laboratory Values	**Normal**	**Acute DIC**	**Chronic DIC**
Fibrinogen	150 to 400 mg/dL (adult)	Decreased	Normal or increased
Fibrin degradation	$<10\ \mu g/mL$	Positive (increased)	Positive (increased)
Platelet count	150,000 to 400,000/mm³ (adult)	Decreased	Normal or increased
Partial thromboplastin time, also known as activated partial thromboplastin time	25 to 35 seconds	Increased	Normal
Prothrombin time	11 to 15 seconds	Increased	Normal
Thrombin time	$1.5 \times$ control value	Increased	Increased

DIC, Disseminated intravascular coagulation

urinary output greater than 0.5 mL/kg/h, and capillary refill less than 2 seconds. Within 24 hours of initiating treatment, the patient verbalizes orientation to time, place, person, and self.
NOC Fluid Balance.

Fluid Monitoring
1. Monitor every 2 hours for increases in HR and RR, decreased BP, and decreasing pulse pressure.
2. Measure urinary output every 2 to 4 hours. Consult the advanced practice provider for output less than 0.5 mL/kg/h.
3. Maintain accurate I&O record. Weigh daily and monitor trends.
4. Increase measurement of vital signs and urine output to at least every 30 minutes for active bleeding. For profuse bleeding, check vital signs at least every 15 minutes. Inspect invasive procedure sites and dressings for bleeding.
5. Monitor CBC daily for significant alterations in Hct, Hgb, and platelets (Table 10-8).
6. Ensure that the patient has typed and cross-matched blood available for transfusion.
7. Monitor coagulation studies (PT, PTT, fibrinogen, FDP/FSP, platelet counts), as appropriate.

Table 10-8	COMPLETE BLOOD COUNT VALUES	
Complete Blood Count Values	**Common Measurement Value**	**Population**
Red blood cells (RBCs)	4 to 5.5 million/mm³	Adult females
	4.5 to 6.2 million/mm³	Adult males
Hemoglobin (Hgb)	12 to 16 g/dL	Adult females
	14 to 18 g/dL	Adult males
Hematocrit (Hct)	37% to 47%	Adult females
Mean corpuscular volume (MCV)	83 to 93 μg³	Adults
Mean cell hemoglobin (MCH)	26 to 34 pg	Adults
Mean cell hemoglobin concentration (MCHC)	31% to 38%	Adults
White blood cells (WBCs)	4500 to 11,000/mm³	Adults
Differential White Blood Cells (Granulocytes)		
Segmented neutrophils (Segs)	54% to 62%	Adults
Band neutrophils (Bands)	3% to 5%	Adults
Eosinophils (Eos)	1% to 3%	Adults
Basophils (Basos)	0% to 0.75%	Adults
Monocytes (Monos)	3% to 7%	Adults
Lymphocytes (Lymphs)	25% to 33%	Adults
Platelets	150,000 to 400,000/mm³	Adults

8. Assess for signs of impending shock if the following signs are noted: increased HR and RR; decreased BP; or pallor, diaphoresis, cool extremities, delayed capillary refill, decreased pulse amplitude, restlessness, or disorientation.
9. Maintain at least one 18-gauge or larger IV catheter for use during shock management, at which time rapid infusion of blood products or IV fluids may be necessary.
10. Evaluate the effects of fluid therapy.

NIC Electrolyte Management; Fluid Management; Hypovolemia Management; Intravenous (IV) Therapy; Shock Management: Volume.

INEFFECTIVE TISSUE PERFUSION (OR RISK FOR SAME)
PERIPHERAL, CARDIOPULMONARY, CEREBRAL, GASTROINTESTINAL, AND RENAL *related to blood loss or presence of microthrombi.*

Goals/Outcomes: The patient has adequate perfusion, as evidenced by peripheral pulses greater than $2+$ on a scale of 0-to-4$+$, brisk capillary refill (less than 2 seconds), BP within the patient's normal range, CVP 2 to 6 mm Hg, and HR regular and less than 100 bpm. The patient is oriented to time, place, person, and self and has urinary output at least 30 mL/h (0.5 mL/kg/h) and oxygen saturation greater than 96%.
NOC Circulation Status.

Shock Prevention
1. Assess and document peripheral perfusion every 2 hours, including temperature, sensation, pulses, and movement in extremities. Perform a comprehensive assessment of peripheral circulation (i.e., check peripheral pulses, edema, capillary refill, and color and temperature of extremities).
2. Monitor vital signs frequently. Evaluate chest pain. Document cardiac dysrhythmias.
3. Monitor BP and assess for early signs of perfusion deficit at least every 2 hours, including dizziness, confusion, and decreased urinary output.
4. Monitor for decreased myocardial or pulmonary perfusion, as evidenced by chest pain, ST segment depression or elevation, T wave inversion, SOB, dyspnea, and decreased oxygen saturation using continuous pulse oximetry.
5. Monitor CVP, observing for both high and low readings. Decreased pressures are indicative of hypovolemia/hemorrhage. Anticipate vasoconstriction with hypovolemia: CO may increase or decrease from normal range of 4 to 7 L/min, depending on cardiac contractility.
6. Monitor GI status by observing tolerance to diet or tube feedings, bowel habits (e.g., constipation, diarrhea), characteristic of stool (e.g., tarry, bloody), and presence or absence of bowel sounds.

NIC Cardiac Care: Acute; Circulatory Care: Arterial Insufficiency; Circulatory Care: Venous Insufficiency; Respiratory Monitoring; Shock Management: Cardiac; Cerebral Perfusion Promotion; Neurologic Monitoring; Peripheral Sensation Management; Fluid/Electrolyte Management; Fluid Management; Vital Signs Monitoring.

IMPAIRED GAS EXCHANGE (OR RISK FOR SAME) *related to loss of oxygen-carrying capacity through hemorrhage or pulmonary microembolus formation.*

Goals/Outcomes: The patient's gas exchange is adequate, as evidenced by Pao_2 at least 80 mm Hg, $Paco_2$ 35 to 45 mm Hg, pH 7.35 to 7.45, RR 12 to 20 breaths/min with normal depth and pattern, oxygen saturation at least 95%, HR 60 to 100 bpm, Svo_2 at least 60%, and orientation to time, place, and person.
NOC Respiratory Status: Gas Exchange.

Respiratory Monitoring
1. Assess respiratory status every 2 hours, noting rate, rhythm, depth, and regularity of respirations. Provide supplemental oxygen as appropriate.
2. Monitor for signs of respiratory failure: restlessness, anxiety, and air hunger indicative of hypoxemia; ABG values for increased $Paco_2$ and decreased pH indicative of hypoventilation; or oxygen saturation less than 95% via pulse oximetry indicative of decreased ventilation. Consult the advanced practice provider if signs of respiratory insufficiency are present.
3. Monitor $Scvo_2$ or Svo_2: steady increase or decrease from the patient's normal level may indicate deterioration.
4. Assess lungs for bibasilar crackles (rales), indicative of pulmonary edema.
5. Monitor the patient's respiratory secretions. Institute respiratory therapy treatments as needed.

6. Monitor for pulmonary embolus, including sharp, stabbing chest pain, dyspnea, pallor, cyanosis, pupillary dilation, rapid or irregular pulse, profuse diaphoresis, and anxiety. Assess the need for supplemental oxygen and consult the physician immediately. Patients with severe pulmonary emboli may require mechanical ventilation. See Pulmonary Embolus, Chapter 4.

7. Assess the patient for changes in sensorium (i.e., confusion, lethargy, somnolence), indicative of inadequate cerebral oxygenation or CO_2 retention (respiratory insufficiency).

NIC Airway Management; Oxygen Therapy; Respiratory Monitoring.

RISK FOR INJURY *related to blood product administration*

Goals/Outcomes: Throughout the transfusion and up to 8 hours after transfusion, the patient does not exhibit signs of a blood transfusion reaction, as evidenced by stable mentation, absence of fever and chills, normal appearance of skin (i.e., no flushing, rash, lesions), and baseline RR, BP, and HR.

NOC Risk Control.

Surveillance: Safety

1. Check blood to be transfused with another professional to ensure that the patient receives the correct blood. Verify the following: patient's name, patient's birthday and hospital number, blood unit number, blood expiration date, blood group, and blood type.

2. Discuss signs and symptoms of potential reaction with the patient and family. Premedicate if there is a history of reaction or antibodies are present.

3. When blood products are being infused, check vital signs every 15 minutes for the first hour. Check the patient frequently throughout the first 15 minutes of the transfusion to observe for signs of an acute hemolytic transfusion reaction, including fever, chills, dyspnea, hypotension, flushing, tachycardia, back pain, hematuria, mentation changes, and shock.

4. Observe for transfusion reactions throughout the transfusion and during the 8-hour period afterward. If a transfusion reaction (Table 10-9) occurs, implement the following:
   - If the transfusion is in progress, stop the infusion immediately.
   - Maintain IV access with NSS.
   - Maintain BP with a combination of volume infusion and vasoactive drugs, if indicated.
   - Monitor HR and ECG for changes. Treat symptomatic dysrhythmias as prescribed by the physician or midlevel practitioner.
   - Administer ordered diuretics and fluids to promote diuresis (urine output approximately 100 mL/h).
   - Obtain blood and urine for a transfusion workup according to institution blood bank protocol.
   - Perform blood cultures if the patient exhibits signs of sepsis.

Table 10-9	ACUTE TRANSFUSION REACTIONS	
Type	**Symptoms**	**Time Frame**
Acute intravascular hemolytic	Fever, chills, dyspnea, tachycardia, hypotension, back pain, flushing, hematuria, shock	After start of transfusion within 5 to 30 minutes
Acute extravascular hemolytic	Fever, elevated bilirubin, unusually low posttransfusion hematocrit and hemoglobin	Usually within 8 hours Delayed: 7 to 10 days
Allergic (mild)	Rash, hives, pruritus	Within 1 hour
Anaphylactic	Dyspnea, shortness of breath, bronchospasms, tachycardia, flushing, hypotension, shock	Within 30 minutes to 1 hour
Febrile	Fever, chills	Within 4 hours
Hypervolemic	Dyspnea, tachycardia, bibasilar crackles, jugular venous distention, possible hypertension, headache	Within 1 to 2 hours
Septic	Fever, chills, tachycardia, hypotension, vomiting, shock, muscle pain, cardiac arrest	Within 5 minutes to 4 hours

5. If an intravascular hemolytic reaction is confirmed, implement the following:
- Monitor coagulation studies, including PT, PTT, and fibrinogen levels (see Table 10-7).
- Monitor renal status by measuring the following: blood urea nitrogen, creatinine, potassium, and phosphate levels.
- Monitor laboratory values for hemolysis: increased lactate dehydrogenase, bilirubin, and haptoglobin.

6. With massive transfusion for severe bleeding, manage hypocalcemia caused by citrated blood, hyperkalemia of uncertain etiology, hypothermia from refrigerated blood, acute respiratory distress syndrome, coagulopathy, and hemochromatosis (iron overload).

NIC Bleeding Precautions; Bleeding Reduction; Blood Products Administration.

ADDITIONAL NURSING DIAGNOSES

The uncontrolled bleeding related to DIC can be terrifying to the patient and significant others, who may fear that the patient will die. Refer to nursing diagnoses in Emotional and Spiritual Support of the Patient and Significant Others, Chapter 2. For patients who manifest activity intolerance, see nursing diagnosis in Prolonged Immobility, Chapter 1. For patients with sepsis or septic shock, see Systemic Inflammatory Response Syndrome, Sepsis, and Multiple Organ Dysfunction Syndrome, Chapter 11.

SELECTED REFERENCES

Abraham J: Romiplostim for treating thrombocytopenia in chronic idiopathic thrombocytopenic purpura, *Commun Oncol* 5:651–656, 2008.

American Association of Blood Banks: *Circular of information for the use of human blood and blood components*, Bethesda, 2013, American Association of Blood Banks. http://www.aabb.org/tm/coi/Documents/coi1113.pdf.

American Society of Anesthesiologists: Practice guidelines for perioperative blood transfusion and adjuvant therapies, *Anesthesiology* 105:198–208, 2006.

American Society of Anesthesiologists Committee on Standards and Practice Parameters: Practice guidelines for perioperative blood management. An updated report by the American Society of Anesthesiologists Task Force on Perioperative Blood Management, *Anesthesiology* 122:1A, 2015.

American Society of Hematology: Red blood cell transfusions: a clinical practice guideline from AABB, *Ann Intern Med* 157:49–58, 2012.

Bickley L: *Bates guide to physical examination and history taking*, ed 11, Philadelphia, 2013, Wolters Kluwer Health/Lippincott Williams & Wilkins.

Gentry CA, Gross KB, Sud B, Drevets DA: Adverse outcomes associated with the use of drotrecogin alfa (activated) in patients with severe sepsis and baseline bleeding precautions, *Crit Care Med* 37:19–25, 2009.

Ghanima W, Godeau B, Cines DB, Bussel JB: How I treat immune thrombocytopenia: the choice between splenectomy or a medical therapy as a second-line treatment, *Blood* 120:960–969, 2012.

Gould S, Cimino M, Gerber D: Packed red cell transfusion in the intensive care unit: limitations and consequences, *Am J Crit Care* 16:39–49, 2007.

Harmon S: Bring on the peanuts: food allergy therapies move closer to approval, *Scientific American* June 30, 2011. http://www.scientificamerican.com/article/food-allergy-therapies/.

Hebert P, Tinmouth A, Corwin H: Controversies in RBC transfusion in the critically ill, *Chest* 131:1583–1590, 2007.

Horvath KA, Acker MA, Chang H, et al: Blood transfusion and infection after cardiac surgery, *Ann Thorac Surg* 95:2194–2201, 2013.

Keating GM: Romiplostin: a review of its use in immune thrombocytopenia, *Drugs* 72:415–435, 2012.

Kelton J, Warkentin T: Heparin induced thrombocytopenia: a historical perspective, *Blood* 112:2607–2616, 2008.

Klein H, Spahn D, Carson J: Red blood cell transfusion in clinical practice, *Lancet* 370:415–426, 2007.

Lee A, Peterson E: Treatment of cancer-associated thrombosis, *Blood* 122:2310–2317, 2013.

Lelubre C, Vincent J: Red blood cell transfusion in the critically ill patient, *Ann Intensive Care* 1:43, 2011.

Marik P, Corwin H: Efficacy of red blood cell transfusion in the critically ill: a systematic review of the literature, *Crit Care Med* 36:2667–2674, 2008.

McEvoy M, Shandra A: Anemia, bleeding, and blood transfusion in the intensive care unit: causes, risks, costs, and new strategies, *Am J Crit Care* 22:eS1–eS13, 2013.

McMahon B: Malignancy-associated thrombosis, *Oncol Issues* 24:20–23, 2009.

Pieracci FM, Barle PS, Pomp A: Critical care of the bariatric patient, *Crit Care Med* 34:1796–1804, 2006.

Robson-Ansley P, Du Toit G: Pathophysiology, diagnosis and management of exercise-induced anaphylaxis, *Curr Opin Allergy Clin Immunol* 10:312–317, 2010.

Rome S, Doss D, Miller K, Westphal J: IMF Nurse Leadership Board: Thromboembolic events associated with novel therapies in patients with multiple myeloma: consensus statement of the IMF nurse leadership board, *Clin J Oncol Nurs* 12(Suppl 3):21–28, 2008.

Sampson HA, Muñoz-Furlong A, Campbell RL, et al: Second symposium on the definition and management of anaphylaxis: summary report—Second National Institute of Allergy and Infectious Disease/Food Allergy and Anaphylaxis Network symposium, *J Allergy Clin Immunol* 117:391–397, 2006.

Simons FE: Anaphylaxis, *J Allergy Clin Immunol* 121(Suppl 2):S402–S407, 2008.

Simons FE: Anaphylaxis: recent advances in assessment and treatment, *J Allergy Clin Immunol* 124:625–636, 2009.

Simons FE, Ardusso LR, Bilo MB, et al: World allergy organization guidelines for the assessment and management of anaphylaxis, *World Allergy Organ J* 4:13–37, 2011.

Weldon B, Yu S, Neale-May T, et al: The safety of peanut oral immunotherapy in peanut allergic subjects in a single center trial, *J Allergy Clin Immunol* 127:AB25, 2011.

Yap C, Lau L, Krishnaswamy M, et al: Age of transfused red cells and early outcomes after cardiac surgery, *Ann Thorac Surg* 86:554–559, 2008.

ABDOMINAL HYPERTENSION AND ABDOMINAL COMPARTMENT SYNDROME

" . . . the end result of a progressive, unchecked increase in intra-abdominal pressure from a myriad of disorders that eventually leads to multiple organ dysfunction."

John Hunt, MD

PATHOPHYSIOLOGY

Intraabdominal hypertension (IAH) occurs when the amount of intraabdominal contents (through edematous bowel or fluid accumulating in the cavity) exceeds the distendable capability of the fascia. The result is an intraabdominal hypertensive state, which can lead to abdominal compartment syndrome (ACS). As the fluid accumulates (because of bleeding, ascites, volume overload, and other causes), the resulting increase in pressure (change in compliance/change in volume) initially affects regional blood flow and results in impaired tissue perfusion, which is then associated with a systemic inflammatory response. The resulting ischemia and inflammatory response further cause capillary leakage and compression of the intraabdominal viscera. If untreated, the continually elevated free fluid and measured pressure begin to compress blood vessels, causing organ dysfunction both inside and outside the abdomen, and lead to ACS. The inflammatory response promotes the release of cytokines, causing vasodilation and cell membrane dysfunction. The cell membrane loses integrity, which causes further inflammation, profound edema, and ultimately cell death. The elevated pressure in the abdominal cavity generated by the severe increase in extravascular fluid load increases the intraabdominal contents (free water) and further impairs intestinal tissue perfusion as compression of the arteries and veins continues. This process underlies the multiorgan effects of rising intraabdominal pressure (IAP). When the IAP rises above critical level, blood flow to the abdominal viscera and organs decreases and ACS is imminent. Although initially described in surgical patients, IAH and ACS also occur in medical patients without abdominal conditions. IAP can be measured easily and reliably in patients through the bladder using simple tools.

RISK FACTORS

Diminished abdominal wall compliance
- Major trauma and burns; acute respiratory failure; abdominal surgery.

Increased intraluminal contents
- Gastroparesis; ileus; pseudoobstruction.

Increased abdominal contents
- Ascites/liver dysfunction; hemoperitoneum/pneumoperitoneum.

Capillary leak/fluid resuscitation
- Acidosis (pH less than 7.2); hypotension; hypothermia (below 33°C [91.4° F]); massive fluid resuscitation; poly transfusion; coagulopathy; sepsis, major trauma and burns.

DEFINITIONS

Bladder pressure reflects the IAP and is measured using the indwelling urinary catheter. The pressure is expressed in mm Hg.

937

Intraabdominal pressure is the pressure within the abdominal cavity. Normal IAP is ~5 to 7 mm Hg, with baseline levels in morbidly obese individuals often ranging from 9 to 14 mm Hg. IAP is considered to be significant when consistently above 12 mm Hg, although a higher pressure often appears to be tolerated in obese individuals. The pressure within the cavity reflects the presence of extravascular fluids, which compress the blood vessels and organs in the abdominal cavity as well as displacing the diaphragm into the thoracic cage, which limits lung expansion. Elevated intrabladder pressure indirectly reflects high pressure within the abdominal cavity.

Intraabdominal hypertension (IAH) is defined by the World Society of Abdominal Compartment Syndrome (WSACS) as a measured IAP of 12 mm Hg or greater, recorded 3 times using standardized measurement methods 4 to 6 hours apart and/or an abdominal perfusion pressure (APP) of less than 60 mm Hg (mean arterial pressure [MAP] − intraabdominal bladder pressure), recorded using 2 standardized measurements 1 to 6 hours apart). These measurements should be evaluated in the context of clinical symptomatology. Increased IAP may reflect a critical finding in patients with multiorgan dysfunction syndrome (MODS) or multisystem failure, which contributes to global hypoperfusion, aggravating the effects of increased IAP (Table 11-1).

Abdominal compartment syndrome is defined as an IAP greater than 15 mm Hg and the onset of new organ failure. ACS is defined as "intraabdominal hypertension with a gradual and consistent increase in the IAP value of [equal to or greater than] 20 mm Hg," recorded by at least 3 standardized measurements taken 1 to 6 hours apart and in

Table 11-1	PRESSURE AND SYMPTOM GRADE FOR INTRAABDOMINAL HYPERTENSION	
Graded Measurement	**Pressure Measurement and Relevance**	**Physiologic Events and Clinical Signs**
Pressure grade I	12 to 15 mm Hg Significant in the presence of organ dysfunction	Cytokine release and capillary leak Third spacing of resuscitative fluid Decreasing venous return and preload Early effects on ICP and CPP Abdominal wall perfusion decreases 42% Marked reduction in intestinal and intraabdominal organ blood flow leading to regional acidosis and free radical formation
Pressure grade II	16 to 20 mm Hg Significant in most patients	Markedly decreased venous return, CO, and splanchnic perfusion Increased SVR, CVP, PAWP Decreased blood pressure, particularly systolic blood pressure, and pulse pressure Decreased TLC, FRC, RV Increased vent pressures, hypercapnia, hypoxia Reduction to 61% of baseline mucosal blood flow and increasing gut acidosis Oliguria, anuria Increasing ICP and decreasing CPP
Pressure grade III	21 to 25 mm Hg Significant in all patients	Hemodynamic collapse, worsening acidosis, hypoxia, hypercapnia, anuria Inability to oxygenate, ventilate, or resuscitate
Pressure grade IV	>25 mm Hg Significant in all patients	Hemodynamic collapse, worsening acidosis, hypoxia, hypercapnia, anuria Inability to oxygenate, ventilate, or resuscitate

If both pressure and clinical symptoms are met for grade III and/or grade IV, patient has abdominal compartment syndrome. CPP: Cerebral Perfusion Pressure. CVP: Central Venous Pressure; FRC: Functional Residual Capacity; ICP: Intracranial Pressure; PAWP: Pulmonary Artery Wedge Pressure; RV: Residual Volume; SVR: Systemic Vascular Resistance; TLC: Total Lung Capacity.

conjunction with at least one new-onset organ dysfunction. ACS can be fatal and often complicates or results in a clinical condition refractory to treatment. The astute clinician suspects IAH and ACS when MODS is evolving and/or the patient presents with persistent lactic acidosis.

Abdominal perfusion pressure is APP 5 MAP 2 IAP. In adults, keeping this greater than 50 to 60 mm Hg significantly improves morbidity and mortality.

Selected definitions from the WSACS:

- Definition 1: IAP is the steady-state pressure within the abdominal cavity.
- Definition 7: IAH is defined by a sustained or repeated pathologic increase in IAP $\geq$ 12 mm Hg.
- Definition 9: ACS is defined as a sustained IAP greater than 20 mm Hg (with or without APP less than 60 mm Hg) that is associated with new organ dysfunction/failure.

Historically, most critical care providers believed that IAH and its more serious evolution, ACS, were solely related to traumatic injury of the abdomen, including surgery. Within the last decade, the understanding of the pathophysiology of IAH and ACS has been enhanced by studies revealing the prevalence in all critical patients: medical as well as surgical and trauma. The progressive conditions have been divided into primary and secondary abdominal hypertension disorders. The causes may differ, but outcomes are similar if either condition remains untreated.

Primary ACS is a condition associated with injury or disease in the abdominopelvic region that frequently requires early surgical or angioradiologic intervention. Any abnormal event that raises abdominal pressure can induce acute IAH, including blunt or penetrating abdominal trauma, abdominal aortic aneurysm, hemorrhagic pancreatitis, gastrointestinal (GI) obstruction, abdominal surgery resulting in retroperitoneal bleeding or secondary peritonitis, and tight closure of abdominal incisions. Primary ACS also includes patients with abdominal solid organ injuries who were initially managed medically and then developed ACS. The condition has been relatively well understood by surgeons and their colleagues but is frequently misdiagnosed and/or untreated until surgical intervention is required.

Secondary ACS includes conditions that do not originate from abdominal injury that creates IAH, including sepsis or any condition prompting capillary leak (e.g., major burns, conditions requiring massive fluid resuscitation). A large multicenter study by Malbrain and colleagues in 2005 found the prevalence of IAH was 54% among medical intensive care unit (ICU) patients and 65% in surgical ICU patients. This was remarkable, as most medical patients are not evaluated for or even considered to have IAH and ACS.

ACS treatments are the same regardless of the cause; however, the caregiver must be very careful in managing secondary ACS. The opportunity for early intervention may be lost because of the subtle development of signs and symptoms of IAH and ACS. The lack of definitive signs often leads to delayed diagnosis and delayed recognition, and an urgent medical condition becomes an emergency surgical situation. Increased organ failure, increased mortality, increased resource use, and longer ICU lengths of stay may result. Similar to sepsis and severe sepsis, the greatest challenge is early recognition and diagnosis. Monitoring all high-risk patients would enable clinicians to trend the IAP, facilitating early, appropriate interventions when the syndrome is more likely to be responsive to medical therapy. The best management strategy is to prevent ACS via early monitoring, early medical interventions, and early surgical decompression if needed.

ASSESSMENT

GOAL OF SYSTEM ASSESSMENT

To rapidly evaluate for significant primary and secondary IAH and correlating reduction of blood flow to other organs

HISTORY AND RISK FACTORS

Patients with a history of abdominal trauma, abdominal surgery, intraabdominal infection, damage control laparotomy with intraabdominal packing, severe infection, sepsis, peritonitis, bleeding pelvic fractures, postoperative bleeding, massive retroperitoneal hematoma, liver transplantation, ruptured abdominal aortic aneurysm, visceral tissue edema, pneumoperitoneum, hypovolemic or vasogenic shock or any patient with aggressive fluid resuscitation, acute ascites, and/or pancreatitis.

VITAL SIGNS AND OTHER VALUES
The following values may be increased
Hemodynamic values: Central venous pressure (CVP), pulmonary artery occlusive pressure (PAOP), systemic vascular resistance (SVR), inferior vena cava (IVC) pressure.
Respiratory: Pleural pressure, peak inspiratory pressure.
Screening lab values: $Paco_2$, serum creatinine, serum blood urea nitrogen (BUN).

The following may be decreased
Respiratory: Tidal volume, Pao_2.
Cardiovascular: Cardiac output (CO), systolic blood pressure (BP), cerebral perfusion pressure.
Renal: Glomerular filtration rate, serum creatinine, serum BUN.

OBSERVATION
Observe for upward trends in respiratory and heart rates (RR and HR, respectively) and decrease in urine output. Signs and symptoms are nonspecific and subtle and may be attributed to other clinical conditions (Table 11-1). Elevated IAP affects the cardiovascular, pulmonary, renal, and neurologic systems.

Cardiovascular: Hypotension may result from decreased CO, which results from IAH-induced vasoconstriction. Signs of shock, including pallor, tachycardia, and cool and clammy skin, may be present. Venous return is diminished caused by compression of the IVC, resulting in loss of compliance (increased IVC pressure) and decreased preload (volume), which further reduces CO. Increased IAP compresses the aorta, resulting in elevated SVR (increased afterload), which reduces CO. The compensatory vasoconstriction affects blood flow to the hepatic and renal veins, leading to renal compromise, oliguria, and hepatic hypoperfusion; if untreated, kidney and liver failure can result.

Pulmonary: Respiratory distress results from the elevated abdominal pressure impeding diaphragmatic movement by forcing the diaphragm upward, which decreases functional residual capacity, promotes atelectasis, and decreases lung surface area. Tachypnea and increased work of breathing may be present. The worsening hypoxemia promotes elevated peak inspiratory pressures, with refractory hypoxemia and a poor P/F ratio, similar to acute respiratory distress syndrome (ARDS). Alternative ventilatory support is often required to maintain oxygenation and ventilation.

Neurologic: Altered mental status results from obstruction of cerebral venous outflow, leading to vascular congestion and increased intracranial pressure . Increased IAP increases intrathoracic pressure, which compresses the veins within the thoracic cavity, making it difficult for cerebral veins to drain properly. The combination of decreased CO and increased intracranial pressure can lead to decreased CPP, which prompts further deterioration in level of consciousness.

Renal: Renal dysfunction results as the increasing abdominal pressure compresses the bladder and urethra as well as the renal arteries and veins. Urine output decreases and serum creatinine and BUN increase, although they may not do so in proportion to each other (BUN/creatinine ratio).

RESEARCH BRIEF 11-1

The findings of this study revealed the mean IAP within 24 hours of ICU admission is an independent predictor of mortality. IAP measurements assist with the identification of patients at increased risk of death in the first 24 hours of admission. This is a time when therapy could save the patient's life. Although no definitive risk factor profile is identified, serial IAP measurements are an excellent indicator when patients have significant evidence of lactic acidosis.

Reintam Blaser A, Sarapuu S, Tamme K, et al: Expanded measurements of intra-abdominal pressure do not increase the detection rate of intra-abdominal hypertension: a single-center observational study. Crit Care Med 42:378-386, 2014.

DIAGNOSTIC TESTS

METHODS OF INTRAABDOMINAL PRESSURE MEASUREMENT

The best method for measurement of IAP is controversial. The most common method is measuring the response of intrabladder compliance to an instillation of 25 mL of sterile fluid by measuring the resulting pressure.

Direct intraperitoneal measurement

The most accurate method requires an intraperitoneal catheter inserted into the abdomen with a fluid manometer or pressure transducer attached to measure the pressure. This method requires expert catheter placement and is highly linked to infection.

Indirect methods

Bladder pressure is commonly used, while other methods are infrequently used. Indirect methods include gastric pressure measurement through gastrostomy or a nasogastric tube, intrarectal pressure measurement using an esophageal stethoscope catheter, or bladder pressure measurement through a urinary catheter.

Bladder pressure measurement: As physical examination is notoriously inaccurate in detecting the presence of IAH, bedside IAP monitoring is essential to both recognizing IAH and avoiding IAP-induced organ failure. An indwelling urinary catheter is connected to either a pressure transducer or a fluid manometer to measure the pressure. Readings are reliable and easier to perform than direct intraperitoneal measurement. More information regarding the different methods to measure IAP, including the pros and cons of each technique, can be found on the WSACS website (www.wsacs.org).

The urinary bladder normally has a compliant wall. Many studies reveal compliance decreases when there is a high presence of intraabdominal fluids, which increases the pressure in the abdominal cavity and compresses the bladder, increasing resistance. When fluid is injected into the bladder pressure system, any decrease in bladder compliance is reflected by increased intrabladder pressure. The procedure is generally easier and safer if a prepackaged closed bladder pressure system is used. If assembling the system without a prepackaged tool, use the urinary/Foley catheter with an aspiration or infusion port:

1. The nurse will connect a fluid-filled pressure system to a transducer, then connect a needle to the distal end of the tubing (farthest from the transducer and after a stopcock).
2. The cable connecting the system to the monitor should allow for visualization of a small pressure (scale either at auto or 30 mm Hg).
3. The connected system will be inserted into the catheter infusion port.
4. After zeroing the system (transducer at the symphysis pubis and the stopcock will be turned off to the patient), the nurse will clamp the catheter drainage system just below the infusion port.
5. Using the stopcock, the system will be turned off to the monitor and 25 mL of sterile fluid (an intravenous [IV] fluid is fine) will be injected rapidly into the infusion port on the urinary catheter. The stopcock will be then turned off to the injecting port, leaving a connected pressure system from patient to monitor.
6. Bladder pressure must be read during end expiration and the patient must be as flat as tolerated to facilitate accuracy. There is no dynamic waveform associated with bladder pressure. One should just observe the level of pressure in the first 10 to 20 seconds after fluid is instilled.
7. A normal value is generally considered between 0 and 5 mm Hg, although levels as high as 15 mm Hg are not unusual in the first 24 hours after abdominal surgery (see Table 11-1). If the pressures are elevated, document and repeat in the next hour using the same techniques. Inform the physician or midlevel practitioner if both measures are elevated.
8. Occlusion is then released and fluid is drained into the urine collection bag. Subtract the amount of fluid from the hourly output.

The measurement of IAP is key to IAH and ACS. The process must be standardized, and definitions are crucial. IAP is measured (in mm Hg) at end expiration; the patient should be supine and refrain (or be controlled) from spontaneous muscle contractions. The midaxillary line is used as the zero reference level for IAP measurement. Methods for continuous IAP measurement also are available. It is advised that IAP monitoring be based on a protocol, known risk factors, monitoring equipment available, and nursing staff experience and should be linked directly to a treatment protocol. Patients with any of the conditions associated with IAH should be monitored using a transvesicular technique at least every 4 hours until IAP decreases to less than 12 mm Hg and the decrease is sustained for at least 24 hours.

RESEARCH BRIEF 11-2

In this retrospective, nonexperimental, observational analysis performed in a large urban trauma center, many risk factors appeared for IAH and ACS. As expected, there was a very strong relationship between polytransfusion and death in patients with ACS. However, what was most significant was that, in the setting where ACS is highly probable, developing and adhering to a protocol for assessing ACS and monitoring IAP were considered essential. Serial measures were not performed, much to the authors' dismay, and the suggestion is that, were they performed according to a protocol, mortality may be decreased.

Harrell BR, Melander S: Identifying the association among risk factors and mortality in trauma patients with intra-abdominal hypertension and abdominal compartment syndrome. *J Trauma Nurs* 19:182–189, 2012.

COLLABORATIVE MANAGEMENT
CARE PRIORITIES
1. Prevent abdominal compartment syndrome
Patients who have a high index of suspicion should have bladder pressure monitoring initiated to identify IAH earlier and possibly avoid decompressive laparotomy, which is the only documented evidence-based therapy for ACS (Box 11-1). Many approaches may be used to

---

Box 11-1 MANAGEMENT OF ABDOMINAL COMPARTMENT SYNDROME

1. Improvement of abdominal wall compliance
   Sedation
   Pain relief (not fentanyl!)
   Neuromuscular blockade
   Body positioning
   Negative fluid balance
   Percutaneous abdominal wall component separation
2. Evacuation of intraluminal contents
   Nasogastric suction
   Rectal tube/enemas
   Gastro/colonic prokinetic agents
   Paracentesis
   Percutaneous drainage of abscess/hematomas
3. Evacuation of periintestinal and abdominal fluids
   Ascites evacuation in cirrhosis
   CT- or ultrasound-guided aspiration of abscess
   CT- or ultrasound-guided aspiration of hematoma
   Percutaneous drainage of (blood) collections
   Ascites evacuation in cirrhosis
4. Correction of capillary leak and positive fluid balance
   Diuretics/colloids/hypertonic fluids
   Hemodialysis/ultrafiltration
   Dobutamine (not dopamine!)
   Ascorbic acid in burn patients

Modified from Ivatury R, Cheatham M, Malbrain M et al: In Vincent JL, editor: *Yearbook of intensive care and emergency medicine*. Berlin, 2008, Springer, Chapter 5.

reduce IAH; all are directed at reducing increased abdominal cavity volume or decreasing compliance.

Therapies include:

- Draining free intraperitoneal fluid: Paracentesis is performed by the advanced practitioner. Some centers may place a peritoneal drainage catheter and leave it in place if abdominal fluid accumulation is persistent and severe.
- Volume replacement with small volumes of higher osmotic gradient intravenous fluids: More highly concentrated IV solutions (e.g., hypertonic [3%] saline, plasma, Hextend, blood products) can sometimes facilitate fluid stabilization within the vasculature for longer periods of time than isotonic solutions.
- Continuous renal replacement therapy: Enables minute-to-minute control of intravascular fluid removal and replacement and more exact fluid management. This technique was thought to benefit the patient by removal of cytokines, but more recent evidence indicates that it may not be of benefit (see Continuous Renal Replacement Therapies, Chapter 6).
- Other options: Include sedation and analgesic management of patients and ultimately the consideration of neuromuscular blockade or chemical paralysis.

2. Perform a decompressive laparotomy to relieve abdominal compartment syndrome

Sudden release of the abdominal pressure may lead to further complications including ischemia-reperfusion injury, acute vasodilation, cardiac dysfunction, and arrest. Arteries and veins within the abdomen are suddenly able to expand to normal size and "refill" with normal blood volume. If the patient has insufficient volume to accommodate the renewed space within the vasculature, hypotension ensues. Patients should be hydrated with at least 2 L of IV fluid, which may include a "cellular protection cocktail," such as 25 g of mannitol 12.5% given along with 2 ampules of bicarbonate/L. IV fluids and vasopressors should be immediately available in case severe hypotension occurs as the abdomen is decompressed.

After opening the abdomen, temporary closure will be applied. The goal is to permanently close the abdomen as soon as possible. For most patients who require emergent opening of the abdomen for ACS, a vacuum-assisted closure device (abdominal wound VAC) attached to a negative pressure device is commonly applied. An open abdomen may precipitate loss of liters of volume. The modified negative pressure wound VAC facilitates open wound fluid management and supports tissue granulation, as well as local perfusion, which facilitate eventual closure of the open wound.

CARE PLANS FOR ABDOMINAL COMPARTMENT SYNDROME AND INTRAABDOMINAL HYPERTENSION

DEFICIENT FLUID VOLUME *related to either active intravascular fluid loss secondary to physical injury or a condition resulting in capillary leak syndrome with third spacing of fluids.*

Goals/Outcomes: Within 12 hours of this diagnosis, the patient is becoming normovolemic, as evidenced by MAP at least 70 mm Hg, HR 60 to 100 beats per minute (bpm), normal sinus rhythm on electrocardiogram (ECG), central venous pressure (CVP) 2-6 mm Hg, cardiac index (CI) at least 2.5 L/min/m², bladder pressure measurements of less than 15 mm Hg, APP at least 60 mm Hg, stroke volume variation (SVV) less than 15%, urinary output at least 0.5 mL/kg/h, warm extremities, brisk capillary refill (less than 2 seconds), distal pulses at least 2+, bladder pressure measurements of less than 15 mm Hg, and APP at least 60 mm Hg. Stroke volume resuscitation, serum lactate, and base deficit are required to evaluate cellular perfusion.

NOC Fluid Balance; Electrolyte and Acid-Base Balance

Fluid/Electrolyte Management

1. Monitor BP at least hourly or more frequently in the presence of unstable vital signs. Be alert to changes in MAP of more than 10 mm Hg. Even a small but sudden decrease in BP signals the need to consult the physician or midlevel practitioner, especially with the trauma patient in whom the extent of injury is unknown.
2. Once stable, monitor BP at least hourly, or more frequently in the presence of any unstable vital signs. Be alert to changes in MAP of more than 10 mm Hg.
3. If massive fluid resuscitation was necessary for either the trauma patient or a patient with third-spaced fluid, the patient is at higher risk for IAH and should be observed closely for signs of decreased perfusion, respiratory distress, and deterioration in mental status.

4. In the patient with evidence of volume depletion or active blood loss, administer pressurized fluids rapidly through several large-caliber (16-gauge or larger) catheters. Use short, large-bore IV tubing (trauma tubing) to maximize flow rate. Avoid use of stopcocks, because they slow the infusion rate. Fluids should be warmed to prevent hypothermia.

5. Measure central pressures and CO continuously if possible, or at least every 2 hours if blood loss is ongoing. Be alert to low or decreasing CVP and PAWP. Be aware that profound tachycardia may be indicative of hypovolemia. Measure central pressures and CO continuously if possible, or at least every 2 hours if blood loss is ongoing. Calculate SVR and pulmonary vascular resistance (PVR) if data is available at least every 8 hours — more often in unstable patients with concurrent thoracic injury, such as pulmonary contusion, smoke inhalation, or early ARDS. ARDS is a concern in patients who have sustained major abdominal injury, inasmuch as there are many potential sources of infection and sepsis that make the development of ARDS more likely (see Acute Lung Injury and Acute Respiratory Distress Syndrome, Chapter 4).

6. Measure urinary output at least every 2 hours. Urine output less than 0.5 mL/kg/h usually reflects inadequate intravascular volume in the patient with abdominal trauma. Decreasing urine output may also signify compression of the renal arteries in ACS.

7. Monitor for physical indicators of arterial hypovolemia, which may include cool extremities, capillary refill greater than 2 seconds, absent or decreased amplitude of distal pulses, elevated serum lactate, and base deficit.

8. Estimate ongoing blood loss. Measure all bloody drainage from tubes or catheters, noting drainage color (e.g., coffee grounds, burgundy, bright red). Note the frequency of dressing changes as a result of saturation with blood to estimate amount of blood loss by way of the wound site.

NIC Electrolyte Management; Fluid Management; Fluid Monitoring; Hypovolemia Management

---

INEFFECTIVE TISSUE PERFUSION: GASTROINTESTINAL *related to interruption of arterial or venous blood flow or hypovolemia secondary to physical injury or any condition resulting in third-spaced fluid or development of ascites.*

Goals/Outcomes: Within 12 hours of this diagnosis, the patient is becoming normovolemic, as evidenced by MAP at least 70 mm Hg, HR 60 to 100 bpm, normal sinus rhythm on ECG, CVP 2-6 mm Hg, bladder pressure measurements of less than 15 mm Hg, APP at least 60 mm Hg, CI at least 2.5 L/min/m^2, SVV less than 15%, urinary output at least 0.5 mL/kg/h, warm extremities, brisk capillary refill (less than 2 seconds), distal pulses at least 2+, SVV less than 15%, urinary output at least 0.5 mL/kg/h, and warm extremities. By the time of hospital discharge, the patient has adequate abdominal tissue perfusion as evidenced by normoactive bowel sounds; soft, nondistended abdomen; and return of bowel elimination.

NOC Tissue Perfusion: Abdominal Organs

Circulatory Care: Arterial Insufficiency

1. Identify patients who are at high risk for IAH.

2. Monitor BP at least hourly or more frequently in the presence of unstable vital signs.

3. Monitor HR, ECG, and cardiovascular status every 15 minutes until vital signs are stable.

4. Auscultate for bowel sounds hourly during the acute phase of abdominal trauma and every 4 to 8 hours during the recovery phase. Report prolonged or sudden absence of bowel sounds during the postoperative period, because these signs may signal bowel ischemia or mesenteric infarction, which requires immediate surgical intervention.

5. Evaluate the patient for peritoneal signs (see Box 3-3, Chapter 3), which may occur initially as a result of injury or may not develop until days or weeks later, if complications caused by slow bleeding or other mechanisms occur.

6. Ensure adequate intravascular volume.

7. Evaluate labwork for evidence of bleeding (e.g., serial hematocrit [Hct]) or organ ischemia (e.g., aspartate aminotransferase [AST], alanine aminotransferase [ALT], lactate dehydrogenase [LDH]). Desired values are Hct greater than 28% to 30%, AST 5 to 40 IU/L, ALT 5 to 35 IU/L, and LDH 90 to 200 U/L.

8. Measure bladder pressure manually: See Diagnostic Tests, Bladder Pressure Measurement, Chapter 11.

9. Prepackaged closed-system bladder pressure monitoring: Complete bladder pressure monitoring systems became available approximately 10 years ago. They remain completely closed throughout injection of fluid into the bladder, making them more useful in preventing catheter-associated urinary tract infections.

10. Assess for changes in level of consciousness, possibly resulting from increased IAP, which may inadvertently affect draining of the cerebral veins.

RISK FOR INFECTION *related to inadequate primary defenses secondary to physical trauma, surgery, underlying infection, temporary closure of abdomen, or insertion of urinary catheter for measurement of IAP; inadequate secondary defenses caused by debilitated condition, decreased hemoglobin, or inadequate immune response; tissue destruction and environmental exposure (especially to intestinal contents); multiple invasive procedures.*

Goals/Outcomes: The patient is free of infection as evidenced by core or rectal temperature less than 37.7°C (100°F); normal white blood cell count and no bandemia; HR less than 100 bpm; orientation to time, place, and person; and absence of unusual redness, warmth, or drainage at surgical incisions and drain sites.
NOC Immune Status; Infection Severity

Infection Protection
1. Note color, character, and odor of all drainage. Report the presence of foul-smelling or abnormal drainage. See Table 3-2 for a description of the usual character of GI drainage.
2. As prescribed, administer pneumococcal vaccine to patients with total splenectomy to minimize the risk of postsplenectomy sepsis.
3. If evisceration occurs initially or develops later, do not reinsert tissue or organs. Place a saline-soaked gauze over the evisceration, and cover with a sterile towel until it can be evaluated by a surgeon.
4. For more interventions, see this diagnosis in Abdominal Trauma (Chapter 3).

NIC Infection Control

ADDITIONAL NURSING DIAGNOSES

Also see Major Trauma, Chapter 3. For additional information, see nursing diagnoses and interventions in the following sections: Hemodynamic Monitoring (Chapter 1), Prolonged Immobility (Chapter 1), Emotional and Spiritual Support of the Patient and Significant Others (Chapter 2), Peritonitis (Chapter 9), Enterocutaneous Fistula (Chapter 9), SIRS, Sepsis and MODS (Chapter 11), and Acid-Base Imbalances (Chapter 1).

DRUG OVERDOSE
OVERVIEW/EPIDEMIOLOGY

Over 2.3 million human toxic exposure cases are reported annually to American poison control centers. Most cases are unintentional, involve a single agent, and can be handled on site with help from a poison control center. Although the overall mortality of these cases is low, over a quarter of them require an emergency department visit and 7.1% result in inpatient admissions.

The type, amount, and route of the agent determine the signs/symptoms, physical presentation, prognosis, management, and outcome of a toxic exposure. Every drug has a threshold for occurrence of serious toxic effects. Drugs of abuse are more dangerous than prescription drugs, as they are uncontrolled and unregulated, with a haphazard nature of administration. The patient's history is often unavailable or of poor quality. Time is critical to successful treatment. A thoughtful and stepwise approach to laboratory testing, medical and nursing interventions, pharmacologic support, and general supportive measures is essential. No organ or body system is protected from the detrimental effects of drug overdose.

INGESTION OF UNKNOWN SUBSTANCES

Many patients with drug overdose present with altered mental status and without a useful or reliable history. Identification of the ingested substance is difficult. Labwork is done for common drugs of abuse, including amphetamines, barbiturates, benzodiazepines, cocaine, opioids, phencyclidine, and cannabinoids. Specific drug levels are available for salicylates, acetaminophen, digoxin, theophylline, iron, and lithium. When one of these drugs is not the offending agent, a number of signs and symptoms should be noted and tests done to determine the list of potential offending agents.

ASSESSMENT

It is beyond the scope of this chapter to include all the drugs and toxins leading to common presenting symptoms, but important clues to the poison may be gleaned from answering the following questions:

- HR and rhythm: Is the patient bradycardic or tachycardic? Is a dysrhythmia present?
- Mental status: Is the patient overall depressed or agitated? Is delirium present?
- Temperature: Is hypothermia or hyperthermia present? Is the patient diaphoretic?
- Seizures: Is the patient having seizures?
- Eyes: Are pupils showing miosis or mydriasis? Is nystagmus present?
- Muscle tone: Is the patient flaccid or rigid? Are dyskinesias present?
- Lungs: If respiratory failure is occurring, is it related to depression, aspiration, edema, hemorrhage, bronchospasm, or cardiac failure? What is the pulse oximetry?
- Arterial blood gas (ABG): Is the pH acidotic or alkalotic?
- Anion gap: If abnormal, is it increased or decreased?
- Blood glucose: Is the patient hyperglycemic or hypoglycemic?
- Psychosocial: Does the patient have a history of psychiatric disorders, drug abuse, or depression? Is the patient on any drugs with narrow therapeutic windows, and is a list of current medications (including over-the-counter drugs) available?

GENERAL TREATMENT OPTIONS: GASTRIC DECONTAMINATION

Gastric decontamination is a general term referring to interventions used to reduce the total bioavailability of a toxin, usually through decreased absorption. Timely administration is essential for success. Best results are obtained if done within an hour of ingestion. If the ingested substance is nontoxic, not amenable to decontamination, or already absorbed, gastric decontamination is contraindicated.

ACTIVATED CHARCOAL

Activated charcoal (AC) is a fine, insoluble, nonabsorbable powder that binds with many toxic drugs to enhance their elimination. A review of the literature yields mixed results on the efficacy of AC. The dose is 25 to 100 g initially. Repeat dosing of half that amount every 4 hours is recommended by the American Academy of Clinical Toxicology if the poisoning involves life-threatening overdoses of carbamazepine, dapsone, phenobarbital, quinine, or theophylline. A combination product of AC and sorbitol is available; the latter component increases the tolerability of charcoal and may help reduce constipation. Contraindications to AC are bowel obstruction or perforation, depressed mental status (unless the airway is protected), delayed presentation, and need for endoscopy. AC does not bind with inorganic ions such as lithium, potassium, and magnesium; with alcohols such as ethanol, methanol, propylene glycol, and isopropyl alcohol; with heavy metals such as iron, lead, mercury, and arsenic; with acidic or alkaline corrosives; or with hydrocarbons.

GASTRIC LAVAGE

Commonly known as "pumping the stomach," gastric lavage is the insertion of an orogastric tube followed by repeatedly instilling and aspirating small quantities of fluid. It is no longer recommended as routine management by American and European toxicology associations. In the rare case that it is used, it must be done as soon as possible, within 60 minutes of the ingestion. When using lavage, the airway must be protected and lavage should continue until the fluid is clear of fragments (it usually requires about 5 L of fluid). Gastric lavage should not be attempted if it delays or interferes with AC administration in appropriate patients.

Large, life-threatening amounts of recently ingested toxin (which may be poorly bound to AC used before lavage) may justify use. Contraindications include the risk or presence of esophageal hemorrhage or perforation, unprotected airways, and caustic or hydrocarbon ingestions.

WHOLE BOWEL IRRIGATION

The administration of a polyethylene glycol-balanced electrolyte solution to rapidly cleanse the bowel may be useful in cases where AC is ineffective, such as with ingestions of iron, lithium, illicit drug packets, and sustained-released tablets. It may diminish the effectiveness of AC, but one study showed that the combination led to decreased absorption of extended-release venlafaxine. Whole bowel irrigation is contraindicated when ileus, GI bleeding, severe vomiting, hemodynamic instability, bowel obstruction, or bowel perforation is present.

GENERAL TREATMENT OPTIONS: EXTRACORPOREAL REMOVAL OF TOXINS

Techniques include all types of dialysis, continuous renal replacement therapy, and plasmapheresis. These methods are most often used to remove methanol, ethylene glycol, lithium, theophylline, salicylates, sotalol, and phenobarbital. Extracorporeal therapies may be used in extreme cases when other management strategies are ineffective for drugs that are not highly protein bound, have a reasonable molecular size, are water soluble (rather than lipid soluble), have a limited volume of distribution, and are not highly charged or ionized. Hemofilters used for continuous renal replacement therapy are often able to accommodate larger-sized molecules than conventional hemodialysis therapy.

ILLICIT AND PRESCRIPTION DRUGS COMMONLY SEEN IN OVERDOSE SITUATIONS

ACETAMINOPHEN

Acetaminophen is one of the most commonly ingested drugs in overdose, and historically it has accounted for the most deaths. Most patients admit taking this drug. Unintentional overdose may occur because of polypharmacy, wherein acetaminophen is contained in one or more other medications being used. Unintentional overdose is more common in children. Signs and symptoms of toxicity vary significantly depending on the dose, time elapsed since ingestion, and whether overdose resulted from acute or chronic ingestion. Toxicity from acute ingestion may be asymptomatic for up to 12 hours. Any person who has ingested greater than 10 g (adult) or 200 mg/kg (child) (or unknown quantity) should be referred to an emergency department.

Routes of administration

Oral (most common); rectal per suppository.

Effects on body systems

Cardiovascular: Hepatic damage may prompt cardiac complications including dysrhythmias, ischemia, and injury (chest pain/pressure, nausea, shortness of breath, T-wave inversion, and ST-segment elevation on ECG).

Respiratory: Bronchospasm (wheezing and difficulty breathing) and tachypnea have been reported as a hypersensitivity reaction or as a side effect of N-acetylcysteine. See the Collaborative Management section that follows.

Neurologic: Coma and seizures.

Hepatic: Acute ingestion will cause hepatic necrosis, which can lead to liver failure. Hypoglycemia, right-sided abdominal pain, and nausea with vomiting may be noted, usually 1 to 2 days after ingestion.

Renal: Acute tubular necrosis with renal failure is seen in some cases but often resolves.

Associated findings: Hypophosphatemia, metabolic acidosis, hypothermia, thrombocytopenia, and hemorrhagic pancreatitis.

COLLABORATIVE MANAGEMENT

Care Priorities

1. Support of cardiovascular and respiratory systems: Supplemental oxygen should be given if ABG values indicate a trend toward respiratory failure. If the patient has an ineffective or absent breathing effort, mechanical ventilation is provided. Serial ECGs monitor for dysrhythmias. Symptomatic ventricular dysrhythmias and bradyarrhythmias are treated per Advanced Cardiac Life Support (ACLS) guidelines.

2. Removing acetaminophen from the patient: N-acetylcysteine (Mucomyst), either orally or intravenously administered, is the drug of choice for acetaminophen overdose. If ingestion occurred within the previous 1 to 2 hours, AC should be administered. It can be given with N-acetylcysteine, either orally or via a gastric tube. N-acetylcysteine prevents systemic toxicity, especially if given 8 to 10 hours after ingestion. Lavage may be used only if less than 1 hour has elapsed since ingestion, but administration of AC and N-acetylcysteine should not be delayed to perform lavage. Acetaminophen levels and liver function tests should be followed closely

3. Treatment of nausea and vomiting: Fluid replacement therapy with lactated Ringer solution or D5NS (dextrose 5% in 0.9% normal saline solution); antiemetics, such as promethazine hydrochloride (Phenergan) or ondansetron (Zofran).

4. Rewarming: Warming therapies (such as warm IV solutions, warm blankets, or water-filled heating blankets) may be used if the patient has significant hypothermia.

5. Treatment of hypoglycemia: Usually done with a bolus of dextrose 50% solution (D_{50}) and continuous infusion of dextrose 5% solution (D_5W), based on serum glucose results. Hypoglycemia occurs because of the potent hepatotoxic effects of acetaminophen.

ALCOHOLS

ETHANOL

Route of administration

Oral.

Effects on body systems

Cardiovascular: Tachycardia, atrial fibrillation, cardiac arrest.
Respiratory: Hypoventilation with acute intoxication, respiratory failure, aspiration.
Neurologic: Confusion, aggressive behavior, irritability, tremors, hallucinations (especially auditory), memory loss, stupor, coma, seizures, loss of deep tendon reflexes.
Renal: May have a large urine output initially; will demonstrate dehydration with low urine output with acute intoxication.
Associated findings: Dry oral mucosa, odor of alcohol on breath, hypoglycemia, hypothermia, lactic acidosis, hypokalemia.

COLLABORATIVE MANAGEMENT

Care Priorities

1. Support of cardiovascular and respiratory systems to prevent collapse: Oxygen supplementation; treatment of ventricular dysrhythmias and bradyarrhythmias according to ACLS guidelines.

2. Fluid/potassium replacement: Manage hypovolemia with IV fluid infusion. Include IV multivitamins in fluid replacement, and provide thiamine to prevent Wernicke encephalopathy. Potassium, calcium, phosphorus, and magnesium should be monitored and supplemented as necessary.

3. Removing alcohol from the patient: As alcohol is metabolized, the blood alcohol level decreases 15 mg/dL/h, according to recent literature (legal limit for driving is less than 100 mg/dL). Coma may occur if the level is greater than 300 mg/dL, but this is influenced by each individual's metabolic process and tolerance. When extreme amounts of alcohol have been absorbed into the system, the liver and kidneys may not be able to break down and excrete the alcohol. Hemodialysis may be used for a life-threatening intoxication.

4. Prevention of emesis: Antiemetics are given, and a gastric tube is inserted and maintained at low continuous suction.

5. Anticipation and treatment of withdrawal: Benzodiazepines are the drugs of choice for treating alcohol withdrawal. Lorazepam, which can be given IV, intramuscularly (IM), orally (PO), or sublingually (SL), is the preferred agent in most alcohol withdrawal protocols. Longer-acting agents such as diazepam are also used, because of the decreased risk of recurrent withdrawal and/or seizures. Oxazepam and lorazepam have a mechanism of metabolism that is less liver dependent and are useful in cases involving cirrhosis. Medications are given as needed for withdrawal symptoms. In patients at high risk for severe withdrawal symptoms or if withdrawal would be dangerous, benzodiazepines may be given on a schedule. If withdrawal is severe and benzodiazepine doses become excessive, barbiturates may be added. Agents that have glutamate-blocking properties, such as lamotrigine, memantine, and topiramate, are showing promise in alcohol detoxification.

6. Treatment of hypoglycemia: A bolus of D_{50} and continuous infusion of D_5W, based on serum glucose. Thiamine should be given with glucose to avoid sudden onset of heart failure and worsening neurologic impairment.

7. Treatment of delirium tremens (DTs): The most severe manifestation of withdrawal, which can result in death. Symptoms develop 48 to 96 hours after cessation of alcohol ingestion and include confusion, disorientation, delirium, agitation, severe diaphoresis, tachycardia, fever, and hypotension. Intubation may be required to protect the airway. Delirium tremens generally resolve within 3 to 5 days. Patients are sedated with benzodiazepines, allowed to rest and sleep, and oriented frequently to reality.

8. Treatment/prevention of seizures: Alcohol withdrawal seizures may occur in a range from the first 6 to 48 hours to late onset at 10 days after abstinence. Benzodiazepines are given to raise the seizure threshold during the withdrawal period. Additional seizure management should reflect institution protocol. If the patient has a history of a primary seizure disorder, an anticonvulsant agent may also be indicated.

9. Prevention of Wernicke-Korsakoff syndrome: Caused by thiamine deficiency and manifested by diplopia (the first real diagnostic clue), confusion, excitation, peripheral neuropathy, severe recent memory loss, impaired thought processes, and confabulation. Prophylactic administration of thiamine is recommended: IM thiamine on admission; supplemental oral thiamine; and multivitamins and multiminerals high in C, B complex, zinc, and magnesium. Multivitamins and minerals are given to prevent malnutrition related to inadequate food intake and malabsorption caused by alcohol's irritating effect on the GI tract. Ingestion of carbohydrates, either orally or parenterally, increases the body's demand for thiamine. Traditionally thiamine has been recommended to be administered before glucose, but evidence supporting a benefit of this practice is lacking. One reason for this may be that thiamine is taken up into the cells more slowly than dextrose, so the order of administration is consequently relatively minor. Thiamine repletion is very important, however, and 100 mg should be administered promptly, via a parenteral route for the first dose in severe cases.

METHANOL AND ETHYLENE GLYCOL
Route of administration
Oral; found in household cleaning and automotive products, especially antifreeze. Methanol poisoning can be associated with illicit distillation of alcohol ("moonshine") or intentional substitution for ethanol.

Effects on body systems
The parent compounds have effects that are similar to ethanol. The metabolites, however, can be extremely toxic.

Formate, a metabolite of methanol, causes retinal injury and edema. Untreated, it can lead to permanent blindness.

Ethylene glycol metabolites target the kidney and lead to reversible acute kidney injury. This compounds the situation by slowing elimination of the ethylene glycol. Hypocalcemia is also a serious sequela of ethylene glycol ingestion.

With both ingestions, a profound anion gap metabolic acidosis develops, which can complicate and accelerate damage from the metabolites ultimately leading to hypoxia and coma or death.

Collaborative Management
Similar to ethanol for hypoglycemia/seizures. Administer bicarbonate if the pH is less than 7.3 and provide thiamine, folate, and multivitamins in all patients. Fomepizole is a specific antidote, followed by hemodialysis if the patient does not respond. In severe cases (pH less than 7.25, high plasma levels of alcohol, kidney injury, or severe electrolyte disturbances), hemodialysis should be done immediately. Ethanol has also traditionally been used as an antidote for methanol and ethylene glycol but, while cheaper, has a worse side effect profile. The preferred IV dosage form has also been removed from the market.

ASPIRIN AND OTHER SALICYLATES
Common Agents: Include Acetylsalicylic acid (aspirin, ASA), Ben Gay topical ointment, methyl salicylate, magnesium salicylate, salicylic acid, bismuth subsalicylate. Ingestion of topical products containing salicylates, including Ben-Gay, salicylic acid (keratolytic), and methyl salicylate (oil of wintergreen), can result in severe salicylate toxicity. One teaspoon (5 mL) of 98% methyl salicylate contains 7000 mg of salicylate (the same as 90 baby aspirins), which is greater than 4 times the toxic dose for a 10-kg child. Salicylate toxicity can occur with use of salicylate-containing teething gels in infants. Use of alternative medicines, herbs, and traditional medicines is increasing, and many of these substances may contain salicylate. Salicylate poisoning should be considered when herbal medicines, including topical oils, have been used.

Routes of administration

Oral, rectal (suppository), topical.

Effects on body systems

Early symptoms/blood levels: Tinnitus, nausea, vomiting, diarrhea, hyperpnea, and vertigo. Signs of toxicity can be seen at therapeutic levels (10 to 30 mg/dL) but are more common at 40 to 50 mg/dL. Adult patients with toxicity usually present with a mixed respiratory alkalosis and metabolic acidosis. Respiratory alkalosis may be transient in children and metabolic acidosis may manifest earlier. Occasionally, patients with mixed acid-base disturbances have normal anion gap metabolic acidosis. Normal anion gap acidosis does not rule out salicylate toxicity. Chronic ingestion of salicylates may result in anxiety with tachypnea, difficulty concentrating, diaphoresis, and hallucinations with agitated delirium. Elderly patients may report a deterioration in functional status or symptoms of pneumonia, caused by the presence of tachypnea and fever.

Later signs and symptoms include the following:

Metabolic: Increased cellular metabolic activity may result in clinical signs and symptoms of hypoglycemia with blood glucose levels that are sometimes normal, caused by a discrepancy between blood and cerebrospinal fluid glucose levels. Intracellular glucose is depleted before blood glucose reflects the change.

Respiratory: Hyperventilation, tachypnea, hyperpnea, noncardiogenic pulmonary edema. Acute lung injury may be seen in pediatric patients and in elderly patients with chronic salicylate toxicity.

Cardiac: Tachycardia and, later, ventricular dysrhythmias (cardiac effects secondary to other factors such as hypovolemia, agitation, and electrolyte disturbances).

Neurologic: Salicylates are neurotoxic. The first manifestation is tinnitus. Later, coma, seizures, and cerebral edema with increased intracranial pressure may be present (see Box 7-1). Hearing loss may occur at serum levels greater than 30 to 45 mg/dL. Central nervous system (CNS) toxicity depends on the amount of drug bound to CNS tissue and is more common with chronic poisoning than with acute ingestions.

Renal: Renal failure secondary to rhabdomyolysis, resulting from muscle breakdown caused by abnormal glucose metabolism. All patients with poisoning are at least 5% to 10% dehydrated. Clearance of salicylate by the kidneys is decreased by dehydration. Hypokalemia and hypocalcemia are prompted by the respiratory alkalosis created by tachypnea and hyperpnea.

Hepatic: Liver dysfunction, hepatitis. Hepatitis manifests in children who ingest doses ≥ 30.9 mg/dL.javascript:showrefcontent('refrenceslayer'); Reye syndrome is a form of pediatric salicylate-induced hepatic disease characterized by nausea, vomiting, hypoglycemia, elevated levels of liver enzymes and ammonia, fatty infiltration of the liver, increased intracranial pressure, and coma.

Hematolgic findings: Hypoprothrombinemia and platelet dysfunction are common. Bleeding may result from inhibition of vitamin K-dependent enzymes or from platelet dysfunction.

COLLABORATIVE MANAGEMENT

Care Priorities

1. Support of cardiovascular system to prevent collapse: Electrical rhythm is monitored. Ventricular dysrhythmias and tachydysrhythmias are treated per ACLS guidelines. When all compensatory mechanisms fail, bradydysrhythmias may occur before cardiac arrest.
2. Removal of salicylates: AC is administered orally or via gastric tube to bind with the substance in the stomach; several doses of AC may be necessary to achieve a 10:1 ratio of charcoal to salicylate. Hemodialysis may be necessary if the substance has been more extensively absorbed. Charcoal hemoperfusion may clear salicylates somewhat but cannot correct acid-base, electrolyte, and fluid problems associated with severe poisoning. Hemodialysis may be necessary if cerebral edema, severe fluid overload, clinical deterioration, or salicylate levels greater than 100 mg/dL occur.
3. Fluid replacement: Replace fluids with lactated Ringer solution or normal saline (NS; 0.9% saline) 20 mL/kg over 1 to 2 hours. Sodium bicarbonate may be added to promote forced alkaline diuresis, even if the pH is normal or mildly elevated. Acetazolamide should not be used.
4. Potassium replacement: See Fluid and Electrolyte Imbalances: Hypokalemia, Chapter 1.

5. Treatment of hyperthermia: A cooling blanket, cool saline infusion, intravascular cooling, or applications of ice may be used.
6. Glucose administration/treatment of hypoglycemia: Blood glucoses should be maintained in the upper normal range (110 to 140 mg/dL). There is a risk of cerebral hypoglycemia even with normal blood glucoses so glucose should be administered to patients with altered mental status even if normoglycemic.
7. Treatment of cerebral edema: Hyperventilation (via mechanical ventilation) or mannitol is used.
8. Respiratory support: Intubation and mechanical ventilation should be avoided if at all possible, but if necessary, high tidal volumes and rates are important to maintain an adequate pH.
9. Treatment of pulmonary edema: Nitrates, morphine, diuretics, potassium replacement, and noninvasive positive pressure mechanical ventilation (NPPV) are possible. Prevention of aspiration: A gastric tube is inserted, and then connected to low suction.
10. Replacement of blood loss: Through delivery of blood and blood products

BARBITURATES
Common agents: See Table 11-2.
Street names
Barbs, downers, ludes, rainbows, red dolls, reds, sleepers, stumblers, tootsies, yellow jackets.

Routes of administration
Oral, IV, IM.

Effects on body systems
Cardiovascular: Hypotension, bradycardia, cardiac arrest.
Respiratory: Hypoventilation leading to respiratory failure and respiratory arrest.
Neurologic: Symptoms may include headache, vertigo, dizziness, lethargy, ataxia, stupor, flaccidity, seizures, absent dolls-eye reflex, coma, loss of deep tendon reflexes, and nystagmus.
Renal: Acute renal failure is possible.
Associated findings: Hypothermia, nausea, vomiting. Patient may experience euphoria and excitability before the normal sedative effects occur. Withdrawal symptoms (tremors and convulsions) may occur.

COLLABORATIVE MANAGEMENT
Care Priorities
1. Removing barbiturates: If less than 1 hour has passed since ingestion, gastric lavage may be initiated (provided there is no delay in the administration of AC). AC is administered orally or via gastric tube to bind with the substance in the stomach, and repeat doses are recommended. Hemodialysis may be considered in severe cases, especially if coma is present, usually correlating with serum levels of 65 to 100 μg/mL. Similar to ASA, sodium bicarbonate can be given to alkalinize the urine and promote elimination.

Table 11-2	COMMON BARBITURATES	
Generic Name	**Common Trade Name**	**Half-life (Hours)**
Amobarbital	Amytal	8 to 42
Secobarbital	Seconal	19 to 34
Pentobarbital	Nembutal	15 to 48
Phenobarbital	Luminal and others	24 to 140
Butabarbital	Butisol	34 to 42
Secobarbital/amobarbital	Tuinal	8 to 42

Note: Withdrawal symptoms can be correlated with the half-life of the drug that was taken. Withdrawal from drugs with shorter half-lives produces more intense symptoms that last for shorter periods; whereas, withdrawal from drugs with longer half-lives produces less intense symptoms that can be prolonged. Moreover, the severity of the withdrawal is directly related to the drug's dosage.

Drug Overdose

2. Support of cardiovascular and respiratory systems to prevent collapse: Electrical rhythm is monitored; bradyarrhythmias are treated according to ACLS guidelines. After fluids are replaced, vasopressor therapy (see Appendix 6), including dopamine and norepinephrine bitartrate (Levophed), may be initiated for hypotension. Mechanical ventilation may be required, depending on the degree of hypoxia and CO_2 retention.
3. Prevention/treatment of seizures: Phenytoin or diazepam may be given.
4. Sedation for withdrawal symptoms: Typically the barbiturate that was ingested is tapered gradually to zero.
5. Prevention of aspiration: A gastric tube is inserted, which is then connected to low suction.
6. Treatment of nausea and vomiting: Antiemetics may be administered.
7. Treatment of hypothermia: A warming blanket is used.

BENZODIAZEPINES
Common agents
See Table 11-3.

Street names
Benzos, BZDs, downers, heavenly blues, qual, robital, stupes, tranx, Valley girl.

Routes of administration
Oral, IM, IV.

Effects on body systems
Cardiovascular: Hypotension, tachycardia.
Respiratory: Respiratory arrest.
Neurologic: Drowsiness, ataxia, slurred speech, coma. Withdrawal may be manifested by seizures.
Renal: Renal failure because of rhabdomyolysis.
Associated findings: Hypothermia.

COLLABORATIVE MANAGEMENT
Care Priorities
1. Support of cardiovascular system to prevent collapse: Electrical rhythm is monitored. Atrial fibrillation or flutter may be treated with digoxin or amiodarone, with initial rate

Table 11-3	COMMON BENZODIAZEPINES	
Generic Name	**Common Trade Name**	**Half-life (Hours)**
Chlordiazepoxide	Librium and others	7 to 28
Diazepam	Valium and others	20 to 90
Lorazepam	Ativan	10 to 20
Oxazepam	Serax	3 to 21
Prazepam	Centrax	24 to 200*
Flurazepam	Dalmane	24 to 100*
Chlorazepate	Tranxene	30 to 100
Temazepam	Restoril	9.5 to 12.4
Clonazepam	Klonopin	18.5 to 50
Alprazolam	Xanax	12 to 15
Halazepam	Paxipam	14

*Includes half-life of major metabolites.
Note: Withdrawal symptoms can be correlated with the half-life of the drug that was taken. Withdrawal from drugs with shorter half-lives produces more intense symptoms that last for shorter periods; whereas, withdrawal from drugs with longer half-lives produces less intense symptoms that can be prolonged. Moreover, the severity of the withdrawal is directly related to the drug's dosage.

control using diltiazem or beta blockers. Severe supraventricular tachyarrhythmias may be treated with adenosine. Hypotension is treated with fluid replacement, followed by dopamine or norepinephrine.

2. Support of respiratory system: Apnea monitoring and mechanical ventilation may be indicated. Flumazenil administration may be considered if hypoventilation ensues. Naloxone may be added if mixed ingestion, including opiates, is suspected.

3. Removing benzodiazepines from the patient: Gastric lavage is initiated if less than 60 minutes after ingestion; AC charcoal is used to bind with the substance in the stomach.

4. Prevention of seizures: Phenytoin is administered.

5. Prevention of aspiration: Gastric tube is inserted, which is then connected to low intermittent suction.

6. Rhabdomyolysis: Seizure activity and breakdown of muscle cause protein to precipitate in the kidneys, leading to renal failure. Creatine kinase levels of five times the upper limit of normal, with possible increases in BUN, creatinine, and urine protein, are noted when rhabdomyolysis is present. Prevention of seizures and aggressive fluid administration are the best means of preventing rhabdomyolysis; fluids are also the main treatment modality. Patients should be monitored closely for hyperkalemia if rhabdomyolysis develops.

7. Treatment of hypothermia: A warming blanket is used if indicated.

8. Flumazenil administration: Sedative and respiratory depressant effects may be reversed by flumazenil. Repeat doses may be necessary, since the duration of action of many benzodiazepines exceeds that of flumazenil. Use with caution, especially in patients with possible multidrug overdose. Flumazenil may precipitate seizures in benzodiazepine-dependent patients and causes arrhythmias in patients who also have high levels of cyclic antidepressants.

BETA BLOCKERS
Common agents
Metoprolol, propranolol, nadolol, atenolol, bisoprolol, carvedilol, sotalol, acebutolol, and nebivolol.

Routes of administration
Oral (for chronic use).

Effects on body systems
Cardiovascular: Bradycardia, hypotension, widened QRS, ventricular arrhythmias.
Respiratory: Depression.
Neurologic: Depressed level of consciousness, seizures.
Other: Hypoglycemia, hyperkalemia, rhabdomyolysis, renal failure, mesenteric ischemia.

COLLABORATIVE MANAGEMENT
Decontamination strategies can be used if 1 to 2 hours since ingestion. ACLS measures, including fluids for hypotension and atropine for severe bradycardia or heart block, may be necessary. IV calcium and glucagon are given to address negative inotropy and chronotropy. Glucose and insulin may be needed for blood sugar and electrolyte imbalances. Beta agonists (vasopressors) such as norepinephrine or epinephrine and sometimes inotropes such as dobutamine or milrinone are often needed to maintain hemodynamics in severe overdose.

CALCIUM CHANNEL BLOCKERS
Common agents
Verapamil, diltiazem, nifedipine, amlodipine, felodipine, isradipine, nisoldipine, and nicardipine .

Routes of administration
Oral (for chronic use).

Effects on body systems
Cardiovascular: Bradycardia, hypotension, widened PR interval, jugular venous distension if heart failure present.

Respiratory: Crackles and edema if heart failure present.
Other: Hyperglycemia (a potential means of differentiating from beta-blocker overdose).

COLLABORATIVE MANAGEMENT

Decontamination strategies can be used if 1 to 2 hours since ingestion. ACLS measures should be initiated, including fluids for hypotension, atropine for severe bradycardia or heart block, and airway and hemodynamic stabilization as necessary. IV calcium is given at high doses in an attempt to displace the overdosed drug and reopen calcium channels, though it is often ineffective. In animal models high-dose insulin has been effective in severe overdose, with or without dextrose depending on blood glucose levels. Other modalities that may be used include glucagon and vasopressors. Electrolytes should be closely monitored and treated accordingly.

CANNABINOIDS

MARIJUANA

Street names

Ashes, ashitshi, Aunt Mary, baby bhang, blanket, blunt, bobo, bomber, boom, broccoli, cheeba, chronic, cripple, dinky dow, Dona Juana, dope, flower tops, gange, giggle smoke, grass, hash, herb, jay joints, jolly green, joy smoke, Maryjane, pot, reefer, roach, skunk, weed.

Sometimes marijuana is combined with other drugs (narcotics, heroin, PCP, LSD, crack, cocaine, alcohol) to achieve a certain high.

Routes of administration

Smoked or ingested most commonly. Less common but presenting as more severely symptomatic is IV use of hashish oil. Cannabinoids contain tetrahydrocannabinol (THC).

Effects on body systems

Cardiovascular: Tachycardia, postural hypotension, atrial fibrillation, and angina.
Respiratory: Minimal effects unless mixed with other drugs.
Neurologic/psychiatric: Euphoria, poor concentration, confusion, somnolence, ataxia, memory impairments, perceptual alterations, mood fluctuations, panic disorders.
Renal: Urinary retention.

COLLABORATIVE MANAGEMENT

Supportive care, benzodiazepines, gastric decontamination measures if ingested recently, IV fluids.

SYNTHETIC CANNABINOIDS

Street names

Aroma, barely legal, bliss, K2, krypto buds, spice, spicestar fire.

Routes of administration

Like bath salts these are relatively recent drugs of abuse (use beginning around 2008), which are composed of a plant/herbal component, such as bay beans, dwarf skullcap, lousewart, red clover, rose, or vanilla, mixed with synthetic cannabinoid derivatives to mimic the effects of marijuana. They are marketed as incense or potpourri (as with bath salts labeled "not for human consumption"), sold via the internet, convenience stores, liquor stores, and head shops, and usually smoked. These synthetic agents bind as full agonists to the CB1 cannabinoid receptor, which is the target receptor, as opposed to THC, which is only a partial agonist, so the effects are more potent and the potential for overdose/toxicity is greater.

Effects on body systems

Similar to marijuana (THC), but more severe. May additionally cause nausea and vomiting, seizures, psychosis, and supraventricular tachycardia.

COLLABORATIVE MANAGEMENT

Supportive care. No antidote is available similar to THC. Some of the synthetic cannabinoids have a longer duration (CP-47, 497) and some shorter (JWH018 and JWH-073). Benzodiazepines for agitation and seizures, antipsychotics for severe or prolonged psychotic symptoms or a comorbid history of psychotic disorder, and IV fluids as needed are given.

COCAINE
Street names
Badrock, base, ball, bazooka, beam, beat, berni, big C, big flake, biscuits, blast, blizzard, blow, bones, boost, bouncing powder, boulders, boy, brick, bump, bunk, C, Cabello, cakes, caine, candy, casper, caviar, chalk, Charlie, chicken scratch, coca, cocaine blues, cocktail, coconut, coke, cola, Colombian, cooking up, cookies, crack, crumbs, cubes, do a line, Damablanca, devil drug, dust, esnortiar, everclear, fatbags, flake, flame cooking, flame throwers, flash, flex, Florida snow, foo, freebase, freeze, G rock, girl, goofball, gravel, happy dust, happy powder, happy trails, hardball, heaven, hell, kibbles 'n bits, king, kryptonite, lady, lady caine, late night, line, love, mama coca, marching dust, marching powder, mojo, monster, moonrocks, mujer and nieve (Spanish words), nose, nose candy, nuggets, onion, P dogs, pebbles, Peruvian, piedras (Spanish word), peace, pimp, powder, press, prime time, ready rock, Roca, rock, rock star, Roxanne, rush, Scott, Scottie, Scrabble, shootin' caine, sleigh ride, smoke houses, smoking gun, sniff, snow, snort, soda, speedball, sporting, stardust, stone, sugar, sweet stuff, teeth, toke, toot, tornado, trails, white horse, white lady, white powder, working bags, Yeyo (Spanish), zip.

Routes of administration
Nasal or IV (cocaine, snow); smoked (crack, rock); cooked; freebased (flame cooking, flame throwers).

Effects on body systems
Cardiovascular: Hypertension; sinus tachycardia and less commonly sinus bradycardia; ventricular dysrhythmias such as premature ventricular contractions, ventricular tachycardia and ventricular fibrillation; myocardial infarction; heart failure; cardiomyopathy; acute endocarditis; and aortic dissection. Intraventricular thrombus, as well as other thrombotic events, have been reported since cocaine enhances thrombus formation. Acute intoxication may result in profound hypotension and shock.

Respiratory: Sharp pleuritic pain, hemoptysis, pneumothorax, bronchospasm, pulmonary edema, and respiratory failure. Both lactic acidosis and metabolic acidosis have been seen.

Gastrointestinal: Vomiting and other GI symptoms are common; if the patient has had a rupture of a cocaine packet in the GI tract, damage can be severe and include GI ulceration and bleeding, as well as ischemia and necrosis.

Neurologic: The degree of CNS stimulation depends on the route and amount of drug taken. Headache, hyperexcitation, paranoia, delirium, hallucinations, tremors, hyperreflexia, and aggression may be seen. Mentation may vary from stimulated, euphoric, and excited states to delirium, stupor, and coma. Seizures are common, usually tonic-clonic, and may last for hours. Initially patients may seem well coordinated, but later may show tremors and fasciculations as their condition deteriorates. CNS ischemia and infarction, intracranial hemorrhage, and strokes have been reported with cocaine intoxication.

Renal: Renal failure can occur and has been related to profound hypotension and rhabdomyolysis. Renal infarction has been reported.

Associated findings: Hyperthermia is common, and rectal temperatures may be elevated to as high as 43°C (109.4°F). Perforated nasal septum, track marks related to IV use, and mydriasis (dilated pupils) occur. "Track marks" on arms and scarring on arms and in hidden locations of the body, including between the toes and in the vessels underneath the tongue.

Indicators of withdrawal: Poor concentration, anergia, anhedonia, bradykinesis, sleep disturbance, decreased libido, intense cocaine craving, depression, and suicidal tendencies.

Indicators of cocaine psychosis: Tactile and visual hallucination and paranoia.

Peak action
- Intranasal: 20 to 60 minutes.
- Oral: 60 to 90 minutes.
- IV: 5 minutes.
- Smoked: less than 5 minutes.

Drug Overdose

Cutting agents

Cutting agents are substances mixed with pure cocaine to increase bulk. Cutting agents are often unknown but may include procaine, caffeine, ephedrine, APAP, theophylline, phencyclidine, amphetamine, quinine, talc, and strychnine, and the clinical effects of a mixed intoxication may vary accordingly. Agents used in the preparation of crack include powdered cocaine, water, baking soda, and lidocaine. Cutting agents can become emboli that shower into cerebral and pulmonary circulation, with subsequent effects.

COLLABORATIVE MANAGEMENT
Care Priorities

1. Support of cardiovascular system to prevent collapse. Electrical rhythm is monitored. Supraventricular tachycardia and ventricular dysrhythmias are managed according to ACLS guidelines. Monitor ECG for ischemic changes or infarction pattern (T-wave inversion or ST-segment elevation or depression).
2. Support of respiratory system: Comatose patients are placed on mechanical ventilation.
3. Identification of route of administration and removing cocaine following oral ingestion: A radiograph of the GI tract may reveal a cocaine-filled condom. Surgery may be performed to remove it. Activated charcoal may be administered to bind with cocaine in the stomach, or a laxative or suppository may be given to facilitate rectal excretion. Flushing cocaine from the circulation using IV ammonium chloride is being investigated.
4. Treatment of hypotension or hypertension: Antihypertensives or vasopressors are administered as indicated.
5. Treatment of volume deficiency: IV fluid replacement is done, such as with lactated Ringer solution or D_5NS.
6. Prevention/treatment of seizures: Diazepam, phenytoin, or phenobarbital is administered.
7. Treatment of hyperthermia: A cooling blanket, ice, and/or acetaminophen is used. Core temperature is the most accurate measurement.
8. Prevention of aspiration: A gastric tube is inserted, then connected to low continuous suction.
9. Rhabdomyolysis: see discussion in Benzodiazepines section.

CYCLIC ANTIDEPRESSANTS

Examples include amitriptyline hydrochloride (Elavil), doxepin hydrochloride (Sinequan), imipramine hydrochloride (Presamine, Tofranil), trimipramine maleate (Surmontil), nortriptyline (Pamelor, Aventyl), and desipramine (Norpramin).

Route of administration

Oral. Overdose has become less common with the much more widespread use of the safer antidepressant class of serotonin reuptake inhibitors (SSRIs) such as fluoxetine, paroxetine, citalopram, escitalopram, and sertraline. Rarely, an SSRI can cause dangerously high levels of serotonin resulting in serotonin syndrome. The condition is often accidental, resulting from when two medications that raise serotonin levels are combined. Offending agents include other antidepressants, pain or headache medications, and St. John's Wort (herbal supplement). Signs and symptoms include restlessness, agitation, confusion, diaphoresis, anxiety, tremors, lack of coordination, and tachycardia.

Effects on body systems

Cardiovascular: Hypotension, sinus tachycardia, supraventricular tachycardia, ventricular dysrhythmias, conduction defects, myocardial infarction, cardiopulmonary arrest. Hypertension has been noted. Monitor ECG for widening QRS complex. Progressive QRS widening signals worsening toxicity.
Respiratory: Respiratory arrest, pulmonary edema, ARDS. Hyperventilation also has been noted.
Neurologic: CNS depression, coma, seizures, delirium, hallucinations.
Renal: Acute tubular necrosis; renal failure secondary to rhabdomyolysis.
Pancreatic: Pancreatitis.
Associated findings: Hyperthermia or hypothermia.

Collaborative management
Care Priorities

1. If the patient is symptom free, monitor for a minimum of 6 to 8 hours, noting vital signs and width of QRS complex.

2. Support of cardiovascular system to prevent collapse: Electrical rhythm is monitored for at least 6 hours to enable assessment for a widening QRS complex, which is a signal of worsening toxicity. Manage supraventricular and ventricular dysrhythmias using ACLS guidelines.

3. Removing cyclic antidepressants: Activated charcoal is administered via gastric tube to bind with the ingested substance in the stomach.

4. Reversal of the effects of the drugs: IV sodium bicarbonate is used. An alternative approach is to promote a state of respiratory alkalosis by increasing respiratory rate via mechanical ventilation.

5. Prevention/treatment of seizures: Phenytoin and diazepam are administered.

6. Respiratory support: Mechanical ventilation is used. Pulmonary edema is treated with nitrates, morphine, diuretics, potassium replacement, and intermittent positive pressure breathing IPPB treatments.

7. Treatment of hypotension: Fluid replacement is carried out, followed by administration of dopamine and norepinephrine as indicated.

8. Treatment of hyperthermia or hypothermia: A cooling or a warming blanket is used as indicated.

9. Prevention of aspiration: A gastric tube is inserted and then connected to low intermittent suction.

DIGOXIN
Routes of administration
Oral/IV.

Digitalis glycosides like digoxin are very serious and potentially life threatening in the event of an overdose; these drugs can accumulate quickly if renal dysfunction develops or worsens. Like tricyclic antidepressants, reports of toxicities are decreasing in frequency as evidence-based use of the drug in heart failure and arrhythmias is decreasing.

Effects on body systems
Cardiovascular: Bradycardia/atrioventricular block with atrial or ventricular ectopy and tachycardia at high levels.
Gastrointestinal: Nausea vomiting abdominal pain.
Neurologic: Lethargy, malaise, weakness, confusion.
Other findings: Hyperkalemia is a marker for severe overdose, and serum digoxin levels are readily available to evaluate.

COLLABORATIVE MANAGEMENT
AC if recent ingestion. Digoxin immune fab is a specific binding antidote that will quickly reverse toxicity. Since it is expensive and whole digoxin levels are unusable after administration, it should be reserved for cases where arrhythmias or other serious signs and symptoms are present and not used to treat moderately elevated, asymptomatic digoxin levels.

HALLUCINOGENS
Street names
Acid, battery acid, blotter, boomers, California sunshine, cids, doses, dots, golden dragon, heavenly blue, hippie, looney tunes, LSD, Lucy in the sky with diamonds, mesc, microdot, pane, purple heart, superman, tab, window pane, yellow sunshine, Zen.

Common agents
Lysergic acid diethylamide (LSD), mescaline (peyote cactus), ketamine (special K, K, ket, kit-kat, super K), morning glory seeds, nutmeg, psilocybin (mushrooms, magic mushrooms, shrooms, magics, blue meanies, liberty caps, golden tops, mushies), phencyclidine (PCP, angel dust, peace pill).

Routes of administration
Oral, IV, nasal, smoked.

Effects on body systems
Effects will depend on the amount and type of drug ingested.
Respiratory: Apnea, respiratory arrest.

Drug Overdose

Neurologic: Hallucinations and paranoid behavior patterns, tremors, seizures, coma.
LSD: Patient may describe tasting or hearing colors or exhibit mental dissociation.
Mescaline: Sense of being followed by moving geometric shapes.
Associated findings: "Track marks" on arms and scarring on arms and in hidden locations
  of the body, including between the toes and in the vessels underneath the tongue. Hy-
  perthermia and diaphoresis. In addition, visual hallucinations may occur. Taking large
  doses of PCP and ketamine can result in coma, seizures, respiratory arrest, and death.
  LSD, mescaline, and magic mushrooms have not been reported to directly cause death.
  Rare fatalities have been a result of accidents, behavior caused by the drug, or plant
  poisoning.

COLLABORATIVE MANAGEMENT
Care Priorities
1. Support of cardiovascular system to prevent collapse. Manage BP and HR/rhythm according to ACLS guidelines.
2. Removing hallucinogens from patient: If oral ingestion was within 1 hour, gastric lavage
   may be attempted, as long as AC therapy is not delayed. AC is administered orally or via
   gastric tube to bind with the substance in the stomach.
3. Prevention of seizures: Anticonvulsants such as phenytoin or diazepam are administered.

OPIOIDS
Common agents
Codeine, fentanyl, heroin, hydrocodone, hydromorphone (Dilaudid), levorphanol (Levo-
Dromoran), pethidine or meperidine (Demerol), methadone (Dolophine), morphine,
opium, oxycodone hydrochloride (Percocet-5, Tylox, Oxycontin), buprenorphine (Subutex),
and oxymorphone (Numorphan). Heroin is the most abused opioid. There has been a steady
increase in abuse of prescription opioids such as morphine.

Street names
China white, Chinese H, dope, dragon, Harry cone, junk, OC, oxy, painkillers, white, white
dynamite.

Routes of administration
Oral, IV, IM, smoked.

Effects on body systems
Cardiovascular: Profound hypotension, bradycardia, cardiovascular collapse, sudden death.
Respiratory: Atelectasis, acute pulmonary edema, infiltrates related to aspiration complica-
  tions, respiratory depression, apnea, hypoventilation, and bronchospasm.
Neurologic: Range from decreased mental alertness to stupor and coma; pinpoint pupils;
  seizures.
Renal: Renal failure has been associated with profound hypotension and rhabdomyolysis.
Associated findings: "Track marks" and scarring on arms and in hidden locations of the
  body, including between the toes and in the vessels underneath the tongue.

COLLABORATIVE MANAGEMENT
Care Priorities
1. Support of cardiovascular system to prevent collapse: Electrical rhythm is monitored;
   bradyarrhythmias are treated per ACLS guidelines. Vasopressor therapy is initiated for
   hypotension after fluids have been replaced.
2. Removal of orally ingested opioids from patient: AC is administered orally or via gastric
   tube to bind with the substance in the stomach.
3. Reversal of opioid effects: Administration of naloxone hydrochloride (Narcan) to manage respiratory depression. After the initial dose of naloxone, the patient's respiratory
   status must be monitored closely, since additional doses may be required. Respiratory depression and coma may occur when the effects of naloxone wear off and the opiate effects
   predominate. The half-life of naloxone is 60 to 90 minutes, and effects last 2 to 3 hours. If
   the narcotic effects last longer than the effects of the naloxone, the patient may slip into
   coma once the naloxone wears off. If persistent respiratory depression is present, a continuous naloxone infusion may be considered.

4. Treatment of drug withdrawal symptoms: Hallucinations are treated with haloperidol (Haldol).
5. Support of respiratory system: Pulmonary edema is treated with diuretics and restriction of IV fluid intake. An individual whose respiratory system is deteriorating is placed on apnea monitoring or mechanical ventilation.
6. Prevention of aspiration: A gastric tube is inserted and then connected to low continuous suction.
7. Prevention/treatment of seizure activity: Anticonvulsant therapy is done, such as phenytoin administration.
8. Rhabdomyolysis: See discussion in Benzodiazepines section.

PHENCYCLIDINE
Street names
Angel dust, mist, PCP, peep, hog, crystal.

Routes of administration
Oral, nasal, smoked.

Effects on body systems
Cardiovascular: Hypertension, hypertensive crisis, tachycardia.
Respiratory: Respiratory depression, respiratory arrest, laryngeal stridor, bronchospasm.
Neurologic: Rage and "superhuman strength" are hallmark signs. Ranges from hyperexcitability, hyperreflexia, muscle rigidity, and paranoid and psychotic behavior to stupor, seizures, and coma. Coma: eyes may be open in a blank stare, nystagmus, and pinpoint pupils.
Renal: Renal failure precipitated by rhabdomyolysis and myoglobinuria.
Associated findings: Hypothermia or hyperthermia, hypoglycemia.

COLLABORATIVE MANAGEMENT
Care Priorities
1. Support of cardiovascular system to prevent collapse: Electrical rhythm is monitored and tachydysrhythmias are treated as previously discussed. Nitroprusside or labetalol may be used for antihypertensive therapy. Nitroglycerin may be given to treat ischemia.
2. Removal of phencyclidine from the patient: No specific antidote is available, although multiple administrations of charcoal to bind with the ingested substance in the stomach are standard practice. Charcoal is ineffective if phencyclidine was smoked, rather than swallowed. The first dose of AC may be accompanied with sorbitol. After ruling out the possibility of rhabdomyolysis, acidification of the urine with ammonium chloride or ascorbic acid to a pH around 5.5 is done.
3. Prevention/treatment of seizure activity: Phenytoin and diazepam are given. Diazepam is administered IV at an initial dose of 2 to 5 mg. May be repeated every 30 minutes until sedation is achieved. Haloperidol may be given 5 to 10 mg IV to control psychosis. Its effects usually occur within 5 to 10 minutes of administration.
4. Respiratory support: Pulmonary edema is treated with diuretics and restriction of IV fluid intake. Persons with hypoxia and respiratory distress require monitoring of pulse oximetry and may require mechanical ventilation.
5. Prevention of aspiration: A gastric tube is inserted and then connected to intermittent low suction.
6. Rhabdomyolysis: See discussion in Benzodiazepines section.
7. Treatment of hypothermia or hyperthermia: A warming or cooling blanket is used as appropriate.

STIMULANTS

AMPHETAMINES
Street names
Crank, crystal meth, ecstasy, ice, methamphetamine, speed, white crosses.

Routes of administration
Oral, IV, IM, intranasal, smoked.

Effects on body systems

Cardiovascular: Tachycardia, atrial and ventricular dysrhythmias, hypertension, myocardial ischemia and infarction, cardiovascular collapse.

Respiratory: Hyperventilation and respiratory failure related to cardiovascular collapse.

Neurologic: Confusion, aggressive behavior, hyperactivity, convulsions, delusions, irritability, tremors, hallucinations, memory loss, stupor, stroke, coma.

Renal: Renal failure related to dehydration and rhabdomyolysis.

Associated findings: Mydriasis, fasciculations, hyperthermia, thrombocytopenic purpura.

Collaborative management

1. Support of cardiovascular and respiratory systems to prevent collapse: Antidysrhythmic agents are given per ACLS guidelines to manage tachycardias. Ischemia is treated with nitrates; myocardial infarction is treated per ACLS guidelines for acute coronary syndromes.
2. Removing amphetamines from the patient: For oral ingestion, AC is administered orally or via gastric tube. Acidification of the urine with ammonium chloride helps clear amphetamine.
3. Treatment of hypertension: Antihypertensives such as nitroprusside or labetalol may be needed to decrease BP.
4. Prevention/treatment of seizures: IV diazepam 0.1 to 0.2 mg/kg is administered slowly and repeated every 5 minutes until sedation is achieved. Lorazepam is an alternative benzodiazepine.
5. Psychosis: Haloperidol 5 mg is given IM or IV. Repeat dose may be required to control behavior.
6. Treatment of hyperthermia: A cooling blanket, antipyretics, and iced IV fluids are used.
7. Treatment of dehydration: Done by fluid replacement, such as lactated Ringer solution and NS continuous IV infusions
8. Anticipation and treatment of rhabdomyolysis: Usually treated with sodium bicarbonate infusion, mannitol, or furosemide (Lasix)

CATHINONES (BATH SALTS)

Street names

Bloom, blue silk, cloud nine, ivory snow, ivory wave, lunar wave, white rush, scarface, sextacy, stardust, vanilla sky, white lightning, and zoom. The energizing and agitating effects mimic other drugs such as amphetamines and cocaine, which raise the level of dopamine, a neurotransmitter, in the brain areas that regulate reward and movement. The surge in dopamine prompts feelings of euphoria and increased energy.

Routes of administration

Oral or nasally insufflated. Less commonly used rectally IV, IM, gingivally, or via inhalation. A recently emerging drug of abuse, bath salts are popular because they are generally cheap, easy to acquire through the internet or at gas stations, convenience stores, liquor stores, or head shops, and have only recently (September 2011) been placed under Schedule 1 as a drug with no medical value and high abuse potential. An easily manipulated chemical structure has been exploited to weaken such control; this chemical family in part led to the Drug Abuse Prevention Act of 2012, which broadened the spectrum and gave a general definition to Schedule 1 substances.

Effects on Body Systems

Body systems effects are similar to amphetamines but less potent. Gastritis, liver toxicity, esophagitis, anorexia, and psychosis have also been associated with ingesting the natural alkaloid in the khat plant. Synthetic cathininones include methylenedioxypyrovalerone (MDPV), methylone, and mephedrone ("drone, meph, meow-meow"), which, in addition to the sympathomimetic toxidrome, have also less commonly been associated with severe hyponatremia and myocarditis.

COLLABORATIVE MANAGEMENT

Primarily supportive; similar to amphetamines.

Table 11-4   MANAGEMENT OF DRUG OVERDOSE/TOXICITIES

Target (toxic) Drug or Class	Treatment or Antidote
Acetaminophen	N-Acetylcysteine
Anticholinergics	Physostigmine
Arsenic, lead, mercury, or other heavy metals	Dimercaprol injection
Benzodiazepines	Flumezanil
Beta blockers	Glucagon, beta agonists
Calcium channel blockers	Calcium intravenous, glucagons
Copper	Trientene
Cyanide	Sodium thiosulfate, sodium nitrite, amyl nitrite, hydroxocobalamin
Cyclic antidepressants	Sodium bicarbonate
Digitalis glycosides	Digoxin immune Fab
Heparin	Protamine
Insulin	Glucagon, dextrose, octeotide
Iron	Deferoxamine
Lead	Succimer, edetate calcium disodium (EDTA)
Methanol/Ethylene glycol	Fomepizole, ethanol
Nitrites	Methylene blue
Opiates	Nalmefene, naltrexone, naloxone
Organophosphate insecticides	Atropine, pralidoxime
Warfarin	Vitamin K (oral or intravenous)

SPECIFIC ANTIDOTES FOR COMMON DRUG OVERDOSES/TOXICITIES

Table 11-4 gives specific drug treatments for a few of the more common and critical drug overdoses not discussed in the preceding section.

CARE PLANS FOR ALL DRUG OVERDOSES

INEFFECTIVE AIRWAY CLEARANCE *related to presence of tracheobronchial secretions or obstruction; decreased sensorium.*

- -

Goals/Outcomes: Chest radiograph normalizes. Within 2 to 24 hours of intervention/treatment, the patient has a patent airway and is free of congestion as evidenced by clear breath sounds over the upper airways and lung fields, RR 12 to 20 breaths/min with normal depth and pattern, Pao_2 at least 90 mm Hg, $Paco_2$ 35 to 45 mm Hg, pH 7.35 to 7.45, and Spo_2 at least 95%.

NOC Respiratory Status: Airway Patency; Aspiration Prevention; Respiratory Status: Ventilation

Respiratory Monitoring

1. Assess for respiratory distress hourly and as needed. Note secretions; stridor; gurgling; shallow, irregular, or labored respirations; use of accessory muscles of respiration; restlessness and confusion; and cyanosis (a late sign of respiratory distress).
2. Suction oropharynx or use suction via endotracheal tube as needed.
3. Administer bronchodilators as appropriate.
4. Monitor ABG values for evidence of hypoxia (Pao_2 less than 90 mm Hg) and respiratory acidosis ($Paco_2$ greater than 45 mm Hg, pH less than 7.35).
5. Monitor respiratory patterns; provide continuous apnea monitoring if available.

6. If the patient has been placed on mechanical ventilation, monitor for indicators of airway obstruction (see Mechanical Ventilation, Chapter 1).
7. Monitor oxygen saturation continuously. Be alert to values less than 95% with response depending on patient's baseline and clinical presentation.
8. Monitor for nausea and vomiting. Evaluate effects of antiemetics.

NIC Airway Management, Aspiration Precautions

HYPERTHERMIA *related to overdose of cocaine, hallucinogens, phencyclidine, salicylates, or cyclic antidepressants.*

Goals/Outcomes: Optimally, within 24 to 72 hours of intervention, the patient becomes normothermic.
NOC Thermoregulation

Safety Alert	*With massive overdose, temperature regulation may never be achieved.*

Temperature Regulation
1. Monitor for hyperthermia: temperature greater than 38.3° C (greater than 101° F), pallor, absence of perspiration, and torso that is warm to the touch. If means are available, provide continuous monitoring of temperature. Otherwise, measure rectal or core temperature hourly, and as needed.
2. Monitor effects of cooling blanket, cooling baths, and ice packs to the axillae and groin.
3. Maintain fluid replacement as prescribed. Monitor hydration status and trend of input and output (I&O).
4. Monitor neurologic status hourly and as needed until stabilized.
5. Monitor vital signs continuously or hourly and as needed until stabilized.
6. Administer and evaluate effects of antipyretic medications.

NIC Fever Treatment; Vital Signs Monitoring; Medication Prescribing

DEFICIENT FLUID VOLUME *related to low intake or losses secondary to vomiting or diaphoresis and shock conditions.*

Goals/Outcomes: Patient remains normovolemic as evidenced by urine output greater than 0.5 mL/kg/h, moist mucous membranes; balanced I&O, BP within patient's normal range, HR less than 100 bpm, stable weight, CVP 8 to 12 mm Hg, and PAWP 6 to 12 mm Hg.
NOC Hydration; Fluid Balance

Fluid Management
1. Monitor hydration status. Note signs of continuing dehydration: poor skin turgor, dry mucous membranes, thirst, weight loss greater than 0.5 kg/day, urine specific gravity greater than 1.020, weak pulse with tachycardia, and postural hypotension.
2. If the patient has a pulmonary artery catheter:
   - Monitor SVR and PVR as appropriate.
   - Monitor CO as appropriate.
   - Monitor PCWP/PAWP and central venous/right atrial pressures.
   - Administer positive inotropic/contractility medications.
3. Evaluate the effects of fluid therapy.
4. Assess for indicators of electrolyte imbalance, especially the presence of hypokalemia. Be alert to irregular pulse, cardiac dysrhythmias, and serum potassium level less than 3.5 mEq/L.
5. Monitor I&O hourly; assess for output elevated disproportionately to intake, bearing in mind the insensible losses.
6. Monitor laboratory values, including serum electrolyte levels and serum and urine osmolality. Note BUN values elevated disproportionately to the serum creatinine (indicator of dehydration rather than renal disease), high urine specific gravity, low urine sodium, and rising Hct and serum protein concentration. Optimal values are the following: serum osmolality 275 to 300 mOsm/kg, urine osmolality 300 to 1090 mOsm/kg, BUN 10 to 20 mg/dL, serum creatinine 0.7 to 1.5 mg/dL, urine sodium 40 to 180 mEq/24 hr (diet dependent), Hct 37% to 47% (female) or 40% to 54% (male), and serum protein 6 to 8.3 g/dL.

7. Maintain fluid intake as prescribed; administer prescribed electrolyte supplements.

NIC Fluid/Electrolyte Management; Surveillance; Hypovolemia Management

DISTURBED SENSORY/PERCEPTUAL PERCEPTION: VISUAL, TACTILE, AUDITORY, KINESTHETIC *related to chemical alterations secondary to ingestion of mind-altering drugs.*

Goals/Outcomes: Within 48 hours of intervention, the patient verbalizes orientation to time, place, and person and is free of abnormal sensory and perceptual experiences.
NOC Cognitive Orientation; Distorted Thought Self-Control

Reality Orientation
1. Establish and maintain a calm, quiet environment to minimize the patient's sensory overload.
2. Assess patient's orientation to time, place, and person. Reorient as necessary.
3. Explain procedures before performing them. Include significant others in orientation process.
4. Do not leave the patient alone if agitated or confused.
5. Administer antianxiety agents as prescribed.
6. If the patient is hallucinating, intervene in the following ways:
   - Be reassuring. Explain that hallucinations may be very real to the patient but they are not real. They are caused by the substance that the patient consumed, and they will go away eventually.
   - Try to involve family and significant others, because the patient may have more trust in them.
   - Explain that restraints are necessary to prevent harm to the patient and others. Reassure the patient that restraints will be used only as long as they are needed.
   - Tell the patient that you will check on him or her at frequent intervals (e.g., every 5 to 10 minutes) or that you will stay at patient's side.

NIC Delusion Management; Environmental Management; Fall Prevention; Surveillance: Safety

RISK FOR VIOLENCE: SELF-DIRECTED AND/OR OTHER-DIRECTED *related to mind-altering drugs or depressed state.*

Goals/Outcomes: Patient, staff, and patient's significant others are free of injury.
NOC Impulse Self-Control

Behavior Management
1. If patient's condition is stable, provide a sitter or auxiliary staff member, such as an orderly or nursing assistant, to observe the patient when he or she is awake.
2. Speak with the patient in a quiet and calm voice, using short sentences.
3. Establish a therapeutic relationship with patient.
4. Encourage the patient to take control over his or her own behavior.
5. Facilitate support by significant others.
6. Limit the number of interventions as much as possible to avoid frequently disturbing the patient.
7. Administer and evaluate effectiveness of sedation to calm patient.
8. Keep all sharp instruments out of patient's room. Follow agency protocol accordingly.
9. Develop appropriate behavior expectations and consequences, given the patient's level of cognitive functioning and capacity for self-control.

NIC Behavior Management: Self-Harm; Substance Use Treatment: Alcohol Withdrawal; Substance Use Treatment: Overdose, Suicide Prevention

ADDITIONAL .NURSING DIAGNOSES

See nursing diagnoses and interventions in the following as appropriate: Nutritional Support (Chapter 1), Mechanical Ventilation (Chapter 1), Hemodynamic Monitoring (Chapter 1), Prolonged Immobility (Chapter 1), Emotional and Spiritual Support of the Patient and Significant Others (Chapter 2), Acute Lung Injury and Acute Respiratory Distress Syndrome

Drug Overdose

(Chapter 4), Acute Respiratory Failure (Chapter 4), Acute Coronary Syndromes (Chapter 5), Heart Failure (Chapter 5), Cardiomyopathy (Chapter 5), Dysrhythmias and Conduction Disturbances (Chapter 5), Aortic Aneurysm/Dissection (Chapter 5), Acute Renal Failure (Chapter 6), Status Epilepticus (Chapter 7), Hepatic Failure (Chapter 9), Acute Pancreatitis (Chapter 9), Fluid and Electrolyte Disturbances (Chapter 1), and Acid-Base Imbalances (Chapter 1). In addition, see Traumatic Brain Injury for Impaired Corneal Tissue Integrity (Chapter 3).

HIGH-RISK OBSTETRICS: HYPERTENSION IN PREGNANCY

Most pregnant women are healthy and rarely in need of critical care. The high-risk obstetric patient presents the unique challenge of caring for the mother and the fetus simultaneously. In most cases, the survival of the mother will take precedence over fetal survival, but the optimal outcome is survival of both. Two basic principles should underlie the care of the pregnant patient. First, maternal anatomic and physiologic changes occur during pregnancy to facilitate adequate blood flow to the fetus and protect the mother after delivery (Box 11-2). The pregnant patient may require hemodynamic monitoring, and the critical care nurse should be

---

Box 11-2   PHYSIOLOGIC ANATOMICAL CHANGES IN PREGNANCY

Body Position
Supine hypotension: After 20 weeks, supine positioning significantly reduces CO and uterine blood flow by compressing the inferior vena cava.

Lateral positioning or hip wedge under right or left hip is recommended to displace the gravid uterus to avoid supine hypotension.

Cardiovascular
Heart rate: 10 to 15 bpm increase from prepregnancy rate by 32 weeks

Blood pressure: 10 to 15 mm Hg decrease from prepregnancy value between 14 and 24 weeks returning to prepregnancy value by 37 to 40 weeks' gestation

Blood volume: 40% to 50% increase by 24 weeks

Stroke volume: 30% increase by 32 weeks

CO: 30% to 50% increase by 24 weeks

Fetal Circulation
More than 10% of maternal CO is diverted into the uterine circulation. Maternal CO increases by at least 25% during pregnancy. Fetal oxygenation is dependent on maintenance of sufficient maternal CO.

Gastrointestinal
Gastric motility: decreased

Gastric emptying time: decreased

IAP: increased

These changes can cause increased risk of aspiration with general anesthesia.

Neck/Throat
Larynx: displaced anteriorly, prompting increased incidence of airway edema and bleeding, leading to failed intubation.

Pulmonary and Acid-Base Balance
Oxygen consumption: increases

Functional residual capacity and volume: decreased by elevated maternal diaphragm, resulting in increased risk of rapid development of hypoxemia and apnea compared with the nonpregnant patient

Acid-base imbalance: respiratory alkalosis

Renal
Glomerular filtration rate: increased by 50% at term

Table 11-5	EXPECTED HEMODYNAMIC CHANGES DURING PREGNANCY, LABOR, DELIVERY, AND POSTPARTUM			
Hemodynamic Profile	Third Trimester Changes Before Labor	Additional Changes During Active Labor	Postpartal Measurements	Normal Values (Before Pregnancy)
Cardiac output	25% to 50% (L/min) (~7.5 L/min)	~10%	To prelabor value in 1 hour; normal in 10 to 14 days	5.0 L/min
Stroke volume	20% to 30% (~75 to 85 mL/beat)	~10%	To prelabor value in 24 hours; normal in 3 to 12 months	65 mL/beat
Central venous pressure Pulmonary artery pressures	Unchanged	Data unavailable	Data unavailable	2–6 mm Hg
Pulmonary artery systolic	Unchanged	Data unavailable	Unchanged	15–25 mm Hg
Pulmonary artery diastolic	Unchanged	Data unavailable	Unchanged	6 to 12 mm Hg
Pulmonary artery wedge	Unchanged	Data unavailable	Unchanged	4 to 12 mm Hg
Systemic vascular resistance	May increase up to 20%	Unchanged	To normal in 3–4 to 12 months	800 to 1200 dynes/sec/cm^5
Pulmonary vascular resistance	May increase up to 25%	Data unavailable	Data unavailable	150 to 240 dynes/sec/cm^5

familiar with the different hemodynamic changes and pressure values in pregnancy and labor as outlined in Table 11-5. Second, the fetus is totally dependent on the mother for all of his or her oxygenation and growth needs, so any intervention performed on the mother will most likely affect the fetus. Despite the unique challenges presented by the critically ill obstetric patient, transfer of the patient to a critical care unit should not be delayed.

Obstetric complications account for less than 1% of intensive care unit (ICU) admissions and less than 0.5% of all deliveries. Despite this relatively low incidence, the acuity of obstetric critical care patients is high because of the unique pathophysiology and the associated clinical disorders. Maternal mortality rates range from 5% to 20% when pregnant women require critical care. Obstetric patients may be admitted into critical care because of complications of obstetric conditions, such as eclampsia, or complications of an underlying medical condition, such as heart disease. Those with obstetric conditions are admitted more frequently and generally have better outcomes than those admitted with underlying medical conditions. The most prevalent indication for obstetric ICU admissions is hypertension in pregnancy. This chapter will focus on the hypertensive complications of pregnancy that may result in admission to a critical care unit.

HYPERTENSION IN PREGNANCY
CLASSIFICATION
Hypertensive disease occurs in up to 22% of pregnancies. The study of hypertension in pregnancy has been hindered by a lack of agreement on a set of definitions to define subsets of the disease. This chapter uses terms recommended by the American Congress of Obstetricians and Gynecologists and endorsed by the National Institutes of Health Working Group on High Blood Pressure to define hypertensive disease in pregnancy (refer to Box 11-3). Of these hypertensive disorders, preeclampsia, eclampsia, and HELLP (hemolysis, elevated liver enzymes

Box 11-3	**CLASSIFICATION OF HYPERTENSIVE STATES OF PREGNANCY**

- Chronic hypertension: Hypertension that is present before pregnancy or develops before 20 weeks' gestation.
- Preeclampsia and eclampsia: A systemic syndrome of hypertensive disease, with proteinuria diagnosed after 20 weeks' gestation. Eclampsia indicates the additional presence of convulsions.
- Preeclampsia superimposed on chronic hypertension: Preeclampsia and/or eclampsia diagnosed in a patient with chronic hypertension.
- Gestational hypertension: Hypertension diagnosed after 20 weeks of pregnancy without proteinuria.

and low platelet count) syndrome were responsible for 30% of obstetric ICU admissions. These conditions, their management, and care will be discussed.

PREECLAMPSIA AND ECLAMPSIA

Preeclampsia is the most common hypertensive disorder of pregnancy, occurring in 6% to 8% of all pregnancies. Preeclampsia is a syndrome that affects both mother and fetus. It is clinically defined as an increase in blood pressure or hypertension of greater than140/90 mm Hg on two occasions at least 4 hours apart or 160/110 mm Hg on two occasions after 20 weeks gestation accompanied by proteinuria in a previously normotensive woman. In the absence of proteinuria, presence of any of the following also confirms a preeclamptic diagnosis: platelet count below 100,000 mm^3, creatinine above 1.1 mg/dL, elevated liver transaminases, pulmonary edema, or cerebral or visual symptoms. Preeclampsia is also known as toxemia, pregnancy-induced hypertension, and preeclamptic toxemia.

Eclampsia is defined as the occurrence of seizures in a woman with preeclampsia who has no known cause for seizure. The seizures of eclampsia are almost always tonic-clonic in nature and are typically self-limited. Eclampsia complicates only 1% to 2% of preeclamptic pregnancies. Eclampsia may develop antepartum (38% to 53%), intrapartum (18% to 36%), or postpartum (11% to 44%) Overall, preeclampsia and eclampsia are responsible for 15% of maternal deaths, mostly from complications resulting from eclampsia.

PATHOPHYSIOLOGY

Preeclampsia has been called the "disease of theories" because true mechanisms behind the pathogenesis remain unclear. Many women with preeclampsia have smaller than normal blood vessels feeding the placenta. However, why this happens to some women and not others is not completely understood. Preeclampsia is characterized by widespread arteriolar vasospasm resulting in increased peripheral vascular resistance. Areas of vasospasm cause breaks or roughened areas in the endothelial layer. These roughened areas trigger fibrin deposition and leakage of intravascular fluid into the extravascular space. Decreased colloid oncotic pressure, a normal physiologic change during pregnancy, also contributes to fluid leakage and proteinuria. These widespread arteriolar vasospasms result in decreased perfusion to virtually all organs, including the placenta, a decrease in plasma volume, activation of coagulation cascade, and alteration in glomerular capillary endothelium. The physiologic process of vasospasm manifests in the development of classic symptoms associated with preeclampsia resulting in decreased blood flow to the major maternal organs such as the kidney, brain, and liver, as well as the placenta. These generalized cyclic vasospasms lead to tissue ischemia and eventually end-organ dysfunction. One of the more common problems related to preeclampsia is pulmonary edema caused by increased capillary permeability. Thrombocytopenia complicates severe preeclampsia in about 7% to 11% percent of women. Abruptio placentae and the release of procoagulants, such as thromboplastin, can result in acute disseminated intravascular coagulation (DIC).

SIGNS AND SYMPTOMS

Most women with preeclampsia do not experience signs other than mild high blood pressure and a small amount of excess protein in the urine. The changes are asymptomatic. Thus, prenatal visits to assess for hypertension and measure urinary protein are scheduled frequently in the last half of pregnancy.

In some cases, preeclampsia can worsen and develop features of severe disease; however, the symptoms may be subtle. Patients should not hesitate to mention concerns about symptoms of preeclampsia to their provider: The increase in severity generally occurs over several days to weeks but may occur more quickly. Features of severe preeclampsia consist of one or more of the following signs or symptoms:

- Blood pressure is greater than 160/110 mm Hg. Women with blood pressures in this range have an increased risk of stroke.
- Abnormal kidney tests (e.g., serum creatinine above 1.1 mg/dL).
- Low platelet count (may be rapidly falling).
- Liver abnormalities (detected by blood tests).
- Pulmonary edema (fluid in the lungs).
- Persistent severe headache.
- Cerebral or visual disturbances (blurred vision, spots or flashes of light, loss of vision, CNS irritability).
- New shortness of breath (caused by fluid in the lungs).
- Pain in the mid- or right-epigastrium (similar to heartburn).
- Oliguria (decreased urine output).
- Intrauterine abnormalities (fetal growth restriction and/or oligohydramnios- decreased amniotic fluid).

Refer to Table 11-6 for more specific changes in physiology.

RISK FACTORS FOR PREECLAMPSIA AND ECLAMPSIA

Demographics: African American and Hispanic women, maternal age over 35 years, and nonsmokers.

Comorbidities: Chronic hypertension, renal disease, obesity, diabetes, vascular disease, connective tissue disease, and maternal infections.

Pregnancy-fetus: Multiple pregnancy (twin, triplet), molar pregnancy, personal history (previous preeclampsia), and family history (mother or sister).

Maternal immunity: History of condom use, fertilization with donor sperm, new sexual partner.

HELLP SYNDROME

HELLP syndrome is an acronym for a unique pregnancy condition representing increased severity of a variant of severe preeclampsia or eclampsia. HELLP syndrome affects 2% to 20% of patients with severe preeclampsia or eclampsia. Maternal mortality ranges from 3.5% to 24%, with perinatal mortality ranging from 10% to 60%. The etiology of HELLP is uncertain. Approximately 10% to 15% of pregnant patients with HELLP syndrome do not have elevated proteinuria of hypertensive disease. The clinical manifestations of HELLP syndrome, which include nausea, vomiting, malaise, flulike symptoms, and epigastric pain, may suggest a multitude of other clinical diagnoses. Misdiagnosis is common and may result in a delay of correct treatment. Any pregnant woman demonstrating clinical manifestations and hemolysis, elevated liver enzymes, and low platelets must be diagnosed with HELLP syndrome. Worsening

Table 11-6	HEMODYNAMIC PROFILES IN OLIGURIC PATIENTS WITH PREECLAMPSIA			
Probable Etiology	**Pulmonary Artery Wedge Pressure**	**Systemic Vascular Resistance**	**Cardiac Output**	**Treatment**
Hypovolemia	Normal to decreased	Increased	Increased	Volume infusion
Spasm of renal arteries	Increased	Normal	Increased	Volume infusion Generalized vasodilation
Spasm of systemic arterial vessels	Increased	Increased	Decreased	Diuresis Arterial vasodilation

of systemic arteriolar vasospasm produces such complications as liver damage, subcapsular hematoma, pulmonary edema, liver rupture, abruption placentae, DIC, and acute renal failure. The HELLP patient should be closely monitored for right upper quadrant pain or shoulder pain because these complaints may be indicative of liver hematoma or liver rupture. The only known treatment for HELLP syndrome is to empty the uterus of the fetus and the placenta.

Diagnostic Tests for Hypertensive Obstetric Disorders	
Test	Findings
Complete blood count	Hemoglobin and hematocrit (Hct) may be elevated (>35 Hct) and steadily rising with severe preeclampsia-eclampsia.
Peripheral blood smear	Schistocytes or burr cells are present with HELLP syndrome.
Urinalysis	Positive for protein spillage
24-hour urine collection	Mild/moderate: 0.3 to 5 g protein with normal urine output. Severe preeclampsia-eclampsia: >5 g protein with low urine output.
Serum albumin	Decreases as urine protein spillage increases; severe: <2.5 mg/dL.
Liver enzymes	Aspartate transaminase, alanine amino transferase, and lactate dehydrogenase are elevated with severe preeclampsia-eclampsia and HELLP syndrome. Bilirubin may be elevated with HELLP.
Renal serum chemistry	Mild-moderate: BUN, creatinine, and uric acid levels may be elevated. Severe preeclampsia-eclampsia: BUN, creatinine, and uric acid will be elevated.
Platelet count	Mild-moderate: <100,000/mm³. Severe preeclampsia-eclampsia and HELLP syndrome: <100,000/mm³
Bleeding time	Prolonged when platelet count is <100,000/mm³.
Fibrinogen	Decreased (<300 mg/dL)
Screening coagulation tests (PT, PTT, thrombin time)	Normal unless the patient develops HELLP syndrome that progresses to DIC, wherein all values are elevated.

CARING FOR THE HYPERTENSIVE PATIENT

COLLABORATIVE CARE

Collaboration between the critical care and obstetrics nurses is necessary in providing safe and comprehensive obstetric critical care for the hypertensive patient. Nurses from each specialty bring unique and complementary knowledge and skills for patient management. Obstetric nurses have experience with fetal heart monitoring and interpretation, and critical care nurses have experience with managing patients requiring invasive monitoring, ventilatory support, and specific critical care procedures. A written protocol should be established to facilitate maternal transfer from the obstetric unit to the ICU or to an institution that can provide the appropriate level of care for both mother and fetus before and after delivery. The protocol should also include planning and support for both obstetric and critical care nurses to work collaboratively to care for the patient. If the baby has been delivered, families may desire unrestricted visitation, or the mother may desire to have the baby remain in her ICU room. The collaborative team should develop a plan of care to address the physiologic, psychosocial, and family needs of the patient. The following guidelines are given to aid the critical care nurse, but optimally, there would be an obstetric nurse as part of the care team for any obstetric patient admitted to the ICU for severe hypertensive conditions.

PROVIDE FETAL SURVEILLANCE

1. Electronic fetal monitoring: All undelivered obstetric patients admitted to the ICU should be placed on electronic fetal monitoring once the infant is viable. An electronic fetal monitor has two external devices, which are strapped to the maternal abdomen. It includes a transducer that records fetal heart rate (FHR) and a tocodynamometer, or "toco," that records uterine activity.

> **Safety Alert** *The use of an electronic fetal monitor requires an obstetrics registered nurse with appropriate training and competency in fetal heart rate interpretation. This can be achieved by having both a critical care and an obstetrics nurse at the patient's bedside. Having a labor nurse "on call" if the critical care nurse notices an abnormal fetal heart rate or the onset of labor is not sufficient and could compromise patient safety.*

2. On admission: Ultrasound, Doppler flow studies, biophysical profile, nonstress test (NST), and amniotic fluid volume studies are ordered to evaluate fetal well-being

3. Fetal nonstress testing: An NST is a frequently ordered noninvasive test to monitor fetal status. NSTs are performed by the obstetric nurse who is trained in the procedure and interpretation of results. This test is used to determine fetal well-being and is reflective of fetal oxygenation and placental function. A reactive NST indicates adequate fetal well-being. A nonreactive NST may indicate a problem with placental functioning or fetal oxygenation and should be followed up with additional testing.

4. Biophysical profile: The biophysical profile uses a combination of NST and fetal parameters observed via ultrasound to measure fetal well-being. The fetus is scored as 0, 1, or 2 for each of 5 parameters: fetal breathing movement, gross fetal movement, fetal tone, amniotic fluid volume, and NST test results.

5. *Amniocentesis:* Withdrawal of amniotic fluid under direct ultrasonography is called amniocentesis. Examination of amniotic fluid can be used to determine fetal maturity in pregnancies less than 34 weeks. An LS (lecithin:sphingomyelin) ratio above 2:1 represents fetal maturity.

POSITIONING OF THE PREGNANT PATIENT

The supine position should be not be used with pregnant women after 20 weeks' estimated gestational age. At that time, the maternal vena cava is compressed by the growing maternal abdomen when the mother lies in a supine position. This effect is called "supine hypotension" and, if left unchecked, will lead to decreased blood return to the heart, decreased maternal BP and CO, and subsequently to decreased blood flow to the uterus, placenta, and fetus. The appropriate position for the pregnant patient is lateral positioning, which avoids the risk of supine hypotension and maximizes blood flow to the uterus, placenta, and fetus. Turning some pregnant women on the left side may improve CO more than the right side. Semi-Fowler positioning with a hip roll tilting the maternal abdomen off of the vena cava is another acceptable position for the pregnant woman in the latter half of pregnancy. If supine positioning is required, manual displacement of the gravid uterus can also alleviate venacaval compression.

MONITORING FOR PRETERM LABOR

Obstetrical hypertensive conditions can increase the risk of preterm labor, which is defined as labor that occurs before 37 weeks' estimated gestational age. Signs and symptoms of preterm labor may be subtle and are likely to go unnoticed by nurses unfamiliar with labor assessment.

1. Routinely screen or observe for the following signs and symptoms of preterm labor:
   * Increase or change in vaginal discharge.
   * Bloody vaginal discharge.
   * Leakage of amniotic fluid.
   * Signs and symptoms of urinary tract infection.
   * Dull backache.
   * Uterine cramping (menstrual-like cramps, intermittent or constant).
   * Pelvic pressure or pain (feeling that the baby is "pushing down").
   * Abdominal cramping with or without diarrhea.
   * If the patient is unconscious, observe for restlessness or nonverbal indications of intermittent pain.

2. If the patient has any signs or symptoms of labor, notify the physician or midlevel practitioner and
   * Position mother in the lateral position (turn to the left or right side).
   * Encourage bladder emptying every 2 hours.
   * Report all new onsets of contractions or any change in contraction pattern immediately to the obstetrician or midlevel practitioner, because cervical examination is the most accurate method for diagnosing preterm labor.

3. Monitor uterine contractions (preterm labor) and fetal status:
- Preterm labor contractions may be infrequent, irregular, and painless or frequent, regular, and painful. Preterm labor, left undetected and untreated, can progress into an emergency delivery of a neonate in the critical care unit.
- Tocolytics are used to stop preterm labor, but they must be started early in the labor process to be effective.

Safety Alert *If frequent, strong, painful uterine contractions continue, notify the obstetrician immediately as placental abruption may be occurring. Placental abruption refers to the detachment of the placenta from the wall of the uterus, which will result in life-threatening maternal hemorrhage and fetal hypoxia. The only definitive treatment of a complete placental abruption is delivery of the fetus by Caesarean section within minutes.*

MANAGEMENT OF PREECLAMPSIA AND ECLAMPSIA

Collaborative management for patients with severe preeclampsia, eclampsia, or HELLP syndrome is basic to stabilize the mother and fetus. Continuous assessment and hemodynamic monitoring of the cardiovascular, renal, central nervous, and pulmonary systems provide early indications of worsening maternal condition. Fetal surveillance may include continuous fetal monitoring, biophysical profile, and fetal lung maturity testing. Delivery of the fetus may be indicated because of the maternal condition or fetal compromise. The goal of the healthcare team is to accurately monitor ongoing organ system dysfunction and prevent further damage leading to end-organ failure and maternal-fetal mortality.

PREVENTION OF ECLAMPSIA/SEIZURE MANAGEMENT

The treatment goals of severe preeclampsia are to prevent seizures, decrease arterial spasms, and effect prompt delivery of the fetus. Magnesium sulfate is the most effective anticonvulsant for preeclampsia, eclampsia, and HELLP syndrome, reflected by results of the Magpie Trial International Study Collaborative.

Safety Alert *Magnesium sulfate is listed as a high-risk medication by The Joint Commission (formerly the Joint Commission on Accreditation of Healthcare Organizations). Obstetric nurses should be familiar with safety recommendations related to the administration of magnesium sulfate to pregnant or delivered patients.*

Mode of Administration: Magnesium is given iv as a loading (bolus) dose followed by a continuous drip.

Action: Magnesium works by decreasing the maternal seizure threshold, and it relaxes the uterine smooth musculature by decreasing or stopping uterine contractions.

Complications: The patient receiving magnesium is at higher risk for postpartum hemorrhage caused by uterine atony (failure of the uterus to contract after delivery).

Excretion: Magnesium is metabolized by the kidneys so a decrease in urine output will cause a subsequent rise in magnesium levels.

Administration of magnesium sulfate
- Administer using an infusion pump. Two nurses should verify the infusion pump settings when magnesium is initiated or dosage changed.
- Magnesium solutions should be premixed and labeled in standard solutions.
- An initial loading dose of 4 to 6 g is given over 15 to 30 minutes followed by a maintenance dose of 2 to 3 g/h.
- Magnesium therapy is continued after delivery for 12 to 24 hours. Side effects of magnesium include flushing, nausea, muscle weakness, headache, and toxicity.
- Serum magnesium levels are drawn 2 hours following the loading dose, then every 6 hours. Serum magnesium levels of 4 to 7 mEq/L are considered therapeutic for prevention of seizure activity.
- Magnesium levels greater than 8 mg/dL are associated with signs of toxicity; refer to Table 11-7.

Table 11-7	CLINICAL EFFECTS OF MAGNESIUM
Serum Magnesium Level	**Signs/Symptoms to Watch for**
1.7 to 2.4 mg/dL	Normal
5 to 8 mg/dL	Therapeutic
8 to 12 mg/dL	Loss of patellar reflexes
10 to 12 mg/dL	Somnolence
12 to 16 mg/dL	Respiratory difficulty and depression
15 to 17 mg/dL	Muscle paralysis
<18 mg/dL	Altered cardiac conduction
30 to 35 mg/dL	Cardiac arrest

- If toxicity is suspected, discontinue infusion, administer oxygen, obtain stat magnesium level, and notify physician.
- The antidote for magnesium toxicity is calcium gluconate 10 mg of 10% calcium gluconate solution IV push IVP or direct IV injection over 10 minutes and should be readily available.
- Control of eclamptic seizures: Accomplished through administration of 4 to 6 g of IV MgSO$_4$ over 5 to 10 minutes. This bolus is followed by a continuous infusion of 2 to 3 g/h. If a patient has a recurrent seizure, another bolus of 2 to 4 g can be given over 3 to 5 minutes. Sodium amobarbitol I (for injection), benzodiazepines, or phenytoin can be used for seizures that are not responsive to magnesium sulfate. Avoid the use of multiple agents to decrease eclamptic seizures, unless necessary. The patient must be closely monitored during magnesium administration. It is recommended that the obstetric nurse be present at the bedside with the critical care nurse to monitor fetal and uterine response during magnesium infusion.

BLOOD PRESSURE CONTROL AND MANAGEMENT

Severe hypertension must be addressed after magnesium infusions. Antihypertensive agents need to be used to keep diastolic BP between 90 and 100 mm Hg. Sudden or extreme drops in maternal BP should be avoided as they may precipitate maternal stroke and/or decreased blood flow to the fetus. Venodilators are often used to lower BP. A drug's effect on the fetus must be considered. Diuretics are used only in the setting of pulmonary edema.

Antihypertensive agents used in pregnancy are chosen because of their ability to avoid vasodilation of placental vessels.

The most commonly used antihypertensives are:

- Hydralazine 5 to 10 mg may be given every 10 to 15 minutes. Maximum dosage: 30 mg.
- Labetalol 20 to 40 mg may be given every 10 to 15 minutes. Maximum dosage: 220 mg.
  - Labetalol should be used cautiously in patients with asthma and cardiac failure.
- Nifedipine 10 to 20 mg may be given every 30 minutes. Maximum dosage: 50 mg.

FLUID MANAGEMENT

Severely preeclamptic patients are easily overloaded with IV fluid, predisposing them to pulmonary edema. Strict observation of I&O is warranted. Total fluid intake is typically maintained at 125 to 150 mL/h. Hemodynamic monitoring may be indicated if pulmonary edema develops. Urine output of less than 0.5 mL/kg/h should be reported to the physician or mid-level practitioner.

A nonglucose solution should always be available as part of a fetal resuscitation protocol, and a bolus of 500 to 1000 mL of lactated Ringer or normal saline is usually given to improve maternal circulating volume and subsequently improve uterine perfusion and fetal oxygenation.

PAIN MANAGEMENT

Medications used in pregnancy are generally limited to classes A and B, to decrease potential negative effects on the fetus. The benefits of medications in classes C, D, and E should be carefully weighed against the risk to the fetus. Butorphanol (Stadol), nalbuphine (Nubain), and fentanyl (Sublimaze) may all be given IM or as an IV bolus/IV push and are commonly given for pain relief during labor.

Safety Alert   *Meperidine (Demerol) and morphine are not often used because of their long half-lives and potential to cause neonatal neurobehavioral depression, which may last several days.*

Neuraxial analgesia techniques (spinal, epidural, or combined spinal-epidural) are commonly used because they are more effective at relieving pain and do not cause respiratory depression in the mother or fetus. Medications used are generally a combination of local anesthetics and opioids, which produce greater pain relief with less motor block than local anesthetics alone. Lumbar epidurals may be given continuously or as a patient-controlled analgesia. Contraindications to neuraxial analgesia include allergy to local anesthetics, administration of low-molecular-weight heparin within 12 hours, coagulation disorders, maternal shock, or infection at the insertion site. Common side effects of neuraxial analgesia include maternal hypotension and itching. Hypotension is generally treated with IV fluid boluses and/or IV ephedrine. Ephedrine is the preferred vasopressor because it causes peripheral vasoconstriction without affecting the umbilical vessels. Loratadine (Claritin) or cetirizine (Zyrtec) may be given to alleviate itching.

DELIVERY OF THE FETUS
Preeclampsia arising at 34 weeks' (or more) gestation is generally managed by delivery. Fetal viability, or the gestational age at which the fetus can survive outside the womb, is generally thought to be 24 to 25 weeks' gestation. After 34 weeks' gestation, the majority of infants will avoid major complications from prematurity. Before 34 weeks, patients with severe preeclampsia-eclampsia require delivery unless the gestational age is less than 26 weeks, wherein attempts to prolong the pregnancy may be initiated. If the mother exhibits signs of HELLP syndrome, such as thrombocytopenia or epigastric or right upper quadrant pain, or has visual disturbances, delivery should be strongly considered regardless of fetal age, since the mother is at risk of life-threatening illness if delivery is delayed. Management of the severely preeclamptic patient will depend on three conditions: maternal status, fetal status, and gestational age. If the pregnancy is at least 34 weeks, delivery is planned as there is little benefit in prolonging gestation. If the pregnancy is 33 to 34 weeks, glucocorticoids are given to the mother to accelerate the development of fetal lung maturity. The glucocorticoids are given intramuscularly in 2 doses 12 hours apart with maximum effect achieved 24 hours after the second dose. Both the maternal and fetal status must be closely monitored. If either deteriorates, definitive steps must be taken regarding plans for delivery. The medical team carefully and constantly weighs the benefits of delivery for the mother versus the risks of preterm delivery for the fetus. The decision to proceed to delivery in a preterm pregnancy should be made in consultation with the obstetrician, pediatrician, critical care physician, and neonatologist (if available).

The following factors should be considered in choosing the best clinical placement for the patient based on availability of equipment, skills, and trained personnel:
- Is continuous electronic fetal monitoring available?
- Are there resources for the administration and monitoring of medications for labor induction or augmentation, anesthesia, and analgesia?
- Are care providers appropriately trained to provide fetal resuscitation?
- Is timely access to operating rooms for an emergency caesarean section feasible?
- Are care providers able to provide maternal hemodynamic/cardiac/respiratory monitoring and treatment?
- Are there resources available for neonatal support should complications arise?

PREPARATION FOR DELIVERY
Labor and delivery of the critically ill obstetric patient may occur either in the labor and delivery unit or the critical care unit, depending on several factors. A multidisciplinary discussion by medical specialists and nursing regarding the pros and cons of critical care versus the delivery room or operating room setting will determine the best placement of the patient for optimal maternal and fetal care during labor and delivery.

Vaginal delivery is the safest method of delivery for the preeclamptic/eclamptic patient with a cervix that is favorable for induction of labor. Caesarean section should be reserved for obstetric indications. The goal of delivery method is to minimize the incidence of complications. If operative delivery is the selected method of delivery, 5 to 10 U of platelets may be ordered preoperatively for a platelet count of less than 50,000 mm³. The patient should be typed and cross-matched for blood and blood products to be used if hemorrhage and/or DIC develops intraoperatively or postoperatively. General anesthesia is typically selected, since regional anesthesia (entering the spine) is generally contraindicated with thrombocytopenia. Because of the potential for difficult intubation caused by airway edema and hyperemia, fiberoptic intubation may be used. The patient will require close observation postoperatively for the first 24 to 48 hours.

EMERGENCY DELIVERY IN THE CRITICAL CARE UNIT

To improve communication and facilitate timely emergency response, the names, specialties, and pager/cell phone numbers of the medical and nursing care team members should be compiled on one sheet of paper or written on one specific white board in all of the units possibly involved in the care of the pregnant critical care patient. The teams would minimally include medical and nursing personnel from critical care, labor and delivery, anesthesiology, neonatology, and possibly nursery and respiratory therapists. Other medical specialists should be added as appropriate for the patient's condition. It is helpful to have core team members communicate every shift to discuss emergency plans, update the plan of care, and discuss any possibility of emergent interventions.

CARE PLANS FOR THE HIGH-RISK OBSTETRIC PATIENT IN CRITICAL CARE

INEFFECTIVE PROTECTION *related to hemodynamic, hematologic, and neurologic changes associated with preeclampsia/eclampsia/HELLP.*

Goals/Outcomes: Within 1 hour of development of severe preeclampsia, eclampsia, or severe HELLP syndrome, the pregnant patient (mother and child) is monitored intensively and prepared for delivery, to avoid life-threatening complications of pregnancy-induced hypertension.
NOC Blood Coagulation; Fetal Status: Intrapartum

Intrapartum
1. Verify HRs of mother and fetus before initiating electronic monitoring.
2. Monitor BP of mother at least every 5 minutes if severe hypertension or seizures have occurred. Monitor FHR for slowing, indicative of fetal distress.
3. Initiate fetal resuscitation measures to treat abnormal fetal heart rhythms, as appropriate. Note response to all supportive interventions.
4. Instruct woman and support person(s) about the need for monitoring and data to be obtained.
5. Keep advanced practice provider informed of significant changes in FHR, interventions for abnormal patterns, fetal response, labor progress, and maternal response to interventions.
6. Administer anticonvulsive medications as ordered to control seizures.
7. Monitor magnesium levels and be alert to hypermagnesemia, decreased respiratory rate and depth, loss of deep tendon reflexes.
8. Assist with application of forceps or vacuum extractor, as needed, during delivery.
9. Monitor the patient closely for hemorrhage if HELLP syndrome is present.
10. Note hemoglobin and Hct levels before and after blood loss, as indicated.
11. Monitor coagulation studies, including prothrombin time (PT), activated partial thromboplastin time (aPTT), fibrinogen, fibrin degradation products (FDPs), fibrin split products (FSPs), and platelet counts as appropriate.

INEFFECTIVE PROTECTION *related to potential for seizures and neurologic complications secondary to eclampsia or HELLP syndrome.*

Goals/Outcomes: Throughout the hospitalization, the patient remains free of seizures and neurologic complications as evidenced by orientation to time, place, and person; normoreactive pupils and reflexes; her normal visual acuity, motor strength, and coordination; and absence of headache and other clinical indicators of increased intracranial pressure.
NOC Risk control

High-Risk Obstetrics: Hypertension in Pregnancy

Seizure Precautions

1. Monitor for and document seizures. Protect the patient from injury by initiating seizure precautions. When the patient is seizing, turn her to the side to promote placental perfusion and prevent aspiration.
2. Assess the patient for initial signs of increased intracranial pressure, including diminished length of consciousness, headaches, abnormal pupillary responses (i.e., unequal; sluggish/absent response to light), visual disturbances, weakness and paralysis, slow HR, and change in RR and pattern. Patient may be experiencing problems related to seizure management, or may experience intracranial bleeding if platelets are extremely low.
3. Monitor trend of Glasgow Coma Scale if the patient has difficulty awakening after seizures. If the patient exhibits signs of magnesium toxicity, consult physician and consider calcium gluconate administration.
4. Increase frequency of neurologic monitoring as appropriate.
5. Assess the epidural site (as appropriate), if the patient received epidural analgesia during labor and delivery. Patients with coagulopathy may develop an epidural hematoma, manifested by sensory or motor deficits, bowel or bladder dysfunction, or back pain. Report problems to the physician immediately. The epidural catheter should remain in place until coagulation studies normalize.
6. Avoid activities that increase intracranial pressure.
7. If initial signs of increased intracranial pressure are noted, consult physician immediately. Signs of impending herniation include unconsciousness, failure to respond to deeply painful stimuli, decorticate or decerebrate posturing, Cushing triad (i.e., bradycardia, increased systolic BP, widening pulse pressure), nonreactive/fixed pupils, unequal pupils, or fixed and dilated pupils. See Traumatic Brain Injury, Chapter 3, for more information about herniation. For additional interventions for increased intracranial pressure, see Box 3-7.

NIC Environmental Management: Comfort; Medication Administration

RISK FOR DEFICIENT FLUID VOLUME *related to active loss secondary to antepartum, postpartum, intraabdominal, or other bleeding.*

Goals/Outcomes: The patient remains normovolemic as evidenced by HR, RR, and BP within 10% of expected normal range; urinary output 0.5 mL/kg/h or greater and absence of epigastric or abdominal pain or tenderness, and frank bleeding resulting from HELLP syndrome.
NOC Fluid and Electrolyte Balance;

Fluid Monitoring

1. Monitor fluid status, including I&O, signs of hypovolemia, including increases in HR and RR, decreases in BP and urinary output, restlessness, and vital signs.
2. Initiate hemodynamic monitoring if necessary to assess shock state and/or manage hemodynamics.
3. Optimize venous return through lateral positioning and/or manual uterine displacement once the patient has a gravid uterus.
4. Monitor hemoglobin and Hct as ordered. Postpartum, the uterus contracts and blood is released into the central circulation as it decreases in size. Despite a normal 500-mL vaginal delivery blood loss, hemoglobin and Hct often increase.
5. Inspect for bleeding from mucous membranes, bruising after minimal trauma, oozing from puncture sites, and presence of petechiae. Maintain patent IV access.
6. Administer supplemental oxygen as necessary for active bleeding.
7. Perform fundus checks and initiate gentle fundal massage to help the uterus remain firm and promote hemostasis.
8. Initiate bleeding control therapy as ordered. Methylergonovine, ergonovine, and carboprost may be used to manage prolonged bleeding or hemorrhage.
9. Replace lost volume with plasma expanders (e.g., albumin, Hetastarch) and/or blood products as indicated. See Table 10-3 for information about blood products.

NIC Shock Management: Cardiac; Cerebral Perfusion Promotion; Fluid/Electrolyte Management

RISK FOR INFECTION *related to inadequate secondary defenses (HELLP syndrome causes liver dysfunction, which may impair the reticuloendothelial system phagocytic activity and portal-systemic shunting); multiple invasive procedures; stress and risks associated with pregnancy, labor, and delivery.*

Goals/Outcomes: The patient is free of infection as evidenced by normothermia, HR less than 100 bpm, RR less than 20 breaths/min, negative culture results, WBC count less than 11,000/mm^3, clear urine, and clear, thin sputum.
NOC Infection Severity

Infection Protection
1. Monitor vital signs for evidence of infection (e.g., increases in HR and RR). Check rectal or core temperature every 4 hours for increases.
2. If temperature elevation is sudden, obtain specimens for blood, sputum, and urine cultures or from other sites as prescribed. Consult advanced practice provider for positive culture results.
3. Monitor CBC, and consult advanced practice provider for significant increases in WBCs. Be aware that a normal or mildly elevated leukocyte count may signify infection in patients with liver dysfunction.
4. Evaluate secretions and drainage for evidence of infection (e.g., sputum changes, cloudy urine).
5. Evaluate IV, central line, and other site(s) for evidence of infection (i.e., erythema, warmth, unusual drainage).
6. Provide routine episiotomy care by spraying the area with warm water at least every 4 hours. Sitz baths are usually not possible with critically ill patients. Ice packs and topical anesthetics may be used to enhance comfort.
7. Provide daily breast care by cleansing the breasts with mild soap and water. Breast engorgement should be managed per physician's orders to help prevent infection and control pain. If left unrelieved, breast engorgement can result in stoppage of lactation. If breast-feeding is planned, breasts can be massaged and milk manually expressed or pumped.
8. Prevent transmission of infectious agents by washing hands well before and after caring for the patient and by wearing gloves when contact with blood or other body substances is possible. Dispose of all needles and other sharp instruments in puncture-resistant, rigid containers. Keep containers in each patient room and in other convenient locations. Avoid recapping and manipulating needles before disposal. Teach significant others and visitors proper hand-washing technique. Restrict visitors with evidence of communicable disease.
9. Administer antibiotics as prescribed. Use caution and reduced dosage when administering antibiotics (especially aminoglycosides) to patients with low urinary output or renal insufficiency.

NIC Medication management;

COMPROMISED FAMILY COPING *related to abnormal circumstances surrounding labor, delivery, and postpartum; creating need for mother to be separated from infant and other family members.*

Goals/Outcomes: The patient and family demonstrate adequate coping behaviors and are facilitated in being together as soon as possible in the postpartal hospitalization.
NOC Surveillance: Safety; Anxiety: Self-Control, Concentration, Coping.

Coping Enhancement
1. Provide regular updates to family members about the condition of both mother and infant.
2. Invite family members to participate in care of the mother as possible.
3. Promote infant-mother bonding by allowing baby visitations in the ICU as soon as mother and infant stabilize. Allow mother to feed baby if possible. Maintain infant safety if mother's condition is marginally stable.
4. Discuss feelings about labor, delivery, and complications with the patient and family members. Relay information about the condition of the infant as often as possible, if mother is unable to visit with the baby.
5. If the infant or mother expires, provide all possible support measures, including pastoral care and referrals to community support groups or professional counseling.

NIC Family Involvement Promotion; Family Process Maintenance; Normalization Promotion

ONCOLOGIC EMERGENCIES

An oncologic emergency is defined as a life-threatening situation occurring as a manifestation of a malignancy or the result of antineoplastic treatment or tumor progression. Such emergencies most commonly arise from the ability of cancer to (1) spread by direct infringement on adjacent structures or metastasize to distant sites leading to thrombosis or hemorrhage; (2) produce abnormal amounts of hormones or cellular products leading to fluid and electrolyte imbalances and organ failure; (3) infiltrate serous membranes with effusion; (4) obstruct vessels, ducts, or hollow viscera; or (5) replace normal organ parenchyma. As more aggressive therapies are used in the treatment of these cancers, side effects are more intense and the use of critical care to manage such side effects will only increase.

Oncologic Emergencies

Early recognition and intervention are essential to enhance positive outcomes. Once an oncologic emergency is recognized, the aggressiveness of management is influenced by the reversibility of the immediate situation, the probability of long-term survival, and the ability to provide effective supportive care.

Oncologic emergencies can be classified as hematologic, structural, metabolic, or side effects from treatment such as chemotherapy, radiation therapy, biologic therapy, surgery, or bone marrow transplantation. Neutropenic sepsis, tumor lysis syndrome (TLS), and superior vena cava syndrome (SVCS) will be discussed in this chapter as examples of oncologic emergencies seen in the critical care arena. When recognized early and managed appropriately, these acutely ill individuals have a high likelihood of recovery. An overview of additional oncologic emergencies, associated causes, and signs and symptoms is given in Table 11-8.

Cancer patients may require intensive care for several reasons: (1) overwhelming infection and sepsis; (2) structural complications of cancer or cancer treatment; or (3) metabolic complications of cancer or cancer treatment. Intensivists sometimes refuse admission to cancer patients needing critical care, which may result in denial of effective care for some deserving patients. A cancer patient may need admission to an intensive care unit for a variety of reasons. The outcomes of patients with hematologic malignancies, previously dismal, have improved over the last 10 years. The previously known indicators of poor outcome are no longer valid in view of recent advances in intensive care. A select group of patients with hematologic malignancies may be offered aggressive therapy for a limited duration and then prognosis can be reassessed. Cancer chemotherapy can produce toxicities affecting all major organ systems. Such patients may be admitted with acute organ dysfunction or years afterward for incidental illnesses. Knowledge of these toxicities is essential for early diagnosis, management, and prognostication in such patients. The postsurgical cancer patient has unique problems; care can range from monitoring alone after major surgery to fully aggressive intensive care for postsur-

Table 11-8	ONCOLOGIC EMERGENCIES DEFINED		
Oncologic Emergency	**Oncologic Causes**	**Definition**	**Signs and Symptoms**
Disseminated intravascular coagulation (DIC) (See Bleeding and Thrombotic Disorders, Chapter 10)	Hematologic: acute Promyelocytic Leukemia, prostate, pancreatic, liver, lung, metastatic cancers	Coagulopathy that develops when the normal balance between bleeding and clotting is disturbed. Excessive bleeding and clotting injures body organs and causes anemia or death.	Petechiae, ecchymoses, hemorrhagic bullae, acral cyanosis, and focal gangrene in the skin and mucous membranes may be evident. Hemorrhages from incisions or catheter or injection sites, GI bleeding, hematuria, pulmonary edema, pulmonary embolism, progressive hypotension, tachycardia, absence of peripheral pulses, restlessness, convulsions, or coma may occur. Laboratory studies reveal a marked deficiency of platelets, low levels of fibrinogen and other clotting factors, prolonged prothrombin and partial thromboplastin times, and abnormal erythrocyte morphologic characteristics.

Table 11-8	ONCOLOGIC EMERGENCIES DEFINED—cont'd		
Oncologic Emergency	**Oncologic Causes**	**Definition**	**Signs and Symptoms**
Neutropenic sepsis	Hematologic: any cancer, bone marrow suppression because of chemotherapy, radiation, or targeted therapies	An abnormally low number of circulating neutrophils (absolute neutrophil count [ANC]) leading to predisposition to infections from endogenous flora from gut or skin. Signs of inflammation are often absent.	Absent: Febrile, infection Mild neutropenia (ANC 1000 to 1500): minimal risk of infection Moderate neutropenia (ANC 500 to 1000): moderate risk of infection Severe neutropenia (ANC <500): severe risk of infection. Symptoms of neutropenia include frequent infections and fevers. Infections can result in diarrhea, oral cavity ulcers, sore throats, burning during urination, and unusual redness around healing wounds.
Malignant pleural effusion	Structural: breast, lung, GI, lymphoma, radiation to the chest wall, cardiotoxic chemotherapy, metastasis	Transudative or exudative in nature; excess fluid accumulates in the pleural cavity, which limits lung expansion and impairs breathing. Chemical (sclerosing agents include tetracycline, bleomycin, talc, etc.) or surgical pleurodesis may be needed in the presence of hemodynamic compromise and recurrence of effusion. Very common, may require thoracoscopic intervention or radiation therapy.	Dyspnea, cough, chest (pleuritic) pain, cyanosis, hypotension, pulsus paradoxus progressing to hoarseness, hiccups, nausea, vomiting, engorged neck veins, distant heart sounds, edema, ascites, hepatosplenomegaly, and hepatojugular reflex.
Spinal cord compression (SCC) (See Acute Spinal Cord Injury, Chapter 3)	Structural: breast, lung, renal, prostate, myeloma, epidural or bony metastasis, sarcoma, multiple myeloma, leukemia, thyroid cancer, lymphoma, melanoma, and GI malignancies	Compressive irregularity, displacement, or encasement of the spinal cord by metastatic or locally advanced cancer. SCC constitutes a true emergency because the initial injury to the spinal cord will lead to permanent loss of neurologic function if the tumor's pressure on the cord is not relieved quickly.	Earliest symptoms are sensory changes such as numbness, paresthesias, and coldness. When neurologic deterioration is rapid and the patient becomes paraplegic, function is rarely regained. SCC is fatal only if it occurs in the cervical region of the spinal cord (C4 and above) and if it results in respiratory paralysis that is uncompensated by mechanical ventilation.

Oncologic Emergencies

Continued

Table 11-8	ONCOLOGIC EMERGENCIES DEFINED—cont'd		
Oncologic Emergency	**Oncologic Causes**	**Definition**	**Signs and Symptoms**
Superior vena cava syndrome	Structural Malignant: lung, lymphomas, breast, mediastinal tumors, metastases from other solid tumors Nonmalignant: Indwelling catheter, thrombosis	Occurs because of obstruction to the blood flow caused by tumors, fibrosis, thrombosis, and direct tumor invasion of great vessels. The treatment depends on the cause, so definitive tissue diagnosis is essential. Lymphoma or small cell carcinoma may respond to chemotherapy and will reduce obstruction. In chemotherapy-resistant tumors, radiotherapy and corticosteroids may provide relief in a significant number of patients.	Facial and upper extremity edema, facial plethora, and tachypnea are most common clinical presentations. May develop slowly and progress to facial edema, venous engorgement, and impaired consciousness caused by brain edema, decreased cardiac output, and upper airway edema. Death can occur from respiratory or circulatory compromise caused by obstruction.
Hypercalcemia (See Fluid and Electrolyte Disturbances, Chapter 1)	Metabolic: lung, breast, prostate, multiple myeloma, renal, head and neck cancers, T-cell lymphomas often caused by metastases. In lymphomas and leukemia there is overproduction of activated vitamin D leading to hypercalcemia.	Most common metabolic complication of malignancies, occurring in 10% to 20% of all cancers. Develops when the rate of calcium mobilization from bone exceeds renal threshold for calcium excretion. Vigorous hydration with intravenous normal saline and furosemide is the standard therapy. Corticosteroids, diphosphonates, mithramycin, and calcitonin can all reduce serum calcium levels by reducing bone resorption of calcium.	Nonspecific: may include polyuria, polydipsia, constipation, lethargy, confusion, nausea, and anorexia progressing to somnolence and coma.

Table 11-8	ONCOLOGIC EMERGENCIES DEFINED—cont'd		
Oncologic Emergency	**Oncologic Causes**	**Definition**	**Signs and Symptoms**
Syndrome of inappropriate antidiuretic hormone (SIADH) (See SIADH, Chapter 8)	Metabolic: oat cell carcinoma of the lung: 80% of cancer cases. Other causes are central nervous system and pulmonary disorders, and pathologic reactions to various drugs.	Abnormal condition characterized by the excessive release of ADH that alters the body's fluid and electrolytic balances. Prognosis depends on the underlying disease, promptness of diagnosis and treatment, and response to treatment. Thus, if a tumor produces abnormal ADH, then surgery, radiation therapy, or chemotherapy may help to reduce tumor size.	Weight gain despite anorexia, vomiting, nausea, muscle weakness, and irritability. In some patients, SIADH may produce coma and convulsions. Most of the free water associated with this syndrome is intracellular. Other significant results include less than normal concentrations of blood urea nitrogen, serum creatinine, and albumin and a concentration of sodium in the urine higher than normal.
Tumor lysis syndrome	Metabolic: most common with hematologic, rapidly growing tumors such as lymphomas, multiple myeloma, leukemias. Also occurs in small cell lung, breast, gastric, choriocarcinoma, testicular, melanoma, and hepatocellular cancer cells, particularly after chemoembolization.	Metabolic imbalance that occurs as a result of high tumor cell kill causing rapid release of normal intracellular products. Hemodialysis is initial treatment of choice to rapidly remove potassium, uric acid, and phosphate from serum, while correcting hypocalcemia.	Rapid change in electrolyte balance, dysrhythmias, altered waveform on electrocardiogram, mentation changes, twitching, cramping, weakness, tetan, oliguria, flank pain, hematuria, weight gain, edema, nausea, vomiting, anorexia, and diarrhea.

Sources: Recommendations for end-of-life care in the intensive care unit: a consensus statement by the American College of Critical Care Medicine. *Crit Care Med* 36:1394-1396, 2008; Guidelines for evaluation of new fever in critically ill adult patients: 2008 update from the American College of Critical Care Medicine and the Infectious Diseases Society of America. *Crit Care Med* 2008 36:1330-1349, 2008; Clinical practice guideline: red blood cell transfusion in adult trauma and critical care. *Crit Care Med* 37:3124-3157, 2009; Dellinger RP, Levy MM, Carlet JM, et al: Surviving Sepsis Campaign: international guidelines for management of severe sepsis and septic shock: 2008 [correction appears in *Crit Care Med* 41(2):580-637, 2013; *Crit Care Med* 2008;36:296-327; National Comprehensive Cancer Network Clinical Practice Guidelines in Oncology, retrieved from www.nccn.org; American Society of Clinical Oncology Practice Guidelines, retrieved from http://www.asco.org; Oncology Nursing Society Practice Guidelines and Resources, retrieved from www.ons.org/ClinicalResources/

gical anastomotic dehiscence, mediastinitis, septic shock, and multiorgan dysfunction. The metabolic and mechanical complications commonly seen in nonsurgical cancer patients are also reasons for admission. Intensive care should be offered to all patients who have a reasonable chance of cure or supportive care of their disease. The intensivist must be able to recognize the potentially reversible critical illnesses among the various groups of cancer patients and discourage admission to terminally ill cancer patients. He or she must also be aware that alleviation of suffering in the last hours of life for a terminal cancer patient is one of the functions of an ICU, once a decision to discontinue aggressive therapy has been made, if there isn't time for transfer to a hospice.

NEUTROPENIC SEPSIS
PATHOPHYSIOLOGY
Neutropenia is defined as an abnormally low level of neutrophils in the blood. The normal level of neutrophils in human blood varies slightly by age and race. Infants have lower counts than older children and adults, and African Americans have lower counts than whites or Asians. The average adult level is 1500 cells/mm^3 of blood. Neutrophil counts (in cells/mm^3) are interpreted as follows:

- Greater than 1000: Normal protection against infection.
- 500 to 1000: Some increased risk of infection.
- 200 to 500: Great risk of severe infection.
- Lower than 200: Risk of overwhelming infection; requires hospital treatment with antibiotics.

Untreated bacteremia in patients with neutropenia is fatal: septic shock is associated with a 50% to 70% mortality rate. Mortality is associated with causative organism, site of infection, and level and duration of neutropenia. The faster the rate of neutrophil count decline and the longer the duration of neutropenia, especially if it lasts longer than 10 days, the greater the risk of infection. Infections in neutropenic patients typically take 2 to 7 days to respond to antimicrobial therapy. Fever (or any inflammatory response related to white cells or cytokines) may not be present in some infected neutropenic patients who are dehydrated or taking steroids or NSAIDs, and the possibility of infection must be considered in any neutropenic patient who is unwell.

ASSSESSMENT: NEUTROPENIC SEPSIS
HISTORY AND RISK FACTORS
Granulocytopenia, immunosuppression, recent cancer treatment, diabetes, organ-related disease, age older than 65 years, indwelling catheters, long hospital stays, loss of skin or mucosal integrity, malnutrition, hypothermia, intubation/mechanical ventilation, aspiration, alcoholism, renal failure, hepatic failure, chronic illness. The risk of death is twice as great for sepsis patients with cancer as for those without and is comparable to the risk observed in sepsis patients who are HIV positive.

THE FOUR STAGES OF SEPSIS
The progression of sepsis is subtle, rapid, and often deadly. It is usually broken down into four stages.

Stage 1
Systemic inflammatory response syndrome (SIRS) describes a systemic inflammation without a defined source of infection resulting from any major insult to the body, such as trauma, burns, or myocardial infarction, in which two or more of the following are present:

- HR at least 90 bpm.
- Body temperature less than 36°C (96.8°F) or greater than 38° C (100.4° F).
- Tachypnea greater than 20 breaths/min or, on blood gas, a Paco$_2$ less than 32 mm Hg.
- WBC less than 4000 cells/mm^3 or greater than 12,000 cells/mm^3 or the presence of greater than 10% immature neutrophils.

Patients with SIRS can be routinely cared for on the medical-surgical floor but should be closely monitored for signs and symptoms of sepsis.

Stage 2
Sepsis is identified by the presence of two of the SIRS criteria in response to pathogenic microorganisms and associated endotoxins in the blood. However, in many cases of sepsis, the actual cause of infection is never identified. The delay in waiting for confirmation of infection can slow the treatment of sepsis; the most effective course of action once SIRS is identified and infection is suspected is to treat the infection and monitor the patient for signs and symptoms of organ failure, which will indicate that the condition has progressed to severe sepsis.

Stage 3
Severe sepsis occurs when a patient who meets the sepsis criteria shows one of the signs and symptoms of organ failure. Once severe sepsis is suspected, the patient requires aggressive treatment in a critical care area.

Stage 4

Septic shock is defined as severe sepsis plus hypotension (a systolic BP less than 90 mm Hg) that does not respond to fluid resuscitation. Septic shock is associated with a high mortality rate. The patient's chances of recovery are significantly reduced if, by this stage of sepsis, she or he has not already been transferred to the ICU.

OBSERVATION: RAPID PROGRESSION IF UNTREATED

Signs and symptoms of infection may be absent because of decreased WBCs.
- General: Fever, hypothermia, chills, pain.
- Neurologic: Confusion, anxiety, restlessness, decreased level of consciousness, coma.
- Pulmonary: Tachypnea, rales, rhonchi, wheezes, dry cough, cyanosis, hypoxia, ARDS.
- Cardiovascular: Tachycardia, hypotension, fluctuating pulse pressure, thready pulse.
- Digestive: Nausea, vomiting, anorexia, decreased GI motility, GI bleed.
- Renal: Decreased urine output, anuria, renal failure.
- Integument: Warm, flushed changing to damp, cool, clammy.

Diagnostic Tests for Neutropenic Sepsis		
Test	**Purpose**	**Abnormal Findings**
Blood cultures (at baseline and every 24 hours if signs and symptoms of sepsis persist)	Check for bacteria or other microorganisms in a blood sample.	Gram-positive cocci: coagulase-negative staphylococci, Viridans streptococci, and *Staphylococcus aureus* Gram-negative pathogens: *Escherichia coli*, *Klebsiella* spp., and *Pseudomonas aeruginosa*. Fungal: *Candida* spp., *Aspergillus* spp. Viral: herpes simplex, respiratory syncytial virus
Cultures (throat, stool, urine, CV catheter, other sites of exudates) before antibiotics to determine pathogen	Determine source of infection.	As above
Chest radiographic examination	Evaluates lung status.	Pulmonary infiltrates, pulmonary edema
Complete blood count	Evaluates composition and concentration of cellular components of blood.	Increased WBC with infection, decreased WBC with sepsis, chemotherapy, radiation, leukemias
Chemistries: electrolytes, liver function tests	Evaluate blood chemistries and liver function.	Increased BUN, creatinine reveal dehydration. Increase to decrease in glucose caused by shock. Increased transaminase, bilirubin, and serum lactate in sepsis caused by shock
Coagulation profile	Examines the factors most often associated with a bleeding problem.	Prolonged PT, PTT
Pulse oximetry, ABGs	Measures oxygenation, acid-base balance.	Respiratory alkalosis followed by metabolic acidosis
Electrocardiogram	Records the electrical activity of the heart.	Tachycardia, arrhythmias

Oncologic Emergencies

COLLABORATIVE MANAGEMENT

Fever (even low grade) is often the only reliable sign of infection in the neutropenic patient. No specific patterns of fever or clinical features can positively distinguish between fever because of infection and one of noninfectious cause. Therefore, all febrile neutropenic patients should be considered for the administration of empirical broad-spectrum antibiotics within 1 hour of presentation. Many patients are outpatients during their cancer treatments, and it is vital to their survival that they and their significant others be educated about early recognition (and timing during treatment) of neutropenia to minimize the risk of sepsis. All healthcare providers should be educated about this potential life-threatening situation and be aware of strategies to minimize risk to patients by systematically and regularly evaluating response to treatment and progress toward desired outcomes.

Because sepsis-related mortality is unacceptably high, the Society of Critical Care Medicine (SCCM) set a quality improvement goal to reduce mortality caused by severe sepsis and septic shock by 25%. Clearer definitions of sepsis, severe sepsis, and septic shock will help in achieving this goal, as will recently updated evidence-based management guidelines for severe sepsis and septic shock. To be effective, these definitions and guidelines need to be applied to the early identification and aggressive treatment of patients who have severe sepsis or septic shock. Early goal-directed therapy to achieve hemodynamic stabilization has been demonstrated to decrease mortality in patients who have septic shock. See SIRS, Sepsis, and MODS, Chapter 11.

CARE PRIORITIES

1. Manage hypovolemia
Once severe sepsis or septic shock has been identified, the highest management priorities are to establish vascular access and initiate fluid resuscitation to improve tissue perfusion. Failure to manage global hypoxia can lead to MODS. Fluid resuscitation guidelines are defined by the SCCM and are a part of early goal-directed therapy (see Sepsis, SIRS, and MODS, Chapter 11).

2. Restore tissue oxygenation
Measurements commonly used are Svo_2 $Scvo_2$, and lactate. Low values indicate several possible causes of poor oxygenation, including inadequate oxygen delivery, high oxygen demand, or inability of tissues to extract oxygen from hemoglobin (see Sepsis, SIRS, and MODS, Chapter 11).

3. Identify and manage the underlying infection
Selection of an appropriate antimicrobial agent, often in the absence of microbiologic confirmation, requires consideration of patient-related characteristics such as drug intolerances, recently used antibiotics, previous infections, underlying disease, and clinical syndrome. Awareness of the prevalence of infections caused by specific organisms can provide clinicians with insight into appropriate empiric antimicrobial therapy. Pathogen resistance patterns in the hospital and community, along with hospital protocols to limit antibiotic resistance, should also be considered.

CARE PLANS FOR NEUTROPENIA

INEFFECTIVE PROTECTION: POTENTIAL FOR LIFE-THREATENING INFECTIONS *related to reduced numbers and activity of WBCs.*

Goals/Outcomes: No fever, no clinical signs or symptoms of sepsis, no growth in blood, excrement, or skin surface cultures

NOC Immune Status

Infection Control
1. Assess for signs and symptoms of infection, sepsis, septic shock.
   - Monitor temperature every 2 to 4 hours.
   - Monitor vital signs frequently for signs of impending shock: increased HR and RR, increased restlessness and anxiety, and cool and clammy skin, followed by a decrease in BP.
   - Monitor WBC and differential for evidence of infection and response to interventions.
   - Auscultate breath sounds for adventitious sounds or diminished breath sounds.

- Observe all dressing sites daily for signs and symptoms of infection.
- Observe all orifices daily for evidence of localized infection.
- Assess areas of localized pain for erythema, swelling, exudate, or rebound tenderness.

2. Control environmental risks of infection.
   - Strict handwashing.
   - Universal precautions.
   - Do not assign neutropenic patients with those known to be infected.
   - Monitor visitors for recent history of communicable disease and institute precautions as needed.
   - Clean all multipurpose equipment between patient use.
   - Live flowers cannot be kept in standing water.

3. Implement patient care routines to minimize infection.
   - Assist with daily bathing, oral, and perineal hygiene; change linens daily.
   - Ensure sleep and nutritional needs are met to promote immune system recovery.
   - Sterile technique for insertion and care of IV catheters.
   - Encourage incentive spirometry or deep breathing and coughing.
   - Encourage ambulation if patient is able or turn every 2 to 4 hours to minimize skin breakdown or atelectasis.

NIC Cardiac Care: Acute; Circulatory Care: Arterial Insufficiency; Respiratory Monitoring; Shock Management: Cardiac; Cerebral Perfusion Promotion; Neurologic Monitoring; Fluid/Electrolyte Management; Vital Signs Monitoring

DECREASED CARDIAC OUTPUT *related to infection or sepsis-induced myocardial infarction*

Goals/Outcomes: The patient will have normal BP and will exhibit signs of adequate tissue perfusion as evidenced by adequate urinary output and normal mental status.
NOC Circulation Status

Hypovolemia Management
1. Monitor I&O hourly. Consult physician for a urinary output less than 0.5 mL/kg/h for 4 consecutive hours. Insert urinary catheter if appropriate.
2. Monitor and document HR, rhythm, pulses, and BP.
3. Evaluate efficacy of volume expansion by closely comparing CVP, PAWP, and CO. Overzealous volume expansion can lead to heart failure and pulmonary edema.
4. Administer diuretics as prescribed in the well-hydrated patient with urine output less than 0.5 mL/kg/h.
5. Assess the patient for volume depletion, including poor skin turgor; dry mucous membranes; hypotension; tachycardia; and decreasing urine output, CVP, and CO.
6. Monitor electrolytes and serum osmolality. A universal increase in electrolytes and osmolality is indicative of dehydration. A universal decrease signals fluid overload.
7. Assess pH (normal range is 7.35 to 7.45) before replacing electrolytes. Acidosis and alkalosis alter electrolyte values. Replace potassium if the pH is outside the normal range.

NIC Electrolyte Monitoring; Fluid Management; Fluid Monitoring; Intravenous (IV) Therapy; Hypervolemia Management; Shock Management: Volume

ACUTE PAIN *related to fever, chills, headaches, myalgias, and arthralgias associated with neutropenia and infection.*

Goals/Outcomes: The patient will not experience chills and will be able to perform activities of daily living without discomfort; temperature will stay below 38° C (100.4° F).
NOC Comfort Level

Pain Management
1. Administer acetaminophen as ordered for fever or mild discomfort.
2. Encourage restful environment.
3. Apply warmth to muscles or joints or cool compress to head as needed.
4. Administer meperidine 12.5 to 25 mg IV or other opiate or benzodiazepine as ordered for chills.
5. Monitor temperature 30 minutes after chill subsides.
6. Bathe the patient and change linens after fever subsides.

Oncologic Emergencies

7. Monitor platelet count as it may decrease with hypermetabolism of hyperthermia.
8. Monitor and document HR, rhythm, pulses, and BP.

NIC Analgesic Administration; Medication Administration; Medication Administration: Intravenous (IV); Heat/Cold Application; Anxiety Reduction; Therapeutic Touch; Music Therapy; Meditation Facilitation

ADDITIONAL NURSING DIAGNOSES

Refer to nursing diagnoses in Emotional and Spiritual Support of the Patient and Significant Others (Chapter 2). For patients who manifest activity intolerance, see that nursing diagnosis in Prolonged Immobility (Chapter 1). For patients with sepsis or septic shock, see Sepsis, SIRS, and MODS (Chapter 11).

SUPERIOR VENA CAVA SYNDROME

PATHOPHYSIOLOGY

The superior vena cava (SVC) is a low-pressure vessel between two immovable bone structures: clavicle and scapula. When mediastinal structures become edematous or mass-occupying lesions are introduced, there is insufficient room and the soft-walled SVC becomes occluded and surrounding lymph nodes become enlarged. SVCS is a disorder defined by internal or external obstruction of the SVC leading to reduced blood return to the right side of the heart. Venous congestion and low CO result.

Complications include laryngeal edema, cerebral edema, decreased CO with hypotension, and pulmonary embolism (when an associated thrombus is present). Potential issues include:
- Failure to establish the correct diagnosis and the underlying etiology.
- Failure to initiate immediate treatment.
- Failure to recognize a thrombus in the SVC.
- Failure to consult a medical oncologist and radiation therapist.
- Failure to expeditiously diagnose and appropriately manage heparin-related complications.

ASSESSMENT

GOAL OF ASSESSMENT

Minimize life-threatening complications of cancer and its treatment through early recognition and effective management.

HISTORY AND RISK FACTORS

Malignancy

Primary intrathoracic malignancies are the cause of SVCS in approximately 87% to 97% of cases. The most frequent malignancy associated with the syndrome is lung cancer, followed by lymphomas and solid tumors that metastasize to the mediastinum. SVCS develops in approximately 3% to 15% of patients with bronchogenic carcinoma, and it is 4 times more likely to occur in patients with right- rather than left-sided lesions. Breast and testicular cancers are the most common metastatic malignancies causing SVCS, accounting for more than 7% of cases. Metastatic disease to the thorax is responsible for SVCS in about 3% to 20% of patients.

Nonmalignant causes

The most common nonmalignant cause of SVCS in cancer patients is thrombosis secondary to venous access devices. Other nonmalignant causes include cystic hygroma, substernal thyroid goiter, benign teratoma, dermoid cyst, thymoma, tuberculosis, histoplasmosis, actinomycosis, syphilis, pyogenic infections, radiation therapy, silicosis, and sarcoidosis. Some cases are idiopathic.

OBSERVATION

Classic symptoms

Patients with SVCS most often present with complaints of facial edema or erythema, dyspnea, cough, orthopnea, or arm and neck edema. These classic symptoms are seen most commonly in patients with complete obstruction, as opposed to those with mildly obstructive disease.

Other associated symptoms

Other associated symptoms may include hoarseness, dysphagia, headaches, dizziness, syncope, lethargy, and chest pain. The symptoms may be worsened by positional changes, particularly bending forward, stooping, or lying down.

Common physical findings

The most common physical findings include edema of the face, neck, or arms; dilatation of the veins of the upper body; and plethora or cyanosis of the face. Periorbital edema may be prominent.

Other physical findings

Other physical findings include laryngeal or glossal edema, mental status changes, and pleural effusion (more commonly on the right side).

Diagnostic Tests for Superior Vena Cava Syndrome

Test	Purpose	Abnormal Findings
Chest radiograph (CXR)	Evaluates lung status at baseline and every 24 hours if signs and symptoms of sepsis persist.	Identify hilar, mediastinal masses, right middle lobe congestion, masses, or nodes between clavicle and scapula.
Spiral chest CT scan with contrast	Further evaluates lung status to help clarify findings from CXR.	Precisely identify location and size of masses around SVC, clarify growth versus compression.
Magnetic resonance imaging of the chest	Provides further data regarding the area of the superior vena cava.	Precisely identifies location and size of masses around SVC.
Doppler ultrasound of the vasculature	Noninvasively assesses the entire vascular tree to identify thrombosis or effects of thrombolysis.	Presence of thrombus or ineffective thrombolysis when therapies are rendered.
Contrast and radionuclide venography	Invasively assesses the entire vascular tree to identify thrombolysis; may be used to validate Doppler ultrasound findings.	Presence of thrombus or ineffective thrombolysis when therapies are rendered.
Complete blood count: platelet count	Evaluates the composition and concentration of the cellular components of blood, particularly platelets.	Declining platelet count may signal the presence of heparin-induced thrombocytopenia or "white clot syndrome." If unmanaged, may lead to extremity gangrene and life-threatening venous thromboembolism.

Oncologic Emergencies

COLLABORATIVE MANAGEMENT

CARE PRIORITIES

1. Provide anticoagulation and thrombolysis

Anticoagulation for SVCS has become increasingly important because of thrombosis related to intravascular devices. In certain situations, the device remains in place. Both streptokinase and urokinase have been used for thrombolysis, although urokinase has been more effective in lysing clots in this setting. Urokinase is given as a 4400 U/kg bolus followed by 4400 U/kg/h; whereas streptokinase is administered as a 250,000 U bolus followed by 100,000 U/h. The use of thrombolytic therapy is controversial for catheter-related thrombosis.

2. Monitor for heparin-induced thrombocytopenia

In particular, one must monitor platelet count and be vigilant should a rapid decline in platelets occur. This suggests the possibility of platelet-induced thrombocytopenia syndrome (white clot syndrome). This rare syndrome may lead to extremity gangrene and life-threatening venous thromboembolism. Management requires urgent discontinuation of heparin and urgent evaluation by a hematologist for appropriate pharmacotherapy. Vascular surgical evaluation may also be indicated.

3. Provide surgical intervention/stenting

Placement of an expandable wire stent across the stenotic portion of the vena cava is an appropriate therapy for supportive care of SVCS symptoms when other therapeutic modalities cannot be used or are ineffective. Use of stents is limited when intraluminal thrombosis is present.

4. Provide radiotherapy and/or chemotherapy

Both radiotherapy and chemotherapy are treatment options for SVCS, depending on the tumor type. The specific drugs and doses used are those active against the underlying malignancy. Radiation therapy is the standard treatment of non–small-cell lung cancer with SVCS. Recent studies suggest that chemotherapy may be as effective as radiotherapy in rapidly shrinking small-cell lung cancer (SCLC). Combination chemoradiation therapy may result in improved ultimate local control over chemotherapy alone in SCLC and non-Hodgkin lymphoma. Retrospective reviews of patients with SCLC have reported equivalent survival in patients with or without SVCS treated definitively with chemoradiation therapy.

> **Safety Alert** *Life-threatening symptoms, such as respiratory distress, are indications for urgent radiotherapy. A preliminary determination of the treatment goal (potentially curative or supportive only) is necessary before initiation of treatment, even in the emergent setting.*

5. Provide additional interventions to assist with maintaining patency of the superior vena cava

Balloon angioplasty is rare but may be considered in patients with SVCS, significant clinical symptoms, and critical SVC obstruction demonstrated by angiography.

CARE PLANS FOR SUPERIOR VENA CAVA SYNDROME

DECREASED CARDIAC OUTPUT *related to reduced venous blood return to the heart.*

Goals/Outcomes: The patient will show evidence of normal tissue perfusion and will not experience upper extremity edema.

NOC Circulatory Status; Tissue Perfusion: Cardiac; Tissue Perfusion: Peripheral; Tissue Perfusion: Pulmonary

Circulatory Care: Venous Insufficiency

1. Monitor I&O hourly. Consult advanced practice provider if urinary output is less than 0.5 mL/kg/h for 4 consecutive hours. Insert urinary catheter if appropriate.
2. Monitor and document HR, rhythm, pulses, and BP.
3. Evaluate efficacy of volume expansion by monitoring CVP and CO. Overzealous volume expansion can lead to heart failure and pulmonary edema, with CVP greater than 20% of normal values and CO less than 5 L/min.
4. Administer diuretics as prescribed in the well-hydrated patient with urine output less than 0.5 mL/kg/h.
5. Assess the patient for volume depletion, including poor skin turgor, dry mucous membranes, hypotension, tachycardia, CVP less than 2 mm Hg, and decreasing urine output.
6. Monitor electrolytes and serum osmolality. A universal increase in electrolytes and osmolality is indicative of dehydration. A universal decrease signals fluid overload.
7. Assess skin and mucous membranes for cyanosis and pallor and skin temperature for signs of change in perfusion.
8. Assist in care of patients receiving therapy to treat SVCS.

NIC Electrolyte Monitoring; Fluid Management; Fluid Monitoring; Intravenous (IV) Therapy; Hypervolemia Management; Shock Management: Volume

IMPAIRED GAS EXCHANGE (OR RISK FOR SAME) *related to decreased blood flow to the lungs.*

- -

Goals/Outcomes: The patient's gas exchange is adequate as evidenced by Pao_2 at least 90 mm Hg, $Paco_2$ 35 to 45 mm Hg, pH 7.35 to 7.45, RR 12 to 20 breaths/min with normal depth and pattern, oxygen saturation at least 95%, HR 60 to 100 bpm, and orientation to time, place, and person.

NOC Respiratory Status: Gas Exchange; Vital Signs Monitoring

Respiratory Monitoring
1. Assess respiratory status every 2 hours, noting rate, rhythm, depth, and regularity of respirations.
2. Monitor for signs of respiratory failure: restlessness, anxiety, and air hunger indicative of hypoxemia; ABG values for increased $Paco_2$ and decreased pH indicative of hypoventilation; or oxygen saturation less than 90% via pulse oximetry indicative of decreased ventilation. Consult advanced practice provider if signs of respiratory insufficiency are present.
3. Monitor Svo_2: steady increase or decrease from patient's normal level may indicate deterioration.
4. Assess lungs for bibasilar crackles (rales), indicative of pulmonary edema.
5. Monitor patient's respiratory secretions. Institute respiratory therapy treatments as needed.
6. Monitor for pulmonary embolus, including sharp, stabbing chest pain, dyspnea, pallor, cyanosis, pupillary dilation, rapid or irregular pulse, profuse diaphoresis, and anxiety. Assess need for supplemental oxygen, and consult advanced practice provider immediately. Patients with severe pulmonary emboli may require mechanical ventilation. See Pulmonary Embolus, Chapter 4.
7. Assess the patient for changes in sensorium (i.e., confusion, lethargy, somnolence), indicative of inadequate cerebral oxygenation or CO_2 retention (respiratory insufficiency).

NIC Airway Management; Oxygen Therapy; Acid-Base Monitoring

TUMOR LYSIS SYNDROME
PATHOPHYSIOLOGY
Tumor lysis syndrome (TLS) is most commonly seen in individuals with rapidly growing tumors that are acutely responsive to chemotherapy because of the rapid release of intracellular contents into the bloodstream, leading to life-threatening concentrations of intracellular electrolytes. If the resulting metabolic abnormalities remain uncorrected, patients may develop acute renal failure and sudden death resulting from a lethal dysrhythmia secondary to hyperkalemia.

The syndrome is caused by rapid lysis of malignant cells resulting in hyperuricemia, hyperkalemia, hyperphosphatemia, hypocalcemia, and an increase in BUN. These abnormalities can occur as early as 6 hours following chemotherapy and in the last 5 to 7 days after treatment. The hyperuricemia is caused by the massive release of intracellular nucleic acids and their metabolism by xanthine oxidase into uric acid. Urate crystals can form in the renal collecting ducts and result in acute renal failure. Similarly, potassium and phosphate are released from the tumor cells, and their excretion is hampered by the hyperuricemia. The best approach to management is to prevent its occurrence by proper hydration. Patients with the diagnosis of rapidly growing lymphoma, uric acid levels of greater than 10 mg/dL, a high blast count in leukemia and a high lactate dehydrogenase level before treatment are at greatest risk of developing TLS.

TLS is also seen in small-cell lung cancer and metastatic breast cancer. Because of clinicians' increased awareness of TLS during the past decade and the use of adequate prophylaxis before initiation of chemotherapy, the number of cases has decreased. Occasionally, TLS occurs following treatment with radiation, glucocorticoids, tamoxifen, or interferon.

ASSESSMENT
HISTORY AND RISK FACTORS
The typical patient at risk for TLS tends to be young (under 25 years of age) and male with an advanced, highly proliferative, high-grade disease (lymphoma, leukemia, etc.), and a markedly elevated lactate dehydrogenase level. Abdominal disease is often present. Comorbid

conditions include renal insufficiency and diabetes. Volume depletion, concentrated acidic urine pH, and excessive urinary uric acid excretion rates may also increase the risk.

TLS most commonly develops during the rapid growth phase of high-grade lymphomas and leukemia in patients with high leukocyte counts; it is less common in patients with solid tumors. The syndrome is often iatrogenic, caused by cytotoxic chemotherapy.

OBSERVATION
Signs and symptoms reflect electrolyte imbalance, coupled with those of acute renal failure. The syndrome is characterized by hyperuricemia, hyperkalemia, hyperphosphatemia, hypocalcemia, and oliguric renal failure (see Fluid and Electrolyte Disturbances, Chapter 1, and Acute Renal Failure, Chapter 6). The diagnosis of TLS is based on the development of increased levels of serum uric acid, phosphorus, and potassium; decreased levels of serum calcium; and renal dysfunction following chemotherapy.

COLLABORATIVE CARE
CARE PRIORITIES
1. Identify patients at risk and initiate prophylactic measures
Patients at risk for TLS should be identified before the initiation of chemotherapy and should be adequately hydrated and given agents to alkalinize the urine. Treatment with allopurinol (IV or PO) may be instituted to minimize hyperuricemia. The recommended dosage of IV allopurinol ranges from 200 to 400 mg/m^2/day. This regimen should be started 24 to 48 hours before initiation of cytotoxic treatment. The dose may be equally divided into 6-, 8-, or 12-hour increments, but the final concentration should not exceed 6 mg/mL.

2. Monitor electrolytes
Serum electrolytes, uric acid, phosphorus, calcium, and creatinine levels should be checked repeatedly for 3 to 4 days after chemotherapy is initiated, with the frequency of monitoring dependent on the patient's clinical condition and risk profile.

3. Provide aggressive, immediate treatment of electrolyte imbalances and acute renal failure
Once tumor lysis is established, treatment is directed at vigorous correction of electrolyte abnormalities, hydration, and hemodialysis (see Fluid and Electrolyte Disturbances, Chapter 1 and Acute Renal Failure, Chapter 6).

CARE PLANS FOR TUMOR LYSIS SYNDROME
FLUID VOLUME EXCESS *related to acute renal failure resulting from hyperuricemia with formation of uric acid crystals lodging in the kidneys.*

Goals/Outcomes: Patient's volume status returns to normal/baseline as evidenced by urinary output at least 0.5 mL/kg/h, stable weight, BP within patient's normal range, HR 60 to 100 bpm, RR 12 to 20 breaths/min, good skin turgor, moist mucous membranes, urine specific gravity 1.005 to 1.025, and CVP 2 to 6 mm Hg. Serum potassium, phosphorus, calcium, uric acid, BUN, and creatinine levels will be within normal limits.
NOC Electrolyte and Acid-Base Balance

Fluid/Electrolyte Management
1. Monitor I&O hourly. Consult advanced practice provider if urinary output is less than 0.5 mL/kg/h for 4 consecutive hours. Insert urinary catheter if appropriate.
2. Monitor electrolytes every 6 to 12 hours during high-risk period.
3. Monitor and document HR, rhythm, pulses, and BP.
4. Administer IV fluids before and after cancer treatment.
5. Administer allopurinol as prescribed to manage hyperuricemia.
6. Administer aluminum hydroxide as prescribed to manage hyperphosphatemia.
7. Administer cation-exchange resins as prescribed to manage hyperkalemia.
8. Assist with renal replacement therapies.
9. Administer diuretics as prescribed in the well-hydrated patient with urine output less than 0.5 mL/kg/h.
10. Monitor electrolytes and serum osmolality. A universal increase in electrolytes and osmolality is indicative of dehydration. A universal decrease signals fluid overload.

11. Assess pH (normal range is 7.35 to 7.45) before replacing electrolytes. Acidosis and alkalosis alter electrolyte values. Replace potassium if the pH is outside the normal range.
12. Teach patients to restrict foods high in potassium and phosphorus and to increase fluid intake.

NIC Electrolyte Monitoring; Fluid Management; Fluid Monitoring; Intravenous (IV) Therapy; Hypervolemia Management; Shock Management: Volume

ADDITIONAL NURSING DIAGNOSES

Refer to nursing diagnoses in Emotional and Spiritual Support of the Patient and Significant Others (Chapter 2). For patients who manifest activity intolerance, see that nursing diagnosis in Prolonged Immobility (Chapter 1).

ORGAN TRANSPLANTATION

Solid organ transplantation remains a viable option for end-stage organ failure. As of May 2014, there were nearly 122,900 people on the United Network for Organ Sharing (UNOS) organ transplant waiting list. The major constraint to meeting the demand for transplants is the availability of donated (cadaver) organs. Dialysis remains the main lifeline for kidney disease and mechanical devices for heart failure are becoming increasingly available throughout the United States. A small number of patients are living at home on mechanical ventilation. In general, those with end stage liver end-stage, pancreatic, and lung disease remain dependent on organ transplantation to sustain life.

Several steps have been taken to alleviate the organ shortage. National laws mandate that families of every appropriate potential donor be offered the option to donate organs and tissues. In addition, the ongoing efforts of the National Organ Donation Collaborative and laws requiring all deaths to be reported to organ procurement agencies have prompted an increase in organ donations. Ongoing efforts of organ recovery coordinators and others to improve public awareness of organ donation will help reduce the shortage, as will use of extended donors.

Nationally, major improvements are being made to optimize organ distribution, improve procurement, and ensure good matches. Inclusion criteria for the waiting list are being standardized using listing criteria for all degrees of sickness (see Box 11-4 for allocation of cardiac organs). UNOS maintains a computerized registry of all patients awaiting organs for transplantations. Organs procured within a region are shared first within that region. If a recipient cannot be found there, UNOS directs the organ to the recipient in another region with the greatest need. Organ recovery coordinators are available 24 hours a day, 7 days a week to arrange serologic testing and organ removal from donors, preserve organs pretransplant, and distribute organs to appropriate recipients.

ASSESSMENT AND DIAGNOSTIC TESTING

GENERAL EVALUATION FOR TRANSPLANTATION

All solid organ recipients require multiple tests to evaluate readiness and appropriateness for transplantation. Health status, including comorbidities, pretransplantation disease processes, and donor matching are evaluated as follows:

LABWORK

- General laboratory assessment profiles including biochemical, hematologic, lipid, hepatic, renal, and thyroid studies, and urinalysis. If findings indicate several organs are impaired, the patient may be inappropriate for transplant, since immunosuppressive drugs can cause renal failure, those with heart disease may have a myocardial infarction in the postoperative period, those with lung disease may be unable to wean from mechanical ventilation, and those with liver disease may be immunocompromised and at higher risk for sepsis and metabolic complications.
- ABO blood typing: Requires duplicate testing for accuracy and safety. Testing includes panel reactive antibody (PRA) and human leukocyte antigen (HLA) testing.
- Virology screening: HIV, hepatitis B and C, herpes, cytomegalovirus (CMV), Epstein-Barr virus (EBV).

Box 11-4   ALLOCATION OF CARDIAC ORGANS

Status 1A

A patient is admitted to the transplant center and has at least one of the following:

A. Mechanical circulatory support for acute hemodynamic decompensation that includes at least one of the following:
  - Left or right ventricular assist device implanted within past 30 days
  - Total artificial heart
  - Intraaortic balloon pump
  - Extracorporeal membrane oxygenator

B. Mechanical circulatory support for >30 days with significant device-related complications such as thromboembolism, device infection, mechanical failure, or life-threatening ventricular arrhythmias

C. Mechanical ventilation

D. Continuous infusion of a high-dose inotrope or multiple inotropes with hemodynamic monitoring

E. Patient does not meet the above criteria but has a life expectancy without a heart transplant of less than 7 days.

Status 1B

A patient listed as status 1B has at least one of the following devices or therapies in place:

A. Left and/or right ventricular assist device implanted for >30 days

B. Continuous infusion of inotropes

Status 2

A patient who does not meet the criteria for status 1A or 1B is listed as a status 2.

Status 7

A patient listed as status 7 is considered temporarily unsuitable to receive a thoracic organ transplant.

From the United Network for Organ Sharing (UNOS) for allocation of thoracic organs. For complete, detailed criteria, see actual policy at www.UNOS.org.

- Other infectious diseases: Syphilis, toxoplasmosis, tuberculosis, resistant bacterial infections including *Burkholderia cepacia.*
- Cancer screening: May include pap smears, prostate examination, prostate-specific antigen, mammogram, colonoscopy, and chest radiography

DIAGNOSTIC TESTING

- Pulmonary evaluation: Oxygenation assessment using pulmonary function testing and chest radiograph.
- Cardiovascular evaluation: Exercise stress test and Doppler imaging for patients with a history of diabetes, coronary artery disease, claudication, cerebrovascular accident.
- Nutritional evaluation: Body mass index (BMI) less than 16 (cachexia) and BMI greater than 30 are associated with poorer outcomes.
- Osteoporosis screening: Osteoporosis may place a patient at higher risk for complications following transplantation, as maintenance medication may increase the severity, which increases the probability of bone fractures.
- Dental examination: Poor oral hygiene may be a source of infection.
- Ultrasound of gallbladder: Presence of gallstones increases the probability of need for cholecystectomy following transplantation.
- Psychosocial evaluation: The patient must be ready to comply with and have an adequate support system to participate in posttransplant medical care and life maintenance activities, including medication management, diet, exercise, and abstinence from substance use and abuse.
- Financial evaluation: The financial burden associated with organ transplantation is significant. The patient must have appropriate resources in place to cover the costs.

ORGAN-SPECIFIC EVALUATION

- Cardiac: Cardiac catheterization (right and left heart), cardiopulmonary exercise testing, cardiac magnetic resonance imaging or positron emission tomography scan, and MVo_2 testing.
- Lung: Computed tomography scan to define the anatomy, ventilation-perfusion scan, 6-minute walk test, ABG, continuous pH testing, smoking cessation readiness, and ability to remain "smoke free."
- Liver: Alpha-fetoprotein, CA 19-9 tumor markers for hepatocellular carcinoma and cholangiocarcinoma. Liver biopsy may be performed to determine staging or presence of disease. Abdominal imaging and GI testing assess portal vein system and hepatic vasculature. A GI evaluation is done to assess for bowel diseases.
  - Alcohol consumption screening: To assess for usage patterns and readiness to stop drinking alcohol. If use persists in a person whose need for liver transplant is directly related to alcohol, he or she is unable to qualify for organ transplantation. A complete battery of tests is performed to determine the cause and acuity of liver failure.
- Kidney: Specific urine testing for preoperative baseline, hypercoagulopathy screen, abdominal imaging for anatomic and renal vessel assessment
- Pancreas: Complete testing referred to in the cardiac section, as well as full assessment of diabetes status. Initial screening includes a hemoglobin A_{1C} test to assess for average blood glucose level over the past 8 weeks.

ORGAN-SPECIFIC CRITERIA FOR TRANSPLANTATION

CARDIAC

Table 11-9 summarizes the selection criteria that patients must meet before they can be considered for cardiac transplantation. Box 11-4 reflects the various statuses of cardiac transplantation patients.

Table 11-9	SELECTION CRITERIA FOR CARDIAC TRANSPLANTATION
Inclusion Criteria	**Exclusion Criteria**
• End-stage heart failure • Refractory and intolerable symptoms; New York Heart Association classes III and IV • Failure of maximal medical treatment (e.g., digoxin, diuretics, vasodilators, ACE inhibitors, beta blockers) • 1-year survival expectancy <50% and poor short-term prognosis or poor functional capacity • Age <60 to 65 years • Left ventricular ejection fraction 20% to 35% • Chronic, unstable angina • Peak O_2 consumption 14 mL/kg/min • Onset of atrial fibrillation • Decreasing cardiac output • Refractory ventricular dysrhythmias • Otherwise good health	Relative • Active substance abuse • Active infection associated with ventricular assist device • Psychological/social issues related to support or finances • Age >65 to 70 years • History of cancer in remission • Absolute • Complicated IDDM with end-organ damage • Poor compliance • Severe obesity • Pulmonary hypertension: PVR >6 Wood units • Comorbid diseases • Active infection (until resolved) and infection with highly resistant organisms that are nearly impossible to eradicate • Irreversible liver and kidney dysfunction • Active peptic ulcer disease • Coexisting cancer • Symptomatic peripheral and cerebral vascular disease • Severe osteoporosis • Amyloidosis

ACE: Angiotensin Converting Enzyme; BMI: Body Mass Index; IDDM: Insulin Dependent Diabetes Mellitus; PVR: Pulmonary Vascular Resistance;

Organ Transplantation

LUNG

Lung transplant candidates generally have a life expectancy of less than 18 months, are dependent on supplemental oxygen, have severe exercise intolerance, are under 65 years of age, and report poor quality of life.

Indications

In adults, irreversible, progressively disabling, end-stage pulmonary disease encompassing a wide variety of etiologies. The majority of lung transplants are performed for chronic obstructive pulmonary disease, followed by idiopathic pulmonary fibrosis, pulmonary hypertension, and cystic fibrosis (CF). Four groupings of lung diseases that may result in transplantation are:

1. Nonbronchiectatic: Obstructive lung conditions or changes in the upper and lower airways NOT resulting from an infectious process, including emphysema, chronic bronchitis, alpha$_1$-antitrypsin disease, and bronchiolitis obliterans syndrome (BOS), a disease associated with chronic transplant rejection. BOS and chronic bronchitis can evolve into bronchiectasis. Most recently, the BODE index was introduced (**B**MI, **O**bstruction of airflow severity, **D**yspnea severity as measured by the modified Medical Research Council dyspnea scale, **E**xercise capacity). Patients scoring greater than 5 on the BODE index should be referred for transplant.

2. Bronchiectatic: Obstructive lung conditions resulting from abnormal dilation and thickening of the walls in the bronchi and bronchioles, which result from recurrent inflammation, leading to mucus retention. Diseases include CF and severe chronic bronchitis, which result in chronic bacterial pneumonia.

3. Interstitial: Restrictive lung disease resulting from chronic inflammation of the lower airways, including idiopathic pulmonary fibrosis, diseases related to occupational exposure to toxins (asbestos, coal, or organic dust, crystalline silica), histiocytosis X, and sarcoidosis. Patients who have been irradiated and/or have undergone chemotherapy for a nonpulmonary condition and who then develop lung disease are considered on an individual basis. Not all centers accept patients with pulmonary fibrosis associated with connective tissue disease.

4. Pulmonary vascular: Pulmonary hypertension resulting from vascular disease that severely increases pulmonary vascular resistance, which leads to right-sided heart failure and chronic hypoxia. Pulmonary hypertension may be primary (idiopathic pulmonary vascular disease) or secondary to a shunt associated with heart disease, thromboembolism, connective tissue disease, or parenchymal disease.

Contraindications

Relative

- Advanced age: Historically, patients older than 65 years of age have a higher mortality rate, but centers vary with candidate acceptance. Generally, the age limit for heart-lung transplantation is 50 years, for bilateral sequential lung transplantation is 60 years, and for single lung transplantation is 65 years.
- Ventilator dependence: A potential contraindication based on length of time on the ventilator because of the potential of developing complications that are absolute contraindications. Patients requiring prolonged mechanical ventilation are at higher risk of infection, development of MODS, muscle atrophy, and other concerns surrounding deconditioning, which impacts success of attaining a functional lifestyle following transplantation.
- Corticosteroid therapy: Low dose is now acceptable, while high dose may be viewed as an absolute contraindication.
- Infection: CF patients may be excluded if infected with the highly resistant organism *B. cepacia* because of inability to eradicate the organism with antibiotics; those with active tuberculosis are generally not candidates, as well as CF patients with *Aspergillus fumigatus*. Infection with nontuberculous *Mycobacteria* is not a contraindication.
- Body weight: Patients with BMI less than 16 likely have a poor nutritional status, which impairs healing. Those with BMI greater than 30 are at higher risk of developing postoperative atelectasis and pneumonia.
- Associated organ dysfunction: Patients with left ventricular systolic or diastolic dysfunction may not be a candidate if disease is severe, as are those with bilirubin of greater than 2 mg/dL and those with connective tissue diseases.

Absolute
- Malignancy within the past 2 years (except cutaneous squamous and basal cell tumors).
- Noncurable, chronic, extrapulmonary infection (e.g., chronic hepatitis B or C, HIV).
- Untreatable advanced organ dysfunction of another body system.
- Current cigarette smoking (must be smoke free for at least 6 months).
- Poor rehabilitation potential (based on evaluation of issues mentioned in relative contraindications).
- Significant psychosocial problems, substance abuse, or history of nonadherence to past medical therapies or disease management programs.

LIVER
Indications
Patients with chronic or acute liver disease who cannot sustain a normal quality of life or have life-threatening complications are probable candidates for liver transplant. Complications that warrant liver transplantation generally include recurrent variceal hemorrhage, intractable ascites, spontaneous bacterial peritonitis, refractory encephalopathy, severe jaundice, and sudden deterioration in status. Reduced-size, split, and living-related liver transplantation continue to expand the number of donors, and yet these efforts still fail to meet the demand for organs.
- Chronic end-stage liver disease: Hepatitis C, hepatitis B, alcoholic cirrhosis, primary biliary cirrhosis, primary sclerosing cholangitis, hepatocellular carcinoma, autoimmune hepatitis, metabolic disease (e.g., Wilson disease, inborn errors of metabolism), and other liver diseases.
- Fulminant hepatic failure (FHF): Severe impairment of hepatic function in the absence of preexisting liver disease. Those who are exposed to or ingest toxins or toxic doses of illicit drugs or medications (e.g., acetaminophen toxicity) are included in this group. Hepatotoxic drugs include acetaminophen (paracetamol), salicylates (aspirin, Pepto-Bismol), methanol (wood alcohol), isoniazid, IV tetracycline, chlorinated hydrocarbons, and sodium valproate. The most commonly involved drug is acetaminophen, and, in some locations, it is the most common cause of FHF. Other diseases that may cause FHF include heart failure, cardiomyopathy, sepsis, shock, cyanotic heart disease, obstructive lesions of the aorta, vascular occlusions, myocarditis, Hodgkin disease, and severe asphyxia.

Contraindications
Relative
- Chronic renal failure (may require a combined liver/kidney transplant).
- Advanced cachexia.
- Large hepatocellular cancers/tumors: More advanced than stage II, as described by the UNOS-modified American Joint Committee on Cancer (AJCC) classification.
- Medication-resistant hepatitis B viral cirrhosis.
- Portal and mesenteric vein thrombosis.
- History of prior cancer not meeting full AJCC cure criteria.
- Active infections.
- MODS.
- Age: Physiologic age, rather than chronologic age, is used.
Absolute
- Spontaneous bacterial peritonitis (or other active infection).
- Active alcohol or other substance abuse.
- Extrahepatic malignancy that does not meet "cure" criteria.
- Severely advanced cardiac or pulmonary disease.
- Extreme psych/social situations that prohibit adherence to immunosuppressive therapies.
- Severe portopulmonary hypertension (moderate and mild pulmonary hypertension are acceptable and sometimes included in the indication criteria).
- Hepatocellular carcinoma lesion(s) greater than 5 cm or more than 3 lesions present.

KIDNEY
Indications
- Chronic end-stage kidney disease.
- Dependency on dialysis or imminent dependence on dialysis.

- Provider and patient to consider transplantation before chronic kidney disease progresses rather than waiting until the advanced stage and an often lengthy wait for a donor.

Relative
- Contraindications are transplant site (facility) dependent.

Absolute
- Active or current malignancy.
- Goodpasture disease or systemic lupus erythematosus (can damage the transplanted kidney).
- Active infection.
- Obesity.
- Significant peripheral vascular disease.
- End-stage diseases of other organs.
- Active systemic vascular disease.
- Noncompliance.
- Active substance abuse.
- Untreated psychiatric illness or mental incapacity.
- Active peptic ulcer disease.
- Limited life expectancy.

PANCREAS

Preexisting advanced renal disease is observed in significant numbers of pancreas transplantation candidates. Many pancreas transplantation candidates may benefit from a combined pancreas/kidney transplant.

- Islet cell: A novel less invasive harvesting of pancreatic cells for transplantation is in limited use. The islet cells are the islets of Langerhans (alpha, beta, and delta). Islet cells are isolated from a donor pancreas or from the patient's own pancreas after the pancreatectomy. The sample is specially processed and then infused into the patient via the portal vein. A neovascularization process takes place. The islet cells begin to produce insulin shortly after transplantation.

Indications
- Type 1 diabetes with chronic poor metabolic control.
- Patients requiring a total pancreatectomy.
- Mean duration of diabetes 23 to 27 years.
- C-reactive peptide less than 0.8 ng/mL.
- Frequent or severe metabolic complications, e.g., hypoglycemia/hyperglycemia and ketoacidosis.
- End-organ failure with numbness of extremities, lethargy, nausea, dizziness, and blurred or poor vision.

Contraindications
Relative
- Evidence of significant secondary complications of type 1 diabetes, including peripheral neuropathy, retinopathy, gastroparesis, nephropathy, and coronary artery disease, which may impede the success of the transplant.
- Persons with type 2 diabetes are seldom evaluated.

Absolute
- Active cancer or history of cancer.
- Severe cardiac, vascular, or pulmonary insufficiency.
- Active/chronic hepatitis B.
- Severe psychiatric or substance abuse issues.
- Although HIV has historically been a contraindication for both candidates and donors, the HIV Organ Procurement Equity Act (HOPE Act) requires the US Department of Health and Human Services to develop criteria for conducting research related to HIV-positive donors donating to HIV-positive candidates. Currently over 20 HIV-positive persons have received an HIV-negative donor organ.

ORGAN DONORS

The mainstay of organ supply is the deceased donor or cadaveric donation. Nationwide, approximately 30% to 40% of all deceased organ donors are trauma patients. Evaluation of the trauma patient as a potential organ donor is critical to maximizing the availability of deceased donor organs for transplantation. Regional transplant centers vary in absolute and relative criteria for excluding potential organ donors. Early criteria limited evaluation to ideal donors aged 10 to 50 years without comorbid conditions. In response to the increasing demand for organs, restrictions have loosened considerably and the donor pool has expanded. Organs are now often procured from patients younger than 10 years and older than 50 years of age. Factors such as hepatitis C or active bacterial infection are no longer absolute contraindications. "Nonideal" donors are often used for specific recipients.

There are relatively few absolute contraindications, and most potential donors are reviewed on an individual or a case-by-case basis. Additional absolute and relative contraindications are assessed for donation of specific organs. Some organs must be transplanted within a very short time following brain death, while other organs can be preserved for much longer periods of time. The following are types of organ donors:

DONATION AFTER BRAIN DEATH

The patient has sustained an irreversible brain injury causing cessation of brain function, including the brain stem. The patient is brain dead but is kept "alive" with respiratory and cardiac support until organ recovery occurs. Brain death is diagnosed by an absence of neurologic function, apnea, irreversibility, and physiologic confirmatory tests.

DONATION AFTER CARDIAC DEATH

Death is declared on the basis of cardiopulmonary criteria (irreversible cessation of circulatory and respiratory function). The patient may have sustained catastrophic brain injury that is not anticipated to progress to brain death (stroke or trauma). If the family members decide to remove the patient from the ventilator to allow for natural death, they may be offered the opportunity for organ donation. Natural death would need to occur within 1 hour of removal from the ventilator. The organs are procured once the patient is pronounced dead. The donation should not hasten the death, and the transplant procurement team enters the operating room after the patient is pronounced dead and is not part of the end-of-life care. All normal care, including palliative measures, occurs until the patient is pronounced. Donation may also be considered if there is an unplanned cardiac arrest.

LIVING DONORS

Living donors are considered for kidney and liver transplants. The evaluation process is critical for living donors. Postoperative care for the donor and donor family must also be clearly defined. Considerations to be assessed include:

1. Risk/Benefit: Is there maximum benefit to the recipient and minimum risk to the donor? It is important NOT to underestimate the risk to the donor.
   - What is the physical and psychosocial health of the donor?
2. Freedom of Choice: Is the potential donor making the decision without pressure or coercion from the recipient or others?
   - The donor should be seen separately in the absence of the prospective recipient.
   - Informed consent is complete, neutral, and not coerced.
   - The donor does not overestimate the benefits of donating.
   - Do the healthcare providers understand donor motivation?
3. Understanding the Costs: Does the donor understand the potential financial costs he or she will incur and the amount of time that will be lost from work?
4. Well-Being: What is the overall state of the donor and family's emotional well-being?
   - Are the donor and family prepared to cope with feelings of anxiety and remorse associated with postoperative pain, postoperative complications, and postoperative depression?
   - Are donors concerned about the recipient?

PAIRED AND CHAIN DONATIONS

Paired donation is an opportunity for a live donation when a direct related donation is not possible. Transplant centers strategically manage a group of potential recipients and potential live donors so that a donor can give to an unrelated person, while the unrelated person's donor can give to their related person. A complex chain of exchanges ("swaps"), if worked out, potentially benefits a larger number of individuals.

LABORATORY AND DIAGNOSTIC TESTS

- Laboratory and diagnostic testing varies from center to center, but general standards are presented below.

GENERAL SCREENING FOR ORGAN DONORS

- Basic laboratory values (e.g., CBC, electrolytes, glucose, ABG).
- ABO blood typing.
- HLA typing.
- Blood cultures.
- Sputum Gram stain, culture, and sensitivities.
- Urinalysis, culture, and sensitivities.
- HIV, EBV, CMV, human T-cell leukemia virus type 1, and hepatitis B and C virus serologies.
- Venereal Disease Research Laboratory test or rapid plasma reagent test.
- Inguinal lymph nodes tested for evaluation of recipient sensitivity.

HEART DONOR

- ECG.
- Chest radiograph.
- Echocardiogram.
- Cardiac catheterization (male older than 40 years or female older than 45 years, or younger if other cardiovascular risk factors present).
- Creatine kinase (CK), CK-MB, and troponin levels.

LUNG DONOR

- ABG on 100% FIO_2; then, serial ABGs.
- Chest radiograph.
- Bronchoscopy.

PANCREAS DONOR

- Serial blood glucose determinations.
- Amylase and lipase levels.

LIVER DONOR

- Liver function tests.
- Liver biopsy for patients with BMI greater than 32, age older than 70 years (older than 60 years if diabetic), past medical history suggestive of liver disease, significant history of alcohol abuse, radiographic studies suggestive of fatty liver infiltration, or positive hepatitis serology.
- PT/INR.
- aPTT.

KIDNEY DONOR

- Electrolytes.
- BUN.
- Creatinine.

PRIORITY/WAITING LISTS/MEDICAL URGENCY DETERMINATION

HEART

Demographics including age, ethnicity, gender, and location, with ABO type, height, weight, diagnosis, and medical urgency, are matched with the donor information (weight, age, distance to transplant center, and need for prospective cross-match). Median time to transplant has been gradually increasing since 2006-2007 when the wait time was at its lowest point for all medical urgency categories. Median time to transplant is longest for status 2 candidates, at almost 20 months. Median time to transplant for status 1A and status 1B candidates was 2.4 months and 6.9 months, respectively, in 2012. The median waiting time for status 1A candidates has not changed appreciably during the last decade, although it has increased for status 1B and status 2 candidates. The median time to transplant among candidates with ventricular assist devices (when listed) was 3 months in 2006-2007 and has since increased to 8.7 months in 2012, the same as for candidates without them.

LUNGS

The Lung Allocation Score (LAS) is a numerical scale (0 to 100) computed from a list of criteria and updated every 6 months. People who are most likely to die before transplantation and have a chance of greater survival after transplantation are the candidates given the highest scores on the list. Along with the LAS, blood type, age, and distance from the donor are used to determine priority for the organ. Also under consideration is the bilirubin level and changes in this level while on the waiting list. A current bilirubin of at least 1.0 mg/dL or an increase by at least 50% during a 6-month time period increases the candidate's risk of dying while on the list. Pediatric and adolescent patients have priority over adults. LAS testing is updated every 6 months.

Since implementation of the LAS, transplant rates have increased for all candidates and are most profound in candidates aged 65 years or older and those in diagnosis group D. Overall median waiting time for candidates listed for lung transplant in 2012 was 4 months and 3.1 months for group D patients. Median months to transplant for group B patients listed in 2011 was 9.7 months. Although 65.3% of lung transplant candidates underwent transplant within 1 year of listing, the percentage of candidates undergoing lung transplant was highly variable based on donation service area (DSA). The variation was from 37.5% to 93.5% for those with at least 10 listings.

KIDNEYS

Living donor allocation/timing is dependent on availability and matching. The waiting time may be less than for a deceased donor. Waiting times can vary from 2 to 5 years for a deceased donor. Recipients must have a glomerular filtration rate of no more than 20 mL/min to be considered. Recipient status is either active or inactive. There is no urgent status. Extended criteria donors are on the rise. Considerations include ABO type, HLA antibodies, crossmatch, and PRAs. PRAs can be tested as frequently as monthly. A new algorithm—Life Years from Transplantation—will attempt to determine the donor and recipient combination that will achieve the greatest survival benefit relative to dialysis.

LIVER

Transplant-appropriate patients are generally determined using the model for end-stage liver disease (MELD) score. Those patients in the ICU with life expectancy of less than 7 days with acute liver failure, hepatic artery thrombosis, primary graft nonfunction, or acute decompensated Wilson disease are considered status 1 and are excluded from other requirements of the MELD score. The overall transplant rate has been gradually declining since 2006. The greatest decline is in candidates with hepatocellular cancer and those aged 18 to 34 years. The decrease in transplant rates reflects the gradually worsening donor shortage. Despite a decline in waitlist registration, the median pretransplant waiting time among active wait-listed adult patients increased from 12.9 months in 2009 to 17.6 months in 2010 and to 18.5 months in 2011. Pretransplant mortality rates decreased in 2012, for the first time in several years.

MELD Score: This score ranges from 6 (less ill) to 40 (gravely ill) and is used to prioritize liver transplant candidates at least 12 years of age. It is predictive of risk of 3-month mortality from liver disease. The number is calculated using a formula that considers three blood studies: bilirubin, which measures liver excretion of bile; INR (international normalized ratio), which measures the ability of the liver to manufacture clotting factors; and creatinine, which measures kidney function. Bile excretion and the ability to synthesize clotting factors are impaired by chronic liver disease. Renal impairment is often associated with liver disease. A numerical scale is used for liver allocation for chronic liver disease only. Status 7 patients are considered inactive.

PANCREAS

Waiting lists and allocation of organs vary by institution and are generally based on time waiting and PRA level. Frequent evaluation is necessary, that is, every 6 months or per program standard. There are four main types of pancreas transplantation:

- Pancreas transplant alone (PTA): Involves patients with type 1 diabetes who generally have severe, frequent hypoglycemia but adequate kidney function.

Organ Transplantation

- Simultaneous pancreas-kidney transplant (SPK): The pancreas and kidney are transplanted simultaneously from the same deceased donor.
- Pancreas-after-kidney transplant (PAK): A cadaveric, or deceased, donor pancreas transplant is performed after a previously performed living or deceased donor kidney transplant.
- Simultaneous deceased donor pancreas and live donor kidney (SPLK): Has a lower rate of delayed graft function than SPK and significantly reduced waiting times, resulting in improved outcome.

Median time to transplant for active candidates listed in 2010-2011 was 19.1 months for PTA and 16.2 months for SPK. The most recent estimate available for PAKs was 36.9 months, for candidates listed in 2008-2009. Waiting times for SPK, PAK, and PTA vary by DSA. In six DSAs, no transplant program performed pancreas transplants in 2011-2012. Organ Procurement and Transplant Network (OPTN) policy allows for local organ procurement organizations to use their discretion in prioritizing SPK or solitary pancreas (PTA or PAK) offers. Lack of national policy likely contributes to the overall geographic variation. The combined pancreas waiting list will treat SPK, PAK, and PTA candidates equally, which may eliminate geographic variations in allocation policy.

PHARMACOTHERAPY
POSTTRANSPLANT IMMUNOSUPPRESSION
Goals of therapy include:
1. Prevent rejection.
2. Improve graft survival.
3. Improve patient survival.
4. Maintain quality of life.

Immunosuppression therapy prevents rejection and is required indefinitely posttransplant. Immunosuppression agents have their own risks: infection, malignancy, and toxicity. Patient compliance to therapy and program compliance also affect rejection. Finding the balance between saving the graft and preventing complications is a lifelong challenge.

LEVELS OF IMMUNOSUPPRESSION THERAPY
Induction
Immunosuppression, usually in high doses, in the initial period of organ transplantation wipes out T cells completely. Commonly used drugs typically consist of corticosteroids and monoclonal and polyclonal antibodies: Orthoclone OKT3, antithymocyte globulin (ATG), basiliximab, daclizumab, alemtuzumab.

Maintenance
A maintenance dose of immunosuppression for transplant patients in stable condition serves to maintain a gradual process of healing and to prevent rejection. The potential for weaning patients off some of their medication therapies is a high priority. Commonly used drugs are corticosteroids, calcineurin inhibitors (CNIs), antiproliferative agents, and mammalian target of rapamycin (mTOR) inhibitors.

Rejection
Immunosuppression, usually in high doses for a patient whose organs are acutely rejecting. Commonly used drugs are corticosteroids and polyclonal and monoclonal antibodies: Orthoclone OKT3, ATG, basiliximab, daclizumab, and alemtuzumab.

Desensitization
Therapies to reduce newly formed or preexisting alloantibodies. Commonly used drugs are IVIG, rituximab, and cyclophosphamide. Plasmapheresis mechanically removes antibodies but does not treat the underlying problem.

CATEGORIES OF DRUGS
Interleukin 1 inhibitors
Corticosteroids are used to treat and prevent organ rejection and to suppress production of cytotoxic T-lymphocytes from noncytotoxic precursor cells. They can be used for maintenance to prevent rejection or as part of an acute rejection protocol. Evidence indicates that steroids

may prevent release of interleukin (IL)-1 and IL-2. IL-1 is released by the macrophages and promotes differentiation of helper T cells. The release of IL-2 promotes differentiation of cytotoxic cells and helps to reduce or prevent edema, to promote normal capillary permeability, and to prevent vasodilation. Side effects are numerous, including mood changes, sodium retention, blurred vision, fragile skin, bleeding, glucose intolerance, increase in appetite and subsequent weight gain, osteoporosis, and "moon face" appearance from an accumulation of fatty tissue on cheeks and upper back.

- Methylprednisolone (Solu-Medrol): A corticosteroid used as an induction agent in doses ranging from 250 to 1000 mg IV at the time of transplantation. Generally, three additional daily doses are administered. The dose is then reduced to 35 mg by mouth (PO) every 12 hours, until the first biopsy is completed or per program protocol. Dosage is reduced by 5 mg per dose until the drug is stopped, or a maintenance daily dose of 10 mg or less is achieved. Methylprednisolone 125 mg IV every 12 hours for three doses is also used before poly/monoclonal antibody therapy for cytokine release syndrome. The drug is tapered to as low a dose as tolerated.

Calcineurin inhibitors

Calcineurin is a protein phosphatase (also known as protein phosphatase 3, and calcium-dependent serine-threonine phosphatase), which activates the T cells of the immune system. CNIs are used to block T-cell activation.

- Cyclosporine (CSA, Sandimmune, Neoral, Gengraf): A CNI used to block the response of cytotoxic T lymphocytes to IL-2, which inhibits the production and release of lymphokines, and stops the generation of cytotoxic and plasma cells. Cyclosporine is metabolized by the cytochrome P-450 enzyme system in the liver, prompting the need for careful monitoring of cyclosporine drug levels. Drug levels may vary when the dosage of cyclosporine or other medications metabolized by the cytochrome P-450 enzyme pathway is modified. Dosage is dependent on the type of transplant, formulation (modified or nonmodified), experience of the practitioner, patient status, and biopsy results.
- Tacrolimus (Prograf): A CNI used to block T-cell activation genes via a similar mechanism to cyclosporine but more potent than CSA. It is also metabolized by the cytochrome P-450 enzyme system in the liver. It is used as a first-line drug or replaces cyclosporine if there are multiple rejections while on cyclosporine. The continuous infusion is dosed based on the type of transplant and peak and trough levels, and then converted to an oral dose administered twice daily when GI function returns following surgery. Trough levels are initially 8 to 15 ng/mL and are maintained at 5 to 15 ng/mL.

Selective T-cell costimulation blocker

Belatacept: A newer immunosuppression drug for the kidney transplant patient that inhibits T-lymphocyte proliferation and production of the cytokines IL-2, interferon γ, IL-4, and TNF α. Belatacept is used as alternative to the CNI drugs and given as an IV infusion of 10 mg/kg before implant on the day of surgery. Another dose is given at 96 hours and then at weeks 2, 4, 8, and 12. Starting at week 16, a maintenance dose of 5 mg/kg is given every 4 weeks.

Antiproliferative agents

Antiproliferative agents are used in maintenance immunosuppression and treatment of rejection to block the proliferative phase of activated T- and B-lymphocyte generation. They are an integral part of most immunosuppression regimens.

- Mycophenolic acid: Mycophenolate mofetile (MMF, Cellcept): Used as a first-line immunosuppressant to inhibit the proliferation of T and B lymphocytes, the production of antibodies, and the generation of cytotoxic T cells. Dosed at 1.0 to 1.5 g every 12 hours IV/PO, no blood level monitoring is required.
- Mycophenolic acid (Myfortic): A delayed-release form of mycophenolic acid with the same indications, efficacy, and adverse effects profile as MMF. Dosing is 720 mg PO every 12 hours.
- Azathioprine (Imuran): Immunosuppressive agent that interferes with gene transcription and used in combination with other drugs to prevent rejection. WBC counts are monitored, and dosage is adjusted accordingly. Maintenance dosage is 1 to 3 mg/kg/day to a maximum of 150 to 175 mg/day. Dosage is decreased or held if WBC count is less than 5/mm^3.

Mammalian target of rapamycin inhibitors

Mammalian target of rapamycin (mTOR), a key regulatory kinase in the process of cell division, is inhibited by these drugs. The mTOR inhibitors improve kidney function when used as a replacement for CNIs associated with higher incidence of renal insufficiency.

- Sirolimus (Rapamune): An mTOR used to inhibit T- and B-lymphocyte activation and proliferation, with added antineoplastic effects. The oral loading dose is 6 mg/day followed by a maintenance dose of 2 mg/day regulated by blood level assessment, divided into 2 doses given every 12 hours. Therapeutic trough blood levels are seen between 8 and 15 ng/mL. The drug is associated with impaired wound healing, so it is not used during induction in the posttransplantation period.
- Everolimus (Certican): Very similar to sirolimus in mechanism of action and side effect profile. Dosage is 0.5 mg to 1.5 mg orally twice daily. The therapeutic drug level range is 3 to 8 ng/mL.

Monoclonal antibodies

Monoclonal antibodies are monospecific antibodies made by fusing the spleen cells from a mouse immunized with a target antigen with myeloma cells. These highly specialized antibodies can detect and bind to the target antigen to purify the substance. Rabbit B cells have been used more recently in the production of monoclonal antibodies.

- OKT3 (Orthoclone): An immunosuppressive monoclonal antibody used to treat organ rejection. OKT3 is a murine (mouse) monoclonal antibody that recognizes and binds the CD3 receptor present on all mature T cells. Anti-CD3 is a homologous antibody that reacts with and blocks the function of the chemical (T3) complex on the surface of the T lymphocytes. The T3 complex is responsible for the T-lymphocyte's identification of a transplanted organ as foreign and the attempts to reject it. OKT3 binds to the T3 antigen on the surface of the T cells, enhancing phagocytosis and entrapment of the cells in the spleen and liver. The T lymphocytes are removed from the circulation by this process in approximately 10 to 15 minutes. Patients are premedicated with acetaminophen, an H_2 receptor antagonist, hydrocortisone, and diphenhydramine to avoid cytokine release syndrome (fever, chills, tremors, pulmonary edema) during the first 2 days of therapy. The dosage is 5 mg given via IV push over 1 minute every day for 10 to 14 days. It is associated with higher infection (especially CMV) and malignancy rates. CD3 levels are measured to maintain adequate levels of OKT3.
- Basiliximab (Simulect): A chimeric (murine/human) monoclonal antibody produced by recombinant DNA technology that is used as an immunosuppressive agent during induction to inhibit IL-2 activation of T lymphocytes. It is not used to treat rejection, but rather to prevent it. The dosage is 20 mg within 2 hours of transplantation surgery and repeated 4 days after transplant. Side effects are rare.
- Daclizumab (Zenapax): Acts similarly to basiliximab. The dosage is 1 mg/kg/dose for 5 doses, the first dose within 24 hours of transplant, followed by 4 doses at intervals of 14 days.
- Rituximab (Rituxan): A monoclonal antibody targeted at the CD20 antigen on B lymphocytes used to prevent and treat humoral rejection. The dosage is 1 dose of 375 mg/m^2 to manage humoral rejection or 375 mg/m^2 every week for 4 doses for posttransplant lymphoproliferative disorder. Patients are premedicated with acetaminophen and diphenhydramine. The drug is started at 50 mg/h and titrated up as tolerated.
- Alemtuzumab (Campath, MabCampath, Campath-1H): A monoclonal antibody used in a very small population of organ transplant patients as induction therapy and to treat rejection. Effective September 4, 2012, Campath is no longer available commercially, but is provided through the Campath Distribution Program free of charge. To receive Campath, the healthcare provider is required to provide written documentation that the patient's condition warrants the treatment. Alemtuzumab has been associated with infusion-related events including hypotension, rigors, fever, shortness of breath, bronchospasm, chills, and rash. Other serious infusion-related events were syncope, pulmonary infiltrates, ARDS, respiratory arrest, cardiac arrhythmias, myocardial infarction, and cardiac arrest.

Polyclonal antibodies

Polyclonal antibodies are antibodies secreted by various lineages of B cells within the body. In contrast, monoclonal antibodies originate from a single cell type. This collection of immunoglobulin molecules has the capacity to identify and purify many different antigens. Each type of molecule targets a specific antigen.

- Antilymphocyte sera (antilymphocytic globulin [ALG] or antithymocyte gamma-globulin [ATGAM or thymoglobulin]): Polyclonal antibody used for induction of immunosuppression and management of rejection. The antilymphocyte antibodies in the sera are useful in the treatment of steroid-resistant rejection and are potent suppressors of cell-mediated immunity. They are directed against many different antigens on the surface of human lymphocytes and affect immunity via reduction of T lymphocytes. When receiving ATGAM or thymoglobulin, patients are premedicated with acetaminophen, an H_2-receptor antagonist, hydrocortisone, and diphenhydramine to help avoid cytokine release syndrome, which may occur during the first 2 days of therapy.

Intravenous immune globulin
Used for desensitization and treatment of humoral rejection. The dosage is 1 to 2 g/kg, started at a low rate (0.05 to 0.06 mg/kg/h) and titrated up as tolerated. Patients are premedicated with acetaminophen and diphenhydramine. Side effects include back pain, headache, chills, fevers, bronchospasms, and hypotension.

Prevention of opportunistic infections
Antibiotics: Antibiotics are used in accordance with Surgical Care Improvement Project (SCIP) guidelines.

Antivirals:
- Valganciclovir (Valcyte): Used for prophylaxis and treatment of CMV, which remains the major cause of morbidity and mortality for cardiac transplantation patients. The dosage for induction is 900 mg every 12 hours for 21 days. For maintenance and prevention, it is given orally at 450 to 900 mg daily for 3 to 6 months following the transplant.
- Acyclovir: Used for prophylaxis against and treatment of herpes virus. The dosage is 5 to 10 mg/kg IV every 8 hours for 7 to 10 days or 200 to 800 mg PO, given as 2 to 5 doses each day, depending on whether managing an active infection or using for suppressive therapy.

Antifungals (Mycostatin, Nystan, Fluconazole): For potential secondary *Candida* infections related to immunosuppression. The dosage is 5 mL for an oral "swish and swallow" or Mycelex as an oral troche 3 times daily following extubation.

Prevention of pneumocystic pneumonia: (Bactrim, TMP/SMX, pentamidine, dapsone)

Management of Side Effects: Antiulcer medications, aspirin, antihypertensive medications, stool softeners, insulin for hyperglycemia, cholesterol-lowering agents, bone-strengthening nutrients (calcium, phosphorus, magnesium), and osteoporosis medications

Pain management
Opiates: Fentanyl is commonly used because it is short acting and, unlike morphine, does not cause histamine-mediated hypotension.

Pretransplant and posttransplant sensitization
Plasmapheresis may decrease sensitization and reduce PRA levels. Positive PRA levels detect circulating HLA and reflect level of sensitization. Elevated PRA levels increase the difficulty of finding an HLA-compatible donor organ. HLA compatibility will enhance graft survival and reduce infection and malignancies related to aggressive immunosuppression. Pregnancy, blood transfusion, ventricular assist devices, or previous transplants can trigger sensitization. Poor outcomes, such as CAD, posttransplant lymphoproliferative disorder, and an increased incidence of rejection, have been associated with pretransplant sensitization.

COLLABORATIVE MANAGEMENT
CARE PRIORITIES
1. Prevent infection
Infection control is paramount because of immunosuppression therapy. Immunosuppressed patients are vulnerable to bacterial (*Staphylococcus, Streptococcus, Klebsiella, Pseudomonas*), viral (CMV, EBV, herpes simplex, varicella zoster,) and fungal (*Aspergillus, Candida, Cryptococcus,*

histoplasmosis, Coccidioides, pneumocystis, and *Toxoplasma gondii*) infections. Prophylactic antibiotics, antivirals, and antifungals are used.

Steps to reduce infection postoperatively and beyond:
1. Isolation. Keep door closed and limit visitors; no employees or visitors with active infection are allowed; avoid taking care of other patients with infections.
2. Carefully monitor for signs and symptoms of infection.

2. Prevent organ rejection

Graft or organ rejection is the leading concern with transplantation. A transplanted organ originates from a donor who is genetically different from the recipient (the exception is a kidney/liver from an identical twin). The organ contains foreign antigens that trigger an immune response in the recipient, which leads the organ to reject that foreign object. Historically, rejection has been classified as hyperacute, accelerated acute, acute, or chronic (Table 11-10). An untreated rejection response results in complete destruction of the organ. Table 11-11 describes the clinical presentation for various types of acute organ rejection.

When the body detects the presence of a foreign substance, the immune system mounts a defense with nonspecific inflammation and phagocytosis. Antibody-mediated (humoral) and cell-mediated immune responses work together to defend after exposure to an antigen. Antibody-mediated immune response stimulates B-lymphocyte activity. When an antigen is encountered, the B-lymphocyte enlarges, divides, and differentiates into a plasma cell that produces and secretes antigen-specific immunoglobulins, or antibodies. The formation of this antigen-antibody complex triggers events that augment the nonspecific responses of inflammation and phagocytosis. Cell-mediated immune response involves T-lymphocytes that recognize a foreign antigen on the surface of the macrophage, bind to the antigen, enlarge, and produce a sensitized clone, which migrates through the body to the site of the antigen. When the sensitized T cell combines with the antigen, chemicals are released that kill foreign cells directly and facilitate phagocytosis and the inflammatory response.
1. Graft-versus-host disease: Applicable to bone marrow transplant, rather than solid organ transplant. A rejection process whereby there is a transplant of functioning allogeneic T cells into an immunocompromised host, such as in a bone marrow transplant.
2. Vasculopathy: A chronic rejection phenomenon seen in the allograft vessels as diffuse disease affecting the full wall thickness of the arteries, rather than solely the intralumen. Atherosclerotic heart disease affects solely the intralumen of the arteries.

DIAGNOSIS AND ASSESSMENT OF REJECTION

Rejection is assessed using various diagnostics and procedures, with transplanted organ biopsy being the most invasive direct assessment. Biopsy provides the means of diagnosing rejection, its severity, and the possibility of response to antirejection therapy. Tiny pieces of tissue are removed for pathologic examination to assess for tissue rejection.

Table 11-10	CHARACTERISTICS OF ORGAN REJECTION BY CATEGORY	
Type of Rejection	**Characteristics**	**Outcome**
Hyperacute	Occurs immediately Antibody-mediated Result of preformed circulatory antibodies	Usually irreversible and untreatable Preventable with crossmatching
Accelerated acute	Occurs 3–5 days after transplant Antibody-mediated Rapid loss of function Fever and oliguria	Irreversible and untreatable Preventable with crossmatching
Acute	Primarily T cell-mediated Possible presence of humoral component Occurs weeks, months, or years after transplant	Treatable and reversible Multiple episodes affect long-term graft survival
Chronic	Develops slowly over months to years Probably a combination of cellular- and humoral-mediated processes	Untreatable, eventually leads to graft loss

Table 11-11	CLINICAL PRESENTATION WITH ACUTE ORGAN REJECTION
Organ	**Clinical Presentation**
Heart	10 to 14 days after transplantation. Indicators include fever, anxiety, lethargy, low back pain, atrial or ventricular dysrhythmias, gallop, pericardial friction rub, jugular venous distention, hypotension, and decreased CO late in rejection.
Lung	Expected during the first 21 days after surgery, with increased frequency and severity 6 to 8 weeks after transplantation Classic rejection: decreased lung ventilation and perfusion alveolar exudate containing desquamated pneumocytes and inflammatory cells Atypical rejection: decreased ventilation without blood flow reduction, ventilation-perfusion imbalances, and respiratory insufficiency with shunting Vascular rejection: increased vascular resistance, decreased blood flow to graft
Liver	4 to 10 days after transplantation. Indicators include malaise; fever; abdominal discomfort; swollen, hard, tender graft; tachycardia; RUQ or flank pain; cessation of bile flow; change in bile fluid from golden to colorless; jaundice; elevated PT, bilirubin, transaminase, and alkaline phosphatase.
Kidney	Occurs in the immediate postoperative period with fever, pain over graft, decreased urine output, and edema with increase in creatinine. Renal scan or Doppler is used for a quick look at blood flow to the kidneys. Patients may even need dialysis for a short time until the kidney functions.
Pancreas	Time of rejection varies. Patient may have hyperglycemia, pancreatitis, or pain over graft. Open biopsy may be necessary to diagnose rejection.

Organ Transplantation

HEART

Biopsy is performed in a cardiac catheterization lab/biopsy lab or surgery. The cannulation site is generally the right internal jugular or sometimes the femoral vein. Biopsy samples are graded according to one of several grading systems. Biopsies are generally performed at 7 and 14 days after surgery and at specified intervals thereafter, and the Biopsy Rejection Scale is used:

Biopsy Rejection Scale	
Grade	**Description**
0R	No evidence of acute cellular rejection
1R	Interstitial and/or perivascular infiltrate with up to 1 focus of myocyte damage
2R	Two or more foci of infiltrate with associated myocyte damage
3R	Diffuse infiltrate with multifocal myocyte damage $+/-$ edema, $+/-$ hemorrhage, $+/-$ vasculitis

The following assist in assessing the transplanted heart for rejection:
- Vital signs and heart sounds: May reveal decreased stroke volume, CO, cardiac tones, and BP and presence of S_3 and S_4 sounds, pericardial friction rub, extrasystole, and crackles.
- Echocardiogram: Used to assess chamber size, wall thickness, ejection fraction, thrombus formation, valve function, and systolic and diastolic function.
- Chest radiograph: Will reveal increased dimensions of the heart late in rejection.
- ECG: Will show presence of atrial and ventricular dysrhythmias and decreased QRS voltage.
- CBC: Will show increased total lymphocyte count.
- Intravascular ultrasound: Used to evaluate vasculopathy of the coronary arteries.
- Blood analysis of rejection: Currently only used to assess cardiac rejection, AlloMap detects the absence of acute cellular rejection in clinically stable heart transplant patients. The test uses a peripheral blood sample <and has replaced biopsies in many institutions. Studies are currently ongoing for lung transplant patients, with studies of other transplant types planned for the future.

LUNG

- Transbronchial biopsy: Not particularly helpful in detecting rejection; the morbidity risk increases with open biopsy.
- Biopsy grading:
  - Grade 0: No acute cellular rejection.
  - Grade 1: Minimal acute cellular rejection.
  - Grade 2: Mild acute cellular rejection.
  - Grade 3: Moderate acute cellular rejection.
  - Grade 4: Severe acute cellular rejection.

The following assist with assessment of the transplanted lung:

- Symptoms: Cough (although it goes away in the initial stages), dyspnea, fatigue, fever, flulike symptoms.
- Chest radiograph: Changes indicative of rejection are noted.
- Leukocyte and absolute T-lymphocyte counts: Rise during rejection.
- Vital signs and hemodynamics: Can change suddenly with increases in PVR, HR, BP, SVR, and CO.
- ABG values: Decrease in Pao_2 and increase in $Paco_2$ occur with rejection. Decrease in pulmonary function tests, change in forced expiratory volume.

KIDNEY

- Renal biopsy: Determines presence, type, and severity of rejection.
- Kidney biopsy grading: (Table 11-12).

The following signs assist in assessment for rejection of the transplanted kidney:

- Symptoms: Fever, pain over graft, edema.

Table 11-12	BANFF DIAGNOSTIC CATEGORIES FOR RENAL ALLOGRAFT BIOPSIES
Acute Active Rejection	
1. Normal	
2. Antibody-mediated rejection: immediate (hyperacute), delayed (accelerated acute)	
3. Borderline changes: No intimal arteritis is present, but there are foci of mild tubulitis.	
4. Acute/active rejection	

Type Grade	Histopathologic findings
IA	Significant interstitial infiltration (>25% parenchyma affected) and foci of moderate tubulitis (>4 mononuclear cells/tubular cross-section or group of 10 tubular cells)
IB	Significant interstitial infiltration (>25% parenchyma affected) and foci of moderate tubulitis (>10 mononuclear cells/tubular cross-section or group of 10 tubular cells)
IIA	Cases with mild to moderate intimal arteritis
IIB	Cases with severe intimal arteritis comprising >25% of the luminal area
III	Cases with transmural arteritis and/or arterial fibrinoid change and necrosis of medical smooth muscle cells

5. Chronic/sclerosing allograft nephropathy	

Grade	Histopathologic findings
I: Mild	Mild interstitial fibrosis and tubular atrophy without Grade 1A or 1B findings or with (specific changes suggesting chronic rejection
II: Moderate	Moderate interstitial fibrosis and tubular atrophy withGrade 1A or 1B findings
III: Severe	Severe interstitial fibrosis and tubular atrophy and tubular loss with Grade 1A or 1B findings
Other	Changes not considered to be because of rejection

- BUN and creatinine values: Will increase from previous 24-hour levels and continue to rise until rejection is reversed.
- 24-Hour urine collection: Will exhibit a change in components (e.g., decreases in creatinine clearance, total amount of creatinine excreted, and urinary sodium excretion; increase in protein excretion).
- Renal scan: Will exhibit decreased blood flow.
- Kidney assessment: May reveal a firm, large kidney that may be tender on palpation.
- Renal scan: Evaluates blood flow to the kidney and rate of excretion of substances into the bladder.

LIVER
Several methods are used to obtain liver samples, including laparoscopic liver biopsy, percutaneous image-guided liver biopsy, and open surgical liver biopsy.

Laparoscopic liver biopsy
With the use of trocars (shafts with 3-sided points), small incisions are made in the abdomen to enable insertion of the laparoscope. Using the monitor to facilitate viewing, the physician uses instruments within the laparoscope to remove tissue samples from one or more parts of the liver. This type of biopsy is used when samples from specific parts of the liver are required.

Percutaneous liver biopsy
A local anesthetic is first administered to numb the area on the body's right side. Through a small incision near the rib cage, a special biopsy needle is inserted to retrieve liver tissue. In some cases, ultrasound or computed tomography may be used to help guide the needle to a specific spot. This biopsy method is often used when the disease process is localized to discrete spots in the liver.

Open surgical liver biopsy
Open liver biopsies are done by a surgeon using a biopsy needle or through surgical excision of a small piece of liver tissue. This is generally used during another surgical procedure, because less invasive techniques are available.

The following signs assist in diagnosis of rejection of the transplanted liver (Table 11-13):
- Symptoms: Light-colored stools, dark-colored urine, jaundice of the sclera or skin, fever, right upper quadrant pain, fatigue, malaise, and pruritus.
- Serum bilirubin level: Total bilirubin will rise in relation to baseline postoperative level.
- Transaminase level: Will increase from baseline; may be markedly elevated early in rejection.
- Alkaline phosphatase level: Will increase from baseline.
- Prothrombin time: Will be prolonged.
- CBC: May reveal decreased platelet count and increased total lymphocyte count.

PANCREAS
Open biopsy is the only means by which a definitive diagnosis can be made.

Table 11-13	LIVER TRANSPLANT DATABASE (LTD GRADING SCHEME)
Grade	**Criteria**
A0	No rejection
A	Rejection without bile duct loss
1	Rejection infiltrate in some, but not all, of the triads confined within the portal spaces.
2	Rejection infiltrate involving all of the triads, with or without spillover into the lobule. No evidence of centrilobular hepatocyte necrosis, ballooning, or dropout
3	Infiltrate in some or all of the triads, with or without spillover into the lobule, with or without inflammatory cell linkage of the triads, associated with centrilobular hepatocyte ballooning or necrosis and dropout

Organ Transplantation

The following signs also assist in the diagnosis of rejection of the transplanted pancreas:
- Symptoms: Pain over pancreas graft; malaise, fever, and hyperglycemia.
- Fasting and 2-hour postprandial plasma glucose: Levels will be increased above normal ranges.
- Serum amylase: Levels may be elevated, indicating presence of pancreatitis, an inconsistent marker of rejection.
- Serum creatinine: Elevated.
- C-reactive peptide (serum and urine): Levels may be decreased.
- Pancreas radioisotope flow scan: Determines organ viability; decreased flow may indicate rejection.

CARE PLANS FOR ORGAN TRANSPLANTATION

RISK FOR INJURY *related to organ rejection related to inadequate immunosuppressant drug levels.*

Goals/Outcomes: Within 48 hours after the transplant, the patient verbalizes accurate information about the signs and symptoms of rejection. Within 72 hours after initiation of medications, the patient and significant others verbalize accurate information regarding the prescribed immunosuppressive agents, the side effects that can occur, and precautions that should be taken.
NOC Immune Status

Environmental Risk Protection
1. Assess patient's knowledge of drug therapy.
2. Provide the patient with verbal and written information for the type of immunosuppressive agent that has been prescribed. Discuss the generic name, trade name, purpose, usual dosage, route, side effects, and precautions.
3. Monitor blood levels as appropriate for drug.
4. Instruct the patient to take medication at designated time(s) each day. Never withhold immunosuppressant without consulting with physician or midlevel practitioner.
5. Monitor for signs of rejection, as appropriate for each specific organ.
6. Reinforce the necessity of regularly scheduled appointments with transplant coordinator. Encourage the patient to bring a significant other to the visit.

NIC Teaching: Disease Process; Teaching: Individual; Teaching: Prescribed Medication, Discharge Planning; Medication Management; Weight Management.

RISK FOR INFECTION (LUNGS AND HEART MOST COMMON) *related to immunosuppression.*

Goals/Outcomes: The patient is free of infection as evidenced by normothermia; absence of erythema, swelling, and drainage of catheter and wound sites; absence of adventitious breath sounds or cloudy and foul-smelling urine; negative results of urine, wound drainage, and blood cultures; WBC count 4500 to 11,000/mm^3.
NOC Immune Status

Infection Protection
1. Patient is to wear a mask when outside his or her immediate living area, in public areas, near construction, or during "cleaning" of environment.
2. Notify the physician or transplant coordinator immediately for a temperature greater than 99.5° F, WBC count increasing, patient complaints of malaise, or any obvious infection. Review bloodwork and radiographs.
3. Perform a thorough physical assessment. Auscultate lung fields every 8 hours, noting presence of rhonchi, crackles, and decreased breath sounds. Inspect graft wound for erythema, swelling, and drainage. Consult physician or advanced practice provider for significant findings.
4. Avoid placement of indwelling catheters; if necessary, remove as soon as possible.
5. Assess and document condition of indwelling IV sites and other catheter sites every 8 hours. Be alert to swelling, erythema, tenderness, and drainage. Consult the physician or advanced practice provider for any of these findings.
6. As prescribed, obtain blood, urine, and wound cultures when infection is suspected.
7. Be alert to WBC count greater than 11,000/mm^3 or less than 4500/mm^3. A below-normal WBC count with increased band neutrophils on differential (shift to the left) may signal acute infection.

8. Record volume, appearance, color, and odor of urine. Be alert to foul-smelling or cloudy urine, frequency and urgency of urination, and patient complaints of flank or labial pain, all of which are signs of renal-urinary infection.
9. Use meticulous aseptic technique when dressing and caring for wounds and catheter sites.
10. Obtain specimens for urine cultures once a week during patient's hospitalization and once a month after hospital discharge.
11. Provide care measures to prevent infection
    - Perform sterile wound dressing changes.
    - Discontinue invasive lines and tubes as soon as possible.
    - Facilitate early extubation.
    - Provide early optimal nutrition.
    - Use a leukocyte filter for blood administration or use leukocyte-reduced blood.

NIC Infection Control; Airway Management; Exercise Promotion and Therapy Medication Management; Respiratory Monitoring; Teaching: Disease Process; Tube Care: Urinary; Vital Signs Monitoring.

IMPAIRED ORAL MUCOUS MEMBRANES *related to treatment with immunosuppressive medication.*

Goals/Outcomes: The patient's oral mucosa, tongue, and lips are pink, intact, and free of exudate and lesions. Patient states that he or she can swallow without difficulty within 24 hours after treatment for altered oral mucous membrane.
NOC Oral Hygiene; Tissue Integrity: Skin and Mucous Membranes

Oral Health Restoration
1. Inspect the mouth daily for signs of exudate and lesions and report abnormal findings to the physician. Teach the patient to perform self-inspection of mouth.
2. Teach the patient to brush with a soft-bristle toothbrush and nonabrasive toothpaste after meals and snacks.
3. To help prevent monilial infection, provide the patient with mycostatin prophylactic mouthwash for swish and swallow after meals and at bedtime.

NIC Oral Health Maintenance; Oral Health Promotion

IMPAIRED SKIN INTEGRITY (OR RISK FOR SAME) HERPETIC LESIONS, SKIN FUNGAL RASHES, PRURITUS, AND CAPILLARY FRAGILITY *related to treatment with immunosuppressive medications.*

Goals/Outcomes: Patient's skin is intact and free of open lesions or abrasions.
NOC Tissue Integrity: Skin and Mucous Membranes

Skin Surveillance
1. Assess for and document daily the presence of erythema, excoriation, rashes, or bruises on patient's skin.
2. Assess for and document the presence of rashes or lesions in the perineal area. Herpetic lesions are common in the immunosuppressed patient.
3. Inspect the trunk area daily for the presence of flat, itchy rashes. Skin fungal rashes are common in the immunosuppressed patient.
4. Teach the patient the importance of daily skin care with water, nondrying soap, and lubricating lotion.
5. Use nonallergenic tape when anchoring IV tubing, catheters, and dressings.
6. Assist the patient with changing position at least every 2 hours; massage areas that are susceptible to breakdown, particularly areas over bony prominences.

NIC Pressure Ulcer Prevention. Additional, optional interventions include Bathing; Bleeding Precautions; Cutaneous Stimulation; Exercise Promotion and Therapy Electrolyte Monitoring; Exercise Promotion: Stretching; Fluid/Electrolyte Management; Infection Control; Infection Prevention; Medication Management; Nail Care; Nutrition Management; Perineal Care; Surveillance; and Vital Signs Monitoring.

Organ Transplantation

SEPSIS, SEPTIC SHOCK, SYSTEMIC INFLAMMATORY RESPONSE SYNDROME, AND MULTIPLE ORGAN DYSFUNCTION SYNDROME

PATHOPHYSIOLOGY

SEPSIS

Sepsis is the most frequent cause of death in hospitalized patients. Although sepsis arises through activation of an innate immune response to a stimulus that represents a danger to the host, it has also been directly related to current treatments rendered to critically ill patients who previously would have died. It accounts for 1,000,000 cases and 200,000 deaths annually in the US alone, but unlike other major epidemic illnesses, treatment for sepsis is nonspecific, limited primarily to support of organ function and administration of IV fluids, antibiotics, and oxygen. There are no approved drugs that specifically target and treat sepsis. Current evidence supports that acute infections worsen preexisting chronic diseases or result in new chronic diseases, which lead to poorer outcomes and increased morbidity in survivors.

Sepsis represents a syndrome, not a disease, and it is difficult to identify because the signs and symptoms are often subtle and evolving and generally mirror the signs and symptoms of other conditions. This clinical diagnostic term used to describe patients who have a continuum of abnormalities in organ function evolved from a 1991 Consensus Conference that defined "sepsis" as documented or suspected infection combined with two or more abnormalities in body temperature, HR, RR, or WBC count. Those individuals with sepsis and evidence of organ dysfunction (cardiovascular, renal, hepatic, or neurologic) were further classified as having "severe sepsis," and those with cardiovascular dysfunction not responsive to fluid were said to have "septic shock." Ten years later the diagnosis of septic shock was expanded to include evidence of inadequate tissue perfusion (low Svo_2, lactic acidosis, wide anion gap). Recently, evidence shows that patients with sepsis or septic shock go on to develop "persistent critical illness" with overt organ dysfunction that may last for weeks or months. These survivors may be disabled by cognitive dysfunction, neuropathies, and other complications.

SYSTEMIC INFLAMMATORY RESPONSE SYNDROME

Frequently the first signs of impending sepsis are identified as SIRS, a state of generalized, uncontrolled inflammation. Inflammation is a complex response initiated by mechanical, ischemic, chemical, or microbial sources. Signs of systemic inflammation such as fever and leukocytosis characterize SIRS. A patient with sepsis presents with at least two of the SIRS criteria: an abnormal body temperature, elevated HR and RR, and an altered WBC count as well as a suspected or proven source of infection. Sepsis is a syndrome consisting of the combination of a systemic inflammatory response and the presence of infection. Risk factors for poor outcome in sepsis include hypothermia, leukopenia, low arterial pH, shock, multiorgan dysfunction, age greater than 40 years, and medical comorbidities. The issues associated with identification are related to this generalized presentation. Almost all acutely ill patients meet SIRS criteria and often have infection, which is not necessarily sepsis. Sepsis with one or more organ dysfunctions is considered severe sepsis.

RESEARCH BRIEF 11-3

The latest definition is that sepsis is a life-threatening condition when the body's response to an infection injures its own tissues and organs. Using this criteria, sepsis cannot be identified until there is organ dysfunction in the primary easily evaluable sixsystems: renal, neurological, hepatic, cardiovascular, respiratory, and coagulation. Other systems may be more difficult to assess; however, any acute dysfunction in this situation must be considered a sign of sepsis.

Czura CJ: Merinoff symposium 2010: sepsis—speaking with one voice. *Mol Med* 17:2-3, 2011.

In some cases, regulatory mechanisms fail and uncontrolled systemic inflammation overwhelms the body's normal protective response. This leads to systemic vasodilation, arterial hypotension, generalized increase in vascular permeability, extravascular fluid sequestration, and increased hematologic cellular aggregation with microvascular obstruction, which greatly accelerates consumption of coagulation products.

SEVERE SEPSIS

Severe sepsis is the compounding of sepsis by comorbid conditions, wherein the inflammatory response to a nidus of infection or inflammation is fulminating and out of control. Severe sepsis has more recently been viewed as endothelial dysfunction resulting from overwhelming inflammatory mediation, in conjunction with profound, unopposed coagulation. The capillary vasculature sustains a significant injury by a cascade of events that ends in capillary occlusion. The more massive the occlusion, the greater the potential for organ failure, as cellular level circulation requires a functional capillary network for delivery of oxygen and nutrients and removal of cellular metabolic waste products. When infection or other injury prompts an initially widespread inflammatory response, or SIRS, the normally smooth surface of microvascular (capillary) endothelium is roughened or damaged by the response. Release of inflammatory mediators prompts vasodilation with increased capillary permeability. Microscopically, the endothelium resembles a road riddled with tiny "potholes." Systemic mediators are released to facilitate healing of the endothelium, which is aimed at "filling the tiny potholes."

The four main factors associated with severe sepsis that may evolve to septic shock are hyperinflammation, hypercoagulation, microvascular obstruction, and increased endothelial permeability. Because endothelial damage is generalized, the extensive or hyperinflammatory response leads to accelerated formation of microclots on the non–smooth capillary endothelium, consuming platelets and inhibiting clot lysis (fibrinolysis). This progresses to uncontrolled alterations in the vascular tone with vasodilation in the large vessels (where BP is measured). Both vasodilation and constriction occur in capillaries, where oxygen delivery takes place.

Stimulated by products of antigen ingestion, activated neutrophils and other humoral mediators combine, activate, and potentiate an ongoing vascular endothelial injury with a concomitant proinflammatory, procoagulating, antifibrinolytic response. Among other mediators, an increased presence of tissue factor persistently stimulates thrombin, which ultimately increases fibrinogen conversion to fibrin and promotes platelet aggregation. Coupled with microvascular clotting, the process limits oxygen delivery and may lead to organ ischemia. Unopposed, this process may lead to a profound consumptive coagulopathy (DIC), diminished distal blood flow, and cell death by activated cellular suicide (apoptosis). The blood flow necessary to maintain tissue oxygenation and aerobic metabolism, nutrient transfer, and metabolic waste removal is profoundly threatened.

Excessive thrombin production and a secondary decrease in endothelial production of plasminogen activator, thrombomodulin, protein C, and other prothrombin and antithrombin mediators, ultimately, activated protein C, illustrate the overwhelming response that separates simple infection from severe sepsis. The endothelial regulation of appropriate blood flow requires a balance of vasodilators (i.e., nitric oxide) and vasoconstrictors (e.g., endothelin). In severe sepsis, when the balance cannot be maintained, the corresponding maldistribution of blood flow and loss of vascular tone at the macro- and microvascular levels result in both ischemia and hyperemia in the cells supplied by the same capillary beds. In addition, myocardial depressant factor is released and may contribute to the loss of the compensatory CO, which is required to keep blood moving through the vascular beds.

SEPTIC SHOCK AND MULTIORGAN DYSFUNCTION SYNDROME

Severe sepsis accompanied by hypotension that does not respond to volume infusion is called septic shock. Impaired perfusion may cause lactic acidosis, oliguria, or acute alterations in mental status. Genetic predisposition and other factors compound severe sepsis, leading to MODS as well as multiple organ failure and may be fatal. MODS is diagnosed when two or more vital organ systems become dysfunctional.

Septic shock is severe sepsis with cardiovascular dysfunction (primary loss of vascular tone) that does not respond to fluid resuscitation and requires vasopressor therapy to maintain MAP above 65 mm Hg. Patients with septic shock often have fluid deficits of 6 to 10 L and need aggressive fluid resuscitation. The cornerstones of therapy for sepsis are volume resuscitation,

Table 11-14	SYSTEMIC INFLAMMATORY RESPONSE SYNDROME (SIRS)
If two or more of the following are present, the patient meets criteria for SIRS:	
1	Temperature >38° C or 100.4°F or <36° C or 96.8°F.
2	Heart rate >90 bpm
3	Respiratory rate >20 breaths/min or $PaCO_2$ <32 mm Hg
4	White blood cell count >12,000 cells/mm^3 or <4000 cells/mm^3 or >10% immature (band) forms

Adapted from Levy MM, Fink MP, Marshall JC, et al: 2001 SCCM/ESICM/ACCP/ATS/SIS International Sepsis Definitions Conference. *Crit Care Med* 31:1250-1256, 2003.

early antibiotic therapy, hemodynamic support with vasopressors as necessary, and glycemic control.

Over the past 30 years, understanding the malignant, destructive, uncontrolled inflammatory, and coagulation process has become the primary focus in the management of patients exhibiting signs and symptoms of severe sepsis that can ultimately result in MODS. The process leading from SIRS to MODS to organ failure is a continuum that often begins with the same event (Table 11-14). SIRS initiates a process of relative hypovolemia. To the unsuspecting practitioner, the early signs of arterial hypoperfusion may be masked by the patient's near normal appearance resulting from compensatory vasoconstriction and increased CO, which maintains a normal BP. If SIRS and/or sepsis is managed aggressively in the early stages, the incidence of MODS is decreased. The American College of Chest Physicians (ACCP)/SCCM Consensus Conference first initiated a suggested approach to the identification of profound and uncontrolled inflammatory response in 1992. These guidelines have been modified and updated several times, with the most recent revisions reflected in the 2012 Surviving Sepsis Campaign International Guidelines (Table 11-15). Some of the more specific recognized signs and laboratory profiles are listed in Table 11-16.

The purpose of the inflammatory response is to protect the body from further injury and promote rapid healing. Vasodilation with increased microvascular permeability, neutrophil activation and adhesion, and enhanced coagulation initially occur in a balanced framework. The vascular response is initiated at the cellular level by histamine, prostaglandins, bradykinin, and numerous other mediators. The term sepsis implies, to many practitioners, an infectious process that has facilitated SIRS. Sepsis is typically not associated with a simple infection requiring antibiotic management to resolve without hospitalization.

In addition to infection, sepsis is associated with multiple injuries in trauma patients and other patients with significant inflammation such as pancreatitis. Critically ill patients with sepsis resulting from infection are often not easily managed, with microorganisms that require considerable skill to control. Microorganisms commonly seen in the critically ill include gram-negative enteric pathogens (e.g., *Escherichia coli*, *Klebsiella* spp., *Enterobacter* spp., *Pseudomonas aeruginosa*), *Staphylococcus aureus*, coagulase-negative staphylococci, *Enterococcus* spp., and *Candida* spp. Antibiotic-resistant bacteria (e.g., methicillin-resistant *S. aureus* [MRSA]) are commonly seen.

The American College of Chest Physicians (ACCP)/SCCM Consensus Conference first initiated one suggested approach to the identification of profound and uncontrolled inflammatory response in 1992. The Surviving Sepsis Guidelines for Management of Severe Sepsis and Septic Shock were first published in 2004, revised in 2008, and recently revised again and published in 2013. The evidence-based update supports components of the overall campaign, but there are other directives that have come under increasing scrutiny. Early identification, antibiotics, and source control as well as initial volume resuscitation remain as the foundation of sepsis management, although the endpoints may not be as clear as they first appeared to be.

KEY POINTS

- Shock is a clinical diagnosis defined by inadequate end-organ perfusion in the setting of hemodynamic instability.
- Definitive treatment is directed at reversing the underlying insult. Goals of supportive therapy include the maintenance of end-organ perfusion.

Table 11-15	ASSESSMENT FINDINGS FOR THE PATIENT WITH SEPSIS IN THE EARLY HYPERDYNAMIC STAGE
Clinical Indicator	**Cause**
Cardiovascular	
Increased HR (>100 bpm)	Sympathetic/autonomic nervous system (SANS) stimulation
Decreased BP (<90 mm Hg systolic, MAP <65 mm Hg)	Vasodilation
CO >7 L/min, CI >4 L/min/m², CVP <8 mm Hg	Hyperdynamic state secondary to SANS stimulation
Svo₂ >80%	Decreased use of oxygen by cells
PAWP usually <6 mm Hg	Venous dilation, decreased preload
SVR <900 dynes/sec/cm⁻⁵	Vasodilation
Strong, bounding peripheral pulses	Hyperdynamic cardiovascular system (keeping in mind that patients with preexisting cardiomyopathy will have minimal elevation in cardiac CO and drop in SVR)
Respiratory	
Tachypnea (>20 breaths/min) and hyperventilation	Metabolic acidosis that leads to decreases in cerebrospinal fluid pH that stimulate the central respiratory center
Crackles	Interstitial edema occurring with increased vascular permeability
Paco₂ <35 mm Hg	Tachypnea and hyperventilation
Dyspnea	Increased respiratory muscle work
Renal	
Decreased urine output (<0.5 mL/kg/h)	Decreased renal perfusion
Increased specific gravity (1.025–1.035)	Decreased glomerular filtration rate
Cutaneous	
Flushed and warm skin	Vasodilation
Metabolic	
Increasing body temperature (usually <38.3°C [100.9°F])	Increased metabolic activity, release of pyrogens secondary to invading microorganisms, release of interleukin-I by macrophages
pH <7.35 Lactic acid >2.5	Metabolic acidosis occurring with accumulation of lactic acid
Hyperglycemia or at times profound hypoglycemia	Release of glucagon, insulin resistance
Neurologic	
Changes in LOC	Decreased cerebral perfusion and brain hypoxia
Fluid	
↑ Fluid retention	↑ ADH, ↑ aldosterone

ADH, Antidiuretic hormone; *bpm,* beats per min; *BP,* blood pressure; *CI,* cardiac index; *CO,* cardiac output; *HR,* heart rate; *LOC,* level of consciousness; *MAP,* mean arterial pressure; *PAWP,* pulmonary artery wedge pressure; *SVR,* systemic vascular resistance.

Table 11-16	ASSESSMENT FINDINGS FOR THE PATIENT WITH SEPSIS IN THE LATE STAGE
Clinical Indicator	**Cause**
Cardiovascular	
Extreme tachycardia with S_3 sound, sinus arrhythmia, and atrial fibrillation with rapid ventricular response	Compensatory attempt by sympathetic nervous system to maintain CO
Profound hypotension	Decreased stroke volume. Diastolic BP may remain high because of vasoconstriction
CO <4 L/min, CI <2.5 L/min/m²	Failure of compensatory mechanisms
PAWP usually >12 mm Hg	Increased left ventricular end-diastolic pressure because of increased residual volume from decreased stroke volume
SVR >1200 dynes/sec/cm⁻⁵	Vasoconstriction
Weak or absent peripheral pulses	Decreased peripheral perfusion because of decreased CO
SvO_2 <60%	Decreased oxygen binding to hemoglobin because of acidosis
Respiratory	
Increased >30 breaths/min (even at late stage) or decreased respiratory rate <12 breaths/min	Metabolic acidosis and acute lung injury lead to tachypnea; whereas, central respiratory center depression can cause hypopnea
Decreased respiratory rate (< 12 breaths/min) and depth	Central respiratory center depression
Crackles, rhonchi, wheezes	Accumulation of lung secretions
Increased FiO_2 required to maintain PaO_2 (possible ARDS)	Ventilation/perfusion mismatch and decreased lung compliance
Renal	
Decreased urine output progressing to anuria	Decreased renal perfusion and tubular ischemia
Low urinary excretion of sodium, with possibly decreased fractional excretion of sodium; if patient develops acute tubular necrosis, sodium excretion typically increases.	Activation of the aldosterone mechanism and release of ADH, which stimulate sodium and water retention
Cutaneous	
Cool, pale skin or cyanosis	Sustained vasoconstriction
Neurologic	
Decreased LOC, coma	Severe hypoxia and metabolic derangements leading to reversible encephalopathy
Hematologic	
Oozing from previous venipuncture sites	Development of DIC caused by stimulation of coagulation process, and fibrinolysis
Acid-Base Status	
pH <7.35; $PaCO_2$ >45 mm Hg, HCO_3 <22 mEq/L (or less than expected)	Mixed acid-base disorder: respiratory acidosis and metabolic acidosis

ARDS, Acute respiratory distress syndrome; *ADH*, antidiuretic hormone; *BP*, blood pressure; *CI*, cardiac index; *CO*, cardiac output; *CVP*, central venous pressure; *DIC*, disseminated intravascular coagulation; *LOC*, level of consciousness; *PAWP*, pulmonary artery wedge pressure; *SVR*, systemic vascular resistance.

- For refractory hypotension, consider the following possibilities: overwhelming systemic inflammatory state, adrenal insufficiency, mixed physiologic condition (e.g., sepsis and congestive heart failure), and neurogenic shock.

ASSESSMENT: SYSTEMIC INFLAMMATORY RESPONSE SYNDROME, SEPSIS, SEVERE SEPSIS, SEPTIC SHOCK AND MULTIORGAN DYSFUNCTION SYNDROME

GOAL OF SYSTEM ASSESSMENT
Evaluate for hypermetabolism, progressive tissue hypoxia, and prevention of organ dysfunction.

HISTORY AND RISK FACTORS
- Multiple presentations to emergency department or physician's office for the same complaint
- Infection, sequential infections, any indwelling catheters, malnutrition, immunosuppression, bone marrow suppression, advanced age (older than 65 years of age), infants
- Recent traumatic injuries or surgical or invasive procedures; presence of intravascular devices or artificial joints
- Chronic health problems (e.g., liver or renal disease, diabetes mellitus, rheumatic heart disease)
- Underlying diseases or conditions such as splenectomy, IV substance abuse

VITAL SIGNS
- Patients may present with tachycardia, tachypnea, hyper- or hypothermia, and hyper- or hypoglycemia. Hypoglycemia is being increasingly recognized and is thought to be related to depletion of glycogen stores, increased cellular glucose use, and/or impaired gluconeogenesis. Criteria for diagnosis of sepsis are evolving.
- SIRS: The 2013 guidelines state that an inflammatory response is associated with sepsis, which is now defined as infection accompanied by two or more of the following signs of systemic inflammation: hypo- or hyperthermia, tachycardia, tachypnea, or elevated or depressed leukocyte count. Decreased $Paco_2$, positive culture, tissue stain, polymerase chain reaction testing, clinical examination, radiologic imaging, or other laboratory findings may support the diagnosis of infection. Older adults may manifest normal or slightly decreased temperature.
- Sepsis: In 2013, the SCCM supported the following definition of sepsis—A documented or suspected infection with some of the following: fever, hypothermia, HR greater than 90 bpm or more than 2 standard deviations (SDs) above the normal for age, tachypnea, altered mental status, hyperglycemia greater than 120 mg/dL in absence of diabetes, leukocytosis, leukopenia, normal WBC count with greater than 10% immature forms (bands), plasma C-reactive protein level more than 2 SDs above normal, and decreased protein C level (see Tables 11-15 and 11-16).
  1. Hemodynamic measurements: The hemodynamic presentation varies with fluid balance and cardiac function of the patient. There is no high-level evidence supporting the most effective MAP for resuscitation of patients with septic shock. When patients experience hypotension, they may decrease their cerebral blood flow (below 50 mm Hg) and different organs are more significantly impacted when BP drops and oxygen delivery is affected The traditional CVP and PAOP are considered static hemodynamic measurements as they are obtained under a single ventricular loading condition and are significantly affected by chamber compliance as well as volume load. The Surviving Sepsis Campaign (SSC) guidelines recommend a CVP range of 8 to 12 mm Hg (spontaneous breather) or 12 to 15 mm Hg (positive pressure breather). There is contradictory evidence regarding use of CVP as a predictor of fluid responsiveness and significant discussion regarding the value of these as stand-alone endpoints. The measurement of CO and in particular stroke volume (SV) is considered currently to influence fluid resuscitation. The reference range for SV is 50 to 100 mL/beat, although a more evidence-based indicator of the SV response to therapy is to note whether it increases by 10% to 15% after a specific therapy. Dynamic methods used to evaluate volume levels and volume responsiveness measure heart-lung

interactions during inspiration. Spontaneous breathers (negative pressure breathing) may be evaluated using pulse pressure variation or systolic pressure variation. Pulse pressure variation, estimated from the arterial waveform, and stroke volume variations, from pulse contour analysis, pulse oximeter plethysmographic waveform, or thoracic bioreactance, have been found to be reliable predictors of fluid responsiveness when patients receive a challenge test, such as passive leg raise. If patients are mechanically ventilated, using the pulse contour analysis, pulse oximeter plethysmographic waveform, or thoracic bioreactance has been found to be reliable in predicting fluid responsiveness when patients receive a challenge test, such as passive leg raise.

2. Monitoring tissue perfusion using a central line with oximeter-based technology.

3. $Scvo_2$: The $Scvo_2$ (reflecting tissue use of oxygen) in early stages may be low to normal. The sample is obtained by measuring a blood sample in the right atrium. The values are generally about 5% to 13% higher than SO_2 levels. Serum lactate levels in conjunction should measure adequacy of tissue oxygenation with methods of monitoring central or local hemoglobin saturation to determine the degree of anaerobic metabolism present and the effects of resuscitation.

   - Tissue metabolic dysfunction: Placement of a central catheter to measure both pressures on ventricular filling, as well as the saturation of hemoglobin after blood has passed the capillaries, may be an important component of monitoring for these patients. Uses of Svo_2 and $Scvo_2$ include:
     - Threats to tissue oxygenation occur, such as a decrease in blood flow from hypovolemia or low CO (relative to tissue demand). The compensatory mechanism is to release more oxygen from hemoglobin (shift to right), which reflects a lower than normal measured $Scvo_2$.
     - In early sepsis, the lower the $Scvo_2$, the more the tissue viability may be at risk. As sepsis progresses, elevated $Scvo_2$ may reflect inability of tissues to utilize oxygen. As sepsis evolves to severe sepsis and septic shock, $Scvo_2$ levels do not fall, but rather increase. Return of $Scvo_2$ to normal may indicate improvement of blood flow, but in late sepsis it may also indicate that shunting is worsening because of vasopressors, microvascular occlusion, obstruction, and other issues interfering with oxygen utilization. The pathologic increase in measured $Scvo_2$ occurs frequently in septic shock. Differentiation from improving status is vital.
   - Declines in $Scvo_2$ ($Scvo_2$) predict the onset of inadequate myocardial compensation and may precede cardiogenic shock, capillary blood flow failure, or arrhythmias, even though vital signs in many patients remain relatively normal. In early compensatory sepsis, the oxyhemoglobin curve shifts to the right often with an $Scvo_2$ as low as 30% to 40%; later, decompensated sepsis frequently presents with cardiac shock features and an Svo_2 that is normal to high, in the presence of significant lactic acidosis.

4. Lactate level: Should be reviewed to assess progress, as increases in $Scvo_2$ are not always indicative of improvement. Although lactate provides a valuable reflection of tissue hypoxia, it cannot be continuously monitored and it changes over time. Lactate is produced excessively when poor circulation and oxygenation prompt cells to initiate anaerobic metabolism. Blood lactate concentrations reflect the balance between lactate production and clearance. The normal blood lactate concentration in physiologically unstressed patients is 0.5 to 1 mmol/L. In critical illness, lactate concentrations of less than 2 mmol/L are considered acceptable. Hyperlactatemia is defined as a mild to moderate persistent increase in blood lactate concentration (2 to 4 mmol/L) without metabolic acidosis. Depending on the hospital or clinical laboratory protocol, lactic acidosis is diagnosed when increased blood lactate levels rise above 3 mmol/L. When patients are at risk of cellular hypoxia, a blood sample to measure the lactate level should be drawn. This may apply to a patient with suspected sepsis, but also to those with sustained tachycardia, tachypnea, hyperventilation, and persistent hypotension.

OBSERVATION AND OTHER ASSESSMENT FINDINGS

- Early signs reflective of systemic inflammatory response syndrome and sepsis: Anxiety, continuous agitation, discomfort in excess of condition. Vasodilation may create a "healthy" flushed appearance of the skin, which may be warm or hot to touch.

- Signs of severe sepsis, septic shock, and multiorgan dysfunction syndrome: Flushed skin that changes to pallor; edema of face, neck, torso, sacrum, and extremities; deteriorating length of consciousness with possible obtundation or unresponsiveness as cerebral perfusion is failing; rales caused by heart failure; respiratory failure requiring endotracheal intubation and mechanical ventilation; oliguria; diminished bowel sounds; and diminished peripheral pulses. Vasodilation may maintain warm-to-hot skin until the patient totally decompensates with cool-to-cold, clammy skin.

Diagnostic Tests for SIRS, Sepsis, Severe Sepsis, Septic Shock and MODS

The diagnosis of the various stages of the continuum of sepsis is based on signs and symptoms, testing for causes of infection, degree of perfusion deficit associated with shock, and presence of organ failure. Treatment should be initiated before laboratory results are available.

Test	Purpose	Abnormal Findings
Complete blood count with white blood cell (WBC) differential	WBC differential evaluates the strength of the immune system's response to the trigger of response and whether infection may be present.	WBC differential: WBC count may be normal, elevated, or decreased. The presence of >10% of bands indicates an inflammatory response. Hematocrit: may be increased from hypovolemia and hemoconcentration.
Blood cultures and antibiotic sensitivity testing of isolates	To identify if a microorganism has moved into the bloodstream to cause a systemic infection, and if so, which antibiotics will be most effective to eradicate the organism.	Possible presence of an organism. Approximately one third of patients with sepsis do not have an identified organism present in the bloodstream.
Culture and antibiotic sensitivity testing of suspect infection sites (e.g., urine, sputum, blood, intravenous lines, incisions)	To identify the original source of the infection.	Results are correlated with blood cultures to validate where the systemic infection causing a massive inflammatory response originated.
Arterial blood gas analysis	Assess for abnormal gas exchange or compensation for metabolic derangements. Initially Pao_2 is normal and then decreases as the ventilation-perfusion mismatch becomes more severe.	pH changes: acidosis may reflect respiratory failure; alkalosis may reflect compensatory tachypnea seen in early stages. Carbon dioxide: elevated CO_2 reflects respiratory failure; decreased CO_2 reflects tachypnea; rising Pco_2 is an ominous sign, since it signals severe hypoventilation, which can lead to respiratory arrest. Hypoxemia: Pao_2 <80 mm Hg Oxygen saturation: Sao_2 <92%
Serum lactate level	Assesses for degree of anaerobic metabolism present. Anaerobic metabolism ensues when capillary beds are unable to effectively perfuse tissues and organs.	Increases to >4 mmol/L indicate the presence of significant capillary occlusion. Normal is <2 mmol/L.

Continued

Diagnostic Tests for SIRS, Sepsis, Severe Sepsis, Septic Shock and MODS—cont'd

Test	Purpose	Abnormal Findings
Blood chemistry or biochemical profile	To screen for changes associated with the stress response. In stress states (e.g., infection, trauma, hypoxia), hormones are released to increase generation of additional glucose from nonglucose products (gluconeogenesis) and create insulin resistance.	Hyperglycemia is common but may improve as the liver fails, since the liver has a key role in gluconeogenesis. If catecholamines (e.g., norepinephrine, phenylephrine) are given to increase blood pressure, this may prolong hyperglycemia, since catecholamines create insulin resistance.
Clotting studies	Assesses for presence of activation of the clotting cascade and for consumptive coagulopathy such as DIC.	Activated clotting cascade reflects decreased platelets (>50% drop over 3 days is an indicator of severe sepsis), increased prothrombin time, increased partial thromboplastin time, increased international normalized ratio, and increased fibrin split products.
Radiographs	Chest radiograph to check for pneumonia or acute respiratory distress syndrome before computed tomography (CT) scanning of the lung. Other radiographs are done to assess underlying condition.	Positive findings help to detect the source of infection or inflammation and the presence of MODS.
CT	Lung CT is more reflective of changes in the pulmonary microcirculation, and most accurately depicts extravascular lung water. Also used to assess for abnormalities such as intraabdominal abscess or perforated viscus.	Positive findings help to detect the source of infection or inflammation and the presence of MODS.
12-lead ECG	To detect dysrhythmias reflective of myocardial ischemia	Ischemic changes (ST depression) may be present as shock progresses.
Biomarkers of sepsis	Presence of various levels of >100 distinct molecules have been suggested to be helpful in the diagnosis of sepsis. Biomarkers are used as part of screening, diagnosis, risk stratification, and evaluating response to therapy.	The ability to use a biomarker varies with each patient and with the stage of sepsis when the value was drawn. There are no universally accepted biomarkers, but the more commonly recognized mediators include tumor necrosis factor, interleukin 6, procalcitonin, and presence of various endotoxins from gram-negative bacteria.

COLLABORATIVE MANAGEMENT

CARE PRIORITIES

Early recognition and therapy are still the cornerstones of acute care of the septic patient. The advent of new technologies and biomolecular testing should improve survival rates and give rise to more accurate incidence statistics. The treatment of severe sepsis and septic shock is an evolving process, and the guidelines continue to be updated. Reduction of septic inflammation may involve several pharmacologic therapies and adjunct therapies. Management of sepsis and septic shock includes respiratory support, aggressive fluid resuscitation, inotropic support, vasopressor therapy, and early antibiotic therapy. In the future less invasive methods of optimizing a patient's fluid status and hemodynamics, along with monitoring the microcirculatory dysfunction common in sepsis, may become more routine.

There are several models available to simplify the identification process. The use of standardized order sets for the management of sepsis should be recommended strongly for better performance in treatment. Standard order sets use serum lactate values because of their relationship to organ dysfunction in sepsis. To reduce mortality rates, sepsis must be identified and treated as early as possible.

Summary of immediate steps: Identify the patient and engage in collaborative practices to begin treatment. Delays in patient identification are often directly related to the nurse's ability to have the appropriate conversation with colleagues on the factors present that are indicative of sepsis. Nurses are crucial to successful patient identification. Broad-spectrum antibiotics are initiated immediately; ideally, after blood cultures are drawn to provide therapy within 1 hour in the setting of severe sepsis, with or without septic shock. Imaging should be done as soon as possible; ideally during the first hour to try to identify and/or confirm the source of infection so necessary steps can be initiated as soon as possible to manage the source. It is crucial to provide aggressive resuscitation within the first 6 hours of diagnosis. As noted, blood cultures should be obtained within 1 hour of recognition, before initiating antibiotics if possible, but delaying antibiotics in lieu of cultures is unacceptable. Large-bore IV access should be secured in preparation for large volume fluid resuscitation, which should be initiated as soon as possible within the first hour of patient identification. Vasopressor therapy with norepinephrine is used to stabilize the patient.

1. Manage the infection immediately, regardless of the ability to obtain blood cultures within 1 hour

Getting broad-spectrum antibiotics on board promptly has been shown to be as important a priority as fluid resuscitation. Delaying therapy could mean the difference between a good and a poor outcome. Once under way, an institution's antibiotic steward, i.e., a knowledgeable physician or clinical pharmacist (PharmD), should be consulted to manage ongoing therapy. Initial antibiotic therapy should not be continued indefinitely. Antibiotics should be administered within 1 hour of the patient presenting with severe sepsis or septic shock and reevaluated daily for appropriateness and need to continue.

2. Manage hypovolemia with intravenous isotonic fluids

IV volume expansion is implemented to maintain adequate ventricular filling pressures and volume, which are compromised by increased capillary permeability and vasodilation. Fluid resuscitation with crystalloids is the preferred fluid replacement strategy. Colloids, such as albumin, may be initiated in patients requiring a large volume of crystalloid to maintain an acceptable MAP. , Adding albumin has not been demonstrated to sustain the MAP, but rather provides a temporary enhancement in certain patients. Hetastarch solutions should be avoided. Current guidelines recommend use of packed red blood cell transfusion and dobutamine drip if Svo_2 remains 70% after initial fluid resuscitation. The initial fluid challenge should be at least 30 mL/kg of crystalloids. Patients with suspected severe hypovolemia resulting in hypoperfusion may require more rapid administration and a larger volume of fluids. The fluid challenge may be continued as long as required to improve hemodynamics. Crystalloid solution such as lactated Ringer or normal saline can be used. Colloids may include albumin and fresh-frozen plasma.

3. Use early goal-directed therapy to prevent or slow patient progression to multiorgan dysfunction syndrome and multiple organ failure

According to current ACCP/SCCM guidelines, the following are points of early goal-directed therapy:

- Immediate fluid resuscitation should be performed if not already done. The goal is to infuse no less than 1 L, or 20 mL/kg, via fluid bolus if tolerated. The rate of fluid infusion should be reduced if filling pressures rise without improvement in overall circulation
- Determining the optimal preload level in sepsis is challenging. A patient who is not considered fluid responsive may be potentially harmed by aggressive fluid resuscitation. In fact, in patients who are not fluid responsive, the volume may exacerbate ARDS, acute

kidney injury, and IAH. Traditionally, CVP and/or PAP monitoring were the methods upon which volume resuscitation was based. Recent evidence, however, negates the value of the CVP (and the PAP) end point, with results indicating that fluid management utilizing CVP-targeted resuscitation significantly contributes to morbidity and mortality. Newer methods to evaluate fluid responsiveness, including systolic pressure variation, stroke volume variation, and passive leg raise techniques, are becoming more widely utilized.

- All blood for labwork for the sepsis profile (serum lactate, blood culture, biomedical profile, CBC with differential, coagulation profile, and biomarkers such as presence of TNF, IL-6, or procalcitonin if available) should be drawn and then repeated every 2 to 4 hours initially to assess for progress.

- Vasopressors are administered for MAP less than 65 mm Hg during fluid resuscitation and after adequate fluid resuscitation. Vasopressors of choice are norepinephrine, epinephrine, and vasopressin. They may be given to augment cardiac contractility and CO. In the late stages of sepsis, positive inotropic drugs may be given with vasodilators such as nitroprusside and nitroglycerin, which decrease preload and afterload by dilating veins and arteries, to assist in the management of terminal heart failure. Given that both vasodilation and vasoconstriction are present throughout the circulation, it is difficult to predict the most effective strategy for support of circulation. Some institutions may use noncatecholamine inodilator medications such as milrinone to provide inotropic support as well as to decrease resistance to ventricular ejection.

RESEARCH BRIEF 11-4

An increased circulating NT-pro-B-type natriuretic peptide plasma level is an independent marker of greater systolic cardiac dysfunction and a better predictor of fluid nonresponsiveness in septic versus nonseptic critically ill patients.

Turner KL, Moore LJ, Todd SR, et al: Identification of cardiac dysfunction in sepsis with B-type natriuretic peptide. *J Am Coll Surg* 213:139-146, 2011.

---

4. If early resuscitation fails, or the patient presents in septic shock or multiorgan dysfunction syndrome, the second group of therapies is instituted in conjunction with or immediately following early goal-directed therapy

- Support ventilation and oxygenation if patient develops acute respiratory distress syndrome. Mechanical ventilation: Intubate and place on low tidal volume, pressure-controlled ventilation if high-flow oxygen or noninvasive positive pressure ventilation fails to stabilize ventilation. If on volume control ventilation, plateau pressure should be on average less than 30 cm H_2O for ventilated patients. Lung-protective ventilation with low tidal volume (6 to 8 mL/kg of ideal body weight) is recommended. Assist control volume- or pressure-controlled ventilation may be initiated (see Mechanical Ventilation, Chapter 1).

- Maintain the Blood Pressure. Vasopressors (e.g., norepinephrine, vasopressin, phenylephrine, epinephrine): May be administered in cases when optimal left ventricular preload fails to restore adequate tissue perfusion (i.e., the initial MAP is very low or MAP is persistently less than 60 mm Hg). If norepinephrine is ineffective, phenylephrine, vasopressin, and high-dose epinephrine may be used. The goal of therapy is to optimize cardiac index by providing a balance among promoting venous return, augmenting cardiac contractility, and creating the ideal level of resistance to ventricular ejection.

- Consider corticosteroids. In stress situations, the normal adrenal gland output of cortisol is approximately 250 to 300 mg over 24 hours. Use of corticosteroids remains controversial. IV hydrocortisone should be given only to adult septic shock patients after it has been confirmed that their BP is poorly responsive to fluid resuscitation and vasopressor therapy and cortisol levels are low. Most important, all patients on chronic steroid re placement, such as those with rheumatoid arthritis taking daily prednisone, have to receive high doses of IV steroids while in shock. Corticosteroids also help to control inflammation (see Acute Adrenal Insufficiency (Adrenal Crisis), Chapter 8). Their use, however, remains controversial.

    - Administer 100 mg of hydrocortisone in an IV bolus, regardless of cortisol level, if the patient's BP is not responding to fluid volume resuscitation and vasopressor therapy,

followed by a continuous infusion of 300 mg in 100 to 250 mL of isotonic sodium chloride solution by continuous IV infusion over 24 hours. Information regarding efficacy of steroids in the setting of sepsis is almost equally divided (pro and con) in the literature. A trial of hydrocortisone is warranted if all other measures have failed.
- An alternative method of hydrocortisone administration is 50 mg as an IV bolus every 6 hours.
- The infusion method maintains plasma cortisol levels more adequately at steady stress levels, especially in the small percentage of patients who are rapid metabolizers and who may have low plasma cortisol levels between the IV boluses.

Treat the Problems
- Provide antibiotics to control infection: Broad-spectrum antibiotic coverage for sepsis (often directed at gram-negative sepsis) should be initiated before identifying a specific microorganism if patients exhibit physiologic changes and positive signs and symptoms. Samples for culturing should be obtained before initiating antibiotics, unless doing so would considerably delay treatment. Obtain at least two blood samples for cultures, one percutaneously and another through invasive IV lines that have been in place more than 48 hours before antibiotic administration. Timely administration of appropriate antibiotics is critical to patient outcome. Choice of antimicrobial depends on the organ and organisms involved. Physicians and midlevel practitioners will prescribe ceftriaxone, zithromycin, or levofloxacin for severe community-acquired pneumonia; whereas hospital-acquired pneumonia may need to be treated with broader-spectrum antibiotics that cover drug-resistant pathogens. Such antibiotics may include ceftazidime, meropenem, vancomycin, and aminoglycosides. The effectiveness of the antibiotics should be reevaluated daily and use should be anticipated for 7 to 10 days. Use of the fewest possible antibiotics reduces the possibility of development of a superinfection with an opportunistic organism including fungus (*Candida*), infection with a resistant organism (MRSA, VRE), or *Clostridium difficile*-Associated Diarrhea. Treatment of infection helps control the inflammatory response.
- Control the source of the infection: Other methods for controlling the source of infection should be weighed carefully for risks and benefits. Identifying the source of infection is critical. Localizing and draining an abscess, removing new pleural fluid collections, and discontinuing infected indwelling catheters are keys to better outcomes.
- Other pharmaceutical agents: For many years, researchers and clinicians have been looking for a miracle medication that will stop the vicious cycle of events that occurs in severe sepsis and leads to MODS. Unfortunately, many of the medications, such as the anti-TNF medications, only affected one of many major cascades involved. Recombinant human activated protein C (Xigris), which had been shown to reduce mortality in patients with an APACHE II score greater than 25 or at high risk of dying from sepsis, was subsequently disproven as an effective agent for widespread use. It is no longer available. Absolute contraindications have always been related to the high risk of bleeding.
- Control blood glucose: Use IV insulin therapy to keep blood glucose below 180 mg/dL, with a target of 150 mg/dL. Use of intensive insulin therapy to lower blood glucose to 80 to 110 mg/dL is no longer recommended, as septic shock patients often become hypoglycemic. (See *Hyperglycemia*, Chapter 8).
- Provide nutrition support: Current SCCM recommendations for enteral feedings/nutrition support in the critically ill include short- and medium-chain fatty acids and branched-chain amino acids administered to stop protein catabolism. The short- and medium-chain fatty acids are absorbed more readily and metabolized more easily than long-chain fatty acids. They may be given orally (e.g., MCT Oil, which is a proprietary name for triglycerides of medium-chain fatty acids), as part of enteral feeding, or via the IV route (e.g., intralipid solutions). Branched-chain amino acid solutions are used in sepsis, as they are metabolized by muscle rather than the liver and can therefore be used in the presence of organ failure. (See Nutrition Support, Chapter 1).

CARE PLANS FOR SYSTEMIC INFLAMMATORY RESPONSE SYNDROME, SEPSIS, AND MULTIORGAN DYSFUNCTION SYNDROME

DEFICIENT FLUID VOLUME *related to active loss from vascular compartment secondary to increased capillary permeability and shift of intravascular volume into interstitial spaces and relative hypovolemia resulting from vasodilation.*

Goals/Outcomes: Within 4 hours of initiation of therapy, the patient is normovolemic as evidenced by peripheral pulses greater than 2+ on a 0 to 4+ scale, stable body weight, urine output 0.5 mL/kg/h or greater, mean BP 60 mm Hg or greater (or within patient's normal range), sustained systolic BP 90 mm Hg or greater (or within patient's normal range), and absence of edema and adventitious lung sounds. SVI is 30 to 40 mL/min /m³, SVV is less than 15%, and $ScvO_2$ or SvO_2 is 60% to 80%.

NOC Fluid Balance; Electrolyte and Acid-Base Balance

Hemodynamic Regulation

1. Monitor hemodynamic pressures, using noninvasive or invasive methods to assess CO, SVI, and SVV if available. If a pulmonary artery catheter is used, PAWP, CO, and SVR are measured. During the early stage of sepsis, filling pressures (PAWP and CVP) may be normal to low, but as biventricular dysfunction occurs, these pressures may increase. If the patient manifests a compensatory increase in CO, the calculated SVR may initially be low, but the calculated value may rise as the CO drops.

2. Initiate early goal-directed therapy to support the CO and BP as prescribed, including IV fluids and positive inotropic agents. Vasopressors are used if inotropic agents and fluid resuscitation fail to stabilize BP (see Collaborative Management, Chapter 11). Fluid replacement therapy is given to maintain a CVP of 2-12 mm Hg or PAWP of 6 to 12 mm Hg. Assess CVP and/or PAWP and lung sounds at frequent intervals during fluid replacement to detect evidence of fluid overload: crackles, wheezing, and increasing CVP and/or PAWP. Current literature does not support the routine use of pulmonary artery pressures in lieu of SvO_2 and $ScvO_2$ when managing septic patients, given challenges associated with cellular oxygenation, which are not reflected unless technology reflective of oxygen delivery, demand, and consumption is used.

3. Assess fluid volume by monitoring BP, peripheral pulses, and urine output hourly. Report failure of early goal-directed therapy to stabilize mean BP to greater than 60 mm Hg or sustained systolic BP to 90 mm Hg or greater or within patient's normal range. Weigh the patient daily; monitor I&O every shift, noting 24-hour trends. Report urine output less than 0.5 mL/kg/h. The patient's weight may actually increase with fluid volume deficit because of a shift of intravascular volume into interstitial spaces.

4. Assess for interstitial edema as evidenced by pretibial, sacral, ankle, and hand edema, as well as crackles on auscultation of lung fields.

5. Position the patient supine with the legs elevated to increase venous return and preload.

NIC Fluid/Electrolyte Management; Hypovolemia Management; Fluid Management; Shock Management: Volume

DECREASED CARDIAC OUTPUT *related to negative inotropic changes in the heart (late stage) secondary to effects of tissue hypoxia, worsening during late septic shock.*

Goals/Outcomes: Within 8 hours of initiation of therapy, the patient has improved CO as evidenced by peripheral pulses greater than 2+on a 0 to 4+ scale, stable body weight, urine output 0.5 mL/kg/h or greater, mean BP 60 mm Hg or greater (or within patient's normal range), sustained systolic BP 90 mm Hg or greater (or within patient's normal range), and absence of edema and adventitious lung sounds. CVP is 2-12 mm Hg (add 3 mm Hg to normal if the patient is on positive pressure ventilation), PAWP is 6 to 12 mm Hg, CO is 4 to 7 L/min, CI is greater than 2.5 L/min/m², and calculated SVR is 900 to 1200 dynes/sec/cm⁻⁵. SVI is 30 to 40 mL/min/m³, SVV is less than 15%, and $ScvO_2$ or SvO_2 is 60% to 80%.

NOC Cardiac Pump Effectiveness; Circulation Status

Cardiac Care: Acute

1. Assess the patient for signs of decreased CO: decreasing BP, increasing HR, decreasing amplitude of peripheral pulses, restlessness, decreasing urinary output, and increasing PAWP.

2. Administer positive inotropic agents (e.g., dobutamine) as prescribed to augment cardiac contractility.

3. If continuous or intermittent CO monitoring is not in place, assess CVP at least every 4 hours. Observe for development of premature ventricular complexes, which may occur with hypoxia, and extreme tachycardia. Dysrhythmias and hypoxia may further reduce CO.

4. Monitor $ScvO_2$ or SvO_2 continuously; report values outside normal range.

NIC Hemodynamic Regulation; Invasive Hemodynamic Monitoring; Fluid/Electrolyte Management

INEFFECTIVE TISSUE PERFUSION: CEREBRAL, RENAL, AND GASTROINTESTINAL *related to hypovolemia secondary to mixed vasodilation and constriction interruption of arterial and venous blood flow secondary to vasoconstriction and thrombus obstruction.*

Goals/Outcomes: Within 24 hours of initiating therapy, the patient has improved perfusion as evidenced by orientation to time, place, and person; peripheral pulses greater than $2+$ on a 0 to $4+$ scale, stable body weight, urine output 0.5 mL/kg/h or greater, mean BP 60 mm Hg or greater (or within patient's normal range), sustained systolic BP 90 mm Hg or greater (or within patient's normal range), and absence of edema and adventitious lung sounds. CVP is 2-12 mm Hg (add 3 mm Hg to normal if the patient is on positive pressure ventilation), PAWP is 6 to 12 mm Hg, CO is 4 to 7 L/min, CI greater than 2.5 L/min/m^2, and calculated SVR is 900 to 1200 dynes/sec/cm^{-5}. SVI is 30 to 40 mL/min/m^3, SVV is less than 15%, and $Scvo_2$ or Svo_2 is 60% to 80%.

NOC Circulation Status

Circulatory Precautions
1. Assess for changes in length of consciousness as an indicator of decreasing cerebral perfusion.
2. Assess for the following signs of decreasing renal perfusion: urine output less than 0.5 mL/kg/h and increased BUN, serum creatinine, and serum potassium levels.
   - Monitor arterial BP continuously for signs of deteriorating circulatory status related to cardiac failure or hypovolemia. Systolic BP will be decreased because of decreased CO, and the diastolic BP may be low secondary to vasodilation or normal to high secondary to compensatory vasoconstriction.
   - Assess peripheral pulses, temperature, color of skin, and capillary refill. With hypoperfusion, pulse amplitude decreases, extremities are cool because of vasoconstriction, skin color is pale or mottled because of decreased perfusion, and capillary refill is delayed.
3. Monitor cellular oxygen consumption (VO_2) as an indicator of tissue perfusion. With sepsis, cellular oxygen delivery is decreased (precapillary vasoconstriction), and thus cellular oxygen use is decreased. Mixed venous blood oxygen saturation (Svo_2) is elevated.
4. Administer vasoactive drugs as prescribed. CVP monitoring using a centrally placed central line or peripherally inserted line is a good alternative. The goal range is CVP of 2 to 6 mm Hg (add 3 mm Hg when positive pressure ventilation is used). Pulmonary artery catheters are associated with high risk and are not used as often for management of septic patients. When in place, SVR and CO can be assessed to determine drug effects. Optimally, SVR will increase to at least 900 dynes/sec/cm^{-5}, CO will be 4 to 7 L/min, and CI will be 2.5 to 4 L/min/m^2. Fluid boluses are administered rapidly to obtain the goal.
5. Assess for evidence of decreasing splanchnic (visceral) circulation, including decreased or absent bowel sounds, elevated serum amylase level, and decreased platelet count.

NIC Cerebral Perfusion Promotion; Circulatory Care; Fluid/Electrolyte Management; Oxygen Therapy; Hemodynamic Regulation; Shock Management; Nutrition Management; Hemodialysis Therapy

IMPAIRED GAS EXCHANGE *related to alveolar-capillary membrane changes secondary to interstitial edema, alveolar destruction, and endotoxin release with activation of histamine and kinins.*

Goals/Outcomes: Within 4 hours of initiation of therapy, the patient's Pao_2 is greater than 80 mm Hg, $Paco_2$ is less than 45 mm Hg, pH is 7.35 to 7.45, and lungs are clear.

NOC Respiratory Status: Gas Exchange; Electrolyte and Acid-Base Balance

Ventilation Assistance
1. Assess for and maintain a patent airway by assisting patient with coughing or by suctioning the trachea as necessary.
2. Assess all ABG values. Be alert to decreasing Pao_2, increasing $Paco_2$, and acidosis (decreasing pH). Monitor the patient for the presence of dyspnea, hypopnea, and restlessness.
3. Listen to breath sounds hourly and with each change in the patient's condition. The presence of crackles may indicate fluid accumulation.
4. If the patient exhibits evidence of inadequate gas exchange (e.g., Pao_2 less than 60 mm Hg while the patient is on 100% oxygen via nonrebreather mask) but mental status remains stable, attempt NPPV. If NPPV fails, prepare for the probability of endotracheal intubation.

5. If the patient has been placed on mechanical ventilation, monitor inspiratory peak and plateau pressures for increasing trends, which may signal decreasing compliance and development of ARDS. As ARDS develops, an increasing FIO_2 (at least 0.50) and increasing levels of PEEP are required to maintain adequate PaO_2 (at least 60 mm Hg) (see Acute Respiratory Distress Syndrome, Chapter 4, and Mechanical Ventilation, Chapter 1).
6. Monitor end-tidal CO_2 trends for changes indicative of development of ARDS, hypoperfusion, and misplacement of the endotracheal tube.
7. Turn the patient every 2 hours to maintain optimal ventilation-perfusion ratios and to prevent atelectasis.

NIC Acid-Base Management: Metabolic Acidosis; Oxygen Therapy; Respiratory Monitoring; Artificial Airway Management; Invasive Hemodynamic Regulation

INEFFECTIVE BREATHING PATTERN *related to decreased lung expansion secondary to central respiratory depression occurring in late shock.*

Goals/Outcomes: Within 2 hours of initiating respiratory support, the patient has an effective breathing pattern as evidenced by normal limits of inspiratory:expiratory ratio (1:1 to 1:2); tidal volume (at least 6 mL/kg); and maximal inspiratory pressures (less than 20 cm H_2O).
NOC Respiratory Status: Ventilation

Respiratory Monitoring
1. Monitor for decreasing respiratory rate, depth, and air movement. Ensure the patient demonstrates adequate air movement by noting presence of breath sounds over all lung fields.
2. Assist the patient into a comfortable position to facilitate respirations. Depending on patient's hemodynamic stability, the optimal position may be a 15 to 30 degrees head of the bed elevation.
3. Assess/measure tidal volume and inspiratory force. Be alert to tidal volume less than 4 mL/kg and inspiratory force less than 20 cm H_2O as indicators of an ineffective breathing pattern.
4. If the patient exhibits respiratory depression/ineffective breathing pattern, prepare for the probability of endotracheal intubation. (See Acute Respiratory Failure, Chapter 4.)

NIC Oxygen Therapy; Mechanical Ventilation

INEFFECTIVE THERMOREGULATION *related to illness with concomitant endotoxin effect on hypothalamic temperature-regulating center.*

Goals/Outcomes: Within 24 hours of initiation of treatment, the patient becomes normothermic.
NOC Thermoregulation

Temperature Regulation
1. Monitor patient's temperature continuously or at frequent intervals. Use temperature probe (rectal, bladder, or esophageal) for continuous monitoring of core temperature. Body temperature can range from 38.3° to 40.6° C (101° to 105° F) in the early stage of sepsis and can be less than 35.6° C (96° F) in the late stage. Patients with immunodeficient states on chronic or high-dose steroid therapy may have a normal or low temperature. Be alert to shaking chills early in sepsis as temperature increases and to profuse chills as temperature decreases late in sepsis. Temperatures up to 103°F may be allowed in the septic patient, as increased temperature may help control bacteremia. The following are weighed for each patient to determine the extent of treatment that should be used to decrease fever (e.g., acetaminophen administration):
    *   Useful effects of a fever: decreased viral and bacterial replication
    *   Harmful effects of a fever: increased cardiac workload and increased oxygen consumption
2. Administer antimicrobials as prescribed. Discuss appropriate antibiotic therapy. Observe for untoward effects, including renal toxicity, ototoxicity, allergic reactions, anaphylaxis, pseudomembranous colitis (*C. difficile*-associated diarrhea), overgrowth of normal flora, and superimposed infectious processes of the skin, urinary tract, or respiratory tract. Large doses of antibiotics may cause the release of endotoxins from dying bacteria, which may potentiate the progression of septic shock.
3. Administer antipyretic agents as prescribed.
4. For patients with hyperthermia, use tepid baths, which decrease body temperature by releasing internal heat. Cooled IV fluids also may decrease core temperature. In addition, a cooling blanket may be prescribed to reduce

the metabolic rate, thereby decreasing myocardial oxygen demand. Avoid "chilling," which will cause shivering and thus increase myocardial oxygen demand and cardiac workload.

5. In the presence of hypothermia, use warm blankets to increase body temperature. Heating devices can damage ischemic cells in peripheral tissues and usually are avoided.

NIC Fever Treatment; Temperature Regulation; Environmental Management

IMBALANCED NUTRITION: LESS THAN BODY REQUIREMENTS *related to increased need secondary to increased metabolic rate.*

Goals/Outcomes: Within 48 hours of initiation of treatment, the patient has adequate nutrition as evidenced by stable weight, serum albumin 3.5 g/dL, prealbumin 20 to 30 mg/dL, retinol-binding protein 4 to 5 mg/dL, urine urea nitrogen 10 to 20 mg/dL, and a state of nitrogen balance as determined by nitrogen studies.
NOC Nutritional Status

Nutrition Management
1. Monitor laboratory findings for serum albumin, prealbumin, retinol-binding protein, and nitrogen studies.
2. Administer nutritional supplements as prescribed.
3. Assess and record weight and nutritional intake daily. Consult with nutritional services for calorie count.
4. Observe for and document areas of tissue breakdown, which may indicate a negative nitrogen state.
5. If the patient is receiving oral feedings, assess for the presence of bowel sounds at least every 8 hours. Paralytic ileus can occur secondary to an ischemic bowel.
6. If the patient is receiving continuous gastric tube feedings, assess for residual feeding at least every 4 hours. (See Nutrition Support, Chapter 1.)
   - Enteral feedings are recommended whenever possible, and the choice of feeding formula is determined based on the individual patient. However, formulas with supplemental omega-3 fatty acids such as gamma-linoleic acid and eicosapentaenoic acid are recommended. Total parenteral nutrition is administered to patients unable to tolerate enteral feedings. Standard total parenteral nutrition solutions are not metabolized well in the septic state. Branched-chain amino acid solutions and short-to medium-chain fatty acid solutions may be used (e.g., MCT Oil or FreAmine HBC).

NIC TPN Administration; Enteral Tube Feeding

ADDITIONAL NURSING DIAGNOSES

Also see nursing diagnoses and interventions in Hemodynamic Monitoring Chapter 1), Acute Lung Injury and Acute Respiratory Distress Syndrome (Chapter 4), Emotional and Spiritual Support of the Patient and Significant Others (Chapter 2), and Bleeding and Thrombotic Disorders: Disseminated Intravascular Coagulation (Chapter 10).

SELECTED REFERENCES

Agarwal R, Schwartz DN: Procalcitonin to guide duration of antimicrobial therapy in intensive care units: a systematic review, *Clin Infect Dis* 53:379–387, 2011.

Aird WC: The role of the endothelium in severe sepsis and multiple organ dysfunction syndrome, *Blood* 101:3765–3777, 2003.

Ait-Oufella H, Maury E, Lehoux S, et al: The endothelium: physiological functions and role in microcirculatory failure during severe sepsis, *Intensive Care Med* 36:1286–1298, 2010.

Alapat PM, Zimmerman JL: Toxicology in the critical care unit, *Chest* 133:1006–1013, 2008.

Amato L, Minozzi S, Vecchi S, et al: Benzodiazepines for alcohol withdrawal, *Cochrane Database Syst Rev* 17:CD005064, 2010.

American College of Obstetricians and Gynecologists: *ACOG optimizing protocols in obstetrics series 4: Key elements for the management of hypertensive crisis in pregnancy (in-patient)*, Washington, 2013, ACOG. http://www.acog.org/Womens-Health/Preeclampsia-and-Hypertension-in-Pregnancy.

American College of Obstetricians and Gynecologists: *ACOG practice bulletin no. 125: chronic hypertension in pregnancy*, *Obstet Gynecol* 119:396, 2012.

Sepsis, Septic Shock, SIRS, and MODS

American College of Obstetricians and Gynecologists: *ACOG practice bulletin no. 33: diagnosis and management of preeclampsia and eclampsia*, Washington, Reaffirmed, 2010, ACOG. http://journals.lww.com/greenjournal/Fulltext/2002/01000/ACOG_Practice_Bulletin_No__33__Diagnosis_and.28.aspx.

American College of Obstetricians and Gynecologists: ACOG practice bulletin number 106: intrapartum fetal monitoring, Washington, 2009, ACOG. http://www.acog.org/Search?Keyword=intrapartum+fetal+monitoring.

American College of Obstetricians and Gynecologists: *ACOG committee opinion 514: Emergent therapy for acute-onset, severe hypertension with preeclampsia or eclampsia*, Washington, 2011, ACOG.

American College of Obstetricians and Gynecologist, Task Force on Hypertension in Pregnancy: Hypertension in pregnancy. Report of the American College of Obstetricians and Gynecologists' Task Force on Hypertension in Pregnancy, *Obstet Gynecol* 122:1122, 2013.

Angus D, Van der Poll T: Severe sepsis and septic shock, *N Engl J Med* 369:2063, 2013.

Arbour R: Clinical management of the organ donor, *AACN Clin Issues* 16:551, 2005.

Association of Women's Health, Obstetric and Neonatal Nurses: *Fetal heart monitoring principles and practices*, Washington, 2003, AWHONN.

Atema JJ, van Buijtenen JM, Lamme B, et al: Clinical studies on intra-abdominal hypertension and abdominal compartment syndrome, *J Trauma Acute Care Surg* 76:234–240, 2014.

Azoulay E, Soares M, Darmon M, et al: Intensive care of the cancer patient: recent achievements and remaining challenges, *Ann Intensive Care* 1:5, 2011.

Barton JR, Sibai BM: Prediction and prevention of recurrent preeclampsia, *Obstet Gynecol* 11:359–372, 2008.

Baumann MH, Ayestas MA Jr, Partilla JS, et al: The designer methcathinone analogs, mephedrone and methylone, are substrates for monoamine transporters in brain tissue, *Neuropsychopharmacology* 37:1192–1203, 2012.

Bienvenu OJ, Neufeld KJ, Needham DM: Treatment of four psychiatric emergencies in the intensive care unit, *Crit Care Med* 40:2662–2670, 2012.

Bronstein AC, Spyker DA, Cantilena LR Jr, et al: 2009 Annual report of the American Association of Poison Control Centers' National Poison Data System (NPDS): 27th annual report, *Clin Toxicol* 48:979–1178, 2010.

Boyd JH, Forbes J, Nakada T, et al: Fluid resuscitation in septic shock: a positive fluid balance and elevated central venous pressure are associated with increased mortality, *Crit Care Med* 39:259–265, 2011.

Boyer E: Management of opioid analgesic overdose, *N Engl J Med* 367:146–155, 2012.

Campbell PT, Rudisill PT: Psychosocial needs of the critically ill obstetric patient: the nurse's role, *Crit Care Nurs Q* 29:77–80, 2006.

Carpenito LJ: *Nursing diagnosis: application to practice*, ed 14, Philadelphia, 2012, Lippincott Williams & Wilkins.

Chalupka AN, Talmor D: The economics of sepsis, *Crit Care Clinics* 28:57–76, 2012.

Chappell LC, Enye S, Seed P, et al: Adverse perinatal outcomes and risk factors for preeclampsia in women with chronic hypertension. A prospective study, *Hypertension* 51:354–364, 2008.

Cheatham ML, Safcsak K: Is the evolving management of intraabdominal hypertension and abdominal compartment syndrome improving survival? *Crit Care Med* 38:402–407, 2010.

Cheatham ML: Nonoperative management of intraabdominal hypertension and abdominal compartment syndrome, *World J Surg* 33:1116–112, 2009.

Christie JD, Edwards LB, Aurora P, et al: Registry of the International Society for Heart and Lung Transplantation: twenty-fifth official adult lung and heart/lung transplantation report, 2008, *J Heart Lung Transplant* 27:957–969, 2008.

Coffier B, Altman A, Pui CH, et al: Guidelines for the management of pediatric and adult tumor lysis syndrome: an evidence based review, *J Clin Oncol* 26:2767–2778, 2008.

Collins JJ: Synthetic legal intoxicating drugs: the emerging 'incense' and 'bath salt' phenomenon, *Cleve Clin J Med* 79:258–264, 2012.

Coppage KH, Sibai BM: Treatment of hypertensive complications in pregnancy, *Curr Pharm Design* 11:749–757, 2005.

Crespo-Leiro MG, Alonso-Pulpon L, et al: Malignancy after heart transplantation: incidence, prognosis, and risk factors, *Am J Transplant* 8:1031, 2008.

Czura CJ: Merinoff symposium 2010: sepsis—speaking with one voice, *Mol Med* 17:2–3, 2011.

De Backer D, Biston P, Devriendt J, et al: SOAP II investigators. Comparison of dopamine and norepinephrine in the treatment of shock, *N Engl J Med* 362:779–789, 2010.

Decker E, Coimbra C, Weekers L, et al: A retrospective monocenter review of simultaneous pancreas-kidney transplantation, *Transplant Proc* 41:3389–3392, 2009.

De Keulenaer BL, De Waele JJ, Powell B, et al: What is normal intra-abdominal pressure and how is it affected by positioning, body mass and positive end-expiratory pressure? *Intensive Care Med* 35:969–976, 2009.

De Laet IE, Ravyts M, Vidts W, et al: Current insights in intra-abdominal hypertension and abdominal compartment syndrome: open the abdomen and keep it open! *Langenbecks Arch Surg* 393:833–847, 2008.

Dellinger RP, Levy MM, Rhodes A, et al: Surviving sepsis campaign: international guidelines for management of severe sepsis and septic shock: 2012, *Crit Care Med* 41:580–637, 2013.

Diffley M, Armenian P, Gerona R, et al: Catecholaminergic polymorphic ventricular tachycardia found in an adolescent after a methylenedioxymethamphetamine and marijuana-induced cardiac arrest, *Crit Care Med* 40:2223–2226, 2012.

Doenges ME, Moorhouse MG, Murr AC: *Nurse's pocket guide (13th edition): diagnosis, prioritized interventions,* and rationales, Philadelphia, 2013, FA Davis.

Dugas AF, Mackenhauer J, Salciccioli JD, et al: Prevalence and characteristics of non lactate and lactate expressors in septic shock, *J Crit Care* 27:344–350, 2012.

Duley L: The global impact of pre-eclampsia and eclampsia, *Semin Perinatol* 33:130–137, 2009.

Elholm B, Larsen K, Hornnes N, et al: Alcohol withdrawal syndrome: symptom-triggered versus fixed-schedule treatment in an outpatient setting, *Alcohol* 46:318–323, 2011.

Flounders J: Superior vena cava syndrome, *Oncol Nurs Forum* 30:E84, 2003.

French D, Smollin C, Ruan W, et al: Partition constant and volume of distribution as predictors of clinical efficacy of lipid rescue for toxicological emergencies, *Clin Toxicol* 49:801–819, 2011.

Fulton HG, Barrett SP, Stewart SH, et al: Prescription opioid misuse: characteristics of earliest and most recent memory of hydromorphone use, *J Addict Med* 6:137–144, 2012.

Funk DJ, Parrillo JE, Kumar A: Sepsis and septic shock: a history, *Crit Care Clin* 25:83–101, 2009.

Gatch MB, Forster MJ, Janowsky A, et al: Abuse liability profile of three substituted tryptamines, *J Pharmacol Exp Ther* 338:280–289, 2011.

Geroulanos S, Douka ET: Historical perspective of the word "sepsis," *Intensive Care Med* 32:2077, 2006.

Ghike S, Aseganonkar P: Why obstetric patients are admitted to intensive care unit? A retrospective study, *J South Asian Feder Obset Gynaecol* 4:90–92, 2012.

Gilbert E: *Manual of high risk pregnancy and delivery,* ed 5, St Louis, 2011, Mosby Elsevier.

Glatstein MM, Alabdulrazzaq F, Garcia-Bournissen F, et al: Use of physostigmine for hallucinogenic plant poisoning in a teenager: case report and review of the literature, *Am J Ther* 19:384–388, 2012.

Gresham C, Wilbeck J: Toxicology in the emergency department: a review for the advanced practice nurse, *Adv Emerg Nurs J* 34:43–54, 2012.

Gupta S, Naithani U, Doshi V, et al: Obstetric critical care: a prospective analysis of clinical characteristics, predictability, and fetomaternal outcome in a new dedicated obstetric intensive care unit, *Indian J Anaesth* 55:146–153, 2011.

Haddad B, Sibai BM: Expectant management in pregnancies with severe preeclampsia, *Semin Perinatol* 33:143–151, 2009.

Hambli M, Sibai BM: Hypertensive disorders of pregnancy. In Gibbs RS, Karlan BY, Haney AF, editors: *Danforth's obstetrics and gynecology,* ed 10, Philadelphia, 2008, Lippincott Williams & Wilkins.

Hansen RN, Oster G, Edelsberg J, et al: Economic costs of nonmedical use of prescription opioids, *Clin J Pain* 27:194–202, 2011.

Harrell BR, Melander S: Identifying the association among risk factors and mortality in trauma patients with intra-abdominal hypertension and abdominal compartment syndrome, *J Trauma Nurs* 19:182–189, 2012.

Hartemink KJ, Twisk JWR, Groeneveld ABJ: High circulating N-terminal pro-B-type natriuretic peptide is associated with greater systolic cardiac dysfunction and nonresponsiveness to fluids in septic vs nonseptic critically ill patients, *J Crit Care* 26:108.e1–108.e8, 2011.

Hazinski MF, Samson R, Schexnayder S, editors: *2010 handbook of emergency cardiovascular care for healthcare providers,* Dallas, 2010, American Heart Association.

Higdon M, Higdon J: Treatment of oncologic emergencies, *Am Fam Physician* 74:1873, 2006.

Hunt S, Haddad F: The changing face of heart transplantation, *J Am Coll Cardiol* 52:587, 2008.

Hutchins S: High-risk and critical care in obstetric issues. In Urden L, Stacy K, Lough M, editors: *Critical care nursing: diagnosis and management,* ed 7, St. Louis, 2013, Elsevier.

In the Know Zone (website). http://www.intheknowzone.com/substance-abuse-topics/cocaine/street-names.html.

Itano J, Taoka K, editors: *Oncologic emergencies. Core curriculum for oncology nursing,* ed 4, St. Louis, 2005, Elsevier Saunders.

Iwashyna TJ, Ely EW, Smith DM, et al: Long-term cognitive impairment and functional disability among survivors of severe sepsis, *JAMA* 304:1787–1794, 2010.

Jabot J, Teboul JL, Richard C, et al: Passive leg raising for predicting fluid responsiveness: importance of the postural change, *Intensive Care Med* 35:85–90, 2009.

Jamaty C, Bailey B, Larocque A, et al: Lipid emulsions in the treatment of acute poisoning: a systematic review of human and animal studies, *Clin Toxicol (Phila)* 48:1–27, 2010.

Jansen TC, van Bommel J, Schoonderbeek FJ, et al: LACTATE study group. Early lactate-guided therapy in intensive care unit patients: a multicenter, open-label, randomized controlled trial, *Am J Respir Crit Care Med* 182:752–761, 2010.

Joint Commission on Accreditation of Healthcare Organizations: National patient safety goals: Effective January 1, 2015. In Jones AE, Shapiro NI, Trzeciak S, et al, editors: Lactate clearance vs central venous oxygen saturation as goals of early sepsis therapy: a randomized clinical trial, *JAMA* 303:739–746, 2010.

Kaukonen KM, Bailey M, Suzuki S, et al: Mortality related to severe sepsis and septic shock among critically ill patients in Australia and New Zealand, 2000-2012, *JAMA* 311:1295–1297, 2014.

Kelsey JJ: Obstetric emergencies in the ICU, in PSAP-VII Book 2, Critical and Urgent Care, *ACCP* 7–19, April 2010.

Kirkpatrick AW, Roberts DJ, De Waele J, et al: Pediatric Guidelines Sub-Committee for the World Society of the Abdominal Compartment Syndrome: intra-abdominal hypertension and the abdominal compartment syndrome: updated consensus definitions and clinical practice guidelines from the World Society of the Abdominal Compartment Syndrome, *Intensive Care Med* 39:1190–1206, 2013.

Kuklina E, Ayala C, Callaghan W: Hypertensive disorders and severe obstetric morbidity in the United States, *Obstet Gynecol* 113:1299–1306, 2009.

Kumar A, Roberts D, Wood KE, et al: Duration of hypotension before initiation of effective antimicrobial therapy is the critical determinant of survival in human septic shock, *Crit Care Med* 34:1589–1596, 2006.

Kumar VV, Oscarsson S, Friberg LE, et al: The effect of decontamination procedures on the pharmacokinetics of venlafaxine in overdose, *Clin Pharmacol Ther* 86:403–410, 2009.

Lam S, Partovi N, et al: Corticosteroid interactions with cyclosporine, tacrolimus, mycophenolate, and sirolimus: fact or fiction? *Ann Pharmacother* 42:1037–1047, 2008.

Lanoxin [package insert], Research Triangle Park, 2012, GlaxoSmithKline.

Leeman L, Fontaine P: Hypertensive disorders of pregnancy, *Am Fam Physician* 78:93–100, 2008.

Legrand M, Dupuis C, Simon C, et al: Association between systemic hemodynamics and septic acute kidney injury in critically ill patients: a retrospective observational study, *Crit Care* 17:R278, 2013.

Levinson AT, Casserly BP, Levy MM: Reducing mortality in severe sepsis and septic shock, *Semin Respir Crit Care Med* 32:195–205, 2011.

Liu V, Moorehouse J, Soule J, et al: Fluid volume, lactate values, and mortality in sepsis patients with intermediate lactate values, *Ann Am Thorac Soc* 10:466–473, 2013.

Long T, Sque M, Addington-Hall J: What does a diagnosis of brain death mean to family members approached about organ donation? A review of the literature, *Prog Transplant* 18:118–125, 2008.

Lowdermilk DM, Perry SE, Alden KR, et al: *Maternity and women's health care*, ed 10, St. Louis, 2011, Mosby Elsevier.

Magee LA, von Dadelszen P: The management of severe hypertension, *Semin Perinatol* 33:138–142, 2009.

Marik PE, Cavallazzi R, Vasu T, et al: Dynamic changes in arterial waveform derived variables and fluid responsiveness in mechanically ventilated patients: a systematic review of the literature, *Crit Care Med* 37:2642–2647, 2009.

Marik PE, Wood K, Starzl TE: The course of type 1 hepato-renal syndrome post liver transplantation, *Nephrol Dial Transplant* 21:478–482, 2006.

Marshall J, Reinhart K: Biomarkers of sepsis, *Crit Care Med* 37:2290–2298, 2009.

Martin D: HELLP syndrome A-Z: Facing an obstetric emergency. In Davidson M, et al, editors: *Old's maternal-newborn nursing & women's health across the lifespan*, ed 9, Upper Saddle River, 2012, Pearson Prentice Hall.

Matthaiou DK, Ntani G, Kontogiorgi M, et al: An ESICM systematic review and meta-analysis of procalcitonin-guided antibiotic therapy algorithms in adult critically ill patients, *Intensive Care Med* 38:940–949, 2012.

Mayer S, Yasir A, Oaqaa KP: Definitions and pathophysiology of sepsis, *Curr Probl Pediatr Adolesc Health Care* 43:260–263, 2013.

Mayr FB, Yende S, Angus DC: Epidemiology of severe sepsis, *Virulence* 5:4–11, 2014.

Manasco A, Chang S, Larriviere J, et al: Alcohol withdrawal, *South Med J* 105:607–612, 2012.

Marshall J, Reinhart K: Biomarkers of sepsis, *Crit Care Med* 37:2290–2298, 2009.

Meierkord H, Boon P, Engelsen B, et al: EFNS guideline on the management of status epilepticus in adults, *Eur J Neurol* 17:348–355, 2010.

Micromedex (website). Retrieved 8 February 2014, http://www.micromedexsolutions.com.

Mohammed I, Nonas S: Mechanisms, detection, and potential management of microcirculatory disturbances in sepsis, *Crit Care Clin* 26:393–408, 2010.

Montoya ID, McCann DJ: Drugs of abuse: management of intoxication and antidotes, *EXS* 100:519–541, 2010.

Mulligan MS, Shearon TH, et al: Heart and lung transplantation in the United States 1997–2006, *Am J Transplant* 8:977, 2008.

Neufeld K, Huberman A, Needham D, et al: *Delirium. Principles and practice of hospital medicine*, Burr Ridge, 2012, McGraw-Hill.

Norwitz ER: *Eclampsia*, UpToDate, Waltham, 2014, Wolters Kluwer, 6 March 2014, http://www.uptodate.com/contents/eclampsia.

Ohler L, Cupples S: *Core curriculum for transplant nurses*, Philadelphia, 2008, Mosby.

Olson KR: Activated charcoal for acute poisonings: one toxicologist's journey, *J Med Toxicol* 6:190–198, 2010.

Orens JB, Estenne M, Arcasoy S, et al: International guidelines for the selection of lung transplant candidates: 2006 update: a consensus report from the Pulmonary Scientific Council of the International Society for Heart and Lung Transplantation, *J Heart Lung Transplant* 25:745–755, 2006.

Oviedo-Joekes E, Guh D, Brisette S, et al: Double-blind injectable hydromorphone versus diacetylmorphine for the treatment of opioid dependence: a pilot study, *J Subst Abuse Treat* 28:408–411, 2010.

Pass S: *Updates in toxicology. Pharmacotherapy self assessment program–critical and urgent care*, ed 7, 2010. http://www.accp.com.

Peake SL, Bailey M, Bellomo R, et al: ARISE. Investigators, for the Australian and New Zealand Intensive Care Society Clinical Trials Group. Australasian resuscitation of sepsis evaluation (ARISE): a multi-centre, prospective, inception cohort study, *Resuscitation* 80:811–818, 2009.

Pearlman BL, Gambhir R: Salicylate intoxication: a clinical review, *Postgrad Med* 121:162–168, 2009.

Pollack W, Rose, L, Denis CL: Pregnant and postpartum admissions to the intensive care unit: a systematic review, *Intensive Care Med* 36:1465, 2010.

Pomfret EA, Fryer JP, Sima CS, et al: Liver and intestine transplantation in the United States, 1996–2005, *Am J Transplant* 7:1376, 2007.

Preisman S, Kogan S, Berkenstadt H, et al: Predicting fluid responsiveness in patients undergoing cardiac surgery: functional preload hemodynamic parameters including the Respiratory Systolic Variation Test and static preload indicators, *Br J Anaesth* 95:746–755, 2005.

ProCESS Investigators, Yealy DM, Kellum JA, Huang DT, et al: A randomized trial of protocol-based care for early septic shock, *N Engl J Med* 370:1683–1693, 2014.

Raghunathan K, Shaw A, Nathanson B, et al: Association between the choice of IV crystalloid and in-hospital mortality among critically ill adults with sepsis, *Crit Care Med* 42:1585–1591, 2014.

Reinhart K, Bauer M, Riedemann NC, et al: New approaches to sepsis: molecular diagnostics and biomarkers, *Clin Microbiol Rev* 25:609–634, 2012.

Reintam Blaser A, Sarapuu S, Tamme K, et al: Expanded measurements of intra-abdominal pressure do not increase the detection rate of intra-abdominal hypertension: a single-center observational study, *Crit Care Med* 42:378–386, 2014.

Repke JT, Sibai BM: Preeclampsia and eclampsia, *OBG Manage* 21:45–55, 2009.

Riddle E, Bush J, Tittle M, et al: Alcohol withdrawal: development of a standing order set, *Crit Care Nurse* 30:38–47, 2010.

Rhyee SH: *General approach to drug poisoning in adults*, 2015, 31 March 2015, www.uptodate.com/contents/general-approach-to-drug-poisoning-in-adults.

Robertson CM, Coopersmith CM: The systemic inflammatory response syndrome, *Microbes Infect* 8:1382–1389, 2006.

Said A, Einstein M, Lucey MR: Liver transplantation: an update, *Curr Opin Gastroenterol* 23:292–298, 2007.

Schorr CA, Zanotti Z, Dellinger RP: Severe sepsis and septic shock; management and performance improvement, *Virulence* 5:226–235, 2014.

Schuetz P, Müller B, Christ-Crain M, et al: Procalcitonin to initiate or discontinue antibiotics in acute respiratory tract infections, *Cochrane Database Syst Rev* 9:CD007498, 2012.

Schwartz BG, Rezkalla S, Kloner RA: Cardiovascular effects of cocaine, *Circulation* 122:2558–2569, 2010.

Shapiro JM: Critical care of the obstetric patient, *J Intensive Care Med* 21:278–286, 2006.

Sibai BM, Barton JR: Expectant management of severe preeclampsia remote from term: patient selection, treatment and delivery, *Am J Obstet Gynecol* 196:514.e1–9, 2007.

Simpson KR: Critical illness during pregnancy: considerations for evaluation and treatment of the fetus as the second patient, *Crit Care Nurs Q* 20:20–31, 2006.

Simpson KR, Creehan PA: *Perinatal nursing*, Philadelphia, 2007, Wolters-Kluwer/Lippincott Williams & Wilkins.

Spiller HA, Ryan ML, Weston RG, et al: Clinical experience with and analytical confirmation of "bath salts" and "legal highs" (synthetic cathinones) in the United States, *Clin Toxicol* 49: 499–505, 2011.

Sprung CL, Annane D, Keh D, et al: Hydrocortisone therapy for patients with septic shock, *N Engl J Med* 358:111–124, 2008.

Steinbrook R: Organ donation after cardiac death, *N Engl J Med* 357:209, 2007.

The ProCESS Investigators: A randomized trial of protocol-based care for early septic shock, *N Engl J Med* 370:1683–1693, 2014.

Thornton M, et al: Bath salts and other emerging toxins, *Pediatr Emerg Care* 30:47–52, 2014.

Turner KL, Moore LJ, Todd SR, et al: Identification of cardiac dysfunction in sepsis with B-type natriuretic peptide, *J Am Coll Surg* 213:139–146, 2011.

United Network for Organ Sharing (UNOS). http://www.unos.org/.

United Network for Organ Sharing: MELD/PELD calculator documentation. http://www.unos.org/waitlist/includes_local/pdfs/meld_peld_calculator.pdf.

Vincent JL, Opal SM, Marshall JC, et al: Sepsis definitions: time for change, *Lancet* 381:774–775, 2013.

Vincenti F, Schena FP, Paraskevas S, et al: A randomized, multi-center study of steroid avoidance, early steroid withdrawal or standard steroid therapy in kidney transplant recipients, *Am J Transplant* 8:307, 2008.

Wacker C, Prkno A, Brunkhorst FM, et al: Procalcitonin as a diagnostic marker for sepsis: a systematic review and meta-analysis, *Lancet Infect Dis* 13:426–425, 2013.

Wanderer JP, Leffert LR, Mhyre JM, et al: Epidemiology of obstetric-related ICU admission in Maryland: 1999-2008, *Crit Care Med* 41:1844, 2013.

Webb SA, Litton E, Barned KL, et al: Treatment goals: health care improvement through setting and measuring patient-centered outcomes, *Crit Care Resusc* 15:143–146, 2013.

Weinberg GL: Lipid emulsion infusion: resuscitation for local anesthetic and other drug overdose, *Anesthesiology* 117:180–187, 2012.

Williams GD, Kirk EP, Wilson CJ, et al: Salicylate intoxication from teething gel in infancy, *Med J Aust* 194:146–148, 2011.

Witcher PM: Promoting fetal stabilization during maternal hemodynamic instability or respiratory insufficiency, *Crit Care Nurs Q* 29:70–76, 2006.

Yarbro C, Wujcik D, Gobel B, editors: *Oncologic emergencies. In Cancer nursing: principles and practice*, ed 7, Sudbury, 2010, Jones & Bartlett Learning.

Zahr NM, Kaufman KL, Harper CG: Clinical and pathological features of alcohol-related brain damage, *Nat Rev Neurol* 7:284–294, 2011.

1

Heart and Breath Sounds

ASSESSING HEART SOUNDS

Sound	Auscultation Site	Timing	Pitch	Clinical Occurrence	End-Piece/ Patient Position
S_1 (M_1 T_1)	Apex	Beginning of systole	High	Closing of mitral and tricuspid valves; normal sound	Diaphragm/ patient supine
S_1 split	Apex	Beginning of systole	High	Ventricles contracting at different times because of electrical or mechanical problems (e.g., longer time span between M_1 T_1 caused by right bundle branch heart block, or reversal [T_1 M_1] caused by mitral stenosis)	Same as S_1
S_2 (A_2 P_2)	A_2 at second ICS, RSB; P_2 at second ICS, LSB	End of systole	High	Closing of aortic and pulmonic valves; normal sound	Diaphragm/ patient supine
S_2 physiologic split	Second ICS, LSB	End of systole	High	Accentuated by inspiration; disappears on expiration. Sound that corresponds with the respiratory cycle because of normal delay in closure of pulmonic valve during inspiration. It is accentuated during exercise or in individuals with thin chest walls; heard most often in children and young adults.	Same as S_2
S_2 persistent (wide) split	Second ICS, LSB	End of systole	High	Heard throughout the respiratory cycle; caused by late closure of pulmonic valve or early closure of aortic valve. Occurs in atrial septal defect, right ventricular failure, pulmonic stenosis, hypertension, or right bundle branch heart block.	Same as S_2

Continued

ASSESSING HEART SOUNDS—cont'd

Sound	Auscultation Site	Timing	Pitch	Clinical Occurrence	End-Piece/ Patient Position
S_2 paradoxic (reversed) split ($P_2 A_2$)	Second ICS, LSB	End of systole	High	Because of delayed left ventricular systole, the aortic valve closes after the pulmonic valve rather than before it. (Normally, during expiration, the two sounds merge.) Causes may include left bundle branch heart block, aortic stenosis, severe left ventricular failure, MI, and severe hypertension.	Same as S_2
S_2 fixed split	Second ICS, LSB	End of systole	High	Heard with equal intensity during inspiration and expiration because of split of pulmonic and aortic components, which are unaffected by blood volume or respiratory changes. May be heard in pulmonary stenosis or atrial septal defect.	Same as S_2
S_3 (ventricular gallop)	Apex	Early in diastole just after S_2	Dull, low	Early and rapid filling of ventricle, as in early ventricular failure, heart failure. Common in children, during last trimester of pregnancy, and possibly in healthy adults >50 years of age.	Bell/patient in left lateral or supine position
S_4 (atrial gallop)	Apex	Late in diastole just before S_1	Low	Atrium filling against increased resistance of stiff ventricle, as in heart failure, coronary artery disease, cardiomyopathy, pulmonary artery hypertension, ventricular failure. May be normal in infants, children, and athletes.	Same as S_3

A, Aortic; ICS, intercostal space; LSB, left sternal border; M, mitral; MI, myocardial infarction; P, pulmonic; RSB, right sternal border; T, tricuspid.

COMMONLY OCCURRING HEART MURMURS

Type	Timing	Pitch	Quality	Auscultation Site	Radiation
Pulmonic stenosis	Systolic ejection	Medium-high	Harsh	Second, ICS, LSB	Toward left shoulder, back
Aortic stenosis	Midsystolic	Medium-high	Harsh	Second, ICS, RSB	Toward carotid arteries
Ventricular septal defect	Late systolic	High	Blowing	Fourth ICS, LSB	Toward RSB
Mitral insufficiency	Holosystolic	High	Blowing	Fifth-sixth ICS, left MCL	Toward left axilla
Tricuspid insufficiency	Holosystolic	High	Blowing	Fourth ICS, LSB	Toward apex
Aortic insufficiency	Early diastolic	High	Blowing	Second, ICS, RSB	Toward sternum
Pulmonary insufficiency	Early diastolic	High	Blowing	Second, ICS, LSB	Toward sternum
Mitral stenosis	Mid-late diastolic	Low	Rumbling	Fifth ICS, left MCL	Usually none
Tricuspid stenosis	Mid-late diastolic	Low	Rumbling	Fourth ICS, LSB	Usually none

ICS, Intercostal space; *LSB*, left sternal border; *MCL*, midclavicular line; *RSB*, right sternal border.

ASSESSING NORMAL BREATH SOUNDS

Type	Normal site	Duration	Characteristics
Vesicular	Peripheral lung	I > E	Soft and swishing sounds. Abnormal when heard over the large airways
Bronchial	Trachea and bronchi	E > I	Louder, coarser, and of longer duration than vesicular. Abnormal if heard over peripheral lung
Bronchovesicular	Sternal border of major bronchi	E = I	Moderate in pitch and intensity. Abnormal if heard over peripheral lung

I, Inspiration; *E*, expiration.

ASSESSING ADVENTITIOUS BREATH SOUNDS

Type	Waveform	Characteristics	Possible Clinical Condition
Coarse crackle		Discontinuous, explosive, interrupted. Loud; low in pitch	Pulmonary edema, pneumonia in resolution stage
Fine crackle		Discontinuous, explosive, interrupted. Less loud than coarse crackles, lower in pitch, and of shorter duration	Interstitial lung disease; heart failure; atelectasis
Wheeze		Continuous, of long duration, high-pitched, musical, hissing	Narrowing of airway; bronchial asthma; COPD
Rhonchus		Continuous, of long duration, low-pitched, snoring	Production of sputum (usually cleared or lessened by coughing or suctioning)
Pleural friction rub		Grating, rasping noise	Rubbing together of inflamed parietal linings; loss of normal pleural lubrication

COPD, Chronic obstructive pulmonary disease.

ASSESSING RESPIRATORY PATTERNS

Type	Waveform	Characteristics	Possible Clinical Condition
Eupnea		Normal rate and rhythm for adults and teenagers (12 to 20 breaths/min)	Normal pattern while awake
Bradypnea		Decreased rate (<12 breaths/min); regular rhythm	Normal sleep pattern; opiate or alcohol use; tumor; metabolic disorder
Tachypnea		Rapid rate (>20 breaths/min), hypoventilation or hyperventilation	Fever; restrictive respiratory disorders; pulmonary emboli
Hyperpnea		Depth of respirations greater than normal	Meeting increased metabolic demand (e.g., sepsis, MODS, SIRS, exercise)
Apnea		Cessation of breathing, may be intermittent	Intermittent with CNS disturbances or drug intoxication; obstructed airway; respiratory arrest if it persists
Kussmaul		Deep, rapid (>20 breaths/min); sighing, labored	Renal failure, DKA, sepsis, shock
Cheyne-Stokes		Alternating patterns of apnea (10 to 20 sec) with periods of deep and rapid breathing. Lesions located bilaterally and deep within cerebral hemispheres.	Heart failure, opiate or hypnotic overdose, thyrotoxicosis, dissecting aneurysm, subarachnoid hemorrhage, IICP, aortic valve disorders; may be normal in older adults during sleep
Central, neurogenic hyperventilation		Rapid (>20 breaths/min), deep, regular. Lesions of midbrain or upper pons thought to be source of pattern.	Primary injury (ischemic, infarction, space-occupying lesion), secondary injury (IICP, metabolic disorders, drug overdose)
Apneustic		Deep, prolonged inspiration, followed by 20 to 30 sec pause and short expiration. Lesion located in lower pons.	Anoxia, meningitis, basilar artery occlusion
Cluster		Irregular breaths occurring in clusters with periods of apnea. Overall pattern irregular. Lesion located in lower pons or upper medulla.	Primary and secondary neurologic injury may produce this respiratory pattern.
Ataxic (Biot)		Irregular deep or shallow breaths. No discernible pattern. Lesion located in medulla.	Primary and secondary neurologic injury may produce this respiratory pattern.

CNS, Central nervous system; DKA, diabetic ketoacidosis; IICP, increased intracranial pressure; MODS, multiple organ dysfunction syndrome; SIRS, systemic inflammatory response syndrome.

Glasgow Coma Scale

Parameter	Patient Response	Score
Best eye opening response (record "C" if eyes closed because of swelling)	Spontaneously	4
	To speech	3
	To pain	2
	No response	1
Best motor response (record best upper limb response to painful stimuli)	Obeys verbal command	6
	Localizes pain	5
	Flexion — withdrawal	4
	Flexion — abnormal	3
	Extension — abnormal	2
	No response	1
Best verbal response (record "E" if endotracheal tube is in place or "T" if tracheostomy tube is in place)	Conversation — oriented $\times$ 3	5
	Conversation — confused	4
	Speech — inappropriate	3
	Sounds — incomprehensible	2
	No response	1

Total Score	Interpretation
15	Normal
13 to 15	Minor head injury
9 to 12	Moderate head injury
3 to 8	Severe head injury
4 to 7	Coma
3	Deep coma or brain death

Cranial Nerves: Assessment and Dysfunctions

Cranial Nerve	Type	Functions	Assessment/Dysfunctions
I Olfactory	Sensor	Smell	Anosmia; cannot distinguish familiar odors; will affect ability to taste; test each nostril separately.
II Optic	Sensory	Sight Visual acuity Visual fields Fundus	Blindness; blurred vision; partial vision; loss of full visual field; distorted vision; test each eye separately; a blind eye does not have a pupillary direct light reflex, but has a consensual light reflex.
III Oculomotor	Motor	Pupillary constriction Elevation of upper eyelid Extraocular movements	Ptosis, diplopia, unequal pupils; abnormal pupillary constriction to light; strabismus; loss of pupillary consensual light reflex.
IV Trochlear	Motor	Downward and inward movement of eye	Diplopia, visual disturbances with downward gaze.
V Trigeminal	Sensory and motor	Sensory: Facial, scalp, anterior two thirds of tongue, lips, teeth, propriocep-tion for mastication, corneal reflex	Loss of corneal reflex; abnormal blinking of eyes.
		Motor: Temporal and masseter muscles (jaw clenching and lateral movement for mastication)	Paresis or paralysis of muscles of mastication, decreased facial sensation; unable to clench teeth or weakly clenches teeth.
VI Abducens	Motor	Lateral eye movement	Eye will not move laterally; cranial nerves III, IV, and VI are tested together for full "6 pointed star configuration" eye movements.
VII Facial	Sensory and motor	Sensory: Taste in anterior two thirds of tongue, proprioception for face and scalp	Loss of taste in anterior two thirds of tongue.
		Motor: Facial expression, lacrimal and salivary glands	Paresis or paralysis of facial muscles, facial droop, cannot open eyes against resistance; reduced or absent saliva and tears.

Continued

Cranial Nerve	Type	Functions	Assessment/Dysfunctions
VIII Acoustic	Sensory	Cochlear division: Hearing	Tinnitus, deafness; test one ear at a time.
		Vestibular division: Balance	Vertigo, nystagmus; nausea, sweating, hypotension, and vomiting can indicate vestibular dysfunction.
IX Glossopharyngeal	Sensory and motor	Sensory: Taste in posterior one third of tongue; pain, touch, heat, cold in tongue, tonsils, soft palate, and pharynx	Loss of taste, pain, touch, heat, and cold in posterior one third of tongue, tonsils, and soft palate.
		Motor: Elevation of the soft palate, movement of pharynx, secretion and vasodilation of parotid glands for saliva; gag reflex	Paresis or paralysis of soft palate and pharynx, dysphagia, dysarthria, loss of gag reflex; coughing with oral intake.
X Vagus	Sensory and motor	Sensory: Muscles of pharynx, larynx, esophagus, thoracic and abdominal viscera; external ear, mucous membranes of larynx, trachea, esophagus, thoracic and abdominal viscera; lungs (stretch receptors), aortic bodies (chemoreceptors), respiratory/GI tract (pain receptors)	Similar to dysfunction of glossopharyngeal; parasympathetic nerve fibers may fail to normally inhibit heart rate; may have slow peristalsis and lack gastric and pancreatic secretions, prompting digestive disorders.
		Motor: Muscles of pharynx, larynx, esophagus, thoracic and abdominal viscera; respiratory/gastrointestinal tract (smooth muscle), pacemaker, and cardiac atrial muscle	Loss of gag reflex and difficulty swallowing; coughing with oral intake; palate may have abnormal arch when patient says "ah"; speech defects (inability to articulate syllables clearly); hoarseness of voice.
XI Spinal accessory	Motor	Sternocleidomastoid and trapezius muscles	Paresis or paralysis of sternocleidomastoid and trapezius muscles; inability to turn head or shrug shoulders.
XII Hypoglossal	Motor	Tongue movement	Paresis or paralysis of the tongue; cannot protrude/ "stick out" tongue from the mouth.

4

Major Deep Tendon (Muscle-Stretch) Reflexes

Reflex	Innervations	Examination Technique	Normal Response
Biceps	C5, C6	Arm partially flexed at elbow, palm down Place thumb or finger on biceps tendon. Strike finger with reflex hammer.	Contraction of biceps muscle Flexion at elbow
Triceps	C6, C7	Arm flexed at elbow, palm toward body, arm pulled slightly across body Strike triceps tendon with reflex hammer above elbow.	Contraction of triceps muscle Extension of arm at elbow
Brachioradialis	C5, C6	Hand resting on abdomen, palm slightly pronated Strike radius with reflex hammer 3 to 5 cm above wrist.	Contraction of brachioradialis muscle Flexion and supination of forearm
Achilles (ankle jerk)	S1, S2	Leg flexed at knee, dorsiflex the foot Strike Achilles tendon with reflex hammer.	Plantar flexion of foot
Quadriceps (knee jerk)	L3, L4	Leg flexed at knee Strike patellar tendon with reflex hammer.	Contraction of quadriceps muscle Extension of knee

GRADING OF DEEP TENDON REFLEXES	
Scale (0 to 4+)	**Interpretation**
4+	Very brisk, hyperactive, repetitive, rhythmic flexion and extension (clonus); indicative of disease
3+	Brisker than average; may be normal for certain individuals or may indicate disease.
2+	Average/normal
1+	Diminished response or low normal
0	No response

Major Superficial (Cutaneous) Reflexes

Reflex	Innervations	Examination Technique	Normal Response
Abdominals			
Above/upper Below/lower	T8, T9, T10 T10, T11, T12	Using tongue blade or wooden end of cotton-tipped applicator, lightly stroke abdomen in each quadrant, outer-to-inner direction, toward umbilicus.	Contraction of abdominal muscles Umbilicus deviates (pulls) toward the stimulus.
Bulbocavernous (male)	S3, S4	Pinch glans penis or apply pressure over bulbocavernous muscle behind scrotum.	Scrotum will elevate toward the body.
Corneal	Cranial nerves V and VII	Using wisp of cotton, lightly touch cornea.	Eyelids will quickly close.
Cremasteric (male)	L1, L2	Lightly stroke inner aspect of thigh.	Testicle on side stroked will elevate.
Gag	Cranial nerves IX and X	Using tongue blade, lightly touch posterior pharynx.	Gagging or retching
Perianal	S3, S4, S5	Stroke tissue surrounding anus with blunt instrument, or examine rectum by gently inserting gloved finger.	Anal puckering with external stimuli Tightening of anal sphincter with internal examination

6 Inotropic and Vasoactive Medication Infusions

Medications	**MEASUREMENTS**				Dosage	Effects
	HR	**PAWP**	**SVR**	**CO**		
Inotropes/ Vasoactives						***Main effect: increase cardiac contractility and change vascular resistance.***
Dopamine hydrochloride	—↑	—	—	—↑	Low dose 1 to 2 μg/ kg/min	Major effect may be to *increase* urine output; may potentiate effect of diuretics.
	—↑	—	—	↑↑	Moderate dose 2 to 10 μg/ kg/min	Major effect is to increase contractility.
	—	—	↑↑	—	High dose >10 μg/ kg/min	Can cause tissue necrosis and sloughing if infiltration occurs.
Dobutamine	—↑	—↓	—↓	↑↑	2.5 to 10 μg/kg/min	Overall effect is improved CO; may cause tachycardia and dysrhythmias as side effects.
Isoproterenol	↑↑	—↓	↓↓	↑↑	2 to 10 μg/ min	Significant increase in myocardial oxygen consumption; can produce ventricular tachycardia and fibrillation.
Epinephrine	↑↑	↑↑	↓↑	↑↑	0.5 to 1 mg IV push for cardiac arrest	May induce ventricular ectopy.
					1 to 4 μg/ min for inotropic support	Can exacerbate myocardial ischemia. Can prompt supraventricular and ventricular dysrhythmias.
					2 to 20 μg/ kg/min	Main effect is vasoconstriction of peripheral blood vessels.
Inamrinone lactate	—↑	↓	↓	↑	Loading dose: 0.75 mg/kg; then 5–10 μg/kg/min	An older "inodilator" medication often used as the first step in managing acute decompensated heart failure.
Milrinone lactate	—↑	↓	↓	↑	50 μg/kg given over 10 min; start infusion of 0.375–0.75 μg/kg/min	"Inodilator" medication used most often as the first step in managing acute decompensated heart failure.

Continued

MEASUREMENTS						
Medications	**HR**	**PAWP**	**SVR**	**CO**	**Dosage**	**Effects**
Levosimendan	—↑	↓	↓	↑↑↑	Loading dose: 24 μg/kg followed by 0.1 to 0.2 μg/kg/min for 24 hours	A calcium sensitizer used to treat patients with acute decompensated heart failure.
Vasopressors						***Main effect: constriction of arteries and veins (vasoconstriction).***
Methoxamine hydrochloride	—	↑	↑↑↑	—	3 to 5 mg	Potent vasoconstrictor: used rarely; increases myocardial oxygen demand.
Norepinephrine	↑↓	↑	↑↑↑	↑	2 to 12 μg/min	Potent vasoconstrictor: contraindicated when hypotension occurs secondary to hypovolemia. Can cause tissue necrosis and sloughing if infiltration occurs. Increased myocardial oxygen demand without increased coronary artery flow can cause myocardial ischemia and infarction.
Phenylephrine	—	↑	↑↑↑	—	100–180 μg/min	Potent vasoconstrictor: may cause dysrhythmias or trigger reflex bradycardia.
Vasopressin	↑	—	↑↑	—	0.02 to 0.1 U/min	Used to augment other vasopressors; higher doses cause marked splanchnic vasoconstriction.
Vasodilators						***Main effect: dilation of arteries and/or veins (vasodilation).***
Sodium nitroprusside	—↑	↓	↓↓	—	Starting dose of 0.5 to 0.8 μg/kg/min; titrate up to 10 μg/kg/min	Drug is photosensitive; keep infusion container protected from light. Thiocyanate (a metabolite of nitroprusside) toxicity can occur after 72 hours. Monitor thiocyanate levels daily, being alert to levels >10 mg/dL and/or signs of metabolic acidosis.
Nitroglycerin	—↑	↓↓	↓	—	Starting dose of 0.5 μg/min; titrate up to 200 μg/min	Absorbed by standard plastic IV tubing. Use special polyvinyl chloride tubing. Ensure that the drug is diluted for IV use

—, No effect; ↑ or ↓ minimal effect; ↑↑ or ↓↓, moderate effect; ↑↑↑ or ↓↓↓, major effect; *CO*, cardiac output; *HR*, heart rate; *IV*, intravenous; *PAOP*, pulmonary artery occlusive pressure; *SVR*, systemic vascular resistance.

Sample Relaxation Technique

Give the patient the following instructions:
1. Sit quietly in a comfortable position. Close your eyes.
2. Relax all your muscles, starting at your feet and progressing to your facial muscles. Focus your attention on one body area at a time while you relax the muscles in that area.
3. Breathe through your nose. As you breathe out, say the word "one" silently to yourself. Become aware of your breathing. Continue this process for about 20 minutes.
4. Do not worry whether or not you are achieving deep relaxation. Maintain a passive attitude and permit relaxation to occur at its own pace. If distractions interfere, see your thoughts floating away like clouds. Continue breathing and repeating the word "one."

A—aortic valve
AACN—American Association of Critical Care Nurses
AAL—anterior axillary line
ABA—American Burn Association
ABG—arterial blood gas
ACC—American College of Cardiology
ACCP—American College of Chest Physicians
ACE—angiotensin-converting enzyme
ACh—acetylcholine
AChR—acetylcholine receptor
ACLS—advanced cardiac life support
ACS—abdominal compartment syndrome
ACT—activated clotting time
AD—autonomic dysreflexia
ADA—American Diabetes Association
ADH—antidiuretic hormone
ADL—activity of daily living
AED—automatic external defibrillator
AEG—atrial electrogram
AF—atrial fibrillation
AHA—American Heart Association
AIDS—acquired immunodeficiency syndrome
AIS—acute ischemic stroke
ALI—acute lung injury
ALP—alkaline phosphatase
ALT—alanine aminotransferase
AM—akinetic mutism
AMA—American Medical Association
AMI—acute myocardial infarction
ANA—American Nurses Association
ANP—atrial natriuretic peptide
APAS—antiphospholipid antibody syndrome
APSAC—anisoylated plasminogen streptokinase activator complex
aPTT—activated partial thromboplastin time
ARDS—acute respiratory distress syndrome
ARF—acute respiratory failure; acute renal failure
ARS—adjective rating scale
ASA—acetylsalicylic acid (aspirin)
ASO—antistreptolysin O
AST—aspartate aminotransferase
AT—antithrombin

AT_1—receptor antagonist
ATGAM—antithymocyte gamma globulin
atm—atmosphere (standard)
ATN—acute tubular necrosis
ATP—adenosine triphosphate
AV—atrioventricular; arteriovenous
AVM—arteriovenous malformation
AVNRT—atrial-ventricular nonreciprocating tachycardia
AVRT—atrial-ventricular reciprocating tachycardia
BAL—bronchoalveolar lavage
BEE—basal energy expenditure
BG—blood glucose
BIS—bispectral index
BMI—body mass index
BP—blood pressure
bpm—beats per minute
BS—bowel sounds
BSA—body surface area
BUN—blood urea nitrogen
C—centigrade; Celsius
Ca^{2+}—calcium
CABG—coronary artery bypass grafting
CAD—coronary artery disease
CAPD—continuous ambulatory peritoneal dialysis
CASHD—coronary atherosclerotic heart disease
CAVH—continuous arteriovenous hemofiltration
CBC—complete blood cell count
CBF—cerebral blood flow
CD—Cotrel-Dubousset
CDC—Centers for Disease Control and Prevention
CDI—central diabetes insipidus
CHF—congestive heart failure
CI—cardiac index
CIE—counterimmunoelectrophoresis
CJD—Creutzfeldt-Jakob disease
CK—creatine kinase
Cl—chloride
CK-MB—creatine kinase–myocardial band
CM—cardiomyopathy
CMV—cytomegalovirus; controlled mechanical ventilation

CNS—central nervous system
CO—cardiac output; carbon monoxide
CO_2—carbon dioxide
COPD—chronic obstructive pulmonary disease
CPAP—continuous positive airway pressure
CPK—creatine phosphokinase
CPP—cerebral perfusion pressure; coronary perfusion pressure
CRRT—continuous renal replacement therapy
CRT—cardiac resynchronization therapy
C&S—culture and sensitivities
CSF—cerebrospinal fluid
CT—computed tomography
cTnI—cardiac troponin I
CVA—cerebrovascular accident; costovertebral angle
CVC—central venous catheter
CVP—central venous pressure
CVVH—continuous venovenous hemofiltration
CVVHD—continuous venovenous hemofiltration with dialysis
CVVHDF—continuous venovenous hemodiafiltration
CXR—chest radiograph
CyA—cyclosporine
DAI—diffuse axonal injury
DCM—dilated cardiomyopathy
DFI—diffusion-weighted imaging (or DWI)
DI—diabetes insipidus
DIC—disseminated intravascular coagulation
DKA—diabetic ketoacidosis
DM—diabetes mellitus
DNR—do not resuscitate
Do_2—oxygen delivery
DOE—dyspnea on exertion
DPAHC—durable power of attorney for health care
DPL—diagnostic peritoneal lavage
DTR—deep tendon reflex
DVT—deep vein thrombosis
EACA—epsilon-(e)aminocaproic acid
EBV—Epstein-Barr virus
ECG—electrocardiogram
ECHO—electrocardiography
EEG—electroencephalogram
EFA—Epilepsy Foundation of America
ELISA—enzyme-linked immunosorbent assay
EMI—electromagnetic interference
EPS—electrophysiologic studies
ESR—erythrocyte sedimentation rate
ET—endotracheal
$ETCO_2$—end-tidal carbon dioxide
ETOH—alcohol
ETT—endotracheal tube

F—Fahrenheit
FAST—focused assessment with sonography for trauma
FDP—fibrin degradation product
FEF—forced expiratory flow
FEV—forced expiratory volume
FHF—fulminant hepatic failure
Fio_2—fraction of inspired oxygen
Fr—French
FRC—functional residual capacity
FSP—fibrin split product
FVC—forced vital capacity
GABA—gamma-(γ) aminobutyric acid
GBS—Guillain-Barré syndrome
GCS—Glasgow Coma Scale
GERD—gastroesophageal reflux disease
GI—gastrointestinal
GKI—glucose-potassium-insulin
G6PD—glucose-6-phosphate dehydrogenase
GU—genitourinary
H_2O—water
HAT—heparin-associated thrombocytopenia
HCM—hypertrophic cardiomyopathy
HCO_3^2—bicarbonate
Hct—hematocrit
HDL—high-density lipoprotein
HELLP—hemolysis, elevated liver enzymes, low platelet count
Hgb—hemoglobin
HHS—hyperglycemic hyperosmolar syndrome
HITT—heparin-induced thrombocytopenia thrombosis
HIV—human immunodeficiency virus
HOB—head of bed
HPO_4—phosphate
HR—heart rate
HRS—hepatorenal syndrome
HSV—herpes simplex virus
HUS—hemolytic-uremic syndrome
HVPG—hepatic venous pressure gradient
HVWP—hepatic vein wedge pressure
IABP—intraaortic balloon pump
IAP—intraabdominal pressure
ICA—internal cerebral artery
ICD—implantable cardioverter-defibrillator
ICH—intracerebral hematoma
ICP—intracranial pressure
ICS—intercostal space
ICU—intensive care unit
IDDM—insulin dependent diabetes mellitus
IE—infective endocarditis
I/E—inspiration/expiration
IER—in expected range
IgG—immunoglobulin G
IHSS—idiopathic hypertrophic subaortic stenosis
IICP—increased intracranial pressure

IM—intramuscular
INR—international normalized ratio
I&O—intake and output
IPD—intermittent peritoneal dialysis; intracranial pressure dynamics
IPPB—intermittent positive-pressure breathing
IRV—inverse ratio ventilation
ITP—idiopathic thrombocytopenic purpura
IV—intravenous
IVP—intravenous pyelogram
JNC VII—Joint National Committee VII
JNC 8—Joint National Committee 8
JT—junctional tachycardia
JVD—jugular vein distention
K⁺—potassium
kcal—kilocalorie
KCl—potassium (K) chloride (Cl^2)
kg—kilogram
KUB—kidney, ureter, bladder
L—liter; lumbar
LAD—left anterior descending (coronary artery)
LAP—left atrial pressure
LDH—lactate dehydrogenase; also abbreviated LD
LDL—low-density lipoprotein
LIS—locked-in-syndrome
LMW—low molecular weight
LOC—level of consciousness
LOS—length of stay
LP—lumbar puncture
LR—lactated Ringer
LUQ—left upper quadrant
LUT—lower urinary tract
LV—left ventricular
LVEDP—left ventricular end-diastolic pressure
LVH—left ventricular hypertrophy
m—meter
M—mitral valve
MAP—mean arterial pressure
MCA—middle cerebral artery
MCL—modified chest lead; midclavicular line
MCS—minimally conscious state
MCT—medium-chain triglycerides
MCV—mean corpuscular volume
Mg²⁺—magnesium
MG—myasthenia gravis
mg—milligram
MI—myocardial infarction
MODS—multiple organ dysfunction syndrome
mOsm—milliosmole
MPAP—mean pulmonary artery pressure; also abbreviated PAM
MRA—magnetic resonance arteriogram
MRI—magnetic resonance imaging

MS—multiple sclerosis
MSO₄—morphine sulfate
MUGA scan—multiple-gated acquisition scan
Na/Na⁺—sodium
NaCl—sodium chloride/saline
NCV—nerve conduction velocity
NDI—nephrogenic diabetes insipidus
NIDDM—non-insulin dependent diabetes mellitus
NG—nasogastric
NHO—National Hospice Organization
nl—normal
NMBA—neuromuscular blocking agent(s)
NPO—nothing by mouth
NRS—numeric rating scale
NSAID—nonsteroidal antiinflammatory drug
NSTEMI—non–ST-segment elevation myocardial infarction
NTG—nitroglycerin
nvCJD—new variant Creutzfeldt-Jakob disease
OT—occupational therapist
OTC—over-the-counter
P—pulmonic valve
PA—pulmonary artery
PAC—premature atrial complexes
Paco₂—carbon dioxide (arterial pressure)
PAD—pulmonary artery diastolic
Pao₂—oxygen (arterial pressure)
PAOP—pulmonary artery occlusive pressure
PAP—pulmonary artery pressure/positive airway pressure
PASG—pneumatic antishock garment
PAT—paroxysmal atrial tachycardia
PAW—pulmonary artery wedge
PAWP—pulmonary artery wedge pressure
PBV—percutaneous balloon valvuloplasty
PCA—patient-controlled analgesia
PE—pulmonary embolus
PEEP—positive end-expiratory pressure
PEG—percutaneous endoscopic gastrostomy
PEJ—percutaneous endoscopic jejunostomy
PET—positron emission tomography
P/F—PaO_2/FiO_2 oxygen (arterial pressure) to fraction of inspired oxygen ratio
PIH—pregnancy-induced hypertension
PJC—premature junctional complexes
PK—pyruvate kinase
PMI—point of maximal impulse
PN—parenteral nutrition
PND—paroxysmal nocturnal dyspnea
PO—by mouth
PO₄—phosphates
PPF—plasma protein fraction
Pplat—plateau pressure
PRA—panel-reactive antibody
PRBCs—packed red blood cells

PSB—protected specimen brush
PSV—pressure support ventilation
PSVT—paroxysmal supraventricular tachycardia
PT—physical therapy; physical therapist; prothrombin time
PTCA—percutaneous transluminal coronary angioplasty
PTH—parathyroid hormone
PTT—partial thromboplastin time
PVC—premature ventricular complex; peripheral venous catheter
PVR—pulmonary vascular resistance
PWI—perfusion-weighted imaging
RAP—right atrial pressure
RBC—red blood cell
RCM—restrictive cardiomyopathy
RDA—Recommended Daily Allowance; Recommended Dietary Allowance
rHuEPO—recombinant human erythropoietin
RLA—Rancho Los Amigos
ROM—range of motion
RPE—rate perceived exertion
RR—respiratory rate
RRT—renal replacement therapy; registered respiratory therapist
rtPA—recombinant tissue plasminogen activator
RV—right ventricle; residual volume
RVP—right ventricular pressure
SA—status asthmaticus
SAH—subarachnoid hemorrhage
SAS—subarachnoid space
SBP—systolic blood pressure
SCCM—Society of Critical Care Medicine
SCI—spinal cord injury
Scvo$_2$—central venous oxygen saturation
SGOT—serum glutamic oxaloacetic acid transaminase
SGPT—serum glutamic pyruvic transaminase
SIADH—syndrome of inappropriate antidiuretic hormone
SIMV—synchronized intermittent mandatory ventilation
SIRS—systemic inflammatory response syndrome
Sjo$_2$—jugular venous oxygen saturation
SOB—shortness of breath
Spo$_2$—pulse oximetry oxygen saturation
SQ—subcutaneous; also abbreviated SC

SS—sensory stimulation
STEMI—ST-segment elevation myocardial infarction
Sto$_2$—tissue oxygen saturation
STSG—split-thickness skin graft
SV—stroke volume
Svo$_2$—mixed venous oxygen saturation
SVR—systemic vascular resistance
T—tricuspid valve
TBSA—total body surface area
TCD—transcranial Doppler
TdP—torsades des pointe
TE—thrombotic emboli
TEA—tranexamic acid
TEC—transluminal extraction catheterization
TEE—total energy expenditure; transesophageal echocardiography
TENS—transcutaneous electrical nerve stimulation
TIA—transient ischemic attack
TIBC—total iron-binding capacity
TIPS/TIPSS—transjugular intrahepatic portal-systemic shunt
TMP—transmembrane pressure
TNA—total nutrient admixtures
TNF—tumor necrosis factor
TOF—train-of-four
TPA—tissue plasminogen activator
TPN—total parenteral nutrition
TSF—triceps skinfold thickness
UF—ultrafiltration
URI—upper respiratory infection
UTI—urinary tract infection
VAD—venous access device; ventricular assist device
VAS—visual analog scale
VC—vital capacity
VCJD—variant (new) Creutzfeld-Jakob disease
VEDP—ventricular end-diastolic pressure
VF—ventricular fibrillation
VLDL—very-low-density lipoprotein
VMA—vanillylmandelic acid
Vo$_2$—oxygen consumption
VS—vital signs/vegetative state
VSD—ventricular septal defect
VT—ventricular tachycardia
Vt—tidal volume
WBC—white blood cell
WNL—within normal limits
WPW—Wolff-Parkinson-White syndrome

Index

Page numbers followed by "b" indicate boxes; "f," figures; "t," tables.

Manual of critical care nursing : nursing interventions and collaborative
Baird, Marianne Saunorus
Seventh edition ID: 19853

Date Due

Sept 21/2017		
July 31, 19		